ISBN 978-0-260-01953-0
PIBN 10922659

FB &c Ltd, Dalton House, 60 Windsor Avenue, London, SW19 2RR.
Company number 08720141. Registered in England and Wales.

For support please visit www.forgottenbooks.com

THE AMERICAN JOURNAL OF THE MEDICAL SCIENCES

EDITED BY

JOHN H. MUSSER, Jr., M.D.

E. B. KRUMBHAAR, M.D.
ASSISTANT EDITOR

NEW SERIES

VOL. CLXV

QUAE PROSUNT OMNIBUS

PHILADELPHIA AND NEW YORK
LEA & FEBIGER
1923

CONTENTS OF VOL. CLXV

ORIGINAL ARTICLES

REVIEWS

PROGRESS OF MEDICAL SCIENCE

THE

AMERICAN JOURNAL OF THE MEDICAL SCIENCES

JANUARY, 1923

ORIGINAL ARTICLES.

EFFECTS OF ACUTE AND CHRONIC PNEUMOTHORAX (A PRELIMINARY REPORT.)[1]

BY J. L. YATES, B.S., M.D.,
MILWAUKEE, WIS.

PHYSIOLOGISTS have cited the interdependence of respiration and intrapulmonary circulation as a nice example of coördinated functions. Indeed, so intimate is this interdependence that the degree of integrity of the pulmonary circulation compared to normal, directly or indirectly measures not alone intrathoracic function but also pleural and pulmonary powers of defense and repair. Consequently the ultimate evaluation of intrathoracic therapeutic procedures can be estimated by the protection and rehabilitation assured to the lesser circulation.

Pneumothorax produces effects common to other forms of pulmonary deflation and compression, either intrinsic, due to exudates, transudates, neoplasms and chronic passive congestion (Drinker), or extrinsic, resulting from pleuritic effusions, mediastinal tumors, aneurysms and the like. Wherever intrapulmonary pressure exceeds intravascular tension a proportion of the blood destined under normal conditions to reach the compressed lung area is immediately diverted to adjacent channels offering less resistance. The capillary network that surrounds the air cells spreads, as its component vascular tubules are thus elongated by overfilling. If air passages are free and lung tissue is elastic, the result is increased inflation in the portion of lung to which extra blood has

[1] Read before the American Association for Thoracic Surgery, June 6, 1921, as part of a symposium on open pneumothorax.

been delivered, a compensatory physiologic emphysema. On the contrary a temporary stoppage of pulmonary circulation produces atelectasis; permanent stoppage causes atrophy in the lung affected. In short, the pulmonary circulation is the most important factor influencing pulmonary inflation, and fluctuation in pulmonary inflation is accompanied by variations in the resistance to blood flow in the pulmonary circulation. The richness of the bronchial arterial blood supply, somewhat proportionate to the size and activity of the lung except in extreme degrees of emphysema and possibly of collapse, can also be measured by the condition of the pulmonary circulation.

The occurrence of compensatory physiologic emphysema in human lungs has long been recognized by clinicians, though it is not always demonstrable post mortem because of failure of blood-pressure at death preceded by a gradual antemortem reduction. The extent of compensatory emphysema depends upon the area of lung compressed and upon the competence of the circulation. Gregoire noted a zone of emphysema about areas of hemorrhagic infiltration due to wounds of the lung which is comparable to similar changes to be found about early foci of bronchopneumonia. Skodaic resonance, so often present above an effusion, was found by Bradford, Soltau and others to be particularly noticeable in the presence of hemothorax and to be due to emphysema in the lung just above that compressed by the bloody effusion. Individuals who have a competent circulation and develop an extensive unilateral pneumonia or pleural effusion regularly show a contralateral emphysema. Surgeons who operated without differential pressure upon soldiers suffering from chest wounds noticed that men in good condition tolerated extensive thoracotomy with comparatively little respiratory distress, whereas those who were in shock were much embarrassed by lesser parietal incisions. Those operators who used positive pressure anesthesia observed that the reëstablishment of a more normal pulmonary circulation through pulmonary inflation usually resulted in improving the individual's general condition. Moreover, during operations, as the extent of pulmonary inflation was varied to give desirable exposure, two other observations were made: The extent of deflation that could be tolerated without distress was greater in the men in better condition, and when complete deflation was possible, the mediastinum instead of becoming convex toward the sound side actually became convex toward the open side. Many surgeons have noticed, when operating without differential pressure to relieve chronic empyema, that as the exudate upon the visceral pleura is incised the underlying lung tends to bulge outward.

The capability of increased pressure in pulmonary circulation to augment inflation in a compensatory fashion explains these reactions. The lung is in effect an erectile tissue. The part played by vasomotor control of the pulmonary circulation remains to be demonstrated.

Experiments are being conducted with the coöperation of Dr. William Thalhimer and Dr. Benjamin Schlomovitz to determine the influence upon defensive pleuropulmonary reactions of varied intrathoracic conditions and among them is artificial pneumothorax. We are unprepared to make final statements, as our observations are incomplete. Results thus far obtained have so direct a bearing upon acute and chronic pneumothorax that they are presentable as a part of this symposium.

Pneumothorax induced by injecting known amounts of air unilaterally into the chests of anesthetized animals produces effects that vary with the type and conditions of the animal and the rate of injection. Cats and dogs, animals of the thin pleura type, have mediastinums that are not air-tight. Man and monkey, thick of pleura, have air-tight mediastinums. Unilateral pneumothorax is possible in man and monkey and impossible in cats and dogs.

If air be injected gradually into the left pleural cavity of a dog, there is a bilateral decrease in the negative pressures, usually greater on the right side (Fig. 1). If the air introduced gradually is insufficient in amount to cause the negative pressure to disappear and then is withdrawn, there is an immediate return to the previous pulse and respiration rates, systemic blood-pressure and negative intrapleural pressure. Increasing pulmonary compression is met with rising blood-pressure and so long as the increment is adequate, respiratory distress, indicated by slower and deeper respirations, does not develop.

A more rapid introduction of air in amounts sufficient to abolish negative pressure leads promptly to respiratory embarrassment as the compensatory blood-pressure rise is insufficient to meet requirements. If more air be injected so as to create increasing positive pressure respiration will cease (Fig. 2). The blood-pressure falls as it becomes inadequate, the rapidity of fall being somewhat proportionate to the extent of compensatory failure. Sudden variations in the negative pressure may occur spontaneously during a period of considerable compression and result from changes in the distribution of blood in the pulmonary circulation (Figs. 1 and 7). These observations offer a probable explanation of the fluttering mediastinum occasionally observed during operations performed without differential pressure. When the air that has caused marked pulmonary compression is withdrawn rapidly, there is a tendency for the negative pressures to increase temporarily beyond normal levels instead of returning to normal as above described (Fig. 2). This transient excess in negative pressures is attributed to a decrease in the amount of intrapulmonary blood, the excess blood having been squeezed out by the compression.

It is soon reaccumulated and normal negative pressures reëstablished. As the animals' hearts become fatigued, the compensatory reactions become less adequate and respiratory distress appears more promptly and with less decrease in the negative pressures (Figs. 3 and 7).

Similar experiments performed upon monkeys produced significant results. If the animal is robust and the air be injected gradually, a positive pressure on the injected side amounting approximately to fifteen times the normal negative pressure may provoke a reduction of but three-fourths of the contralateral negative pressure (Fig. 4). So long as the blood-pressure rises sufficiently there is no respiratory distress. If, however, the animal be feeble or both feeble and fatigued, the reaction to unilateral pulmonary compression is similar to that of the dog (Fig. 5). In other words, with inadequate powers of cardiac compensation, compensatory contralateral emphysema does not occur and the animal reacts as if the pneumothorax were bilateral.

The effects of chronic pneumothorax have been studied only in the monkey. Apparently the compensatory emphysema is distributed irregularly through the contralateral lung and is present in patches even in the lung subjected to compression. This is because of irregularities in the distribution of blood. Although simple of explanation upon the basis of hydraulics, it may indicate the effects of vasomotor control. There is a thickening of the visceral pleura due to proliferation of the mesothelial cells of the serosa and the subserous elements which is very significant. Air is irritating to serous membranes and the long-continued effects of compression in the presence of an irritant makes for decreased pulmonary elasticity and therefore curtails normal respiration.

The following conclusions are based upon personal clinical experiences in caring for over two hundred soldiers suffering from intrathoracic injuries and upon many animal experiments not cited here. The list includes about one hundred and twenty-five soldiers upon whom open thoracotomy was performed. Differential pressure was used in ninety-three; the remainder were operated upon at the Ambulance de l'Ocean under ether anesthesia according to the teachings of Duval. During convalescence the progress in intrathoracic repair was studied when possible with fluoroscope and roentgen-ray pictures. All who died came to necropsy. There has thus been provided unusual opportunity to study the effects of acute and chronic pneumothorax and to compare the death rate, amount of distress and the duration of disability following thoracotomies performed with and without differential pressure. Experiments of the type cited in this communication have served to explain and to substantiate previous clinical and experimental observations.

Acute pneumothorax is dangerous in so far as it interferes with the pulmonary circulation. The extent of the danger is determined by the integrity of the circulation, chiefly by the latent energy of the myocardium. Since reserve myocardial energy cannot be estimated accurately and is quite essential to life during a period of stress, open thoracotomy should be performed with some form of differential pressure. Thus alone may the degree of pulmonary deflation required for the intrathoracic operation be permitted to develop gradually, be controlled so as not to become excessive and allowed to be as transient as possible. The operation is incomplete until full pulmonary inflation is both obtained and maintained. The latter is possible only when suitable one-way primary drainage is used. Gas-oxygen positive pressure analgesia as developed by Gwathmey is simple, safe and satisfactory, and, in the absence of a negative pressure cabinet, is the best method now available.

Chronic pneumothorax, as well as chronic pulmonary compression by the pleuritic effusions inevitable after thoracotomy, must be avoided if surgeons would assure to patients the best chances for rapid, comfortable and complete recovery.

Experiments. Aspirating needles or small trocars attached to bromoform manometers were inserted obliquely through the third or fourth interspace so that only the tips entered the pleural cavity and were placed posteriorly and above the heart. The connection on the left side, provided with a two-way cock, permitted air to be injected or aspirated with a graduated piston syringe. Blood-pressure was recorded from a femoral artery by means of a mercury manometer. Fairly deep surgical anesthesia with ether was maintained throughout the experiments and as nearly as possible at the same depth. The possibilities for error were recognized, likewise the constancy thereof, so that they were held to be negligible since relative accuracy was sufficient for the purposes at hand.

The diagrams have all been reconstructed from kymographic tracings in the same way and are directly comparable. Time is measured as abscissas; 1″ equals two minutes; the ordinates indicate pulse, 1″ equals 160 beats; blood-pressure, 1″ equals 50 mm. Hg; intrathoracic pressure, right and left, 1″ equals 4 mm. bromoform; the amount of air injected or aspirated, 1″ equals 50 cc. The line marked ⊕ indicates atmospheric pressure.

Figure 1, *Dog* 5, *Observation* 1. The observation was begun with 100 cc of air already in the chest. A total of 300 cc was injected in thirteen minutes, which reduced negative pressures one-half and did not produce respiratory distress. The air was withdrawn at the same rate. The increased blood-pressure sufficed to provide compensation. Just before the total amount of air had been injected the negative pressure on the left side fell abruptly and quite as promptly returned to its proper level, an expression of a fluctuation in the pulmonary circulation. At the end of the experiment normal conditions were reëstablished.

Figure 2, Dog 5, Observation 2. A total of 400 cc of air was injected in eleven minutes, causing respiration to cease, and then it was withdrawn in two minutes. The dog was able to compensate temporarily with increasing blood-pressure until 350 cc had been

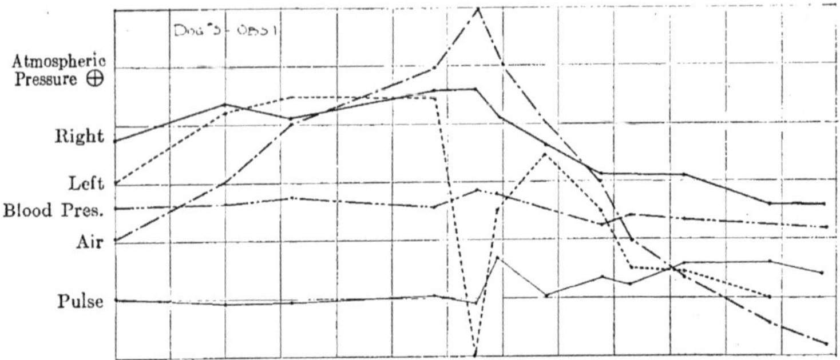

Fig. 1.—Abscissa, 1″ two minutes; ordinate, 1″ 160 beats; blood-pressure, 1″ 50 mm. Hg; intrathoracic pressure, right and left, 1″ 4 mm. bromoform; air injected or aspirated, 1″ 50 cc; atmospheric pressure ⊕.

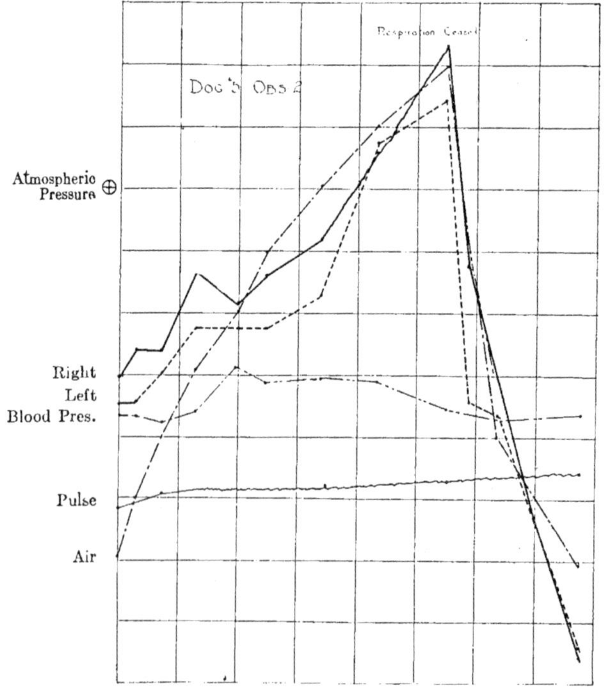

Fig. 2.—Abscissa, 1″ two minutes; ordinate, 1″ 160 beats; blood-pressure, 1″ 50 mm. Hg; intrathoracic pressure, right and left, 1″ 4 mm. bromoform; air injected or aspirated, 1″ 50 cc; atmospheric pressure ⊕.

injected even though there was positive intrathoracic pressure. Rapid removal of the air protected the blood-pressure from a material fall. The intrathoracic negative pressures at the end of the experiment were twice as great as at the start.

Figure 3, *Dog* 5, *Observation* 5. Between observations 2 and 5 two experiments were done. In each a cessation of respiration resulted when 350 cc were injected in three minutes. A repetition of the experiment shown in Fig. 2 proved that now 300 cc injected in five minutes caused respirations to cease, whereas before it required 400 cc in eleven minutes. There is now a decided fall in blood-pressure as compared to a slight fall in the former instance. A comparison of Figs. 2 and 3 shows the striking reduction in powers of compensation due chiefly to cardiac fatigue.

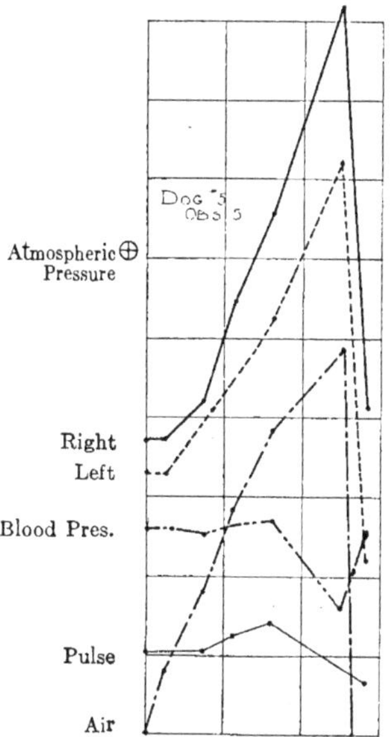

Fig. 3.—Abscissa, 1″ two minutes; ordinate, 1″ 160 beats; blood-pressure, 1″ 50 mm. Hg; intrathoracic pressure, right and left, 1″ 4 mm. bromoform; air injected or aspirated, 1″ 50 cc; atmospheric pressure ⊕.

Figure 4, *Monkey* 17. An injection of 150 cc of air in five minutes fell just short of provoking serious respiratory distress, though the fall in blood-pressure showed that to be imminent. The blood-pressure promptly rose with aspiration. The significant fact is that a positive pressure on the left side nearly five times as great as the amount of normal negative pressure reduced the right-sided negative pressure by only three-fourths. At the time when the left-sided pressure was atmospheric and equivalent to an open thorax, the negative pressure on the right side was reduced by about one-half and respiration was unembarrassed. This explains why a thoracotomy can be performed without differential pressure in animals with a competent circulation in which the mediastinum is air-tight.

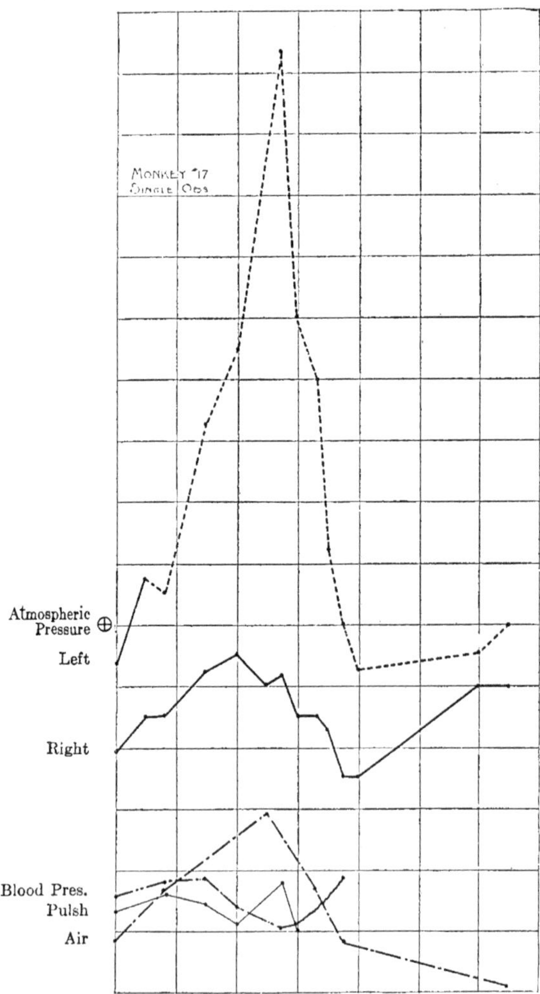

Fig. 4.—Abscissa, 1″ two minutes; ordinate, 1″ 160 beats; blood-pressure, 1″ 50 mm. Hg; intrathoracic pressure, right and left, 1″ 4 mm. bromoform; air injected or aspirated, 1″ 50 cc; atmospheric pressure ⊕.

Figure 5, *Monkey* 16, *Observation* 1. An injection of 150 cc in six and a quarter minutes caused respirations to cease, and in spite of prompt aspiration artificial respiration was required to save the animal's life. The striking feature of this experiment is to be seen in the changes in intrathoracic pressures. Fifty cc of air in the left caused no change in the right side. Between 50 cc and 100 cc the right-side pressure rose rapidly but less rapidly than the left, and after 100 cc they rose even more abruptly. Monkey 16 responded more like a dog than like Monkey 17. Monkey 16 was an undernourished animal, unusually vicious and restive, and at the time the experiment was performed was considerably exhausted from fighting with its companions.

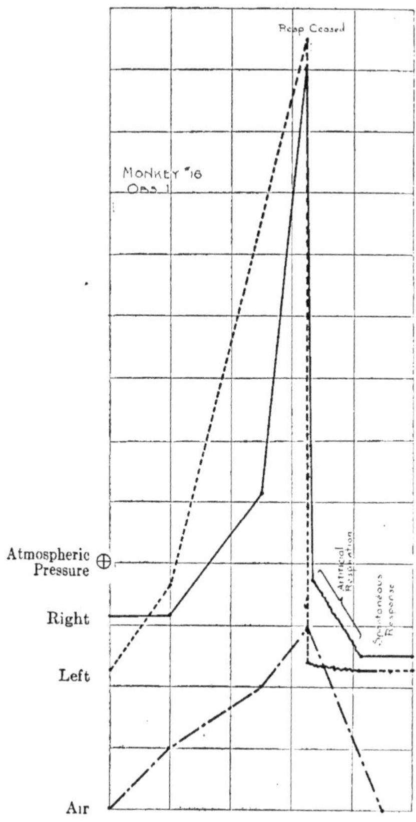

FIG. 5.—Abscissa, 1″ two minutes; ordinate, 1″ 160 beats; blood-pressure, 1″ 50 mm. Hg; intrathoracic pressure, right and left, 1″ 4 mm. bromoform; air injected or aspirated, 1″ 50 cc; atmospheric pressure ⊕.

Figure 6, *Monkey* 16, *Observation* 2. 150 cc of air injected in eleven minutes brought on respiratory distress. The more gradual injection of a smaller amount of air showed a more normal response in the intrapleural pressures and that respiration is temporarily possible in the presence of bilateral positive pressure.

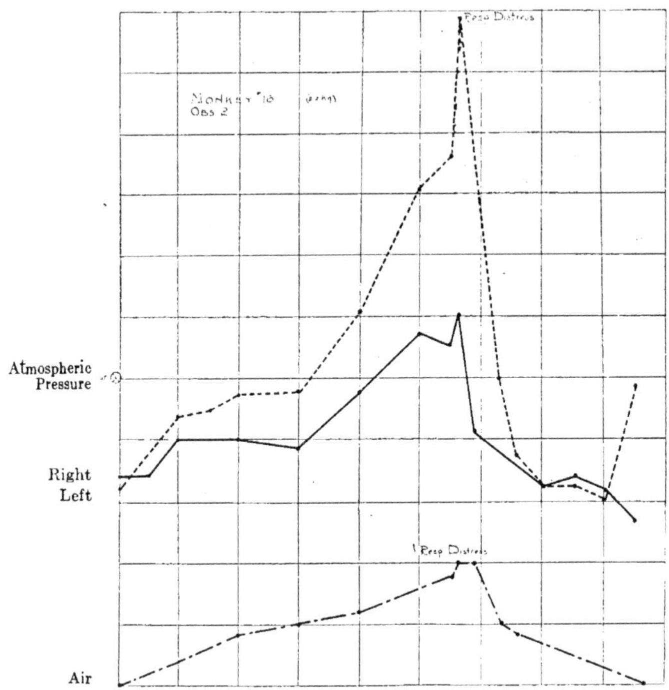

Fig. 6.—Abscissa, 1″ two minutes; ordinate, 1″ 160 beats; blood-pressure, 1″ 50 mm. Hg; intrathoracic pressure, right and left, 1″ 4 mm. bromoform; air injected or aspirated, 1″ 50 cc; atmospheric pressure ⊕.

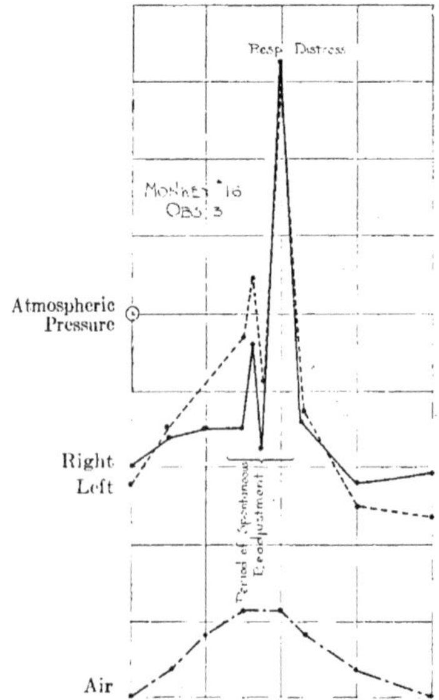

Fig. 7.—Abscissa, 1″ two minutes; ordinate, 1″ 160 beats; blood-pressure, 1″ 50 mm. Hg; intrathoracic pressure, right and left, 1″ 4 mm. bromoform; air injected or aspirated, 1″ 50 cc; atmospheric pressure ⊕.

Figure 7, Monkey 16, Observation 3. An injection of 60 cc of air in 3 minutes provoked cardiac instability that was followed after a minute by respiratory distress. A comparison of Figs. 5 and 7 shows an effect of fatigue similar to that illustrated in Figs. 2 and 3. The marked and sudden fluctuations in the intrathoracic pressures that occurred spontaneously are probably the cause of the "fluttering mediastinum."

REFERENCES.

Bradford: Quart. Jour. Med., 1919, **12**, 127; War Medicine, 1918, **2**, 10; British Med. Jour., 1917, **2**, 141.
Drinker: Jour. Exp. Med., 1921, **33**, 695.
Gregoire: Presse méd., 1917, n. s., **65**, 673; 1919, p. 355.
Gwathmey: Laboratory of Surgical Research of A. E. F., Boston Med. and Surg. Jour., 1919, **180**, 403.
Soltau: War Medicine, 1918, **2**, 1.

ANEURYSM OF THE HEPATIC ARTERY.[1]

BY JULIUS FRIEDENWALD, M.D.,
BALTIMORE,
AND
KARL H. TANNENBAUM, M.D.,
CHICAGO.

(From the Gastro-Enterological Clinic of the Department of Medicine, University of Maryland.)

ANEURYSM of the hepatic artery is an exceedingly uncommon affection. Crisp in a study of 591 cases of aneurysm in general in 1847 does not refer to a single case of hepatic aneurysm. Mester in 1895 was only able to record 20 instances collected from literature and added a case of his own; Grunert in 1904 collected 36 cases; Schupfer in 1906, 38 cases, and Rolland in 1908, 40 cases. Weiss in 1921 described a case from McCrae's clinic in Philadelphia, which had previously been studied by McCrae himself, and was able to add 14 additional cases from literature, making 55 cases in all. Since then we have collected 9 additional cases not previously reviewed, and have added a case of our own, making 65 cases in all.

The following chart presents briefly an outline of the principal data of all the cases so far observed in literature. The scheme followed is that of Rolland, from whose chart we have abstracted the record of many of the first 40 cases.

[1] Presented at the Meeting of the Association of American Physicians, Washington, May 3, 1922.

							ize.		of death.	ogy.	Symptoms.	appearance.
1	1809	Wilson	Lectures on blood, etc., before Royal College of Surgeons, 1819, p 379 (specimen now in Surgeons' Hall, Edinburgh)				Resembles heart in size and shape	Left branch intrahepatic	Rupture	(?)	(?)	(?)
2	20	Saint-Vincent	Arch gén. de Chir., 1909, 122	51	M.	One	(?)	Main trunk	Rupture into peritoneal cavity	(?)	None	Abdomen filled with blood.
3	21	Pitcairn	Specimen in Museum of Surgeons' Hall, Edinburgh, 36–296 (evidently unpublished)	48	M.	One	Hen's egg	Main trunk	Rupture into peritoneal cavity	(?)	None	(?)
4	1833	Sestie	Bull. de la Soc. Anat., tome **8**, 30	?	F.	One	Hazelnut	Right branch, extrahepatic	Exhaustion	(?)	"Chronic painful affection of liver"	Gangrene of gall-bladder.
5	1834	Stokes	Dublin Med. Jour., **5** 401	35	M.	One	Large orange	Main trunk, extrahepatic	Rupture into peritoneal cavity	(?)	Jaundice; hematemesis; slight pain; gall-bladder palpable	Abdomen filled with blood, due to rupture, aneurysm pressed on gall-bladder.
6	1834	Jackson	Med. Mag., Boston, **3,** 115	22	M.	One	Pullet's egg	Main trunk, extrahepatic	Rupture into hepatic duct	(?)	Pain; jaundice	Phthisis pulmonalis; old carotid aneurysm.
7	1855	Lebert	Anat. Path., **2,** 322	30	F.	One	Pigeon's egg	Main trunk, extrahepatic	Rupture into gall-bladder; marasmus	Embolic (?) typhoid and rheumatism	Pain; slight jaundice; hematemesis; melena; anemia	Old mitral endocarditis, old and recent pericarditis, enlarged liver; aneurysm did not rupture
8		Lebert	Quoted by Uhlig., Krankheiten der Arterien	. .	M.	One	Hazelnut	Right branch	(?)	(?)	Gastric disturbance	(?)
9	1856	Ledieu	Jour. de méd. Bordeaux, p. 125	54	F.	One	Hazelnut	Main trunk, just above the origin of the pyloric artery	Albuminuria and general dropsy	(?)	None caused by aneurysm	Aneurysmal cavity quite occluded by very firm coagulum; cirrhosis of liver.
10	1856	Babington	Dublin Med. Jour.	25	F.	One	(?)	Main trunk	Rupture into duodenum	(?)	Sudden hematemesis; melena; epigastric pain	Blood in intestines.
11	1848	Wallmann	Virchows Arch., **14,** 389	36	F.	One	Child's head	Main trunk, 7 mm. above subdivision	Rupture into peritoneal cavity	(?)	Very severe paroxysmal pain; no fever, enlarged liver and spleen	Gall-bladder much distended.
12	1868	Uhlig	Inaug. Diss., Leipzig, 1868	48	M.	One	Goose's egg	Left branch, extrahepatic	Rupture into peritoneal cavity	Infective (osteomyelitis); atheroma (?)	Severe pain	Abdomen filled with blood.
13	1868	Kaufman	Inaug. Diss., Leipzig, 1868	48	M.	One	Goose's egg	Main trunk	Rupture into abdominal cavity	Arteriosclerosis	Attacks of abdominal pain; died in one attack	Enlarged liver; enlarged spleen; atheroma of arteries.

14			Specimen in George's Hospital Museum (mentioned by Rolleston, Diseases of Liver, 1904, p. 44)					extrahepatic	Rupture into peritoneal cavity	aorta	hospital	[illegible]erent to small intestines.
15	1871	Quincke	Berl klin Wchnschr., p 349	25	M.	One	Chestnut	Right branch, intrahepatic	Exhaustion from loss of blood	Infective	Severe pain; hematemesis; melena; jaundice; fever	Pneumonia; no rupture found.
16	1875	Standhartner	Berl. d Wiener allg. Krankenheit.	23	M.	Two	(1) Walnut (2) Small nut	(1) Right branch; (2) left branch	Rupture of larger aneurysm into peritoneal cavity	Infective (?)	Icterus; high fever (not due to aneurysm)	Suppurative mediastinitis; pleurisy; pneumothorax.
17	1877	Ross and Osler	Canadian Med. Jour., **6**	21	M.	One	Small lemon	Right branch, extrahepatic	Pyemia	Infective (?)	Those of pyemia	Double pleurisy; abscesses of liver.
18	1878	Borchers	Inaug. Diss., Kiel, 1878	17	M.	Two	(1) 2.2 cm. (2) 2.5 cm.	Intrahepatic	"Amputation of femur"	Infective (?) (osteomyelitis); trauma (?)	Pain; icterus; hematemesis; melena; fever	Ruptured into hepatic duct.
19	1878	Irvine	Trans. Path. Soc., London, **29,** 128	45	M.	One	Small almond	Left branch, intrahepatic	Hemorrhage into stomach	Infective	Slight pain; hematemesis; melena	Stomach adhering and communicating with abscess of liver; early cirrhosis of liver.
20	1880	Drasche	Wien med Wchnschr., No. 37–39	27	M.	One	Hazelnut	Right branch, 1 to 5 cm. beyond division	Rupture into peritoneal cavity	(?)	Severe pain; hematemesis; melena	Abdomen filled with blood.
21	1880	Heschl	Quoted by Drasche	56	F.	One	Pigeon's egg	Main trunk just before division	Tuberculosis	(?)	None	(?)
22	1883	Weinlechner	Aerztl. allg. Bericht. der k. k. Krankenh zu Wien	Young	M.	One	(?)	Main trunk	Rupture into peritoneal cavity	Infective (?)	Sudden death	Recent osteomyelitis of femur.
23	1883	Chiari	Prag med. Wchnschr., No. **4**	33	M.	Three	Largest 2 to 1 cm.	Cystic artery	Rupture into gall-bladder	Cholelithiasis	Hematemesis; melena	Fistula between gall-bladder and duodenum.
24	1886	Caton	Clin Soc. Trans., **19,** 275	40	M.	One	1 inch in diam.	Main trunk, extrahepatic	Rupture into common duct	(?)	Intense pain; jaundice; hematemesis; melena; fever	Other organs healthy.
25	1892	Hale White	British Med. Jour., Jan , 1892, p. 223	18	M.	Two	(1) Tangerine orange (2) Slightly smaller	Right branch, extrahepatic; left branch, intrahepatic	Rupture of (1) into peritoneal cavity	Infective (?)	Pain; jaundice; hectic temperature	Pneumonia; empyema.
26	1892	Sachs	Deutsch. med. Wchnschr., **20,** 443	60	M.	One	(?)	(?)	Rupture into portal vein; aneurysmal varix	(?)	(?)	Numerous gastric ulcers; portal thrombosis.
27	1893	Sauerteig	Inaug. Diss., Jena, 1893	31	M.	Two	(1) Apple (2) Cherry	(1) Right branch, extrahepatic (2) left branch, intrahepatic	Rupture of (1) into cystic duct	(?)	Severe pain, jaundice; fever; hematemesis; melena; enlarged liver	Operated on for cholelithiasis.
28	1893	Ahrens	Inaug. Diss., Greifswald, 1893	32	F.	One	Hen's egg	Main trunk	Rupture into peritoneal cavity	Infective	Collapse	Phlegmonous inflammation of leg; hematoma of hepatoduodenal ligament.

No.	Date.	Author.	Publication.	Age.	Sex.	Number.	Size.	Position.	Immediate cause of death.	Etiology.	Symptoms.	Postmortem appearance.
29	1894	Schmidt	Deutsch. Arch. f. klin. Med., **52,** 536	46	F.	One	(?)	Right branch, intrahepatic	Rupture into hepatic duct	Cholelithiasis; 13 stones	Pain; hematemesis, melena; jaundice	Perforations between gall-bladder and duodenum.
30	1894	Niewerth	Inaug. Diss., Kiel, 1894	19	M.	Two	(1) 1.8 to 3 cm. (2) cherry	(1) At the point of division; (2) main trunk	Rupture of (1) into gall-bladder and peritoneal cavity	Atheroma of hepatic artery	Partial obstruction of [illegible]el, intense colic; tumor palpable	Cirrhosis of kidney; atheroma of aorta, etc.
31	1895	Mester	Ztschr. f. klin. Med., **28,** 93	42	M.	One	5 to 3.5 cm.	Right branch, intrahepatic	Rupture into hepatic duct	Trauma (kick of horse)	Pain; fever; hematemesis; melena; jaundice; operation by [illegible]licz; died in five days	Fatty degeneration of heart; bronchopneumonia; anemia.
32	1896	Sainton Bernard's Thesis 1897	Soc Anatom., Paris, May	46	M.	One	Large orange	Main trunk	Rupture into peritoneal cavity	Diffuse atheroma	Slight j[illegible]; collapse; pain	Atheroma of aorta, etc.
33	1897	Hansson	Centralb f die Grenzgeb d. Med u Chir, **I,** 299	14	M.	One	Hen's egg	Right branch, intrahepatic	Rupture into hepatic duct	Infective (?) (osteomyelitis	Hematemesis; melena	(?)
34	1900	Sacquepee	Zentralb f. Path Anat, **II,** 748	44	M.	One	Orange	Intrahepatic	Rupture into peritoneal cavity	Syphilitic endarteritis	Sudden collapse	Cirrhosis of liver.
35	1901	Brion	Deutsch Aerzte Zeitung, No. 18	15	M.	Four	Cherry to pea size	Intrahepatic	Rupture and hemorrhage	Typhoid fever	Sudden pain; [illegible]ver; [illegible]; icterus	Necrotic areas in liver.
36	1902	Sommer	Prag. med Wchnschr., **27,** 469	28	M.	One	(?)	Main trunk	Perforation into common duct	Infective	Icterus, pain; hematemesis; melena	Pneumonia, no atheroma.
37	1902	Sommer	Prag med Wchnschr., **27,** 469	65	F.	One	(?)	Point of origin of gastroduodenal artery	Rupture into duodenum and peritoneum	Trauma (fall)	No icterus; pain; fever; hematemesis	No atheroma.
38	1903	Kehr	[illegible]. med Wchnschr, p 1861	29	M.	One	Hen's egg	Right branch, extrahepatic	(Recovery after operation)	Pleurisy	Pain; jaundice; hema[illegible]	Aneurysm perforated into cystic [illegible].
39	1904	Grunert	Deutsch Ztschr. f. [illegible]r, **21,** 158	21	M.	One	Apple	Main trunk	Detected at operation for infection of gall-bladder (Habs, operator)	Infected gall-bladder; pneumonia	Hemorrhage; icterus; pain	Operation; gall-bladder full of infected bile; died [illegible] days after operation.
40	1904	Sojecki	Inaug. Diss., Wurzburg, 1904	36	M.	One	(?)	Main trunk	(?)	Syphilis	(?)	(?)
41	1904	Riedel	Verhandl. Deutsch. Gesellsch. f. Chir.	31	M.	One	Apple	Right branch	Rupture into hepatic duct	(?)	Colic; icterus; hematemesis; tumor in gall-bladder region; operation	Hemorrhage; aneurysm contains numerous clots.
42	1905	DeVecchi	Bull. d. Science Med. di Bologna,	83	M.	One	Cherry	Right branch, extrahepatic	Cerebral hemorrhage	Gallstone	None caused by aneurysm	Jaundice; cerebral hemorrhage; granular kidney; gall-stones.

43	1905	Libman	Proc. Path. Soc. News, 1905, **5**, 49	24	M.	One	Large	Right branch, intrahepatic	Acute endocarditis; pneumonia; streptococcic; septicemia	Infection	Only abdominal symptoms were diarrhea; poor appetite; cramp-like pain in abdomen; in addition mitral stenosis; acute endocarditis; mycotic aneurysm of right femoral artery; operated on for aneurysm of leg; streptococcic septicemia	Pneumonia in both lungs; vegetations in heart; several branches of superior mesenteric artery has several aneurysms, two the size of walnut, two the size of a bean; liver large and congested; fatty
44	1905	Schultze, 38	Ziegler's Beiträge, 38	57	M.	One	Apple	Main branch	Rupture into common duct	Gallstones	Colicky pain; jaundice; hematemesis	Hemorrhage into the bowel.
45	1906	Allessandri	Bull. d. Accad. med. di Roma, **32**, 63	22	M.	One	Hen's egg	Right branch, extrahepatic	Rupture into common duct	Infection (pneumonia)	No pain; no fever, jaundice; melena; liver enlarged; gall-bladder palpable, operation; tamponed aneurysm	Death six days after operation; hemorrhage.
46	1906	Livierato	Gazz. d. Osp. Milano, **27**, 593	28	M.	One	....	Main trunk	Rupture into peritoneal cavity	Infection (pneumonia)	Severe pain; vomiting; collapse	Double pneumonia; thrombosis of hepatic artery; liver healthy.
47	1906	Waetzold	München. med. Wchnschr., **43**, 2167	44	M.	Several	Largest a cherry, others smaller	Right branch, intrahepatic	Rupture into peritoneal cavity	Syphilitic endarteritis and periarteritis	Pain in liver region; those of cirrhosis of liver	Cirrhosis of liver; parenchymatous nephritis; endocarditis of aortic valve, necrosis of liver area.
48	1906	Schupfer	Gaz. d. hôp., Aug. 26, No. 102	38	M.	One	Hen's egg	Main trunk	Rupture into gall-bladder	Infection	Icterus; hematemesis	Hemorrhage into gall-bladder
49	1907	Bickhardt and Schuman	Deutsch. Arch. f. klin. Med., p. 289	69	F.	One	Child's fist.	Right branch	Rupture into duodenum	Arteriosclerosis	Pain; pulsating tumor; vomiting, icterus, fever, hematemesis; osteomyelitis, pain; sudden hemorrhage, vomiting	Rupture and hemorrhage into peritoneal cavity, atheroma of aorta, hemorrhage into peritoneal cavity; swelling of liver cells; small abscesses of kidneys; coxitis.
50				10	M.	One	Hen's egg	Right branch	Rupture into peritoneal cavity	Embolic		
51	1908	Rolland	Glasgow Med. Jour., **69**, 342	46	F.	Three	(1) 25 cm. by 15 cm. (2) pea (3) barleycorn	Main trunk, intrahepatic	Rupture into abdominal cavity	Diffuse atheroma	Sudden pain in abdomen with collapse	Abdomen filled with blood; cardiac hypertrophy, chronic hepatitis
52	1908	Reichmann	Virchows Arch., **104**, 71	26	M.	One	Pigeon's egg	Right branch	Rupture into abdominal cavity and bowel	Embolic	Colicky pain, fever	Thrombosis of aneurysm of hepatic artery
53	1909	Tuffier	Presse méd., No. 18	72	M.	One	Goose's egg	Main trunk	Operation, ligation of artery	Obliteration, endarteritis	Icterus, pruritus; tumor in gall-bladder region	Patient died five days following operation; thrombus of artery partly calcified.

ate.	Author	Publication.	Age.	Sex.	Number.	Size.	Position.	Immediate cause of death.	Etiology.	Symptoms.	Postmortem appearance.
1909	Bode	Beitr. klin. Chir.	23	M.	One	Walnut size	Right branch, intrahepatic	Operation, gastroenterostomy (Garre); death after eight days; rupture into duodenum	Trauma	Hematemesis, intense pain	Congestion and necrosis of small areas of liver.
1912	Dean and Falconer	Edinburgh Med. Jour., **8**, 124	22	M.	One	$1\frac{1}{2}$ to $1\frac{1}{4}$ inches, multilocular	Main trunk	Rupture into hepatic duct	Infection pneumonia	Icterus; hematemesis; melena; colicky pain; tender in epigastrium and gall-bladder region	Rupture and hemorrhage; necrosis of area in right lobe of liver.
1912	Friedman	Med. Rec., Sept. 21, p. 522	35	F.	One	S-shaped; six inches in length	Main trunk	....	(?)	Alcoholic subject; pain; pulsation in liver region; systolic murmur and pulsation over liver; diagnosis made during life and confirmed by operation	
1913	Merkel	Virchows Arch., **214**, 289	56	M.	One	Hen's egg, 5 cm. long, 3.3 cm. wide	Main trunk	Carcinoma of stomach; operation, resection with gastrojejunostomy; sudden death ten days after operation	Trauma	None pointing to aneurysm	Hepatic artery entirely thrombosed and calcified; liver intact due to collateral circulation; chronic nephritis; chronic peritonitis.
1913	Fleckenstein	Inaug. Diss., Giessen, 1913	41	F.	One	Twice size of man's fist	Main trunk	Acute intestinal obstruction due to incarceration of intestine	Arteriosclerosis	Severe pain in abdomen	Aneurysm with many adhesions to the liver and portal vein; hepatic artery sclerosed.
1915	Baruch	Beitr. z. klin. Chir., **95**, 502	36	M.	One	Size of fist	Main trunk	Operation, pressure with tampon; died one day following operation from shock	Incipient arteriosclerosis	Jaundice; hemorrhages; fever; anemia	Hemorrhage into peritoneal cavity.
1916	Teacher and Jack	Glasgow Med. Jour., p. 277	43	M.	Three	(1) 4 by 25 cm. (2) very small (3) size of a walnut	Branch of hepatic artery intrahepatic	Rupture into abdominal cavity, chronic cardiac and nephritic disease	Probably syphilitic	Those of chronic nephritis with edema of extremities and cardiac disease; temp. to 102°; pain in liver region; died suddenly.	Intraperitoneal hemorrhage; periarteritis nodosa; thrombosus of aneurysm; chronic nephritis.

61	1919	Anderson	Tenn. Med. Jour., **12,** 32	32	M.	One		Branch of hepatic artery, intrahepatic		Syphilis	Previous history of aneurysm of radial artery; pain; collapse; operation; laparotomy; 2 qts. of blood removed; sutures and packing; recovery; antisyphilitic treatment later; aneurysm of hepatic artery	
62	1919	Kading	Deutsch. Ztschr. f. Chir., **150,** 82	35	M.	One		Intrahepatic, branch of hepatic artery		Trauma	Shot through liver and pleura; hematothorax; pain in liver region; faintness; hematemesis; melena; 1st operation nothing accomplished; 2d operation a few days later (Sudeck); ligated hepatic artery; recovery	
63	1920	Hogler	Wien. Arch. f. inn. Med., **1,** 509	51	M.	One	Walnut	Cystic branch of hepatic artery	Rupture into cystic duct; hemorrhage	Atheroma	Diagnosis made during life; systolic murmur over liver; colic; pain; hematemesis	Thrombosis of aneurysmal sac.
64	1926	McCrae	International Clinics, **3,** 1	50	M.	One	2 cm. by 3 cm.; middle size of plum	Main trunk at point of division into the terminal branches	Rupture into abdominal cavity	Panarteritis of branches of hepatic artery	Acute abdominal pain; fever 100° to 102°; jaundice, tenderness in gallbladder area; died while taking anesthetic for exploratory incision	Chronic diffuse nephritis; granular degeneration of pancreas; obliterative endarteritis of small vessel of liver; aortitis; dissecting aneurysm of thoracic aorta and aneurysm of the left iliac artery.
	1921	Weiss	Am. Jour. Med. Sci., **161,** 859									
65	1922	Friedenwald and Tannenbaum	Am. Jour. Med. Sci., **165,** 11	48	M.	One	5 cm. by 4½ cm.; small orange	Extrahepatic	Rupture and hemorrhage into abdominal cavity	Panarteritis and atheroma of the hepatic artery and its branches	Jaundice; anemia; emaciation; hemorrhage; pain at termination	Endarteritis and atheroma of hepatic artery and its branches; rupture of aneurysm and hemorrhage into peritoneal cavity.

Case History. H. L. F., male, married, aged forty-eight years, a merchant by occupation, consulted us on May 9, 1921, with the complaint of jaundice. His family history is essentially negative. His father died from nephritis; his mother is still alive and is well; two brothers and two sisters are living and are enjoying good health; while one brother died of nephritis.

Personal History. The patient's general health has always been excellent. He has had measles twice, but gives no history of any other infectious diseases or other illnesses. There was a small cyst removed five years ago from the outer surface of the upper gum in the midline by extracting the four central incisors and curetting the jaw. Healing proceeded normally following the operation and this affection has never since given him the slightest discomfort. The teeth are replaced by a removable bridge.

The patient was rejected from life insurance last fall on the ground of the finding of albumin in the urine. This was inconstant however, and was not revealed in two succeeding examinations. At that time the patient says nothing else abnormal was revealed.

Present Illness. About three months ago the patient began a course of dieting, being under the impression that he was too obese. He lost 12 pounds in weight in three weeks, and then began to feel a "bit out of sorts." He had indigestion following this occasionally, but of a mild type, and was affected with a slight diarrhea, but not with pain. The patient discontinued his reduction cure. He did not, however, feel quite up to normal, though he had no real complaint or discomfort. Eight weeks ago he began to notice a slight jaundice, which has gradually since been increasing. There has never been any pain and nothing abnormal was further revealed with the exception of a rather marked itching of the skin, bitter taste in the mouth, together with some loss of appetite, weakness, drowsiness and gradual loss of 18 more pounds in weight. The stools have never been clay colored, but are rather the reverse, darker than normal.

Physical Examination. The patient is a rather stout, well-developed man with a moderately deep jaundiced skin and sclerotics.

Head is of normal contour. Cheeks and eyes do not seem particularly sunken. Everywhere a marked degree of jaundice. Pupils round, regular and equal; moderately contracted; react somewhat slowly to light and accommodation. Extraocular movements are good. Ears and nose apparently normal.

In the mouth four upper incisors are missing and are replaced by a removable bridge. Beneath this is a well-healed scar of the operation on the gums, which leaves a rather marked depression in the center of the upper jaw, just beneath the septum of the nose. There is no infiltration of the gums about the scar. There is considerable dentistry. The tongue is coated with a brownish fur and protrudes in the midline; no tremor. The posterior pharynx is moderately injected. The tonsils are small and normal in appearance. The neck is short and thick; no glands are palpable. The thyroid is not enlarged.

Thorax. The thorax is well formed; is rather broad and deep; some suggestion of barrel-shaping; expansion is good. The lungs are clear throughout to percussion and auscultation, except that the area of the liver dulness reaches up to just above the fourth rib, to the right, compressing the right lung slightly. The heart is not enlarged. The sounds are clear and of normal relative intensity. No murmurs can be made out. There does not appear to be any palpable degree of peripheral sclerosis. The pulses are of good volume and equal in force and rhythm.

Abdomen. The abdomen is full and thick walled. The edge of the liver can be palpated almost as far down as the umbilicus. The liver itself is rather smooth and not particularly tender to pressure and no nodules can be detected. The gall-bladder and spleen are not palpable. The lower abdomen is apparently normal.

Extremities. The extremities are normal. No glandular enlargements can be detected anywhere. The knee reflexes are present and are moderately active and equal throughout.

Laboratory Examinations. Total red count 4,200,000; hemoglobin 60 per cent; color index 0.71. Total leukocyte count 7500. Differential count: Polynuclears 57 per cent; small mononuclears 58 per cent; large mononuclears 3 per cent; eosinophils 1 per cent; basophils 1 per cent. Morphological examination negative with the exception of evidences of a secondary anemia. Serum bile tinged. The urine is of a specific gravity of 1025; presents a large bile ring and a few hyaline casts, but is otherwise negative.

The gastric contents; 60 cc obtained after an Ewald meal. Total acidity 34; free HCl 24; bile tinged; no blood.

Stool. The stool is almost tar colored, containing a few undigested meat fibers; no parasites; large quantities of blood.

Duodenal drainage according to the Lyon method revealed a markedly turbid bile which flowed freely; no gall-bladder bile obtained. Cultures showed numerous colonies identified as the colon bacillus. Fractional analysis of the pancreatic ferments according to the Einhorn method revealed an imperfect steapsin and trypsin digestion.

Roentgen-ray Examination. Stomach is of cow-horn type held to the right under the gall-bladder region; deformity surrounding the pylorus, suggesting a mass in the upper right quadrant. The liver is enlarged. Chest roentgen-ray is negative.

Diagnosis. On account of the age of the patient, his loss of flesh, absence of pain, jaundice, blood in the stools, diminution in pancreatic ferments, and the roentgen-ray findings, the diagnosis was made of carcinoma of the pancreas, though the possibility of a stone lodged in the ampulla could not be entirely ruled out.

Clinical Notes. The patient was admitted in the Union Memorial Hospital, for further observation and possibly for operation, on May 15, 1921.

May 16, 1921. Patient was examined last night and appeared in good condition when last seen at 11 P.M. At 3 A.M., while on the commode, but before his bowels had moved, he had a sudden fainting attack. He lost consciousness and his pulse became imperceptible. This was associated with a very severe pain in the right hypochondrium just to the right of the epigastrium. The patient was revived after the administration of camphorated oil, although his pulse remained very weak and his respiration rapid; he was extremely pale and shocked. The pain in the epigastrium continued, though less severe than at the onset. Half an hour after the collapse the patient had a profuse bowel movement, but there were no evidences of blood clots or hemorrhage. Following this there was a second partial collapse, which was again relieved by the administration of camphorated oil.

During the remainder of the night the patient remained in a more or less shocked state, but had improved somewhat by morning. The pain in the epigastrium gradually subsided until now there is but little remaining. The medication consisted in the application of an ice cap to the epigastrium; morphine gr. $\frac{1}{8}$, every four hours. Nothing was allowed by mouth with the exception of crushed ice. The pulse during this entire period did not exceed 90 beats per minute, and the rate this morning was 76; yet the pulse is extremely weak, and the patient appears exsanguinated. The temperature is subnormal, 96.8°; respirations, 22. There is no evidence whatever of any lung complication. A transfusion of 500 cc of whole blood was given in the afternoon; no reaction was noted. At night the patient feels and appears much improved. The bowels have not been evacuated during the day. There is neither nausea nor vomiting. Nothing abnormal can be detected on palpation at the site of the pain. The abdomen is soft; there is neither tenderness nor rigidity. The attack remains unexplained.

May 17, 1921. Patient had a comfortable night; slept brokenly. Pulse is of good quality, about 50 per minute. Temperature 97°, respirations 20. He is allowed a slightly increased diet together with water. He was nauseated once in the afternoon, but did not vomit; there are frequent eructations following the ingestion of fluids. Large amounts of flatus are expelled. The bowels have not been evacuated in spite of a water and glycerine enema. The temperature rose to 100° in the evening. The patient has voided but 250 cc of urine since the attack, now almost forty-eight hours. He is perspiring almost constantly. His condition appears improved, although there is still no explanation of the attack, except the possibility of an internal hemorrhage not uncommonly observed in jaundiced individuals.

May 18, 1921. The patient passed a comfortable night. He has been annoyed at times by hiccoughing. He has voided urine very well since midnight. Some blood-tinged mucus has been expectorated this morning, due apparently to a general oozing from the nasopharynx rather than from a single bleeding-point; a slight cough has appeared this afternoon. An examination revealed the abdomen to be soft without tenderness. The borders of the liver extend to the umbilicus, and up to just above the fourth rib.

The lung is much compressed in this area but is resonant. A very loud coarse to-and-fro rub is heard over the whole front of the right chest, extending through to the back. Calcium lactate was prescribed in an effort to control the bleeding. The patient appeared quite comfortable and in an improved condition, except for the rub over his right lung. The patient has been ordered for operation in the morning.

May 19, 1921. A comfortable night was passed by the patient. At 8 A.M. his temperature was 98°, pulse 86, respiration 20. At 8.15 he suddenly uttered a cry, became pulseless and died. The diagnosis of hemorrhage was arrived at, the cause of which was not ascertained.

Autopsy Report. May 19, 1921. A partial autopsy only was permitted. The peritoneal cavity was opened through a high right rectus incision. The peritoneum was everywhere of dull appearance, the normal glistening quality being absent. About 2 liters of blood escaped on incising the cavity. Blood clots in large amounts were removed from the right side of the abdomen. The stomach and duodenum were inspected and found to be normal in appearance. The liver was much enlarged, and somewhat of a pale yellowish color, apparently fatty. The gall-bladder was slightly distended and contained a dark viscid bile but no stones. A mass was observed attached to the inferior surface of the liver posteriorly and adjacent to the gall-bladder. It appeared to be just anterior to the common duct. The mass was about the size of a small orange and presented a perforation on its anterior surface from which blood oozed following manipulation. The mass, together with the pylorus, part of the duodenum, portion of the abdominal aorta with the celiac axis and common bile duct, was removed.

The mass is an aneurysm of the hepatic artery. It is 5 cm. in length by 4.5 cm. in width and shows a perforation in its anterior surface 1.5 cm. in length from which it is evident the blood has escaped into the peritoneal cavity. The hepatic artery widens as it enters the aneurysmal sac, having a diameter of 2.5 cm. at this point. The interior of the aneurysm is partly filled with clotted blood extending into the branches of the hepatic artery. The jaundice noted can be easily explained on the basis of pressure of the aneurysm against the hepatic and common ducts.

A microscopic examination made by Dr. Standish McCleary is as follows: Sections made from the sac adjacent to the point of rupture show laminated fibers lying upon a much thickened hyaline intima. The medium as such has disappeared and is represented by an atheromatous mass containing many fat-laden phagocytes. There is also present a deposit of minute masses of calcium. The adventitia is thickened and has attached to its outer surface a thin layer of normal hepatic tissues. There is not the slightest suggestion of a luetic process in the tissue. Sections were also made from several of the smaller branches of the hepatic artery, and all show well-advanced endarteritis and in some cases early changes in the media.

Pathology. According to Mester, aneurysms of the hepatic artery may be divided into two groups, the extra- and the intra-hepatic forms. Of these, according to this author, the extrahepatic is four times as frequent as the intrahepatic, while Rolland following the same classification finds it three times as frequent. In one collection of all cases previously recorded, in addition to our own case, numbering 65 cases in all, there were 45 extrahepatic and 18 intrahepatic, while in 2 both intra- and extrahepatic aneurysm were noted, as was observed in Sauerteig's and Hale White's cases, in which the right branch revealed an extrahepatic aneurysm and the left branch an intrahepatic.

In 60 of our 65 cases the main trunk was involved in 29 instances, the left branch in 6 and the right in 23; in 2 instances the aneurysm was noted as a part of the cystic artery (Chiari and Hogler). Two aneurysms were observed in 5 instances (Standhartner, Sauerteig, Borchers, Hale White, Niewerth). In Chiari's, Rolland's, and Teacher and Jack's cases there were three and in Waetzold's several. Aneurysms usually form adhesions to surrounding tissues, hepatic duct, cystic duct, gall-bladder, common duct, or surface of the liver, and finally rupture occurs into the organs to which there has been adhesions or into the peritoneal cavity which may thus be the immediate cause of death; usually repeated hemorrhages, however, occur, the blood causing a coagulum in the sac which seals the opening temporarily.

Of the 65 cases rupture of the aneurysmal sac occurred in 45 while 13 remained unruptured. The rupture was most commonly noted into the peritoneal cavity. In 33 instances of this series it occurred into the abdominal cavity, in 21 into the bile passages and in 4 into other organs, the stomach in 1, the duodenum in 2 and the portal vein in 1. When in intrahepatic aneurysms rupture occurs into the abdominal cavity, it takes place through the liver and is accompanied by a stripping of Glisson's capsule. Sacquepee was the first to note the importance of rupture of an intrahepatic aneurysm as the cause of rupture of the liver. Similar observations have been reported by Waetzold, Wilson and Rolland.

Occasionally the aneurysm may undergo spontaneous healing as was noted in Ledieu's case where the patient died of renal disease and in whom an aneurysm of the hepatic artery was demonstrated, occluded by a thrombus and which had not produced any symptoms whatsoever.

In Merkel's case the patient died ten days following a resection of the stomach and gastrojejunostomy. At autopsy an aneurysm of the hepatic artery the size of a hen's egg was discovered entirely thrombosed and calcified which too had not produced any symptoms.

The aneurysmal sac is usually single, though in 2 cases (Borchers and Niewerth) it was divided into two parts.

In 10 cases of this series the aneurysm itself was not the immediate cause of death (Lestie, Heschl, Ledieu, Ross and Osler, Grunert, DeVecchi, Libman, Quincke, Merkel, Fleckenstein).

The size of hepatic aneurysms varies from that of a barleycorn (Rolland) to a child's head (Wallmann), the average being that of a hen's egg. The extrahepatic forms are usually larger than the intrahepatic.

Etiology. This disease is more common in males than females. According to Hogler the incidence in males to females is as three to one, and according to our own observations as four to one.

Of the 63 cases in which the sex is recorded 50 were males and 13 females. The ages of the individuals affected range between the fourteenth year (Hansson) and eighty-third year (DeVecchi); the average age of the 63 cases is thirty-eight years; the average age of the males being thirty-six and females forty-four years; females are evidently as a rule affected in a later period in life. According to Rolland occupation plays but an insignificant role in the etiology of this affection, the disease being met with in individuals following the most diverse vocations.

As etiological factors in the production of this disorder infectious processes play a very significant role. Of these, strangely septic endocarditis, typhoid fever, pneumonia, osteomyelitis are far more frequent than syphilis. In many instances infective emboli are probably the cause, following such infections as endocarditis and suppurative processes. In a small proportion of cases syphilis is a factor. According to Grunert 73 per cent of the 36 cases collected by him were due to infectious processes.

Trauma has been considered in some instances as a causative factor in the production of these aneurysms, which may not only act from without but also from within, as by the direct injury against the arterial wall by gallstones.

In a number of instances of aneurysm embolism occurred as a result of endocarditis, while a certain number of cases were directly due to such infections as pneumonia, typhoid fever, osteomyelitis, pleurisy and empyema. In a not inconsiderable number atheromatous changes of the aorta and other vessels were observed. In vegetative endocarditis emboli may be thrown off and caught in the arteries. Such vegetations ordinarily contain staphylococci and streptococci. At the position of the embolic thrombus there is at first an exudative inflammation produced, then an acute periarteritis with destruction of the media and the adventitia, and the intima bursts. As the result of these lesions, there is a bulging of the vessel and in the wall of the dilatation all layers of the arterial wall are to be found.

In Chiari's and Niewerth's cases atheroma was noted in the hepatic artery itself, but was also observed in many of the other bloodvessels, so that certain local conditions must be at hand to determine the production of the hepatic aneurysm. In some instances this may be in the form of a cholelithiasis on account of which direct injury to the weakened artery must be considered. In syphilis there is an intense endarteritis with visible damage to the arterial wall together with changes in the surrounding connective tissue. This affection was present in Sacquepee's, Waetzold's, Rolland's, McCrae's, Teacher and Jack's, Anderson and Sojecki's cases. Trauma as a cause of aneurysm was noted by Mester, Sommer, Sauerteig, Brion, DeVecchi, Merkel, Bode and Kading. In Sommer's case the patient fell in the dark and injured himself in the abdomen. In Mester's case a kick in the abdomen by a horse was noted as the cause. In Brion's case the patient was subjected to frequent pressure on the abdomen with bars of iron during his work.

In this series of 65 cases a definite causative factor was noted in 50 instances. Of these a general infection was observed in 7; typhoid fever in 2; pneumonia in 5; pleurisy with empyema in 1; osteomyelitis in 3; arteriosclerosis in 12; cholelithiasis in 5; syphilis in 7; trauma in 8 cases.

Symptoms. The symptoms most frequently observed in aneurysm of the hepatic artery are pain, hemorrhage, icterus, enlargement of the liver, fever, fluctuating tumor in the region of the gall-bladder, marked anemia, emaciation, together with attacks of syncope, dizziness, headaches, weakness and indigestion. All of these symptoms are rarely present in any individual case and ordinarily there are but few, in many instances the patient dying after a single attack of pain followed by hemorrhage without having had any previous symptoms whatever.

Pain. Of the symptoms noted above, pain is rarely absent and but few cases are recorded in which this symptom is not noted as an early and important sign. According to Schupfer it occurred in 70 per cent of his cases. It was present in 39 of the 49 cases of this series in which symptoms are recorded (79 per cent). Pain was extremely moderate in Stokes's and Irvine's cases and was entirely absent in Lebert's, Standhartner's, Ross and Osler's, Chiari's, Hansson's, Allessandri's, Schupfer's, Tuffier's, Baruch's and our cases. In the case reported by us pain occurred but twice during the stage of hemorrhage at the very termination of the affection. The pain is usually paroxysmal, is of great severity, resembling biliary colic and is localized in the epigastrium and right hypochondrium in the region of the gall-bladder, descending according to Hogler

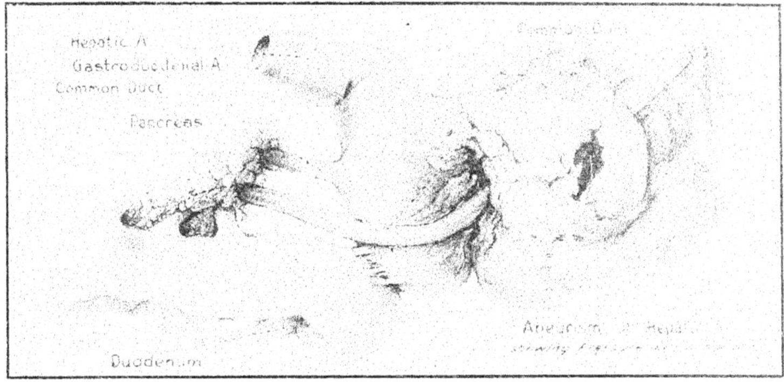

Fig. 1

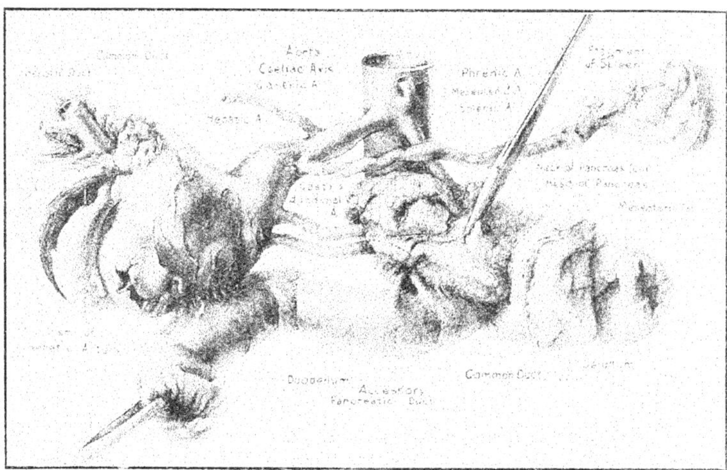

Fig. 2

toward the lower abdomen and back. It occurs rarely in the upper left quadrant (Irvine's case). In the intervals between the paroxysms pain is ordinarily absent.

The cause of the pain in the intrahepatic aneurysms is pressure on the liver capsule; in the extrahepatic forms to pressure of the aneurysmal sac on the hepatic plexus of nerves. During the attack of pain tenderness on pressure is observed in the epigastrium and right hypochondrium.

Hemorrhage. Hemorrhage is a frequent symptom of this affection and is not uncommonly noted in the form of hematemesis or melena, or as both. Hemorrhages occurred in 31 of the 49 cases in which symptoms were recorded (63 per cent). They indicate rupture of the aneurysm, are often massive, intermittent, recur at irregular intervals, and are usually the immediate cause of death. The hemorrhages may take place into the abdominal cavity or bile ducts, or into the gastrointestinal tract. Gastric and intestinal hemorrhage is frequently occasioned in these cases as a result of the rupture of the aneurysm into the biliary tract. In Irvine's case, however, rupture occurred into the stomach; in Sommer's and Babington's into the duodenum and in Reichmann's into the intestine. Bleeding frequently checks itself by the rapid filling of the bile passages with blood. Even though moderate, hemorrhage usually occurs following the colicky pain and is associated with constitutional signs of weakness, rapid pulse and anemia.

Jaundice. According to Grunert, icterus was noted in 64 per cent of the cases of hepatic aneurysm and according to Schupfer in 62 per cent and to Rolland in 40 per cent. In this series of 49 cases in which symptoms were recorded, it occurred in 27 instances (55 per cent). It may be temporary or permanent and is usually increased with the attacks of the pain, though jaundice without pain has been observed in a number of instance. (Tuffier's, Baruch's, and our own cases). Temporary jaundice was noted by Quincke, Lebert and Mester. The jaundice is caused by the pressure of the aneurysm on the biliary passages or it may be due to hemorrhage from the aneurysm into the larger biliary passages producing obstruction by the formation of clots. The recurrent forms of jaundice are produced according to Bickhardt and Schuman by the latter condition.

Fever. A rise in temperature is occasionally noted. It occurred in 16 of this series of 49 cases, in which symptoms were noted (32 per cent), though in some of the cases it may be explained by causes other than those due to the aneurysm.

It may rise as high as 103° or 104° and usually occurs with the paroxysms of pain and may be associated with chills. Fever was first noted by Quincke in his case and occurred in Standhartner's, Ross and Osler's, Borchers's, Caton's, Hale White's, Sauerteig's, Mester's, Hansson's, Brion's Sommer's, Allessandri's, Reichmann's, Baruch's, Teacher and Jack's and McCrae's cases.

The rise in temperature has been compared by Quincke with that accompanying biliary colic and is probably due to infection or in some instances to the absorption of the blood following hemorrhage.

Tumor Formation with Enlargement of the Liver. Marked enlargement of the liver has been noted in a number of instances, especially where the aneurysm had become massive. It was present in Sauerteig's, Wallman's and our cases. Distention of the gall-bladder was recorded in the cases of Stokes, Niewerth and Allessandri. In Stokes and Allessandri's cases it was due to pressure on the bile ducts and to the retention of bile in the gall-bladder and in Niewerth's it was produced by hemorrhage into the gall-bladder.

A palpable mass representing a hepatic aneurysm noted in the region of the liver was observed in the cases of Riedel, Bickhardt and Schuman and Tuffier. In Riedel and Tuffier's cases the tumor was nonfluctuant, while in Bickhardt's it fluctuated several days before death. While a nonpalpable mass was revealed in the cases of Friedman and Hogler, a visible pulsation was noted over the region of the liver associated with a systolic murmur. These signs lead to a correct diagnosis.

In addition to the symptoms already noted others more general, such as indigestion, anemia, emaciation, weakness, dizziness and fainting attacks have frequently been observed.

Diagnosis. The diagnosis of this affection is usually exceedingly difficult, as is evidenced by the fact that in but 2 cases of the 65 collected was the diagnosis correctly made during life except in those instances in which exploratory incisions were performed. The signs of colic resembling those of cholelithiasis, hemorrhage and icterus must be considered, especially when following upon such infectious diseases as pneumonia, typhoid fever and acute endocarditis. The diagnosis becomes more positive if a pulsating tumor is evident in the region of the liver exhibiting a systolic bruit.

In the differential diagnosis, cholelithiasis, duodenal ulcer and pancreatic carcinoma must be considered. In cholelithiasis there is usually an absence of hemorrhage and always of a pulsating tumor. On the other hand gallstones and aneurysm of the hepatic artery may occur in the same individual as was noted in Chiari's, Schmidt's, Grunert's and DeVecchi's cases, which may render the diagnosis even more difficult.

In duodenal ulcer the pain is not usually of the violent gall-bladder type, jaundice is usually absent and the roentgen-ray findings are ordinarily sufficiently suggestive to clear up the diagnosis. In carcinoma of the pancreas there is usually an absence of severe abdominal pain and large hemorrhages are unusual.

The average duration of this affection is from four and one-half to five months, the shortest being two months, as was noted in Borcher's case, and the longest eight and one-half months, as in Mester's case.

Treatment. Zesas,[2] who carefully reviewed the literature of this subject in 1910, concludes that ligation of the hepatic artery in cases of aneurysm is the only rational method of treatment and

[2] Fortschr. der Med., 1910, **28**, 1313.

maintains that there should be no delay in performing this operation once the diagnosis is established. Hogler very recently likewise arrives at a similar conclusion and points to the fact that Kehr was the first to perform this operation with recovery of his patient, establishing this operation as a justifiable surgical procedure. Previous to this period 3 cases were operated on with fatal results (Sauerteig, Niewerth, (Heller, operator), Mester, (Miculicz, operator), in none of which was the artery ligated.

On the other hand there has been considerable controversy regarding the propriety of ligating the hepatic artery in cases of aneurysm. Baruch refutes the advisability of performing this procedure from his experiments on thirty animals, and maintains that necrosis of the liver may result in consequence; according to his observations the more centrally the ligature is placed the less liable is this complication to ensue. Behrend[3] has also arrived at a similar conclusion from his experimental work on animals and has demonstrated that ligation of the hepatic artery terminates fatally, the interruption of the circulation resulting in an acute yellow atrophy of the liver with large areas of necrosis. Zesas, however, maintains, in opposition to this view, that animal experimentation differs in many respects from the actual conditions observed in human beings in whom on account of the length of duration of the affection sufficient time has elapsed for a collateral circulation to have thoroughly established itself.

Since the first successful operation performed by Kehr in 1903, 9 other cases have been subjected to surgery, the case of Riedel, Grunert (Habs, operator), Allessandri, Tuffier, Friedman, Merkel, Baruch, Anderson and Kading; of these but 3 recovered, the cases of Friedman, Anderson and Kading.

Finally it is interesting to note that of the 13 cases on whom operations were performed, on but 8 was the diagnosis correctly made at operation, the cases of Kehr, Grunert, Allesandri, Tuffier, Baruch, Friedman, Anderson and Kading.

Conclusion. It may be well to again draw attention to the fact that aneurysm of the hepatic artery is a rather rare affection, but 65 cases in all having been recorded; that the main symptoms of the diseases are colicky-like pain occurring in the region of the gall-bladder, hemorrhage and jaundice and occasionally a pulsating tumor exhibiting a systolic bruit; that ligation of the hepatic artery is the only rational method of treatment.

[3] Surg., Gynec. and Obst., 1920, **31**, 182.

FIBRILLATION OF THE AURICLE RETURNED TO NORMAL RHYTHM.

By Louis Faugeres Bishop, M.D.,

PRESIDENT OF THE GOOD SAMARITAN DISPENSARY AND CONSULTANT IN HEART AND CIRCULATORY DISEASES AT THE LINCOLN HOSPITAL, NEW YORK.

It would seem advisable to study a few electrocardiograms of cases illustrating the return to normal rhythm in hearts which have been the seat of fibrillation of the auricle but were later normal in their auricular function. Some of the people with hearts of this type are under observation at the present time.

An excellent example is that of a man with extremely advanced circulatory disease, which is shown by an enormous enlargement of the heart, the maintenance of a terrific blood-pressure, the recurrence at various times of all the cardiac symptoms of heart failure, namely, dyspnea, edema, congestion of the lungs, liver and kidneys, and occasionally fibrillation of the auricle.

This man, nevertheless, now presents a fair appearance of health and a regular heart as the result of being put on a strict regimen. The only specific treatment he has been given for his fibrillation is digitalis. His normal rhythm is therefore a part of the natural history of the ups and downs of the auricle.

Another illustration of auricular fibrillation of an entirely different character is that of a man who developed cardiac disease as a result of long-standing, continued nervous strain and overwork. He had symptoms of angina pectoris. At the time of his examination he had auricular fibrillation. His heart is now regular as a result of his being put under a strict regimen.

The histories of the other cases are herewith described in detail with the electrocardiograms illustrating the return of rhythm to normal after auricular fibrillation.

Case I (LPIB).—A tall, stout man, single, aged forty-one years, weighing 200 pounds, came to the office complaining of palpitation. He had no precordial pain. His family history was negative and his personal habits were very good. He kept his bowels regular by daily doses of Russian oil. He gave a history of malaria seven years ago and rheumatism when thirteen years old, which, however, was apparently without cardiac involvement. He had had an attack of palpitation similar to his present one ten years ago. His present attack of cardiac palpitation followed influenza which he had four weeks previously. The attacks were best relieved by taking aromatic spirits of ammonia.

No marked abnormalities were found on physical examination. There were no heart murmurs and the pulse was regular on auscultation. The systolic blood-pressure was 120 and the diastolic

95. The blood picture was normal in every respect. Urinalysis showed no albumin and no sugar, but there were some leukocytes. It had a specific gravity of 1030. The Wassermann reaction was negative.

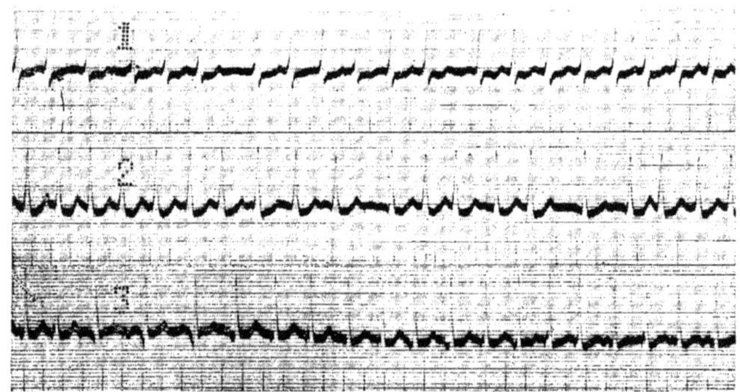

Fig. 1 (*a*).—Electrocardiogram showing auricular fibrillation, April 7, 1919.

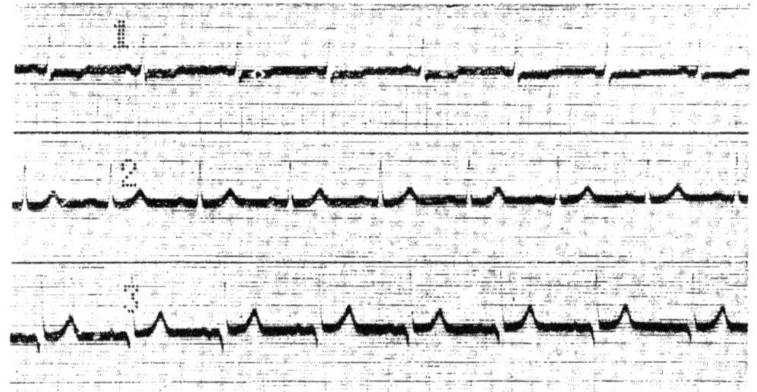

Fig. 1 (*b*).—Electrocardiogram showing return to normal rhythm without specific treatment, April 8, 1919.

Case II (LISD).—A minister, aged forty-seven years, weighing 185 pounds, came for examination because of precordial pain on exertion. This pain occasionally extended down his left arm. His first attack of pain came on suddenly about a year previous to his coming here. He never had any attacks at night, but slept very well.

His family history was negative. His personal habits were excellent. Aside from recurring attacks of tonsillitis, he had had no former illness.

On examination a systolic murmur was heard several times over the aortic area, but no more definite signs were found. His systolic blood-pressure was usually 140 and his diastolic 100. The blood picture was entirely normal and the Wassermann reaction was negative. Urinalysis revealed a faint trace of albumin and an occasional hyaline cast. The specific gravity varied between 1008 and 1028.

Under routine treatment with fortnightly doses of castor oil and careful dietary restrictions the symptoms have been greatly relieved during the succeeding two years.

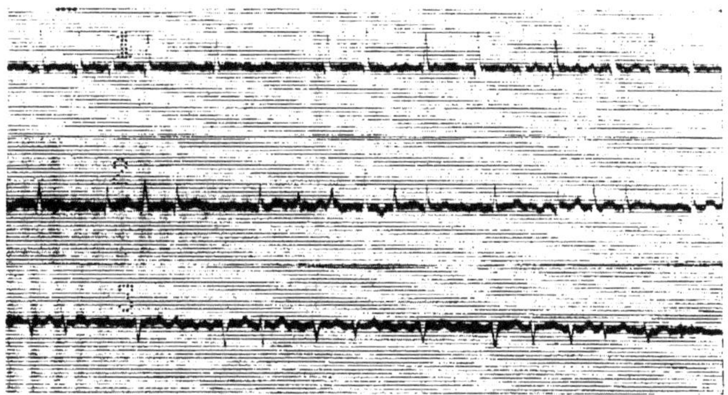

FIG. 2 (*a*).—Electrocardiogram showing auricular fibrillation, April 20, 1918.

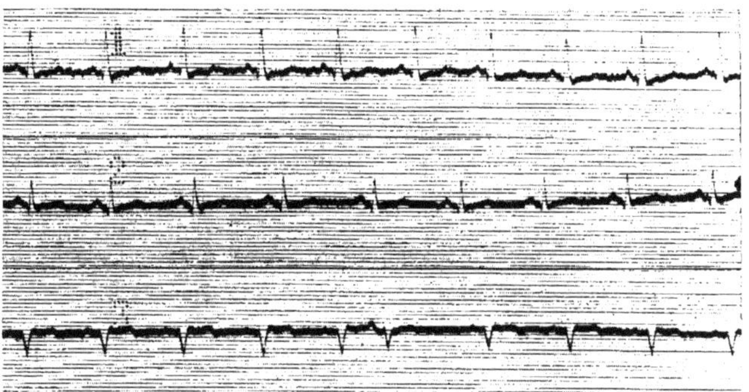

FIG. 2 (*b*).—Electrocardiogram showing return to normal rhythm without specific treatment, March 22, 1921.

CASE III (LOSL).—This man was a physician, aged forty-eight years, short and weighing 172 pounds. He complained of occasional skipping of the heart, giving him a peculiar feeling and a little dull pain. These symptoms had occurred during the preceding five years and seemed to have some relation to the eating of shellfish and green peppers, as well as to excessive tobacco smoking. His family history was negative aside from the death of one brother from tuberculosis. His appetite was good and his bowels were regular, due, no doubt, in some part to the fact that he took plenty of daily exercise.

The only illness he had had was pneumonia when at college and occasional attacks of grip.

Physical examination on several occasions showed a soft systolic murmur both at the apex and over the aortic area. While under observation he suffered from an attack of auricular fibrillation, which was also verified by the electrocardiogram. The blood-pressure varied between systolic 115-130 and diastolic 90-95. On our advice his tonsils were removed. Following the attack of fibrillation $\frac{1}{2}$ gr. of digitalis was given b. i. d. A week later the heart was greatly improved.

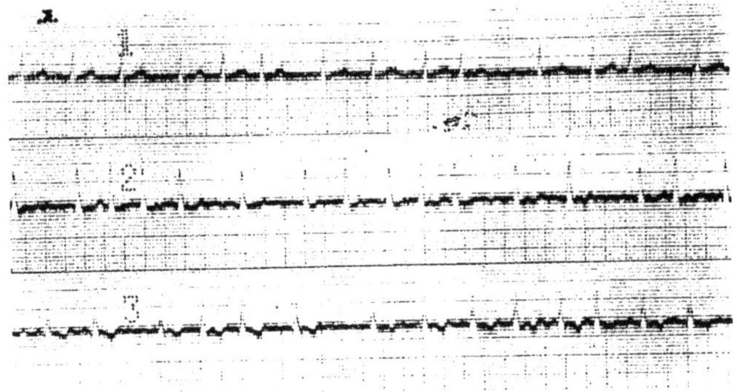

FIG. 3 (*a*).—Electrocardiogram showing auricular fibrillation, January 18, 1919.

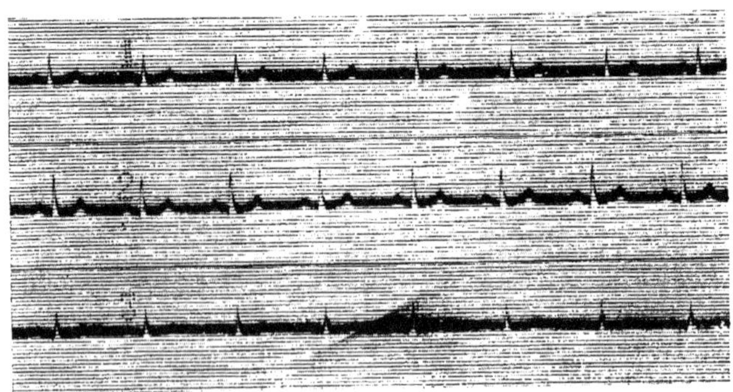

FIG. 3 (*b*).—Electrocardiogram showing return to normal rhythm, January 20, 1921.

The first urine examination showed a specific gravity which varied between 1024 and 1028. There was a faint trace of albumin, and in one specimen sugar to the extent of 1.6 per cent was found. Exactly two years later the urinary findings were entirely normal. The blood Wassermann was negative. The red and white cell counts and the hemoglobin were normal.

During the two years which have elapsed since this patient was in the office he has had only four or five heart attacks, all of which were of very short duration. Since his tonsillectomy he has felt much better, but is unable to say whether this has had anything to do with the relief from heart attacks.

Under the regimen of fortnightly doses of castor oil he has had entire relief from his attacks and is able to exercise and go hunting as much as he wishes. He has noticed that the attacks usually follow either overeating or excessive use of tobacco.

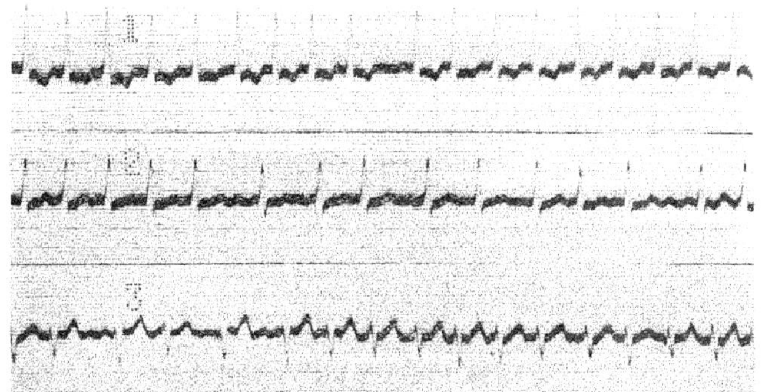

FIG. 4 (*a*).—Electrocardiogram showing auricular fibrillation, October 16, 1920.

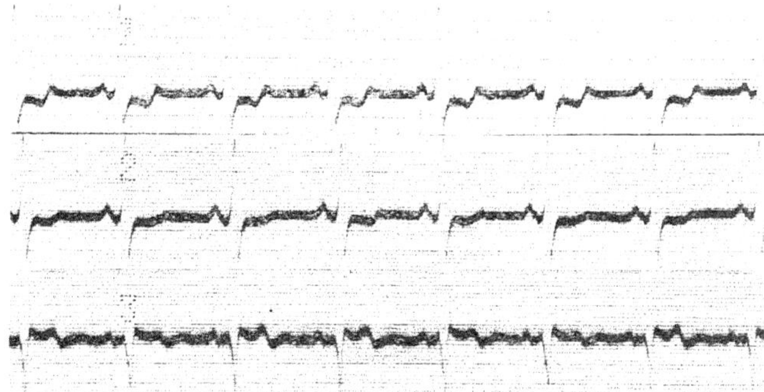

FIG. 4 (*b*).—Electrocardiogram showing return to normal rhythm, December 15, 1920.

CASE IV (IBIP).—A man, aged fifty-three years, weighing 175 pounds, single, came to the office complaining of dyspnea on exertion, pain and high blood-pressure. His personal habits were good. He abstained from tobacco, tea and coffee. His history revealed several attacks of rheumatism, measles and two attacks of pneumonia, twenty and five years ago respectively. His family history was negative except that his father died of Bright's disease.

His present complaint was of apparently rather short duration, having commenced three or four months previous to examination.

His heart was found to be very much enlarged, with a soft apical systolic murmur and marked accentuation of the aortic sound. His blood-pressure was very high, ranging between 250-220 systolic and 140-120 diastolic. The blood examination showed a very definite anemia with 80 per cent hemoglobin and 4,200,000 red blood cells. The Wassermann reaction was negative. Urinalysis revealed a marked amount of albumin with a moderate number of hyaline and granular casts. The specific gravity was 1015.

The first electrocardiograms showed the heart-rate to be regular. Under slight digitalis therapy the last tracings gave only a moderate sinus arrhythmia.

A month ago he complained of slight precordial pain on exertion.

This is a contribution to the natural history of fibrillation of the auricle, with particular reference to the emphasis of the importance of a careful appraisal of results of treatment in these people.

A CASE OF HEART-BLOCK AND AURICULAR FIBRILLATION WITH POSTMORTEM SPECIMEN; COMMENT ON THE ETIOLOGY OF FIBRILLATION.

By Selian Neuhof, M.D.,

Cardiologist, Broad Street Hospital; Attending Physician, Central and Neurological Hospital; Associate Physician, Lebanon Hospital, New York.

M. S., female, aged eighty years, was admitted to the ward August 7, 1920. Except that she entered the hospital acutely ill and that she had been in normal health prior to admission, no history was obtainable which threw any light upon her present illness.

The house physician made the following notes: "Shortly after admission the pulse-rate was around 150 and very irregular. The patient was cyanotic. She was given 1 dram of tincture of digitalis and $\frac{1}{100}$ gr. nitroglycerin every five minutes for one hour. (The total amount of the tincture thus administered was $1\frac{1}{2}$ ounces.) After a short time the cardiac rate dropped to forty per minute and gradually became slower until the rate was twenty-eight per minute. It remained at that rate for a few days, again gradually to increase to forty per minute. Upon admission she had an attack lasting two or three minutes, during which time breathing almost entirely ceased, and the pulse and heart action were scarcely perceptible. These spells were rather frequent during the first two days; they became less frequent, to disappear entirely on the fourth day." The patient died November 15, 1920.

I examined the patient for the first time about one week after admission. The heart action then was slightly irregular, the rate forty-five per minute. On the succeeding days and until the time of death, the ventricular rate remained between forty and fifty per minute. There were no cardiac murmurs. There was no edema of the legs. There were a few mucous rales at both bases. The patient was fairly comfortable and not very dyspneic. I took the first electrocardiogram two weeks after admission (August 21) and then another on November 10 (Fig. 1), one week before death. Both were alike and showed auricular fibrillation and heart-block (Fig. 1). As a terminal illness the patient developed lobar pneumonia, with fever ranging to 104° F.; during this period the pulse varied from forty to sixty-five per minute.

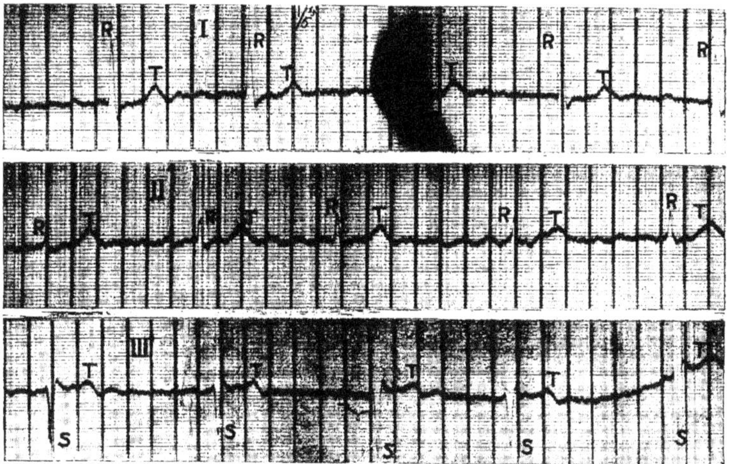

FIG. 1.—Typical section of a long electrocardiogram showing auricular fibrillation and heart-block. The ventricular action is slightly arrhythmic and the predominating rate is forty-six per minute.

Because the patient, a city ward, died without leaving relatives or friends, the heart could not be obtained for several weeks after her death. A bit of ventricular musculature was then excised, hardened and sectioned to discover whether the heart could still be used for microscopic study; it was found that the musculature was in too poor a state of preservation for such purpose. The gross pathology, however, was quite apparent, and it is questionable whether microscopic examination would have added anything of importance. The heart was slightly enlarged. The wall of the left ventricle was slightly thicker than normal; the right ventricle was abnormally thin toward the apex. The right ventricular cavity was somewhat dilated. There were small areas of thickening on the mitral cusps. There was surprisingly little interstitial fibrous change throughout the entire musculature. The auricles were not enlarged or thickened. The region of the sino-auricular node—the pace-making area at the junction of the soperion vena cava and the right auricle—showed no macroscopic change; the artery of that node was not visible or palpable.

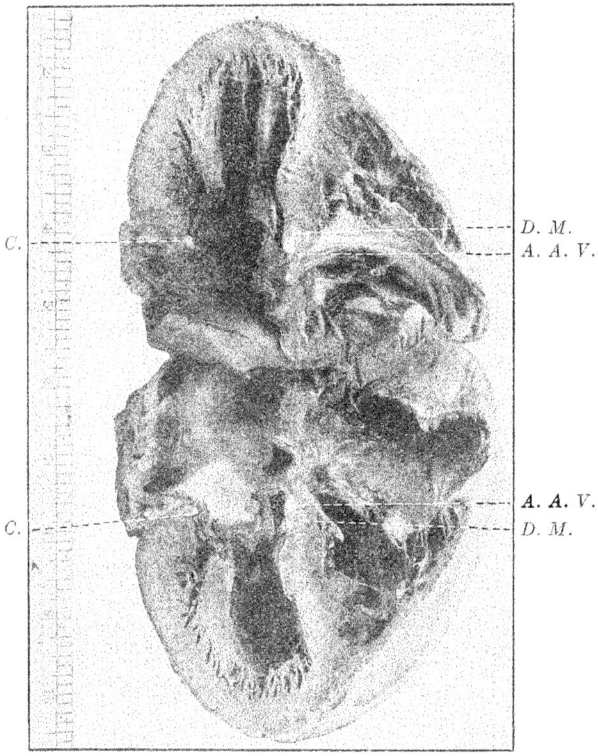

Fig. 2.—Photograph of the heart showing sclerosis of the coronaries (*C.*) and of the artery of the auriculoventricular node (*A. A. V.*). The artery is surrounded by a zone of degenerated musculature (*D. M.*).

The chief pathologic changes (Fig. 2)—undoubtedly the ones that finally caused the cardiac disturbance—were found in the coronaries, in the artery of the auriculoventricular node (the node of Tawara) and in the musculature surrounding the node. The coronary was thickened and sclerosed, although slightly patulous. The artery supplying the auriculoventricular node (the beginning of the auriculoventricular conduction system, the normal conveyer of impulses from auricle to ventricle) was completely calcified. The artery is seen occupying a position somewhat lower than the normal site of the node, but surrounding the artery (and probably as the result of its calcification) may be seen a distinct zone of degenerated musculature (Fig. 2), which undoubtedly includes the node, either partly or entirely.

Comment. It is of great pathologic and clinical importance, especially in those suffering from what I may term impending "coronary failure," to note how long the final pathologic "insult" can hold-off before complete occlusion of the coronaries or their subsidiaries occur. Undoubtedly the calcifying process in the coronary, and particularly in the artery of the node, had been going on for many years, yet the patient at the time of her death was eighty years old and had lived in cardiac comfort until sudden heart failure supervened; in all probability this resulted from final complete closure of the calcified artery supplying that node. This patient is but another illustration of the fact that the *slow* process of intracardiac arterial disease had never at any time sharply interfered with the factor of safety of the heart, and that ample time had probably been given for the establishment of coronary anastomosis; for, contrary to older teachings, it is now known that the coronaries are not end-arteries and that many deeply situated anastomoses exist.

Before proceeding to the clinical aspect of the case it may perhaps be well to recall certain pertinent physiologic attributes of the cardiac musculature. One of these is cardiac irritability. This does not depend upon the strength of the stimulus. It is, however, considerably influenced by other factors, especially by the state of nutrition of the cardiac musculature at the time of stimulation. Cardiac tissue is refractory to all stimulation during its period of contraction, hence the heart is irritable in the physiologic sense during its diastolic or resting period alone. Conduction, another important attribute, varies considerably in different parts of the heart; it is best in the specialized tissues—the sinoauricular node (the rhythm center) and the junctional tissue (the auriculoventricular conduction system).

The chief clinical interest in our case centers in the occurrence of heart-block and auricular fibrillation, but especially in the etiology of the latter. The heart-block is the cause of the slow ventricular activity. This is readily explicable from the gross pathologic changes—the calcified nodal artery and the myocardial changes in and near the atrioventricular node (Fig. 2). These focal changes undoubtedly destroyed the conducting function of the atrioventricular node. The massive digitalis therapy—1½ ounces of the tincture within one hour—may have been a factor in continuing the slow ventricular activity, although there is a definite note of the house physician stating that there were attacks of apnea with scarcely perceptible heart action (Stokes-Adams syndrome) upon admission. Nor does it seem probable that digitalis, even in such massive doses, could have had continued depressant action upon the ventricles during the remainder of the patient's life, approximately three months.

Regarding the auricular fibrillation we have no exact data as to its onset, except that the rapid and irregular pulse at the time of admission was probably indicative of this type of arrhythmia. Whether it had been present before hospital admission we do not know; from the obtainable history, however, there is no evidence of any prior attack of dyspnea or heart failure. Toxic causes (such as are encountered, for example, in exophthalmic goiter), reflex disturbances of the rhythm center from gastrointestinal disease, emotional disturbances, etc., need no consideration here as etiologic factors of the auricular fibrillation.

The possible causes of auricular fibrillation with heart-block in our case may perhaps best be discussed under the following headings:

1. Structural changes in the pace-maker.
2. Primary nutritional disturbances in the pace-maker.
3. Interference with and blocking of the normal spread of auricular impulses from a normally functionating pace-maker.

1. *Structural Changes in the Pace-maker.* Several observers (Cohn and Lewis,[1] Falconer and Dean,[2] Draper,[3] H. Freund[4] and others) had previously made careful serial microscopic examinations of the pace-maker and of the pace-making area in cases of auricular fibrillation with and without heart-block, and had ascribed decided etiologic significance to more or less extensive pathologic changes in the sinoauricular node. Such changes—usually degenerative and sclerotic in nature—where marked can undoubtedly cause auricular fibrillation. In some cases of auricular fibrillation, however, the sinoauricular nodal region was found normal or almost so. Hence where marked sclerotic changes are absent other causes for this arrhythmia must be sought. As above mentioned, macroscopic examination showed no evidence of any gross or extensive change in the pace-maker in our specimen.

2. *Primary Disturbances in the Pace-maker.* This would here refer practically to calcification and consequent occlusion of the artery of the pace-maker or to occlusion of one of the coronaries which occasionally gives off a branch to this node. The former change was absent in our case. Regarding the latter, while the coronaries were thickened and sclerosed they were still patulous, and hence would scarcely have interfered sufficiently with the arterial supply to the pace-maker, even assuming that a branch of the latter was given off by one of the coronaries.

3. *Interference with and Blocking of the Normal Spread of Auricular Impulses from a Normally Functionating Pace-maker.* Porter

[1] Auricular Fibrillation and Complete Heart-block, Heart, 1912–13, **4**, 15.

[2] Observations on a Case of Heart-block with Intermittent Attacks of Auricular Fibrillation, Heart, 1911–12, **3**, 247.

[3] Pulsus Irregularis Perpetuus with Fibrosis of the Sinus Node, Heart, 1911–12, **3**, 13.

[4] Klinische und Pathologisch-anatomische Untersuchungen über Arrhythmia perpetua, Deutsch. Arch. f. klin. Med., 1912, **106**, 1.

(quoted by Garrey) considers that "fibrillary contractions may be due to interruption of the contraction waves." Working independently, Garrey[5] and Mines[6] have shown experimentally that if the auricles be thrown into a state of fibrillation by direct faradization (the usual method), and if then a portion of auricular tissue (*e. g.*, the auricular appendix) be temporarily clamped off, fibrillation will continue in the remainder of the auricular tissue. When the clamp is removed the entire auricle again fibrillates. They have also found that if the auricle be incised trouser-fashion, so that sufficiently broad auricular strips remain connected by sufficiently broad auricular bridges and then the auricle be faradized anywhere, contraction of the various auricular strips will continue long after faradization has ceased. Garrey calls such contractions "circus contractions," for he assumes that such an excitation wave travels in a continuous circuit and that the impulse spreads from fiber to fiber. In the experimentally slit auricle these circus excitation waves are irregularly and sinuously blocked because of the difference in refractory periods of the incised fiber groups and because impulse conduction is interfered with. Thus while the circus excitation as an excitation impulse continues, the auricular strips are actually contracting at varying times and with varying energies. The result is incoördinate contraction, the irregular auricular tremor characteristic of fibrillation. Garrey also points out that "circus waves" are different from the normal in that the latter are large waves with rapid spread of the excitation; the reverse is true of "circus waves." Lewis and his co-workers[7 8 9 10] have recently corroborated Garrey's observations in a series of experimental and clinical papers.

The theory of Garrey and Mines seems to explain some clinical entities in which auricular fibrillation occurs frequently and in which an auricular mass as such may act as a factor. Thus in rheumatic mitral stenosis in which auricular hypertrophy and distention is common, and in cardiosclerosis in which accompanying sclerotic changes in the musculature are not infrequent, simple mechanical interference with the propagation of a "circus wave" may finally throw the auricle into fibrillation. My tentative interpretation in such instances is that there occurs mechanical hindrance to the spread of the excitation wave similar to what happens in the experimentally slit auricle; the excitation wave

[5] The Nature of Fibrillary Contraction of the Heart: Its Relation to Tissue Mass and Form, Am. Jour. Physiol., 1914, **23**, 397.

[6] On Dynamic Equilibrium in the Heart, Jour. Physiol., 1913, **46**, 349.

[7] Observations upon Flutter and Fibrillation, Heart, 1920, **7**, 127, 191.

[8] Observations upon Flutter and Fibrillation, Heart, 1921, **8**, 83.

[9] Further Observations upon the State of Rapid Reëxcitation of the Auricles, Heart, 1921, **8**, 311.

[10] A Demonstration of Circus Movement in Clinical Flutter of the Auricles, Heart, 1921, **8**, 341, 361.

cannot spread evenly and ripple-like because auricular conductivity and irritability are interfered with by the diseased or distended auricular strips; hence the excitation wave is irregularly and sinuously blocked and fibrillation results.

In addition to pathologic or mechanical changes in the auricular musculature, and excluding all toxic causes, it is of clinical importance to attempt a correlation of the theory of "circus waves" to disease primarily found not in the auricles but in the ventricles. It is, for example, no uncommon experience to find auricular fibrillation as a temporary or agonal arrhythmia with or without slow ventricular action in cases of coronary disease during an attack of occlusion (coronary failure), with or without pulmonary edema. Such sudden disturbance in intracardiac circulation with resultant impaired nutrition in the auricular musculature would seem sufficient to interfere with and impair the normal physiologic rhythmic excitation wave in the latter by producing local differences in the refractory periods and conduction time of the auricular excitation wave; thus a pathophysiologic basis for auricular fibrillation would be laid. In our case there was coronary disease with occlusion, the ventricles were beating automatically (heart-block) and the auricles were fibrillating. The possible influence of digitalis has already been discussed. Ordinarily in heart-block with coronary disease the auricles beat regularly and approximately at a normal rate. The assumption in such cases is that auricular nutrition is not sufficiently damaged to prevent the normal spread of impulses and excitation waves. Where auricular fibrillation occurs with heart-block the assumption seems fair that auricular disease or at least poor coronary circulation (coronary failure) so damages the entire intracardiac nutrition—auricles as well as ventricles—that auricular excitation waves are irregularly blocked similar to the blocking of the experimental "circus waves." As a result the auricles are thrown into that state of fibrillary contraction we designate clinically as auricular fibrillation.

THE ARSENICAL TREATMENT OF CHRONIC INFECTIOUS ENDOCARDITIS.*

By Joseph A. Capps, M.D.,

CHICAGO.

(From the Medical Clinic, St. Luke's Hospital, Chicago).

By the term "chronic infectious endocarditis" we refer to the group of cases known also as chronic malignant, or ulcerative

* Read at the Meeting of the Association of American Physicians, Washington, D. C., May, 1922.

endocarditis, running a course of three months to two or more years. This group is sharply distinguished from the chronic rheumatic endocarditis by the fact that the latter is associated with polyarthritis and by bacteria-free blood. It is convenient to separate this group also from the acute forms of infectious endocarditis, which present the clinical picture of acute septicemia. The organisms grown from the blood of these acute cases are the virulent strains of hemolytic streptococcus, pneumococcus, or gonococcus, while the organisms found in the blood of the chronic infectious type are the less virulent Streptococcus viridans or closely allied pneumococcus.

The diagnosis of chronic infectious endocarditis is somewhat difficult to make, because the patient is often up and about and may consult the physician only after weeks of malaise, weakness, slight fever, palpitation and loss of weight. Sometimes the occurrence of daily fever and sweats suggests tuberculosis; occasionally the development of abdominal tenderness and enlargement of the liver leads to a diagnosis of cholecystitis; frequently a high fever, enlarged spleen, and leucopenia simulate typhoid fever; or, in the absence of fever, the rapid pulse, sweats and loss of weight resembles a thyrotoxicosis. Later the true nature of the affection is revealed by the appearance of cardiac murmurs and emboli. When the emboli reach the brain, transitory loss of consciousness and motor symptoms may ensue; when they go to the spleen the organ becomes large and tender; when they affect the kidney, blood and albumin appear in the urine. Upon these findings the clinical diagnosis may be made, but the final proof rests with the recovery of Streptococcus viridans or pneumococcus, or rarely influenza bacillus in blood cultures. Skillful technic on the part of the bacteriologist and repeated examinations of the blood are essential in obtaining positive cultures. Even then according to Libman the majority of cases will yield negative results.

The purpose of this paper is to enter into a discussion of symptomatology only so far as it affects the diagnosis of the disease. The diagnosis established, our interest is in the prognosis and the result of various methods of treatment.

A review of the literature (Table I) brings out the frequency of an earlier and supposedly a healed rheumatic endocarditis. The mitral valves are most often involved, but the aortic may also be inflamed, either alone or in combination with the mitral valves. Blood cultures were not taken by the early observers and are not recorded by many recent writers. The positive cultures obtained show a marked preponderance of Streptococcus viridans, next in frequency the pneumococcus and a few scattered instances of influenza and staphylococcus.

TABLE I

Author.	No. of cases.	Duration of illness.	Blood cultures.	Organisms.	Specific treatment.	Deaths.	Recovery	Remarks.
1. Harbitz, 1899	16	4 to 8 mos.	.....	Pneum. 4 Strept. 9 Others 3	....	16	0	All came to postmortem; noted healing process often.
2. Bartel, 1901	22	....	.....	....	....	22	0	Noted healing valve lesions.
3. Lenhartz, 1904	16	3 to 7 mos.	.....	Pneum. staph.	....	16	0	
4. Osler, 1909	10	4 to 13 mos.	3 + 3 0	Strept. 2 Staph. 1	....	10	0	
5. Billings, 1909	14	3 to 14 mos.	All +	Strep. vir. 14	Autog. vaccine Ant. strep. serum	13	1	One well after seven years; thinks vaccine and serum useless.
6. Latham and Hunt, 1910	1	15 mos.	+	Coccus	Autog. vaccine by mouth	0	1	Thinks vaccine valuable.
7. Schottmüller, 1910	5	....	.....	....	....	5	0	Reports 1 recovery; case died later.
8. Jochmann, 1912	7	....	Some +	Strep. vir.	Autog. vaccine Ant. strep. serum	5	2	1 died on vaccine and serum. 1 well on vaccine and serum. 1 well on no vaccine and serum.
9. Libman, 1912–1920	150	3 to 18 mos.	+	Strep. vir. 95% Influenza 5%	....	146	4	
10. Christian, 1918	2	....	±	Strep. vir.	....	1	?	1 living; too recent.
11. Starling, 1920	38	3 to 14 mos.	.....	....	....	35		Recoveries all recent cases.
12. Horder,		....		Strep. vir.	....			

Harbitz and Bartel both made important observations in large series of necropsies in chronic infectious endocarditis. They described even in these fatal cases evidences of healing of the valve lesions and suggested that recovery was possible.

In 1909, Osler stimulated a fresh clinical interest in the subject. Until the year 1885 he had seen only the acute types of septic endocarditis, all terminating in death within three months. From 1885 to 1909, he observed 10 cases of chronic infectious endocarditis, running a course from four to thirteen months and all ending fatally. He drew a clear picture of the condition, emphasizing the frequency of a previous rheumatic infection, the daily remittent fever, the petechiæ, the occurrence of emboli in the brain, kidney and retina, and the occasional development of characteristic painful nodular swellings under the skin. In six of his patients blood cultures were taken, three of which were negative, two showed streptococcus and one staphylococcus.

Soon after Osler's publication Billings reported 14 cases of the chronic type. The notable feature of his contribution was the success in securing positive cultures from the blood in every case, an achievement made possible by frequent and repeated efforts in taking cultures. In 11, Rosenow found pneumococcus and in 3 Streptococcus viridans, which may be considered as identical. Some of this series were treated by autogenous vaccines, and some by antipneumococcic and antistreptococcic sera. One patient of the 14 recovered, but she had received no specific therapy. Billings concludes that vaccines and serum therapy are of no value in treatment.

Schottmüller states that 1 of his 5 cases recovered, but this patient subsequently died of the disease (Libman).

Latham and Hunt record an interesting case with apparent recovery after fifteen months. Blood cultures six times yielded a growth of Gram-positive cocci and later they became negative. They attributed this result to administration of autogenous vaccine by mouth.

Jochmann says that in his experience chronic infectious endocarditis is caused almost exclusively by Streptococcus viridans, whereas the acute type is usually due to Streptococcus hemolyticus. He reports 7 cases with 2 recoveries. Three cases were treated with antistreptococcus serum, 1 of which recovered and 2 died. The other recovered patient received no specific therapy.

Libman (1912) as a result of a very extensive clinical and bacteriological experience states that the organisms responsible for chronic infectious endocarditis are Streptococcus viridans in 95 per cent and influenza and gonococcus together in 5 per cent of cases. He describes a large series with typical clinical picture, but in the "bacteria-free" stage. He believes healing of the valves does occur, "although the evidence of complete recovery from the clinical side is still very meagre." "Nearly all cases in which we found bacteria in the blood went on to fatal termination with bacteria still in the blood. In but few cases did the blood cultures become negative and these patients also succumbed."

In a recent discussion (1920), however, Libman refers to 4 recoveries in a group of 150 well observed cases.

Starling recently referred to 38 cases of chronic infectious endocarditis, no mention being made of blood cultures. Three of these patients he considered had recovered, but sufficient time had not elapsed to settle this point.

Sir Thomas Horder in a discussion of 150 cases that had come under his observation says that the diagnosis of chronic infectious endocarditis rests on a triad of symptoms, viz., active endocarditis of chronic type, occurrence of emboli, and the recovery of streptococci in the blood. On any two of these symptoms the diagnosis may be made with reasonable certainty. Only 1 patient in his series recovered.

Münzer's case deserves mention because of his experiments with collargol injections which proved to be of no value.

Oille, Graham and Detweiler have made an interesting study of 8 mild cases of this disease. Three of the group developed arthritis, 3 had hematuria, 1 only exhibited a large spleen and none had petechiæ. In all, however, there was a distinct heart murmur and in every case the authors succeeded by the Rosenow method in growing Streptococcus viridans in blood cultures. The cases were so recent that the final outcome could not be included in the table. But the striking success in obtaining positive cultures in such mild types of the disease should be a stimulus to more intensive bacteriological studies in all suspected cases.

A summary of the results obtained in the combined series of Table I is as follows:

Of 419 cases reported 12 patients recovered, or less than 3 per cent.

Two of the 12 patients who recovered received vaccine. The remaining 10 cases received no specific treatment.

It is altogether probable that spontaneous recovery does occur in chronic infectious endocarditis, far more often than these statistics would indicate. The testimony of pathologists is that healed ulcerative lesions of the heart valves are not infrequently encountered at necropsy in persons dying of some other affection. Libman in particular has emphasized the likelihood of recovery in many cases that are never diagnosed.

Personal Observations. During the past twelve years we have treated all of our cases of chronic infectious endocarditis with daily injections of sodium cacodylate (usually intravenously), continued over a period varying from seven weeks to four months. In many of these patients we failed to find bacteria in blood cultures,

TABLE II. OUTCOME OF CASES TREATED WITH ARSENIC

Name.	Period of observation.	Previous duration.	Prev. rheum.	Valves affected.	Temperature.	Blood.	Emboli.				Blood cultures.	Organisms.	Treatment.	Outcome.
							Spleen.	Kidneys.	Skin.	Elsewhere.				
R. T. L.	11½ yrs.	1 mo.	0	Mitral	99 to 100	H = 60 R = 3,020,000 W = 6,000 to 10,000	++	Alb. Blood casts	++	0	2 pos. 1 neg.	St. vir.	Sod. cacod. 10 wks.	Recovery
M. C.	5 yrs. 1 mo.	4 mos.	+	Mitral	97 to 100	H = 65 R = 4,100,000 W = 7,000	+	Blood casts	0	0	1 pos. 3 neg.	St. vir.	Sod. cacod. 4 mos.	Recovery
C. H. R.	yrs.		0	Mitral and aortic	98 to 101	H = 80 R = 4,800,000 W = 4,000 to 10,000	+	Alb. Blood casts	+	0	1 neg. 1 pos. 1 neg.	St. vir.	Sod. cacod. 7 wks.	Recovery
L. M.	2 yrs. 3 mos.	2 mos.	+	Mitral	97 to 101	H = 50 R = 3,420,000 W = 7,000	++	Alb. Blood casts	+	0	2 pos. 1 neg.	St. vir.	Sod. cacod. 2 mos.	Recovery
M. P.	5 mos.	9 mos.	0	Mitral	98 to 101	H = 64 R = 3,200,000 W = 9,000, to 10,000	+	Alb. Blood	+	Cutan. nodes	3 neg. 1 pos.	St. vir.	Sod. cacod. 12 wks.	Death
J. F.	15 wks.	10 wks.	0	Mitral	100 to 103	H = 84 R = 4,100,000 W = 12,000 to 18,000	+	Alb. Blood casts	+	Cutan. nodes Retina Hemipleg.	6 pos.	St. vir.	Sod. cacod. 3 mos.	Death
M. T.	6 mos.	8 mos.	+	Mitral	97 to 100.4	H = 76 R = 4,300,000 W = 7,600	+	Alb. Blood casts	+	0	2 neg. 1 pos. 3 neg.	St. vir.	Sod. cacod. 12 wks.	Improving
F. B.	[illegible]					H = 85		Alb.	0	Cerebral		St. vir.	Sod. cacod. 3 mos	Improv-

although the other clinical findings were sufficiently characteristic for making the diagnosis. But for the purpose of determining the results of a specific therapy it seemed best to limit the present study to those cases alone in which the clinical evidence was corroborated by positive cultures from the blood. Eight cases were proven up by blood cultures and these are described in Table II.

The clinical features of these cases are so similar to the excellent descriptions of Billings, Osler and Libman that little detailed comment is called for.

Two of our patients died, and 6 survive. The duration of the disease in the fatal cases was six and thirteen months respectively.

The observation of the 6 surviving cases extends over periods of eleven years and six months, five years and one month, five years, two years and one month, six months and three months respectively. As the infection runs such a chronic course we can draw no conclusions from the last 2 cases. The remaining 4 cases having remained in good health for two years and more may be reasonably classified as recoveries.

The only specific therapy attempted was the prolonged use of sodium cacodylate in daily doses of 1 to 4 grains. The drug was pushed until a strong garlic odor was expelled with the breath. The preparations sold in the market in ampoule form are not very dependable, so that it is advisable to make a fresh preparation every few days of a reliable drug. No untoward effects were observed in any case. If the bowels became loose the dose was decreased for two or three days. Rest in bed was insisted upon during the period of treatment.

The results of blood cultures were of especial interest. Streptococcus viridans was the organism found in all cases.

In 1 fatal case six consecutive cultures were positive. In the second fatal case three negative cultures were followed by one positive.

All the healed cases showed the disappearance of bacteria from the blood during recovery. But it is never safe to give a good prognosis from negative cultures alone, since patients frequently die under these conditions.

Experimental Work. The experiments of Allison upon the effect of arsenic, in the form of a watery solution of salvarsan, diarsenol and arsenobenzol on streptococcus have an important bearing on the rationale of this treatment. "These preparations" he asserts "possess a distinct bactericidal power against virulent strains of streptococci in vitro in dilutions up to 1:3000, and an *inhibiting* power for at least twenty-four hours in weaker solutions. They possess bactericidal action against streptococci also in the blood stream of experimental animals. They produce no untoward effects on animals where large doses were frequently repeated. They possess hopeful possibilities for the treatment of streptococcus infections in human subjects as shown by limited human experience."

Our own experience with the arsenic treatment inclines us to believe that the drug in the ordinary dosage is "inhibiting," rather than bactericidal, and that it should, therefore, be given over a long period in order to bring about the death of the organisms.

We have employed cacodylate of soda because of its apparent safety, but other forms of arsenic may prove superior.

BIBLIOGRAPHY.

1. Harbitz: Deutsch. med. Wchnschr., 1899, **25**, 121.
2. Bartel: Wien. klin. Wchnschr., 1901, p. 1004.
3. Lenhartz: Die Septoschen Erkrankungen, Wien., 1904, p. 434.
4. Osler: Quart. Jour. Med., 1909, **2**, 219.
5. Billings: Arch. Int. Med., 1909, **4**, 409.
6. Latham and Hunt: Proc. Royal Soc. Med. Clin. Sec., 1911, 14.
7. Schottmüller: München. med. Wchnschr., 1910, p. 880.
8. Jochmann: Berl. klin. Wchnschr., 1912, **49**, 436.
9. Libman, E.: Am. Jour. Med. Sci., 1912, **144**, 313.
   Libman: Discussion, British Med. Jour., 1920, **2**, 301.
10. Christian: Internat. Clinics, Phila., 1918.
11. Starling: British Med. Jour., 1920, **2**, 304.
12. Horder: British Med. Jour., 1920, **2**, 301.
13. Münzen: Verhandl. d. Kong. f. inn. Med., 1921, p. 241.
14. Oille, Graham and Detweiler: Jour. Am. Med. Assn., 1915, **65**, 1159.
15. Allison: Jour. Med. Res., 1918, 38, 1, 56.

THE FATE OF ARSENIC AFTER INTRAVENOUS OR INTRATHECAL INJECTION.*

By R. D. Rudolf, M.D.,

and

F. M. R. Bulmer, M.B.,

Toronto, Canada.

The question of the fate of salvarsan, using the term salvarsan as a group one for all such arsenical preparations, after its intravenous injection is a large one and the work that is here presented only goes a very little way toward answering it. After its administration, arsenic certainly soon appears in the urine and in the feces and probably is chiefly got rid of by these routes,. It is equally certain that in the body it is not equally distributed: certain tissues hold most of it and others scarcely take it up at all. We have so far only studied the question thoroughly as regards the liver and the spinal cord and find that the drug lodges in the former largely in proportion to the amount placed in the blood and is apparently not taken up by the nervous tissues in any

* Read at the meeting of the Association of American Physicians, Washington, D. C., May, 1922.

recognizable amount. A few preliminary experiments would suggest that the drug also lodges largely in the long bones and in the lungs.

Several observers have found arsenic in the spinal fluid after intravenous administration, but McIntosh and Fildes[1] failed to detect it in the brain. No work has been yet done, as far as the writers are aware, in analyzing the spinal cord after intravenous injection of the drug.

In reviewing the literature regarding experiments with arsenic it seems that the usual test employed has been the Marsh one, which is now obsolete for the quantitative estimation of small amounts of the drug.

The method employed by the writers is a modification of the Gutzeit test as described in the Transactions of the International Congress of Applied Chemistry in 1912. The principle of the test depends on the formation of arsine from arsenic compounds in the presence of nascent hydrogen. Iron as ferric ammonium alum is added to the material to be tested, which causes a steady and regular evolution of hydrogen, although it inhibits the production of arsine. The inhibitory action of the iron is offset by the addition of stannous chloride to the material. The advantage of this method is that for each test a new set of standards is made under exact conditions as to the materials being examined. The lowest amount of arsenic that can be estimated in this way is 0.001 mg., as arsenic trioxid, and the highest is 0.02 mg. From this the percentage of arsenic in any quantity of material can be easily calculated.

The method used for the separation of arsenic from the organic material was as follows. The material to be tested was treated with hydrochloric acid and potassium chlorate. This causes the arsenic present in the material to be ionized into solution. The material is filtered and in the filtrate the arsenic is in solution. The filtrate is then treated by the co-precipitation method. This is done by neutralizing the filtrate with ammonia, and the addition of ammonia until this is 2.5 per cent in excess. Sodium phosphate and magnesia mixture are next added, resulting in a precipitation, the arsenic being thrown down in the precipitate. The precipitate is dissolved by acid and the arsenic further reduced by the addition of potassium iodide.

The following are sources of difficulty and possible error in the determination of small amounts of arsenic:

1. *Reagents*. One of the greatest troubles is the difficulty of obtaining arsenic-free chemicals. Special acid must be procured, as the ordinary so-called chemically-pure acids always contain arsenic. Likewise a special arsenic-free zinc must be used. In

[1] Jour. Am. Med. Assn., April 14, 1917, p. 1147.

all tests where chemicals have a trace of arsenic a control on the reagents must be run through with the test and the amount of arsenic in the control is then subtracted from the reading of the results.

2. *Glassware.* Ordinary glassware usually contains arsenic which is set free when in contact with acids, different amounts at different times. Thus it is impossible to blank glassware. Hard glass, however, is usually arsenic-free. In all our work *pyrex* glassware was used, each piece being tested before being employed.

3. *Filter Paper.* All filter papers at our disposal contained arsenic, some as high as 0.001 mg. per paper, others a mere trace. Fortunately, each paper of a brand held the same amount of arsenic, and this, therefore, could be subtracted from the readings.

4. *Special Precautions.* Needles and glassware must be carefully washed before being used. This is specially necessary when needles have previously been used for the administration of arsenic.

On account of the rather poor results obtained by clinicians in spinal syphilis after intravenous and intrathecal administration of arsenic-containing drugs much controversy has arisen as to whether arsenic has any special effect on the virus of syphilis when in the spinal cord. We have attacked the problem by giving arsenic medication to animals and then analyzing the cord tissues to find if the drug really reached them at all.

On giving a normal rabbit a dose of phenarsenamine proportional to what is given to man no arsenic could be demonstrated in the cord one hour after intravenous injection, although it was very evident in the blood and the liver. This experiment was repeated several times with the same result. Next the dose was increased in a series of animals as much as eight and nine times. The rabbit getting the smallest amount would have a relatively high therapeutic dose while the one receiving the largest amount had sufficient to produce profound degenerative changes in the liver. All the rabbits were killed one hour after the intravenous injection. Fig. 1 is a graph representing the result of these experiments. It will be seen that the amount of arsenic in the blood rises steadily with the dose; that in the liver rises slowly at first, and later very rapidly, but none is shown in the tissues of the spinal cord. The dose in the lowest animals corresponded to 0.8 gm. in a man and in the highest 5.6 gm. in a man.

It is not surprising that no arsenic appears in the spinal cord when one considers the nature of its tissues. McIntosh and Fildes[2] found that the factor governing the passage of dyes into the brain after intravenous injection was their solubility reaction. This, they state, is a peculiar and not a general lipoid one. It corresponds to a solubility in chloroform and in water or perhaps their partition

[2] Loc. cit.

coefficient in these liquids. In all probability the same holds good for the spinal tissues owing to their composition. Thus from a solubility point of view, no arsenic would be expected to lodge in the spinal cord after intravenous injection and this is just what the above experiment shows.

Failing to detect arsenic in the cord after intravenous injection, the writers next tried the intrathecal route. The first problem was, would the arsenic if introduced into the lower part of the spinal canal diffuse upward? The following experiment would suggest at least that it does not do so to any extent. A glass tube

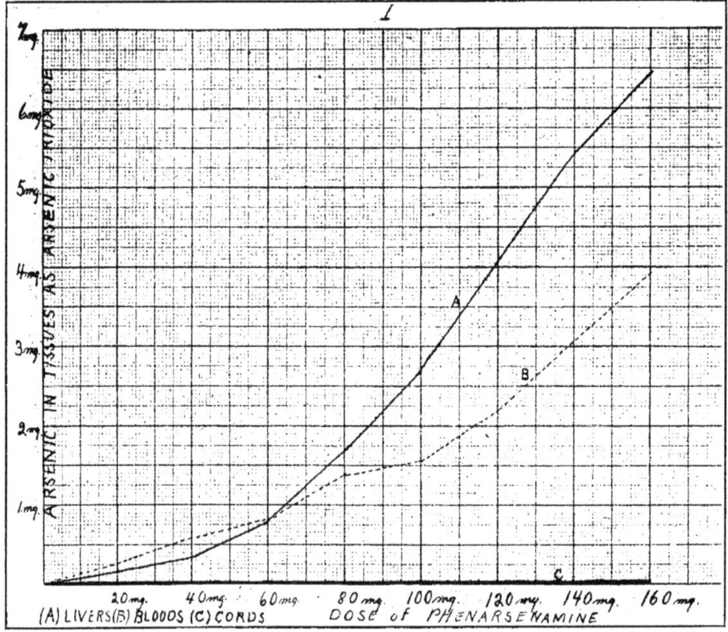

FIG. 1.—Graph.

was filled with 100 cc of water. The vertical column of water measured 53 cm., 10 cc were withdrawn and replaced at the lower end by 10 cc of water containing 1 mg. of arsenious acid. The experiment was repeated using different time intervals, and at the end of the time 10 cc of the fluid were withdrawn from the highest part of the tube and 10 cc from the lowest. Analysis showed that nearly all the arsenic remained in the lowest part of the tube. The experiment was repeated with phenarsenamine with the same result. Fig. 2 shows the results after 6 mg. was injected at the bottom of the tube, and the fluid analyzed twenty-four hours later.

Theoretically it does not seem likely that drugs injected into the spinal theca should enter the cord tissues as there is normally no circulation in that direction. The writers found that in order to get any arsenic into the cord in this way it was necessary to inject a very large amount. After 1.25 mg. of phenarsenamine in 1 cc of saline solution was injected into the spinal theca arsenic was found in the spinal cord at the end of one hour, the lower part of the cord showing a considerable amount and the upper a mere trace. And this, too, while the spinal canal was more or less horizontal. The results are seen in Fig. 3. It will be seen in this figure that no arsenic appeared in the cord after injection of 18 mg. phenarsenamine intravenously. The amount of arsenic in the control must in all cases be subtracted from the readings.

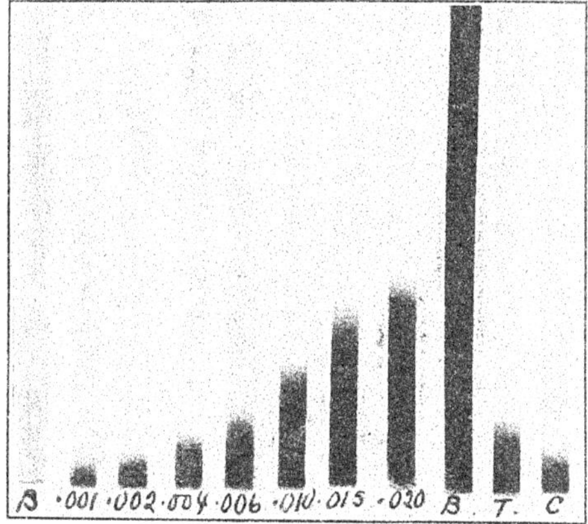

Fig. 2.*—Diffusion experiment, using phenarsenamine. Time twenty-four hours: B, 10 cc from bottom of tube; T, 10 cc from top of tube; C, control of reagents.

In the above experiments it must be remembered that not only was a very large amount of arsenic injected into the theca but that this was done under considerable pressure.

Rabbits receiving sufficient arsenic intrathecally to show in the cord at death if permitted to live all suffered paralysis after the injection. This paralysis seemed to improve somewhat but up to the time that they were killed, one hour later, nothing like complete recovery took place. In order to determine if the paralysis was due to pressure or to the arsenic two rabbits of the same litter were treated as follows: One was given 0.75 cc saline solution intrathecally and the other a similar amount of saline containing 1.25 mg.

* In the illustrations here given the first column is always a blank of the reagents used in the actual test and the next seven show the stains produced by different amounts of arsenic in milligrams as enumerated underneath. The remaining columns show the stains produced by the arsenic in the tissues analyzed, one being always a control of the reagents used in the extraction of arsenic from organic material in a suitable form for analysis.

of phenarsenamine. The animal that received the pure saline showed weakness in the hind limbs but within an hour this had disappeared. The rabbit that received the phenarsenamine intrathecally showed a profound paralysis in the hind quarters. In thirty minutes this had somewhat lessened and the animal was able to draw up the limbs. Two hours later the paralysis was much less but the animal had developed a general tremor. In six hours the animal could hop. Twenty-four hours after the injection profound paralysis had set in, with incontinence of feces. Next day the weakness had reached the fore limbs; the animal was weak and died forty-nine hours after the injection, apparently of paralysis of the respiratory system. This experiment shows that very grave results followed if arsenic gets into the spinal cord in sufficient amounts to be detected by analysis.

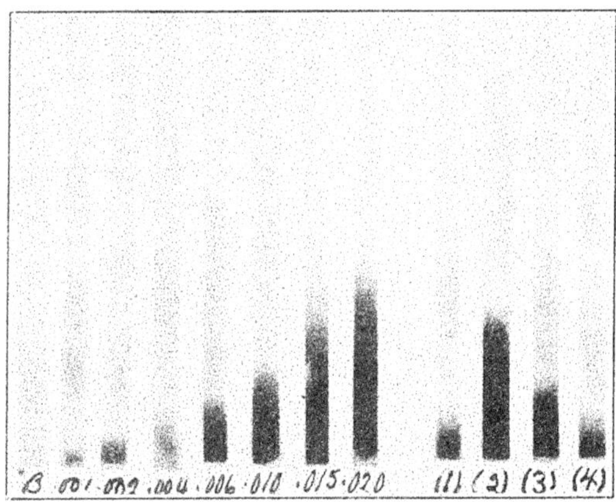

Fig. 3.—Analysis of spinal cords after administration of phenarsenamine: 1, Intravenous injection of 18 mg.; 2, lower half of cord after 1.25 mg. intraspinally; 3, upper portion of same cord; 4, control cord; no arsenic given to animal.

We next tried whether a solution of arsenic in blood serum would induce the deposition of arsenic in the cord. Many experiments were done with serum prepared in the manner proposed by Swift and Ellis. Both cats and rabbits were used in the work, with the same results. Fig. 4 shows the findings in a series of cats. The Swift-Ellis serum used was always prepared from the cat it was afterward given to. In each case the cat was given 75 mg. of phenarsenamine intravenously, an enormous dose when compared to the therapeutic one. An hour later the animal was bled, the blood centrifuged and the blood serum obtained placed in the ice box over night. Then it was diluted to 40 per cent with normal saline, inactivated for a half hour at 57° C. and then used as described. As will be seen from Fig. 4 there was no arsenic found in any of the cords after the blank of the reagents had been subtracted. It will also be noted that the Swift-Ellis serum showed only a trace of arsenic which of itself would account for the finding of no arsenic in the cords after its intrathecal use. Each of the animals preparatory to our making the serum received a far higher dose of arsenic intravenously than is ever given therapeutically.

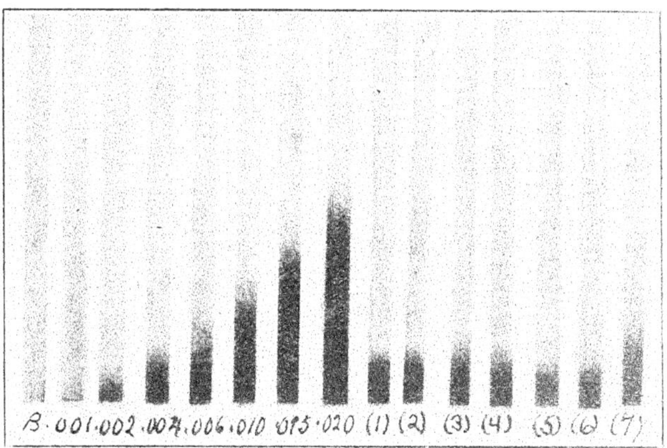

FIG. 4.—Analysis of spinal cords after administration of phenarsenamine and Swift-Ellis serum: 1, Intravenous injection of .25 cc Swift-Ellis serum; 2, intraspinous injection of .25 cc Swift-Ellis serum; 3, no Swift-Ellis serum given (In 1, 2, and 3 cats have had 75 mg. phenarsenamine intravenously); 4, control cord; 5, control of reagents; 6, one cc serum prepared from control cat after Swift-Ellis method only cat received no arsenic; 7, one cc Swift-Ellis serum from cat 2.

When one considers the small amount of arsenic, if any, that reaches the cord after intravenous administration, even when this is supplemented by intrathecal injection next day, it seems unlikely that any possible good effects in the treatment of cerebrospinal syphilis by either the intravenous use of salvarsan or this enhanced by intrathecal injection of arsenic-containing blood serum can be due to the presence of any of the drug in the cord, but must be explained in some other way.

The writers desire to record their gratitude to Professor L. Joslyn Rogers for much skilled advice in regard to the technic here used, and also to Professor V. J. Harding for constant assistance.

Conclusions. 1. When arsenic is injected intravenously little if any of it reaches the central nerve tissues.

2. When it is given in therapeutic doses intrathecally none of it can be detected in the spinal cord.

PNEUMOTHORAX IN TUBERCULOSIS.

By J. J. Singer, M.D.,
(Instructor in Clinical Medicine.)

(From the Department of Internal Medicine, Washington University Medical School.)

It is not the purpose of this paper to go into the literature of the many methods and investigations in pneumothorax, but to merely give a short description of one of the methods used and the various kinds of lung conditions which seem to be benefited by this procedure.

For many years new and startling cures have been foisted on the public, and so positive have been the claims of most of the discoverers that even Congress has investigated certain cures. From many years of experience with the various cures it is conceded that rest and proper diet offer the most in the line of cure.

In discussing the various factors which constitute rest, one must consider pneumothorax in this light. It is my opinion that the beneficial effect of pneumothorax is primarily the rest given to a diseased lung. Conversely, overactivity of the lung during exercise increases the diseased process.

The mechanical factor of rest as produced by pneumothorax—that is, placing the air cushion between the lung and the chest wall—is very simple. As we breathe, air is forced into the lungs through the bronchial tree. The bronchial tube represents the line of least resistance, and thus the air is forced into the alveoli of the lungs (Fig. 1). As the bronchial tubes simply represent the conduction channels of the air, it therefore becomes a relatively simple matter to close the line of conduction by pressure on the lungs. In this condition the tubes in the opposite lung being the line of least resistance, air will then be forced into them and thereby give the desired rest to the diseased lung (Fig. 2).

Pneumothorax Apparatus. This consists of a stand upon which an upright is fastened. On the upright portion a manometer is placed. Two 500 cc bottles are arranged on the base, one upright, *B*, and one inverted, *D*. The height of the upper bottle is adjustable, as seen in the illustration. The upright portion of the instrument contains clips in which various test-tubes for the necessary solutions are kept *K*, also a hand bulb, *L*. The tube *A* connects with a two-way valve *F*, so that the current or pressure can be directed from the bottle *B* or to the manometer through the tube marked *G*. This apparatus is placed in a covered box. The apparatus is portable, its weight being twelve pounds.

The *modus operandi* of the instrument is as follows: By connecting the hand bulb to the upright bottle after disconnect-

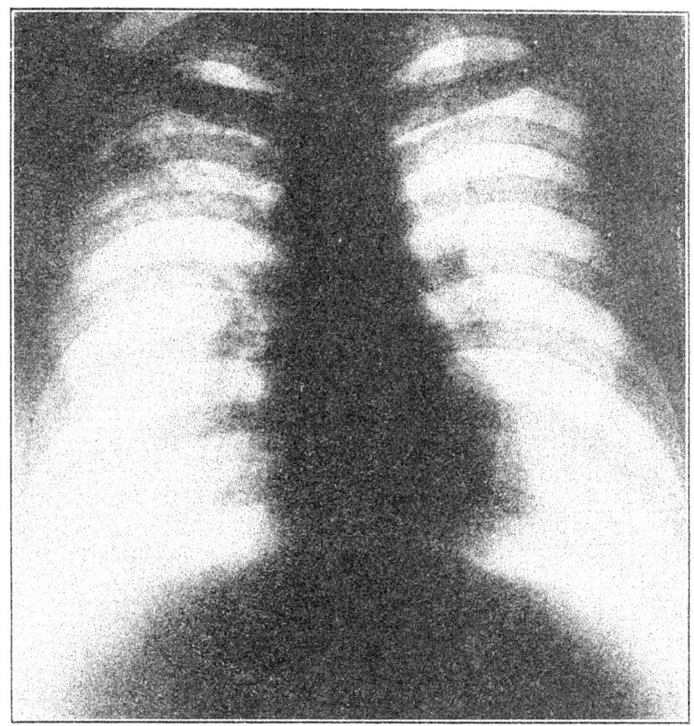

PLATE I.

Shows evidence of tuberculosis in the right upper lung down to the fourth rib. This patient (Mr. W.) had repeated hemorrhages in the month previous to examination. Temperature 101°, with persistent cough. After several pneumothorax injections the condition of the lung is shown in Plate II.

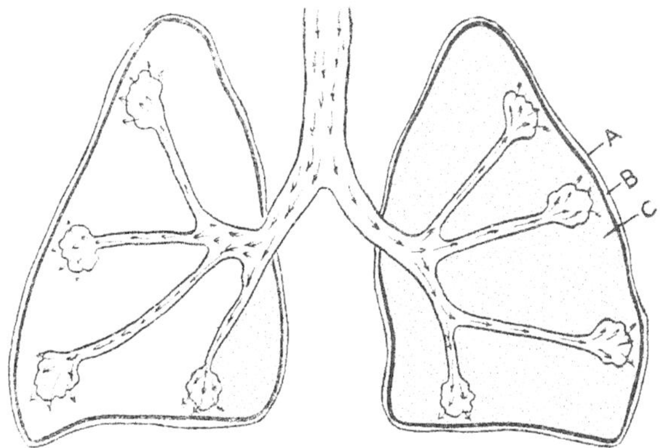

Fig. 1.—A schematic drawing showing the trachea with the bronchial tree and alveoli. *A* represents the parietal pleura, *B* represents the normal pleural cavity and *C* represents the lung. The arrows show the course of the air breathed. Note the equal distribution in both lungs.

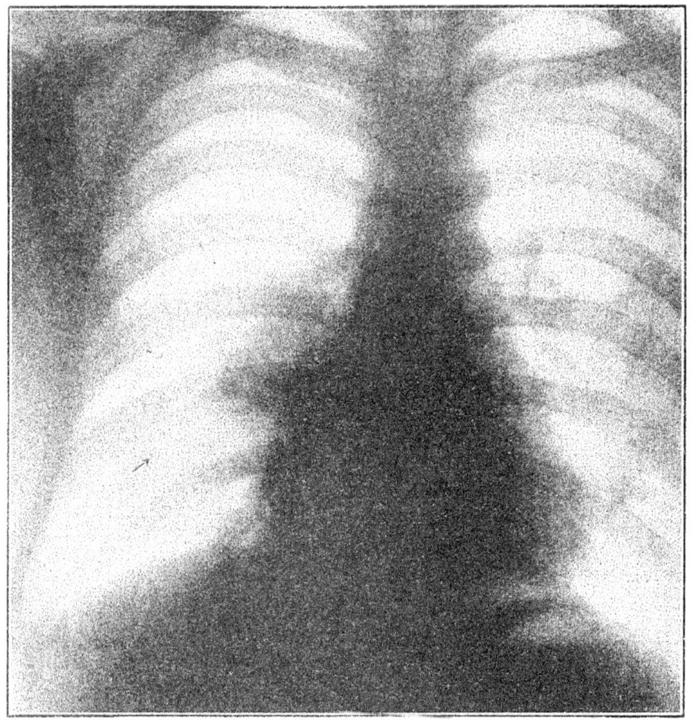

PLATE II.

Note the complete collapse of the lung about the hilus on the right side. There was a complete cessation of hemorrhages from April 9, 1920, as injections up to date. It has been necessary to refill the lung with air every three or four weeks. Note the relative freedom from tuberculous infection in the left lung. This complete compression is not usually seen on account of adhesions which are usually present in most lungs.

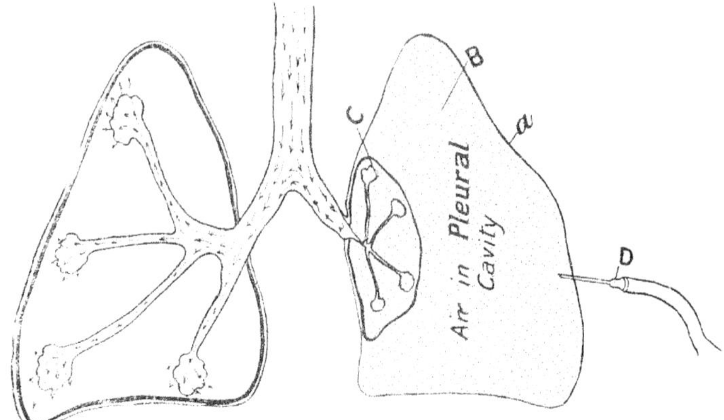

FIG. 2.—A schematic drawing shows how the introduction of air into the pleural cavity *B* compresses the bronchial tree, so that the air currents are directed into the opposite lung. Note the size of the pleural cavity *B* after air is injected. The pressure of the air against the lung closes the bronchial tree of the side.

ing the tube at *A*, air is forced into the same; this forces the water through *C* into the upright bottle *D*. By connecting the tube at *A* and closing the valve at *F* the water will remain in *D*: By opening the valve at *F* the water slowly drips from *D* into *B*. This

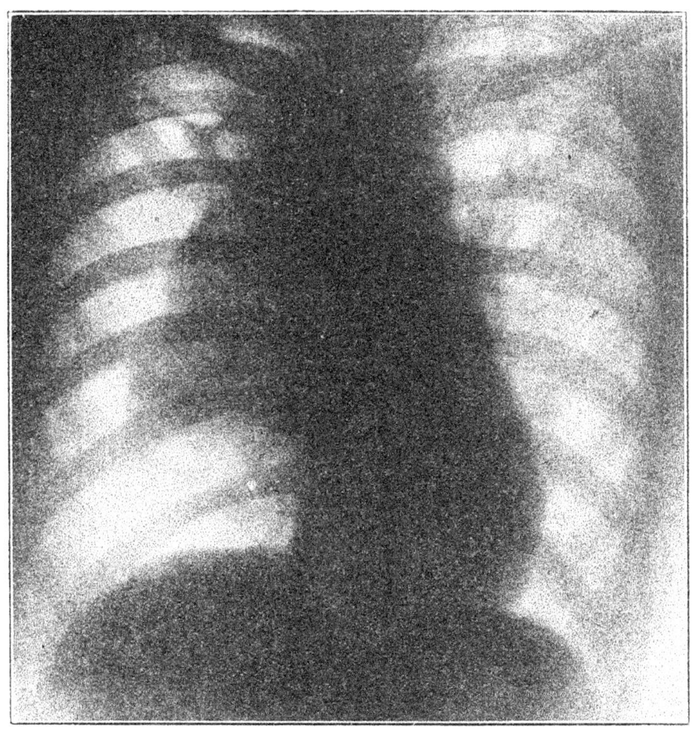

PLATE III.

Plate III is the plate of a patient (F. R.) who had tuberculosis in both lungs, and owing to severe and repeated hemorrhages and the hopelessness of her condition it was decided to do a pneumothorax on the side which seemed to be less affected. It will be noted in the second interspace on the left side that there is a dense, dark, annular shadow, and there are also areas of dense fibrosis; the right lung has been partially collapsed, but the adhesion seen between the first and the second rib shows why the complete collapse could not be effected. It is in this class of adhesions that Jacobaeus recommends cauterization through the thoracoscope. We can also note the annular shadow, which is not compressed. These particular shadows have been described as localized pneumothoraces. Formerly this type of shadow was considered by most men as evidence of cavities, but it was noted that the physical signs of cavities did not exist in these cases. (Lawrason Brown.)

forces the air into *B*, through *A*, on through the tube and through the needle *J* and into the chest cavity. The air is filtered through sterile cotton before being admitted into the chest. To register the pressure in the chest, the valve *F* is connected with the manometer, and by noting oscillations as varying negative during inspiration and expiration one will know when the needle is in the pleural cavity. Until one is sure that the needle is in the pleural cavity he should not connect the air in *B* with the needle *J*. During the operation the pleural pressure should be taken from time to time, so that as soon as the positive pressure is noted great care can be used in the introduction of more air, as the adhesions might be torn and hemorrhages occur, and collapse of the patient might result.

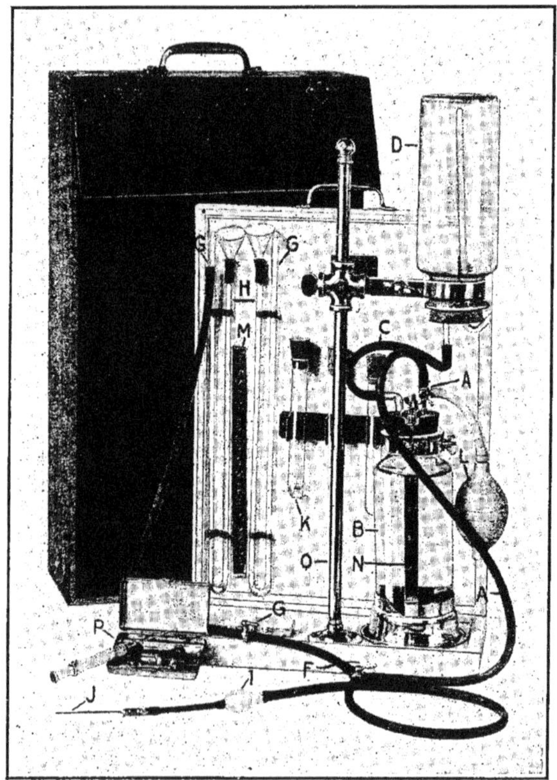

FIG. 3.—This drawing represents the portable pneumothorax apparatus which is used in our work. Its simplicity is such that similar instruments can be made by anyone who possesses any mechanical skill. The outfit shown weighs twelve pounds, and occupies very little space. (See text of the article describing the method of operation.)

The site of injection should be swabbed with tincture of iodin and alcohol. We use novocain, 0.5 per cent, as a local anesthetic on the skin and pleura. The location of the puncture, of course, depends on the physical signs and roentgen findings. When possible the axillary line is used, as there is less muscle and fat tissue at this site.

The first treatment is usually the most severe, as most patients fear the operation and the sensation of pain seems to be most acute at this time. It is very seldom that any untoward symptoms result, except a slight pain in the shoulder of the side treated. This is due to reflex irritation of the pleura. Occasionally patients become dizzy and nauseated. Frequently fluid collects (hydropneumothorax) in the chest cavity, but it is rarely of any importance, although at times it may become infected (pyopneumothorax).

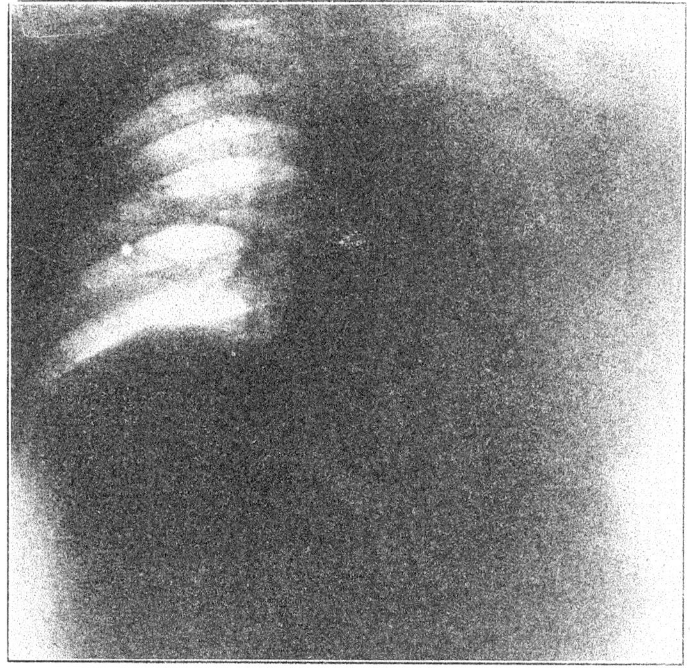

PLATE IV.

Plate IV is that of a patient (M. S.) admitted November 1, 1920. This dense shadow in the chest so obliterated the markings in the lung that it was impossible to tell by physical signs or the roentgen ray whether this was due to fluid or complete consolidation. Thoracentesis done at this time gave dry tap, and a diagnostic pneumothorax was done.

The amount of air injected varies with the pressure recorded. Occasionally 100 cc will register a positive pressure. This is due to the air being injected in a pocket in the pleura. At the next treatment, which should be done in a few days, more air should be injected so that a gradual pressure on the adhesions will result. If this does not occur after several injections it is best to discontinue the treatment.

Jacobaeus[1] recommends the use of an electrocautery needle inserted through a trocar between the ribs to sever the adhesions between the lung and the chest wall. Previous to this operation he inserts an instrument, called the thoracoscope, in between the ribs and finds the adhesions. Occasionally hemorrhages result with fatal results. So far as I know no one in this country uses this method.

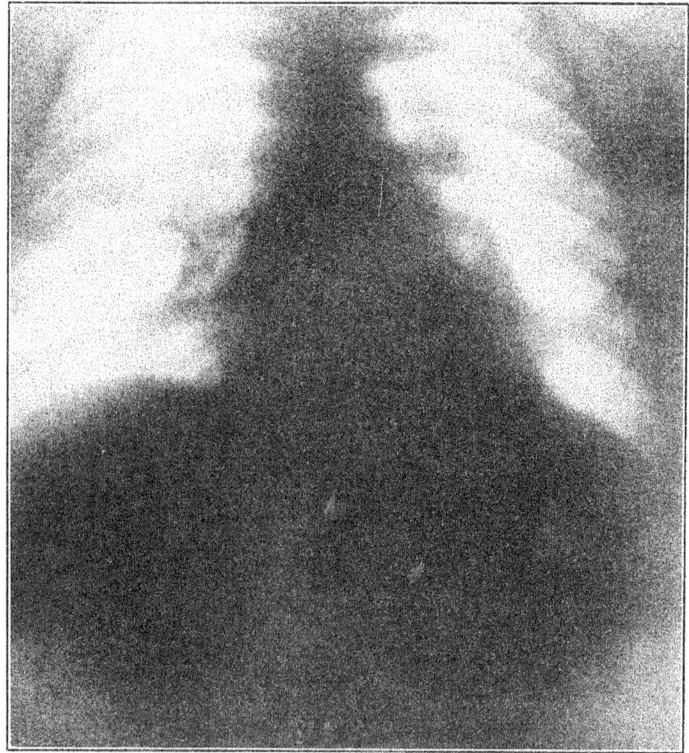

PLATE V.

Plate V shows the same patient after several fillings with air; this was taken on December 10, 1920. Note the almost complete collapse of the lung with the cavity between the third and fifth interspace, which was not compressed. One can readily see by comparing Plates IV and V how important the diagnostic pneumothorax is, as without this procedure described no true interpretation of the lung could be made.

However, the time may come when surgery of the chest will be much more safe than it is today and the surgeon will not hesitate to remove the adhesions from the lung, and it may be as simple a matter as removing adhesions within the abdomen.

[1] Beiträge zur Klinik der Tuberculose, 1915, **35**, 137.

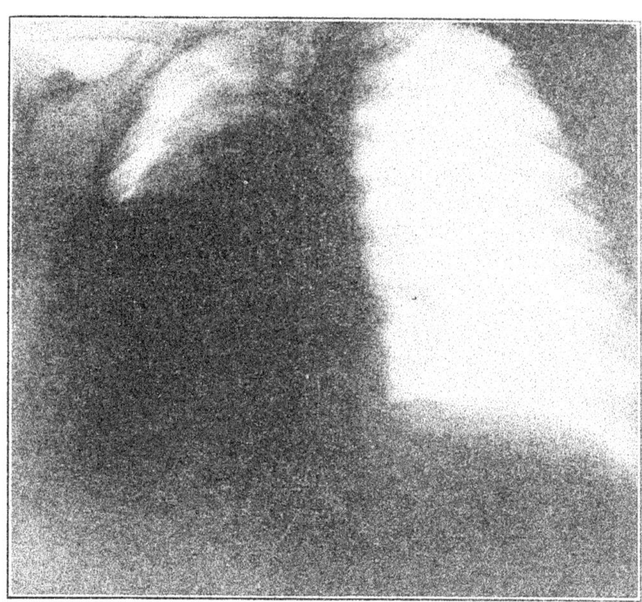

PLATE VI.

Plate VI which was taken on the same patient on March 15, 1921, showed evidence of fluid, "hydropneumothorax." The lung is shown partially collapsed, with fluid in the base of the pleural cavity and air above the fluid.

Complication of serous effusion occurs in one-third of the cases.

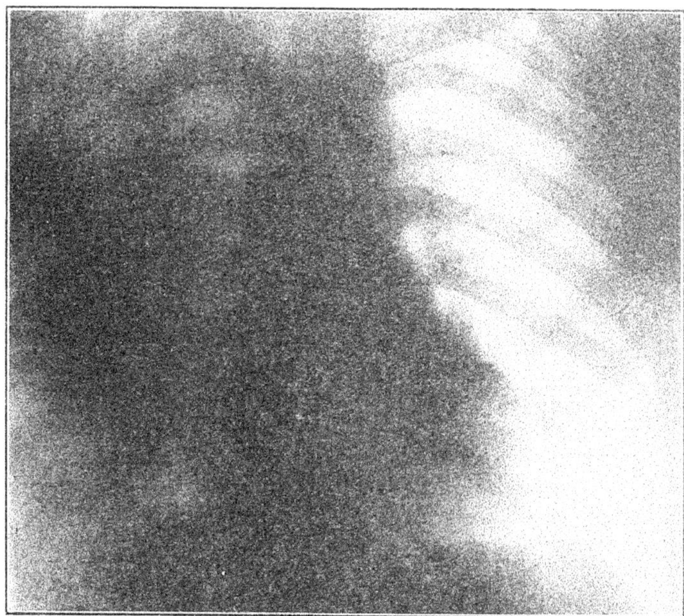

PLATE VII.

Plate VII is that of a patient (R. B.) admitted December 18, 1920. The entire right chest was more or less obliterated by a dense shadow. The physical signs were such that no definite character of his lung can be made out. Comparing this shadow with the one in Plate IV, one sees a striking resemblance. After a diagnostic pneumothorax was done (see Plate VIII) note that the shadow was due to fluid.

The collapse of the lung need not be complete to obtain beneficial results. It is not at all unusual for patients to say they have less cough and that fever is less after the first injection. How much benefit is due to imagination I do not know. However, after more or less collapse most of the patients are improved objectively. The illustrations will show varying degrees of compression in which satisfactory symptomatic results have occurred.

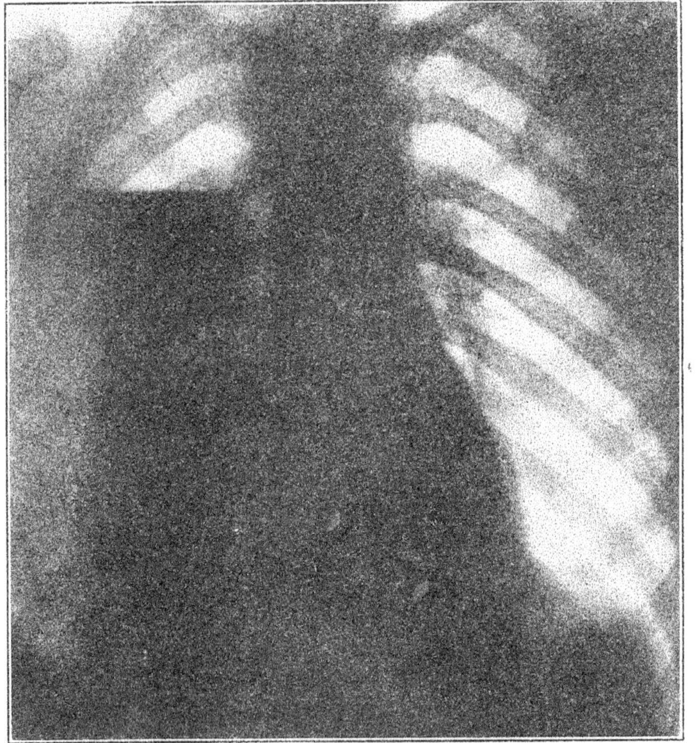

PLATE VIII.

Plate VIII shows the condition of the chest after the introduction of 200 cc of air. The fluid level is easily seen at the junction of the introduced air.

Pneumothorax can be done in the physician's office provided one has the facilities for proper roentgenological examinations and the proper facilities for sterilization. Most patients can take the pneumothorax sitting in a chair or on a stool, and are able to leave within a few minutes after the operation. The entire treatment can usually be done in ten minutes.

Spontaneous Pneumothorax. The danger of spontaneous pneumothorax is great, as the sudden filling up of the pleural cavity with air through a tear in the lung compresses the lung and pushes the mediastinum with its vessels into the opposite chest cavity. The sudden pressure occurs before the compensatory mechanism of the body can adjust itself to this condition. When a spontaneous pneumothorax occurs the patients are usually in a state of body collapse—marked dyspnea, cold, clammy skin, and occasionally the patient dies. Spontaneous pneumothorax occurs in tuberculosis fairly frequently, so that compression gradually done will

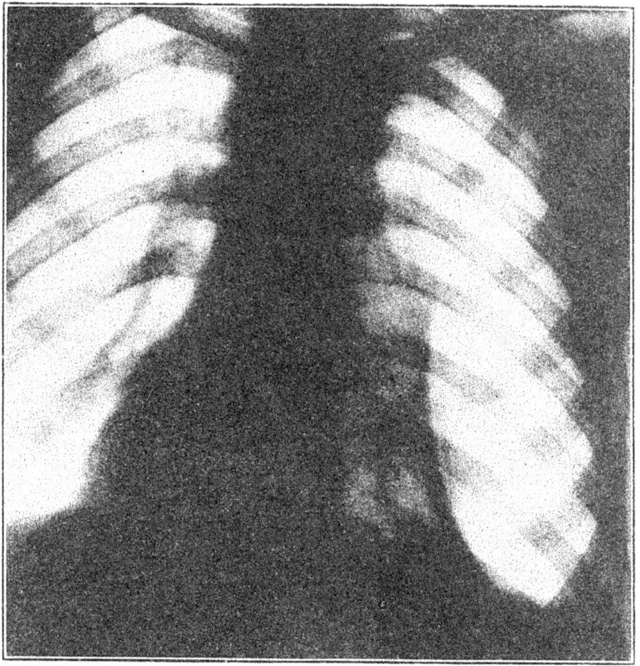

PLATE IX.

Plate IX shows the chest after removal of practically all of the fluid. It will be noticed that the lung had not reëxpanded. This condition is due to the dense adhesion which extends vertically through the chest; this condition will always remain as a chronic pyopneumothorax unless a radical operation is done, in which the ribs are removed and the adhesion severed. This was not done in this case because it proved to be tuberculosis.

prevent in many instances a spontaneous collapse. By reversing the pneumothorax outfit described in this paper and connecting the chest cavity through the needle *J* to the bottle *D*, which is filled with water, the air is extracted from the pleural cavity until a normal manometer pressure is noted.

Diagnostic Pneumothorax. It has been suggested by Fishberg[2] that the diagnostic pneumothorax will bring certain extrapulmonary

[2] Jour. Am. Med. Assn., 1921, **76**, 581.

masses into better view. "In about 50 per cent of cases of malignancy of the lung, pleural effusion" (serous, sanguineous or purulent) takes place and diagnosis is then rendered more difficult. When this takes place the entire one-half of the affected side of the chest is obscured in the roentgen plate by a dense homogeneous shadow and the usual roentgenographic report is pleural effusion. By the removal of several hundred cubic centimeters of this fluid and injecting nitrogen or air the extrapulmonary condition can be readily noted.

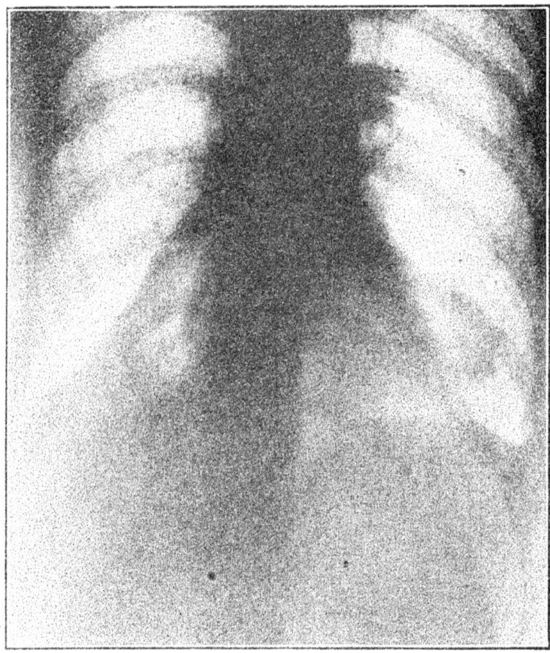

PLATE X.

Plate X is of a patient (A. S.) taken December 17, 1920. It will be noted that the dense shadow extends from the hilus on the right side downward and blending with the diaphragm, and it is three-quarter inches wide. The physical signs and history warrant a diagnosis of bronchiectasis. The patient would bring up two or three times a day from eight to twelve ounces of purulent sputum. This condition followed an attack of influenza. For two years she was unable to lie down in bed on account of severe paroxysms of coughing and the sensation of smothering.

In using the diagnostic pneumothorax we find that when fluid is present in the pleural cavity only one or two operations are necessary to determine lung detail.

Pneumothorax in Other Chest Diseases. Pneumothorax is indicated in severe bronchiectasis, abscess of the lung and empyema emptying into a bronchus.

Severe bronchiectasis may be benefited by pneumothorax. It is simply marvellous to see the improvement following the collapse of the lung. Patients who have been bringing up purulent sputum from four ounces to a pint, and who have found it impossible to lie down in bed, after the second injection will have little or no sputum and be able to lie down in any position. Occasionally, however, in bronchiectasis we have very dense adhesions which

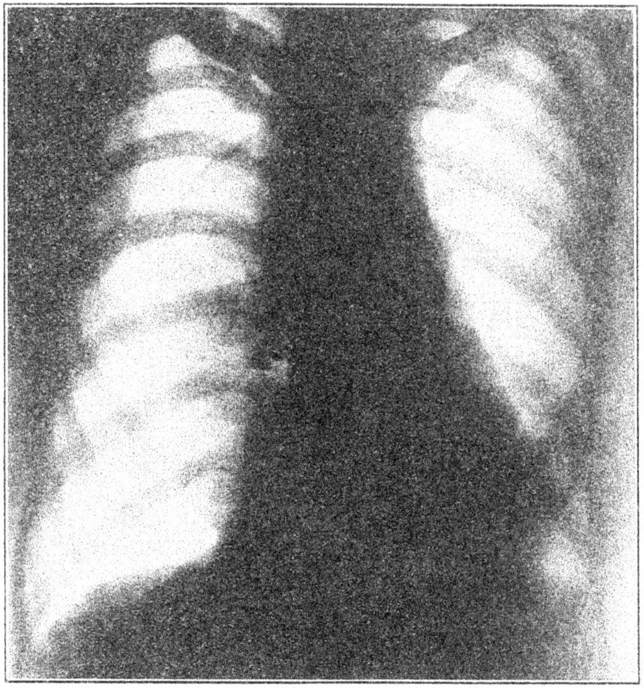

PLATE XI.

Plate of the same patient taken November 13, 1921, shows a collapse of the lung following artificial pneumothorax. In this case compression was done on account of the severe hemorrhages which occurred two weeks previous to the introduction of artificial pneumothorax. One can note in the base of the lung the collapse of the bronchiectatic area. Since the operation patient has had no hemorrhages, and is able to lie down without coughing and bringing up only an ounce or two of purulent sputum daily. Apparently the bronchiectatic cavities are all collapsed.

prevent collapse of the lung. In these cases surgery is indicated. The procedure used in bronchiectasis is the same as described before in the early part of this paper.

In cases of abscess of the lung, when patients are bringing up purulent sputum and when there is a connection between the abscess cavity and a bronchus, good results may be obtained in this condition.

Empyema with bronchial fistula, especially in tuberculosis, can be treated by this method. The pressure of the air forced into the cavity will force the fluid through the bronchus, and this can then be expectorated.

Conclusion. 1. The most suitable cases are one-sided tuberculosis or moderately advanced cases with proper compensatory lung tissue.

2. Cases with hemorrhages are especially benefited by pneumothorax.

3. Bronchiectasis, lung abscess and tuberculous empyema are frequently very much improved.

4. As a diagnostic measure of the lung condition it offers considerable.

I wish to thank Dr. George Dock and Dr. Albert Taussig for their kindness in supervising this work.

THE SURGICAL NEUROSES OF THE THYROID GLAND.[1]

By John Rogers, M.D.,
NEW YORK.

The conditions which result from an apparently overacting thyroid gland were formerly classified as neuroses. These disorders can be defined as abnormalities in the functions of one or more parts of the nervous system for which there are no corresponding demonstrable nerve lesions. The manifestations of hyperthyroidism are of this character and should be designated as neuroses because that terminology helps to direct attention not only to the probable locality and manner in which the thyroid product acts, but to the general nature of the disturbance. It seems to be traceable to certain alveoli which differ from those of the normal thyroid, and if the duration and intensity of the process is sufficient morphologic changes occur in other organs. To prevent these, and to relieve or cure the antecedent neuroses, experience has proved the necessity of surgery. But operative treatment alone should be regarded as fulfilling only a small part of the indications, for these neuroses are essentially the same as all others, that is, dependent in all probability upon some preceding defect or deficiency in the nervous biochemistry. Either the nerve tissue itself is "weak," which means that the nutritional chemistry of the nerve elements is not as sound and vigorous as it should be, or else that there is a defect or deficiency in the metabolic processes

[1] Read before the Surgical Section of the Buffalo Academy of Medicine, March 1, 1922, and the Philadelphia County Medical Society, May 11, 1922.

of the viscera upon which the nervous nutrition depends. The deficiency may be a congenital and inherent, or an acquired error, or it may be secondary and related to the so-called vitamin or deficiency diseases with which some of the thyroid neuroses present many analogies. Certainly the administration of minute doses of thyroid material or of iodin can occasionally produce remarkable results. Thus, many of these hyperthyroid neuroses are strongly suggestive of some primary weakness or defect in the nutrition, especially of the involuntary nervous system, and of changes in the thyroid which are secondary. That is, many individuals seem to possess "weak nerves," and conditions which require their active functionation necessitate a corresponding thyroid activity, and this organ, of evident importance for the nervous nutrition, then fails or "overacts." These cases are generally characterized by the presence of neuroses which precede, and later accompany, the recognizable hyperthyroid symptoms, and usually show only a small or insignificant "goiter."

Others, and they probably constitute the majority of the hyperthyroid cases, seem to originate not in "weak nerves" but in a "weak" thyroid, and this has a very close relationship to the gland's ability to obtain or to metabolize iodin. A deficiency of this element in the ingesta seems to be a common cause of "goiter," or, more correctly speaking, of simple hypertrophy which, certainly in animals, may be accompanied by more or less evident signs of hypothyroidism. As the feeding of iodin to these animals is followed by a disappearance of all symptoms, the hypertrophy seems to represent an attempt to compensate or to supply some deficiency. In man a lack of iodin in the ingesta is not so easily demonstrable, and there also seem to be other variables. For the simple hypertrophy of the thyroid, which is so common in growing children, especially during adolescence, does not always subside with the administration of iodin. Indeed, too large or too frequently repeated dosage may even be followed by increased hypertrophy or by the development of adenomatous or cystic changes.

The latest determinations place the iodin content of the normal human thyroid at 0.5 mg. per gram of fresh gland substance.[2] The hyperthyroid gland seems unable to hold this amount, and the severity of the symptoms is more or less proportionate to the thyroid's lack of iodin. Feeding this element generally increases the disturbance, though it may prove inert or temporarily beneficial. In the latter case the gland usually first enlarges and gives a sensation of constriction or pressure, and if then the iodin is continued there follows an exacerbation of the process which may be dangerous. Rarely a very small amount of iodin, especially if combined with

[2] Zunz: Arch. Int. Physiol., 1921, **16**, 288.

adrenal feeding, as will be described later, may prove curative. That is, there may be an abundance of available iodin, but the thyroid cannot without assistance from other organs metabolize it. The gland is not independent and its unaided functional capacity is limited.

Clinical observations are not entirely trustworthy but they seem to show that the great majority of the hyperthyroid disturbances begin rather gradually and run a more or less recognizable course. There is the not inconsiderable group which, as stated above, apparently start with "weak nerves" or ill-defined neuroses, with an irritable and then a constantly rapid pulse. The enlargement of the thyroid is then and thereafter slight or inconspicuous. These cases generally present a much less favorable surgical prognosis than the other more common group, which seem to start with a "weak" thyroid. The latter, as it gives the first noticeable symptom, is apparently the primary lesion. In these cases there is an initial simple hypertrophy which can be reasonably regarded as an attempt to compensate or to supply demands which exceed the gland's functional capacity. These demands apparently emanate from every organ, and especially from the nervous system, and in each seem to pertain to the chemistry which promotes that organ's functional activity. For in recognizable hypothyroidism the chief symptoms may be of deficient functionation in almost any part of the body, and any or all of these symptoms can often be relieved by the right kind of thyroid feeding. Then, after the appearance of the hypertrophy, unusual or excessive functionation in other organs or groups of organs is regularly followed by increase in the size of the "goiter," and cessation of this activity by its shrinkage.

The gland when overactive is well known to accelerate metabolism and to be intimately connected with oxidation. It is not the only factor in this process, but its importance is shown by Kocher's "cachexia strumipriva," which is irremediable unless Kendall's thyroxin should prove efficient. Because of these evident relationships the chief if not the only function of the thyroid apparently is the promotion through the process of oxidation of the organism's chemical reactions. Or more briefly and less accurately, the gland's purpose seems to be the "production of energy." To fulfil this duty the organ must have available a certain minimum amount of iodin, and it must possess a certain minimum amount of epithelium which is capable of functioning. The functional capacity of the epithelium, and the factors which regulate its nutrition and so its functional capacity, or the multiplication or atrophy of its epithelium, can only be surmised. But they evidently are variable and even more important than the circulating iodin.

The conditions, then, under which the first signs of the hyperthyroid neuroses develop are almost always those requiring an excessive expenditure of one or another kind of energy. This may be to resist acute or chronic infections, or to endure pregnancy and labor, or to sustain muscular exertion, or most often to withstand an unfavorable environment. An inefficient thyroid, then, responds to those demands for its "production of energy" by simple hypertrophy. Coincident with, or following, this evidence of an attempt at compensation there are usually pallor, more or less headache and lassitude or weariness, and signs of deficient gastrointestinal activity. These are the signs of ordinary fatigue and cannot be differentiated from that common condition except by the presence of the "goiter." When the goiter is perceptible the symptoms are generally accepted as those of hypothyroidism. If the causes which induce the excessive (and this varies with each individual) expenditure of energy persist, the preceding quiet pulse-rate becomes "irritable" and then constantly rapid, and with this phenomenon there occur the usual increased, or perhaps "unchecked," vasomotor, cutaneous, respiratory and gastro-intestinal activity or evidences of hyperthyroidism. The exophthalmos, if it occurs, generally appears last. Its origin is unknown, but this symptom adds materially to the gravity of the prognosis.

An unfavorable environment is one of the most common causes for provoking expenditure of energy, and many individuals, in all probability, by avoiding this environment because of the symptoms it excites, seem to have their disturbance arrested midway between hypothyroidism and typical hyperthyroidism. These cases form the rather large group which give the so-called "mixed" or coexisting signs of both hypo- and hyperthyroidism. If it can be accepted that the disease starts in an initial simple hypertrophy, apparently to compensate for an expenditure of more energy than the normal gland can supply, and passes through a hypo and then a mixed hypo and hyper stage and finally into typical hyperthyroidism, then the gland should be treated at least with conservatism. The hyperthyroid condition in following this course gives strong evidence of originating in a "weak" thyroid which "overacts" not because of a primary and vicious functionation, but because the gland's epithelium, under "strain" or demands which are excessive, fails in its power to metabolize iodin.

The initial simple hypertrophy may at any time, especially if the conditions are those which require much expenditure of energy, be complicated by the development of a cyst, or cystadenoma, or a "toxic adenoma." Apparently, the demand upon the thyroid for functionation is accompanied by congestion which may obstruct an alveolus and lead to a "retention" cyst or cause an intraglandular hemorrhage with a reactive and often encapsulated epithelial proliferation. The epithelium in and immediately around the damaged area seems to have less than the normal functional capacity, and its iodin metabolism, therefore, becomes faulty. The resultant general symptoms are the same as those of ordinary hyperthyroidism, except that these cases less often develop the highest metabolism tests and less often show marked exophthalmos. But some, especially the multiple toxic adenomata, may show all of these signs.

The symptoms of the typical hyperthyroid neuroses are traceable chiefly to abnormal or "unchecked" activity in the functions performed by the autonomic or parasympathetic nerves. This group might be more generally appreciated if it were designated by the name of its most prominent member, or as the vagus system. The flushed and moist skin, the usually low blood-pressure, the overacting rather than the merely rapid heart, the lacrimation and salivation, the abnormal hunger and the frequent bowel movements, are all referable to these nerves. That is, the accepted symptoms of an overactive thyroid are those of overactivity in the autonomic or vagus, and not in the sympathetic system. A great many cases, however, show only a simple tachycardia and practically nothing else except a thyroid enlargement and some vague "nervousness." These symptoms certainly may indicate the existence of a hyperthyroidism, but they do not necessarily prove that the thyroid product stimulates or acts through or upon the cardioaccelerator, or at least one of the sympathetic nerves, and much less all of the group.

While testing the effects upon dogs of various derivatives of the thyroid it was found that noncoagulable extracts excite immediate and definite responses. The most active of these preparations seemed to be a slightly hydrolyzed aqueous extract which was designated as the thyroid "residue" because it consisted of what remained, after the removal by boiling in dilute acid and alkali, of all coagulable material. Another extract made with 95 per cent alcohol, then evaporating the alcohol and adding water, was nearly but not quite as active. Each was standardized to contain 0.05 mg. of iodin per cc. The responses which these noncoagulable extracts provoked were vasodilatation, apparently through stimulation of the vasodilator nerve terminals, an increase in the salivary flow and a vigorous stimulation of the flow of the gastric and pancreatic secretions.[3] There was also some stimulation of the gastric and intestinal peristalsis. A dose of atropin which, of course, paralyzes the terminals of the vagus, prevented or stopped this stimulation. After section of the vagus just above the diaphragm and degeneration of its peripheral fibers, the injection of the noncoagulable thyroid extracts produced little or no effect. Thus, at least in the case of the stomach and pancreas, the noncoagulable extracts of the thyroid apparently act through and upon the terminal

[3] Am. Jour. Physiol., 1916, **39**, 345; Ibid., 1919, **48**, 79.

filaments of the vagus. They may also produce more or less diuresis. In the kymograph tracings there was no thyroid derivative which would cause any appreciable degree of tachycardia. This seems to mean that the product of the thyroid does not stimulate the cardioaccelerator nerve nor, for that matter, any other part of the sympathetic system.

These particular nerve endings are, of course, activated or stimulated by epinephrin; therefore, experiments were next carried out with derivatives of the adrenal gland (all of which contain at least traces of epinephrin), and it was found that a slightly hydrolyzed aqueous extract made like that from the thyroid and designated as the adrenal "residue" (because it contained all that remained after removal of the coagulable materials) prevented or stopped the stimulation excited by the noncoagulable derivatives of the thyroid. The coagulable derivatives of the adrenal gland, like the nucleoprotein material, contain only faint traces of epinephrin, while the noncoagulable are quite rich in this substance; they all excite vasoconstriction or raise the blood-pressure in proportion to their epinephrin content. They all also stop or prevent the stimulation by the noncoagulable thyroid derivatives of the stomach and pancreas. But these effects, though apparently brought about by direct excitation of the functions believed to be performed by the terminal filaments of the sympathetic are not those of epinephrin. At least, a dose of adrenalin which is equivalent to the epinephrin content of the adrenal nucleoprotein material, or to the noncoagulable derivatives of the entire gland, shows comparatively slight inhibitory powers. That is, the supposed active principle of the adrenal gland is not nearly as vigorous an antagonist of the thyroid derivatives as are at least some of the materials which can be extracted from the whole adrenal gland. Because the adrenal nucleoproteins and the slightly hydrolyzed aqueous extract (adrenal "residue") produced so marked an inhibition of the gastrointestinal functionation, apparently through stimulation of the sympathetic nerves, their effects were next tested, in comparison with commercial adrenalin, upon the iodin content of the dog's thyroid. The noncoagulable extracts given hypodermically are followed by severe and sometimes fatal reactions. Therefore, crystals of commercial adrenalin and the adrenal nucleoprotein material and the adrenal residue were fed over a period of six weeks by mouth. The dosage of each was standardized by its epinephrin content. One thyroid lobe was removed from each animal at the beginning of the experiment and the other at the close. It was then found that the thyroid lobe in the dogs which were fed adrenalin showed, as compared with the control animals, a practically negligible gain in iodin. Those fed the adrenal nucleoprotein material showed an average gain of about 50 per cent while those fed the adrenal residue gained about 75 per cent.[4]

It is well known, as stated previously, that in cases of excessive activity of the thyroid the gland contains per gram of gland substance less than the normal amount of iodin, and the greater the loss in iodin the more severe seem to be the symptoms. Therefore, because the feeding of derivatives of the *entire* adrenal gland results in a gain in the thyroid's iodin, it is reasonable to believe in some inhibitory effect of the adrenals upon the thyroid, probably through the intermediation of the latter's sympathetic nerve supply.

The impulses discharged from the sympathetic, as determined by electrical and chemical tests, produce vasoconstriction and, in general, inhibition of gastrointestinal activity. Those from the autonomic or vagus system, on the other hand, excite, as a rule, vasodilatation and increased gastroenteric functionation. As the thyroid product, both clinically and experimentally, seems to have a selective and stimulating affinity for the autonomic or vagus terminals, its part in the production of chemical energy can be briefly described as that of "drive." The adrenal product, by its corresponding effect upon the opposing or sympathetic terminals, can then be supposed, by its inhibition of functional activity, presumably through each organ's metabolism, to act as the opposing automatic "check." Hence, theoretically and because of the effects of adrenal feeding upon the thyroid's iodin content, any excess of thyroid activity "drives" the adrenals into activity, probably through their vagus nerve supply, and then the adrenal product returns in the circulation and, probably through the sympathetic terminals, automatically "checks" the thyroid.

Any break in this chain should lead to the development of a vicious circle. Its most vulnerable link ought to be in the terminals of the vagus, or sympathetic, nerves. It is presumable that either the latter or the vagus (autonomic) endings may have their functions interrupted or destroyed by bacterial or other poisons or, as clinically seems common, by fatigue. In the experimental fatigue of voluntary muscles which can be induced by electrical stimulation of their nerve supply, the first effects are those of failing vigor in the contractions due to failure in the function of the nerve ending. When this failure becomes marked the injection into the circulation of noncoagulable derivatives of the thyroid or adrenal glands quickly restores the muscular vigor. If, however, the fatigue is continued until there is no contraction, that is until the function of the nerve ending is destroyed, then the thyroid and adrenal extracts are without effect.[5]

These findings seem to have some significance in the origin of

[4] Am. Jour. Physiol., 1918, 45, 97.

[5] Ibid.

the thyroid neuroses and their treatment, for fatigue should be capable of interrupting the functions, also, of the involuntary nerve terminals, and if the sympathetic supply of the thyroid fails the gland should lose its automatic "check" and then ought to overact. Clinically, however, when fatigue appears to originate the disturbance, at the outset it seems to affect both the vagus "drive" and the sympathetic "check." The accompanying symptoms are those called hypothyroidism. Later, with a continuation or intensification of the fatigue, the sympathetic becomes conceivably more intensely affected, and the ultimate result is lack of check upon the gland and hyperthyroidism. Furthermore, the fatigue experiments mentioned above suggest that organ therapy can be helpful only when the involuntary nerve terminals are capable of at least some functionation; hence, also, the need of rest.

In the differential diagnosis of the thyroid neuroses an evident excess of activity or of "drive" in all or a majority of organs indicates, in the presence of at least a perceptible "goiter," an excess of thyroid product or hyperthyroidism and a lack of drive the opposite condition. We know nothing of a corresponding hypo- or hyperadrenalism. Nevertheless an excess of drive can theoretically mean only a deficiency of the normal check, which may be in the sympathetic and not in the adrenal portion of the chromaffin system.

But in what seems to be the intermediate stages of the disease, or the so-called mixed hypo- and hyperthyroid disturbances, when the hyper symptoms are beginning and advancing from, or perhaps receding into, the primary failure, it is necessary to study the history and the general nutrition and then judge whether more organs are overacting than underacting. If there is only a tachycardia and "nervousness" without any flushed, moist skin and evidence of gastrointestinal activity, the signs of lack of drive predominate over those of its excess, and the condition is one more of hypo- than hyperthyroidism. Just what this means cannot at present be definitely stated, and there is no mechanical test which alone is conclusive. The calorimeter, in my experience, is often more useful in these doubtful cases for proving the existence of hypo- rather than hyperthyroidism, for it not infrequently shows a metabolism which is even 20 per cent or 30 per cent above normal, yet this may be promptly reduced by the *right kind* of thyroid feeding. In the absence of any better explanation it can be imagined that the "mixed" symptoms are traceable not so much to a failure of inhibition in the thyroid as to a failure in varying degrees and in different organs of the sympathetic "check" mechanism with a presumable increase in their metabolism which should be reflected in the calorimeter. There is a general belief, however, that the product of the hyperthyroid gland may vary in both quantity and quality. An alteration in the quality of the thyroid secretion might then stimulate some and not all parts of the autonomic system; or it might lead to an imperfect adrenal product (as the thyroid seems to be needed by all organs) and this to imperfect inhibition, which would then be expressed as "overactivity" or imperfect balance in some other viscera. In whatever way the complicated disturbance may be interpreted the fact remains that not infrequently in the early or mild or atypical cases of apparent hyperthyroidism the "feeding" of some thyroid derivative will relieve or cure and not intensify the condition. As the administration of iodin may rarely accomplish the same result, there are thus some reasons for believing in a poor quality rather than a mere excess of quantity of secretion.

The materials commonly available for thyroid feeding are prepared by different methods of desiccation of the whole gland, and lately there have been added the nucleoprotein substance which can be extracted from the fresh organ and also an alcoholic extract and a slightly hydrolyzed aqueous extract spoken of previously as the thyroid "residue." As there seemed to be great variations in the clinical reactions of patients to these different preparations our laboratory recently tested the effects upon three groups of dogs of the products of several of the best-known manufacturers. The first group consisted of normal animals, the second were thyroidectomized, and the third, to denervate the organ, had the gland transplanted into the spleen, where, at the close of the experiment, it was later demonstrable. The dosage of thyroid material was standardized so that each animal received by mouth daily an amount which contained approximately 2 mg. of iodin. After feeding one preparation of the entire desiccated gland for a few days the urine of all the dogs, especially those which had been thyroidectomized, showed the presence of glucose. Feeding the similar product of another manufacturer was followed by the appearance of albumin in the urine of the thyroidectomized dogs and in those which had the thyroid transplanted into the spleen. Still another desiccated product caused albumin in the urine only of the dogs with the spleen transplant, or both sugar and albumin. That is, all of the desiccated products regularly caused gross changes in the urine of the thyroidectomized dogs, or in those with a presumably denervated thyroid, and one product seemed to cause albuminuria even in the normal dogs. On the other hand, the preparations like the nucleoprotein material and the thyroid residue made from fresh glands showed no gross ill effects. Hence, as dogs are very tolerant of thyroid feeding it is presumable that a cautious therapeutic test for the existence of hyperthyroidism by the oral administration of the *usual dried gland substance,* though much more harmless than the hypodermic administration of adrenalin, would at least not be positive. But the derivatives like the thyroid nucleoprotein material, which are made from the fresh gland, seem to be free of toxic effects in animals, and clinically in the border-line cases will often relieve and not intensify the "mixed" symptoms.

When an apparently hyperthyroid condition can be improved or slowly cured by feeding a more or less "nontoxic" thyroid derivative, there is no proof that the original diagnosis was wrong. It is only probable that the popular conception of the disease is wrong. The product of the thyroid epithelium is apparently not excreted, but in some disintegrated form returns to its source and is there recombined. If the epithelium is "weak," it may not be able to recombine a badly disintegrated product, but might be able to utilize a material which is nearer to the normal. The ingestion in comparatively minute amounts of some "nontoxic" thyroid derivative could not materially increase in the circulation the quantity of the pathological thyroid product and might act toward the thyroid epithelium like a specific predigested food.

The tachycardia, which is so constant and characteristic in hyperthyroidism, because of its relationship to the cardioaccelerator nerve, seems to have given origin to the prevailing and apparently erroneous belief that the thyroid acts through or upon the sympathetic nerves. As stated previously, there is no derivative of the thyroid which, experimentally and within the usual laboratory period of two or three hours, will excite this symptom. It only occurs after a rather prolonged treatment with thyroid feeding, and then is apparently an accompaniment of the generally increased metabolism. It may signify an increased metabolism of the cardiac musculature, but evidently is not due to direct stimulation of the cardioaccelerator nerve by the thyroid product.

The peculiar disturbance excited in the doubtful or mixed hypo- and hyperthyroid cases by the injection of adrenalin is of unknown significance. It proves nothing. Because the evidence points toward some primary failure in the thyroid, it would be far more reasonable and much less injurious in guessing at which extreme predominates, to administer some nontoxic derivative of the thyroid. If then, in spite of every attempt to relieve the needs for the production of energy, the signs of too much "drive" upon the viscera persist and are not relieved or are aggravated by cautious thyroid feeding, there is need of surgery.

As stated previously, the ultimate cause of the hyperthyroid neuroses seems to be traceable to certain pathologic alveoli in the diseased gland, for if this abnormal tissue can all be removed, as it can be in some encapsulated "toxic adenomata," the manifestations of hyperthyroidism quickly subside. If it cannot all be removed the immediate relief seems to be more or less in proportion to the amount excised. But to obtain this kind of a result the diseased part of the thyroid must be excised before the neuroses have produced at least pronounced changes in the viscera.

The location and extent of the hyperplasia can only be estimated by the consistency and contour of the gland and by the comparative size and apparent vascularity of the two lobes and the isthmus. For surgical purposes these observations can be expressed diagrammatically as representing three types of hyperthyroid glands, although each is capable of transformation into any of the others.

1. The symmetrically enlarged thyroid of even consistency, vascularity and contour throughout the entire organ. This gland contains, presumably, the hyperplastic tissue equally distributed in all parts and is usually accompanied by the signs of typical hyperthyroidism, and often the worst forms of exophthalmic goiter.

2. The asymmetrically enlarged thyroid in which one lobe is greater in size than the other and generally more dense and vascular, and thus can be more or less surely presumed to contain most, if not all, of the hyperplastic tissue, for the latter contains less colloid and more cells and bloodvessels than the normal tissue. The accompanying neuroses in this type of hyperthyroid gland are usually less severe than in the first, and the exophthalmos may be only perceptible on the side of the enlarged lobe.

3. The thyroid of the "toxic adenoma" type. This gland may be slightly or considerably enlarged, but contains an evidently circumscribed tumor. The accompanying neuroses are usually less severe than in either of the two preceding types of hyperthyroid glands, and are seldom accompanied by exophthalmos. But it is possible for a nontoxic adenoma, or one containing no hyperplasia, to occur in a hyperplastic thyroid which may even be not noticeably enlarged. Furthermore, a comparatively normal thyroid containing a single toxic adenoma can develop, usually under conditions which force the patient to expend much energy, other toxic adenomata, and in addition hyperplasia in the intervening, comparatively normal tissue.

That is, almost any of these three types of thyroid, which seem to represent the initial changes in the gland, can alter into any other and be accompanied by any or all of the hyperthyroid neuroses or symptoms and by the subsequent visceral lesions.

Some if not all of the toxic adenomata seem to originate in a congestion, presumably to promote functionation, and then there occurs a localized hemorrhage. Others apparently begin like a retention cyst. These peculiar alveoli, with their thickened epithelium, seem, of course, to represent a multiplication of the secreting structure of the thyroid with a corresponding increase in the gland's functional activity. Occasionally, and that, too, without any treatment, the hyperplastic alveoli are evidently capable, though slowly, of returning to the normal. The recovery, however, is more frequent after cutting down the circulation by the ligation of one or more of the superior or inferior thyroid vessels. Hence it is reasonable to believe that the chief stimuli which cause the gland to "overact" reach it through the blood. The same inference can be drawn from the congestion of the organ, which is evident during exacerbations of hyperthyroidism. These surgical aspects of the diseased gland can be readily understood from the accompanying rough diagrams. (Figs. 1, 2, 3).

To be reasonably sure of operative success all, or the major part of the hyperplastic alveoli, must be excised. This is comparatively simple in the second and third types of diseased gland. The

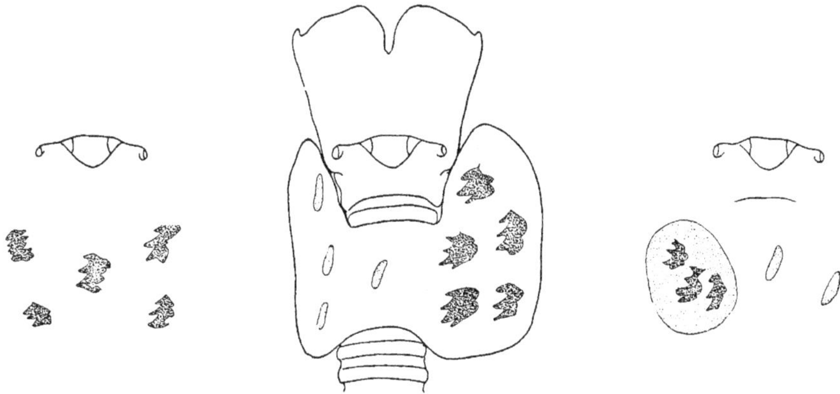

FIG. 1 FIG. 2 FIG. 3

FIG. 1.—The symmetrically enlarged thyroid of even consistency, contour and vascularity. The hyperplastic alveoli are presumably distributed throughout all parts of the gland. Ligation of the four chief vessels is the safest and best operation.

FIG. 2.—Asymmetrically enlarged thyroid. Excision of all or the greater part of the diseased alveoli yields the best surgical result. But relapse or recurrence of hyperthyroidism must be constantly kept in mind and prevented by the right kind of thyroid feeding.

FIG. 3.—Thyroid of the toxic adenoma type. The diseased and generally encapsulated alveoli should be treated by enucleation of the tumors and by ligation of the two superior vessels. There should be no extensive resection of simply hypertrophied tissue. Normal alveoli are represented by the oval shaded patches in the thyroid; hyperplastic alveoli by the darker shaded patches with irregular outline.

removal of the lobe which apparently contains all or most of the pathologic tissue, or the enucleation of a toxic adenoma, fulfils these surgical indications. But it is always wise at the same time to tie both superior vessels, if only because of the unavoidable uncertainty as regards the extent of the hyperplasia. When, however, the goiter is like Type 1, that is, when there is reason to believe the hyperplasia is evenly distributed throughout all parts of the entire organ, the problem is much less simple. The common procedure is to excise four-fifths or five-sixths of the gland or to leave an amount which is more or less equivalent in size to that of the normal organ. This is probably unwise, as the prognosis for the operative result is uncertain, or at least more uncertain than it should be. In the hands of the average surgeon there is, in the first place, grave danger of the acute postoperative toxemia; and it is worth noting in considering the gland's pathologic physiology, that the greater the amount of the *uniformly* hyperplastic thyroid which is removed the greater seems to be the danger of this violent toxemia. If a considerable amount of diseased tissue remains, the remote result may be bad but there is less risk of an immediate fatality. In the next place, whether little or much hyperplastic tissue remains, to restore health this must ultimately become normal. If it does become normal there must also apparently be enough of the gland to supply the required amount of "drive" or the hyperthyroidism will recur. There seems to be great variations in the amount of thyroid which different individuals require. To meet these uncertainties in the first type of hyperplastic gland, or that in which the diseased alveoli seem to be evenly distributed through the whole organ, I have practised in over four hundred cases the ligation, at intervals of a week or more, of first the two inferior thyroid vessels and then the two superiors. The inferior arteries can be reached most easily by a three-inch vertical incision along the posterior border of the lower end of the sternomastoid muscle. The guide is the outer edge of the scalenus anticus. After dividing the fascia over the latter, the incision is deepened by blunt dissection in front of the phrenic and behind the internal jugular and common carotid. The inferior thyroid can then be readily felt or seen as it passes upward and inward along the inner border of the scalenus anticus. Its double ligation, without section, seems practically all that is necessary. The postoperative pain is very slight, but after the ligation of the two superior vessels the pain and dysphagia are always quite severe, and are no inconsiderable factors in the following and inevitable "exacerbation" of the disease. A week or ten days later there need be no hesitation in tying through the usual collar incision the two superior vessels. This operation of quadruple ligation is by no means ideal, but experience shows that it involves no danger of a subsequent atrophy of the gland and the consequent irremediable myxedema. Especially in the presence of marked exophthalmos, it involves much less postoperative danger and much less risk of a therapeutic failure than the usual extensive excisions. The recovery to the normal, or to the hypothyroid asthenia of convalescence, which seems to be the primary disturbance, is usually quite gradual and may be complicated by the development of one or more toxic adenomata which were possibly unrecognizable in the original diffuse hyperplasia. Under these conditions there will be need of a third operation to enucleate or excise the more localized disease. But this is not an uncommon occurrence after the radical operations, especially when they are preceded by the preliminary ligations. In all of these hyperthyroid cases, however, surgery should be regarded as only a part of the treatment.

After any operative interference the persistence of the symptoms of too much visceral, cutaneous and vasomotor drive should be regarded as indicating some failure in the normal check mechanism which is supposed to aid the thyroid epithelium to retain or metabolize the necessary iodin. As adrenal feeding experimentally increases the content of this element in the dog's gland, it is reasonable to administer by mouth 10 to 15 drops of the adrenal "residue" (as at present it seems the most efficient adrenal derivative) every three or four hours. When the gastrointestinal tract is very active, the 1 gr. tablets, containing in each 10 per cent of the adrenal nucleoprotein material, are sometimes more helpful. It is also reasonable to add a very small amount of iodin, preferably in the form of 3 or 4 drops of the official tincture, in a half-glass of water once daily. But if it should be followed by any swelling of the thyroid or by a feeling of pressure or constriction the dose of iodin should be postponed or stopped. If iodin is continued under these conditions there is danger of aggravating the symptoms.

As convalescence approaches, and in the more ideal operations or those in which all or most of the hyperplasia has been excised, it may appear within a few days, the hyper symptoms change to hypo, or too little drive. There is pallor, lack of appetite and lack of intestinal activity, and the heart and respiration become quiet. The indications in this stage then are those of the probable original disturbance, or hypothyroidism. There is indicated thyroid feeding, and the least "toxic" or the most commonly helpful is the thyroid nucleoprotein material. One-grain tablets containing 2 per cent or 5 per cent of this substance can generally be given every three or four hours and continued indefinitely. Occasionally, especially if there is marked inactivity in the gastrointestinal tract, the thyroid residue in 5 to 10 minim doses at the same intervals may prove more beneficial. Experimentally, this preparation is a most vigorous stimulant for the gastric and pancreatic secretions. At the same time, and for a long period, the patient should be relieved from all conditions which require expenditure of energy. But his or her thyroid gland, even under the most favorable circumstances, should always be regarded as "weak" or prone to fail in its "drive," and so give rise first to the hypothyroid neuroses, which should be met by feeding, preferably, some nontoxic thyroid derivative to prevent the process from advancing or relapsing into the more serious hyper disturbance.

The acute or subacute postoperative toxemia, which is generally regarded as an exacerbation of the preëxisting hyperthyroidism, is accompanied by a dry skin and by nausea and vomiting and constipation or signs of gastroenteric failure. If it lasts long enough there is enlargement of the liver and spleen and jaundice. The rising pulse and temperature are accompaniments of any toxemia. The thyroid in these conditions shows almost a complete absence of colloid from the alveoli, which, instead, are filled with a mass of cells and granular material. The condition seems, therefore, to be one which is not the result of too much thyroid product and, clinically, the failure of the gastrointestinal tract and probably the liver supports this assumption. For these reasons I have not hesitated, whenever the postoperative course becomes threatening, to administer hypodermically 20 to 30 minims of the liquid thyroid residue every four to six hours.* This treatment does not increase the pulse-rate but rather lowers it, and also the temperature, and relieves the evident failure in the abdominal viscera and thus seems to have saved several of these very dangerous cases.

Summary. 1. The hypo- and hyperthyroid conditions are interchangeable and are manifested by neuroses chiefly of the autonomic group of nerves.

2. The hyperthyroid neuroses do not represent a primary and vicious overactivity of the gland, but seem to develop secondarily from some preceding deficiency in the biochemistry either of the involuntary nervous system or of the thyroid.

3. The hyperthyroid symptoms are traceable to certain "hyperplastic" alveoli in the gland. When all, or the greater part, of these alveoli can be excised the symptoms quickly subside to those of the initial and underlying hypothyroidism.

4. If the hyperplastic alveoli are scattered diffusely and evenly throughout the entire "goiter" the safest and best surgical treatment is to ligate first the two inferior thyroid arteries and later the superior vessels.

5. The convalescence after any surgical intervention may require weeks or months of treatment with adrenal feeding and iodin to support the "check" upon the thyroid, or with thyroid feeding in the form of some "nontoxic" thyroid derivative to correct the primary hypothyroidism and to prevent its relapse into the secondary hyper disturbance.

* The thyroid and adrenal preparations mentioned above were originally made and tested in the Department of Experimental Therapeutics, Cornell Univ. Med. College. They can now be obtained from Schieffelin & Co.

THE INFLUENCE OF OLIGURIA ON NITROGEN RETENTION IN THE BLOOD.*

By O. H. Perry Pepper, M.D.,
PHILADELPHIA.

The influence which a marked reduction in the quantity of urine may have on the excretion of nitrogen, and so indirectly on the level of nitrogen in the blood, does not seem to receive adequate recognition. The principle is well known, but it has not been sufficiently applied, and certain points which it seems to make clear have therefore been left in confusion and uncertainty. It is in the problems of nephritis that these principles find their most important application.

In acute nephritis, for example, there is often a decrease in urinary output, a failure to excrete sodium chlorid and a moderate rise in the level of the various fractions of the noncoagulable protein of the blood. In such cases it is frequently assumed that there is impairment of the urea-excreting function of the kidney, as well as interference with the elimination of water and salt. Some even dignify these cases with the name "mixed nephritis." When the evidence is examined, however, one cannot help being impressed by the fact that the nitrogen retention may in some instances be the result solely, or in large part, of the interference with water elimination and that the urea-excreting function of the kidney may be entirely unimpaired. If this view is accepted, a number of apparently contradictory observations become barmonized. Let me review certain of the facts touching on this matter and let me employ urea as representative of the group forming the noncoagulable protein of the blood.

It is the function of the kidneys to maintain the normal composition of the blood and under normal conditions normal kidneys accomplish this result. Under abnormal conditions, however, even normal kidneys may not be able to perform this task and may fail to keep pace with the demands made upon them. For example, an unusual formation of urea may temporarily exceed the kidneys' excreting capacity, and an increase in the blood urea nitrogen will occur. Such an unusual increase in urea content may result from a variety of causes, such as excessive protein diet, rapid destruction of body protein as perhaps in certain acute infections and intoxications, experimental introduction of urea, etc. It is obviously a fallacy to assume, on the basis of such an increased blood urea nitrogen that there is any insufficiency of renal functional capacity. Other evidence is required. Furthermore, the

* Read before the Section on Medicine of the College of Physicians of Philadelphia, March 27, 1922.

blood urea nitrogen may increase simply from rapid concentration of the blood, as when water is lost to the body so rapidly that the concentration of urea nitrogen in the blood rises despite the activities of normal kidneys. This may occur, for example, from diarrhea, sweating or even from diuresis of urine of low concentration.

Even the normal kidney has a limit to the amount of solids which it can excrete in a given amount of urine, and for urea in the human this maximal concentration is put down by Ambard[1] at 5.6 per cent. This high figure, however, was only obtained after feeding large amounts of milk casein and permitting but little water intake. MacLeod,[2] alone, apparently puts it at a higher figure, but it is possible his statement is made in reference to the urine of dogs. Cushny[3] says, "These limits of concentration appear to be fixed by the energy which the kidney can bring to act against the osmotic resistance." He gives the upper limit of urea concentration in human urine at from 4 to 5 per cent. Up to this limit, which, however, is seldom reached, the rate of urea excretion per unit of body weight has been shown by Austin, Stillman and Van Slyke[4] to increase in the normal approximately in a simple direct proportion to the blood urea concentration, and secondly, in proportion to the square root of the rate of volume output of urine per unit of body weight as long as the volume rate remains within ordinary limits. There is apparently a limit above which a rise in the urine volume to any height fails to further accelerate urea excretion. Also, there may be a limit above which a rise in the blood urea concentration will fail to increase excretion. So it is clear that the rate of excretion of urea is limited by the kidneys' concentration ability, which is often reduced in disease of the kidney, and by the amount of urine excreted, which is markedly reduced in still other types of renal disease.

Ambard logically points out that if the concentration maximum is known, the least amount of urine required to permit the excretion of any stated amount of urea is also known. This he terms the "volume obligatoire." Thus, for example, if the level of urea production remains at about its usual level of 30 gm. per day the least amount of urine in which normal kidneys could excrete this would be about 500 cc.

When we turn to the consideration of nitrogenous retention in the blood in kidney diseases we find at once that the various factors which may play a part in bringing about an increase of blood urea nitrogen are not clearly differentiated in most writings of today,

[1] Physiologie Normale et Pathologique des Reins, 2d edition, Masson & Cie, Paris, 1920.

[2] Physiology and Biochemistry in Modern Medicine, 3d edition, St. Louis, Mosby, 1920.

[3] Secretion of Urine, London, Longmans, 1917.

[4] Jour. Biol. Chem., 1921, **46**, 91.

nor is sufficient weight placed on the reduction in the quantity of urinary output.

In acute or chronic nephritis with edema there is quite constantly a diminution of the amount of urine—perhaps due to factors leading to a retention of water in the tissues or to a failure of the kidney to secrete the water. Such urine as is passed is high colored, concentrated and shows a high specific gravity and usually a high concentration of urea and other substances. If there is complete anuria then all of the water, urea and other substances which do not leave the body by other routes must remain in the body. If the oliguria is sufficiently marked as to make it impossible for the kidney to concentrate into it all the urea presented to the organ for excretion, then the excess urea must either be retained or otherwise disposed of. Thus an increase of blood urea nitrogen will occur with perhaps no impairment of the kidneys' ability to concentrate, and resulting simply from a diminished output of water which may have its fundamental cause in tissue retention.

This aspect of the production of nitrogen retention was emphasized by French writers—Legueu, Chabanier, Widal, Weill, Ambard and others—in the literature just before the war. They recognized two types of nitrogen retention: The first with a less than maximal concentration of urea in the urine; the second not dependent on interference with the excretion of urea, but partially, at least, due to the output of an insufficient amount of urine. There has been little application of these principles to actual conditions.

Thus, for example, the kidneys normally excrete urea at a concentration of about 2 per cent, and various workers in this field, including MacLean and deWesselow[5] and Weiss,[6] consider a concentration of 2 per cent as indicative of a fairly efficient urea excreting function of the kidney. At a concentration of 2 per cent the average daily output of urea is excreted in about 1500 cc of urine in the twenty-four hours. Now if for any reason the urinary quantity is reduced to less than a third while the urea production remains at its former level, then the kidney, no matter how normal, must fail to excrete the whole amount of urea even if a concentration approaching the maximum of 5.6 per cent is reached. It is apparent, therefore, that the oliguria of acute nephritis must of itself sometimes lead to a failure of urea excretion, due simply to the urinary quantity being inadequate to carry off the amount of urea produced. This would be true even if the urea production were no greater than usual; but there is reason to believe that it may be considerably increased in many instances coincident with the onset of the acute nephritis.

With a failure of excretion some retention occurs, and that this is usually not more evident may, in part, be due to its gradual

[5] British Jour. Exper. Path., 1920, **1**, 1.
[6] Jour. Am. Med. Assn., 1921, **76**, 298.

development and to the dilution of the blood by retained fluid, and there may occur even at low levels some compensatory elimination of urea by bowel.

Undoubtedly in many cases even of acute nephritis there is some direct interference with nitrogen excretion, but in many instances the degree of retention which occurs can be explained simply on the disturbed water secretion. Some of the so-called mixed cases, supposedly exhibiting evidences of interference with both water and nitrogen elimination, can be explained on this evidence and properly classed among those showing simply interference with water elimination.

In experimental nephritis in animals the occurrence of an increase in the blood nitrogen in instances with supposedly purely tubular lesions has led to some confusion, for the nitrogen retention should perhaps be explained, at least in part, on the oliguria alone and in part by the increased protein breakdown due to the toxic agent employed. For example, MacNider[7] employs uranium nitrate and considers that it produces in the dog's kidney an acute tubular lesion without degeneration in the vascular tissue. When such an acute tubular injury is produced in a dog whose kidney already shows a naturally developed glomerulonephropathy with histologically well-preserved tubular epithelium, the acute injury is expressed by a rapid reduction in the elimination of phenolsulphonephthalein and by a retention of blood urea and creatinin. These animals become acutely anuric and die, and the kidneys show an early edema and necrosis of the tubular epithelium without the development of any acute injury to the glomeruli. From these experiments MacNider concludes that the inference appears allowable, that all of these substances, phenolsulphonephthalein, urea and creatinin, are eliminated by the renal epithelium, and he concludes that this and other evidence tends to minimize the importance of the glomerulus as a functional unit and to emphasize the relative importance of the tubular epithelium.

However, in the four protocols given by MacNider to illustrate the experiments in which naturally nephropathic animals were given an acute kidney injury from uranium or mercuric chlorid an abrupt cut-down in urine output dates from the administration of the nephrotoxic agent, and in the absence of figures giving the urea concentration in the urine it is difficult to say whether these protocols indicate any true impairment of the urea-excreting function of the kidney or whether they simply show the results of the diminished output of urine. It must, however, be remembered that the dog is said to be able to concentrate the urea in the urine to over 10 per cent. Further investigations along these lines are greatly needed.

[7] Arch. Int. Med., 1920, **26**, 1.

On the other hand, that the concentration ability of the kidney for urea may be well preserved in acute nephritis is well evidenced by the figures given in a recent article by Rabinowitch[8] concerning the urea concentration test. He gives his results in 50 cases, of which 6 are put down as having had acute nephritis. Of these 6 cases, 1 concentrated urea in the urine to 4.04 per cent, 1 to 3 per cent and 2 to 2.79 per cent, while of the remaining 44 cases of chronic nephritis only 3 showed a concentration of 3 per cent or over. The total amount of urine for the twenty-four hours is not given, so it is impossible to judge whether any increase in blood urea nitrogen might be attributed to the oliguria.

This aspect of the matter also touches upon the question of the interpretation of functional tests. For instance, there are certain cases in which, with some nitrogen retention, the phthalein elimination remains high. This may in part be explained by the greater concentration ability of the kidney for the dye, so that while a kidney may be able to excrete a normal percentage of phthalein in a very small amount of urine, the rate and volume of urine in the twenty-four hours will be too low for the kidney to secrete all the day's urea. Furthermore, in the so-called urea concentration test the amount of urine passed must be sufficient for the excretion of the urea administered before any conclusions concerning the functional efficiency of the kidneys can be drawn from any rise in the blood urea nitrogen. And it is to be remembered that fluids are stopped for six to twelve hours before the test. The same applies to the use of any "formula" or index based upon the excretion of urea. For example, Weiss points out that in certain cases of mixed chronic nephritis (nitrogen and salt and water retention) the test, in spite of distinct clinical and functional evidences of nephritis, at times fails to demonstrate the degree of renal inefficiency which he assumes is present. He does not, however, discuss the possibility that there may, in fact, be little or no interference with urea excretion and that the retention of nitrogen is due to a simple oliguria, although in one case of chronic parenchymatous nephritis with 29 mg. of blood urea nitrogen, there was a urea concentration of 4.2 per cent in the urine. The total daily output of urine is not given, so that no conclusions can be drawn. Nor in the earlier work on the urea concentration test by Addis and Watanabe[9] and MacLean and de Wesselow[10] are figures given which apply to the question in hand.

Prognostically there is, it would seem, a considerable difference in the significance of the two types of nitrogen retention. As a rule a true impairment of the concentration power of the kidney is a serious and permanent thing, while, as is well known, those cases of nephritis with no other manifestation than edema often recover with little or no residual renal damage. If it is true that there are

[8] Arch. Int. Med., 1921, **28**, 827.
[9] Jour. Biol. Chem., 1916, **28**, 251.
[10] Loc. cit.

cases of acute or subacute nephritis in which the nitrogen retention is only a secondary manifestation of the water retention, then these cases should have a better prognosis than those with the other type of nitrogen retention.

In the treatment of nephritis an appreciation of these principles is important, for they supply a basis for understanding what can be expected of the kidneys in a given condition. They emphasize the importance of maintaining polyuria when the concentration ability is diminished and of decreasing, if possible, the urea production to an amount which the concentration maximum and the amount of urine, indicate that the patient can dispose of. We can do little or nothing therapeutically toward raising the concentration ability of the kidneys, but we can, by avoiding passive congestion and body dehydration, make sure that the kidneys shall have every opportunity to excrete water; and by reducing the protein of the diet and by avoiding tissue destruction as far as possible, we can lower the demands placed upon the nitrogen-excreting function of the kidney and so avoid one factor which undoubtedly favors nitrogen retention in the body.

PERSISTENT LEUKOCYTOSIS IN THE EARLY STAGES OF THROMBOANGIITIS OBLITERANS.

By Henry M. Thomas, Jr., M.D.,
BALTIMORE, MD.

The thorough clinical and pathologic studies of thromboangiitis obliterans made by Leo Buerger during the past fifteen years leave no doubt of the fact that such a separate and distinct disease entity exists. Occurring, as he has pointed out, in young male Jews, it affects usually the lower extremities, but not uncommonly also the upper, starts as an inflammation of the walls of the smaller arteries and veins and subjacent tissues and more or less slowly leads to thrombosis of the larger arteries. It gives rise to a clinical syndrome that is, as a rule, definitely characteristic.

Commenting upon the symptomatology of the disease, Buerger says: "Severe nonlocalizable shooting pains in the calf or foot, attended with difficulty in walking, or possibly with tender calf muscles with or without vasomotor symptoms, and coldness in the foot with or without obliteration of the dorsalis pedis and posterior tibial pulses, may be the only symptoms. It is only when we compare the history with its further clinical course and pathology, that we can relegate certain indefinite signs to the onset of the affection. In most instances, however, the patient will not seek advice for such initial symptoms, either because they are not sufficiently severe to require the attention of a physician or because they are incorrectly regarded as rheumatic in origin, possibly due to trauma, to cold, the presence of flat or weak feet, or because they are explained on the basis of some other minor ailment."

Recently a patient, a Jewish physician, consulted Dr. Llewellys F. Barker, stating that he had suffered from intermittent pains in the legs on exertion, which he could convince himself were symptoms of the "physician's usual neurasthenia," were it not for the simultaneous presence of a persistent leukocytosis. He requested that a general diagnostic survey be made in the hope that somewhere in the body something might be found that would explain the pains in the lower extremities and the continued leukocytosis. The case has so many points of interest that at the suggestion of Dr. Barker I have compared it with other similar cases in the records of the Johns Hopkins Hospital, and have decided that, owing especially to the persistent leukocytosis, it should be placed on record in the literature.

Case History. Married man, aged forty-four years, white, a Jewish physician.

Complaint. Aching and pain in the hips and thighs increasing to disability on walking; continuous numbness of the left foot.

Family History. Father died, aged sixty-three years, of angina pectoris; mother died, aged sixty-three years, from apoplexy during diabetes; one brother died at forty-five years from Bright's disease; three brothers and five sisters living and well. Wife has congenital heart disease; two children living and well; no miscarriages. No history of tuberculosis, of mental disease or of cancer in the family.

Past History. He has always been well, except for a fracture of two ribs (followed by a pleuritis) in 1909, until the present illness. Habits: tea used in moderation; no alcohol; fifteen to twenty cigarettes a day for many years.

Present Illness. The patient regarded himself as healthy until August, 1918, when after eating heartily at a barbecue, where he had also one drink of "white lightning," he awoke at 3 a.m. with an excruciating pain and a sense of constriction in his lower chest. His brother-in-law said that in this attack his face was black, and a physician who saw him reported that "from the neck up he looked like a man with apoplexy." He was given morphin twice, three-quarters of a grain in all. The physician diagnosed his condition as "angina pectoris." After remaining in bed for ten days, during which he had slight fever (100° to 101°) and tachycardia (pulse 110 to 120), the pain gradually subsided. A little later he consulted Dr. Evan Evans, who had an electrocardiographic tracing made which showed auricular fibrillation. Dr. Evans also stated that there were evidences of sequelæ of influenza in the left lung, confirmed by roentgen ray. A dull ache in the lower chest persisted, as did neuralgic pains in the left shoulder and arm.

In April, 1921, owing to a sudden illness of his wife, our patient made a hurried railroad trip to visit her, and after a day or two began to have severe pains in his hips and legs after exertion. In four or five days these pains became so severe that he could not get about except in a taxicab.

On returning to his home and resting his condition improved somewhat, but in less than a week the symptoms underwent exacerbation. He could not walk to the office, one block away, without stopping two or three times to rest. As he walked the "ache" grew more and more intense, rising finally to "real pain." He could not move the thighs, but was forced to "swing his trunk"; soon he felt that he must stop and sit down or he would fall down. As a matter of fact he admits that he has never fallen.

At about this time a blood examination was made and the white cell count found to be 22,000 per cmm. Some abscessed teeth were discovered and removed; later on the tonsils were found to be badly infected, and they were removed on July 9, 1921. After this the pains in his shoulder and arm entirely disappeared, but the condition in the legs grew steadily worse.

Another white cell count was made in August, 1921, and showed 18,000 leukocytes. Wassermann tests made by two different men were negative.

Three days before reaching Baltimore the patient, after riding three hours in an automobile, on trying to walk was forced to sit down with his legs straightened out before him no less than three times in the course of four blocks. The pain was, he stated, excruciating. In walking two blocks from the hotel to Dr. Barker's office on the day of consultation he was obliged to stop now and then and lean against buildings. When he is quiet he feels perfectly well. He has tried to make himself think that his symptoms are all due to nervousness, but the persistent leukocytosis and the severe pains convince him that there must be something radically wrong with him. Libido has been much lessened during the past year and potentia has been poor, though ejaculatio has been normal.

Physical Examination. On November 2, 1921 (Dr. Norman B. Cole). Patient is a man, aged forty-four years, lying quietly, without dyspnea. He is ten pounds under his calculated ideal weight. Skin normal. Muscular development and tone fair. Moderate canities, beginning calvities. Contour of the face normal. Eyes protrude slightly. There is a moderate Dalrymple sign, a slight von Graefe, a negative Rosenbach. Convergence well maintained. Pupils equal and regular, reacting equally and promptly to light. Slight hippus. Scleræ moderately injected. Nasal ventilation normal. Dental occlusion largely maintained by dentures (superior and inferior); considerable retraction of the gums; recently treated for pyorrhea. The tongue is protruded in the midline without tremor; it is moist and with a slight yellowish-white coat. The right tonsillar fossa is empty and the left shows a small tag of tonsil. Pharynx negative. External ears and canals negative. No tenderness over paranasal sinuses or mastoids. No struma. No general glandular enlargement.

Chest well formed. Expansion good and symmetric. Lungs negative except for a few moist rales in the lower left back. Left border of cardiac dulness just lateral from the nipple line in the fifth left interspace on direct percussion. Apex beat feebly palpable in the same locality. Heart rate 96, regular; no heart murmurs; second aorta sound slightly louder than second pulmonic. Blood-pressure: 122 systolic and 78 diastolic. No tremor of the outstretched fingers. Palms dry and warm. Radial pulsations equal and synchronous; radial walls not palpable; brachials not visible; temporals not tortuous. Just in front of the medial condyle of the right elbow a small gland is palpable, due to an earlier infection of the hand.

Abdomen normal in contour; no tenderness; no abnormal masses; no muscle spasm. Liver and spleen not palpable. Hirci and crines pubis rather sparse. Crines of the transverse type. Phallus and gonads normal.

No edema of the shins. Knee-jerks equal and active. Ankle-jerks are equal. Babinski, Gordon and Oppenheim tests negative. No bathyanesthesia. Cremasteric and abdominal reflexes normal. Deep reflexes in arms normal. Chvostek sign negative.

Slight external hemorrhoids present. Tone of rectal sphincter normal. Prostate normal.

No pulsation can be felt in the A. dorsalis pedis, the A. tibialis posterior or in the A. femoralis on either side.

Laboratory Findings (Dr. H. M. Thomas, Jr.). The blood, the stomach contents, the feces and the urine were examined.

Blood Examination. Red blood cells, 5,080,000; hemoglobin, 85 per cent, Sahli; white blood cells, 17,300; color index, 0.85.

Differential count in a stained smear of the white corpuscles showed polymorphonuclears, 59.5 per cent; eosinophils, 1.5 per cent; basophils, 0.5 per cent; small mononuclears, 30.5 per cent; large mononuclears, 3 per cent; transitionals, 4 per cent; basophilic myelocytes, 1 per cent.

No poikilocytosis nor anisocytosis of the red cells. Platelets normal. Blood-Wassermann reaction negative.

Analysis of the Stomach Contents. 40 cc recovered; free HCl 28 acidity per cent, combined acid 38 acidity per cent; total acid 66 acidity per cent. Microscopically, no yeast cells. Neither Oppler-Boas bacilli nor sarcinæ present.

Stool Examination. Dark brown, formed; occult blood, negative; microscopically, an occasional striated muscle fiber seen. No ova or parasites seen.

Examination of the Urine. Reaction acid; specific gravity, 1002 to 1025; no albumin; no sugar; no Bence-Jones body. Microscopically, negative for casts and red blood cells. A few calcium oxalate crystals seen, also numerous shreds of mucus. Phenolsulphonephthalein test: output in two hours, 67 per cent.

Roentgen-ray Reports (Dr. F. H. Baetjer):

Paranasal Sinuses. Frontals, ethmoids and antra clear.

Lateral Skull. Sella of normal size and shape and of the open type. Frontal and sphenoidal sinuses clear. Calvarium negative.

Lumbar Spine. Shows a little sharpening, especially of the upper edge of the third lumbar vertebra, and there are slight spurs on the crests of the ilia.

Impression (Dr. Baetjer): Spine and scaroiliacs practically negative.

Roentgenoscopic Report of Chest and Abdomen. Heart of normal size; slightly globular in shape. Pulsations normal. Aorta not dilated. Lungs not remarkable. Diaphragm smooth. Swallowing normal. Maximal degree of visceral ptosis and hyperactive gastro-intestinal tract.

Orthopedic Report (Dr. George E. Bennett). Impression: We are at a loss to give an explanation of the patient's symptoms from a bone or joint standpoint. There is some evidence, however, of shortening of the hamstring tendons, but we believe that these changes are secondary to some general systemic disturbance. The back gives one the impression that there may possibly be an anomaly of the fifth lumbar, but this is not definite.

Laryngologic Report (Dr. Harry R. Slack, Jr.). Impression: there is no focus of infection in the nose, throat or ears to account for an arthritis.

Neurologic Report (Dr. H. M. Thomas, Jr). The patient appears to have had an arthritis in his shoulder, which was relieved by having an abscessed tooth and the infected tonsils removed; but since then this curious disability in his legs has become worse. The history sounds like that of an intermittent claudication, but I do not remember having seen a case in which the pain and cramp were in the thighs and not at all in the muscles below the knees. He has a contraction of the hamstring muscles, and their consistency seems to me to be unusually firm. No other neurologic findings were important. The circulation in the legs is certainly disturbed, and I must acknowledge that I could not feel the pulses at the ankles, or, indeed, in the femoral arteries, though perhaps careful search on repeated examination may reveal them.

Psychiatric Report (Dr. John R. Oliver). Normal findings.

Dental Report (Dr. H. H. Streett). Partial upper and lower dentures. Nonsuppurative pyorrhea with absorption of alveolar crests and damage to central tissues. Radiographs negative. Find nothing to indicate a focal factor.

Basal Metabolism Estimation (Dr. J. T. King, Jr.). The CO_2 output is 3.5 per cent below the expected for the patient's age and sex, indicating a normal metabolic rate. Resting pulse varied from 80 to 88, and the patient took the test comfortably.

Electrocardiographic Report (Dr. E. W. Bridgman). Impression: normal cardiac mechanism. Inverted *T*-waves in the first two leads. The inversion of the *T*-wave in leads I and II suggests either that there is a myocardial weakness or that there has already been administered a physiologic dosage of digitalis.

Polygraphic Tracings (Dr. Norman B. Cole). Jugular vein and brachial artery yield normal curves.

Diagnosis. 1. Thromboangeitis obliterans with intermittent claudication.

2. Persistent leukocytosis with relative lymphocyte increase.

3. Slight myocardiopathy with history of auricular fibrillation, but none now. Slight changes in electrocardiogram.

4. Slight thyreopathy with eye signs and slight tachycardia, but normal basal metabolic rate.

5. Slight undernutrition (ten pounds), with visceroptosis, slight gastric hyperacidity and hypermotility of the gastrointestinal tract.

6. Nonsuppurative gingivitis.

7. Chronic tabagism.

Subsequent History. On November 7, 1921, the patient was admitted to Johns Hopkins Hospital for further observation. While there his white blood count was 19,400 on Nov. 8, 1921, and on one occasion the left posterior tibial artery was felt to pulsate.

As the patient was to spend a few days in New York, he was advised to see Dr. Leo Buerger and Dr. Emanuel Libman while there. In a letter to Dr. Barker, Dr. Libman reported as follows: "My opinion is the same as yours, namely, that he is suffering from a thromboangiitic disease of the veins and arteries. I am not sure that the case belongs to exactly the same group as that which Buerger describes. In other words, I am not sure that a microscopic examination of fresh lesions would show the typical miliary foci with giant cells which Buerger considers characteristic of the early lesions of the disease which he investigated. It would be interesting to know whether the chest attack, which he had some time before the pains in the lower extremities began, was due to an embolus in the distribution of the pulmonary artery.

"The leukocytosis is interesting. I have not particularly noted it as occurring in cases of Buerger's disease. I have discussed this question with Dr. Buerger, and he tells me that he has made no definite studies concerning the leukocyte count in the disease."

A letter from the patient dated January 1, 1922, states that on restriction of his physical activities, cutting off tobacco and performing circulatory gymnastics outlined for him he has been doing very satisfactorily. The leukocytosis persists; a blood count made soon after arriving home at the end of November showed 18,300 white blood cells; another made on December 31, 1921, showed 14,700.

Discussion. The case is, it is believed, one of thromboangiitic disease of the arteries and veins supplying both lower extremities. The patient is a full-blooded Jew, born in the United States; his parents were citizens of Austria-Hungary. He has smoked cigarettes to excess for many years. After a sudden attack, in 1918, of auricular fibrillation (which subsided) he was well until April, 1921, when he first became troubled with severe pains in the lower extremities on walking. It was then found that he had a white blood count of 22,000. The pain in the legs and numbness of the left foot increased during the next seven months and the leukocytosis persisted. The rather widespread distribution of the vascular disorder with a comparatively low grade of cyanosis without rapid blanching on change of position of the leg left us in doubt as to the exact diagnosis. There was evidently obstruction to the arterial flow in the vessels of both lower extremities. Whether this is or is not due to true thromboangiitis obliterans the subsequent course of the disease alone can decide, though we think it probable.

Arterial thrombosis not associated with any acute infection, not associated with any wasting disease and not secondary to syphilis or arteriosclerosis has led for many years to much speculation as to the factors concerned in its etiology. Mendel called attention to the susceptibility to a second attack of thrombosis and termed the condition "thrombophilia." Before him Erb had pointed out the susceptibility of young male Jews to dysbasia angiosclerotica (or intermittent claudication), and mentioned alcohol and tobacco as contributory factors. More recently the careful and complete studies of Leo Buerger have established the fact that there exists an infectious disease of unknown etiology which produces inflammatory lesions of the vessel walls and perivascular tissues, and subsequently leads to thrombosis with gradual involvement of the larger vessels. There are still many writers who dispute the infectious nature of this process, whereas others claim that typhus fever is a constant precursor.

As Buerger has pointed out, the disease is rarely seen by the physician until its later stages, since only in them, as a rule, are the symptoms of a nature severe enough to lead the patient to consult a doctor. In the case here recorded the patient, a doctor himself, was soon impressed by the persistent leukocytosis and proceeded on an exhaustive but unsuccessful search for a causative focus of infection. It seems now fairly clear that the infectious process in Buerger's disease is located in the vessels supplying the extremities; and it seems altogether likely, from the study of the case here reported, that if an opportunity were afforded for study of the leukocyte count early in cases of thromboangiitis obliterans a persistent leukocytosis would be revealed.

In 2 of the other 5 cases studied at the Johns Hopkins Hospital a positive Wassermann reaction was obtained, and in 1 the disease had already existed several years. The fourth case had been affected long enough to produce gangrene of a toe, although subjective symptoms were noted only five months before admission to the hospital. The absence of a leukocytosis in these atypical or long-standing cases is not, therefore, to be considered as evidence on this point.

Conclusion. A case is reported of thromboangiitis of the vessels supplying the legs, similar in many respects to Buerger's disease, and the existence in the patient of a well-marked and persistent leukocytosis is emphasized. It would seem probable that a leukocytosis may be found to occur frequently in the early stages of thromboangeitis obliterans; if this be verified the fact would lend weight to Buerger's contention that the process is infectious in nature.

REFERENCES.

1. Buerger, L.: Thromboangiitis Obliterans: a Study of the Vascular Lesions Leading to Presenile Spontaneous Gangrene, Am. Jour. Med. Sci., 1908, **136**, 567.
2. Mendel, F.: Ueber "Thrombophile" und das Frühaufstehen der Wochnerinnen und Laparotomierten, München. med. Wchnschr., 1909, **56**, 2149.
3. Erb, W.: Ueber Bedeutung und praktischen Wert der Prüfung der Fussarterien bei gewissen, anscheinend nervösen Erkrankungen, Mitt. a. d. Grenzgeb. d. Med. u. Chir., Jena, 1899, **4**, 505.
4. Erb, W.: Ueber Dysbasia angiosclerotica (intermittierendes Hinken), München. med. Wchnschr., 1904, **51**, 905.
5. Erb, W.: Zum Kapitel der angiosklerotischen Störungen der unteren Extremitäten (intermittierendes Hinken, etc.), Deutsch. med. Wchnschr., 1906, **32**, 1895.
6. Buerger, L.: The Pathology of the Vessels in Cases of Gangrene of the Lower Extremities Due to So-called Endarteritis Obliterans, Proc. New York Path. Soc., 1908–9, n. s., **8**, 48.
7. Buerger, L.: The Veins in Thromboangiitis Obliterans with Particular Reference to Arteriovenous Anastomoses as a Cure for the Condition, Jour. Am. Med. Assn., Chicago, 1909, **52**, 1319.
8. Buerger, L.: Is Thromboangiitis Obliterans Related to Raynaud's Disease and Erythromelalgia? Am. Jour. Med. Sci., 1910, **139**, 105.
9. Buerger, L.: Cases of Thromboangiitis Obliterans, Med. Record, New York, 1914, **86**, 860.
10. Buerger, L.: Recent Studies in Thromboangiitis Obliterans, Proc. New York Path. Soc., 1914, **14**, 108.
11. Buerger, L.: Is Thromboangiitis Obliterans an Infectious Disease? Surg., Gynec. and Obst., 1914, **19**, 582.
12. Buerger, L.: Recent Studies in the Pathology of Thromboangiitis Obliterans, Jour. Med. Research, 1914–15, **31**, 181, 5 pl.
13. Buerger, L.: Concerning Vasomotor and Trophic Disturbances of the Upper Extremities, with Particular Reference to Thromboangiitis Obliterans, Am. Jour. Med. Sci., 1915, **149**, 210.

14. Buerger, L.: The Pathological and Clinical Aspects of Thromboangiitis Obliterans, Tr. Coll. Phys., Philadelphia, 1916, 3 s., **38**, 214.
15. Buerger, L.: The Pathological and Clinical Aspects of Thromboangiitis Obliterans, Am. Jour. Med. Sci., 1917, **154**, 319.
16. Buerger, L.: Pathology of Thromboangiitis Obliterans, Med. Record, 1920, **97**, 431.
17. Meyer, W.: Thromboangiitis, Med. Record, 1917, **92**, 262.
18. Meyer, W.: Etiology of Thromboangiitis Obliterans (Buerger), Jour. Am. Med. Assn., 1918, **51**, 1268.
19. Meyer, W.: Further Contribution to the Etiology of Thromboangiitis Obliterans, Med. Record, 1920, **97**, 425.
20. Goodman, C.: Thromboangiitis, Med. Record, 1917, **92**, 261. Presenile Gangrene: Thromboangiitis Obliterans: Further Confirmation of its Relation to Typhus Fever, Ibid., p. 275.

INJURY OF THE SPINAL CORD IN BREECH EXTRACTION AS AN IMPORTANT CAUSE OF FETAL DEATH AND OF PARAPLEGIA IN CHILDHOOD.*

By Bronson Crothers, M.D.

NEUROLOGIST TO CHILDREN'S HOSPITAL, BOSTON; ASSISTANT IN NEUROLOGY, AND IN PEDIATRICS HARVARD MEDICAL SCHOOL, BOSTON, MASS.

I. **Introduction.** Injuries of the spinal cord, or of the vertebral column, due to breech extraction, are frequently discovered by pathologists. On the other hand, such injuries are rarely reported by obstetricians, and disability from such accidents is rarely recognized by those who see older children.

The obvious inference is that serious damage to the spinal cord during delivery is inconsistent with prolonged life.

From a theoretic standpoint any such conclusion is most surprising for several reasons. In the laboratory young animals survive cord transection with great regularity and for indefinite periods, and on the whole show less evidence of shock than adults of the same species.

Babies frequently survive the severe operations necessitated by spina bifida and often live for long periods, even if the operation involves destruction of a considerable portion of the cord.

Many soldiers lived for indefinite periods after receiving wounds which, in addition to severing the cord, injured the lung.

It seems as if some peculiarly fatal factor must be involved if the general impression that obstetric cord injury is inconsistent with prolonged life is well founded, yet it is hard to see what it can be.

One of the most obvious explanations is that the injury to the cord is always high enough to involve the medulla or the phrenic nerves. This theory is untenable, because there is considerable reliable pathologic and clinical evidence against it.

* Read in abstract before the December, 1921, Meeting of the New England Pediatric Society.

It is also conceivable that trauma to the cord is always accompanied by such severe injury to the spine and muscles that babies almost inevitably perish from traumatic shock. A very casual study of the spinal column at birth suggests that this is an unlikely explanation, as the infantile vertebræ have no such elaborate interlocking bony processes as those seen in adult spinal columns. Furthermore, there is good reason to believe that babies, during a period of several years, can suffer severe cord injuries without serious shock or gross damage to the spine.

If no adequate reasons exists for believing that all babies with traumatic cord lesions die early, and if such injuries can be shown to be common, it is reasonable to suppose that some of them survive and are not properly classified.

These theoretic considerations are of absolutely no interest unless it can be proved that a fair number of such cases are now living with definite signs which can be logically referred to accidents during breech deliveries.

Before reporting cases it is necessary to review, very briefly, certain papers in order to show the development of the present standards of diagnosis of severe cord injuries and to consider a few studies of obstetric traumata.

II. **Bastian's Law.** Up to 1890, as Riddoch points out, clinicians were observing with interest and understanding the spectacular experiments of physiologists on "spinal" animals. Very generally they accepted the obvious conclusion that reflex activity might be expected below the level of a cord transection in man. In that year Bastian, apparently exasperated by the tendency to draw conclusions from the study of laboratory animals and to apply these conclusions to man, collected a number of cases and overwhelmed the clinicians who were influenced by laboratory results. His observations, more or less misinterpreted and misquoted, led to very general acceptance of the theory that reflex activity was practically negligible below the level of cord transection in man. Even Sherrington apparently accepted this point of view.

This polemic paper of Bastian's, destined to exert a profound influence on neurologic progress for a quarter of a century, begins with the following statement:

"The physiologist, by reason of his observation on certain of the lower animals, seems to have instilled into the minds of clinical observers the notion that when the spinal cord is absolutely cut off from communication with the encephalon the reflexes dependent on the spinal cord below the point of section will, in the course of a very short time—that is, as soon as the immediate effects of shock resulting from the operation have subsided—exhibit themselves in an exaggerated manner."

He follows this belligerent opening with reports of cases of cord transection, most of whom died within a few days or dragged out prolonged existences made miserable by bed-sores or cancer. There is no reason to doubt the accuracy of Bastian's observations, though the following extracts from his case records show his state of mind and incidentally reinforce the present standards of diagnosis.

Among the records is one from a colleague. The patient "died of exhaustion in connection with bed-sores and bladder troubles." The record shows that although knee-jerks had been absent and anesthesia present for a month, "involuntary contractions of the legs, causing them to be completely flexed,. are more marked—they move at the least irritation of the skin." In another case, where a fracture-dislocation at the sixth cervical vertebra caused the lesion, the report by Tooth shows that on the twentieth day sole reflexes were present and a feeble knee-jerk was obtained. Postmortem examination proved the lesion to be a practically complete transection. In regard to this case Bastian observes: "This is not a very conclusive case, I merely quote it for what it is worth, it at least suffices to show that there was no exaggeration of reflexes."

Largely as a result of this paper, supported by another by Bowlby in the same year, clinicians for twenty-seven years have taught that cord lesions in man did not allow reflex activity at all comparable with that observed in animals similarly injured. As generally understood, Bastian's law is as follows:

High thoracic or cervical transections produce paralysis of the legs and abdominal muscles and anesthesia and loss of tendon-jerks. The bladder is at first atonic, but later empties itself partially. That is, transections in man cause, essentially, flaccid paralysis and incontinence of urine.

It is clear enough, on careful reading of Bastian's paper, that nothing in the case reports, or in his own conclusions, justifies the statement that permanent flaccidity always follows cord transections in human beings. In fact, there are numerous contradictions to any such assertion. But the tradition was started and, in spite of sporadic protests, it was generally accepted. As a result the diagnosis of cord transection is not made, as a rule, in the presence of reflex activity of the legs.

III. **Study of Cord Transections Due to War Wounds.** The work of Head and Riddoch forces an absolute abandonment of the so-called Bastian's law. These writers were able to study the results of lesions produced cleanly and suddenly in young men, who were at once picked up and cared for under practically ideal scientific conditions. Riddoch states that "any light that has been thrown on the innate functions of the cord is due not only to the unique cases at our disposal but principally to the attitude of mind induced by the monumental work of Sherrington."

The cases thus observed are all entirely convincing, as the degree of damage to the cord was observed at operation or postmortem and the clinical notes were made by accurate observers. Therefore the results may be taken as conclusive. In healthy men cord lesions amounting to high physiologic transections cause the following signs:

First Stage. Muscular flaccidity with toneless skeletal muscles, anesthesia, dry, easily damaged skin and retention of urine and feces.

Second Stage. After a few weeks reflexes appear. At first nocuous stimulation of the soles causes various toe movements. Later a variety of flexor responses can be elicited by stimulation of any part of the leg or lower abdomen. With severe stimulation both legs and recti abdominis share in a vigorous mass reflex, which is accompanied by evacuation of the bladder. The easy elicitation of this mass reflex, accompanied by sweating, from stimulation of the legs or abdomen is characteristic of the stage of reflex activity. Tendon-jerks and other signs of extensor excitability are later signs. The bladder becomes "automatic," emptying itself at definite degrees of pressure without other stimulation, or at lower pressures when the mass reflex is evoked. In adults a definite coitus reflex can be obtained on genital stimulation.

Third Stage. If sepsis of serious importance supervenes, the reflex activity subsides or even disappears and sometimes never returns. Obviously sepsis occurring prior to the second stage may prevent the occurrence of reflex activity of any kind.

Naturally, Bastian, working with cases complicated by sepsis or malignant tumors, saw few evidences of reflex activity. Further he apparently started with distrust of the physiologist deep in his being. Head and Riddoch, profoundly impressed by physiologic data, had an opportunity to work with men whose wounds practically duplicated laboratory lesions. Their results confirm the physiologic workers while explaining the results of Bastian.

IV. **Obstetric Cord Lesions.** Bruns quotes C. Ruge as authority for the statement that injury of the vertebral column was found in 8 out of 64 babies dying during or after breech deliveries. I have not been able to find Ruge's original paper. However, Warwick, who has published reports on a series of autopsies on the newborn, states that all cases of vertebral damage in her series were accompanied by cord laceration, so it seems fair to assume that serious cord injuries may have been present in Ruge's cases. In 136 infants in whom the central nervous system was examined Warwick discovered cord injury in 3. If, as seems probable on clinical grounds, this injury occurs almost exclusively with breech extractions, Warwick's figures show a very high proportion of such injuries, as not over 10 of her cases were likely to have been breech deliveries.* Moreover, as her series is made up of cases

* In a personal communication Warwick states that the three cord injuries occurred in babies delivered by version.

of all sorts, worked up by different people, it is entirely possible that the whole cord was not examined in every case. The fact that all her cases had cervical lesions suggests the same possibility.

The most striking article is one by Stoltzenburg published in 1911. This observer found gross lesions of the spinal column in 9 out of 75 babies dying of asphyxia, 8 followed breech extraction. In other words, over 10 per cent of the "asphyxial" deaths in her series followed injury of the spinal column during breech extraction. The cords showed no gross evidence of laceration.

In one large obstetrical clinic in this country similar findings are common, though published reports are not at present available.

Clinically the evidence is definite enough that paralysis due to cord transection at birth has long been known. In a recent article Kooy reviewed the literature and reported that, except for his own case, he found no record of any child surviving severe cord injury more than six months. His own case lived nine years, with almost complete anesthesia, incontinence of urine and feces and spasticity of the legs. The lesion was attributed to violence incident to a very difficult version and extraction. The pathologic examination showed a low thoracic lesion with one ventral pyramidal tract still intact.

Burr recently reported 2 cases, 1 confirmed by autopsy. Both babies were born by breech extraction and both died within five months. One showed reflex activity on pinprick but no tendon reflexes. The autopsy in this case showed that the cord was a mere fibrous band between the fourth cervical and first thoracic segments. The other child showed anesthesia and flaccid paralysis suggesting a complete cervical transection. No reflexes were obtained.

Beevor reports a baby, born by a difficult breech extraction, who showed paralysis of the muscles of one arm, and of the chest, abdomen and legs. Anesthesia corresponded. At autopsy evidence of fracture-dislocation of the third cervical vertebra was found, and below the level of the lesion, practically complete destruction of the cord, presumably as a result of hemorrhage and fibrous tissue formation.

Friedman, in an analysis of 2000 cases seen in the neurologic service at the Children's Hospital, Boston, found only 1 diagnosed as cord injury due to dystocia. His case showed flaccid paralysis and anesthesia. Again a history of breech extraction was obtained.

From this cursory review of the literature several conclusions can be drawn: In the first place cord lesions, as a consequence of breech extractions, are not infrequent. Second, they are usually recognized only when accompanied by flaccid paralysis and anesthesia—that is, when the clinical picture conforms to the so-called Bastian's law. Third, in the reported cases the babies almost invariably died after a few weeks or, at most, a few months of life. Fourth, in the light of the work of Head and Riddoch it seems entirely likely that such babies will show high degrees of reflex excitability provided the lesion is not high enough to involve the medulla or the phrenic nerves or low enough to destroy the lumbar enlargement. The routine care of a baby provides cleanliness and reasonable freedom from chance infection. Under these favorable circumstances indefinite existence seems quite possible.

CASE REPORTS.

CASE I.—*Obstetric Lesion with Widespread Cord Destruction. No Reflex Activity.* J. B., a male baby, two weeks of age, was seen in the neurological out-patient department in November, 1920.

The mother had had several children without any trouble. This baby was delivered by a thoroughly competent doctor, who referred the case with a note giving the following history: The child presented by the breech. Great difficulty was occasioned by the extension of the right arm. During the manipulation necessary to free this the child became weak and rapid extraction, with considerable force, was necessary. Asphyxia required attention. For the next few days he showed tension at the fontanelle and strabismus, and he had convulsions. These signs cleared up, leaving paralysis as at entrance.

When I first saw him he was in a wretched condition. His skin was dry and he was nursing poorly. His right arm was hanging at his side with inward rotation at the shoulder, extension at the elbow pronation and flexion at the wrist and tight flexion of the fingers. Feeble motions at the wrist and of the fingers were possible. Deviation of the hand to the ulnar side was apparently due to weakness of the supinator longus.

No signs suggested cranial nerve lesions, the pupils were equal and reacted, the fontanelle was level and the left arm appeared normal.

The remainder of the body showed flaccid paralysis of the abdominal muscles and of both legs.

Urine dribbled from the urethra, pressure on the abdomen caused evacuation of the bowels and a free flow of urine. Sensation was as shown in the chart. The black area (on the accompanying chart) was absolutely anesthetic, the shaded area more doubtful, but almost certainly involved.

A tentative diagnosis of hemorrhage into the cord as a result of avulsion of some of the upper roots of the brachial plexus was made. Roentgen-ray study showed no evidence of dislocation or fracture. Lumbar puncture showed cloudy yellow fluid under slight pressure. Unfortunately no manometer was used but the sinking of the fontanelle, as fluid flowed from the needle, apparently ruled out obstruction at the site of injury. Microscopically abundant changed red cells were found.

The question of surgical intervention was considered. The possibility of relieving pressure by laminectomy did not seem worth taking risks for, as lumbar puncture had demonstrated that there was no obstruction to the flow of fluid past the point of injury.

Since entrance to the department the condition of the baby has not improved appreciably. The bladder and rectum became, at six weeks, "automatic." Absolutely no other evidence of reflex activity has occurred in twelve months. The arm is slowly improving with fairly free motion at the fingers, the wrist and the elbow, but inward rotation and pronation persist as in ordinary obstetric paralysis, due to plexus injury. The skin is still dry but intact.

The abdomen and legs show extreme muscle atrophy. Anesthesia is as at entrance.

Comment. The lesion here is obviously one of the cord. Possibly two lesions exist, one of the plexus and one of the cord. The type of arm palsy, with the equal pupils, rather suggests a peripheral origin for the arm paralysis. To me a more logical explanation is that avulsion of some of the cervical roots caused a hematomyelia, which resulted in an almost complete destruction of the lower thoracic and lumbar cord. Such a lesion would explain the striking and persistent flaccidity of the abdomen and legs. Beevor's case, quoted above, showed a quite comparable pathologic and clinical condition.

Treatment is of course purely negative. It is interesting, however, that no catheter was necessary in this or in subsequent cases.

Prognosis is entirely hopeless, as far as I can see.

CASE II.—*Obstetric Transection with Reflex Activity.* F. Y., a girl of three years, was transferred to the neurological department from the clinic of the Harvard Infantile Paralysis Commission, to which she had been referred by her physician.

She was the fourth child. Five years before her birth her mother had infantile paralysis involving one leg. Delivery at eight months was required as a result of nephritis in the mother. A difficult accouchement forcé was done and considerable difficulty was encountered in the version and extraction of the child. For weeks the baby was very ill and was not expected to live from day to day. Gradually she gained strength and seemed to thrive, but has never sat up or attempted to stand. She has never been conscious of movements of the bowels or emptying of the bladder. She has never had any serious acute illness.

When she entered the neurological out-patient department May 9, 1921, the physical examination was as follows:

She was a cheerful, intelligent child, lying comfortably with legs abducted and semiflexed at hips, partly flexed at knees and extended at ankles. The upper extremities and head and chest were normal throughout. The abdomen was moderately distended and the muscles of the abdominal wall were flaccid. No voluntary movements were seen below chest. Development of legs was normal. The skin was clear and moist.

Reflexes were as follows: knee-jerks were difficult to get and when obtained were atypical, as the adductors contracted strongly and the quadriceps only slightly. They were the same on the two sides. Ankle-jerks were very much more lively than the knee-jerks. Attempts to obtain clonus led to curious responses. Occasional typical sustained ankle or patellar clonus was elicited in the usual way. Irritation of the skin over any part of either leg or just above the symphysis led to clonus of the whole lower extremity, sometimes spreading across and involving the opposite side. This manifestation was usually followed on further stimulation by abrupt strong flexion reflexes, including urination.

Stroking or gentle pressure on the sole of the foot caused Babinski's phenomenon and occasionally strong extension suggesting the extensor thrust in laboratory animals. Chaddock's, Gordon's and Oppenheim's reflexes were present.

Definite flushing of the skin on stroking was present, ending sharply at the upper border of anesthesia.

Roentgen rays of the spine were negative.

No important changes have taken place since she was first seen.

Comment. This child shows anesthesia and absence of voluntary motion below the chest, corresponding with the signs to be expected from a severe lesion at the seventh dorsal segment. The flaccid paralysis of the recti abdominis suggests that several segments are almost completely destroyed. The legs show lively reflex activities, chief among which are the flexion reflex as described by Head and Riddoch and extensor phenomena suggesting the extensor thrust of the spinal animal. Vasomotor disturbances and the automatic bladder and rectum conform to the picture of transverse lesions as now understood. The prominent extensor phenomena suggest that the lesion may not be absolutely complete.

Obstetrical injury can be assumed in view of the history of the difficult extraction of a premature baby.

Prognosis as to the restoration of functional communication with the brain seems hopeless. Later on, orthopedic apparatus may possibly be fitted which may make some locomotion possible.

(This child was again seen in May of 1922. At that time there was slight but definite sensation over legs and abdomen. Orthopedic apparatus was fitted and muscle training begun. After a few weeks definite voluntary movements appeared. The child in October walks with apparatus and support though all motions are very slight. However, enough motion and sensation are evident to warrant hope of some functional recovery after four years of anesthesia and paralysis. There is also consciousness of sphincters though no real control has been obtained.)

CASE III.—*Obstetric Transection with Reflex Activities.* E. T., a girl, born February 9, 1919, was seen in February 1921, and repeatedly since then.

She is the only child of healthy parents, born with great difficulty, with forceps to the after-coming head. No asphyxia or convulsions followed. For a few months she was very weak, moved very little and was not expected to live. Then she seemed to thrive, except for the fact that she could not sit alone until over a year old, and has never attempted to stand. According to the mother she controls her rectal sphincter but not her bladder.

When I saw her first she was a very cheerful, active child as far as head, chest and arms went. Below the line shown in the chart she was absolutely a reflex mechanism. Anesthesia was complete. On the left she retained control of the upper segments of the rectus abdominis. The rest of the abdominal wall was flaccid and without reflexes. The back showed marked weakness below the ribs and she tended to slip forward unless supported.

The legs were in semiflexion at hip, knee and ankle. Reflexes were as follows: knee-jerks and ankle-jerks present—not active. No clonus. Babinski and associated phenomena present. Painful stimulation caused active, quick flexion of hip, knee, ankle and toes, with inconstant urination. The receptive field for this reflex extended over both legs and for a short distance above the symphysis. By gentle, steady pressure occasional typical extensor thrusts could be elicited.

In general the muscles showing these reflex activities were not spastic—in fact, they gave the impression of flaccidity when not active. While under observation in the wards the child showed no signs that she was conscious of reflex activities or of urination or defecation, and she was not in any way upset by lumbar puncture, which showed no abnormality of fluid or pressure.

Attempts to measure the activities of the bladder, after the method of Head and Riddoch, failed, as the child urinated at once when the catheter was introduced. Genital manipulation caused an extreme flexion response.

Flushing of the skin below the level of anesthesia was marked. The skin was soft and moist.

The development of the legs was normal. Roentgen rays showed no abnormality of the spine.

Comment. This child shows a picture of reflex activity practically identical with that seen in laboratory animals and one that is quite comparable to that described in man. The lesion is probably due to hemorrhagic softening of the cord over several of the lower thoracic segments, and presumably is the result of manipulations during delivery.

The mother of this child had been assured that the appearance of reflexes meant later control of muscles. Of course, this prognosis is not justified. In fact it is entirely likely that any severe infectious disease will result in loss of activity.

Fitting of orthopedic apparatus may allow a certain amount of activity later.

CASE IV.—*Obstetric Transections with Reflex Activity.* M. P., a boy of thirteen months, was brought to the hospital in May, 1921, because he could not walk or sit up. He has been followed in the out-patient department since entrance.

He was the first child of healthy parents. A friend of the mother, who helped at the delivery, gave the following account of the procedure: The mother was etherized and the doctor started on a breech extraction. Four people held the mother in bed while the operator, with his feet braced against the side of the bed, pulled. Suddenly, he said, "Something broke." Immediately afterward the child was born, apparently dead, but after a few hours, without efforts at resuscitation, he began to cry. For the next week he seemed likely to die at any moment, but gradually began to nurse well. Since then he has done well, except for inability to sit up. No definite bladder or rectal disturbances have been noticed. The legs are said to have shown movement for many months.

Physical examination shows a well-nourished, evenly developed baby, perfectly comfortable, lying with legs extended. The head and arms seem normal and the chest muscles of respiration seem to be acting normally. The abdomen is protuberant. No voluntary motion noticed in the legs.

Sensory examinations shows anesthesia below the nipple line.

No vasomotor changes are obvious. The skin is clear and moist.

The abdominal and lower back muscles are flaccid and without reflexes. The muscles of the legs are relaxed and passive motion shows no evidence of spasticity or contractures. Both legs show definite lowering of muscle tone, and knee-jerks and ankle-jerks cannot be elicited. No ankle-clonus.

Reflex activity occurs as follows: on stroking the foot or lower leg on either side Babinski's phenomenon appears. Nocuous stimulation, as by pinch or pinprick, changes the character of the response abruptly, and the whole flexion reflex, including evacuation of the bladder, is started. On severe stimulation this reflex is shared by the opposite leg. The receptive field of this reflex appears to extend from just above the symphysis to the toes. In addition the crossed extension reflex can be easily elicited at times, that is, flexion of the stimulated leg and extension of the other.

Roentgen rays show no abnormality of the spine.

Comment. As a basis for discussion of the symptoms of transverse lesions this child is most satisfactory. First, there is no question as to the possibility of rupture or other cord lesion resulting from the spectacular method of delivery. Second, the absence of deep reflexes would reconcile Bastian's followers to the diagnosis. Third, the reflex activities show great similarity to those seen in the physiologic laboratory, or in war hospitals where Head and Riddoch did their work.

The lesion is evidently in the lower thoracic region, with its upper border about the fifth segment, extending down, as suggested by the flaccid abdominal wall, to the tenth.

Case V.—*Obstetric Injury to the Cord with Signs of Incomplete Cervical Transection.* E. H., a girl of twelve, seen in consultation with Dr. R. W. Lovett, and Dr. F. R. Ober, of Boston, on October 24, 1921.

She is the only child of healthy parents.

She was delivered at full term by a well-known and competent obstetrician. The child presented by the breech. A gauze fillet was used to get traction in the groin. The left arm was extended and required some force for its release. As far as I could gather from the very clear account of both parents no unusual force was used and no anesthetic was used or needed. Afterward, in response to questions, the nurse said the delivery was "done too quickly."

After birth the child showed the following signs:

1. Sunken, almost closed left eye without evidence of any local trauma.

2. The left arm was abducted and externally rotated at the shoulder, sharply flexed at the elbow and hyperextended and supinated at the wrist so sharply that the back of the hand lay on the extensor surface of the forearm.

3. Respiration was noticeably shallow and rapid.

4. Both legs were flaccid.

5. Pinprick over the left arm, body and legs produced no reaction, either sensory or motor.

For the next two and a half years the parents noticed no change. Nutritional disturbances were overcome by careful regulation of diet.

At two and a half years she was operated on for contractures of the adductors and gastrocnemii. Prolonged orthopedic treatment was persistently carried out until she was able to walk at four and a half years. Since then several operations have corrected deformities at wrist and ankle.

At six years, for the first time, she was able to control her sphincters enough to wear ordinary clothing. Since then this control has gradually improved until it is adequate, except on rare occasions.

She now goes to school, dresses herself, combs her hair and, in general, leads an active life, though stiffness of gait and an awkward, weak left arm handicap her more or less. Mentally she is obviously unusually bright. She has never had convulsions.

Physical examination shows a well-developed, alert girl, standing erect in plaster jacket.

Her expression is normal, except that there is definite narrowing of the left palpebral fissure and a small left pupil. No disturbance of any cranial nerve is present. She has no speech defect. She has no involuntary movements of arms or legs.

The neck and throat are normal.

The thorax is asymmetric with absence of movement over the upper left chest. The spine shows a sharply circumscribed scoliosis of the lower cervical and upper thoracic spine, with convexity to the left. There is extreme atrophy of the sternal portion of the pectoralis major and of the intercostals on the left, particularly those between the upper six or seven ribs.

The left arm shows some atrophy of the big muscles about the shoulder, which is held higher than the right. All motions are possible at the shoulder-joint. The upper arm shows strong flexor muscles and a rather weak triceps. The lower arm shows weak flexors and stronger extensors. Functional balance results from tendon transplantation done a number of years ago. The hand shows practically complete atrophy of the small muscles, which, however, retain a very little power, enough to give a distinct functional value to the extremity.

The right arm is and always has been, efficient, but the hand is distinctly thin as compared to the strongly muscled upper arm and forearm.

The abdomen and lower back appear normal.

The legs show moderate spasticity with more marked signs on the left. Various tenotomies and persistent after-care have corrected deformities.

Sensory changes are definite. The evidence for diminished power to discriminate between heat and cold over the area shown in the chart is conclusive. Tubes at 120° and 45° F. were used. Pain sense is less definite, and I thought the element of fear entered. Touch and muscle sense are not impaired. Vibration is well recognized.

Visceral examination shows no abnormality beyond the intrathoracic signs due to the asymmetry of the chest.

Comment. The signs at birth were consistent with an oblique lesion with its upper angle at the seventh cervical segment on the left.

The later course of the case shows that permanent changes in the anterior horn cells have occurred on the left from the seventh or eighth cervical to the sixth or seventh thoracic and probably in some cells of the eighth cervical segment on the right. The spastic legs can be accounted for by partial destruction of the pyramidal tracts, while the sensory changes may be produced by a hematomyelia destroying the central gray matter or by interference with fibers higher up. As a result of the anterior horn destruction and consequent paralysis of thoracic respiration on the left a compensatory expansion of the right chest has caused a scoliosis. The pupillary changes and the enophthalmos are accounted for by involvement of the sympathetic fibers before emergence from the cord.

From the standpoint of diagnosis there is no difficulty about the case, once it is recognized that obstetric accidents can affect the cord; but it is significant that thirteen successive consultants, including neurologists, pediatricians and orthopedists regarded this case as one of cerebral palsy, and several gave the gloomiest forecasts as to mental development. During the past year our experience at the Children's Hospital with the other cases here reported has kept us on the lookout, and the diagnosis was made in the office of Dr. Lovett and Dr. Ober before I saw the child. A moment's consideration shows that the combination of partial flaccidity of the arm, spasticity of the legs and sensory changes with ocular signs could not be accounted for by any combination of cerebral lesions consistent with life and intelligence.

As far as other possibilities are concerned the history rules them out. Only a traumatic lesion could explain the steady improvement and the present condition.

Discussion. 1. *Pathologic Data.* There is every reason to suppose that pathologic statistics underestimate the frequency of cord injuries. As far as I know no considerable series of autopsies has been reported where the entire cord has been examined. It is fair to assume, therefore, that low thoracic injuries are often overlooked. Furthermore, it seems possible that certain serious lesions might be passed over if routine sections of the hardened cord were not examined.

Physiologically there is a certain amount of pertinent evidence. In the first place, young animals recover from "spinal shock" more rapidly than older ones of the same species. This can be demonstrated easily by comparing the time within which a decapitated kitten begins to show reflexes with the longer period required by the adult cat.

Experience with decerebrate animals also has some bearing on the problem. Ordinarily an animal decerebrated by midbrain section shows a very constant rigidity for many hours. Sometimes this rigidity fails or the animal dies suddenly. Often the only reason appears to be a thin film of blood over the medulla. It is possible that clots from an intracranial hemorrhage might cause a block of physiologic impulses in the cord. Such a situation, as in one baby I have recently seen, might lead to a diagnosis of cord injury where the real trouble was intracranial.

Further evidence on the question of asphyxia will be considered in connection with obstetric data.

2. *Clinical Data.* The fact that so few previous cases have been reported needs explanation.

In the first place it is obvious that the diagnosis of cord transection is almost never made where reflexes are lively. Of course the work of Head and Riddoch, now universally accepted, will lead to recognition of many hitherto unsuspected cases.

But a more important element enters into the situation. There is so much emphasis laid on the difficulties of focal diagnosis in neurologic disease in infancy that examination is entered on in a spirit of perfunctory despair. Naturally, when knee-jerks, plantar reflexes and sensory signs are regarded as hopelessly confused accurate study is regarded as a rather fatuous procedure.

On the other hand if one looks upon an infant as a rather simple physiologic problem many clues are found. It seems to me that failure to recognize neurologic disorders in babies usually depends on failure to look for gross changes in sensation, for abolition of voluntary activity and for strikingly abnormal reflexes rather than on inaccuracy in detailed examination.

Differential diagnosis is relatively simple if the possibility of cord lesion is borne in mind. In the newborn infant brachial palsy, intracranial hemorrhage and spina bifida are the important alternatives. Pure peripheral brachial palsy is usually obvious enough. Intracranial hemorrhage, if severe or if accompanied by clots in the vertebral canal, may be indistinguishable. Obviously if there is serious intracranial pressure the cerebral condition is the one to watch. Spina bifida, if not obvious, demands roentgen-ray study.

It is a striking fact that roentgen-rays are regularly negative in my series. A possible explanation of this unexpected finding will be given later.

The various atrophies, infantile paralysis, spinal injuries in infancy and so on require a good history rather than any very refined physical examination.

Examination of the spinal fluid in young infants may reveal evidence of hemorrhage, but of course does not localize the lesion. Possibly combined cistern and lumbar puncture, as used by Ayer, might give valuable information where pressure on the cord is suspected.

Treatment is restricted, primarily, to avoidance of contractures and prevention of infection. One thing seems fairly clear: The bladder, if left alone, will take care of itself without dangerous overdistention or urinary sepsis. The fact that trophic changes are not evident in most of the cases renders timely assistance by optimistic orthopedic men more or less promising.

Prognosis is of course discouraging, but there is no evidence to prove that improvement may not be hoped for. Naturally mental development is not in any way threatened.

3. *Obstetric Considerations.* The obstetrician does not fear cord injury in breech extractions. In the text-books there is no suggestion that well-conducted obstetric maneuvers can damage the cord. Asphyxia is the single recognized danger. To prevent this asphyxia speed in extraction is regarded as essential.

In discussing the subject of asphyxia two grades are distinguished: the livid and the pallid. The first is regarded as unimportant, the second as extremely dangerous. I get the impression that pale asphyxia is thought of as the final stage of blue asphyxia. It is hard to see any reason for believing that there is any such thing as "pale asphyxia." Physiologically, asphyxia stays asphyxia until the blood recovers a sufficient amount of circulating oxygen. Clinically, pure asphyxia, as in choking or in conditions like chlorine gas poisoning, produces cyanosis which persists until adequate relief is given or death ensues.

On the other hand, collapse and death, with pallor and failure of respiration, occur in patients after traumatic shock and in cases suffering from intracranial pressure.

If breech babies do not die of oxygen deprivation what kills them? As far as I know the literature is silent. It is legitimate, therefore, to speculate.

In considering possible causes it is of course necessary to pay special attention to factors which occur only in breech delivery.

Traction on the neck, sharp bending of the spinal column and traction on the brachial plexus all occur in head deliveries.

The two possible forces which appear to operate only in breech cases are:

1. Traction exerted over the entire length of the vertebral column.

2. Direct pressure on the head, resulting from uterine contraction or due to direct suprapubic pressure by the operator or assistant.

The first factor would offer a logical explanation of cord rupture. The spinal column of the infant is obviously extensible. In head presentations the extension takes place only between the head and the shoulders, and presumably the cord can adapt itself to this degree of stretching. In breech deliveries, however, the total increase in length is greater as the column may give at every space throughout the length of the spine.

The spinal cord of the baby is firmly anchored below by the cauda equina. Above in the cervical region short, heavy, almost horizontal roots fix it firmly in place. Its upper end, of course, is continuous with the medulla.

If the spinal column becomes too long one of two possible accidents may occur. The cord may give, with resultant hemorrhage or even rupture, or the cord may hold and herniation of the medulla into the foramen magnum may result. These serious results may theoretically occur without gross bony injury discoverable by roentgen ray.

In the first case more or less definite blocking of physiologic impulses will occur, as in the clinical cases here reported. It is also possible that combinations of various forces may favor avulsion of the brachial plexus roots from the stretched cord.

On the other hand if the cord does not yield the medulla must be pulled down. Just at this moment pressure on the head increases, often to an extreme degree. Theoretically such a combination of forces might cause fatal medullary pressure with vasomotor collapse or extreme vagus stimulation. The logical result would be collapse of just the type which obstetricians call asphyxia pallida.

If these entirely theoretic considerations are reasonable it is clear that the procedure in breech extractions may be based on wrong foundations.

There is some clinical experience that is relevant. Potter, who believes that version is a reasonable method of delivery in practically all cases, pays no attention to ordinary degrees of blue asphyxia. He even cuts the cord before beginning extraction if it is in his way. On the other hand by thorough dilatation, maintenance of flexion, lack of hurry, gentle traction and moderate suprapubic pressure he avoids the combination of severe traction and extreme pressure so often seen in extractions. A further fact, which may be of vital importance, is that he does version as a matter of choice, and, therefore he does not have the uterus contracted down on the head as it is when an ordinary breech delivery is under way. In spite of his apparent lack of fear of asphyxia, his fetal death-rate is not tremendous. It is certainly against all theories in the text-books that a man who deliberately disregards the single cause of death should not kill a very high percentage of his babies.

I have discussed the obstetric bearings at some length elsewhere. It seems quite certain that the traction and suprapubic pressure sometimes exerted in breech deliveries are extremely likely to favor herniation of the medulla.

Without any valid evidence from the obstetrical point of view I believe that there is good reason for investigating the pressure changes within the cranio-vertebral cavity. From a theoretic point of view it seems probable that these change are of as great importance as the chemical changes in the blood,

Conclusions. Five cases are reported in which crippling depends on injuries to the spinal cord apparently caused by breech extraction. In making the diagnosis pathologic, clinical and physiologic facts are considered.

Four of these cases showed conclusive evidence of practically complete transection. In transections the following syndromes may be expected:

1. High cervical transections are probably all fatal on account of the proximity of the lesion to the phrenic nerves and the medulla.

2. Transections below the fatal level, if accompanied by enough hemorrhage to destroy the cells of the lower segments, result in anesthesia and permanent flaccidity below the lesion.

3. Transections confined to a few segments and not involving the lumbar enlargement will show in succession the following syndromes:

(*a*) Anesthesia with flaccid paralysis. After a few days or weeks the flaccid paralysis will be modified. The infant will then show:

(*b*) Anesthesia, as before, a zone of flaccidity corresponding with the destroyed anterior horn cells, and below this zone, reflex activity of distinctive type. During this stage the bladder and rectum become "automatic."

(*c*) On theoretic grounds it seems likely that this stage of reflex activity will last only so long as severe infection is avoided.

One child showed evidence of an incomplete lesion. She showed flaccid paralysis dependent on destroyed cells and, lower, spasticity from tract involvement, with sensory disturbances and sphincter disorders proportionate to the involvement of cells and tracts.

It is evident that the vast majority of obstetric spinal-cord injuries are caused by maneuvers incident to breech extractions.

From a theoretic consideration of the forces at work in extractions it seems justifiable to suggest that traction on the cord, when combined with suprapubic pressure or uterine contractions on the head, may cause collapse or death from herniation of the medulla through the foramen magna.

If this possibility can be proved by suitable laboratory or clinical studies, it will be proper to challenge the statement, now almost universally accepted, that asphyxia is the only important cause of fetal death in breech extractions.

BIBLIOGRAPHY.

1. Ayer, J. B.: Arch. Neurol. and Psychol., 1920, **4**, 529.
2. Bastian, H. C.: Med. Chir. Trans., London, 1890, **73**, 90.
3. Beevor, C. E.: Brain, 1902, **25**, 85.
4. Bowlby, A.: Med. Chir. Trans., London, 1890, **73**, 310.
5. Bruns, L., Cramer and Ziehen: Handbuch der Nervenkrankheiten im Kindesalter, Berlin, 1912, p. 296.
6. Burr, C. V.: Am. Jour. Dis. Child., 1920, **19**, 472.
7. Crothers, B.: Med. Clin. North America, March, 1922.
8. Head, H., and Riddoch, G.: Brain, 1917, **40**, 188.
9. Kooy, F. H.: Jour. Nerv. and Ment. Dis., 1920, **52**, 1.
10. Potter, I. W.: Am. Jour. Obst. and Gynec., 1921, **1**, 560.
11. Riddoch, G.: Brain, 1917, **40**, 264.
12. Sherrington, C. S.: Integrative Action of the Nervous System, New Haven, 1906, p. 247.
13. Stolzenburg: Berl. klin. Wchnschr., 1911, No. 37, p. 1741.
14. Warwick, W.: Am. Jour. Dis. Child., 1921, **21**, 488.

VISCERAL ADHESIONS AND BANDS: NORMAL INCIDENCE.

SECOND PAPER.*

By John Bryant, M.D.,

BOSTON

At the last annual meeting of the Gastro-enterological Association, the writer presented the first of a series of papers on visceral adhesions, based upon a study of 297 unselected postmortem sections of all ages and both sexes. This paper was entitled "Visceral Adhesions and Bands. A Preliminary Report."[1] Its object was to indicate the scope, methods, and some of the conclusions arrived at as a result of the investigation being reported upon.

The object of the present communication is to make available in tabular form what may be called a standard of expectation of frequency of visceral involvement by adhesions in both sexes. This standard is given for all ages, and for four separate age periods. The tables themselves are comparable to and based upon the same original material as a table indicating the frequency of visceroptosis in unselected material at all ages, which was presented at the last annual meeting of the American Medical Association under the title "Visceroptosis: Normal Incidence. A Preliminary Report."[2]

There exists in the literature no series of cases with which the present can be compared. Therefore, although it is realized that greater accuracy might have been obtained from the study of a larger number of cases, the present results are offered in the belief that they will prove reasonably reliable, and in the hope that they may at least stimulate other workers to prove their accuracy or otherwise by reporting larger series of cases.

With regard to the tables themselves, it may be explained that the two main age groups "Below Forty" and "Above Forty" include the two other age subdivisions of "Fetal" and "Senile." Thus the age of forty becomes a proven dividing line between youth and age. The column entitled "No. of Obs." appearing in Table I, might better have been entitled "Actual Frequency," since the figures in this column represent in each case the number of positive findings with reference to the total number of cases in each sex group. In Table VI, the column "No. of Obs." indicates the total number of viscera involved by adhesions in the given age-sex group. In

* Read at the Annual Meeting of the Gastro-enterological Association, Washington, May 2, 1922.

Original data for this article obtained in 1912–1914 through the courtesy of Professors Pick and von Hansman, of Berlin, Professor Frankel, of Hamburg, and the students then working in their Institutes of Pathology.

[1] Bryant: Am. Jour. Med. Sci., 1922, **163**, 75.

[2] Bryant: Jour. Am. Med. Assn., 1921, **77**, 1400.

Table VIII, the same column, "No. of Obs." indicates the total number of actual adhesions present in each age-sex group, the number of different types of adhesions that are present in any age-sex group being indicated in the main column of the table. In Table VII, under "Legend" appear for the sake of brevity the expressions "2 to 8 Adhesions Present" and "8 or More Adhesions Present." It might have been more correct and more explicit to have used the phrases "Two to Eight Viscera Involved by Adhesions" and "Eight or More Viscera Involved by Adhesions." With these exceptions, it is hoped that the Tables will prove reasonably self-explanatory.

NO. OF OBS	VISCERA INVOLVED	SEX	PERCENTAGE FREQUENCY (10 20 30 40 50 60 70 80 90 100)
62	OMENTUM	MALE	34.4
33		FEMALE	28.2
67	PERITONEUM	MALE	37.2
46		FEMALE	39.3
3	RIGHT KIDNEY	MALE	1.7
4		FEMALE	3.4
31	LIVER	MALE	17.2
19		FEMALE	16.2
130	GALL BLADDER	MALE	72.2
75		FEMALE	64.1
101	DUODENUM	MALE	56.1
74		FEMALE	63.2
1	SMALL INTESTINE	MALE	0.6
2		FEMALE	1.7
5	TERMINAL ILEUM	MALE	2.8
6		FEMALE	5.1
36	APPENDIX	MALE	20.0
11		FEMALE	9.4
4	CAECUM	MALE	2.2
3		FEMALE	2.6
57	ASCENDING COLON	MALE	31.7
31		FEMALE	26.5
31	HEPATIC FLEXURE	MALE	17.2
14		FEMALE	12.0
144	TRANSVERSE COLON	MALE	80.0
82		FEMALE	70.1
4	SPLENIC FLEXURE	MALE	2.2
3		FEMALE	2.6
19	DESCENDING COLON	MALE	10.6
7		FEMALE	6.0
13	SIGMOID FLEXURE	MALE	7.2
2		FEMALE	1.7
0	RECTUM	MALE	NONE
3		FEMALE	2.6
0	ADNEXA	MALE	NONE
14		FEMALE	12.0

	TOTAL CASES	TOTAL OBSERVATIONS
MALE -	180	708
FEMALE -	117	429
BOTH SEXES	297	1137

TABLE I.—Visceral involvement by adhesions. Percentage frequency in relation to sex and age. All ages.

A glance at Table I indicates that, in the average case coming for examination, the transverse colon may be expected to be involved by adhesions more often than any of the other viscera; 7 women and 8 men out of every 10 presumably have some involvement of this structure by congenital or acquired adhesions. The gall-bladder and duodenum come next in order of frequency of involvement, these viscera being followed in frequency in the order named by the peritoneum, omentum, ascending colon, and hepatic flexure. The appendix, liver, and descending colon are also involved by adhesions sufficiently often to attract attention on a graphic chart. A study of Table I also indicates that although the difference in the rate of involvement of the two sexes for any given organ seldom varies by as much as 10 per cent, neither sex has an excess of involvement of all the viscera studied. Thus, in the first group of the three viscera

VISCERA INVOLVED	SEX	PERCENTAGE FREQUENCY (10 20 30 40 50 60 70 80 90 100)
OMENTUM	MALE	5.6
	FEMALE	6.3
PERITONEUM	MALE	16.7
	FEMALE	43.8
RIGHT KIDNEY	MALE	NONE
	FEMALE	6.3
LIVER	MALE	5.6
	FEMALE	NONE
GALL BLADDER	MALE	88.9
	FEMALE	68.8
DUODENUM	MALE	55.6
	FEMALE	50.0
SMALL INTESTINE	MALE	NONE
	FEMALE	NONE
TERMINAL ILEUM	MALE	5.6
	FEMALE	25.0
APPENDIX	MALE	5.6
	FEMALE	12.5
CAECUM	MALE	NONE
	FEMALE	NONE
ASCENDING COLON	MALE	11.1
	FEMALE	NONE
HEPATIC FLEXURE	MALE	11.1
	FEMALE	6.3
TRANSVERSE COLON	MALE	105.6
	FEMALE	68.8
SPLENIC FLEXURE	MALE	5.6
	FEMALE	NONE
DESCENDING COLON	MALE	5.6
	FEMALE	6.3
SIGMOID FLEXURE	MALE	NONE
	FEMALE	NONE
RECTUM	MALE	NONE
	FEMALE	NONE
ADNEXA	MALE	NONE
	FEMALE	NONE

	TOTAL CASES	TOTAL OBSERVATIONS
MALE -	18	58
FEMALE -	16	47
BOTH SEXES	34	105

TABLE II.—Visceral involvement by adhesions. Percentage frequency in relation to sex and age. Fetal (12 to 55 cm.)

most often involved by adhesions, the male percentage of involvement is higher than the female with regard to the transverse colon and gall-bladder, but lower than the female with regard to the duodenum. Also, the male percentage of involvement is greater as regards the omentum, ascending colon, appendix, and hepatic flexure, but lower for the peritoneum.

A study of Tables II to V inclusive, allowing a consideration of progressive age changes in both sexes, reveals, as would naturally be supposed, more facts of interest than can be obtained from the consideration of a single mixed-age table. Furthermore, a study of these tables is sufficient to give a basis for inference concerning the congenital or acquired character of the adhesions found involving any individual viscus.

A careful preliminary study of all the available data, when arranged by successive age decades, caused the age of forty to be taken as a definite point sharply dividing youth and age; this is from

VISCERA INVOLVED	SEX	PERCENTAGE FREQUENCY (0 10 20 30 40 50 60 70 80 90 100)
OMENTUM	MALE	18.2
	FEMALE	11.5
PERITONEUM	MALE	30.7
	FEMALE	27.9
RIGHT KIDNEY	MALE	1.1
	FEMALE	6.6
LIVER	MALE	6.8
	FEMALE	13.1
GALL BLADDER	MALE	69.3
	FEMALE	67.2
DUODENUM	MALE	52.3
	FEMALE	60.7
SMALL INTESTINE	MALE	1.1
	FEMALE	1.6
TERMINAL ILEUM	MALE	2.3
	FEMALE	6.6
APPENDIX	MALE	18.2
	FEMALE	4.9
CAECUM	MALE	2.3
	FEMALE	NONE
ASCENDING COLON	MALE	19.3
	FEMALE	16.4
HEPATIC FLEXURE	MALE	17.0
	FEMALE	11.5
TRANSVERSE COLON	MALE	70.4
	FEMALE	59.0
SPLENIC FLEXURE	MALE	2.3
	FEMALE	NONE
DESCENDING COLON	MALE	5.7
	FEMALE	3.3
SIGMOID FLEXURE	MALE	5.7
	FEMALE	NONE
RECTUM	MALE	NONE
	FEMALE	1.6
ADNEXA	MALE	NONE
	FEMALE	4.9

	TOTAL CASES	TOTAL OBSERVATIONS
MALE	88	284
FEMALE	61	181
BOTH SEXES	149	465

Table III.—Visceral involvement by adhesions. Percentage frequency in relation to sex and age. Below forty years of age.

the point of view of adhesive processes within the abdomen. Having arrived at this point in the study, the material at hand was arranged as shown in the tables, in the two main age groups "Below Forty" and "Above Forty," further indication of the relation of age to adhesions being gained by utilizing the two subgroups, "Fetal" and "Senile." Obviously, in the point of total cases, the fetal and senile groups are too small to be more than suggestive; but they are at least suggestive.

The most striking fact about Table II, based upon a study of the fetal group, is that it should be possible to make any table worth showing at all, graphically, since it has for the most part been considered that adhesions in the fetus are the exception rather than the rule. The second striking fact about this table, is that the percentages should run so high for the viscera which are chiefly involved. It is for example rather startling to find 105 per cent of the transverse colons in this fetal group of 18 males involved by

VISCERA INVOLVED	SEX	PERCENTAGE FREQUENCY (0–100)
OMENTUM	MALE	50.0
	FEMALE	46.4
PERITONEUM	MALE	43.5
	FEMALE	51.8
RIGHT KIDNEY	MALE	2.2
	FEMALE	NONE
LIVER	MALE	27.2
	FEMALE	19.6
GALL BLADDER	MALE	75.0
	FEMALE	60.7
DUODENUM	MALE	59.8
	FEMALE	66.1
SMALL INTESTINE	MALE	NONE
	FEMALE	1.8
TERMINAL ILEUM	MALE	3.3
	FEMALE	3.6
APPENDIX	MALE	21.7
	FEMALE	14.3
CAECUM	MALE	2.2
	FEMALE	5.4
ASCENDING COLON	MALE	43.5
	FEMALE	37.5
HEPATIC FLEXURE	MALE	17.4
	FEMALE	12.5
TRANSVERSE COLON	MALE	89.1
	FEMALE	82.1
SPLENIC FLEXURE	MALE	2.2
	FEMALE	5.4
DESCENDING COLON	MALE	15.2
	FEMALE	8.9
SIGMOID FLEXURE	MALE	8.7
	FEMALE	3.6
RECTUM	MALE	NONE
	FEMALE	3.6
ADNEXA	MALE	NONE
	FEMALE	19.6

	TOTAL CASES	TOTAL OBSERVATIONS
MALE	92	424
FEMALE	56	248
BOTH SEXES	148	672

TABLE IV.—Visceral involvement by adhesions. Percentage frequency in relation to sex and age. Above forty years of age.

demonstrable adhesions, this statement being explained by the fact that many of the cases under consideration presented more than one definite band involving the transverse colon. Incidentally, the method of recording the presence of these adhesions may be indicated by the following example: a fetus presents one adhesive band running from the gall-bladder across the duodenum to the transverse colon, and another band running from the ascending to transverse colon; this case would be recorded as having a total of five viscera involved by adhesions, that is the gall-bladder, duodenum and ascending colon once each, and the transverse colon twice. As in Table I, sex differences in the rate of involvement are conspicuous in Table II. Thus whereas the transverse colon, gall-bladder, and duodenum are involved more often in the male than in the female fetus, the peritoneum, terminal ileum, appendix and omentum are more frequently involved in the female than in the male fetus.

VISCERA INVOLVED	SEX	PERCENTAGE FREQUENCY (0–100)
OMENTUM	MALE	64.7
	FEMALE	50.0
PERITONEUM	MALE	35.3
	FEMALE	55.6
RIGHT KIDNEY	MALE	NONE
	FEMALE	NONE
LIVER	MALE	29.4
	FEMALE	33.3
GALL BLADDER	MALE	76.5
	FEMALE	50.0
DUODENUM	MALE	47.1
	FEMALE	50.0
SMALL INTESTINE	MALE	NONE
	FEMALE	5.6
TERMINAL ILEUM	MALE	NONE
	FEMALE	NONE
APPENDIX	MALE	11.8
	FEMALE	11.1
CAECUM	MALE	NONE
	FEMALE	NONE
ASCENDING COLON	MALE	35.3
	FEMALE	33.3
HEPATIC FLEXURE	MALE	29.4
	FEMALE	11.1
TRANSVERSE COLON	MALE	88.2
	FEMALE	100.0
SPLENIC FLEXURE	MALE	NONE
	FEMALE	11.1
DESCENDING COLON	MALE	35.3
	FEMALE	16.7
SIGMOID FLEXURE	MALE	23.5
	FEMALE	11.1
RECTUM	MALE	NONE
	FEMALE	NONE
ADNEXA	MALE	NONE
	FEMALE	22.0

	TOTAL CASES	TOTAL OBSERVATIONS
MALE	17	81
FEMALE	18	83
BOTH SEXES	35	164

TABLE V.—Visceral involvement by adhesions. Percentage frequency in relation to sex and age. Senile (over seventy years.)

As one studies Tables II to V with reference to the relationship of progressive age to visceral involvement by adhesions, several points of interest are brought to the attention. Among these points of interest may be mentioned the fact that the rate of involvement for any given viscus may either increase or decrease with age in both sexes. Also, the relative frequency of involvement of any special viscus with regard to sex may vary at different periods. One or two examples may be given.

The terminal ileum shows in both sexes a decreasing involvement by adhesions with progressive age, the rate being distinctly highest in the fetus. Incidently, this finding is diametrically opposed to the dictum of Lane; he has stated that bands about the terminal ileum represent crystallization of lines of force which increase with age, this crystallization resulting from efforts of the organism to support a sagging viscus. The omentum in both sexes is increasingly involved with progressive age; the same progressive increase with age is evident as regards the adnexa of the female, and the sigmoid in both sexes.

The sigmoid flexure is a conspicuous example of a viscus progressively involved with increasing age. No involvement occurs in the fetus in either sex. Below the age of forty in the male there is an involvement of but 5.7 per cent. The rate increases to 8.7 per cent in the male above forty, and the figure for the senile male rises sharply to 23.5 per cent of involvement. The figures for the female with regard to increased age involvement are less striking but the same in character.

The female adnexa present another striking example of what one must look upon as adhesive processes of degeneration. Here, the involvement is but 4.9 per cent below the age of forty, as contrasted with a rate of 19.6 per cent for the female group above forty years of age, and a rate of 22 per cent for the female senile group.

The peritoneum is an example of a viscus varying with age in its relative frequency as to sex involvement. Thus, although the rate is much higher in the female than the male fetus, the figures are reversed in the group below forty years of age; the figures are, however, reversed again in the group above forty years of age; furthermore, the peritoneum becomes increasingly more involved in the senile female, but less involved in the senile male group.

It is believed that even the few examples given above are sufficient to prove that in any study of the subject of visceral adhesions and bands, both age and sex factors must be carefully considered before any reliable results can be arrived at.

In general, the problem of visceral adhesions may be approached from at least two main points of view. The first, is that of the involvement of the individual viscera by adhesive processes either congenital or acquired; this is the point of view from which Tables I to V inclusive have been considered. The second point of view from which the problem of viscera adhesions may be approached, is that of the actual adhesions themselves. For example, the congenital band frequently found running from the gall-bladder down across the duodenum to the transverse colon, if studied from the first point of view, would be considered under the three separate headings of gall-bladder, duodenum and transverse colon. On the other hand, if studied from the second point of view of the adhesive process itself, this congenital band would be considered as a single distinct structure. It is from this second point of view that Tables

VI, VII, and VIII approach the subject of visceral adhesions, from three particular angles.

The object of Table VI is to indicate the surprising increase in the average number of viscera involved by adhesions with increasing age, in both sexes. It will be seen that below the age of forty the average number of viscera involved does not exceed 4 per case, whereas above the age of forty the average rate of involvement is nearer 5 than 4 per case. Reducing this question to percentage

NO. OF CASES	NO. OF OBS.	AGE	SEX	AVERAGE NUMBER OF VISCERA INVOLVED (0–10)	INCREASE OVER FOETAL RATE PERCENTAGE (0–80)
18	58	FOETAL	MALE	3.2	
16	47		FEMALE	2.9	
88	284	BELOW 40	MALE	3.2	NONE
61	181		FEMALE	3.0	3.4
92	424	ABOVE 40	MALE	4.6	43.8
56	248		FEMALE	4.4	51.7
17	81	SENILE	MALE	4.8	50.0
18	83		FEMALE	4.6	58.7

TABLE VI.—Average number of viscera involved by adhesions in relation to sex and age.

increase above the fetal rate of involvement, it is shown that whereas there is practically no percentage increase below the age of forty, the increase after this age averages about 50 per cent for both sexes. It is difficult to explain this striking 50 per cent increase on any other basis than that of some increasing degenerative tendency to adhesions, possibly based upon decreased resistance to the irritative and infective trauma to which all viscera are exposed in varying and progressive degrees at all ages in both sexes.

94.4
87.5
82.9
85.2
77.2
69.6
76.5
55.6

TABLE VII.—Variation in complexity of adhesions present in relation to sex and age.

The relation of age to the complexity of adhesions or the number of viscera involved in any single adhesive process is clearly shown in Table VII. From this one learns that the adhesions found in the fetus are relatively uncomplicated in character, and that complexity is practically a synonym for age. In other words, the increasing complexity of adhesions with age seems to be an indication of the decreasing resistance of the viscera to the trauma of all kinds to which they are subjected throughout life.

It has been shown in Tables VI and VII that the age of forty is critical in relation to the average number of viscera involved, and in relation to the complexity of the adhesions themselves. A study of Table VIII leads to the conclusion that the total variety of adhesions present in any age group also increases with age, but that the marked increase occurs in the thirty–forty-year decade, or ten years before the onset of the two other age changes just referred to.

In summarizing these various age changes, it may be said that the distinguishing characteristics of such congenital or developmental adhesions as are found in the fetus are firstly, the limited average number of viscera involved, and secondly the simplicity and absence of variety in type of the adhesions themselves. The acquired and degenerative adhesions of age, are on the contrary characterized

NO. OF CASES	NO. OF OBS.	AGE	SEX	ACTUAL NUMBER OF DIFFERERENT ADHESIONS PRESENT (0, 5, 10, 15, 20, 25)
18	58	FOETAL	MALE	10
16	47		FEMALE	8
10	26	BIRTH-2 YRS.	MALE	8
8	16		FEMALE	5
12	30	2–10	MALE	10
11	30		FEMALE	9
11	36	10–20	MALE	10
1	2		FEMALE	1
13	48	20–30	MALE	11
11	38		FEMALE	11
24	86	30–40	MALE	20
14	48		FEMALE	15
23	104	40–50	MALE	23
16	77		FEMALE	18
31	142	50–60	MALE	23
15	59		FEMALE	14
21	97	60–70	MALE	20
7	29		FEMALE	8
17	81	70–80	MALE	19
18	83		FEMALE	25

TABLE VIII.—Total number of variations in types of adhesions present in relation to sex and age.

by the large average number of viscera involved in any given process, the great increase in the variety of adhesions found, and the strikingly increased complexity of the adhesions themselves.

Conclusions. 1. The transverse colon is more frequently involved by adhesions than any other abdominal viscus. Seven women and 8 men out of every 10 persons presumably have some involvement of this viscus by congenital or acquired adhesions. Next in order of frequency of involvement come the gall-bladder, duodenum, peritoneum, omentum, ascending colon, hepatic flexure, appendix, liver and descending colon.

2. Within a range of variation not usually exceeding 10 per cent, the rate of involvement of a given viscus may be greater in the male or in the female, and this relative rate of involvement with regard to sex may further vary with age.

3. The rate of involvement by adhesions, is for several viscera higher in the fetus than at later ages, as for the transverse colon in the male and the terminal ileum in the female.

4. The rate of involvement by adhesions increases rapidly with progressive age for certain other viscera, as for the sigmoid flexure in the male and the adnexa in the female.

5. The age of forty is critical in both sexes with reference to the average number of viscera involved by adhesions in any given case. After the age of forty, there is a sudden increase of involvement by about 50 per cent in both sexes, the increase being somewhat more marked in the male than in the female.

6. Complexity is practically a synonym for age, with regard to the number of viscera involved in any given adhesive process. This increase in complexity amounts to over 200 per cent after forty years of age.

7. Variety in the character of the adhesions present also increases with age. A sudden marked increase of nearly 100 per cent occurs in the thirty–forty-year decade, or ten years earlier than the onset of the marked increase with regard to the average number of viscera involved, and the onset of the increase in the complexity of the adhesions themselves.

8. The distinguishing characteristics of congenital or developmental adhesions, are simplicity and lack of variety in type.

9. The distinguishing characteristics of acquired adhesions, are complexity and variety in type.

IS THE STOMACH A FOCUS OF INFECTION?

By Nicholas Kopeloff, Ph.D.,

Department of Bacteriology, Psychiatric Institute, Ward's Island, New York.

The relation of focal infection to systemic disease, and more particularly to the psychoses, has been the subject of considerable controversy. Before establishing that a focus of infection is the etiologic factor in a systemic disease or in a psychosis, it must first be proven that the bacteria in any organ involved are not merely fortuitous but actually constitute a focus of infection. Periapical abscesses and tonsil infections are generally conceded to belong to the latter category. However, the question is at once raised whether the stomach is a focus of infection in the same sense. The present investigation is concerned with a critical analysis of the relevant facts, as determined by the Rehfuss method of fractional gastric analysis, and the writer wishes to emphasize that there is no attempt made to discuss whether or not the stomach is a focus of infection when other criteria are employed.

It has been quite generally recognized that acidity is the most important factor in influencing the bacterial content of the stomach. That is to say, the higher the acidity the fewer the numbers and types of bacteria present. The fractional method of gastric analysis makes possible a bacteriologic study of the stomach, which includes not only the active cycle of digestion but the resting phase as well. So far as could be ascertained no quantitative bacterial studies employing this method have heretofore been reported. In fact very little data concerning the types of bacteria in the stomach at different stages of digestion have appeared in the literature beyond the work of Cotton.[1] He claims that: "The stomach and duodenum are very frequently the seat of secondary foci. . . . The bacteria invade the stomach wall and appear to interfere with the secretion of hydrochloric acid, so necessary to digestion. Cultures of the stomach contents will reveal the presence of various types of streptococci and frequently of various types of colon bacilli. The chemical examination of the stomach contents will show either a very low secretion of hydrochloric acid, or, in many cases, its entire absence during the test meal." Upon the administration of autogenous vaccines the acidity of the stomach is increased and the bacteria disappear.

The first criticism which can be advanced against such a position is that these conclusions are based upon single determinations by the Rehfuss method of fractional analysis. The writer has shown[2] that repeated analyses carried out on the same individual within a short period of time yield different acidity curves. In other words the same subject may show a low, high and intermediate acidity on three separate analyses carried out within a single week. This holds true likewise for the average fasting contents. Obviously therefore, it is not valid to base any conclusions on a single determination. Before entering into a discussion of further objections, it would be more appropriate to present the data upon which they are based.

Bacteriologic studies of fractional gastric analyses carried out repeatedly on psychotic patients and normal individuals have shown that in only one-half the instances was there any correlation between high acidity and low bacterial numbers or *vice versa*. In other words there was evidently still another factor operating which precluded any such simple explanation as that wherein acidity alone determined the bacterial count of the stomach. Upon

[1] The Defective Delinquent and the Insane, Princeton University Press, p. 201. New York Med. Jour., 1920, **111**, 672, 721, 770.

[2] Kopeloff, Nicholas: Individual Variation as Influencing the Rehfuss Fractional Method of Gastric Analysis, Jour. Am. Med. Assn., 1922, **78**, 404.

close observation it became appare that the amount of saliva swallowed by a patient during the vo-and-one-half hour period necessary for the complete gastric an ysis by the fractional method was of considerable significance. or example, the bacterial counts made on all the gastric fractio varied from 0 up to 100,000 per cubic centimeter, depending up the individual. Only one patient consistently showed a comete absence of bacteria on repeated analyses. It is of particu r interest that this was a case of profound depression. In fac she refused food and often fasted for as much as forty-eight hers at a time. It is furthermore of importance to note that her cretory activity was greatly reduced. Her mouth was usually ceedingly dry, and it was difficult to stimulate any flow of sa va. The conclusion, therefore, was that the absence of saliva us the limiting factor, so far as her bacterial content was concened. It might perhaps be mentioned in passing that her gastri acidity was not abnormally high.

The major problem under invest ation, namely, the relation of focal infection to the psychoses, emands a thorough investigation of the gastrointestinal tract order to establish whether or not it is to be considered a focus f infection. Obviously it is essential to determine whether the acterial flora, and especially the pathog[illegible] thereof, are rue stomach bacteria in the same s[illegible] bnormal condtion in the stomach permits of th[illegible] consequent mtiplication; or whether this fl[illegible] resultant of such cmparatively external factors [illegible] va.

[illegible] estly impossible complety to prevent the swallowing [illegible] a during the course of a actional gastric analysis, in [illegible] determine its relative valu as a factor influencing the [illegible] al content of the stomach. he method finally devised [illegible] ever, proved effective in reducin the swallowing of saliva to minimum. The procedure consied in placing an ordinary dental suction tube, which was attach to a running-water vacuum pump, in the subject's mouth thughout the analysis. The subject was continually reminded to nove this tube freely about in the mouth (*cavum oris*) and also t expectorate as frequently as possible. In order to reduce the largeamount of saliva necessarily swallowed when the Rehfuss tube is itroduced, the dental suction tube was kept in the mouth for one-hlf hour prior to the swallowing of the Rehfuss tube. An addedprecaution was to have the subjects brush their teeth with paicular care and rinse with chlorazene solution the night before nd morning of the analysis; the mouth was again rinsed with hlorazene solution followed by successive portions of sterile watr before the aseptic dental tube was inserted. The standard Ewald test meal consisted of 35 gm. of sterilized toast and 250 cc of sterile tea. The Rehfuss

close observation it became apparent that the amount of saliva swallowed by a patient during the two-and-one-half hour period necessary for the complete gastric analysis by the fractional method was of considerable significance. For example, the bacterial counts made on all the gastric fractions varied from 0 up to 100,000 per cubic centimeter, depending upon the individual. Only one patient consistently showed a complete absence of bacteria on repeated analyses. It is of particular interest that this was a case of profound depression. In fact, she refused food and often fasted for as much as forty-eight hours at a time. It is furthermore of importance to note that her secretory activity was greatly reduced. Her mouth was usually exceedingly dry, and it was difficult to stimulate any flow of saliva. The conclusion, therefore, was that the absence of saliva was the limiting factor, so far as her bacterial content was concerned. It might perhaps be mentioned in passing that her gastric acidity was not abnormally high.

The major problem under investigation, namely, the relation of focal infection to the psychoses, demands a thorough investigation of the gastrointestinal tract in order to establish whether or not it is to be considered a focus of infection. Obviously it is essential to determine whether the bacterial flora, and especially the pathogenic members thereof, are true stomach bacteria in the same sense that some abnormal condition in the stomach permits of their presence and consequent multiplication; or whether this flora is a natural resultant of such comparatively external factors as food and saliva.

It is manifestly impossible completely to prevent the swallowing of all saliva during the course of a fractional gastric analysis, in order to determine its relative value as a factor influencing the bacterial content of the stomach. The method finally devised however, proved effective in reducing the swallowing of saliva to a minimum. The procedure consisted in placing an ordinary dental suction tube, which was attached to a running-water vacuum pump, in the subject's mouth throughout the analysis. The subject was continually reminded to move this tube freely about in the mouth (*cavum oris*) and also to expectorate as frequently as possible. In order to reduce the large amount of saliva necessarily swallowed when the Rehfuss tube is introduced, the dental suction tube was kept in the mouth for one-half hour prior to the swallowing of the Rehfuss tube. An added precaution was to have the subjects brush their teeth with particular care and rinse with chlorazene solution the night before and morning of the analysis; the mouth was again rinsed with chlorazene solution followed by successive portions of sterile water before the aseptic dental tube was inserted. The standard Ewald test meal consisted of 35 gm. of sterilized toast and 250 cc of sterile tea. The Rehfuss tube and syringe were sterilized as well as the test-tubes in which the samples were collected. The attempt therefore was made to have all conditions as aseptic as the circumstances would permit. In this way counts made on the bacteria would be a true approximation of the numbers and kinds actually present in the stomach and could be satisfactorily compared with previous results obtained where saliva was present in greater amount. The acidity of each fraction was obtained by titration, using methyl orange and phenolthalein as indicators, while the hydrogen ion concentration was determined colorimetrically, using the Clark and Lubs indicators. One cubic centimeter of each fraction was plated in triplicate at once upon withdrawal, on both glucose meat-infusion agar and lactose meat-infusion agar, to which brom-cresol purple was added. Since the subjects were not in bed during these analyses, as is customarily the case, but sat upright in chairs, their stomachs emptied in somewhat less than the usual time.

In Table I are presented the bacteriologic and chemical results obtained with a psychotic patient (diagnosed manic-depressive:

TABLE I.—COMPARISON OF GASTRIC FRACTIONS WITH SALIVA REMOVED AND NOT REMOVED—MANIC SUBJECT.

M. Sl.	Saliva not removed.			Saliva not removed.			Saliva removed.		
	Bact. per 1 cc.	TA.	p^H.	Bact. per 1 cc.	TA.	p^H.	Bact. per 1 cc.	TA.	p^H.
F.C.	15,500	5	2.8	...	...	...	2	12	2.8
¼ hour	380	11	2.7	310	35	2.9	5	23	2.5
½ "	78	41	2.2	5100	37	3.0	8	52	1.7
¾ "	5	46	1.8	925	41	2.8	2	70	1.4
1 "	60	25	2.5	2800	28	3.0	0	71	1.3
1¼ hours	800	18	2.7	110	36	2.2	1	42	1.5
1½ "	215	25	2.3	95	43	1.9	1	29	1.7
1¾ "	55	6	2.7	12	45	1.8	32	12	2.0
2	110	28	2.7	5400	10	3.7	*	2	3.0
2¼	48,000	9	2.7	3200	9	4.3	*		
2½ "	46,000	10	2.7	6800	16	3.5	*		

TA., total acidity; p^H., hydrogen-ion concentration (inverse); F.C., fasting contents; * stomach empty.

manic). The first two main headings, "Saliva NOT Removed," are for the fractional gastric analyses carried out at two different times with the technic employed in previous work.[2] Under the final heading, "Saliva REMOVED," appear the data obtained with the modified technic herein described. In the first column of figures giving bacteria per cubic centimeter, where saliva was not removed, we see that the fasting contents contained 15,500 bacteria per cubic centimeter. During the process of digestion the numbers are considerably lower until two and one-quarter

In Table II are given the results obtained in a healthy normal individual, in order to show clearly that the mental condition did not unduly affect the conclusion previously arrived at. Here, again, are seen practically the same points as were brought out in the previous case. Thus where saliva is not removed, as in the first column, the fasting contents contain 700 bacteria per cubic centimeter while the last two fractions contain 51,000 and 58,000 bacteria per cubic centimeter respectively. The intermediate fractions vary between 250 and 1050 bacteria per cubic centimeter. In the second column of bacterial numbers where saliva was not removed, there is a variation from 550 to 1200 bacteria per cubic centimeter. Comparing this with the third column, where saliva *was removed*, a striking decrease is evident. There is a variation from 38 to 300 bacteria per cubic centimeter. In other words, the *highest* bacterial count where saliva was removed is lower than the *lowest* bacterial count in the second column where saliva was not removed, and very slightly higher than the lowest bacterial count in the first column where saliva was not removed. The conclusion is therefore corroborated that the saliva is one of the most important single factors influencing the bacterial content of the stomach. In the first column where saliva is not removed, as with the previous subject, it is seen that the bacterial count for the fasting contents is lower than in the last two fractions, showing that there could not have been any multiplication of bacteria in the interdigestive phase. The same fact may be observed in the final column where saliva was removed. The second column is an exception to the rule, but may easily be explained on the basis that somewhat more saliva was swallowed with the Rehfuss tube than is ordinarily the case. It is furthermore obvious that there is no correlation between bacterial numbers and variation in acidity as measured either by titration or hydrogen-ion concentration, which points to the greater importance of saliva as a limiting factor.

Similar results were obtained with other psychotic patients (also manic-depressive: manic). It is scarcely necessary to discuss these results in detail, since the data which corroborate the points already emphasized are published elsewhere.

An important consideration, however, is that these patients had a very low acidity and would be ... type of subjec[t] therefore in which bacteria mi[ght] ... a f... ...nd make t[he] stomach a focus of infection ... fr... ...sults whe[re] saliva is removed such is far fro[m] ... ca...

It must be remembered that ... ...as ... carried out on a normal individual is ... ...h ... ...nt on

[3] Kopeloff, Nicholas: The Fractional ... A... ...d to the Psychoses, State Hospital Quarterl[y] ... 7, ...

a manic patient i quite another. The difficulties must truly be seen to be appre ated. The continual conversation must perforce induce a ser s of swallowing reflexes, which tend to carry saliva down the ophagus despite any devices for removal of saliva. The atte pt, therefore, to remove saliva during the course of analysis n such a patient could scarcely be put to a severer test or m t with less response. Consequently the data take on an added gnificance when they so definitely point to the observation that t removal of saliva is accompanied by a striking reduction in bact al count. The conclusion, therefore, is that saliva influences t bacterial content of the stomach.

A qualitative st y of the types of bacteria found in the saliva, and by the fracti al method of analysis, in the stomach serves as additional evid ce in support of these findings.[3] The organisms found most fr uently have been streptococci, yeasts, staphylococci, members f the lactic-acid and aërogenes groups. It was found that t re was no correlation between the degree of acidity and the s cies or numbers of bacteria found. Streptococci were associa d as frequently with stomachs having high acidity as with t se having low acidity. The toast contained many yeasts and me bacteria. The other bacteria noted were almost invariabl be found in the saliva, so that there remains no question but th the bacterial flora of the stomach is a resultant of purely external ctors, food and saliva.

Therefore, Cott 's[1] contention that the stomach is a focus of infection finds no bstantiation after a critical inspection of the fundamental facts. His conclusions are based upon results obtained by the Rehfuss m hod, and therefore are open to the following objections: (*a*) Re ated analyses by the Rehfuss method on the same individual ld different curves and little constancy in bacterial species; *b*) no correlation can be established between low acidity and h h bacterial numbers or species, since it has been shown th a dity is not the limiting factor in determining the bacterial c nt t of the stomach during a fractional analysis by the Rehfuss m hod (*c*) saliva is the most important factor in influencing the ba erial content of the stomach (without gastric lesions), although e bacterial content of the food ingested must be considered.

Should the obje on be raised that the bacterial content of the stomach is an aca mic one, the burden of proof falls on him who rts that it is pssible to determine infection in the lining of mach wall. Removal of the stomach is the only positive known f proving whether or not such infection exists.
T of otaining the knowledge in such a manner could ed worth while from the standpoint of treat- nfection in the stomach (without lesions) Cotton from results obtained by the Rehfuss

hours have elapsed, when there is a tremendous increase. It may be mentioned, parenthetically, that the unsterilized toast usually given contained an average of about 600,000 microörganisms per gram. The acidity in the stomach is generally sufficient to decimate a large proportion of the original number of bacteria ingested, which would be approximately 50,000 per cubic centimeter of total gastric contents. In the second column of bacterial numbers the fasting contents were unfortunately not obtained, but the remaining figures, while higher than those in the first column, have much the same general proportions, namely, the last few fractions show the highest bacterial counts. Contrast these two columns with the column of bacterial figures where saliva *was removed*. Here the first number is 2 and the last, which is the highest, is 32. The results speak for themselves. In other words, based on the last fraction in the first column where saliva was removed, this represents only 0.007 per cent of the bacteria found in the former fraction. Such a striking reduction makes the conclusion irresistible, namely, that bacterial numbers in the stomach at any one time depend almost entirely upon the saliva swallowed (where the bacterial content of the food may be disregarded).

Several other interesting points may also be noted. The most important of these bears on the relation of the active digestive cycle to the interdigestive phase. In other words it would naturally be expected that the greatest multiplication of bacteria and maximum numbers would be attained in the "interdigestive" phase when the stomach is relatively at rest and the secretion of acid is at a minimum. Accordingly, therefore, the fasting contents should show the highest bacterial count. But such is not the case. As a matter of fact the last fractions, whether saliva be removed or not, contain a far greater number of bacteria. Unquestionably the secretion of acid during the actual process of digestion, together with the natural motility of the stomach, should materially reduce the numbers present at the outset. Contrary to this inference the numbers are actually increased, and this is additional evidence that the continual swallowing of saliva (which contains millions of bacteria per cubic centimeter) is in reality the factor which determines the bacterial content of the stomach. The mere act of swallowing the Rehfuss tube is alone responsible for carrying down considerable saliva, and this is probably why the bacterial count on the fasting contents is as high as it is. Furthermore, it has been observed that toward the end of the analysis, when the stomach is almost empty, it becomes necessary to manipulate the tube considerably in order to obtain the fraction, and therefore a large increase in bacterial numbers would naturally accompany this procedure. Occasionally it will be found necessary to manipulate the tube during some stage of the analysis, which almost invariably results in an increase in the number of bacteria. Again, the fact that the bacterial numbers where saliva was removed were so small as to be negligible is significant when it is noted that the secretion of acid is without much influence, *i. e.*, only two bacteria appear where the total acidity is as low as 12 and as high as 70. All these considerations mentioned point to the fact that the saliva is the most important single factor in influencing the bacterial content of the stomach under the conditions employed. No attempt is made here to underestimate the importance of gastric acidity in influencing the numbers and kinds of bacteria. If anything, these data corroborate from another aspect the bacteriologic findings of previous investigators who claim that gastric acidity is sufficient to control the development of bacteria in the stomach. There are two important factors to be considered in this connection: (*a*) the actual concentration of hydrogen ions and buffer salts, and (*b*) the element of time. Bacteriologic studies which have been concerned with mathematical aspects bring out this latter point very clearly. In other words, while it is possible to find a great number of bacteria in the stomach at one particular moment, the continued limiting effects of acidity will soon be manifest, and it will be seen that in only very few cases, and chiefly where organic lesions are present, may the stomach be regarded as a focus of infection. However at any particular time it is possible to find numbers of bacteria, and it is the contention borne out by these data that at such time the saliva is the more important factor. It is scarcely necessary to add that the finding of bacteria may or may not be of significance, depending upon the numbers and types found; still it is generally conceded that large numbers would be expected in such stomachs as might be considered foci of infection.

TABLE II.—COMPARISON OF GASTRIC FRACTIONS WITH SALIVA REMOVED AND NOT REMOVED—NORMAL SUBJECT.

S. My.	Saliva not removed.			Saliva not removed.			Saliva removed.		
	Bact. per 1 cc.	TA.	p^H.	Bact. per 1 cc.	TA.	p^H.	Bact. per 1 cc.	TA.	p^H.
F.C. . . .	7,000	15	3.0	12,000	20	2.7	97	14	3.0
¼ hour . .	1,050	17	3.0	550	25	2.6	300	16	3.0
½ " . . .	700	30	2.8	1,700	39	2.6	40	22	2.4
¾ " . . .	780	42	2.7	1,400	62	1.6	180	38	1.9
1 " . . .	1,000	50	2.6	1,800	76	1.6	138	45	1.7
1¼ hours . .	1,050	37	2.6	1,100	73	1.5	115	49	1.7
1½ " . .	250	39	2.3	600	65	1.4	38	52	1.7
1¾ " . .	450	47	1.6	800	45	1.6	43	49	1.7
2 " . .	750	25	2.1	1,000	22	2.4	70	35	1.8
2¼ " . .	31,000	7	4.5	600	21	2.4	300	15	4.2
2½ " . .	58,000	4	5.0	900	30	1.9	*	7	4.4

TA. total acidity; p^H, hydrogen-ion concentration (inverse); F.C., fasting contents; Bact., bacteria; * stomach empty.

In Table II are given the results obtained on a healthy normal individual, in order to show clearly that the mental condition did not unduly affect the conclusion previously arrived at. Here, again, are seen practically the same points as were brought out in the previous case. Thus where saliva is not removed, as in the first column, the fasting contents contain 7000 bacteria per cubic centimeter while the last two fractions contain 31,000 and 58,000 bacteria per cubic centimeter respectively. The intermediate fractions vary between 250 and 1050 bacteria per cubic centimeter. In the second column of bacterial numbers, where saliva was not removed, there is a variation from 550 to 12,000 bacteria per cubic centimeter. Comparing this with the third column, where saliva *was removed*, a striking decrease is evident. There is a variation from 38 to 300 bacteria per cubic centimeter. In other words, the *highest* bacterial count where saliva was removed is lower than the *lowest* bacterial count in the second column where saliva was not removed, and very slightly higher than the lowest bacterial count in the first column where saliva was not removed. The conclusion is therefore corroborated that the saliva is one of the most important single factors influencing the bacterial content of the stomach. In the first column where saliva is not removed, as with the previous subject, it is seen that the bacterial count for the fasting contents is lower than in the last two fractions, showing that there could not have been any multiplication of bacteria in the interdigestive phase. The same fact may be observed in the final column where saliva was removed. The second column is an exception to the rule, but may easily be explained on the basis that somewhat more saliva was swallowed with the Rehfuss tube than is ordinarily the case. It is furthermore obvious that there is no correlation between bacterial numbers and variation in acidity as measured either by titration or hydrogen-ion concentration, which points to the greater importance of saliva as a limiting factor.

Similar results were obtained with other psychotic patients (also manic-depressive: manic). It is scarcely necessary to discuss these results in detail, since the data which corroborate the points already emphasized are published elsewhere.[3]

An important consideration, however, is that these patients had a very low acidity and would be precisely the type of subjects therefore in which bacteria might gain a foothold and make the stomach a focus of infection. Judging from the results when saliva is removed such is far from being the case.

It must be remembered that a fractional gastric analysis carried out on a normal individual is one thing and when carried out on

[3] Kopeloff, Nicholas: The Fractional Method of Gastric Analysis as Applied to the Psychoses, State Hospital Quarterly (New York), 1922, 7, 326.

a manic patient is quite another. The difficulties must truly be seen to be appreciated. The continual conversation must perforce induce a series of swallowing reflexes, which tend to carry saliva down the esophagus despite any devices for removal of saliva. The attempt, therefore, to remove saliva during the course of analysis on such a patient could scarcely be put to a severer test or meet with less response. Consequently the data take on an added significance when they so definitely point to the observation that the removal of saliva is accompanied by a striking reduction in bacterial count. The conclusion, therefore, is that saliva influences the bacterial content of the stomach.

A qualitative study of the types of bacteria found in the saliva, and by the fractional method of analysis, in the stomach serves as additional evidence in support of these findings.[3] The organisms found most frequently have been streptococci, yeasts, staphylococci, members of the lactic-acid and aërogenes groups. It was found that there was no correlation between the degree of acidity and the species or numbers of bacteria found. Streptococci were associated as frequently with stomachs having high acidity as with those having low acidity. The toast contained many yeasts and some bacteria. The other bacteria noted were almost invariably to be found in the saliva, so that there remains no question but that the bacterial flora of the stomach is a resultant of purely external factors, food and saliva.

Therefore, Cotton's[1] contention that the stomach is a focus of infection finds no substantiation after a critical inspection of the fundamental facts. His conclusions are based upon results obtained by the Rehfuss method, and therefore are open to the following objections: (*a*) Repeated analyses by the Rehfuss method on the same individual yield different curves and little constancy in bacterial species; (*b*) no correlation can be established between low acidity and high bacterial numbers or species, since it has been shown that acidity is not the limiting factor in determining the bacterial content of the stomach during a fractional analysis by the Rehfuss method (*c*) saliva is the most important factor in influencing the bacterial content of the stomach (without gastric lesions), although the bacterial content of the food ingested must be considered.

Should the objection be raised that the bacterial content of the stomach is an academic one, the burden of proof falls on him who asserts that it is possible to determine infection in the lining of the stomach wall. Removal of the stomach is the only positive method yet known of proving whether or not such infection exists. The advantage of obtaining the knowledge in such a manner could scarcely be considered worth while from the standpoint of treatment. Therefore, infection in the stomach (without lesions) has been diagnosed by Cotton from results obtained by the Rehfuss method. Two possibilities are open: The first is that the infection is secondary and has been brought by means of the blood stream and lymph channels, and the second is that it results from the swallowing of infected material. In either event if the infection is "hidden" in the living stomach wall, the gastric contents upon withdrawal will not show the bacteria in question. On the other hand, if the bacteria from the focus are being actively discharged into the stomach contents, then if the infection has come by way of the blood or lymph stream the number of bacteria found in the gastric contents should not be decreased by cutting off the flow of saliva. However, such is not the case, and it has been shown that the removal of saliva reduces the bacterial content. Consequently it must be inferred that the bacteria in the gastric contents are introduced by the swallowing of saliva. It naturally follows then that there should be a multiplication of microörganisms when the stomach is at rest. However, it has been previously shown[2] that no such multiplication exists even in stomachs having a low acidity. No question is raised here with regard to the stomach being a focus of infection where organic lesions are present, for undoubtedly ulcers and other similar conditions may well act as foci of infection. The chief concern is whether the stomach is a focus of infection where there is no indication of organic lesions, or where no other criteria than the Rehfuss method for establishing such infection has been used, as in cases reported by Cotton,[1] which have yielded to treatment with autogenous vaccines. Since the bacterial flora of the stomach have been shown in this paper to be the resultant of external factors, such as food and saliva, the results obtained by the Rehfuss method of fractional gastric analysis cannot be considered adequate criteria for determining whether or not the stomach is a focus of infection. Consequently no validity can be attached to the conclusion based upon the use of this method that the stomach bears an etiologic relationship to the development of systemic disease or a pyschosis.* Studies concerning the presence and elimination of foci of infection (teeth and tonsils) in psychoses are now in progress, and in the near future a report will be made on a group of functional psychoses all showing infected teeth and tonsils. In one-half of the group the foci of infection were removed, the remaining half of the group were not operated upon and therefore could be regarded as "controls."

The staff have been very generous in their assistance, particularly Dr. C. O. Cheney, and Mr. E. J. Kennedy has rendered invaluable aid in the laboratory.

Summary. 1. A quantitative as well as a qualitative study was made of the bacteria found in the stomach at different stages

* N. Kopeloff and C. O. Cheney.: Studies in Focal Infection; Its Presence and Elimination in the Functional Psychoses. Am. Jour. Psychiatry, Oct., 1922.

in the digestive process, employing the fractional method of gastric analysis.

2. The device used for the removal of saliva during gastric analysis was a dental suction tube. This made possible a comparison of gastric fractions contaminated and uncontaminated by saliva.

3. Bacterial counts showed a striking reduction in numbers in gastric fractions when saliva was inaccessible. The highest number of bacteria per cubic centimeter in a psychotic patient (manic-depressive: manic) where saliva was *not* removed was 48,000; where saliva *was* removed the highest number found was 32. Similar results were obtained with a normal individual and with other manic patients.

4. These data take on an added significance when it is remembered that the swallowing of saliva is particularly difficult to control in manic patients. Furthermore it is important to note that this reduction in numbers of bacteria when saliva is removed occurs alike with patients having a very low gastric acidity and those of a more normal type.

5. There is no correlation between high acidity in the stomach and low bacterial numbers, or *vice versa*. Streptococci were found associated with high as often as with low gastric acidity, cousequently there seems to be no reason to attach undue importance to their presence or therefore to consider the stomach a focus of infection. This means that another factor, the saliva, is of greater importance in determining the bacterial content within certain limits.

6. The fact that the bacterial count on the "fasting contents" is usually considerably lower than during the process of digestion indicates that little or no multiplication of bacteria takes place when the stomach is relatively at rest.

7. The microörganisms found in the different gastric fractions with greatest frequency are: Yeasts, staphylococci, streptococci and members of the lactic-acid and aërogenes groups. Almost invariably these are found in the saliva of the same patient or in the food given. Consequently they cannot be regarded as constituting a true bacterial flora of the normal stomach.

8. From these various considerations it may be inferred that the stomach is not acting as a focus of infection but merely as a receptacle for the bacteria poured into it. This is in agreement with the bacteriologic investigations of others to the effect that gastric acidity is sufficient to prevent bacterial development.

Conclusion. The bacterial content of the stomach is influenced by the saliva. The Rehfuss method of fractional gastric analysis cannot be considered an adequate criterion in determining whether the stomach is a focus of infection.

REVIEWS.

A Dictionary of Dental Science. By L. Pierce Anthony, D.D.S., Associate Editor of the *Dental Cosmos*. Pp. 324; 23 plates. Philadelphia and New York: Lea & Febiger, 1922.

The author's long experience in dental literary work has well fitted him to produce this, as far as we know, the first purely dental dictionary in the English language. The book defines all words likely to be met by the dentist in medical works of interest to him, and in addition many technical dental words are found that are not included in medical dictionaries. In view of the ever-increasing contact between the two professions the book should be valuable for the physician as well as the dentist. I.

Pulmonary Tuberculosis. By Maurice Fishberg, M.D., Clinical Professor of Medicine, University and Bellevue Hospital Medical College; Chief of the Tuberculosis Service, Montefiore Hospital for Chronic Diseases, and of Bedford Hill Sanatorium for Incipient Tuberculosis. Third edition, revised and enlarged. Pp. 891; 129 engravings and 28 plates. Philadelphia and New York: Lea & Febiger.

Books descriptive of a single disease are so frequently written by a specialist with the object of exploiting some special views or method of treatment, that they are generally viewed with suspicion by the general practitioner. Unfortunately many works on tuberculosis devote too much space to one phase of the disease, while other equally important aspects are treated briefly and casually. This too-frequent failing has been avoided in the third edition of this unusually well-balanced work, which has been improved by the addition of several chapters dealing with certain phases of this disease frequently disregarded, while the other chapters have been largely rewritten or amplified so as to present the more recent views and researches. While it is impossible to agree fully with all the views of this author, there is no recent work which presents the subject of tuberculosis in such a convenient form, from such a sane viewpoint, and at the same time contains so much information of equal value to the general practitioner and to those physicians who are specially interested in this disease. C.

Modern Methods in the Diagnosis and Treatment of Renal Disease. By Hugh MacLean, M.D., D.Sc., Professor of Medicine, University of London and Director of the Medical Clinic, St. Thomas's Hospital. Pp. 102; 4 illustrations. Philadelphia and New York: Lea & Febiger, 1922.

To those of the medical profession interested in the study of kidney disease no more thorough and comprehensive volume of its size has been placed before the reader. Concentrated in a comparatively few pages are all the important facts that have to do with the diagnosis and treatment of renal disease. This concentration of the subject matter is of particular value to the practitioner because in the past few years in many ways our conception of nephritides has very materially changed and many new studies have appeared which have to do with the determination of the function of the kidneys. The author deals with first the chief functions of the kidney, then goes on and discusses the kidney in disease, the significance of albumin and casts, blood examinations and other tests to determine renal function. He describes the proper examination of patients to determine renal inefficiency and has a series of illustrative cases. He also writes upon the importance of determining the condition of the kidney in certain surgical lesions and concludes with some observations on the dietetic treatment of nephritis. All these phases of urinary pathology and diagnosis are treated most sensibly. The book is well rounded out, well proportioned and can be heartily recommended to the practitioner of medicine. M.

Advanced Suggestion. By Haydn Brown, L.R.C.P. (Edin.), F.R.S.M. Pp. 402. New York: William Wood & Company, 1922.

This is the second edition, a review of the first one having appeared in this journal a few years ago. Inasmuch as there have been very slight changes, with the exception of the addition of three chapters, the original review is herewith reprinted.

"On page 230, in a chapter on 'A Study in Morbid Growths,' appears the following paragraph: 'I have myself, at will—knowing how to act and what to expect—obtained unquestionable results by psychotherapy in dealing with examples of organic disease and abnormal growth, which could not be exceeded by radium in similar cases.'

"On the next page, paragraph 8 reads as follows: 'I have indisputable proof of organic disorder and the development of newgrowth having been originated by suggestion. In one such case I have reversed the causative impression, and the newgrowth has regressed and disappeared.'

"A further reading of this chapter denotes that the author has the belief that cancer can be cured by psychotherapy, or, as he calls it, neuroinduction. He prefers the latter to suggestion, for neuroinduction to him implies 'the accurate conveyance of reliable sensations and conclusions, and their correct interpretation; it is a true sense demonstration and elucidation, both physically and mentally.'

"The author in his introduction to the chapter 'Study in Morbid Growths,' which contains the paragraphs mentioned above, makes the following naïve statement: 'I wrote the following eight and a half pages some time before finishing this book and I offered it to two of the leading medical journals. It was declined—for what reason I shall probably never know; but I can only think, in all charitableness of heart, that the time was not ripe for it.' He later mentions specifically the *British Medical Journal* as one journal which refused to publish his views.

"It is hardly necessary to say any more about this book on *Advanced Suggestion*. The astonishing part is that such a work as this should be put on the market by a reputable publisher and that the author is a Fellow of the Royal Society of Medicine."

A further surprising fact is that this book has reached its second edition, from which it is a justifiable conclusion that the medical public will buy anything that appears in book form.

TREATMENT OF INJURIES OF THE PERIPHERAL SPINAL NERVES. By SIR HAROLD J. STILES, K.B.E., F.R.C.S. (EDIN.), Regius Professor of Clinical Surgery, University of Edinburgh; and M. F. FORRESTER-BROWN, M.S., M.D., formerly Surgeon, Edinburgh War Hospital. Pp. 178; 67 illustrations, of which 33 are in color. Oxford Medical Publications, 1922.

THIS monograph has as its object "to place at the disposal of the general surgeon who may be called upon to deal with an occasioual case of peripheral nerve injury, the experience which has been gathered from the exceptionally abundant material provided by the Great War." The authors have had an unusually large experience in this field of work and in this book attain their object. It cannot be looked upon as an exhaustive treatise on the subject nor has it been intended to be. The reviewer has no criticism to offer of either the text or the illustrations, both of which are good. Undoubtedly, the general surgeon may find himself in a position of having to do peripheral nerve surgery, in which event he will find this book useful. The reviewer believes, however, that the general surgeon is not the one to do this work if others are available who have made a special study of neurologic surgery. Peripheral nerves are in reality prolongations of the central nervous system, and it requires more than written directions to handle its lesions properly. The reviewer was pleased to see the stress laid upon anatomy in this monograph. It is unquestionably true that the surgery of lesions of the peripheral nerves require an exact knowledge of the anatomy of the part in question. It is hoped that we will soon begin to hear of the end-results of the various operative procedures used in treating nerve injuries, especially in the Great War. Then will we really learn the value of each procedure. R.

De Arte Phisicali et de Cirurgia of Master John Arderne, Surgeon of Newark. Dated 1412. Translated by Sir D'Arcy Power, K.B.E., M.B. (Oxford), F.R.C.S.; from a transcript made by Eric Millar, M.A. (Oxford). Pp. 60; 14 illustrations. New York: William Wood & Company, 1922.

Master John Arderne, of Newark, was born in 1307, and became an operating surgeon, whose practice lay among the nobility, wealthy landowners and the higher clergy. He was a sound, practical surgeon and taught that wounds should heal without suppuration. He cut boldly and invented the operation for the cure of fistula, which, after falling into disuse for nearly five hundred years, is now universally employed. His medical treatment, on the other hand, was that of his time, employing spells, herbs and nasty or innocuous substances. The present work consists of a photographic reproduction of an illustrated manuscript of Arderne's works, with a translation and notes by Sir D'Arcy Power. The illustrations are very quaint and the many medicinal treatments are amazing; the surgical sections are of much greater interest.

As the first research study in medical history of the Wellcome Historical Medical Museum, the book should be well received and should be of value to those interested in early surgery and in the history of medicine. P.

Aids to Bacteriology. By William Partridge. Fourth edition. Pp. 276. New York: William Wood & Company, 1922.

In this new edition the author has made many additions, bringing his book well abreast of the times. Preparations of more recent media have been incorporated and the H-ion method of titration is suggested, but the reader is referred to other sources for its technic.

The different typhoid vaccines and the Dreyer agglutination test have been added to the section on typhoid; and the anaërobes have been brought up to date by the inclusion of those isolated from wounds and soil during the war, with comments on wound antiseptics. Among the filtrable viruses, additions have been made to the foot-and-mouth disease, trench fever and typhus fever—also the Proteus X-9 agglutination test. The fermentation reactions of the common yeasts have been tabulated.

In all, the book must be considered as a manual. As such, it will be of assistance to the laboratory diagnostician in the determination of pathogenic bacteria—Trichomycetes, Blastomycetes, Hyphomycetes and Protozoa alike. J.

MANUAL OF PHYSIOTHERAPEUTICS. By THOMAS DAVEY LUKE, formerly Physician, Peebles Hydropathic, Peebles, N. B.; Assistant Physician, Smedley's Hydropathic, Matlock; some time lecturer at the Edinburgh University. Second edition. Pp. 480; 210 illustrations. New York: William Wood & Company, 1922.

THIS work is a revised edition of the author's *Manual of Natural Therapy*, published in 1908. The practitioner will here find adequate descriptions of the theory and technic of therapy by means of heat, light, baths, massage, electricity and other physical agents. The fundamental defect of the work—shared by the majority of books and papers upon this subject—consists in the too ready acceptance of unproved dicta. Indeed there is probably no field in medicine which more richly deserves a thoroughgoing investigation from the standpoint of modern physiology than the field of physiotherapy, and until such an investigation is forthcoming we need feel no surprise that the claims of the osteopath and chiropractor remain unrefuted in the public mind. However, despite the fact that in reading this book one is here and there reminded of these less legitimate schools of therapy, the book, on the whole, is well arranged and compares favorably with other standard works on physiotherapeutics. A.

BASAL METABOLISM: ITS DETERMINATION AND APPLICATION. Edited by FRANK B. SANBORN, M.S. Pp. 282. Boston: Sanborn Company, 1922.

THIS volume is intended to supply physicians and technicians with a reference book that will be a guide in making basal metabolism tests and in interpreting the same. The editor has prepared some original articles which deal with the fundamental principles while the remainder of the book consists of compilations of abstracts and original papers by various authors, each dealing with a different phase of the subject. The result of this is much repetition.

A description is given of the various types of indirect calorimeters, without comment on the merits of each type. It seems to the reviewer that a few words on the advantages and disadvantages of the open and closed types might have been given and a spirit of impartiality still maintained. This book will find a place with those who wish a digest of this subject without going into the voluminous literature. J.

CANCER OF THE BREAST AND ITS TREATMENT. By H. SAMPSON HANDLEY, M.S., M.D. (LOND.), F.R.C.S. (ENG.), Hunterian Professor of Surgery and Pathology in the Royal College of Surgeons of England; Surgeon to the Middlesex Hospital and to Its Cancer Charity, and Lecturer to Its Medical School. Second edition. Pp. 404; 82 illustrations. New York: Paul B. Hoeber, 1922.

THE present edition contains new chapters on Radiologic Treatment, on Recurrence and Its Operative Treatment, on Paget's Disease of the Nipple, on Lymphangioplasty, and on Injury as a Causative Factor in Carcinoma. Chapter IX has been rewritten.

The work contains, as one would surmise, a complete review of the author's researches on dissemination, which he concludes is proven for cancer of the breast. Should it prove to be true for all the carcinomata, the surgery of malignant disease for the first time is placed upon a rational basis, and a criterion is provided by which variations in surgical technic can be judged.

The importance of pathology in the approach to the operative treatment of cancer is emphasized, for technical work must be guided and checked at every step by a first-hand pathologic knowledge. The type of operation which the author performs, therefore, is based upon such information, and important facts are discussed in planning the skin incision, removal of the permeated area of deep fascia, etc.—all of which are of the utmost importance.

The work is distinctly a review of the author's own ideas and technic. No mention is made of the type of operative procedure successfully carried out by other surgeons, if such procedure does not accord fully with the theory of permeation. He believes roentgen-rays are suitable, especially for prophylactic irradiation, covering a wide area, or for the treatment of multiple scattered deposits in the parietes. Radium should be given the preference if the recurrence is single, or if nodules are only present in one or several limited areas. With all its limitations, radium has secured a definite position in the treatment of breast cancer, relieving pain, prolonging life, and in single recurrences it presumably may complete the cure of the disease.

The chapter on Lymphangioplasty describes the method of performing this operation, and the benefits, as well as cases suitable for this measure are discussed. The chapter on Injury as a Causative Factor in Carcinoma alludes to many facts of importance from the medicolegal standpoint. S.

PHYSIOLOGY AND BIOCHEMISTRY IN MODERN MEDICINE. By J. J. R. MACLEOD, Professor of Physiology in the University of Toronto; assisted by R. G. PEARCE, A. C. REDFIELD and N. B. TAYLOR and others. Fourth edition. Pp. 992; 243 illustrations. St. Louis: C. V. Mosby Company, 1922.

THE presentation to the public of the fourth edition of the author's well-known text-book follows most appropriately the important work on pancreatic extracts that has recently appeared from his laboratory. One looks eagerly to find if it has been included and is rewarded on pages 713 to 715 with a modest but satisfactory account of "insulin" and its effects.

Important additions have also been made in the section devoted to the circulation of the blood. In the chapters on the electrocardiogram are to be found, in addition to the usual subject-matter, a full description of the "triangle method," Lewis's concept of the "bicardiogram" and the "circus-movement" hypothesis of auricular flutter, the last properly credited to Mines. Space forbids to do more than mention other subjects that have been rewritten, such as the output of the heart, intracardiac pressure, acid-base equilibrium, capillary circulation, etc. Considering that only two years have elapsed since the appearance of the third edition, the authors seem to have amply realized the function of the volume, "To describe not merely what already has been achieved in the clinical applications of physiology, but also to anticipate where this application is likely soon to be made and to prepare the way by describing the physiologic principles that may be involved." In spite of the limitations acknowledged in the preface, one cannot but be surprised at the total omission of a consideration of the special senses, the spleen and other organs of internal secretion.

K.

PROGRESS

OF

MEDICAL SCIENCE

MEDICINE

UNDER THE CHARGE OF

W. S. THAYER, M.D.

PROFESSOR OF MEDICINE, JOHNS HOPKINS UNIVERSITY, BALTIMORE, MARYLAND

AND

ROGER S. MORRIS, M.D.,

FREDERICK FORCHEIMER PROFESSOR OF MEDICINE IN THE UNIVERSITY OF CINCINNATI, CINCINNATI, OHIO,

Cardiac Gallop Rhythms.—LeBard (*Arch. d. mal. du cœur,* 1922, **15**) contributes an exhaustive study of gallop and triple cardiac rhythm. Acoustic differences between the various types (he recognizes three) are drawn with a fine distinction that is not usually attempted by American clinicians: (I) The presystolic (or mesodiastolic) gallop rhythm of the "nephritic heart" is described as representing not only the gallop sound that occurs shortly before the first heart sound, but others that extend forward into mesodiastole and which may be actually nearer the preceding second sound than the succeeding first sound. The author points out that wherever this sound occurs, however, it is a phenomenon of telediastole. The presystolic gallop is generally believed to be due to auricular contraction. (II) The protosystolic gallop is due, he believes, to a dissociation of the valvular and the muscular elements of the first sound. It is compatible with a long period of compensation and is in this respect different from the presystolic or mesodiastolic gallop, which is an indication *per se* of cardiac strain. The author does not differentiate this type of split first sound from the reduplication that may occur in normal hearts in the erect posture, and does not describe the effect of posture upon this type of gallop. (III) The protodiastolic gallop is rare, but the author has had several instances of it. It differs radically from the first two types, from the clinical point of view, though it resembles the mesodiastolic gallop closely in its acoustic properties. The protodiastolic gallop gives a more powerful, palpable, and sometimes visible, apical

thrust and is associated with jugular collapse; the other types are synchronous with a jugular wave. He presents tracings which show that this type of gallop definitely precedes auricular contraction and is, therefore, a physiologic entity.

The Toxicity and Parasiticidal Action of Arsenicals as Influenced by Their Rate of Excretion.—Voegtlin and Thompson (*Jour. Pharm. and Exp. Therap.*, 1922, **20**, 85) have studied in albino rats the rate of excretion of three groups of arsenical compounds, the trivalent arsenoxides, arsenobenzene derivatives (the arsphenamin group), and pentavalent arsenicals, and have compared the rates of excretion with the factors of toxicity and parasiticidal action. They find considerable variation in the rate of excretion in different individuals of the same species. The trivalent oxide compounds, which are more toxic and also more active therapeutically, show the slowest rate of excretion; the comparatively nontoxic and therapeutically less active pentavalent compounds are excreted with the greatest rapidity, while the arsenobenzene derivatives occupy an intermediate position. The ratio between urinary and fecal excretion of different drugs shows great variation, from 80 to 90 per cent of the pentavalent compounds being excreted through the urine, while 82 per cent of injected arsphenamin leaves the body through the feces. The authors believe that the evidence indicates that the chemical constitution, in so far as it is responsible for the physical properties of an arsenical, determines its rate of excretion and, therefore, its toxicity and parasiticidal action. In the next paper of the series, Voegtlin, Dyer and Miller (*Jour. Pharm. and Exp. Therap.*, 1922, **20**, 129) show that if the removal of arsenicals from the body is prevented, by means of complete ligation of the ureters, bile duct, or both (depending upon the type of drug and its relative urinary and fecal excretion), their toxicity and parasiticidal activity is greatly enhanced. When the ureters alone were ligated this effect was marked only in those drugs chiefly excreted through the kidneys; and in the same way ligation of the bile duct alone caused a great increase in the toxicity and trypanocidal activity of arsphenamin and neoarsphenamin, which are largely excreted in the feces. The authors conclude that their experiments offer direct proof of the theory that the toxicity and therapeutic value of arsenicals is governed by the rate of excretion from the body, and that Ehrlich's chemical theory of organotropism and parasitotropism is disproved. Retention of arsenicals by the tissues of the host is, therefore, a necessary requisite for drugs of practical chemotherapeutic value, but the retention must be followed by such a chemical change, effected by the tissues, as ultimately to lead to the formation of arsenic in a form which can be easily excreted.

The Apparent Role of Immunity in the Genesis of Neurosyphilis.—The present status of our knowledge on this important subject is summed up by Keidel (*Jour. Am. Med. Assn.*, 1922, **79**, 874). He points out the applicability to neurosyphilis of the "laws of progression and of inverse proportions," *i. e.*, that various tissue groups are not equally susceptible and reactive to syphilitic infection, and that an inverse quantitative relationship exists in the intensity of consecutive reactions to infection. Thus, the incidence and gravity of neurologic reaction is regulated by the antecedent tissue reactions in other parts of the body, so that patients who show only mild reactions to early syphilis are more liable to neurosyphilis than those who have severe secondary lesions. The author points out, however, that the influence of natural immune reactions may be greatly altered by the factor of antisyphilitic treatment. It is shown that in early syphilis a short course of intensive treatment predisposes the patient to neurosyphilis while prolonged courses of adequately intensive, continuous treatment greatly reduce the incidence of neurologic damage. Another modifying factor in women is pregnancy, which tends to suppress the lesions of syphilis, particularly neurosyphilis, and to induce latency.

Effects of Antisyphilitic Therapy as Indicated by the Histologic Study of the Cerebral Cortex in Cases of General Paresis.—SOLOMON and TAIT (*Arch. Neur. and Psych.*, 1922, **8**, 341) have had the unusual opportunity of studying histologically the brains of 27 cases of general paresis which had been more or less intensively treated during life. For purposes of comparison, the brains of 15 untreated cases were also studied. So far as parenchymatous, true vascular or neuroglia changes are concerned, no conclusions could be drawn because of the nature of the pathology of these structures in general paresis. The critical finding of diffuse plasma cells in the perivascular and pial infiltration could be fairly accurately compared in the treated and untreated groups. It was found that plasma cells were few and infrequent in most of the treated patients, and this was so uniformly the case that it was often possible to predict from the histologic picture whether or not the patient had been treated. Also both lymphocytic perivascular infiltration and pial infiltration were strikingly less in the treated than in the untreated group. Neither the age of the patient, the clinical variety of the psychosis, its duration, nor the kind and amount of treatment given seemed to have any distinct bearing on the amount of cellular inflammatory reaction. They conclude that antisyphilitic treatment of paretics does affect the histologic picture and that this is probably an evidence of lessened chronicity of the process.

Glucose-tolerance Test.—BEELER, BRYAN, CATHCARD and FITZ (*Jour. Metab. Res.*, 1922, **1**, 549), by the aid of the stomach tube, found that there was great variation in the absorption of glucose ingested for the purpose of determining tolerance. Administration of the glucose intravenously corrected this error, but added to the complication of the procedure. The writers suggest, therefore, that the glucose be administered by mouth, as usual, and that at the end of an hour, the stomach should be completely emptied. The amount of glucose recovered in the stomach contents should be subtracted from the amount originally given and the amount absorbed per kilo body weight thus calculated. Interpretation of the resulting blood-sugar curve may then be based upon a knowledge of the approximate amount of glucose which was able to influence that curve. Other factors of error, such as variation in the speed of absorption from the small intestine and increase of blood volume by absorption of fluid may be safely disregarded.

SURGERY

UNDER THE CHARGE OF

T. TURNER THOMAS, M.D.

ASSOCIATE PROFESSOR OF APPLIED ANATOMY AND ASSOCIATE IN SURGERY IN THE UNIVERSITY OF PENNSYLVANIA; SURGEON TO THE PHILADELPHIA GENERAL AND NORTHEASTERN HOSPITALS AND ASSISTANT SURGEON TO THE UNIVERSITY HOSPITAL.

Recognition of Congenital Syphilitic Inflammation of the Long Bones.—TURNBULL (*Lancet*, 1922, **1**, 1239) believes that syphilis in the fetus or in infants may give rise to inflammation in the diaphysis at a distance from the epiphysis or in the periosteum. Much more commonly, however, it causes inflammation in the diaphysis at its junction with the epiphyseal cartilage; that is to say, in the metaphysis and in the epiphyseal cartilage itself. Congenital syphilitic disease of bone is not a general systemic condition, but is due to the local presence of spirochetes. The older the child, the fewer are the portions of bone affected. In the fetus the infection tends to be widespread, but it is not necessarily universal. The femur, tibia, humerus and ribs are sites of election.

Pyelography.—KIDD (*Brit. Med. Jour.*, 1922, **1**, 748) considers it unwise to try to do both kidneys at one sitting. It is a mistake to employ too large a ureteral catheter. The author makes use of a No. 5½ Charriere. Sterilization of catheters with hot formalin vapor helps to avoid implanting infection in the kidney. It is quite a useless procedure to measure the amount of urine coming away, with the idea that this will give information as to whether the renal pelvis is a large one or a small one and as to how much fluid to inject before taking a picture. This is the bedrock difficulty in pyelography. This method of clinical research is indicated particularly in cases of severe abdominal pain of doubtful origin, to determine the nature of abdominal tumors and to complete the diagnosis in many cases of hematuria and pyuria.

Hyperplasia of the Rudimentary Lymph Nodes of the Prostate.—FUKOSE (*Surg., Gynec. and Obst.*, 1922, **25**, 131) says that small, primitive or rudimentary lymph nodes occur normally throughout the prostate in the form of very small aggregations of lymphocytes located beneath the glandular and duct epithelium, most marked toward the outlets of the ducts. They are analogous to the rudimentary lymph nodes found in other organs as the liver, kidneys, uterus, etc. Hyperplasia of these rudimentary lymph nodes of the prostate occurs chiefly in chronic hyperplastic prostatitis and in primary carcinoma of the prostate. In both conditions the hyperplasia is essentially an inflammatory one, due to chronic infection or irritation and possesses the same significance that such hyperplasiæ have in other parts of the body. In the absence of chronic inflammation a hyperplasia of the primitive lymph nodes of the prostate occurs in the lymphatic constitution and may be found also in other generalized diseases of the lymphoid system as Hodgkin's disease, lymphocytoma and leukemia. In both the inflammatory and noninflammatory hyperplasias, well-developed germinal centers may be produced in the hyperplastic node. Other evidences of functional activity by these hyperplastic nodes are shown in the metastasis of pigment, tubercle bacilli and carcinoma cells to them.

Malignant Neoplasms of the Extrahepatic Biliary Ducts.—RENSHAW (*Ann. Surg.*, 1922, **76**, 205) says that cancer of the bile ducts as a clinical and pathologic entity was not recognized previous to the middle of the nineteenth century. Malignancy of the bile ducts, while less common than that of the gall-bladder, is not uncommon. The ratio in a series of 104 cases of malignancy of the biliary ducts and gall-bladder was 1 to 4. Carcinoma is the most common type of neoplasm found. Gall stones would seem to be of greater etiologic importance than is generally considered. About two-thirds of the cases occur between the ages of fifty and seventy years. A diagnosis of malignancy of the ducts is uncertain. After a diagnosis of obstructive jaundice has been made exploration is generally advisable. From the standpoint of slowness of growth and rarity of metastasis, surgical treatment should be favorable.

Air Embolism following Various Diagnostic or Therapeutic Procedures in Diseases of the Pleura and the Lung.—SCHLOEPFER (*Johns Hopkins Hosp. Bull.*, September, 1922, p. 321) emphasizes that complications may follow various diagnostic and therapeutic procedures. The sudden release of a great amount of fluid in emaciated people with a neurotic constitution may cause a similar clinical picture. Because of its slightness and short duration with lack of localized cerebral symptoms and serious sequelæ, this condition is considered to be due to shock. Chronic myocardial lesions or an insufficiency of the adrenals may cause sudden death during the performance of one of these operations on the chest wall. A similar clinical picture is seen in embolism of the pulmonary artery. Death accompanied by these signs may occur also in a few cases of emboli in the brain following thrombosis of pulmonary veins. It was demonstrated by experiments that we do not have a pleural reflex even in the normal pleura, which would explain these complications. They are proved by the accidents in pneumothorax therapy to be due to air emboli. The pathologic condition of the lung and of the pleural sheaths is the same in all these cases. The lung tissue shows in a circumscribed area a condition which is partly an infiltration, partly an induration of the tissue where the bloodvessels, especially the veins with their weaker walls, are fixed in a distended position.

An Experimental Study of the Ureter after Nephrectomy.—LATCHEM (*Jour. Urol.*, 1922, **8**, 257) finds that in the normal ureter after nephrectomy no attempt is made toward obliteration of the lumen by disappearance or atrophy of the mucous membrane; there is a noticeable atrophy of the muscular coat. Hydronephrosis developed in every case following the production of complete obstruction of the ureter, the condition progressing to complete destruction of the substance of the kidney unless the obstruction was removed. The ureter after complete obstruction becomes a hydroureter by distention of the ureteral lumen with the retained urine. Hypertrophy of the muscular layers, chiefly of the circular, occurs. In the hypertrophic hydroureter or pyoureter with drainage of its contents after nephrectomy, the mucous membrane remains intact and the muscular coat gradually atrophies. In hypertrophic hydroureter or pyoureter with complete obstruction to drainage of the ureteral contents after nephrectomy, the mucous membrane remains intact and the muscular coats remain hypertrophic. Absorption of the contents of a distended ureter is very limited if it occurs at all. If infection is present in the contents of the ureter, it may spread through the wall and give rise to periureteral infection and abscess formation.

Some Experiences with the Meltzer-Lyon Test in Gall-bladder Disease.—Cutler and Newton (*Surg., Gynec. and Obst.*, 1922, **35**, 146) think that there is still much to be proven before the so-called Meltzer-Lyon test can be accepted as of value in aiding diagnosis, for it is only in the experimental stage. The test depends upon the law of contrary innervation, which must be proven before the test is accepted. At the present time evidence would seem to show that syphonage is the principal factor in the dejection of bile into the duodenum. It is the authors' opinion that dark bile comes from the gall-bladder, for dark bile has never been found in cholecystectomized cases. The contentions of Einhorn and Meyer, that the dark color is due to reëxcretion of the salt or to destruction of red blood cells in the liver, with the production of excess iron, must bear further study. The authors' experience has given the distinct impression that the test is not of dependable diagnostic aid.

Tuberculosis in Children from the Standpoint of the Surgeon.—Brown (*Boston Med. and Surg. Jour.*, September 28, 1922, p. 470) says that at present there are no accurate statistics in Massachusetts as to the number of nonpulmonary cases of tuberculosis and this lack is due to failure of hospitals and physicians to report their cases. Surgery in tuberculosis is and should be the exception and that it should always be made only an incident in the general and necessarily prolonged treatment. In children operations for spinal immobilization are not advisable, and without the proper postoperative care in adults do not give the results claimed. Ambulatory and supportive treatment both in adults and children have not given satisfactory results. The ideal treatment for children is recumbency, for at least two to three years, followed by carefully observed and protected weight-bearing for two years more. For adults in selected cases the operation for spinal immobilization may be advisable if it can be followed by at least six months of recumbency and a year or more of supportive treatment. In Massachusetts there are no hospitals, however, with equipment or personnel which can adequately carry out the prolonged treatment of recumbency and heliotherapy.

PEDIATRICS

UNDER THE CHARGE OF

THOMPSON S. WESTCOTT, M.D., AND ALVIN E. SIEGEL, M.D.,
OF PHILADELPHIA.

Dried Milk Powder in Infant Feeding.—CLARK and COLLINS (*Public Health Reports*, 1922, **40**, 2417) studied 319 infants. Of these, 241 were under observation a sufficiently long time to furnish reliable data for use in tabulating weights. No infant was included in the tabulation of results unless there was a record of weighing for at least four weeks; but in most cases the observations extended over a much longer period. Those babies fed on grade "A" milk were included in a group called Group I. In Group II there were those infants fed on reconstituted whole-milk powder. Considerable difficulty was experienced by the workers to gain the consent of the mothers to place infants on the reconstructed milk made from skimmed-milk powder and butter fat, for which reason Group III comprised a far smaller number. It was difficult to educate the mothers to this new form of infant-feeding. It was also difficult to get them to use this preparation, as the failure to procure a perfect emulsion made a certain collection of fat in the top of the bottles which did not appeal to them. In all age classes the infants fed on a modification of cows' milk made distinctly less progress as measured by gain in weight than those fed on a modification made from whole-milk powder. The difference was especially marked in the younger group—from one to three months old. The infants fed on a modification reconstructed from unsalted butter and skimmed-milk powder increased less rapidly in weight in the older groups and in the total groups; but in the younger age group the gain in weight closely approximated that of infants on whole-milk powder for about eleven weeks. After the twelfth week on this diet the rate decreased and the weight curve approached that of Group I. Because the weight curves for Group I were consistently below those for Group II for all age groups, the authors felt safe in concluding that the infants fed on whole-milk powder gained in weight more rapidly than did those fed on cows' milk. On account of the small number in Group III no definite conclusions were attempted. As regards scurvy, they feel that protection is dependent upon the antiscorbutic content of the particular dried milk used. The dried milks vary in this way in just the same manner that fresh milks do. To safeguard against the developing of this condition, orange juice or some similar material rich in antiscorbutic vitamine should be given routinely. The relation of the diet to rickets is much more complicated. It has been shown that some of the dried milks are as rich in antirachitic factor as cows' milk. A complete examination was made in 200 of these infants enrolled for this study and special attention was directed toward the incidence of rickets. One of the important points brought out by these examinations was the frequency and the similar distribution of this disorder in the different feeding groups. A number of these infants undoubtedly presented a slight degree of rickets at the time of enrollment, but on account of the relatively short period of observation of the individual cases it was impossible to state with positiveness the effect of dried-milk feeding on the course of this disorder. It is important to note that the infants studied were recruited from homes of varied economic and hygienic status, and were fed on milk products containing fat in the usual percentages. This seems to indicate that other factors than the deficiency of fat-soluble vitamine must be taken into consideration in any attempt to determine the true cause of rickets. The writers feel as a result of their observations that dried-milk powders and their remade products, such as were used in this study, are safe for infant-feeding, and in some cases seem to have distinct therapeutic effect.

Rabbit Hair Asthma in Children.—Ratner (*Am. Jour. Dis. Child.*, 1922, **24**, 346) says that rabbit hair as an etiologic factor in the production of asthma would at first hand appear to be of little practical significance. As a matter of fact, its distribution is widespread, and it should be placed second to horse hair as a causative agent in the keratin group of asthma. Desensitization of this group of cases has not been successful, but the removal of the hair is easily accomplished, and avoiding the hair relieves the patient of all symptoms. In attempts at desensitization, the writer calls attention to certain dangers inherent in this form of treatment, and adrenalin should always be kept on hand to combat any emergency that may arise. Dosage undoubtedly plays a large part in the production of attacks. Human beings are capable of showing what might be called temporary desensitization. Eczema, vomiting, angioneurotic edema, urticaria and conjunctivitis may all occur as direct result of contact with animals besides the classic symptoms of asthma. In the way of prophylaxis it is recommended that rabbit hair and all fine dust-producing substances be kept out of pillows, mattresses, clothing and toys that are used for infants and young children. Those suffering from chronic coryza should be studied from the standpoint of their being potential asthmatics.

The Food Requirements of Children: Percentage Distribution of Calories.—Holt and Fales (*Am. Jour. Dis. Child.*, 1922, **24**, 290) emphasize the importance of the balanced ration. The protein need of the growing child is very important and there seems to be a fairly general understanding of the amount required. All evidence seems to indicate than when 15 per cent of the theoretical total caloric need is supplied by protein, the nutritive needs in protein are met. The amount of fat required is still a subject of debate, but it seems reasonable and desirable that the amount of fat given the growing child should be equal to the amount of protein. Since fat has two and a quarter times the caloric value of protein, equal amounts of fat and protein would supply calories in the proportion of 2.25 to 1. When the protein furnished is 15 per cent of the total calories, an equal amount of fat would furnish about 35 per cent of the total calories. The remaining caloric need of 50 per cent would then be supplied by the carbohydrate.

When this distribution is deviated from, to any marked degree, for a long period of time, or when the proper balance of the diet is disturbed, various undesirable results may follow. If the protein is reduced much below 15 per cent of the caloric requirement, the nutritive need may not be met. If the fat given supplies much less than 35 per cent of the total caloric requirement, it usually happens that the caloric intake is excessive in carbohydrate and digestive disturbances usually follow. If the fat supplies too high a proportion of the total caloric requirements the fat tolerance of the child may be exceeded, and digestive upset may result. High fat with low protein forms a food from which constipation is likely to result. Low fat with high carbohydrate is apt to cause diarrhea.

Studies on Experimental Measles.—Duval and D'Aunoy (*Jour. Exper. Med.*, 1922, **36**, 239) obtained defibrinated human blood from measles cases at the stage of high temperature. This was inoculated into experimental animals. Their results show that an active transmissible virus exists in the blood of measles patients during the eruptive stage of the disease. The virus produces in rabbits after intravenous injection a specific reaction analogous in all essential features to that of the human infection. Repeated passage of the virus of measles through rabbits seems to increase its virulence. It is a noteworthy fact the pneumonia, so common in the fatal cases of human measles, was not evident in any of these experimental animals. The authors believe this to be of considerable significance, especially in elucidating the direct etiologic factor of the fatal pneumonias so often present in human measles cases. Apparently such infections in man can be explained purely on the basis of the destruction of normal defense barriers by the specific excitant of the infectious disease, and the lack of host resistance to the ordinary pyogenic bacteria.

Defects in School Children.—Bruce (*Brit. Med. Jour.*, 1922, **2**, 346) found that 58 per cent of the crippling existing at five years of age in 15,605 school children was due to rickets, and usually to rickets of the more severe type. The next most frequent cause of crippling was tuberculosis, which caused 9 per cent of the total crippling. He found comparatively little pulmonary tuberculosis. Routine medical inspection revealed no evidence of definite pulmonary tuberculosis, and only 7 suspected cases of the large total of 15,605 children examined. Chronic bronchitis was responsible for 6 per cent of the crippling found at this age. Mental deficiency comes next in the order of frequency, with 6.3 per cent, after nervous disorders with a percentage of 7.4. The cases of anemia and malnutrition, which account for 3.9 per cent of the total crippling, are those which showed no symptoms of other disease. In some of the cases a tuberculous family history could be elicited. The remaining 9 per cent of crippling was due to eye conditions, mostly strumous ophthalmia, a few cases of heart disease resulting from scarlet fever or rheumatism and other congenital and acquired deformities.

DERMATOLOGY AND SYPHILIS

UNDER THE CHARGE OF

JOHN H. STOKES, M.D.,

MAYO CLINIC, ROCHESTER, MINN.

Ulceration of the Female Genitalia.—Planner and Remenovsky (*Arch. f. Dermat. u. Syphilol.*, 1922, **140**, 162) describe cases illustrative of gonorrheal, aphthous and typhoid ulcerations of the female genitalia and of ulcerative lesions associated with erythema nodosum. The gonorrheal ulcer is the occasional sequel of perforation of a concealed Bartholin abscess through the labium, with involvement of the connective tissue, resulting in ulceration suggesting soft chancre. The gonococcus can be cultivated from the discharge from the ulcer base. It is often difficult to demonstrate the sinus-like connection with the gland. The authors insist that the term aphthous should be reserved for lesions of the vulva, in which no distinct etiologic factor can be recognized. The vaginal mucosa as well as the vulva may be involved and the eruptive outbreak preceded by a chill and high fever. Successive crops may occur, each associated with the same constitutional manifestations. Lesions of this type have been associated with erythema nodosum and with outbreaks of stomatitis. Bacteriologic investigation gives no characteristic findings. The authors describe a case of necrotic ulcer of the genitalia, associated with typhoid fever, in which typhoid bacilli were repeatedly recovered from the discharge from the lesions. The fourth group described includes 4 cases of tumor-like and ulcerative lesions of the genitalia, in 2 of which patients had demonstrable tuberculosis, and in 3 of which the lesions of erythema nodosum, associated with purpura and arthritic manifestations, were present. A similar case has been described by Jadassohn in 1904.

Hematogenous Distribution of Trichophyta.—Bruusgaard. (*British Jour. Dermat.*, 1922, **24**, 150) discusses the hematogenous distribution of trichophytic organisms and describes a case of kerion celsi in an elderly man, in which erythema multiforme-like lesions appeared upon the extremities. From these lesions tissue was obtained, in which it was possible to demonstrate the presence of trichophytic spores in the bloodvessels. Cultures from the fresh tissue showed the organism to be Trichophyton gypsum. The work of Bloch, Guth and others have shown that the deep pustular trichophyton infection of the skin is not infrequently associated with the development of eruptions, often follicular in character and general in distribution or nodular and localized on the extremities in certain cases, which strongly suggest a hematogenous distribution of the infecting agent. Immediately following the appearance of the Bruusgaard report, Pasini (*Arch. f. Dermat. u. Syphilol.*, 1922, **140**, 369) refers to Jessner's report in the same journal (1921) of the cultivation of Trichophyton gypsum from the blood of a boy, aged ten years, with an extensive lichenoid trichophytid of the body. He states that Ambrosoli has also succeeded in cultivating Trichophyton gypsum directly from the blood in a boy, aged eleven years, with kerion of the scalp, just at the time the patient was developing a lichenoid trichophytid. It appears that this group of observations substantiates the hitherto theoretical conceptions of the hematogenous trichophytic origin of the so-called trichophytids. Apart from its independent interest as an immunologic and bacteriologic fact, the direct cultivation of the responsible organism from the blood in an eruption clinically so closely homologous with certain tuberculids, is a point of much significance and encourages the belief that improved cultural methods and earlier observation of cases will ultimately conclusively demonstrate the presence of tuberculosis bacilli in the circulation of patients with certain types of tuberculids. Moreover, as Bruusgaard remarks, these observations remove the deeper trichophyton infections from the domain of purely local to that of systemic disease.

Intramuscular Administration of Arsphenamin.—The revival of interest in intramuscular injection as a mode of administering arsphenamin derivatives is expressed in several recent articles. Voegtlin, Dyer and Thompson (*Am. Jour. Syph.*, 1922, **6**, 576) cite Ehrlich's beliefs that intravenous use of these drugs should be regarded only as a means of avoiding the pain and inconvenience of the intramuscular technic. They quote Craig and Harrison as demonstrating a better effect of the latter method on the Wassermann, and cite also Voegtlin and Smith's demonstration of the superior trypanocidal effect of intramuscularly as compared with intravenously administered arsphenamin. The authors have conducted an experimental study of a derivative of arsphenamin closely related to neoarsphenamin (French trade name *sulpharsenol*), which they find is much less productive of local irritation even than neoarsphenamin when injected subcutaneously. Its trypanocidal effect is only slightly less than that of neoarsphenamin, its toxicity about equal to that of neoarsphenamin. It is very soluble and stable in solution, and produces little or no local irritation in the rat or rabbit in concentrations as high as 20 per cent in distilled water. The rate of excretion of the arsenic is about the same as that of arsphenamin and neoarsphenamin. The authors urge a more extended clinical trial of the drug as well suited to the needs of the general practitioner and possessing the advantages of intramuscular use without the disadvantages.

Comparisons of Arsphenamin and Neoarsphenamin.—The clinical differences between arsphenamin and neoarsphenamin, particularly with respect to therapeutic effectiveness, are illuminated by the report of Voegtlin and Miller (*Public Health Reports*, 1922, **37**, 1627) on a series of comparisons of the parasitic value of the two drugs. The trypanocidal index was used because of its greater dependability as compared with the variability of syphilitic infections in experimental animals. The authors compared thirteen lots of arsphenamin and fifteen lots of neoarsphenamin of different manufacture, most of them recent products. The trypanocidal power of arsphenamin is remarkably constant in contrast with the very great variability of neoarsphenamin. Both drugs showed a considerable variability in toxicity, with a distinct reduction as compared with the products made two years ago. The authors point out the very interesting parallel relation between increased toxicity and increased therapeutic effectiveness, which seems to indicate that the reaction-producing power of a given lot of the drug is by no means necessarily a reason for discarding it. The comparison between the two drugs is certainly distinctly in favor of arsphenamin as the more constant and dependable preparation. The wide use of neoarsphenamin would seem then to be a matter of convenience rather than of intrinsic merit.

OPHTHALMOLOGY

UNDER THE CHARGE OF

EDWARD JACKSON, A.M., M.D.,

DENVER, COLORADO,

AND

T. B. SCHNEIDEMAN, A.M., M.D.,

PHILADELPHIA.

Ill-effects of the Arsenobenzols.—MEYNIARD (*La clin. ophthal.*, August, 1922, p. 319) calls attention to the occurrence of fatal or grave accidents from the arsenobenzols, notwithstanding that these substances have been in use now for more than ten years and the technic of their employment greatly improved. These ill-effects may be due to the administration of an ill-preserved product, polluted water, excessively warm syringe, faulty sterilization, failure of preliminary fasting and resting, contraindications overlooked, injection pushed too rapidly. [Improper hydrion concentration.—ED.] Very frequently, however, accidents occur in spite of every precaution; these are then usually attributed to intoxication, an occurrence which unfortunately is still inevitable in the present state of our knowledge; or to inferior quality of the agent, responsibility for which rests upon the manufacturer, as it is impossible for the physician to gauge the exact composition of the medicament. It is to be hoped that chemical and biologic standardization of these substances may be rigorously carried out before they are furnished to the practitioner.

Hereditary Optic Atrophy (Leber's Disease).—LAGRANGE (*Arch. d'ophthal.*, September, 1922, p. 530) concludes that it has not been proven that Leber's hereditary optic atrophy is due to defective development of the skeleton (optic foramen, sphenoidal cells) acting mechanically upon the retrobulbar portion of the optic nerve. Fischer has drawn attention to the relations which may exist between the development of the endocrine system and hereditary optic atrophy; but his hypothesis of the mechanical effect exerted by an overgrown hypophysis or an enlarged sella turcica upon the adjacent optic nerve is unsatisfactory. In fact, in this disease the semeiology (white atrophy of the papilla, which is never one of stasis and always preserves its sharp contour with symptoms of retrobulbar neuritis) is clearly a syndrome, the opposite of that caused by intracranial tumors (papillary stasis) and in particular to juxtachiasmatic growths (temporal hemianopsia). In a case observed by the writer the blood presented a notable anomaly: Retarded coagulation with feebly retractile clot. It is remarkable that this particularity is precisely the stigma of hemophilia; now hemophilia and Leber's disease are comparable by their common character as hereditary diseases; the retarded coagulation in hemophilia may be considered as a simple stigma rather than as a symptom of pathogenic value. Without denying the numerous influences which may favor the occurrence of Leber's disease, in particular the associated influence of chronic intoxication, nor unmindful of the obscurities which surround the pathogeny of this hereditary malady, early endocrine opotherapy deserves a place as a treatment of choice.

Primary Intraneural Tumor (Glioma) of the Optic Nerve.—VERHOEFF (*Arch. Ophthal.*, 1922, **51**, 120, 239) publishes a histologic study of eleven cases of intraneural tumors of the optic nerve. His conclusions are that the most common tumors of the optic nerves are gliomas—in fact the only primary intraneural tumors of this nerve that have been observed. These tumors are composed of three main types of neuroglia which may grade into one another. Some tumors consist of all three types; rarely does one consist of a single type. Tumors, in which so-called spindle cells predominate, contain the largest and most conspicuous neuroglia fibers. The spongy structure often displayed by these tumors, which at times has led to a diagnosis of myxoma, myxoglioma or myxosarcoma, is not the result of myxomatous degeneration, but is produced by excessive vacuolization of a neuroglia syncytium. Cysts of various sizes, which also often occur in these tumors, are due to the same process. The tumor is probably essentially congenital in origin and dependent upon some abnormality in the embryonic development of the neuroglia of the optic nerve. The growth stimulates proliferation in all contiguous neuroglia tissue, and thus causes the latter to take on the character of tumor tissue. The theory that tumors of the optic nerve stem are related in origin to neurofibromas of the peripheral nerves is, at present, founded on insufficient evidence, but cannot be dismissed as impossible.

The Influence of Trauma Upon the Onset of Interstitial Keratitis.—BUTLER (*Brit. Jour. Ophth.*, September, 1922, p. 413) concludes that an attack of interstitial keratitis may be precipitated by an accident to a cornea which is disposed to the disease by syphilis or tubercle; such trauma may be very slight, even the instillation of drops or the irritation of a general anesthetic. The attack in the injured eye is liable to be followed by the same disease in the uninjured eye, or the injury to one eye alone may cause interstitial keratitis in the other eye; in fact is it not possible that in every case of interstitial keratitis the disease is precipitated by some slight trauma?

The Lachrymal Fluid.—Rotth (*Klin. Monats. f. Augenhk.*, April-May, 1922, p. 598) discusses the question whether the properties of the tears vary according as the stimuli which calls them forth is different. His conclusion is that the index of refraction of the fluid secreted under the same stimulus varies within wide limits in the same person as also in different individuals; these variations in all probability depend upon the admixture of varying amounts of conjunctival secretion. When the tests are made with anemic conjunctivæ results are more uniform; in this case it is the secretion of the lacrymal gland alone. The index of such portions as are gathered after different stimuli also varies considerably, but the average values are quite concordant,. showing that the lachrymal secretion from various stimuli is chemically identical in healthy eyes.

Ocular Complications of Pneumonia and Bronchopneumonia.—Villard (*Annal. d'oculist.*, October, 1922, p. 746) observes that of the various complications occurring in the course of pneumonia and bronchopneumonia, the ocular complications are the least known. He has been unable to find any mention of their occurrence in any work which he has consulted except two short paragraphs in the French *Encyclopedia of Ophthalmology*. From a lengthy study of the subject, he draws the following conclusions: In the course, or during the decline of pneumonia and bronchopneumonia there may supervene upon the part of the ocular apparatus an entire series of complications, rare indeed, but not so exceptional as to justify their entire neglect in classic works. The ocular complications are both extra- and intrabulbar. Among the former the least common are those which affect the conjunctiva, optic nerve and motor nerves, while the most frequent affect the cornea. These keratids may arise in the course of pneumonia, but more frequently complicate a severe bronchopneumonia, especially those occurring in the course of measles. They may take the form of an ordinary hypopyon keratitis, interstitial keratitis or a true keratomalacia; the prognosis is extremely unfavorable, resulting ordinarily in the loss of vision of the affected eye; in all probability, such keratids are due to an exogenous infection from the fingers or handkerchiefs soiled by expectoration in patients whose resistance has been lowered by the pulmonary affection. The intrabulbar complications may affect the iris, retina, the media and the deeper membranes of the eye. On the part of the iris there occurs exceptionally a true iritis, or more commonly, inequality of the pupils, the larger one corresponding to the side of the affected lung. Ophthalmoscopic examination shows inflammatory lesions of the retina, described by the author under the name "septic retinitis;" the lesions resemble tuberculosis of the retina and have a favorable prognosis. The media and deep membranes are at times gravely affected by lesions described under the name "metastatic ophthalmia;" this occurs in two forms: More rarely as a plastic iridochoroiditis, but most frequently as a suppurative iridochoroiditis, *i. e.*, a true panophthalmitis; this last affection is of endogenous origin, due to embolism of pneumococci which invade the vessels of the retina or perhaps those of the uveal tract.

PATHOLOGY AND BACTERIOLOGY

UNDER THE CHARGE OF

OSKAR KLOTZ, M.D., C.M.,

DIRECTOR OF THE PATHOLOGICAL LABORATORIES, SAO PAULO, BRAZIL,

AND

DE WAYNE G. RICHEY, B.S., M.D.,

ASSISTANT PROFESSOR OF PATHOLOGY, UNIVERSITY OF PITTSBURGH, PITTSBURGH, PA.

The Bacteriology of Human Cystic Bile.—In a series of 408 specimens of human bile, submitted by the surgeon at the time of cholecystostomy or recovered from the removed, intact gall-bladder shortly after operation and cultured, routinely, on plain serum broth with subsequent segregation of colonies on human blood-agar plates, isolation on slants and identification on appropriate carbohydrate fermentation "sets," RICHEY (*Penn. Med. Jour.*, 1922, **26**, 4) found pathogenic microörganisms in 173, or 44 per cent. The types of bacteria isolated fell within well-known groups, of which Bacillus coli was the most frequent (27 per cent), although due significance was given to Bacillus typhosus (7.4 per cent) and Bacillus paratyphosus (1.8 per cent) as well as to the other members of the colon-typhoid group. The Bacillus mucosus capsulatus group was responsible for 11.5 per cent of the positive cultures. Green streptococci (11.5 per cent) occurred twice as frequently as hemolytic streptococci (5.6 per cent), while staphylococci comprised 13.4 per cent. The author believes that the types of bacteria isolated, their relative incidence and usual habitat can be made to corroborate the statement of the experimental investigators that the two most important portals of entry of bacteria to the gall-bladder are the hematohepatogenous and the hematogenous, of which the former is the more frequent and important.

Complement-fixation in Typhoid Fever.—Although typhoid fever was one of the first diseases in which the phenomenon of complement-fixation was demonstrated, the field has not been explored extensively since the original endeavors of Bordet and Gengou. HADJOPOULOS (*Jour. Infect. Dis.*, 1922, **31**, 226) applied this test to 50 cases of typhoid and over 100 control cases. The complement-fixations were controlled by blood cultures and agglutination tests. Fresh human serum was placed in six pairs of small test-tubes in doses of 0.01, 0.02, 0.03, 0.04, 0.05 and 0.1 cc respectively. The left-hand series of tubes received 0.5 cc salt solution each and served as controls for the hemolytic value of serum in question. The right-hand tubes received 0.5 cc of the bacillary antigen each. After incubation at 37° C. for thirty minutes, 0.5 cc of 0.5 per cent suspension of sensitized sheep cells was added to all tubes. To those serums which were deficient in hemolytic value, a typhoid negative serum of high hemolytic value was added and the test carried on as usual. As a nucleus for antigen, eight or ten vaccines were collected from various sources. By enriching this from time to time with strains from cases with a positive blood culture and negative complement-fixation, an antigen was obtained which would detect at least 80 per cent of cases in all stages of disease from the first to the fifth week. In 50 cases of typhoid and over 100 control cases it was found that the percentage of positive blood cultures was higher during the first week than the complement-fixation or agglutination tests, but, with the beginning of the second week the blood-culture curve fell abruptly, the immune reaction curves rose steadily, the fixation curve always preceding. During the fourth week of the disease the agglutination curve reached its peak at 88 per cent, tending to fall thereafter, whereas the complement-fixation curve, from the fourth week and on, stood at 100 per cent. The pathologic conditions giving rise to nonspecific complement-fixation, excepting 1 case of typhus, clinically also could be differentiated from typhoid. On the other hand, nonspecific agglutination occurred in almost 100 per cent of acute infectious diseases as typhus, malaria, miliary tuberculosis, acute mastoiditis, acute appendicitis and influenza, that could not be easily differentiated from typhoid without further clinical and laboratory data. The authors believe that "In the course of typhoid infection the formation of complement-fixing antibodies is one of the earliest and most constant immune manifestations."

The Incubation Period of Typhoid Fever.—It is recognized generally that the incubation period of typhoid fever cannot be determined accurately, as a rule, as the exact date of infection is not known. Miner (*Jour. Infect. Dis.*, 1922, **31**, 296) has analyzed eleven reported typhoid fever epidemics in which the time of infection could be definitely established and in which, therefore, the distribution of the incubation period could be determined. By calculating the results of the various investigators with mathematical precision, it was found that the results were consonant with the belief that the length of the incubation period depends in part on the virulence of the infection and is extremely variable, ranging from three to thirty-eight or forty days. The mean incubation period in the different epidemics varied from 7. ± 0.26 to 19.5 ± 0.31, whereas the means for those due to infected food, in which the dose was in all probability more massive, were 7. ± 0.26 and 9.54 ± 0.39.

The Meiostagmin Reaction.—"The meiostagmin reaction (*meion*, small; *stasso*, drop) is the name given to a phenomenon, which involves a lowering surface tension during incubation when a diluted serum, containing certain antibodies, is mixed with its specific lipoid-containing antigen. First employed by Ascoli, working with alcoholic extracts of typhoid bacilli, the reaction was later applied by Ascoli and Izar to the diagnosis of certain malignant tumors with rather indifferent success. Like similar physicochemical reactions the method has not been used extensively by physicians, although several investigators have reported conflicting findings which have served to throw doubt on the procedure as to its efficacy. Recently Gouwens (*Jour. Infect. Dis.*, 1922, **31**, 237) conducted over eleven hundred tests in a study of this reaction, using almost two hundred different mixtures of rabbit serum and antigen. The serum was obtained from animals immunized against Bacillus paratyphosus B, and the antigens were prepared from homologous and several heterologous organisms, as well as from the liver of a healthy rabbit immune to Bacillus paratyphosus B. In making the tests it was found that the Du Nouy surface tension apparatus gave readings with the biochemical mixtures employed, which were as accurate as those obtainable with the more cumbersome and slow drop weight apparatus, while the sources of experimental error were less than those involved in the use of the Traube stalagmometer. The spontaneous surface tension changes and the limits of experimental error were as great as when relatively dilute serum was used as when the serum was diluted only 1 : 20, the blood serum being responsible for the relatively large error. The meiostagmin reaction did not reveal the presence of antibodies in Bacillus paratyphosus B immune rabbit serum of high titer regardless of the dilutions in which the serums and antigens were employed or of the solvents used in the preparation of the antigens.

The Hydrogen-ion Concentration of Joint Exudates in Rheumatic Fever and Other Forms of Arthritis.—In order to compare the reactions of the exudates in certain arthritic diseases and to determine whether an acidity occurs in the inflamed joints in acute rheumatic fever sufficient to permit the liberation of free salicylic acid following salicylate therapy, Boots and Cullen (*Jour. Exper. Med.*, 1922, **36**, 405) ascertained the hydrogen-ion concentration of 26 joint fluids including 16 from patients with acute rheumatic fever, 7 of undetermined origin and 2 with bacterial arthritis. In each instance the fluid was aspirated by means of a Luer syringe, care being taken throughout the entire determination to prevent the fluid from coming in contact with air. When large quantities of fluid were available both electrometric and colorimetric p^H determinations were made, although only the colorimetric method was used in the majority of cases. The electrometric measurements were conducted at 38° C. in the Clark cell, in a hydrogen atmosphere containing CO_2 at the tension existing in the joint fluid, while the colorimetric determinations method was that described by Cullen for the determination of the p^H concentration of blood. The joint fluids in the acute rheumatic fever patients were never frankly purulent, being viscous, slightly to definitely turbid and usually of a pale yellowish green color. The exudates contained considerable fibrin, forming soft clots on standing. Bacteriologically they were all sterile by ordinary culture methods. The fluids from the cases with arthritis of undetermined origin were indistinguishable from some of these exudates. It was found that, "With the exception of the joint exudates of the 2 patients with bacterial arthritis, the reactions were all slightly alkaline and approximated the normal reaction of blood," varying between p^H 7.27 and 7.42 in acute rheumatic fever and between p^H 7.33 and 7.47 in those arthritides of undetermined origin. The exudate from the knee-joint infected with Staphylococcus aureus was p^H 6.69 and from the one with Streptococcus hemolyticus, p^H 6.19, both being distinctly acid. The effusion from the patient with anasarca of myocardial insufficiency was p^H 7.34. The authors state that they have evidence to show that the exudates in experimental arthritis of animals inoculated with green streptococci are also acid and from their results "It would seem that if green streptococci were growing in the joint fluids of rheumatic fever patients, one would expect those fluids to be acid," which, as they have shown, is not the case. They conclude that "Since a definitely acid medium is necessary for the liberation of free salicylic acid and since all of the joint fluids from patients with acute rheumatic fever were slightly alkaline, no free salicylic acid could possibly exist in such joint fluids following the administration of salicylates."

HYGIENE AND PUBLIC HEALTH

UNDER THE CHARGE OF

MILTON J. ROSENAU, M.D.,

PROFESSOR OF PREVENTIVE MEDICINE AND HYGIENE, HARVARD MEDICAL SCHOOL, BOSTON, MASSACHUSETTS,

AND

GEORGE W. McCOY, M.D.,

DIRECTOR OF HYGIENIC LABORATORY, UNITED STATES PUBLIC HEALTH SERVICE, WASHINGTON, D. C.

The Use of Semilogarithmic Paper in Plotting Death Rates.—Whipple (*Public Health Reports*, 1922, **37**, 1891) emphasizes the advantage of semilogarithmic paper (vertical scale based on logarithms, horizontal arithmetical) and presents graphs showing the movements of many diseases since 1870. Pneumonia remains relatively constant, save for large excursions due to epidemic influenza. Tuberculosis has shown a steady decline, interrupted by a rise due to influenza also, but the present mortality stands at about one-fourth that of 1870. Typhoid fever shows a decline in deaths from 100 per 100,000 to less than 3 in the same population unit. Diphtheria and scarlet fever have shown irregular, but, on the whole, marked declines, but this does not hold for measles or whooping-cough. Bright's disease, cancer and diseases of the circulatory system have been steadily increasing.

Preparation and Administration of Arsphenamine and Neoarsphenamine.—The U. S. Public Health Service (*Public Health Reports*, 1922, **37**, 1867) issues a series of instructions on the administration of the newer arsenicals. In general, the preference is given to arsphenamine over neoarsphenamine. High dilutions of the drugs are recommended and special stress is laid on the proper alkalinization of the arsphenamine. Slowness of injection is urged as being highly important in preventing reactions. Detailed instructions are given covering preparation of solution and injection. (Reprints may be had by addressing the Surgeon-General, U. S. Public Health Service, Washington, D. C.)

The Posture of School Children in Relation to Nutrition, Physical Defects, School Grade and Physical Training.—Sterling (*Public Health Reports*, 1922, **37**, 2043) states: "The posture of school children cannot be said to depend entirely, or even chiefly, on any one condition. The following conclusions seem to be confirmed by the facts noted in this study: (1) While good nutrition is a contributing factor to good posture, it is by no means an indispensable condition. (2) Defective vision, adenoids and bad tonsils tend to have an unfavorable effect on a child's posture. (3) When the hygienic conditions in a school are not of the best, and health measures are inadequate, there is a moderate decrease of good posture and increase of poor posture from the first to the fifth grade, inclusive. This is not believed to be a necessary accompaniment of school life, but a condition that may be easily remedied by coöperation of the health and education authorities. (4) In planning exercise with a view to the promotion of good posture, it is suggested that setting-up exercises be simple and vigorous and play full of energy and vim. Formless, jellyfish gymnastics, or stupid, silly games, played half-heartedly, have little place in the proper physical development of the growing child."

Typhus Fever in Boston and a Review of the Newer Methods of Diagnosing Typhus.—Shattuck (*Am. Jour. Trop. Med.*, 1922, **2**, 225) states that the small number of cases of typhus, and of probable typhus, found in the records of the Boston City Hospital, covering the period of the past ten years, points to the conclusion that the typhus problem there has not been significant from the diagnostic standpoint. Nevertheless, the potential epidemiologic significance of typhus, and particularly of atypical cases, requires that all cases of possible typhus be studied with the greatest care in order to arrive, if possible, at a satisfactory diagnosis. Under the head of possible typhus are included a considerable group of cases having eruptions or temperature curves suggestive of typhus. This group is composed of two classes of cases: (1) Undiagnosed infections; (2) diagnosed infections, in which the diagnosis is not adequately supported by facts when recent advance of knowledge is taken into consideration. Careful investigation of all cases in which typhus might seem a possible diagnosis would perhaps show that typhus fever is in reality more common in Boston than it appears to have been in recent years. A Widal reaction positive in the dilutions generally used for diagnosis is commonly present in typhus fever and, therefore, it is not, *per se*, an obstacle to the diagnosis of typhus. The proteus reaction of Wilson, Weil and Felix is not infallible, but a very valuable aid to diagnosis. The proteus reaction to be of value must be adequately controlled. Not only should controls be performed with the test, but it would seem necessary from time to time to check, with known typhus serum, the agglutinability of the culture used for the test. For interpretation of the results of the test, all known facts regarding it should be borne in mind and clinical evidence should be taken into consideration. Probably the surest means of diagnosing typhus fever during life is by means of histologic examination of excised bits of skin. Pathologic changes developing in the guinea-pig after inoculation, with material containing the virus of typhus, are believed to be constant, but may be difficult to demonstrate. Somewhat similar lesions due to other causes may perhaps lead to error. Guinea-pig inoculation may be used for diagnosis. The point of greatest importance for diagnosis in the blood picture is the almost constant absence of leukopenia in typhus and its nearly constant presence in typhoid. The cerebrospinal fluid shows an increase of cells which may be slight or marked. Failure to recognize this fact may lead to erroneous interpretation of the findings. Other changes usually found in this fluid are less important. Wiener's color reaction is very easily performed and seems to warrant further trial. Other tests and diagnostic points have not been shown to have considerable value.

The Relative Parasiticidal Value of Arsphenamine and Neoarsphenamine. — VOEGTLIN and MILLER (*Public Health Reports*, 1922, **37**, 1627) describe the technic of determining in an experimental way the therapeutic activities of members of the arsphenamine group, and conclude as follows: "The results obtained in this investigation confirm previous data from this laboratory to the effect that arsphenamine of different manufacture is fairly uniform in parasiticidal power, whereas neoarsphenamine shows great variations. The toxicity of the average commercial arsphenamine and neoarsphenamine manufactured at the present time is considerably lower than that of preparations found on the market two years ago. The technic of the trypanocidal test as elaborated in this laboratory during the last few years is described in detail."

The Weil-Felix Test for Typhus Fever.—HOLT-HARRIS and GRUBBS (*Public Health Reports*, 1922, **37**, 1675) have employed the agglutination test for typhus, using certain strains of the Proteus group in connection with maritime quarantine procedure and find it of great value. A positive reaction is regarded as diagnostic, and a negative one after three to seven days constitutes very strong evidence against the disease.

Notice to Contributors.—All communications intended for insertion in the Original Department of this JOURNAL are received only *with the distinct understanding that they are contributed exclusively to this* JOURNAL.

Contributions from abroad written in a foreign language, if on examination they are found desirable for this JOURNAL, will be translated at its expense.

A limited number of reprints in pamphlet form, if desired, will be furnished to authors, *providing the request for them be written on the manuscript.*

All communications should be addressed to—

DR. JOHN H. MUSSER, JR., 262 S. 21st Street, Philadelphia, Pa., U. S. A.

THE

AMERICAN JOURNAL

OF THE MEDICAL SCIENCES

FEBRUARY, 1923

ORIGINAL ARTICLES.

A CLINICAL INVESTIGATION OF TROPICAL SPRUE.[1]

By Bailey K. Ashford, M.D., Col. Med. Corps, U. S. A.

INSTITUTE OF TROPICAL MEDICINE AND HYGIENE, SAN JUAN, PORTO RICO.

The symptomatology of sprue is a complex. The principal factors in the production of this complex are, on the one hand, glandular insufficiency, and, on the other, colonization in the digestive tube of a superimposed specific organism, *Monilia psilosis*, the latter bringing out the typical clinical picture we know as sprue.

Instead of rehearsing a list of symptoms commonly observed, let us first analyze the results of a long, clinical study of the disease as it exists in Porto Rico, and then group the phenomena according to their source.

The usual sequence of events is about as follows:

1. Physiologic glandular deficiency due to one or more of the following conditions:

(*a*) Hereditary depression of cellular vitality.

(*b*) Long-continued exposure to a tropical climate.

(*c*) Lack of healthful exercise, lack of sufficient sleep, frequent pregnancies, long-continued lactation, irregular hours of eating and monotonous and ill-prepared or indigestible food.

(*d*) An ill-balanced diet in which inordinate quantities of vitamine-less cereal foods, sweets and lard or vegetable oil are preferred to fresh garden products, meat and butter fat.

(*e*) Previous wasting diseases, such as enterocolitis in childhood, dysentery, malaria, tuberculosis, syphilis and others of chronic course, especially those in which the appetite fails, or the nature of

[1] Published with permission of the Surgeon-General U. S. Army, who is not responsible for any opinion expressed or conclusions reached herein.

the disease suggests a long-continued restriction of normal alimentation.

2. The gradual development of the symptom-complex resulting from this condition in which are prominent:

(*a*) Asthenia.

(*b*) Acid dyspepsia.

(*c*) Excess of intestinal gas.

(*d*) Constipation with or without occasional attacks of indigestion and "loose bowels."

(*e*) Reduction in size of the liver.

(*f*) Loss of appetite and weight.

(*g*) "Nervousness" with palpitation of the heart, pains in the body, depression of spirits, sleeplessness and mental hebetude.

(*h*) Pallor.

(*i*) Disorders of menstruation.

(*j*) Pigmentation of skin, chiefly over the malar prominences and forehead.

3. The gradual or abrupt development of sore tongue or large white, frothy movements, or both, with a pronounced increase in all of the symptoms of glandular deficiency above recounted. In the characteristic picture of tropical sprue, *Monilia psilosis* can usually be demonstrated, in contrast with the preliminary condition in which this organism is usually absent, unless it has effected a foothold, but has not yet succeeded in completing the sprue syndrome. It is in these borderland cases between incomplete sprue and the syndrome of glandular insufficiency that clinical diagnosis is practically impossible without a positive laboratory finding. This difficulty is increased by a subjective sensation of slight burning in the tongue without visible lesions, common to both conditions. When, in addition to this, constipation alternates with loose bowel movements, the confusion is complete. Very little difficulty is experienced in diagnosing a fully developed classical case of sprue, but such a case will have reached a point in which pancreas, intestinal glands and liver are apt to be in a state of partial atrophy from which recovery is slow and laborious, no matter what treatment is employed.

While the above is the usual trend of events in the unfolding of the sprue picture, the exceptions to the rule are most striking and far from rare. Many times, perhaps in a third of my cases, there has been no reasonable doubt that food deficiency played no part whatsoever. Moreover, a goodly number of these showed no evidence of a previous glandular deficiency. A relatively small class of acute cases, recent arrivals from the North, in which, after a sharp attack of gastroenteritis, the full sprue syndrome appeared, is the culminating fact which demonstrates that sprue is not necessarily dependent upon either food deficiency or glandular insufficiency.

On the other hand, about 12 per cent of our cases of sprue were negative, mycologically and serologically. Such were usually old chronic cases, often in a state of cachexia, or those in whom the tongue lesions and characteristic diarrhea, once prominent, were quiescent at the time of examination. The cachectic cases are to be considered practically as in a state of extreme glandular atrophy the result of sprue, and no surprise need be exhibited in finding no traces of the organism that produced the condition. The cases of undoubted sprue in a state of quiescence, while far more apt to give a positive blood reaction, are not much less apt to make a positive mycologic finding difficult if not well-nigh hopeless. While both of these classes are perfectly understandable from a scientific point of view, and for a like reason occur in syphilis and tuberculosis, they seem to furnish the scanty material from which men of excellent standing in the practice of medicine of the temperate zone draw the sweeping conclusion that *Monilia psilosis* has nothing to do with the production of sprue, even that there is no such disease as sprue at all. When we reflect that only 1.5 per cent, at most, of tropical people living in endemic zones have been found to harbor *Monilia psilosis* without showing its characteristic effects and contrast this with the fact that 87.6 per cent of our sprue patients are heavily infected with it, it does not seem necessary to enter into any further controversy with those who are probably not in a position to argue the point they themselves raise.

We are now prepared to consider the data which have been collected personally since 1908.

A few words are necessary before entering into these details in order to comprehend the scope of the work and the significance of certain necessary symbols.

Sprue was first announced to be a disease of Porto Rico by the writer in the summer of 1908. Hence the study from that time until the close of 1913 was purely clinical and epidemiological. In 1914, *Monilia psilosis* was identified as the direct cause of the disease, and from that date until 1917 studies were focussed on the mycologic study of tongue scrapings and feces in connection with only such a number of clinical cases as could be personally followed throughout their entire course. On return from France in 1920, where the writer engaged in the military operations of our land forces in the Great War, a series of clinical cases, checked upon by serologic study of the Laboratory of the Institute of Tropical Medicine and Hygiene of Porto Rico, was completed. In 1921, another series was undertaken and completed, checked upon by both mycologic and serologic examination by this Institute, and further contrasted with cases of pure glandular insufficiency, half of which were examined serologically and mycologically and found negative for *Monilia psilosis*.

Whereas the cases of the series 1908–1913 and 1914–1917 were complete as far as outstanding signs and symptoms were concerned, particularly regarding the state of the tongue and feces, no fixed questionnaire had been adopted for all cases.

In 1920, however, a set of questions was prepared covering all of the usual phenomena clinically observed in sprue, and these same questions were propounded with fair regularity to all patients, whatever might be their affection, in the series of that year.

The questionnaire was amplified and rigidly observed in all cases for 1921, and by comparing the condition in sprue with that seen in glandular insufficiency and in other affections, a very clear picture of what we know as sprue is revealed.

The order of these questions was necessarily peculiar for practical purposes of history taking, but it will be conserved in this work.

The symbols used for brevity will also be adhered to for the same reason and the key to these tables is herein displayed.

Symbols Used in Classifying Pathologic Conditions in this Text.

D = *Digestive system.*

1 = Subjective burning in tongue without demonstrable evidence thereof. Ranges from slight irritation to sensation of burning.

1 = Burning in tongue with evident lesions on tip or tip and edges. Ranges from redness to excoriation.

1 = Raw tongue resembling a piece of raw beef.

2 = Acid gastric dyspepsia with fulness after eating, rawness and the belching up of a hot acrid fluid.

3 = Excessive intestinal gas.

4 = "Loose bowels," or "attacks of indigestion," alternating with constipation.

4 = Diarrhea, generally light in color, gaseous and lienteric, but the symbol also denotes bilious, mucous watery and particolored movements.

4 = Typical white, frothy stools of classical sprue.

5 = Constipation.

6 = Abdominal pain referable to intestine.

7 = Small liver.

7 = Unusually small liver.

8 = Nausea.

9 = Vomiting.

10 = Heat and burning in rectum.

11 = Heat and burning in vagina.

12 = Loss of appetite.

12 = Complete anorexia.

13 = Excess of saliva.

N = *Nervous system.*

1 = "Nervousness," ranging from nervous irritability to nervous excitability.

2 = Asthenia.

3 = Sleeplessness, fitful sleep, nightmare.

4 = Pains in trunk and limbs, ranging from a feeling of muscular soreness on overexertion to definite neuralgia and neuritis, general or localized.

5 = Palpitation of the heart, cardiac irregularity.

6 = Psychic depression.

7 = Tingling, burning and coldness of hands and feet, a tendency for upper and lower extremities to go to sleep.

8 = Forgetfulness. Mental hebetude.

P = *Unclassified.*

1 = Sallowness to pallor.

1 = Extreme pallor.

2 = Vertigo.

3 = Dysmenorrhea.

4 = Amenorrhea.

5 = Headache.

6 = Subcutaneous extravasation of blood without apparent cause or on slight contusion.

7 = Brown pigmentation resembling nut stains on skin. Usually symmetrical and most common and prominent over malar prominences, cheeks and forehead.

8 = Excessive menstrual flow, to menorrhagia.

9 = Irregular menstruation.

10 = Scanty menstrual flow.

G 2 = Loss in weight.

This bizarre grouping of signs and symptoms, including all of the usual phenomena accompanying sprue, may seem unsystematic and inexact. It should be remembered, however, that it is necessary to consider the psychologic attitude of the sick man in making up a questionnaire, in order to allow the patient himself, with least amount of what he would consider obstruction, to expand the picture he would like to draw. The sense of good order and exactness of the physician may appear to suffer thereby, but in the long run much more information is obtained.

Therefore, once adopted, this order of questioning has been followed throughout the series of 1920–21. Although it can now, and will be later, simplified and increased in scope, it did not seem justifiable to make these changes until the series under analysis were completed.

Indefiniteness is not a rare quality in the average patient when relating what he feels that is abnormal, no matter what the disease or condition may be; but the average patient suffering from sprue, beyond his tongue and bowel symptoms, is notoriously indefinite in rehearsing his wretchedness. He hardly knows how to express himself, hardly realizes what it is that makes him a sick man, beyond his unruly "stomach," his loose bowels and his sore tongue. It is all very well to say that in history-taking one should not ask leading questions, but with most sprue patients I have seen, one would never find out what they had if clear questioning is not employed. It should be borne in mind that mental confusion and forgetfulness in sprue is a feature of the disease, so that it is well to begin by saying, "Now tell me all that you can about what ails you.' Then proceed to ask question after question, in the order given, carefully pinning the man or woman down to as exact and uncolored statement of fact as may be possible. This being concluded, a physical examination on the table is to be made, and finally all clinical laboratory analyses bearing on the individual case, including mycologic and serologic examinations for moniliasis.

Exclusive of laboratory work, the primary examination of each case requires for its thorough accomplishment not less than half an hour and often much more.

It seems hardly necessary to say that answers to questions in the taking of the history should embrace the entire period from which the patient has suffered from his affection and are not to be confined to symptoms on the day of his first visit. This is needful to avoid a negative of characteristic phenomena which generally occur only from time to time and which may constitute an important part of the evidence upon which the clinical diagnosis of sprue may be justified.

Series of 1908–1913. This period corresponds to the clinical and epidemiological study, begun in 1908, which culminated in the identification of *Monilia psilosis*. These cases, therefore, possess no laboratory guide or check and only very clear pictures of classical sprue were so regarded. Among the doubtful cases many more must have been included, but, as the writer was depending chiefly upon Manson's work on *Tropical Diseases*, no departure from the criterion therein expressed of what should constitute an unquestioned clinical entity was permitted. The cardinal symptoms, sore tongue, gastric disorder, excess of intestinal gas and diarrhea, were faithfully recorded in all, but the importance of the remainder of the signs and symptoms, found in the questionnaire above detailed, were not appreciated and were only noted when the patient happened to mention them in his personal narrative. Therefore, for statistical purposes, all save these cardinal symptoms must be discarded.

Series of 1914–1917. (Mycologic Series.) This series began with the discovery of a pathogenic yeast-like budding fungus, later designated by myself *Monilia psilosis,* in the scrapings from the inflamed tongue of a young Porto Rican boy. Within a short time, in three more cases, the same organism was recovered, one from a child of two or three years whose only symptom was a raw tongue, one from a young woman with a life history of gastrointestinal derangement and an incipient tuberculosis, and one from a continental American in the last stages of uncomplicated acute sprue, from which he later died. These four cases were studied mycologically for some months with uniform mycologic findings; later some twenty more cases were added and the tedious mycologic study repeated; finally, the series was continued to include a total of 476 assorted cases of which 246 were clinically sprue.

A mycologic study of tongue scrapings and feces was made in 448 of the 476 cases; in 225 cases of clinical sprue, of which 75 per cent were positive for *Monilia psilosis*, and in 223 cases not clinically sprue, of which 1.3 per cent were positive for this organism.

TABLE 1.—CONSOLIDATED TABLE SHOWING RELATIVE FREQUENCY OF CARDINAL SYMPTOMS OF SPRUE IN ALL FOUR SERIES (1572 CASES)

	All our series.[2]	Percentage.
D 1	494	31
1	303	19
1	319	20
All 1	1116	71
2	1259	80
3	1329	84
4	531	34
4	258	17
4	426	27
All 4	1215	77

TABLE 2.—RELATIVE PROPORTION OF CASES OF COMPLETE AND INCOMPLETE SPRUE IN A TOTAL OF 1309 CASES.

	Series 1914–17.	Series 1920.	Series 1921.	Total.	Per cent.
Both D 1 and D 4	158	285	370	813	62
One or the other	24	140	171	335	26
Neither D 1 nor D 4	8	78	75	161	12
Total	190	503	616	1309	100

Explanation of Graphs. The panels in each fan are rounded off at their broad extremity and bear a number corresponding to symbols already explained in this text. The lines within each panel stand for the percentage of cases which the clinical phenomenon or phenomena, represented by the symbol, bear to the total cases in this series. Each line within the panel represents 5 per cent or major fraction thereof. No lines appear where less than 7 per cent of the cases showed the phenomenon.

[2] The separation of cases suffering from sore tongue into three degrees (D 1, *1* and **1**) and of those with diarrhea into D 4, *4* and **4**, was not consistently carried out in the 1920 series, but as the total number of cases of sore tongue and diarrhea yielded a percentage to total cases of sprue almost identical with corresponding totals in 1921, the relative number in each one of the three groups under D 1 and D 4, 1920, has been calculated from the percentage in 1921.

The important point in interpreting these fans is to remember that 453 of the 616 cases of sprue and 124 of the 259 cases of glandular insufficiency were examined in the laboratory, the first being all

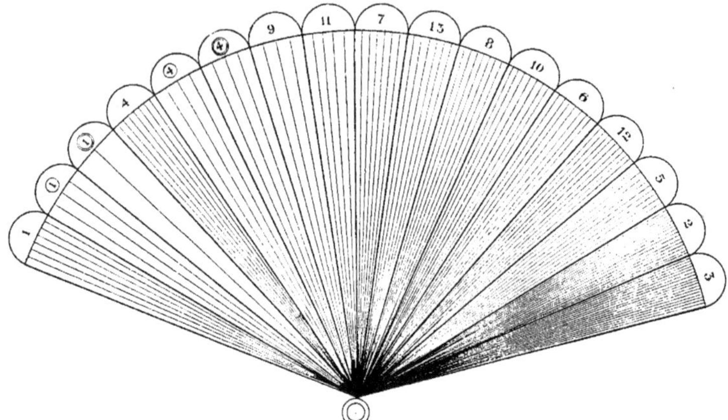

FIG. 1.—Series 1921; 616 cases. Digestive symptoms. Sprue.

positive for *Monilia psilosis,* the second all negative. The examinations in laboratory were only made *once* in 98 per cent of these cases. Had time and personnel as well as constancy on the part of

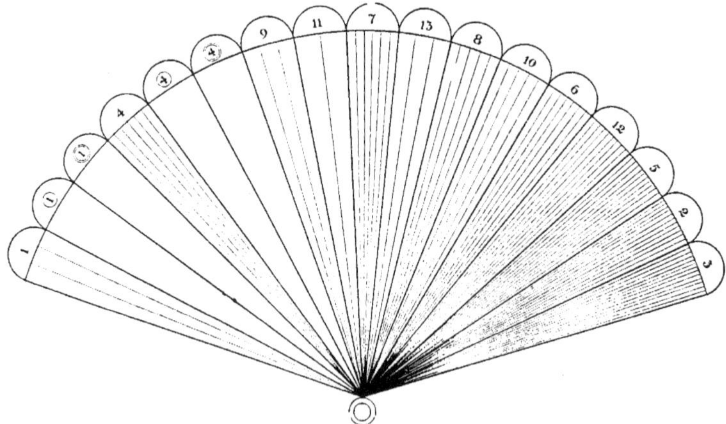

FIG. 2.—Series 1921; 259 cases. Digestive symptoms, glandular insufficiency in Porto Rico.

the patients permitted, a much higher percentage of positive results in the sprue series might have been obtained. As to the series of cases of glandular insufficiency, mycologic study of the feces daily for a continued period would have undoubtedly revealed a stray colony now and then, as *Monilia psilosis* is a widespread fungus in Porto Rico and frequently must pass through the intestinal canal as

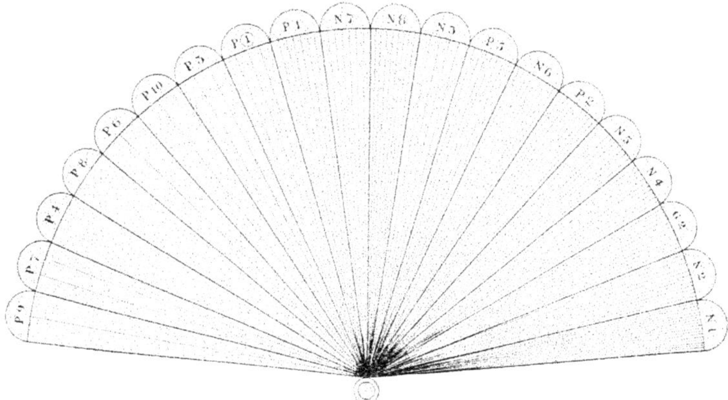

FIG. 3.—Series 1921; 616 cases. Assorted symptoms. Sprue.

a *voyageur*, or, as Anderson so well expresses it, "like so much waste food," but without colonizing. When it colonizes in the intestinal tract then we may expect its pathogenic effect. The best way to bring out the presence of an infection by *Monilia psilosis* is to sow

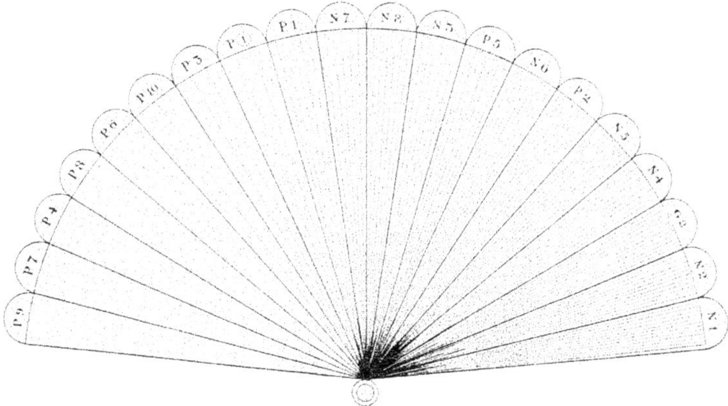

FIG. 4.—Series 1921; 259 cases. Assorted symptoms, glandular insufficiency in Porto Rico.

in Sabouraud agar Petri plates by Anderson's method, *i. e.*, by making a hundred separate points of contact with a platinum loop soiled in the feces and taking a percentage of positive colonies.

This series was intended to be purely a clinical versus mycologic study, but in 1916–1917 the feasibility of applying the complement-deviation test for diagnosis became evident and 88 of the 225 cases

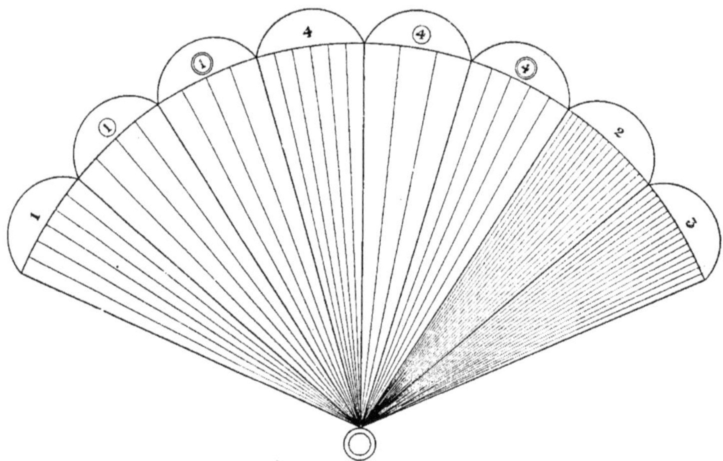

FIG. 5.—All series; 1572 cases. Sprue.

of sprue were thus examined. In this way 20 cases which had been mycologically negative were shown to be serologically positive,

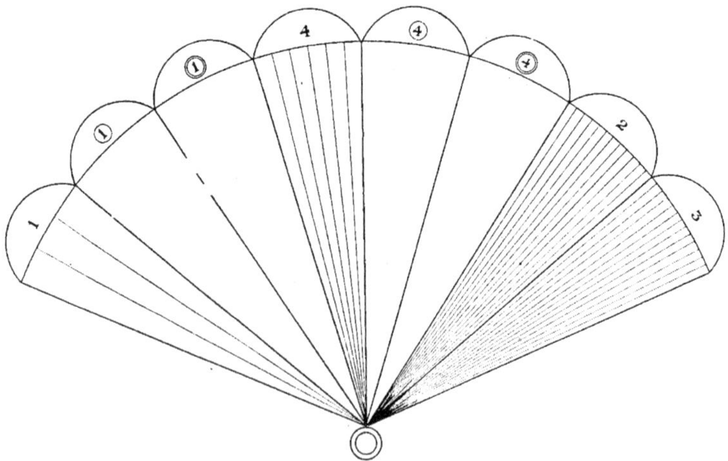

FIG. 6.—Series 1921; 259 cases. Glandular insufficiency in Porto Rico.

raising the percentage of positive laboratory findings to 84 per cent. Had all of the 225 been available for this blood test this rate would have probably been above 90 per cent.

The tabulation of clinical phenomena is as in the preceding series. No questionnaire was adhered to, save as concerns the tongue symptoms, acid gastric dyspepsia, excessive intestinal gas and diarrhea (D 1, *1*, **1**, 2, 3, 4, *4*, **4**).

In this series the individual grouping of the four cardinal symptoms of sprue was consolidated in 211 cases, 84 per cent of which were confirmed by laboratory finding.

Cases with typical raw tongue and frothy, white diarrhea, 92, or 48 per cent.

Cases with typical raw tongue, with or without diarrhea, 101, or 53 per cent.

Cases with tongue raw at tip and edges, with or without diarrhea, 22, or 11 per cent.

Cases in whom only a sensation of burning was felt, with or without diarrhea, 44, or 22 per cent.

Cases with both sore tongue and diarrhea, 158, or 83 per cent.

Cases with one or the other of above symptoms, 24, or 13 per cent.

Cases with neither one nor the other, 8, or 4 per cent. Total, 190.

In the spring of 1917 these studies were abruptly suspended by the Great War, which scattered the group of men who formed the Institute of Tropical Medicine throughout the armies of the United States, and for a period of three years the writer was unable to take up the tangled skein of tropical sprue. But such was the spirit of the Institute that the other members kept the work alive. Adding valuable confirmatory data to the investigation begun in 1908, Drs. Gutierrez Igaravidez, Dr. González Martinez and Dr. Carl Michel, each separately, the first while in the training camp of the 2d Brigade of the 81st Division, the second in his personal work and at the close of the war in Paris and Barcelona, and Dr. Michel in the laboratory and later in the United States, kept up a persistent and brilliant campaign to extend the application of what was up to that time known.

In 1920 the writer returned to Porto Rico, thanks to the scientific spirit of his military chief, to complete this series of studies, and since that time, with the same technicians who had for ten years diligently kept up the laboratory work, this investigation has been going forward. It is difficult to estimate the value of the work of these technicians, Messrs. José Loubriel and Figueroa, who throughout a period of these three years had become as expert as ourselves in the routine laboratory methods of revealing the presence of *Monilia psilosis*, mycologically and serologically. Up to 1917, the writer had personally accomplished every step in this mycological laboratory work in each case, even to the preparation of media, the technicians then in training duplicating this work under my supervision in order to familiarize them thoroughly with every possible laboratory situation. Dr. Michel and Dr. González trained them in the special serology of moniliasis. The object, on my part, was to continue these investigations by permitting our technicians to render the laboratory reports in cases of which they knew nothing clinically and free me for the clinical study and treatment of a larger series of cases in order to submit each case of sprue to the severe test of a laboratory analysis to determine the presence or absence of *Monilia psilosis* in which I, the interested party, would be eliminated. In the meantime I continued research laboratory work in *Monilia psilosis* and its congeners and with Drs. Gutierrez and González, supervised the clinical laboratory work.

Series of 1920. This was principally a clinical versus serologic study, mycological investigations being employed only from time to time for corroboration, or in certain cases, but not systematically, in which a typical case of sprue had been reported as negative serologically.

In all, 503 cases of sprue, out of a total of 1267 patients examined, were found. In contemplation of these figures it must be remembered that I was dedicating practically my entire attention to sprue, and the majority of those who came for examination were either sent to me from all over the Island by other physicians as cases suspicious of, or positive for, that disease, or were persons who had themselves come to believe that they were suffering from sprue, whose complete clinical picture had by this time become almost universally recognized by laymen throughout the Island.

Series of 1921. The development in medical science of the recognition of a syndrome of glandular insufficiency came to put the finishing touches upon this study of sprue in Porto Rico, and we believe, all of us of the Institute, and an ever-increasing number of observing practitioners in these tropics, that it may be accepted with a fair degree of certainty that the veil of mystery which has enshrouded tropical sprue has at last been rent in twain.

It is curious how the forces of our little group in the Institute of Tropical Medicine have complemented one the other. At the very outset of the modern work on sprue, back in 1914, Dr. Gutierrez Igaravidez stoutly maintained that the underlying cause of sprue was a glandular disturbance. Dr. W. W. King, who was one of the founders with us of the Porto Rico Anemia Commission for the study of uncinariasis and later of the Institute, believed that whatever sprue might be, *Monilia psilosis* seemed to have something to do with its manifestations. Dr. González Martinez, without commenting upon the conception of an intestinal moniliasis, silently worked out the specific serological reaction and became gradually more and more convinced of the importance of this fungus in its etiology, finally taking a stand publicly in defense of this conception. All have persistently and dispassionately sought the light while always remaining loyal to the Institute.

While I am only reporting my own personal work, I do not wish to leave the idea that no other work on sprue has been accomplished here. The others, members of the Institute, have their case records and will some day, it is to be hoped, express their own experiences and opinions regarding this disease.

In this series of 1921 the study made was for the purpose of comparing clinical, mycological and serological data, as well as for separating out the cases of glandular insufficiency.

TABLE 3.

	Clin. sprue confirmed by laboratory, 385 cases.		Clin. sprue not examined in laboratory, 163 cases.		Clin. sprue negative in laboratory, 68 cases.		Total sprue, 616 cases.		Clin. not sprue and negative in laboratory, 238 cases.		Cases of glandular insufficiency, 259 cases.	
	No.	Per cent.	No.	Per cent.	No.	Per cent.	No.	Per cent.	No.	Per cent.	No.	Per cent.
D 1 . .	128	33	70	43	29	43	227	37	38	16	44	17
1 . .	57	15	41	25	24	35	122	20	6	3	6	2
1 . .	39	10	24	15	9	13	72	11	1	½		
All 1 . .	224	58	135	83	62	91	421	68	45	18½	50	19
2 . .	326	84	145	88	64	94	535	86	108	45	162	62
3 . .	337	87	147	90	65	95	549	89	138	58	169	65
4 . .	154	40	65	40	25	37	244	39	62	26	76	29
4 . .	67	17	35	21	21	30	123	20	21	9	19	7
4 . .	62	16	38	23	20	29	120	19	7	3		
All 4 . .	283	73	138	85	66	96	487	79	90	38	95	37
5 . .	176	45	78	48	42	62	296	48	97	40	140	54
6 . .	135	35	78	48	78	70	261	42	31	34	92	35
7 . .	94	24	55	34	27	40	176	28	52	22	61	24
7 . .	23	6	15	9	10	15	48	8	11	5	11	4
8 . .	153	39	64	39	37	54	254	41	59	25	69	26
9 . .	76	19	39	24	25	37	140	23	33	14	40	15
10 . .	141	36	68	42	44	65	253	41	53	22	62	24
11 . .	47	20	32	20	19	28	87	14	17	7	19	7
12 . .	153	39	72	44	46	68	271	44	74	31	96	37
12 . .	26	6	9	5	4	6	39	6	6	2	19	7
13 . .	121	31	50	31	33	48	204	33	37	16	43	16
N 1 . .	255	66	106	65	60	88	521	84	121	50	168	65
2 . .	235	60	103	63	54	80	392	63	109	45	156	60
3 . .	171	45	81	50	47	69	164	26	75	31	94	36
4 . .	208	54	86	53	50	73	344	55	92	39	133	51
5 . .	184	47	80	49	46	68	310	50	86	36	127	49
6 . .	191	50	72	44	53	78	316	51	82	34	113	43
7 . .	125	32	59	36	48	70	233	37	56	24	75	29
8 . .	158	40	71	44	46	68	275	44	67	28.	89	34
P 1 . .	127		57	35	28	41	212	34	56	24	78	30
1 . .	82		39	24	16	23	137	22	36	15	42	16
All 1 . .	209		96	59	44	65	349	56	92	39	120	46
2 . .	189		76	46	45	66	310	50	95	39	120	46
3 . .	39	10	10	6	7	10	56	9	13	5	22	8
4 . .	17	4	2	1	6	9	25	4	7	3	10	4
5 . .	145		70	43	37	54		41	77	32	109	42
6 . .	36	9	16	10	11	16	63	10	11	5	17	7
7 . .	47		14	9	17		78	13	12	5	14	5
8 . .	19	5	5	3	3	4		4	10	4	10	4
9 . .	16		5	3	9	13	30	5	7	3	9	3
10 . .	21	5	11	7	1	1		5	14	6	16	6
G 2 . .	214	55		56	50	73	356	57	186		104	40

The questionnaire was here placed rigidly in force and its data are considered as reliable as ordinary human observation can make them. In this table, separate classification of the phenomena observed in 259 cases of glandular insufficiency has been made. Table of clinical phenomena observed in 616 cases of sprue, in 238 cases which were clinically not sprue and negative by laboratory methods, and in 259 cases of glandular deficiency, giving the number of cases suffering from the condition denoted by each symbol and the percentage this number bears to the total number in each group. Of the cases listed as cases of glandular insufficiency, 124 were examined by laboratory methods and were negative. These 124 cases are also included under "cases clinically not sprue and negative in laboratory" in column 5. The remaining 135 were clinically cases of glandular insufficiency but were not examined by laboratory methods although entirely similar to the 124 which were so examined.

In table 3 it will be noted that the clinical picture in the cases which were negative in the laboratory was more vivid than in those which were positive. This obtains in every series and results from a combination of two factors: (1) The cases of complete sprue confirmed by the laboratory were augmented by a number of incomplete cases which lowered the intensity of the composite picture; (2) severe and cachectic cases are often negative when chronic and quiescent, *i. e.*, when, at the time of examination, they are bereft of active inflammatory changes in the mucosæ. In fact, very cachectic or very chronic cases, or those in which active symptoms of sprue are temporarily in abeyance, are frequently negative, mycologically or serologically, or both, as occurs in syphilis and tuberculosis, and for the same reasons. The increased number of sore tongues and diarrheas in these cases does not necessarily refer to the condition at the time of examination, but to the past history as well.

The severe type in purely clinical cases without laboratory examination in this table is due to the fact that such cases were so clearly sprue that no serologic examination could be urged for diagnostic purposes in certain persons who strongly objected thereto, or in those whose physical condition made the effort palpably unjustifiable, from the standpoint of the patient.

The most interesting feature of this table is the comparison which can be made between identical symptoms in sprue, on the one hand, and glandular deficiency on the other. In making this comparison it should be remembered that:

1. Of the 616 cases of sprue, 453 were examined by laboratory methods and 85 per cent yielded a positive finding for *Monilia psilosis*.

2. Of the 259 cases of glandular deficiency, 124 were examined by laboratory methods and all were negative for *Monilia psilosis* the rest were not examined in the laboratory.

All of the phenomena in the syndrome of glandular insufficiency were more frequent and, clinically, far more vivid in sprue, generally about double that of the former condition. But the salient point is found in that in sprue the tongue lesions are over fifteen times, and the frank diarrhea over five times, as frequent as in glandular insufficiency. In fact, the strictly classical raw tongue and white, frothy diarrhea were never found in glandular insufficiency. The graphic exposition of the clinical difference between these two conditions can be better appreciated by reference to the fans prepared to illustrate the point.

TABLE 4.—LOSS OF WEIGHT IN SPRUE AND GLANDULAR INSUFFICIENCY.

Loss in weight.	Clin. sprue confirmed by laboratory, No. of cases.	Clin. sprue not examined in laboratory, No. of cases.	Clin. sprue negative in laboratory, No. of cases.	Total sprue, No. of cases.	Glandular insufficiency, No. of cases.
Under 10 lbs. . .	3	2	1	6	7
10 to 15 " . .	19	4	1	24	5
16 to 20 " . .	11	5	1	17	2
21 to 30 " . .	18	4	4	26	2
31 to 40 " . .	11	1	2	14	
41 to 50 " . .	4	2	4	10	1
51 to 60 " . .	1	1	. .	2	
Number weighed .	67	19	13	99	17
Average loss . .	24 lbs.	25 lbs.	31 lbs.	. . .	15 lbs.

TABLE 5.—GENERAL RÉSUMÉ OF ALL FROM SERIES CONTAINING 1595 CASES OF SPRUE.

	Series 1908–13.	Series 1914–17.	Series 1920.	Series 1921.	Total.	Per cent.
Cases of sprue without laboratory examination .	230	21	88	163	502	32
Sprue confirmed by laboratory methods . . .	. . .	189	379	385	953	60
Same negative by laboratory methods . . .	. . . .	36	36	68	140	8
Total sprue . . .	230	246	503	616	1595	100
Cases suspicious of sprue but not examined in laboratory[1]	328	. . .	. . .	. . .	328	
Cases definitely not sprue, negative by laboratory examination	. . .	226	180	238	645	
Carriers	. . .	1	6	3	10	
Cases definitely not sprue not examined in laboratory; not classified . .	3159	3	578	782	4519	
Total	3717	476	1267	1639	7097	

[1] All of the "cases suspicious of sprue" were so diagnosed clinically, as these studies were made previous to the discovery of the causal organism.

TABLE 6.—TABLE OF CLINICAL PHENOMENA OBSERVED IN 942 CASES OF SPRUE CONFIRMED BY LABORATORY METHODS GIVING THE NUMBER OF CASES SUFFERING FROM THE CONDITION DENOTED BY EACH SYMBOL AND THE PERCENTAGE THIS NUMBER BEARS TO THE TOTAL NUMBER IN EACH GROUP.

	1914–17, 178 cases.		1920, 379 cases.		1921, 385 cases.		Total.	
	No.	Per cent	No.	Per cent.	No.	Per cent.	No.	Per cent.
D 1	39	22	. .	. .	128	33		
1	20	11	. .	. .	57	15		
1	99	56	. .	. .	39	10		
All 1	158	89	231	60	224	58	603	65
2	146	82	300	78	326	84	772	82
3	160	90	319	83	337	86	816	87
4	39	22	. .	. .	154	40		
4	6	3	. .	. .	67	17		
4	114	64	. .	. .	62	16		
All 4	159	89	246	64	283	73	688	73
7	66	37	80	28	117	30	263	28
P 1	90	50	178	46	209	54	477	50

TABLE 7.—TABLE OF CLINICAL PHENOMENA OBSERVED IN 149 CASES OF SPRUE, NEGATIVE ON LABORATORY EXAMINATION, GIVING THE NUMBER OF CASES SUFFERING FROM THE CONDITION DENOTED BY EACH SYMBOL AND THE PERCENTAGE THIS NUMBER BEARS TO THE TOTAL NUMBER IN EACH GROUP.

	1914–17, 45 cases.		1920, 36 cases.		1921, 68 cases.		Total.	
	No.	Per cent.	No.	Per cent.	No.	Per cent.	No.	Per cent.
D 1	9	20	. .	. .	29	43		
1	5	11	. .	. .	24	35		
1	23	51	. .	. .	9	13		
1	37	82	35	97	62	91	134	90
2	32	71	28	77	64	94	124	83
3	36	80	34	94	65	95	135	90
4	8	18	. .	. .	25	37		
4	1	2	. .	. .	21	30		
4	32	71	. .	. .	20	29		
All 4	41	91	34	94	66	96	141	95
7	9	20	10	27	27	40	46	30
P 1	11	24	12	37	44	64	67	45

TABLE 8.—TABLE OF CLINICAL PHENOMENA OBSERVED IN 481 CASES OF SPRUE, NOT EXAMINED IN LABORATORY, GIVING THE NUMBER OF CASES SUFFERING FROM THE CONDITION DENOTED BY EACH SYMBOL AND THE PERCENTAGE THIS NUMBER BEARS TO THE TOTAL NUMBER IN EACH GROUP.

	1908–13, 230 cases		1920, 88 cases.		1921, 163 cases.		Total.	
	No.	Per cent.	No.	Per cent.	No.	Per cent	No.	Per cent.
D 1	34	15	..	..	70	43		
1	56	24	..	..	41	25		
1	166	28	..	..	24	15		
All 1	156	67	78	88	135	83	369	77
2	152	65	65	75	145	88	362	75
3	153	66	78	88	147	90	378	78
4	64	27	..	..	65	40		
4	39	17	..	..	35	21		
4	74	32	..	..	38	23		
All 4	177	78	71	80	138	84	386	80
7	..	...	..	..	70	43		
P 1	..	..	..	..	96	60		

TABLE 9.—GRADE OF SPRUE IN 1470 CASES.

Grade.	Series 1908–13.	Series 1914–17.	Series 1920.	Series 1921.	Total.	Per cent.
Light	9	32	81	80	202	14
Moderate	38	72	265	269	644	44
Severe	38	90	157	237	522	35
Cachectic	20	52	..	30	102	7
Total	105	246	503	616	1470	100

TABLE 10.—CARRIERS.

		1	6	3	10	

Percentage of carriers to 645 cases definitely not sprue and examined in laboratory = 1.5.

Percentage of carriers to 1093 cases of sprue, 0.9.

NOTE.—In constructing the graphs the percentages for D 11 and P 3, 4, 8, 9 and 10 are calculated from the number of women in the series. This makes an apparent discrepancy with the table of total percentages.

THE TOTAL CIRCULATING VOLUME OF BLOOD AND PLASMA IN CASES OF CHRONIC ANEMIA AND LEUKEMIA.[1]

By Norman M. Keith, M.D.,

MEDICAL DEPARTMENT, UNIVERSITY OF TORONTO, TORONTO, CANADA, AND DIVISION OF MEDICINE, MAYO CLINIC, ROCHESTER, MINN.

Since the introduction of methods for the determination of blood volume applicable to clinical study, numerous estimations have been made in cases of chronic anemia. The volumes obtained in a given type of anemia, for example in pernicious anemia, have varied markedly even when the same investigator employed a single method. Corroboration or disproof of such results is important because of the well-recognized fact that in health the blood volume is remarkably constant. Therefore, shortly after Keith, Rowntree and Geraghty introduced the dye method for estimating blood and plasma volume, they made determinations in a few cases of chronic anemia. The early results indicated that both plasma and blood volumes might be little altered. Later, in a study of one case of pernicious anemia, the plasma volume was found to be definitely greater than in the normal controls, although the total blood volume was not increased. Subsequent estimations by the writer in a series of 14 cases of chronic anemia confirmed the original findings. Several cases showed but little deviation from the normal, while others showed a distinctly high plasma volume. Repeated determinations in these latter cases gave constantly high plasma values, although the total blood volume was not uniformly increased. Similar variations in total plasma were observed in 10 cases of chronic leukemia with this difference, that in cases of leukemia with high plasma contents the total blood volume was more often increased. Repeated determinations made periodically in individual cases in this series revealed distinct volume changes. The object of the present communication is to emphasize the fact that in chronic anemia and leukemia variations occurring in blood and plasma volume should be considered in evaluating the blood picture and other clinical findings.

Methods. The blood and plasma volumes were determined by the dye method introduced by Keith, Rowntree and Geraghty.[2]

[1] Read before the American Society for Clinical Investigation, Washington, D. C., May, 1922.

[2] *Relation of Blood Volume to Body Weight and Body Surface.* Dreyer and Ray believe that the blood volume in mammals is proportional to body surface and not to body weight. Accordingly they consider that the practice of expressing the blood volume in percentage of body weight is misleading, particularly when comparing individuals in any given species that differ greatly in weight. In order to ascertain by the dye method whether in normal adults the relation between blood volume and body surface was more constant than that between blood volume and body weight, data were obtained from ten persons in our previous series of normal male controls.

Comparison of this indirect method with other procedures has been made repeatedly by Whipple, Harris, and others. Whipple concludes from his experiments that the dye method gives remarkably constant results for total plasma, but considers that the value obtained for total circulating blood is higher than the amount actually present. That the absolute values for whole blood obtained by the dye method may be slightly higher than the actual amount of blood present seems probable on theoretical grounds. As yet there is no one method, not even any of the many modifications of the original Welcher direct method, that is free from obvious error. However, relative changes in blood volume can be definitely determined by the dye method. The hemoglobin estimations were made on venous blood by Palmer's modification of the Haldane method. Contrary to some workers, I have found that the 20 per cent standard hemoglobin solution will keep satisfactorily for several months provided the proper precautions are followed. Centrifuge tubes graduated to 10 cc containing 0.01 gm. of dry sodium oxalate were used for the hematocrit reading. The hematocrit tubes were then centrifugalized for twenty minutes at a speed of three thousand revolutions each minute. It should be noted that after centrifugalizing leukemic blood the line of demarcation between the red and white cell layers may be distinct or it may be scarcely perceptible. The erythrocyte and leukocyte counts were made in the usual manner, Hayem's solution and 1 per cent acetic acid being used as diluents. The basal metabolic rate[3] was determined in the leukemic patients by the gasometer method of Tissot.

The surface area was estimated according to the height and weight formula of Du Bois. The greatest variation in weight was 56.1 and 90.4 kg. and in height 162.5 and 183.1 cm. The average number of cubic centimeters of blood for each kilogram was 84.7 and the number of liters of blood for each square meter averaged 3.16. In considering the extreme variations from these average figures, the percentage deviations were slightly less marked when computed according to surface area than to body weight. But if the percentage deviation of each individual determination from the general mean were averaged, the values derived from surface area were more constant. Similar results were obtained when the plasma volume in 29 normal males was compared to body weight and body surface. The average values for plasma volume in these normal persons were 48 cc for each kilogram and 1 78 liters for each square meter. Although these results, limited to normal adults, showed no marked difference, whether the blood and plasma volume were computed as a function of the body weight or surface area, still the deviation from the average was distinctly less when the surface area was considered. These findings seem to indicate that the blood volume is a function of the body surface rather than of body weight. Further study of this question is desirable before a positive conclusion can be made. I am at present carrying out an investigation which includes normal persons exhibiting greater variations in age, weight and height, and also different species of animals. The blood and plasma volumes are expressed in relation to body weight, except in the cases of leukemia; in these the results are expressed both in relation to body weight and body surface.

[3] Boothby and Sandiford. (I am indebted to Dr. W. R. Campbell, University of Toronto, for the basal metabolic-rate determinations made in Toronto.)

TABLE 1.—PERNICIOUS ANEMIA.

Case.	Date.	Age and sex.	Weight, kg.	Hemoglobin, per cent.	Hematocrit, erythrocytes, per cent.	Erythrocytes.	Leukocytes.	Plasma, cc.	Plasma, cc, for each kg.	Blood, cc.	Blood, cc, for each kg.
'27 H. W. B.	July 12, 1919	63	..	35	..	1,200,000	13,000				
	Oct. 9, 1919	M.	52	16	6	...	...	4069	78	4330	83
	Oct. 18, 1919	..	51	26	12	...	...	4068	78	4610	88
	Nov. 21, 1919	..	46	23	..	704,000	3,400				
	Dec. 7, 1919	..	..	..	..	672,000	2,200				
24 W. R.	Aug. 10, 1919	56	..	..	..	1,800,000					
	Sept. 27, 1919	M.	..	25	..	1,200,000	1,500				
	Nov. 14, 1919	..	46	23	8	1,050,000	1,300	3580	78	3900	85
	Dec. 12, 1919	..	..	21	..	974,000					
	Dec. 30, 1919	..	47	33	15	1,062,000	2,200	3460	73	4070	87
	Jan. 12, 1920	..	47	29	..	1,000,000	2,200				
	Mar. 1, 1920	..	..	60							
	Mar. 17, 1920	..	47	84	34	2,800,000	4,900	3300	70	5000	106
	April 5, 1920	..	47	84	..	3,200,000	3,200	...	..	...	
	April 16, 1920	..	51	88	32	...	...	3200	62	4705	92
23 C. M.	Dec. 31, 1919	55	51	32	..	1,470,000	7,600				
	Jan. 5, 1920	M.	51	46	21	1,990 000	...	3395	66	4295	84
26 C. H.	Mar. 13, 1920	44	65	62	24	2,700,000	3,600	3950	60	5300	81
	April 7, 1920	M.	63	80	33	...	2,800	3480	55	5195	82
01 R. G.	April 12, 1920	41	52	47	17	1,500,000	4,400	3135	60	3825	73
	April 27, 1920	M.	..	34	..	1,300,000					
	May 17, 1920	..	..	22	..	1,130,000	5,600				
	June 7, 1920	..	47	26	10	900,000	...	3265	69	3630	77
	July 14, 1920	..	..	28	..	870,000	5,200				
	Aug. 19, 1920	..	..	90	..	2,472,000	3,000				
'02 E. H.	May 22, 1920	52	46	50	..	1,600,000					
	June 1, 1920	F.	46	35	13	1,000,000	5,000	2555	55	2935	64
	June 26, 1920	..	..	25	..	770,000	4,000				
	July 5, 1920	..	..	19	..	600,000					
18 S. B.	June 12, 1920	57	46	16	..	650,000	6,800				
	June 26, 1920	F.	45	41	20	2,150,000	...	3660	81	4575	102
	July 22, 1920	..	49	80	..	3,300,000					
	Aug. 27, 1920	..	..	71	..	3,170,000	5,400				
	Oct. 27, 1920	..	..	22	..	1,000,000	6,000				
'85 G. A. McK.	April 27, 1921	53 M.	62	69	27	2,100,000	7,400	3680	59	5040	81
66 W. S.	May 4, 1921	39 M.	70	46	20	2,040,000	4,200	3655	52	4570	65
16 E. L.	May 17, 1921	63	60.5	37	18	1,650,000	3,700	3800	63	4635	77
	May 19, 1921	M.	..	40	20	2,150,000	7,000	3800	63	4740	79
29 G.	June 6, 1921	53 M.	52	36	16	1,480,000	1,200	3265	62	3875	74
50 F. U.	June 18, 1921	45 F.	40	44	17	1,340,000	4,000	2965	74	3575	89

Chronic Anemia. This group includes 12 cases of pernicious anemia, one of severe secondary anemia and one of Banti's disease (Tables 1 and 2). In 6 cases of pernicious anemia the values for plasma volume were high, ranging from 66 to 81 cc for each kilogram of body weight. The corresponding values for blood volume were

77 to 106 cc for each kilogram; only two patients had a blood volume above normal. In general, the highest plasma values were in patients with low hemoglobin percentages, although no absolute relationship could be demonstrated. The highest plasma volume, 81 cc for each kilogram, calculated on the basis of cubic centimeters of plasma to body weight was found in Case S. B., when the hemoglobin was 41 per cent. In several patients changes in the hemoglobin percentages were associated with definite variations in plasma volume. In Case W. R. (Chart 1) the rise in hemoglobin from 23 to 88 per cent, an increase in weight of 5 kg., and general clinical

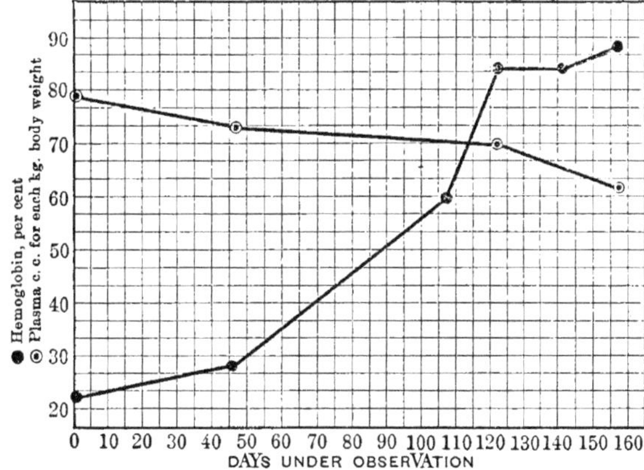

CHART I

improvement were associated with a definite decrease in plasma, 78 to 62 cc for each kilogram. A similar though smaller decrease in plasma was observed in Case C. H. P. with a distinct rise in the hemoglobin percentage. The converse findings were observed in Case R. G., a fall in hemoglobin, 47 to 26 per cent, being accompanied by an increase in plasma, 60 to 69 cc for each kilogram. Smith made repeated blood-volume determinations in a single case of pernicious anemia using the carbon monoxid method. He noted that the blood volume increased as the hemoglobin percentage fell. In the remaining 6 cases of the series of pernicious anemia the plasma volume varied from 52 to 63 cc for each kilogram and the blood volume from 64 to 82 cc for each kilogram. The findings in the last 6 cases are similar to the findings Bock noted in his series of 7 cases of pernicious anemia.

Two volume determinations made within a month in the case of Banti's disease (Case L. J., Table 2), gave practically identical results. The secondary anemia was not marked and the patient was up and around. Both the plasma and blood volumes were distinctly increased. In the last case (Case H.) the patient was suffering from severe secondary anemia, the hemoglobin being 20 per cent. The amount of plasma, 60 cc for each kilogram, was not strikingly increased, while the total amount of blood, 69 cc for each kilogram, was low.

TABLE 2.—SECONDARY ANEMIA.

Case.	Date.	Age and sex.	Weight, kg.	Hemoglobin, per cent.	Hematocrit, erythrocytes, per cent.	Erythrocytes.	Leukocytes.	Plasma, cc.	Plasma, cc, for each kg.	Blood, cc.	Blood, cc, for each kg.
26850 L. J.	Nov. 12, 1919	27	..	65	..	3,400,000	7800				
Banti's disease	Dec. 4, 1919	M.	57	71	26.4	...	..	4115	72	5605	98
	Dec. 29, 1919	..	55	..	26.4	...	..	4000	73	5435	99
H.	Dec. 10, 1919	M.	70	17	10.0	..	..	4250	61	4700	67
Secondary anemia	Dec. 20, 1919	..	70	20	14.0	...	..	4210	60	4880	69

In pernicious anemia great variations in the blood volume have been reported. Smith used the carbon monoxid method and found that the blood volume in this disease might be increased or decreased below the normal level. In one case variations in volume were presented which bore a definite relation to changes in the clinical course of the disease. Such results may possibly be explained by plasma volume changes as noted in the present series. Quincke, Lindeman, and Denny (Table 4) have determined the blood volume in pernicious anemia by methods based on the concentration of the red blood corpuscles before and after transfusion. The findings noted by Lindeman are open to criticism as he reports some exceedingly low values, much lower than those of other observers. The varied results of both Lindeman and Denny may not be due so much to technical inaccuracies inherent in the methods themselves as to the uncertain fate or distribution of the normal cells after their introduction into the circulation of a diseased person.

The fact that Bock, who used the dye method, failed to find in 7 cases of pernicious anemia a single plasma volume above the normal, may possibly be explained by mere chance or by the clinical condition of the patients at the time the estimations were made. As I have noted, in only one-half of the present series of cases was the amount of plasma increased, while in the other half the findings were practically within normal limits. The high plasma content often found in this study would lead one to the conclusion that in chronic anemia the variations in plasma volume are much greater in latitude than in the normal person. The exact significance of this increase is difficult to ascertain. We know that following acute hemorrhage, with considerable loss of erythrocytes, the depleted circulation can be readily augmented by an increase in the plasma fraction due to an inflow of fluid from the tissues. Thus, the total circulating volume of blood becomes adequate by a relative increase in the plasma volume. The subsequent increase in blood volume to the normal level is brought about by the rapidly increasing number of erythrocytes. This early mechanism of a rapid inflow of fluid into the circulation after hemorrhage may fail because of the lack of tissue fluid, or inability of the smaller vessels to take up fluid, even when present in sufficient amount. Such a condition was found in cases of hemorrhage associated with traumatic shock. Now, early in a slowly progressing anemia the usual mechanism for maintaining an adequate blood volume may be called into play with a resulting high plasma content. Since the subsequent increase in erythrocytes does not occur, however, the total blood volume is reduced. In order, then, to maintain a normal or high blood volume in such cases there must necessarily be an increased plasma content. The actual proof in certain cases in this study of a high plasma volume would indicate the possibility of such a reaction. There is often a tendency to hemorrhage in chronic anemia. This may be a possible factor in causing variations in plasma volume.

Chronic Leukemia. Is the dye taken up by the leukocytes in leukemic blood? If this occurred to any extent the increased dilution of the dye would give estimations of plasma volume much too great. It had previously been demonstrated *in vitro* that little or none of the dye is taken up by the erythrocytes or leukocytes in normal blood. This observation was confirmed by Harris. A similar experiment was carried out on leukemic blood. This consisted in adding a known amount of dye to equal quantities of whole leukemic blood and plasma.

In Case J. F. (Table 3), November 28, 1919, the total leukocyte count was 44,000 for each cubic millimeter. December 2, two samples of blood were rendered incoagulable by 0.1 gm. of sodium citrate[4] and 0.01 gm. of sodium oxalate. The tube containing the oxalated blood was centrifugalized and the plasma pipetted off. To Tube "A," containing 8 cc of citrated whole blood, was added from an accurately graduated 1 cc pipette, 0.03 cc of a 1.5 per cent solution of vital red. The tube was gently shaken for eight minutes in order to insure a thorough mixing of the dye and blood. To Tube "B" containing 8 cc of oxalated plasma was also added 0.03 cc of a 1.5 per cent solution of vital red. After Tube "A" was centrifugalized[5] and the hematocrit reading taken, the plasma was pipetted off and compared in a Duboscq colorimeter with the plasma dye mixture from Tube "B." The readings were $\frac{A}{B} = \frac{7.0}{9.0}$. Therefore, Tube

[4] Sodium citrate was used as anticoagulent because in this amount it has no toxic action.

[5] Three thousand revolutions each minute for twenty minutes.

TABLE 3.—CHRONIC LEUKEMIA.

Case.		Date.	Age.	Sex.	Weight, kg.	Height, cm.	Hemoglobin, per cent.	Hematocrit, erythrocytes and leukocytes, per cent.	Erythrocytes.	Leukocytes.	Plasma, cc.	Plasma, cc, for each kg.	Plasma, liters, for each sq. m.	Blood, cc.	Blood, cc, for each kg.	Blood, liters for each sq. m.	Basal metabolic rate, per cent.
		SPLENOMYELOGENOUS.															
26828	J. F.	Sept. 17, 1919	44	M.	..	..	50	..	2,600,000	326,000							
		Oct. 15, 1919	..	..	..	..	45										
		Oct. 24, 1919	..	..	..	..	..	..	1,728,000	153,000							
		Nov. 4, 1919	..	..	..	..	..	..	...	..	..	..	..	..	..	..	+57
		Nov. 8, 1919[1]	..	..	..	..	20	..	896,000	230,000							
		Nov. 18, 1919	..	..	64	181	47	22	1,888,000	..	5000	77	2.74	6400	100	3.52	
		Nov. 26, 1919	..	..	65	..	59	28	2,513,000	45,000	5710	88	3.12	8000	123	4.37	
		Dec. 2, 1919[2]															
		Dec. 7, 1919	..	..	..	..	..	..	2,911,000	46,000							
		Dec. 19, 1919	..	..	67	..	68	30	3,040,000	9,200	5405	80	2.90	7720	115	4.17	
		Jan. 13, 1920	..	..	71	..	74	32	4,100,000	96,000	4820	67	2.64	7090	100	3.73	
		Feb. 27, 1920	..	..	..	..	81	39	...	32,000	4705	..	..	7715			
		Mar. 19, 1920	..	..	..	..	..	..	...	..	..	..	..	..	..	..	+43
A175501	A. T.	Mar. 4, 1921	43	F.	51	150	91	41	...	..	3345	65	2.32	5670	111	3.93	+36
		May 18, 1921	..	..	..	..	..	..	3,980,000	135,600							
A186558	H. A. S.	Mar. 17, 1921	55	F.	51	161	71	43	2,660,000	176,000	3050	60	2.05	5360	105	3.55	+37
A273047	A. K.	Mar. 18, 1921	49	M.	68	175	71	37	2,640,000	177,000	4580	67	2.53	7270	107	4.01	+36
A356322	C. C. K.	May 9, 1921	18	M.	56	169	46	26	2,210,000	97,000	3975	70	2.42	5370	96	3.29	+44
		May 13, 1921	..	..	56	..	46	27	2,110,000	156,000	3925	70	2.42	5375	96	3.29	+47
A315316	J. S.	May 10, 1921	30	F.	53	156	48	47	2,700,000	514,000	3680	69	2.50	6945	131	4.63	+59
		LYMPHATIC.															
A355667	C. S.	April 21, 1921	50	F.	56.6	159	79	43	3,590,000	394,000	2910	51	1.87	5105	90	3.27	+51
A354070	W. C.	April 22, 1921	55	M.	61	172	87	40	5,010,000	88,000	4195	68	2.44	6990	114	4.06	+ 9
A342995	H. T.	April 22, 1921	66	M.	71	165	88	38	4,760,000	87,000	3845	54	2.18	6200	87	3.50	+44
A258636	J. H. K.	May 25, 1921	61	M.	55.5	169	76	42	4,100,000	112,000	3295	57	2.02	5590	102	3.44	+12

[1] Severe internal hemorrhage, esophageal (?)
[2] Experiment *in vitro* in regard to dye being taken up by the leukocytes.

"A" contained 128.6 per cent as much dye for each cubic centimeter as Tube "B." The amount of plasma in the blood in Tube "A" as shown by the hematocrit was 6.15 cc. Thus, if 0.03 cc of dye is diluted in 6.15 cc of plasma, 1 cc of dye is diluted in 205 cc of plasma. In Tube "B" 0.03 cc of dye is diluted in 8 cc of plasma, thus 1 cc of dye is diluted in 266 cc of plasma. Therefore, there should be $\frac{266}{205}$ or 129.7 per cent of dye in Tube "A." Colorimeter reading, as calculated from hematocrit data, was 129.7 per cent. Colorimeter reading observed was 128.6 per cent.

In the foregoing experiment the calculated and observed values agree so closely that the amount of dye lost from the plasma must be negligible. This experiment is offered as evidence that the leukocytes in splenomyelogenous leukemia have no special tendency, during the short period of a blood-volume determination, to take up the dye, vital red, from the circulating plasma.

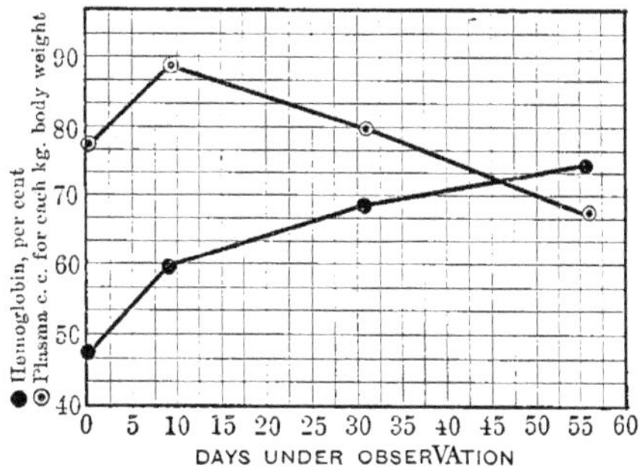

Chart II

In 10 cases of chronic leukemia (Table III), 6 were splenomyelogenons and 4 lymphatic in type. Each showed considerable variation in the plasma and blood-volumes, although the most marked changes occurred in the cases of splenomyelogenous leukemia. No exact relation between plasma volume, hemoglobin percentage or leukocyte count was noted. Detailed studies in Case J. F. are of interest: following a severe internal hemorrhage, probably esophageal in origin, the patient's hemoglobin fell to 20 per cent. Ten days later, with the hemoglobin at 47 per cent, the plasma and blood volume were definitely high, the plasma amounting to 77 cc for each kilogram. The patient continued to improve rapidly and on the next examination, within nine days, the hemoglobin rose to 59 per cent while the plasma volume reached the very high mark of 88 cc for each kilogram. On three subsequent determinations the plasma volume showed a gradual decrease, while the hemoglobin percentage rose from 59 to 81 (Chart 2). During this period of rapid recovery, the patient received several roentgenray treatments and as a result the leukocyte count on one occasion

100 to 123 cc for each kilogram, during the entire period of observation, November 18, 1919, to February 27, 1920.

In Case C. C. K., two determinations made within a few days gave almost identical results. Here again both the plasma and total blood were increased. In the 4 other cases the plasma amounted to from 60 to 69 cc for each kilogram, while the blood volume varied between 105 and 131 cc for each kilogram. The striking feature, therefore, in these cases is the consistently high plasma volume.

In considering the data of the 4 cases of chronic lymphatic leukemia there was only 1 case (Case W. C.) in which the plasma volume was noticeably increased. The amounts of plasma observed in Cases C. S., H. T., and J. H. K., were within normal limits.

The basal metabolic rate was determined in all of the 10 cases of leukemia. In the splenomyelogenous group the rates were all definitely elevated. On the other hand, in cases of lymphatic type, two were raised while two had rates of +9 and +12. The highest plasma volume, 68 cc for each kilogram, was in Case W. C., with the rate of + 9. No absolute relationship, therefore, was found to exist in this small series between plasma or blood volumes and the basal metabolic rates.

Clinicians have long believed that certain cases of leukemia are plethoric. The presence of a large volume of circulating leukocytes also suggests the possibility of an increased total volume of blood. That the leukocytes may possibly play such a part is supported by frequent high cell volumes obtained *in vitro* in the hematocrit tube (Table 3). Few actual blood-volume determinations have been made in leukemia.

Plesch and Oerum each report a single case having a normal blood volume. Kammerer and Waldmann, using the Behring tetanus antitoxin method, made determinations on 4 cases, two lymphatic and two splenomyelogenous in type. In one of the latter the blood volume was high. Behring also reports the finding of an increased volume in 2 cases of leukemia (Table 4). The results recorded in this series indicate that in certain cases the plasma volume is high and that this is more often associated with an increased blood volume than in chronic anemia. It is difficult to correlate the large amount of plasma with any one other clinical or laboratory finding common to the disease. The enlarged spleen and liver were considered as possibly having a casual relation. This idea was given added support because of the finding of a large plasma volume in the case of Banti's disease (Case L. J., Table 2). Giffin and Haines are at present making determinations before and subsequent to splenectomy in such cases. If a previous high plasma volume should still persist after splenectomy, then the enlarged spleen could be definitely ruled out as an etiologic factor. The relation of an enlarged liver to a high plasma content is obviously more difficult to appraise.

TABLE 4.—PREVIOUS DETERMINATIONS IN PERNICIOUS ANEMIA AND CHRONIC LEUKEMIA.

PERNICIOUS ANEMIA.

Author.	Method.	Cases.	Plasma, cc, for each kg., extremes.	Blood, cc. for each kg., extremes.	Blood, per cent of body weight, extremes.	Remarks.
Smith	Carbon monoxid	7	...	49—117	4.9—11.7	
Oerum	Carbon monoxid	1	...	...	5.1	
Plesch	Saline infusion	1	...	37.5	3.96	
Behring	Tetanus antitoxin	2	...	...	9.6—11.7	
Quincke	Erythrocytes before and after transfusion	2	...	...	4.3— 5.0	
Lindeman	Hematocrit before and after transfusion	11	...	26—60	2.4— 5.8	
Denny	Oxygen capacity of blood before and after transfusion	10	...	...	5.1— 9.7	
Keith, Rowntree and Geraghty	Vital red	2	54—72	66—81	7.0— 8.7	
Bock	Vital red	7	38—59	44—72	4.3— 7.3	
		LEUKEMIA.				
Plesch	Saline infusion	1	...	51.6	5.4	Type of leukemia (?)
Behring	Tetanus antitoxin	2	...	...	10.5—11.5	Type of leukemia (?)
Kammerer and Waldemann	Tetanus antitoxin	2	...	83—86	8.7— 9	Lymphatic leukemia.
	Tetanus antitoxin	2	...	93—110	9.7—11.5	Myelogenous leukemia.

Summary. 1. Wide variations in blood and plasma volume have been observed in 24 patients presenting definite evidence of chronic disease of the blood-forming organs. These variations were sometimes noted in the same patient.

2. In certain cases of chronic anemia there was a striking increase in the volume of plasma; in others, a normal plasma volume. In all cases the blood volume was normal or reduced.

3. In cases of chronic anemia no exact relationship could be determined between the amount of plasma and the hemoglobin percentage, although in individual cases these varied somewhat inversely with one another.

4. An experiment *in vitro* on the blood of a patient with splenomyelogenous leukemia failed to show that any appreciable amount of the dye, vital red, is taken up by the leukocytes.

5. In chronic leukemia the blood volume is almost invariably increased. The plasma volume often reaches a high value, especially in the splenomyelogenous type.

6. In chronic leukemia no definite relationship could be demonstrated between the basal metabolic rate and the variations in blood or plasma volume.

BIBLIOGRAPHY.

1. von Behring, E.: Meine Blutuntersuchungen. Beitr. z. Exper. Therap., Berlin, Hirschwald, 1911, **12,** 115.

2. Bock, A. V.: The Consistency of the Volume of the Blood-Plasma. Arch. Int. Med., 1921, **27,** 83-101.

3. Boothby, W. M., and Sandiford, Irene: Laboratory Manual of the Technic of Basal Metabolic-rate Determination. Philadelphia, Saunders, 1920.

4. Denny, G. P.: Blood Volume in Pernicious Anemia. Arch. Int. Med , 1921, **27,** 38–44.

5. Dreyer, G., and Ray, W.: The Blood Volume of Mammals as Determined by Experiments upon Rabbits, Guinea-pigs and Mice and its Relationship to the Body Weight and to the Surface Area Expressed in a Formula. Proc. Roy. Soc. London, 1910, **82,** 545–546.

6. Du Bois, D., and Du Bois, E. F.: Clinical Calorimetry. Tenth Paper. A Formula to Estimate the Approximate Surface Area if Height and Weight be Known. Arch. Int. Med., 1916, **17,** 863–871.

7. Harris, D. T.: The Value of the Vital-red Method as a Clinical Means for the Estimation of the Volume of the Blood. British Jour. Exper. Path., 1920, **1,** 142–158.

8. Kämmerer, H., and Waldmann, A.: Blutmengebestimmungen nach v. Behring und andere quantitative Untersuchungen der Blutbestandteile. Deutsch. Arch. f. klin. Med., 1913, **109,** 524–559.

9. Keith, N. M., Rowntree, L. G., and Geraghty, J. T.: A Method for the Determination of Plasma and Blood Volume. Arch. Int. Med., 1915, **16,** 547–576.

10. Lindeman, E.: A New Method for Estimating Total Blood Volume in Anemias. Preliminary report. Jour. Am. Med. Assn., 1918, **70,** 1209–1210.

11. Lindeman, E.: The Total Blood Volume in Pernicious Anemia. Jour. Am. Med. Assn., 1918, **70,** 1292–1297.

12. Oerum: Quoted by Plesch.

13 Palmer, W. W.: The Colorimetric Determination of Hemoglobin. Jour. Biol. Chem., 1918, **33,** 119–126.

14. Plesch, J.: Hämodynamische Studien. Ztschr. f. exper. Path. u. Therap., 1909, **6,** 380–618.

15. Quincke, H.: Weitere Beobachtungen über perniciöse Anämie. Deutsch. Arch. f. klin. Med., 1877, **20,** 1–31.

16. Smith, H. P., Arnold, H. R., and Whipple, G. H.: Blood Volume Studies. VII. Comparative Values of Welcher, Carbon Monoxide and Dye Methods for Blood Volume Determinations. Accurate Estimation of Absolute Blood Volume. Am. Jour. Physiol., 1921, **56,** 336.

17. Smith, J. L.: The Blood in Disease. Tr. Path. Soc. London, 1900, **51,** 311–329.

A CASE OF MULTIPLE MYELOMA.

By Guthrie McConnell, M.D.,
CLEVELAND, OHIO.

(From the Department of Pathology of the Cleveland City Hospital.)

Inasmuch as cases of multiple myeloma are still uncommon, this one has been reported. For the opportunity of so doing, thanks are due to Dr. Paryzek and to the residents and interns under whose care the patient came. When compared with the others that have been reported, this particular one is interesting in that it is so thoroughly typical of the classic form.

Case Report.—Patient I. N., colored man, aged forty-nine years. Admitted to the Cleveland City Hospital the first time on January 9, 1921, when the following notes were obtained:

Previous History. Born in Mississippi. Influenza two years ago. Chancre thirty years ago and also one attack of gonorrhea. Had "chills and fever" once or twice a year until 1919. He claimed to have had night-sweats for the past eight to ten years, but no hemoptysis or loss of weight. No skin lesions or sore-throat. No loss of power in the extremities.

Present Illness. Began December 12, 1920, when the patient had to go to bed on account of severe precordial pains which radiated through the chest and were made worse by exertion. Remained in bed practically all the time. Finally brought to the hospital in January, 1921. On admission his chief complaint was that he felt "sore all over," but particularly throughout the abdomen and in the lumbar region.

Physical Examination. No cough; marked hoarseness. Holds chest rigid and breathes with difficulty. Movement is distinctly painful, but by moving very slowly and carefully is able to change his position.

Ear, nose and head showed nothing abnormal. Pupils slightly unequal and irregular and reacted sluggishly to light. Teeth in good condition. Mucous membranes appeared normal. No glandular enlargement in the neck. Jugular vessels slightly distended. Slight tracheal tug. Chest is flattened abnormally in its anteroposterior dimension. The sternum is not perfectly straight, is unduly flexible, particularly at the junction of the manubrium and the gladiolus, at which point there is a moderately soft mass about 2.5 cm. in diameter. Ribs also are unduly flexible and show many small, round or oval areas in which the bone is quite soft. (These softened areas are quite tender to pressure.) Many small nodules, apparently subperiosteal, are found.

Both clavicles are somewhat enlarged, particularly in the middle third, where they are quite soft and where a crackling sensation is noted on pressure. In these areas no solid bone can be felt, and there is evidently a lack of support to the shoulder girdle. The acromion processes on both sides show a very similar condition, and in the left scapula there is a large tumor mass that is comparatively safe.

Lungs resonant throughout. Breath sounds normal.

Heart: Diffuse visible precordial activity to right and left of the sternum. Systolic thrill palpable over apex and aortic area.

The sounds at the apex are accompanied by a systolic murmur heard best at the aortic area. Aortic second sound increased. Pulse rate, 90; good rhythm and volume. Arteries tortuous.

Abdomen: Slight tenderness of the liver, which extends three finger-breadths below the costal margin. Spleen not palpable.

External genitalia: Negative. No enlargement of the prostate.

Extremities: Show nothing abnormal.

Neurological: Reflexes normally active. No Babinsky, clonus or ataxia. No sensory changes. No lesions of the cranial nerves.

Blood: Red blood cells, 4,720,000; white blood cells, 7200; hemoglobin, 80 per cent; polynuclears, 58; small, 30; large, 7; transitionals, 5; myelocytes, 0.

Blood-pressure: Systolic, 175; diastolic, 100.

Spinal fluid: Clear. Increased pressure. 20 cc obtained. Globulin present. Ten cells present; mononuclear.

Wassermann negative with both blood and spinal fluid.

Lange colloidal gold test negative.

Temperature: Lowest, 36°; highest, 37.4°.

Pulse: Lowest, 70; highest, 102.

Respiration: Lowest, 18; highest, 25.

Urine, January 24, 1921: 1008. Albumin present. Sugar, 0. A few casts. Bence-Jones protein positive.

January 26 1921: 1008. Albumin present. Sugar, 0. No casts. Bence-Jones protein positive.

Roentgen-ray report, January 26, 1921: Marked dilatation of the aorta with transverse position of the heart. Multiple areas of destruction of bones; most marked in ribs and clavicles, the anterior portion of the ribs being almost completely destroyed as far as the bony structure is concerned. There is also considerable involvement of the scapulæ, upper portion of the humeri, upper spine and skull. Of the skull the bones that show the most involvement are the parietal, frontal and malar. Also some involvement of the lower jaw and a few small areas in the femurs.

After remaining a few weeks in the hospital the patient felt better and decided to return home. His improvement continued to some extent and he attempted to work, but the old symptoms reappeared and he had to go back to bed.

The patient was readmitted to the hospital on July 7, 1921. At this time his condition was distinctly worse. The palpable nodules were more numerous and larger. Softened areas were present in the skull; the sacrum on the right side was thickened and the head of the right femur was distinctly enlarged but not softened. No enlargement of the lymph nodes was found.

Blood, July 6, 1921: White blood cells, 7000; hemoglobin, 85.

July 17, 1921: Polynuclears, 63; small, 22; large, 8; transitionals, 3; myelocytes, 4.

July 18, 1921: Red blood cells, 3,900,000; white blood cells, 7800; hemoglobin, 68.

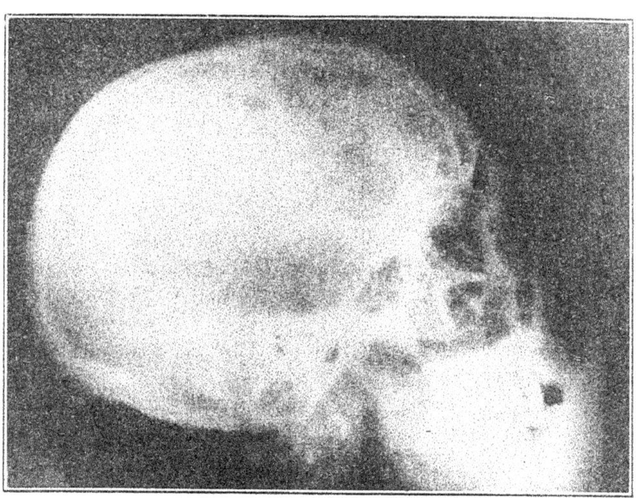

FIG. 1.—Roentgen-ray of skull showing many areas of softening.

Blood-pressure: Systolic, 190; diastolic, 100.
Urine, July 7, 1921: Casts, +; sugar, 0; specific gravity, 1011.
July 13, 1921: Albumin, ++; casts, ++.

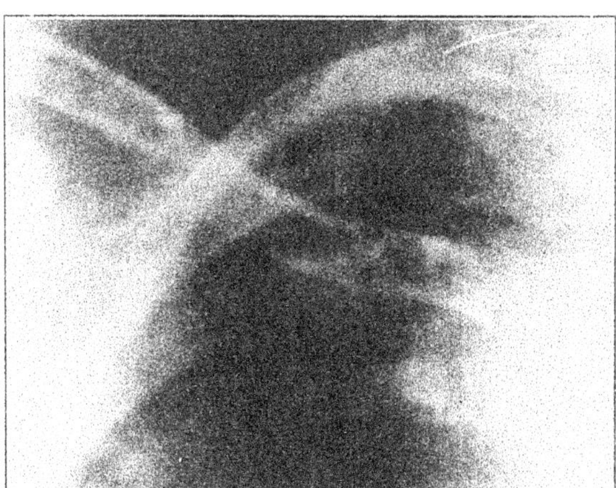

FIG. 2.—Roentgen-ray of right clavicle and ribs showing involvement.

July 18, 1921: Albumin, ++; casts, +.
July 19, 1921: Albumin, +++; casts, +.

Bence-Jones protein: large amount present constantly.

Feces and spinal fluid were not examined.

Blood Wassermann negative.

On August 26 he died, but unfortunately no relative could be located in order that a permit for an autopsy could be obtained until the following day, when it was performed twenty-nine hours after death.

I. N. (autopsy twenty-nine hours after death).

Clinical Diagnosis. Multiple myeloma. Chronic aortitis with dilatation and elongation of ascending portion of the arch. Generalized arteriosclerosis. Cardiac hypertrophy.

Anatomical Diagnosis. Multiple myeloma. Bronchopneumonia, bilateral. Edema of the lungs. Chronic parenchymatous nephritis with acute changes. Mesenteric adenitis, tuberculous. Atheroma of the aorta.

Body that of a much emaciated adult negro of about fifty years of age. Slight rigor. The chief peculiarity lies in the condition of the bones. There evidently has developed a growth within the marrow cavities causing an atrophy of the bony tissue with softening and in some cases fracture of the bone. This is particularly noticeable in both clavicles, which are much enlarged in their middle portions, crackly to the touch and no longer continuous. Similar conditions were present in the upper portion of the sternum and in many of the ribs, several of the latter showing multiple lesions. In the skull several small areas of softening were present. The upper portions of the two humeri were distinctly enlarged, as was the upper portion of the right femur. No areas of softening were noticed in the above long bones.

On opening into the canal of the left humerus the marrow was a dark-brownish red and very soft. Apparently no definite structure.

No change was found in the marrow of the right tibia.

On incising the masses found in the sternum and in the ribs they were found to be quite soft, pale gray, with numerous minute areas of congestion or hemorrhage. They appeared to be distinctly encapsulated by a thin membrane which was probably the stretched periosteum. No fragments of bone were found within the tissue. The impression was that of a central mass undergoing expansile growth with subsequent atrophy of the surrounding bone. According to the autopsy findings the following bones were involved: skull, cervical vertebræ, both scapulæ, both clavicles, sternum, most if not all of the ribs, both humeri, both iliac bones and the upper portion of both femurs, particularly the right. The forearms and hands, legs and feet showed no changes.

With the exception of several of the mesenteric, there was no enlargement of the lymph nodes in general nor metastatic growths in any of the organs.

Microscopic Diagnosis. Myeloma of bone-marrow of the humerus, of the rib and of the sternum. Fibrous myocarditis with calcification in the walls of the vessels. Emphysema and congestion of the lungs with extensive calcification of the alveolar walls. Chronic interstitial nephritis with extensive calcification. Pigmentation, congestion and calcification in the spleen. Slight calcification in the pancreas. Cloudy swelling of the liver. Fibrous tuberculosis of the mesenteric lymph node.

Heart: Distinct calcification of the elastic membrane of the larger arteries accompanied by degenerative changes of the subintimal tissues. One portion shows a very extensive replacement of muscle fibers by large masses of dense connective tissue. In these masses are many particles of lime, as evidenced by the irregularity of outline and deep staining by hematoxylin. Capillaries filled with blood.

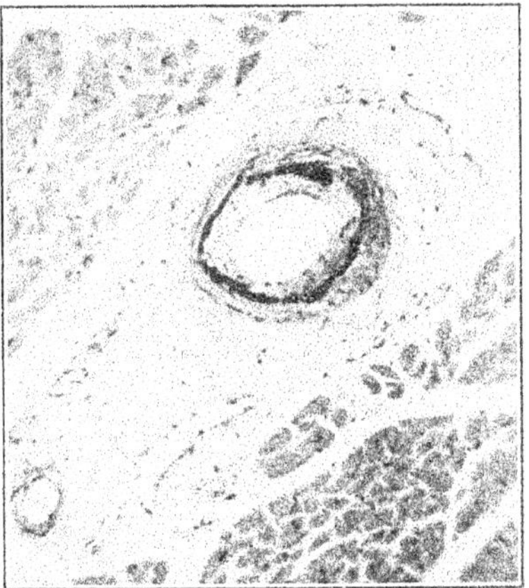

FIG. 3.—Heart showing deposits of lime.

Lung: The conspicuous feature is the very widespread calcification of the alveolar capillary vessels. In many instances the wall has been replaced by a large mass of lime salts in which no remnants of tissue are visible. Fragments are found occasionally lying within the alveoli, possibly misplacements due to the cutting of the tissues. The walls of the larger bloodvessels also show similar infiltration. In some areas there is tremendous congestion with the escape of blood into the alveoli.

Kidneys: Very great loss of tubules with replacement by a very marked widespread formation of dense fibrous tissue. Many of the glomerular tufts have undergone fibrous changes as a result apparently of capsular proliferation. Widespread infiltration by lymphocytes. Numerous tubules contain hyaline material. Some thickening of the bloodvessel walls but no calcification. In the fibrotic areas of the cortex particularly there is a widespread calcification, masses lying not only in the connective tissue but within the tubules as well.

Adrenal: Shows no definite lesion other than an area in which there are numerous small masses of rather large cells containing round or oval, deeply staining nuclei, surrounded by a distinct zone of protoplasm. No calcification.

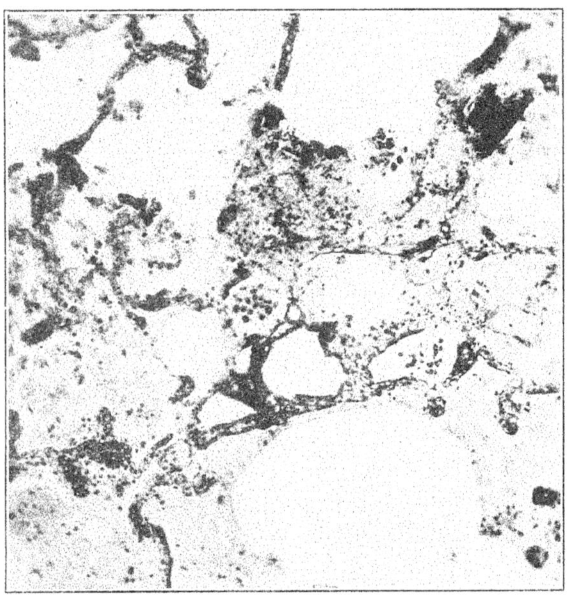

FIG. 4.—Lung showing deposits of lime in the alveolar walls.

Liver: Epithelium swollen and cloudy. Blood sinuses distended. No cellular infiltration. No calcification.

Spleen: Large masses of lime salts in the walls of the large bloodvessels. Some pigmentation and congestion.

Pancreas: Epithelial changes, probably postmortem. Some very slight calcification in the walls of a few of the large vessels.

Mesenteric lymph nodes: Show many irregular areas of fibrosis with some necrosis in which are many typical Langhans giant cells. No calcification.

Lymph node: Shows a very distinct fibrosis but no areas of degeneration or giant-cell formation. Apparently a chronic fibrosis. No calcification.

Marrow (from the left humerus): Section shows two very distinct types of tissue. One of them is composed of broad bands of homogeneous material, suggesting degenerated fatty tissue, the meshes of which are engorged with blood. Practically no white cells are present in the above area. There is then a very abrupt change into an area in which there are myriads of white cells and very few erythrocytes. These cells occupy the blood spaces and enclose round clear spots evidently where fat has been dissolved out. Under the oil-immersion two types of large cells are found to predominate. In one the nucleus is round or slightly oval, stains quite deeply and is surrounded by a narrow but distinct zone of cloudy but nongranular protoplasm that stains a very faint blue. In the second type the nucleus is distinctly larger, contains much less chromatin and consequently does not stain so deeply; is very definitely vesicular. It is surrounded by a large amount of protoplasm, which although nongranular appears distinctly cloudy. In many instances the nuclei are eccentrically situated in the cell.

Although the majority of the cells conform to these two types there are many variations. There are very large cells with very densely staining nuclei and there are many small cells with vesicular nuclei. Throughout the tissue are many large mononuclear cells with a granular eosinophilic protoplasm. Here and there are found multinucleated cells many times larger than the surrounding cells, conforming to the characteristics of the megakaryocyte. No mitotic figures noted.

Tumor from rib: The tumor mass is sharply delimited by a definite band of connective tissue which probably is the result of condensation. Beyond this is muscle tissue which in a few places shows infiltration by the tumor cells. Throughout the section are many very minute capillaries, all of which show a complete endothelial wall. There are no places in which blood spaces, formed by the cells themselves, were noted, an arrangement that explains the absence of metastasis.

Under the oil-immersion it is quite evident that the two varieties of cells already mentioned are but variations of one type.

The cells are large and more or less polygonal as a result of mutual pressure; the nuclei, as a rule, are eccentrically placed in a large amount of a cloudy but nongranular protoplasm. The nuclei differ greatly in their staining. As a rule the smaller ones stain the more deeply. As they become larger there appears to be less chromatin, but what is present is arranged mainly in small irregular masses around the periphery of the nucleus, leaving a comparatively clear central area.

In many cells the nucleus has definitely broken down into small fragments, and there are others in which no trace of the nucleus can be seen.

An occasional granular eosinophilic mononuclear cell is found and some show a definitely pinkish protoplasm, but no granules are evident. No typical megakaryocytes were found, although there were a few cells with two or three nuclei, but their characteristics were those of the tumor cell. No definite fibrils could be distinguished between the individual cells.

Tumor from the sternum in every respect appeared similar to that from the rib.

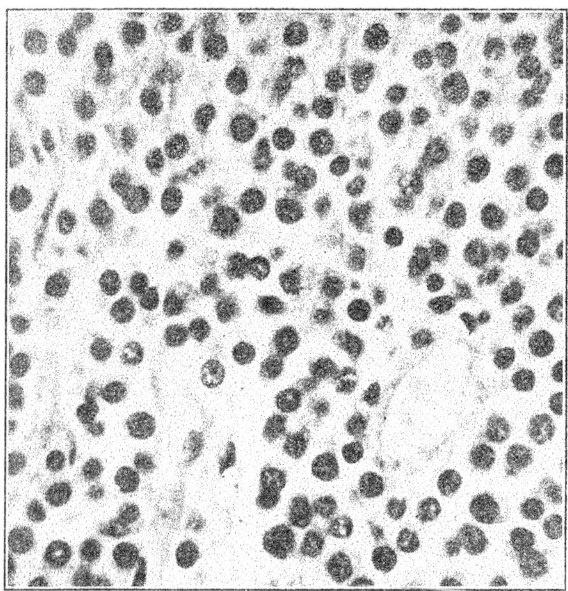

FIG. 5.—Tumor mass from the sternum. Oil-immersion.

From the morphologist's point of view the interesting feature of these tumors is the origin of the cells composing them. A classification based entirely on morphology is very unreliable, yet many observers who have reported such cases have considered them as "plasma-cell" tumors on account of their resemblance to that cell. Others classify them as atypical derivatives from the neutrophilic myelocytes. That they originate primarily within the bone-marrow seems to be undisputed, as examinations of the tissues and blood in these cases show no source outside of the marrow, although in a very few instances myelocytes have been found in the blood stream. All the evidence tends, however, to show that the multiple myeloma is a disease that occurs *de novo* in the marrow and is not an instance of metastases from some single primary tumor.

According to most hematologists the parent cell in the bone-marrow is the myeloblast; from it both the leukocytes and the erythrocytes develop. Although the myeloblast is nongranular its descendants are the granular myelocytes and polymorphonuclear leukocytes. The plasma cell, on the other hand, is supposed to be derived from the nongranular lymphocyte, which is not considered to originate within the bone-marrow. Although there is a certain similarity between the myeloma cell and the plasma cell the resemblance may not be very striking. The tumor cell is distinctly larger, there are great variations in the size and staining reactions of the nuclei, and the protoplasm, although seldom granular, is definitely cloudy and takes a neutrophilic tinge.

Vance[1] in discussing multiple myeloma states: "There is no doubt, however, that these cells, diverse as they are, are derivatives of the undifferentiated cell of the bone-marrow or myeloblast, which is the ancestor of both the leukocyte and the erythrocyte." He holds that the cells in his case all took their origin from the cells in the bone-marrow, although the oxydase test was negative.

Forman and Warren[2] say that "Since it has been established definitely that the oxydase reaction is characteristic of myeloid cells the application of this reaction to the cells of a myeloma ought to be of great service in identifying these tumors." In the case they report they used this method and found oxydase granules not only in cells morphologically like the myeloid type but also in many of the cells which in size, shape and staining closely resembled the plasma cell. Although most of the cells gave the reaction there were some that did not. The question arose, therefore, as to whether or not such cells had matured sufficiently to contain the granules.

Beck and McCleary[3] found in their case that the indophenol blue test showed oxydase granules, thus indicating that the cells belonged to the myeloid group, although the morphology was that of the plasma cell. Jacobson[4] reports a case of "multiple myeloma of the plasma cell, nongranular, nonoxydase type."

Mallory[5] states quite emphatically where the myeloma cell does not belong but does not classify it. "The type cell of this tumor has not yet been determined. Evidently it does not belong to the myeloblast series of cells because it does not differentiate like them. Moreover the myeloma is never associated with myelogenous leukemia. The only other cells peculiar to the bone-marrow are the erythroblast and the megakaryocyte. Possibly it arises from one of these cells. It is claimed by some writers that there exists in the bone-marrow another peculiar kind of cell which they call the bone-marrow plasma cells, and that from it this tumor arises. Time alone will tell." Mallory makes no mention of the oxydase reaction as a method of determining the myeloid origin of the cell.

MacCallum[6] divides the myelomas into two kinds: One composed

[1] Am. Jour. Med. Sci., 1916, **152**, 693.
[2] Jour. Cancer Research, 1917, **2**, 79.
[3] Jour. Am. Med Assn., 1919, **72**, 480.
[4] Jour. Urology, April, 1917.
[5] Pathologic Histology, 1914, p. 338.
[6] Pathology, 1916, p. 775.

of lymphoid cells and another composed of myeloid cells. In the former the "cells are nongranular, mononuclear, have a basophilic protoplasm and are very similar to the plasma cell, with which they are regarded by most writers as identical." In the second type the cells correspond with the myeloblast.

Ewing[7] in classifying myeloma according to different observers gives four groups: (1) Plasmocytoma; (2) erythroblastoma; (3) myelocytoma, adult and embryonal; (4) lymphocytoma. "Whether such varied interests are actually represented in the scope of multiple myeloma or whether we have to deal with varying grades of anaplasia in a single cell or origin remains to be determined. At present the data seem to favor the former alternative."

Hoping that some definite information might be obtained by means of the oxydase reaction, portions of two tumor masses which had been hardened in formalin were frozen, sections made and stained according to the method given by Forman and Warren.[8] Although the reaction took place no definite conclusion could be drawn because only a very small percentage of the cells showed blue granules. Scattered through the tumor tissue were granular cells occurring either singly or in small masses, intimately intermingled with other cells which showed no reaction. There were also many large areas in which none of the cells reacted. In order to bring out the nuclear structure, safranin was used as a counterstain and proved to be very satisfactory, but no definite differences could be determined between those cells giving the oxydase reaction and those that did not. Examinations made of the sections stained by eosin and hematoxylin revealed no areas in which the cells differed distinctly from neighboring groups.

There would seem to be several explanations as to why such a condition should exist. As several observers have suggested it may be that the great majority of the cells, although myelogenous in origin, had not reached that point of development in which granules appear. It is a well-recognized fact that the connective-tissue tumors may represent all the different stages of development and that they remain in that particular stage. A round-cell sarcoma does not eventually become of the spindle-cell type. In the myeloma we are dealing with tumors of varying degrees of malignancy. In those in which practically all the cells contain oxydase granules the development may have been more complete than in those which show little or no reaction.

Although we know that the myeloma develops within the bone-marrow, nothing is known as to the fate of the original marrow cells. It could be assumed that many of them remain more or less physiologically active in spite of being imbedded in masses of tumor cells. In this case scattered cells and cell groups might be considered as

[7] Neoplastic Diseases, 1919, p. 289.
[8] Loc. cit.

remnants of the original tissue, consequently the fact that some of the cells contain blue granules and others do not has little bearing as to the origin of the non-reacting cells. As there were no metastases in this case there was no way of determining whether or not the granular cells were actually neoplastic or not.

From the morphologic viewpoint the cells in this tumor resemble plasma cells much more closely than any other type. It being accepted rather generally that the plasma cell is a derivative of the nongranular lymphocyte, such growths, therefore, would have to be considered as lymphatic in origin, but histologists do not consider the bone-marrow as playing a part in the formation of lymphocytes. Such being the case it does not seem permissible to consider any of the primary myelomas as being either true plasma cell or lymphocytic tumors.

Accepting the view that we are dealing with anaplastic stages of a single cell, the oxydase reaction becomes nothing more than a method of determining the stage of development of any particular myeloma. By analogy to the sarcoma the earlier the stage the more malignant. It would be interesting if comparisons could be made in this respect between various cases.

An interesting feature in the case here reported is the presence of lime deposits in the heart, lungs, kidneys, spleen and pancreas. As a result of the expansile growth of the individual tumor masses there occurs a great destruction of the bone which causes a large amount of lime salts to be set free. These salts are carried through circulation and deposited in the different organs, particularly in the walls of the vessels. In the lung there were large areas in which the alveolar walls were represented by a network of lime deposit.

Vance[9] gives references to three cases in which deposits of calcium were found in the viscera.[10]

Blatherwick,[11] as a result of his chemical investigations of a case of myeloma, reports that the analyses of the feces and urine showed an abnormally increased calcium excretion.

From the clinical side there is nothing unusual in this case, excepting possibly its being a colored man. As in the majority of instances the patient was about fifty years old. There was nothing suggestive in the previous history as far as any etiologic factor was concerned. The initial lesions in the ribs, clavicle and sternum, with subsequent involvement of more distant bones, is typical, and the duration of the disease, eight months, is rather characteristic, as it seems to be unusual for a patient to live more than about one year after the appearance of symptoms.

[9] Loc. cit.

[10] Bender: Deut. Zeit. f. Chir., 1902, **65**. Scheele and Herxheimer: Zeit. f. klin. Med., 1904, **54**. Tschislowitsch and Kolesnikoff: Virchows Arch., 1909, **197**.

[11] Am. Jour. Med. Sci., 1916, **151**, 432.

ON OCCUPATIONAL SENSITIZATION TO THE CASTOR BEAN.

By Harry S. Bernton, A.B., M.D.

Associate professor of hygiene, the school of medicine, Georgetown University, Washington, D. C.

The literature affords numerous examples of poisoning with the castor bean and with its products. Thus the toxic action resulting from the ingestion of the whole bean, accidental or otherwise, and even from the medicinal use of castor oil has been recorded. Especially noteworthy is the toxalbumin found in the residue of the castor beans after the removal of the oil. Stillmark, in 1889, termed this toxalbumin "ricin" and regarded it as a globulin. Osborne, Mendel, and Harris,[1] however, have ascribed the toxic action of the castor bean to the protein fraction which is an albumin, coagulable at 60° to 70.° Ricin ranks among the most powerful of the vegetable poisons when injected directly into the bloodstream. It, also, has the property of agglutinating red blood cells extravascularly. Injected subcutaneously into rabbits, ricin proves fatal in a dose of 0.0005 mg. per kilogram of body weight. At the point of injection, a localized area of necrosis results. If applied to mucous surfaces, a severe inflammatory reaction ensues.

The meal, which is the fat-free residue of the castor bean, has poisoned cattle when mixed with fodder. The use of the meal as a fertilizer has not been without danger to man and beast. Exposure to its dust has caused irritation of the nasal and conjunctival mucous membranes. It is obvious, therefore, that the careless handling, in the industries, of the castor beans and of the castor meal is fraught with grave consequences. Kobert[2] lists the following signs and symptoms of ricin poisoning in man: Nausea, vomiting, stomachache, colicky pains, diarrhea, at times bloody evacuations, tenesmus, headache, fever, hot skin, burning sensation in the throat, thirst, clammy perspiration, small and rapid pulse, cramps in the legs, dilatation of pupils, cyanosis, and anuria.

The case, herein recorded, presents features which have not been mentioned in the literature. The symptom-complex warrants the diagnosis of protein sensitization, occupational in origin, due to the castor bean. The subject is that of a white male, aged twenty-seven, a chemist by occupation and engaged in the "Drug, Poisonous, and Oil Plant Investigations of the Bureau of Plant Industry of the U. S. Department of Agriculture." He has always enjoyed good health and has had no operation performed on the nose or throat. Employment in the Bureau dates back to 1913. Prior to 1916, there had been no sensitiveness to dust of any kind. In 1916, after three years of service, the subject noticed that exposure to dust was accompanied by itching of the eyes, lachrymation, sweating of the forehead, sneezing, and coryza. The sneezing would be continuous for fifteen to twenty minutes. The administration of atropine and the use of adrenalin-spray did not control the symptoms. The attacks of sneezing were more frequent and severe in the spring, April to May, and in the fall, the latter part of August and September. There was no family nor personal history of asthma or of hay fever. During the eighteen month period from December, 1917, to July, 1919, the subject was free of symptoms. In this interval, he was in the military service and was assigned to a serological laboratory. After his discharge from the army, there was a return of symptoms with the resumption of his former duties in the Bureau of Plant Industry. The symptoms were, however, aggravated by attacks of asthma during the night. Severe sneezing spells during the day inevitably ushered in attacks of asthma during the night. Frequently he was aroused out of a sound sleep by asthmatic attacks.

In November, 1921, the subject was afflicted with the usual attacks of sneezing while working with the short ragweed. During the night, the attack of asthma was of exceptional severity so that he felt as if "he were going to die." He was incapacitated from work for the two following days.

In virtue of the history of perennial hay fever, more prominent in the spring and in the fall, cutaneous tests were performed (November 15, 1921) with the hope of discovering the sensitizing agent. The materials employed were as follows:

Right forearm: Control decinormal NaOH solution, pollen-extract of red top, timothy, June grass, cocklebur, ragweed (short), cosmos, ash, dandelion, dock, sweet vernal, willow and black walnut.

Left forearm: Alcoholic saline extract of the pollen of ragweed (short) A, chenopodium album, ragweed (short) B, sodium hydrate extract of the pollen of ragweed (short), pollen of chenopodium ambrosioides and pollen of ragweed (short).

The cutaneous tests proved negative with all the above-mentioned pollens and pollen extracts.

The second series of cutaneous tests was prompted by the suspicion of the subject that the dust of the castor bean was the specific exciting cause. He recalled that, in 1916, investigations of the castor oil were undertaken in the Bureau and the extraction of the oil from the beans formed a new part of the routine of the laboratory. Coincident with this investigation, symptoms of irritation of the nasal mucosa appeared. There was a constant exposure to the dust of the fat-free meal. This, when dry, consisted of a fine, dirty-white, amorphous powder. The slightest inhalation of the powder while at work brought on attacks of sneezing.

The pouring of the meal into bags by an associate in one end of the laboratory inevitably produced sneezing in the subject, while engaged in reading or writing at his desk at the other end of the laboratory. Even the necessary moving about of the sacks of castor beans by charwomen in the early morning hours caused sneezing of the subject upon first entering the room. Invariably emptying the sacks or stumbling into them, with or without the knowledge of the subject, gave rise to symptoms. The severity of the attacks of sneezing was determined by the amount of dust afloat.

Accordingly on November 18, 1921, cutaneous tests were performed with the castor meal. Decinormal sodium hydrate solution was employed as a solvent. Other materials were added for control observation.

The details of the second series of skin tests follow: Five drops of decinormal sodium hydrate solution were placed one-half inch apart on the anterior aspect of the left forearm. A slight superficial scratch was made through each drop with a fine needle. The first drop just below the end of the elbow served as a control. The test materials were then applied in the following order to each drop of alkali by means of the flattened end of a tooth pick: Control of sodium hydrate solution, castor meal powder, pollen of ragweed (short), horse serum protein, and castor meal powder. Within fifteen minutes, wheals developed at the site of drops, numbers 2 and 5, to which the castor meal had been applied. The wheals were irregular in outline, showing numerous pseudopods, the upper one measuring 17 mm. and the lower one 10 mm. in greatest diameter. At the end of the half-hour, the entire forearm was one erythematous patch. The lymphatic trunks on the inner aspect of the upper arm appeared as reddish streaks. Moreover, wheals were formed approximately 7 mm. in diameter at the site of the other drops.

It is to be emphasized that every precaution had been taken to prevent the inhalation of the fine particles of organic matter during the transfer from bottle to the arm. Obviously, dust formation was impossible when once the test material became moistened with the sodium hydrate solution. The development of a constitutional reaction at the end of fifteen minutes was, indeed, a surprise. The conjunctivæ became engorged. Lachrymation and coryza were profuse. An attack of sneezing added to the discomfort. The subject felt nauseated and experienced a sensation of weakness in the abdomen. There was, also, moderate flushing of the face and perspiration of the forehead. Full recovery was made within half-hour of the onset of the reaction. Absorption, therefore, of the minutest amount of castor meal solution from two superficial abrasions on the forearm reproduced the clinical symptoms ordinarily occasioned by the exposure to large doses of the dust of the castor meal.

Thirty-five minutes after the above test had been begun on the left arm, the following materials were employed in similar manner on the anterior aspect of the right forearm: Control of sodium hydrate solution, pollen of ragweed (short), horse serum protein and chicken feather protein. These tests proved negative. It will be recalled that the sodium hydrate solution, the ragweed pollen, and the horse serum protein each gave a delayed reaction with the formation of a 7 mm. wheal on the left arm. Undoubtedly, the delayed reaction was an expression of the increased circulation of lymph in response to a powerful local irritant. The negative cutaneous reaction of the same materials on the other arm indicated a lack of sensitiveness on the part of the subject to them.

It became a matter of interest to determine quantitatively the degree of sensitiveness to the castor meal. Accordingly, 1 gm. of the fat-free meal was treated with 100 cc of a 12 per cent alcoholic saline solution. The mixture was shaken for forty-eight hours, centrifuged, and the supernatent fluid was pipetted off. The fluid, representing the stock solution of 1:100, was clear and colorless. Dilutions were made from the stock as high as 1:1,000,000. Cutaneous testing with the varying dilutions of the soluble proteins was completed in two trials on December 15, and 18, 1921.

A definite wheal, 3 mm. in diameter, was produced by a drop of the protein extract in the dilution of 1:250,000. No reaction was obtained with the higher dilutions. The wheals, produced by the lower dilutions, gradually increased in size; the stock solution formed a wheal 17 mm. in diameter which made its appearance in five minutes. No constitutional effects were noted on these two occasions.

The attempt was next made to establish which protein constituent of the fat-free meal might be the sensitizing agent.

Four preparations were used, which were obtained in the following manner: The fat-free castor meal was extracted with a 10 per cent sodium choloride solution. The mixture was filtered. The filtrate, designated A, was a deeply straw-colored fluid. The residue, designated B, was a mealy powder. Solution A was then boiled and filtered. The filtrate, C, was a light straw-colored fluid, and the residue, D, after washing and drying, consisted of a light brownish crystalline powder.

On February 3, 1922, the above mentioned test materials, A, B, C, and D, were applied to the anterior surface of the left forearm. The smallest possible drops of liquids, A and C, which would adhere to the under surface of the corks, were deposited on the skin and a superficial scratch through the epithelial layers was made with a fine needle. Powders B and D were each mixed on the skin with a drop of decinormal sodium hydrate solution and the usual skin scratch was made. The amount of the powders used was such as could be gathered on the flattened tip of a toothpick.

Two minutes after the application of the test materials, the subject experienced itching at scratch marks A and C, which were bathed with the liquid reagents. Soon wheals appeared at A and C, and at B and D. Five minutes later, constitutional effects were in evidence. The subject complained of itching at both wrists and in both palms. He seemed restless. The palms began to sweat. This was followed by itching and perspiration of the forehead. Within fifteen minutes, the constitutional effects were most marked. The subject sneezed eight times in succession; he complained of nausea and then vomited four times. The conjunctivæ were injected. The face was flushed. The temporal arteries became prominent. The pulse was full and bounding. The subject stated that his heart thumped violently. The general reaction was so acute that it necessitated the subcutaneous administration of 1 cc of adrenalin solution. This happily brought relief.

The cutaneous reactions were read at the end of twenty minutes. The wheals produced at A measured 15 mm., at B 10 mm., at C 12 mm., and at D 15 mm. Solutions A and C, as previously mentioned, were the first to produce a local response and the induration about these two scratch marks persisted over night.

It would seem as if the protein constituent chiefly concerned in causing the local reaction were soluble in 10 per cent sodium choloride solution and non-coagulable—a globulin in character; and that the reactions obtained with powders B and D were secondary to the intense local irritation. This cannot be stated with certainty. Cutaneous testing with each protein fraction at different times might have cleared up this point. The subject, however, was averse to further tests.

It is of interest to note that, despite the presence of the toxalbumin in the castor meal, cutaneous tests in other individuals have proven negative. Eleven asthmatic and six hay fever patients have been tested with the same specimen of meal, and the cutaneous tests have in all instances been negative.

Furthermore, five other associates of the subject have been engaged in castor bean investigations in the laboratory. They have been exposed to the organic dust even more intimately than our subject. This was particularly true during the war when the exigency demanded intensive study. Only one of the five workers showed a slight tendency to sneezing while engaged in the work. This tendency was only transitory. During this period, the subject was in the military service and did not suffer from the specific symptoms.

The danger to workmen resulting from exposure to the castor bean in the industries has been emphasized by Kobert. Curiously enough, no mention has been made by him of any symptoms comparable with those of the case described. Kobert[3] has prepared a "Ricinusheilserum" for rendering workmen, who handle the pressed cake, immune to the poisonous constituent. The use of the "Ricinusheilserum" in relieving inflammation of the eyes is recommended.

In this connection, the following statements from two of the largest castor-oil manufacturers in this country are noteworthy: "We know by experience that the dust from the whole castor beans and also from the castor pomace, after most of the oil is extracted, is effective on people that are subject to asthma. People that work in our factory are troubled more of less until they get what you might call acclimated." The second statement reads: ". . . up to the present time we have never noted anything of this kind among our employees. However, in the handling of castor beans in our plant there would be only one man that would be likely to come in contact with this dust, as the beans are all received in bags and the bags are opened and emptied into a trap-door receiver. After that they are handled by machine conveyers until they reach the presses, so that the only man that would come in contact with this dust would be the man who cuts the bags at the time they are emptied; as this is done in a large open space, and the bag being cut at the place of emptying, this man would not be likely to be affected by the dust."

Sensitization to organic dust in occupation has been recognized as a cause of asthma and of perennial hay fever. Its mechanism, however, is not fully understood. Thorough investigation of the occupational history of patients assumes great importance. Cutaneous tests with the suspected materials not only determine the diagnosis, but also expedite treatment. They may in some cases indicate the advisability of change of occupation. Thus Walker[4] records the case of a jewel polisher who became sensitized to boxwood dust. Several inoculations with boxwood protein enabled the patient to continue at his work, freed from symptoms of perennial hay fever. Peshkin[5] cites a case of a pharmacist who developed bronchial asthma because of an acquired sensitiveness to the powder of ipecac. Relief from asthma followed a change in occupation. In the experience of Rackemann,[6] a coffee worker with a positive skin reaction to coffee dust and eight professional bakers with positive skin reactions to wheat proteins are included.

In our subject, desensitization with a protein extract of the fat-free meal was considered. The inherent poisonous qualities of the substance, however, discouraged the attempt, despite the successes of Ehrlich.[7] The latter established an immunity in white mice toward the toxic effects of ricin by feeding and by subcutaneous injections of preparations of the toxin. On March 3, our subject was transferred to another laboratory at his request. To date he has enjoyed entire freedom from attacks of sneezing or of asthma.

Summary and Conclusions.—1. A chemist acquires in course of his occupation a sensitiveness to the dust of the castor bean.

Attacks of sneezing and of asthma are the clinical manifestations of this sensitiveness.

2. The fat-free castor meal produces an urticarial wheal at the site of a superficial scratch on the forearm.

3. A cutaneous reaction is obtained with a drop of the protein solution of the meal in a dilution of 1:250,000.

4. Symptoms of protein intoxication result from the absorption of extracts of the castor meal from skin abrasions.

5. The presumptive evidence indicates that the globulin fraction possesses antigenic properties.

6. Exposure to organic dust in industries may cause an acquired sensitiveness. Cutaneous testing with the suspected material is of value in diagnosis and treatment.*

* It is a pleasure to record my thanks to Dr. W. W. Stockberger, Physiologist in Charge of Drug, Poisonous and Oil Plant Investigations of the Bureau of Plant Industry of the U. S. Department of Agriculture, and to the members of his staff for many courtesies.

REFERENCES.

1. Osborne, Mendel and Harris: A Study of Proteins of Castor Beans, Am. Jour. Physiol., 1905, **14**, 259.
2. Kobert, R.: Lehrbuch der Intoxicationen, Stuttgart, 1902, pp. 695–703.
3. Kobert, R.: Erste ärztliche Hilfe, bei Vergiftungen, Ztschr. f. ärztl. Fortbild., 1905, **23**, 737.
4. Walker, I. Chandler: Frequent Causes and the Treatment of Perennial Hay-fever, Jour. Am. Med. Assn., 1920, **75**, 783.
5. Peshkin, M. Murray: Ipecac Sensitization and Bronchial Asthma, Jour. Am. Med. Assn., 1920, **75**, 1133.
6. Rackemann, Francis M.: Skin Tests with Foreign Proteins in Various Conditions, Am. Jour. Med. Sci., 1922, **163**, 87.
7. Ehrlich: Deutsch. med. Wchnschr., 1891, **17**, 976.

THE DIAGNOSIS OF OBSCURE CHRONIC ABDOMINAL CONDITIONS.*

By J. Louis Ransohoff, M.D.,
CINCINNATI, OHIO.

The diagnosis of chronic abdominal disorders is, as a rule, far more difficult than the diagnosis of acute lesions of the same variety. The very nature of the acute case with its more or less stormy onset has, as a rule, something characteristic of its causation. All the exact methods of the last decade have not made the diagnosis of the chronic abdomen a sinecure. Even the roentgen ray, so widely heralded that most of our patients request its use before submitting to an operation, not infrequently leads us into error.

The typical chronic cases are usually easy to recognize. It is

* Read before the Birmingham Surgical Society, January 28, 1922.

the obscure case of one kind or another which intrigues and puzzles the most expert diagnostician. The obscure cases under consideration are the more common intra-abdominal conditions with atypical symptoms, leaving out of consideration the surgical rarities which we occasionally encounter. Fortunately, particularly in large clinics, the so-called exploratory laparotomy is fast finding its way into the discard. The well-regulated hospital requires a preoperative diagnosis written on the operative record, and this to be written before the completion of the operation. We are fast graduating from the custom of seeing a patient from the country at five o'clock one afternoon (still, of course, speaking of the chronic cases) and operating on him the next morning, so as to save the visiting doctor an extra trip to town.

An exact diagnosis, permitting an ordinary incision instead of a tremendous exploratory opening and a minimum of handling, ensures a rapid recovery, and not only a low mortality rate but an equally low morbidity rate. I am confident that the mortality of the so-called exploratory laparotomy is appallingly large.

There is a German medical proverb which reads, "The most common is usually there:" The most common is, of course, the appendix, and numberless cases of obscure abdominal symptoms are due to chronic appendicitis.

In the early days of gastroenterostomy, before more accurate methods of diagnosis, particularly the exact interpretation of the roentgen rays, came into general use, gastroenterostomy was frequently done without a demonstrable lesion of the stomach, trusting that a drainage of the stomach would heal the ulcer, which frequently was not even present. It is only after the lapse of years that we have been brought to realize how disastrous and harmful this operation is in the absence of a demonstrable gastric or duodenal lesion. Occasionally we still see the results of these unnecessary gastroenterostomies, where a gastroenterostomy has been done and the true cause of the abdominal symptoms, either the inflamed appendix or the chronic gall-bladder, has been allowed to remain, the patients being only the worse for their operative interference. The obverse of this picture I shall discuss later, that is, the frequent removal of the appendix when a gastric or duodenal ulcer or some pelvic disease is at fault.

The more chronic abdominal cases which come under observation the fewer true gastric or duodenal ulcers are seen. The greater the number of clinical gastric ulcers studied the more are found to be due to extragastric intra-abdominal lesions. To quote from Smitties: "The close simulation of the symptomatology of uncomplicated gastric ulcer by disease of other abdominal organs would appear to suggest that the clinical manifestations associated with ulcers are often the evidence of abdominal or other constitutional derangement, in the course of which ulcer is only an incident or an end-result. It is within the experience of all who have had reliable training that laparotomy often fails to disclose gastric ulceration in patients presenting all the so-called characteristic symptoms of ulcerations."

It is these cases, which Moynihan has grouped under the name of "appendix dyspepsia," which form a group of particular interest. As a rule they present no history of definite attacks or inception of the disease. There is a gradual letting down of the entire organism—a loss of the feeling of well-being. There is more or less abdominal distress and pain which, as a rule, comes on after the taking of food. This distress or pain rarely approaches in severity that due to gastric or duodenal ulcer, and there is not the definite relation of pain to the taking of food. For instance, instead of the relief from pain which in gastric ulcers follows the taking of food there is, as a rule, an accentuation of pain following the ingestion of food. Unlike gastric and duodenal ulcer this pain has not the regular time for occurrence. The situation of the pain is very like that of gastric and duodenal ulcer, that is, around the epigastrium or just above the umbilicus. The pain is, as a rule, increased by exercise, which is a very characteristic symptom. Vomiting is frequent, usually at irregular intervals, and often without relation to the intake of food. Flatulence, belching and heartburn are the most distressing and constant symptoms.

In a few cases vomiting of blood is present, and in these it is almost impossible to make a differential diagnosis from clinical gastric ulcer. Why or wherefore this vomiting of blood occurs is difficult to determine. In all probability it is due to the presence of very minute toxic ulcers or erosions in the stomach which are too superficial to be discovered by roentgen ray and too small to make themselves evident by the palpation of the stomach during operation. It is in these cases that the inexperienced surgeon is tempted to do a pyloric exclusion and gastroenterostomy without the true evidence of gastric ulceration, when the removal of a diseased gall-bladder or appendix will solve the entire situation.

Case I.—J. L., aged twenty-nine years, has had for five years some pain in the abdomen, often incapacitating him for work. Pain has followed taking of food, but he occasionally has hunger pains and pronounced loss of weight. Frequent vomiting, the vomiting occurring irrespective of taking food. At times he has vomited large amounts of blood. There is tenderness in the epigastrium and marked tenderness over the appendix region, with some rigidity. Wassermann negative. Occult blood in stool. Roentgen ray shows slight irregularity in the duodenum and an adherent appendix, its tip pointed upward.

Diagnosis. Duodenal ulcer and chronic appendicitis.

Operation, May 20, 1920. Gas-oxygen anesthesia, upper right

rectus incision, the appendix was found chronically inflamed, its tip adherent to the omentum, which was in turn adherent to the anterior surface of the duodenum. The adhesions were separated and the appendix removed. The duodenum where the omentum was adherent showed no ulceration. The peritoneal abrasion in the duodenum was repaired with a fine silk suture and the wound closed. Recovery uneventful and there has been no recurrence of the symptoms.

The abdominal tenderness in appendicular dyspepsia is, as a rule, of great interest. There is usually marked tenderness in the epigastrium, though rarely the same exquisite tenderness of the gastric or duodenal ulcer. A very characteristic sign is that pressure over the appendix region, frequently causing pain in the epigastrium, the same pain of which the patient is suggestively aware. If a careful and gentle examination is made in many instances there is a superficial rigidity of the right rectus, even in the absence of localized pain, tenderness on pressure or deep rigidity of the abdominal muscles. I have found this superficial abdominal rigidity a very important diagnostic sign in the differentiation of intra-abdominal conditions. In making this examination the pressure must not be sufficient to cause any pain sensation. Only the lightest and most gentle touch must be used. In many instances it has proved of greater value than the tenderness or deep rigidity.

The symptoms of appendix dyspepsia are so variable and, as a rule, so atypical that only by repeated examination and frequent taking of the history can a diagnosis be arrived at.

The question how morbid changes in the gall-bladder and appendix induce symptoms in other viscera and distant parts has been ably discussed by Rolleston, who divides the causes into reflex, mechanical, toxic and infectious.

"*Reflex*. Irritation in the appendix or gall-bladder may cause hypertonus of the stomach and spasm of or failure to relax on the part of the pyloric or ileocecal sphincter, leading to gastric or ileal stasis and so to excess of acid or to toxemia. . . . Hurst has seen visible spasm of the middle of the stomach when the appendix is manipulated under the roentgen ray. . . . In the case of chronic appendicitis failure of relaxation of the ileocecal sphincter is thought by Hurst to be commoner than spasm. Cecal stasis from inhibition of peristalsis or from enterospasm (spastic constipation) may be due to chronic appendicitis. Appendicitis may reflexly lead to increased frequency or inhibition of micturition through an irritated focus in the spinal cord (Mackenzie), and chronic irritation of the appendix may be responsible for cardiac irregularities.

The reflex pain in the epigastrium, which is so common in the appendix and gall-bladder dyspepsia, has given rise to some discussion. Mackenzie maintains that it is in the peripheral termination of the sixth and seventh dorsal nerves in the abdominal wall, and that this depends on the irritated focus in the spinal cord, whereas Hurst argues that the pain is visceral, in the pyloric end of the stomach and due to the hyperperistalsis. They both, however, agree that the epigastric tenderness is due not to pressure on the stomach but to the irritated focus in the spinal cord, which causes an exaggerated sensory effect when the skin, and especially the muscles and the underlying subperitoneal tissues, are pressed on. Very often the appendix when removed shows little naked-eye change to correspond with the prominent symptoms that then disappear. Microscopic examination may be necessary to reveal the evidence of past inflammation in its walls, especially fibrosis in the submucous coat, and often, as I have seen in many sections, the changes are very slight.

Mechanical. Pericholecystic adhesions may embarrass the movement of the stomach, interfere with the passage of food through the pylorus or even lead to the hour-glass stomach. . . . Pericecal adhesions may cause intestinal stasis and so toxemia, and the same result, only in a more marked degree, may be produced by an appendix adherent across the lower part of the ileum.

The appendix adherent in the pelvis explains a very interesting and apparent paradox in the symptomatology of chronic appendicitis. Most cases are more comfortable and have less frequency of pain when the bowels have moved well. This is a most common feature of chronic ileocecal appendicitis or retrocecal appendicitis. There are, however, occasional cases in which the pain is less when the bowels are constipated. In this class of cases the cause is as follows: the appendix is adherent by the tip in the pelvis; the loaded cecum releases the adherent appendix and relieves the pain. On taking a laxative and emptying the cecum the latter tends to draw high up in the abdomen and so increase the pain.

The toxic and infectious origin of gastric symptoms in diseases of the appendix and gall-bladder are more easily understood and depend upon the absorption of septic contents, the same as in any other source or focus of infection.

As Munsell has said, "It is a group of symptoms and perhaps signs which point so strongly to organic gastric or duodenal disease that it is only by the most careful examination or by the fortunate supervention of definite appendicular symptoms that a correct diagnosis is possible."

A typical case of this kind is as follows: CASE II.—A doctor in a neighboring city has complained of pain in the abdomen for eleven years. This pain centered in the umbilicus and was of an irregular nature. There was an increase of the pain after taking food and an accentuation after exercise. During this eleven years the pain has intermitted for several months at a time and was usually restarted by an overindulgence in food or an indulgence in alcohol. He was treated for nervous indigestion for many years, and finally sought the advice of one of the most prominent stomach men in the country. A very careful examination was made, including roentgen-ray and fractional gastric analysis. The gastric analysis showed increase in the free and combined acids. As far as could be learned the roentgen-ray picture showed what was thought to be a gastric ulcer on the lesser curvature. He was put on the Sippy treatment and temporarily improved, and was advised if the pain recurred to submit to an operation.

In February, 1921, the pain was of unusual severity, started at the umbilicus and radiated toward McBurney's point. I saw him at this exceedingly opportune time, during an exacerbation of the symptoms. His temperature was normal, his pulse slightly accelerated and there was marked tenderness and rigidity over the epigastrium. There was vomiting which contained no blood and a marked rigidity and tenderness over McBurney's point. On pressure over McBurney's point the tenderness was referred to the epigastrium. I advised him to come to the city, where further examination was made. Gastric analysis showed hyperacidity. Roentgen-rays revealed gastric hypermotility without evidence of gastric or duodenal disease, and a long irregularly filled appendix with its tip pointed toward the pylorus. Fluoroscopically the cecum was immobile and tender to pressure.

A diagnosis of appendicitis was made and an operation done. A very long appendix, about nine inches in length, was removed with a stricture and adhesions about the middle and the tip pointing toward the pylorus. Postoperative recovery was uneventful and the patient has been completely relieved of his symptoms.

This is characteristic of a group of cases in which the occurrence of acute supervening symptoms point definitely to the diagnosis. The sufferers from chronic appendicular dyspepsia lead the lives of invalids and have travelled the rounds from doctor to doctor with the usual diagnosis of chronic nervous indigestion.

The comprehensive diagnosis and treatment of these cases is made much more difficult by the frequency of associated true disease of the appendix, gall-bladder and stomach. It is probable that the association of these diseases is not only clinical but more probably pathologic. According to Deaver's view, in which I concur, the appendix, which is so frequently affected alone, so far as pathologic and clinical evidence is concerned, is usually the first offender, involving the other organs by sepsis, toxins or reflex nervous phenomena. In many instances the timely removal of the diseased appendix may prevent the formation of gastric or duodenal ulcer. The roentgen-ray examination, so valued in the diagnosis of lesions of the stomach and duodenum, frequently leaves us in the lurch in the diagnosis of chronic appendicular conditions, and is right about as often as it is wrong. If the appendix is not seen at all it is interpreted as being constricted so that the barium meal cannot enter, or it is said to be retrocecal, and according to the views of many observers, nearly all retrocecal appendices are pathologic, and conversely an irregular filling defect may be interpreted as being irregular fibrous bands constructing the appendicular lumen.

What is important in these cases is the tenderness of the filled cecum under the fluoroscope and the absence of cecal and appendicular motility. That is, the seemingly fixed immobile cecum is apt to be the seat of pericecal adhesions due to infection of the appendix. A fixed shape and anchorage of the appendix seen on several plates at different times is strongly suggestive of appendicular change, as the normal appendix changes its form and position during the digestion of food, moving with the cecum.

There are some cases of appendicular or gall-bladder dyspepsia simulating gastric ulcer in which, due to the reflex pyloric spasm, there may even be a simulated roentgen-ray picture of gastric or duodenal ulcer. When there is the slightest doubt it is wise to have the roentgen-ray examination repeated after a two-day or three-day interval. A gastric or duodenal lesion once shown on the roentgen-ray.plate or once visualized on the fluoroscope can be shown again if it is present. If, on the other hand, the second or third roentgen-ray place fails to disclose the lesion it is certainly not there. A case of this kind is rather interesting:

Case III.—Male, aged thirty-six years. Six months before I saw him he began to have severe pains in the epigastrium accompanied by vomiting. The pain came on with increased severity after taking food and was increased by exercise, so that the man was unfitted for work. There was no vomiting of blood. Gastric analysis showed slight hyperacidity. There was slight tenderness just to the right of the umbilicus and over the appendix region; no occult blood in the stool. Wassermann negative. Roentgen-ray examination, October 15, disclosed a filling defect in the lesser curvature of the pylorus, with pyloric spasm and an irregularly filled appendix. Roentgen-ray diagnosis: appendicitis and gastric ulcer. We were not satisfied that the case was truly one of gastric ulcer, so three days later a second roentgen ray of the stomach was made, and although the spasm was present the filling defect could not be shown. Also at this time, under the fluoroscope, pressure over the cecum caused epigastric pain with an increased gastric peristalsis. Clinical diagnosis: Chronic appendicitis. Operation, October, 1921, gas-oxygen anesthesia, right pararectal incision, inspection of the pylorus, gall-bladder and duodenum revealed no abnormality. The appendix was adherent and buried in the wall of the cecum, ileocecal in position; removed in the usual way. Operative recovery uneventful. In the two months since operation the patient has regained his normal weight and is free from all symptoms.

That too much reliance must not be placed on a single series of roentgen-ray examinations is also shown by the following case:

CASE IV.—Mrs. T., aged fifty years, referred from a neighboring city with a diagnosis of cancer of the stomach. She had always been in good health until six months before, when she began to have pains in the abdomen, loss of weight and vomiting. She brought roentgen-ray plates with her, which evidently showed a pyloric obstruction. Examination disclosed a rather thin, fairly well-nourished woman. In the right side of the abdomen was a tender mass, the size of a fist, which could be moved from the epigastrium to the right iliac fossa. We thought we had to deal with a movable kidney. Roentgen-ray examination showed hyperperistalsis of the stomach. Under the fluoroscope the mass was seen to be a cecum mobile. The irregularly filled appendix was seen retrocecal. The kidneys were in their normal place. Diagnosis: cecum mobile and chronic appendicitis. Operation, November, 1921, gas-oxygen anesthesia, right pararectal incision. The cecum was found freely movable with the appendix adherent to its posterior surface. The appendix was removed and the cecum anchored. Postoperative recovery was uneventful and she has been free of her symptoms ever since.

The reason for the misreading of the first series of plates was probably the position in which they were taken, that was flat on the back instead of in the upright position, so that the contour of the barium meal was due to the pressure of the loaded stomach on the spinal column.

After appendicitis the most frequent cause of ulcer symptoms without the presence of an ulcer is gall-bladder inflammation with or without stone.

For one who looks only for the classic signs of gall-bladder disease —pain, colic and jaundice—many cases will entirely escape detection and will be consigned to that unknown land of chronic dyspepsia and nervous indigestion. Long-continued gastric indigestion in a woman past forty years is always more or less suggestive of gall-bladder disease, although the more we see of gall-bladder disease the less important is the age factor and the more cases we see in young individuals. The constant indigestion, gas eruptions, vomiting at irregular intervals and constant epigastric distress are always suspicious. This epigastric distress may never reach the point of pain, but is, as frequently, more a fulness or sense of weight.

There are a few cases, and one in particular has come to my notice, in which the only single symptom was backache located between the shoulder-blades. There was absolutely no indigestion and no vomiting. The only symptom she had to suggest gall-bladder disease was a slight rigidity of the right side of the epigastrium with an interference with deep inspiration on pressure. In this case the roentgen ray helped us by showing eight very small stones. Cholecystectomy was done and the recovery was uninterrupted, with a complete disappearance of the symptoms.

Gastric analysis is little help, as either a hyperacidity or a subacidity may be present. A very positive sign is the interference with deep inspiration when pressure is made over the gall-bladder region. With the patient flat on his back, his knees flexed, firm pressure is made under the right costal arch and the patient is requested to take a deep breath. In the presence of gall-bladder inflammation, even of a minor degree, the breath is stopped with a sharp catch, short of full inspiration. If this is present on the right side and absent on the left this sign almost invariably points to gall-bladder or liver inflammation. I have never found the so-called tender points in the region of the scapula or spine of much assistance.

The roentgen ray in these cases as frequently leaves us in the lurch as otherwise, and for the benefit of our diagnostic acumen it is perhaps just as well, as we are forced occasionally to make a diagnosis on our unassisted powers of observation.

A rather interesting and not common extragastric lesion which may closely simulate gastric ulcer is epigastric hernia, the rarity of which is evidenced by Coley's statistics; among 3383 cases of hernia only 3 were of the epigastric variety. The large ones are very easy to recognize. Occasionally, however, they are only of minute size, and only the most careful palpation of the linea alba above the umbilicus may disclose their existence, and then only if the examiner is on the lookout. These cases frequently have excruciating pain, closely simulating that of gastric ulcer. The pain may be of such severity as to interfere with the patient's activity. There may also be periodic attacks of vomiting, absolutely independent of the intake of food. They rarely, however, show the emaciation and evidences of chronic invalidism following gastric or intra-abdominal disease. The lesion begins as a small protrusion of subperitoneal fat through a transverse slit in the linea alba. In very early cases there is frequently no true sac but simply a protrusion of subperitoneal fat. Moschcowitz reports two cases in which there was not even a protrusion of subperitoneal fat. There was in these cases merely a small slit in the viscera through which protruded a single large vessel. The vessel was tied off and the slit closed and the pain in both cases was relieved. The second degree contains a true empty small sac and a third a small piece of usually adherent omentum. They are rarely of sufficient size to contain intestine, though Gatewood has reported a case in which there was an intestinal strangulation. It is, however, only the small epigastric hernias which particularly interest us, because of the difficulty of diagnosis and because of the symptoms they present out of all proportion to their size. The cause of the symptoms is probably the drag on the parietal peritoneum, and a very frequent sign is the increase of pain after exercise. We have had several cases of this kind in all of which the recovery was complete after operation.

Lewisohn, in speaking of these cases, sounds a timely warning, which is not to be certain, in the presence of epigastric hernia, that the symptoms are entirely due to the hernia. In his service at Mt. Sinai Hospital he has seen several cases in which the symptoms persisted after an operation for epigastric hernia and in which further investigation and subsequent operation disclosed intra-abdominal lesions.

. We have been speaking thus far of symptoms of gastric and duodenal ulcer which are due to less serious intra-abdominal lesions. The reverse side of the picture is equally obvious and neither so simple nor so pleasant. That is the numberless cases in which an appendix or gall-bladder operation has been done without relief when the trouble is elsewhere, as a rule, either a pyloric or duodenal ulcer. I venture to say that all of us have more than once made this mistake and have still more frequently done so without having had the opportunity of knowing it—this because of the frailty of human nature, and patients are prone to seek elsewhere when an unsuccessful operation has left them unbenefited. It is only by the most painstaking care and the weighing of every scintilla of diagnostic evidence that we can avoid making these diagnostic errors, and when our diagnostic means fail then and then only should we make a so-called exploratory laparotomy.

One of the most important factors in the diagnosis of all chronic cases, abdominal or otherwise, is the search for syphilis. This has been particularly brought to my attention by the occurrence of several distressing experiences. There is no symptom-complex of any intra-abdominal disease which cannot be simulated by syphilis. In a recent communication Salzer has reviewed the records of 150 consecutive private patients who presented themselves for examination for chronic conditions. As a matter of routine a Wassermann was taken in every one of these individuals. These cases were in no wise venereal cases but represented the ordinary run of cases which seek the assistance of the internist for chronic conditions. Of these 150 cases 24 showed a positive Wassermann, and of these 24 cases only 5 gave a definite history of syphilitic infection. Of these 24 cases 6 had undergone abdominal operations, from which they had been absolutely unrelieved of their symptoms. Of these 6 all had had appendix operations in addition to one kidney operation, two ovarian operations and 1 in which three distinct operations had been done for abdominal adhesions, besides numerous sacrifices of teeth and tonsils. It is only of late years that we have come to appreciate the protean aspects of congenital syphilis. The opportunity of examining a large number of men in the army undoubtedly threw a great light on this subject. What is important to bear in mind is that congenital syphilis may exist without any of the so-called stigmata for which we have been taught to seek, and undoubtedly many of these cases with obscure abdominal symptoms are of congenital origin.

Several experiences of my own have led me to the taking of

Wassermanns in all chronic abdominal conditions. Three of these cases are of particular interest.

Case V.—Female, aged thirty-two years, has been troubled for years with frequent gastric disturbances—pain after eating, flatulence, tenderness in the epigastrium and hyperacidity. Roentgen-ray examination was entirely negative except for a slight increase in tenderness over the cecum and the fact that the appendix could not be shown. She was seen in consultation with a reliable internist who made the diagnosis of appendicular dyspepsia and advised operation. Through a long pararectal incision, under gas-oxygen anesthesia, the entire abdomen was explored and nothing abnormal was found except a slightly inflamed retrocecal appendix, of normal size, without adhesions. The appendix was removed in the usual way and the abdomen closed without drainage. Postoperative recovery was uneventful, and for some time, as is very often the case, the symptoms were entirely relieved, only to recur with increased severity. Some months later a blood examination was made and a 4-plus Wassermann was found. The history taken with this lead pointed definitely to congenital infection. Treatment improved the condition and entirely relieved her abdominal and gastric symptoms.

Case VI.—This case represents a class of parasyphilitic diseases with a definite symptom-complex of cholecystitis. The man when first seen had been suffering for three years with obscure symptoms of indigestion, with infrequent attacks of nausea and vomiting. There was no history of definite gall-stone colic. There was, however, a marked tenderness over the gall-bladder, which was somewhat distended and interference with inspiration on deep pressure. Roentgen-ray examination was negative except of a prolapsed and dilated stomach. Constipation had been marked for several years. Gastric analysis showed nothing unusual. March 23, 1917, incision over the gall-bladder region revealed a distended gall-bladder without any adhesions. Normal pylorus and duodenum. The appendix was slightly adherent but otherwise normal. The appendix was removed and the gall-bladder drained. Postoperative recovery was uneventful. This man was not relieved of his symptoms in any way. Three years later he was seen by an internist, having passed out of my hands. A Wassermann was taken, which was found to be positive. Antisyphilitic treatment was instituted and recovery from his gastrointestinal symptoms was prompt.

That a typical picture of gastric or duodenal ulcer can be simulated by syphilis is well known. This may either be due to a true gumma of the stomach, demonstrable syphilitic lesions in extragastric organs or by producing changes in the central and sympathetic nervous systems. Eusterman has reported a series of 23 cases and Smitties a series of 21 cases, all presented on clinical, roentgen-ray and serologic studies. The symptoms are typical of gastric or duodenal ulcer, including pain, loss of weight, vomiting and hematemesis. If a syphilitic history is obtainable a lead to a diagnosis is easily established; but even in the absence of a history a Wassermann is essential. If the Wassermann is negative and the history, nevertheless, points to syphilis a provocative salvarsan injection should be made and another Wassermann taken. These cases are, as a rule, diagnosticated and treated by the internist, and rarely fall into the hands of the surgeon. I venture to say that if the routine taking of Wassermanns were done a large number of gastric operations would be found unnecessary. The case which follows is what I consider a classic case of syphilis with symptoms of gastric ulcer:

Case VII.—W. M., aged thirty-nine years, service of Dr. Morris, Cincinnati General Hospital, admitted November 23, 1921, complain of pain in the stomach and loss of weight, the pains in the stomach having been more or less constant and relieved by the intake of food. During the last attack he vomited blood. The general history is not germane to the case, except marked tenderness in the epigastrium. No tumor mass to be felt. Wassermann 4-plus positive. Roentgen ray shows nothing abnormal except marked gastric hypermotility. Gastric analysis: free acid, 35; combined, 14; total, 49. Stool, occult blood. In view of the positive Wassermann and history of syphilis, salvarsan and mercury treatment were instituted and rapid improvement made. He was discharged in a month from the date of admission free from pain and eating house diet, apparently cured.

Now just a word on the reverse side of this syphilis question: A positive Wassermann and a positive history of syphilis do not necessarily mean that the symptoms complained of are necessarily syphilitic. This is particularly important when malignant disease, particularly of the mucous membranes, is suspected. This is all the more misleading since cancer, particularly of the mucous membrane, is not infrequently engrafted on a previous syphilitic basis. If syphilitic treatment is instituted in these cases, not only is valuable time lost, but the cancerous lesion is frequently relighted to renewed activity by the administration of salvarsan.

Conclusions. 1. Many cases of clinical gastric and duodenal ulcers are due to extragastric intra-abdominal lesions.

2. A single series of roentgen-ray plates is frequently misleading, and if there is the slightest doubt a complete reëxamination is essential.

3. In the successful treatment of chronic abdominal disease an exact diagnosis is essential, and except as a last resort, so-called exploratory operation should not be made.

4. In all cases of chronic abdominal diseases a diligent search for syphilis should be made before any operation is done.

THE DIAGNOSIS OF SPLEEN FUNCTION.

By Morris H. Kahn, M.A., M.D.,
NEW YORK.

Introduction. The functional activity of various organs in the body has received ample study both clinically and experimentally. Where the organs are accessible either by means of their physiologic effects, especially where they produce an obtainable secretion, chemical tests have been developed. In the case of the organs of internal secretion, their functions are becoming better understood and tests for these are now available. As the spleen has no external secretion and no known internal secretion the results of its actions cannot be studied directly.

Tests of the functional activity of the spleen are in a comparatively undeveloped state. There are essential difficulties which this organ presents in the study of its physiology. This is especially the case because the spleen is part of a system. It is part of the lymphatic system of the body, and its function is supplemented by the lymphatic glands, while it may compensate to a degree for their various activities or deficiencies.

In considering the functional diagnosis of the spleen, therefore, it must be kept in mind that the organ is essentially a lymphatic structure. Its function is related not alone to that, but also to the function of the blood and blood-forming organs and to the liver; its roles in immunity and infection, in the metabolism of iron and in its relation to special blood diseases, have become subjects of considerable study in recent years.

The spleen function would naturally vary in different individuals, depending upon the rapidity of a disease process in the spleen, the acuteness of the disturbance of its function and the compensatory functioning of the rest of the lymphoid and hemopoietic systems.

Structure of the Spleen. The histologic details of the spleen are important as an indication of its function. The splenic artery subdivides as it enters the hilus of the spleen into numerous branches. These carry with them a covering of the capsular connective tissue, dividing the spleen by trabeculæ. Each branch supplies a section of the spleen and the final subdivisions terminate in minute capillaries. Immediately upon emerging from the connective tissue the arterioles give off minute branches which end abruptly and are surrounded by a more or less compact mass of lymphocytic cells called the lymph follicle or Malpighian body. These seem to be held together by a fine network enmeshing them, which in its turn is connected with trabecular connective tissue and a few elastic fibers around the capillary. This region is called the white pulp of the spleen.

After the follicular capillaries are given off, the central artery, leaving the follicle, becomes narrower and enters the red pulp as an arteriole, or modified capillary, with characteristic three coats. These arterioles are called pulp arteries. They have a constant diameter of 6 to 8 μ and are characterized by distinct thickness of the wall and a layer of endothelium with long nuclei which sometimes project into the lumen, which is filled with red blood cells. This arteriole breaks into a minute brush of terminal vessels, the so-called penicilli of Ruysch. These end in the spleen sinuses or lose themselves in the reticulum of the spleen pulp. The spleen sinuses are a dense plexus of capillary spaces, each varying from 10 to 40 μ in diameter. On one side they are in contact with the arterial capillaries and on the other with the veins. The assumption is that the blood entering the pulp from the arterial side must pass through the spleen sinuses to be led off through the veins. The walls of the sinuses contain stomata which permit this transmigration.

The veins are in direct contact with the stomata of the sinuses. They possess only an endothelial coat and some fine fibrillar connective tissue. These veins pass through the trabeculæ and join to form the splenic vein at the hilus.

The capillaries of the spleen, therefore, are either in contact with the sinuses which in turn are connected with the veins or end directly in the pulp in contact with the pulp cells. Injection methods corroborate this, in that the coloring matter finds its way through the vessels and in places also through unwalled spaces.

Most authors believe that there are no intraparenchymatous lymph channels, but that these occur only under the serous coat of the capsule of the spleen.

Hemolymph Glands and Accessory Spleens. The hemolymph glands are a special type of structure closely related to the spleen. They are more frequent in the embryo and may be considered as embryonic remains. After splenectomy they increase in size, containing many large red blood cells free in the meshes of the reticulum and filling up the lymph channels between the follicles.

They occur in the sheep and only inconstantly in other animals. They are found in the human body placed in the retroperitoneal fat and in the prevertebral region of the neck.

The hemolymph glands are not related to the lymphatic vessels, but are interposed in the circulatory system. The artery entering it carries with it trabeculæ from the capsule, which it leaves finally as an independent capillary, while the trabecular system is connected with the reticulum. Here, also, there occur lymph follicles. The capillaries are of similar structure to those of the spleen with prominent endothelial nuclei and thick adventitia. The venous capillaries terminate either in the lacunar spaces (venous blood sinuses) or open free into the lymphoid tissue. The venous lacunæ are filled with red blood cells which give the color to the glands.

The blood must necessarily pass into these spaces or into the lymphoid tissue before being taken up by the veins.

The red blood cells of the hemolymph glands are detained in the lymphoid tissue and the network to undergo phagocytic absorption. Both the anatomical structure and cytologic changes indicate a close functional resemblance to the spleen. The hemolymph glands permit of better study of the destructive changes of the blood than the spleen itself. They show migration of the red blood cells into the red pulp more clearly than the spleen and in that way assist the study of the spleen function. A supernumerary spleen or hemolymph glands may enlarge and assume the pathologic function of the spleen[1].

Accessory spleens occur more frequently in south Europeans than in north Europeans because of the greater frequency of tropical diseases. They also occur after splenectomy and hemolytic jaundice. This organ is analogous to hypertrophy of the remainder of a partially extirpated spleen.

Cellular Structure of the Parenchyma of the Spleen. In the red pulp the connective-tissue fibers and the other connective-tissue elements form a thick network. In the meshes of this network lie the parenchyma of the spleen and the sinus spaces. The cellular elements of the reticulum are distinct macrophages.

Von Ebner[2] distinguishes the varieties of pulp cells according to their morphology without reference to their origin, as: (1) Small mononuclear lymphocytes; (2) mononuclear, polymorphonuclear and multinuclear leukocytes; (3) nucleated red blood cells; (4) adult red blood cells; (5) large cells inclosing red blood cells or pigment granules (phagocytes); (6) free pigment granules; (7) giant cells with polylobular nuclei (megacaryocytes) occurring only in young animals; and (8) blood platelets.

The leukocytes (2) are in the majority. The lymphocytes (1) are next and the phagocytes (5) are next.

In the embryo the spleen tissue is mainly white pulp surrounding the trabeculæ and vessels. This reduces with age, and in the adult the spleen consists mainly of red pulp. The spleen follicles resemble lymph nodes in structure with a central zone of large lymphocytes showing mitosis. The periphery of the follicle consists of small lymphocytes and areas of lymph tissue radiating into the red pulp and also large mononuclear leukocytes (pulp cells or splenocytes). The lymphocytes of the Malpighian bodies may be inactive or may assume an active role as macrophages; in the latter capacity they may absorb protoplasm, red blood cell granules or the remains of other leukocytes. They also occur in many lymph glands and in bone-marrow.

Granulated leukocytes (myeloid reaction) are frequent in the red pulp under normal conditions and to a less degree in the Malpighian bodies. Eosinophilic leukocytes are also abundant wherever there is much red-cell destruction. These facts speak for the monophyletic theory of the origin of blood cells.

Most hematologists, however, subscribe to the heteroplastic theory of the formation of granular cells. They agree that eosinophilic polymorphonuclear leukocytes develop chiefly from undifferentiated mononuclear cells within the bone-marrow and in smaller numbers within certain special tissues of the organism, particularly lymphoid tissues. Whether this development is a direct transformation from lymphocytes or is the result of maturation from metastic bone-marrow tissue is undecided. There is no conclusive evidence in favor of the theory of direct transformation of neutrophilic polymorphonuclears into eosinophils either in the blood stream or in the general tissues.[3]

The presence of nucleated red blood cells (erythroblasts) in the bone-marrow as well as in the spleen tends to establish the latter as an erythropoietic organ. There is an increase in nucleated red blood cells in the spleen in various types of anemia and infectious diseases. This occurs together with an increase in myeloid reaction.

Red blood cells that are brought by the splenic vessels and have entered the pulp may be absorbed by erythrophages or destroyed and hemolyzed in the pulp, or may return to the circulation. The erythrophages are large pigment-containing cells in the spleen, the pigment being derived from the breaking down of red cells in the parenchyma. Megacaryocytes in the spleen occur in many animals, but only in young human beings. They seem to have a relation to blood platelets, occurring often after bleeding and in the region of the Malpighian bodies. Little is known of their relation to human pathology.

To sum up, the parenchyma of the spleen consists of a mass of cells. It is possible that the Malpighian follicles are the physiologic place of origin of the functionating cells produced in the spleen. It is asserted that the different regions of the spleen have different functions.

This is supported by the fact that exposure of rats to the roentgen-ray first destroys the cells of the follicles and the pulp elements remain unchanged until after much longer exposure. The different reaction of pulp and follicle in the leukemias also supports this theory. In myeloid leukemia the pulp shows hypertrophy, whereas in the lymphatic form the follicle shows hypertrophy.

The Fate of Injected Foreign Bodies. In the white pulp of the spleen one finds red blood cells lying among the lymphocytes. These show that the arterial capillaries open upon the spleen pulp. However, the other belief is that these cells as well as the leukocytes of the spleen pulp were formed there. Both leukocytes and red blood cells are known to pass through the wall of the capillaries by means of diapedesis.

Experimental intravenous injections of India ink, cinnabar pigments and chicken red blood cells were made into dogs. Five minutes after, the dogs were killed and the foreign body was not found in the sinuses of the spleen but in the parenchyma and especially in the peripheral zone of the Malpighian body. This implies that the India ink travels by way of the follicle capillaries into the red pulp. A small lodgment of transfused chicken red blood cells was found among the many red blood cells of the parenchyma and relatively few in the sinus spaces. Most of all the foreign red blood cells occurred in the periphery of the follicles and in the meshes of the reticulum between the lymph cells. This shows that the foreign red blood cells entered the parenchyma through the open ends of the arterial capillaries. After that the cells might return by way of the spleen sinuses.[4]

Venous Stasis in the Spleen. Venous stasis in the spleen is another means of analyzing the function of its sinus spaces. After experimental ligation of the splenic veins there is a distinct exudation of red blood cells into the spleen sinuses and pulp. In an earlier stage only the sinuses fill with the red blood cells, whereas the pulp or parenchyma shows only edema. In from two to twelve hours the red blood cells absorb first from the parenchyma, whereas the congestion of the sinus spaces remains for a long time and the pigment content after such an experiment is no greater than normal.[5] It may be that the red blood cells gather in the spleen sinuses to return unchanged to the circulation.[6 7] This is contradicted however by the following experiments.

Ligation of the splenic veins in dogs gives an increase of venous pressure. Electrical stimulation of the efferent nerves of the spleen increases the venous blood-pressure still further. If the nerves are, however, cut infarction of the spleen takes place within twenty-four hours. These experiments show that red blood cells which have exuded and lodged in the parenchyma of the spleen after venous stasis find great difficulty to return into the general circulation.[8]

Another belief opposes this view of the direct transmigration of red blood cells from the sinus into the parenchyma. According to this the stasis of the sinus produces edema of the parenchyma, and the edema prevents the invasion of the parenchyma by formed elements; the stasis of the sinus also hinders the circulation in the arterial capillaries and forces the blood from the capillary toward the parenchyma.[9]

Methods Available for the Study of Spleen Function. The following methods have been utilized for the study of the various functions of the spleen:

1. Cytologic analyses of the blood.
2. Chemical analyses of the blood.
3. Resistance of the red blood cells.
4. Relation of hemoglobin to hematin and biliary pigments.
5. Relation of the spleen to iron metabolism.

6. Effects of splenectomy.
7. Effects of spleen feeding.
8. Effects of roentgen rays.
9. Clinical signs of functional disturbance of the spleen.

Cytologic Analyses of the Blood. From the cytologic analyses of the peripheral blood the condition of blood formation and blood destruction can be told only in extreme cases.

Megalocytes are considered young red blood cells prematurely emitted into the circulation, as after severe hemorrhage. Grawitz considers these cells the degenerative forms, their size being due to imbibition of water.[10]

Eppinger considers microcytes also newly formed cells, but Biernacki considers their form due to deficient blood plasma.[11]

Poikilocytes are degenerating cells; the megaloblasts, mitotic figures and erythroblasts indicate bone-marrow stimulation. Polychromatophilia indicates aging of the red blood cells. Basophilic stippling, according to Grawitz and Naegeli, is a sign of degenerative changes.[12] Others believe that the stippling is a caryolytic phenomenon and the cells are analogous to the nucleated reds, indicating an excessive production and output of red blood cells. These have the same resistance to hypotonic solution as normal cells. A granulofilamentous substance occurs in red blood cells as a postvital phenomenon.[13] High color-index occurs in pernicious anemia and usually indicates an accelerated regenerative function of the bone-marrow.

The Dualistic and Monophyletic Theories. It is generally believed that the white blood corpuscles of mammals come from two distinct sources, the lymphocytes and mononuclears from the spleen and lymphatic glands and the granular leukocytes from the bone-marrow. Ehrlich was probably the first to bring into prominence this dualistic theory.[13]

French writers particularly, on the other hand, support the monophyletic theory of the genealogy of blood cells from a single type.[14] Rieux describes three phases of cellular development:[15]

1. A process of specific differentiation. This is fundamental. The primary embryonal mesenchymatous cells out of which the blood is developed are totally undifferentiated. By differentiation the mother cell gives rise to three main forms of blood cells:
   (*a*) Erythroblast, which is the head of the hemoglobin series.
   (*b*) Myeloblast or leukoblast, which heads the myeloid series.
   (*c*) Lymphoblast, which gives rise to the lymphoid series.
2. A process of proliferation and multiplication by karyokinesis.
3. A process of maturation and of aging by ontogenesis, which is common to all blood cells and is the natural consequence of their fundamental quality as they are mobile and migratory cells.

The nucleus and the protoplasm both partake of these processes. As the nucleus is spherical in the young cells, with a tendency toward polymorphism as it grows older, it may show pyknotic degeneration and expulsion as in the red blood cells. The protoplasm which is very fine in the young cells becomes coarser and takes on acid-staining properties as it grows older. These facts can conveniently be schematized in the following genealogical tree:

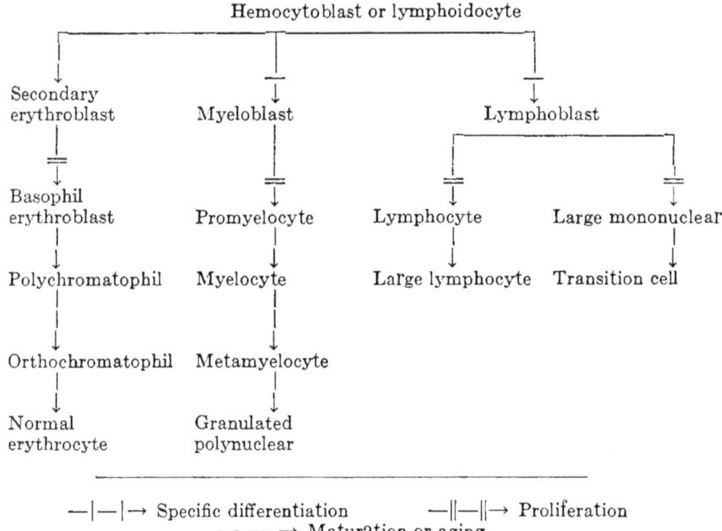

Thus, then, the differentiation of these primary cells once established and their proliferation observed the daughter cells present cytologic characteristics, fixed and specific, by which we can tell the type and age of the blood cells.

The two theories of the significance of mononuclear leukocytes are: (1) That they are an earlier stage of granular leukocytes and (2) that they are a form of lymphocytes.

Normet, after much experimentation, concluded that the mononuclear leukocyte is capable of directly or indirectly producing an eosinophil cell and even red blood cells, and that it is the cell of origin of all the blood cells.[16]

The white blood cell is the most primitive, derived from the mesenchyme cell. The earliest blood cell discovered in the fetus is the white, and the red cells are probably derived from the white cells. The earliest heart was possibly a lymphatic heart, circulating white blood, which merged later with the venous heart, leaving among other evidence the lymphatic connection of the thoracic duct with the venous system. Animals which have only one kind of blood have white blood. The fetal blood cell is produced by the lymphoid and adenoid structures of the body, including the liver and spleen.

Classification of Spleen Functions.

1. Blood formation.
2. Blood destruction.
3. Role in iron metabolism.
4. Regulating influence on blood-producing organs.
5. Function concerned with digestion.
6. Cholesterinogenic function.
7. Internal secretion of the spleen.
8. Detoxicating function.

Blood Formation. There is no doubt that the spleen is a lenkopoietic organ. The studies of the venous blood of the spleen and especially its white-blood-cell content lend support to our knowledge of its blood-forming function.[17] The venous blood of the spleen shows many more (seventy times as many) white blood cells than the splenic artery and many more than the vein of any other organ of the body.[18] This abundance of white blood cells occurs especially a short time after a meal. The number of polynuclears is greater in the splenic vein than in the artery, whereas a larger number of mononuclear cells are brought by the artery.[19]

Ehrlich obtained definite data of the influence of splenectomy on the white blood cells. He concluded that the spleen of the guinea-pig plays a subordinate role in the production of white blood cells.[20] Its absence is compensated for by the function of the lymph glands. The characteristic change is an increase of eosinophil cells the second year after splenectomy, and lymphocytosis during the first year. Audibert and Vallet,[21] Port,[22] and the recent work of Dubois[23] accord with these results, as also do the findings of Noguchi[24] and Bayer[25] in a case of splenectomy in man.

The focus of origin of the lymphocytes is the spleen follicle. They circulate from here through the red pulp together with the blood. The presence of myelocytes in the spleen suggests the possibility of their origin there; if not normally, under pathologic conditions.

Blood platelets are not present physiologically in the liver, lymph glands or bone-marrow, but they are in the blood channels of the spleen. Following splenectomy a remarkable increase of these elements takes place in those organs. This speaks for the seat of normal production in the spleen, a function which the organs take on vicariously.[26] There has been found a transitory but distinct increase in the blood platelets in the circulation following splenectomy.

In certain conditions, after many infectious diseases, in anemia and in some other pathologic conditions, changes take place in the spleen pulp and in the interfollicular regions that resemble myelogenous leukemia. Ehrlich[27] first described this and found that when blood crises took place the bone-marrow elements were held back in the spleen where they underwent proliferation, thus essentially acting as metastases from the bone-marrow. This myeloid tissue is more abundant in the embryonic spleen and it is conceivable that the rudiments of this take on sudden growth under a special stimulus in the above conditions.[28]

The thickness of the capillary walls of the spleen is greater than in any other vascular organ, and they are supplied with nerves, implying a close association of the organ with the vegetative nervous system.

Elliott and Kanavel[29] have shown that the intramuscular injection of epinephrin contracts the spleen one-third size. According to Hartmann and Lang,[30] dilatation of the spleen is caused by the action of epinephrin on the twelfth and thirteenth dorsal root ganglia, the semilunar ganglion or on some terminal structure in the spleen itself. Constriction can result from the response of a mechanism in the dorsal root ganglia or from a structure in the spleen.

Frey's[31] adrenalin test for the hemopoietic function of the spleen consists of a subcutaneous injection of 1 mg. of adrenalin. Normally after twenty minutes a distinct increase of the leukocytes in the peripheral circulation takes place with particular increase of lymphocytes, *i. e.*, a relative lymphocytosis. There may be a still further increase in one hour. In disease of the spleen, especially in Banti's disease or fibroadenie of the spleen, the increase of lenkocytes is slight or absent, with no relative lymphocytosis. This reaction is negative after extirpation of the spleen in dogs.[32]

Sanguinetti[33] does not agree with the hypothesis that the increase in white blood cells after adrenalin comes in large degree from this organ. The same dose of adrenalin will in one case produce contraction of the spleen and in another none, although in both cases the increase of white corpuscles in the circulation is nearly doubled. A better hypothesis, according to him—based on observations showing that cold increases the leukocytes while the heat scatters them—is that the increase after adrenalin must be ascribed in large part to changes of capillary circulation. For the present it must be believed that the properties of the blood elements themselves, such as specific gravity and viscosity, determine their special distribution in the capillary regions. This belief is strengthened by the cell modifications and the changes of leukocyte formulæ occurring in the veins and capillaries produced by adrenalin.

Freidberg[34] finds no effect on the white blood cells of children upon stimulation of the vegetative nervous system. He finds a marked similarity between the pilocarpin and the epinephrin blood pictures which leads to the supposition that these blood reactions are not dependent on the specificity of the ingested drugs but are rather a general form of reaction of the hemopoietic organs to nonspecific stimuli.

It has been written[35] that the visceromotor centers in the cord may be stimulated by percussion so that one may at random either contract or dilate the spleen. These reflexes are known respectively as the splenic reflex of contraction and dilatation. Normally the reflexes are of short duration, not in excess of two minutes. It has been determined empirically that the excitation of the reflex of contraction is effected by concussion of the second lumbar spine and the countersplenic reflex of dilatation by concussion of the eleventh dorsal spine. A pleximeter is placed on either spinous process and then struck a series of moderately vigorous blows with a plexor.

The attempts of Scalas[36] to elicit the splenic reflex in 9 children and 10 adults were practically negative. After percussion of the spine in 5 children there was a slight increase in mononuclears and transitional cells in the blood. But in no instance was a febrile attack elicited in malarial cases, nor did the parasites appear in the blood.

Blood Destruction. Eppinger[37] summarizes the theory of spleen function so far as it concerns blood destruction somewhat as follows: There is a double way open for the red blood cells after entering the splenic artery to gain entrance into the pulp structure. One way is through the pulp artery of the spleen sinus and the other way is directly into the pulp along unchannelled paths. Those which go the first way leave the spleen unchanged; those, however, which go the second and invade the tissue are probably ripe for degeneration to take place and, after more or less time in the pulp, are destroyed. Those of these, however, that find their way into the sinus perhaps later become destroyed by the macrophages. The pulp substance serves, therefore, as a place where the red blood cells are discarded and undergo destruction and phagocytosis by the macrophages.

One normal function of the spleen, therefore, is the capacity for selection of which red blood cells are to undergo destruction and which are to continue in the circulation. They may be somehow injured by the contact with the spleen tissue and continue to suffer degeneration in their course through the liver.[38]

Von Kölliker[39] showed that the red blood cells undergo changes immediately on entering the parenchyma of the spleen. They become smaller, darker staining, and finally break up into small granules. He expressed the belief that this constituted physiologic pigment metamorphosis of the red blood cells.

Virchow[40] showed that phagocytic cells containing red blood cells and pigment exist wherever there is extravasated blood, and also in chronic inflammations, in the lymph glands, the bone-marrow and after blood transfusion. Perls[41] by a staining reaction definitely proved the iron content of these cells. Metchnikoff[42] later definitely established the phagocytic power of these cells and called them macrophages, laden as they were with red blood cells.

These have been believed to be destructive of the red blood cells and capable of decomposing their hemoglobin.[43 44]

The spleen loses its power to produce red blood at birth and the liver at about the fifth fetal month, but the spleen retains its power for a limited production of white cells throughout its life. This is shown by a relative increase in the white cells and hematin in the splenic veins over other veins in the body.

The spleen also assumes the function of the destruction of worn-out red cells. This function depends upon: (1) An active cellular change, such as phagocytosis; and (2) a chemical change as by means of lysis, or by diminution of the resistance of the red blood cells to lytic influences. It seems that a cellular function of the spleen predominates in its blood-destroying mechanism.

Some investigators hold that phagocytosis is of itself sufficient to account for blood destruction. The spleens of different species show that this function is subject to wide variation. The number of corpuscles ingested in the large spleens of the rat, dog and guinea-pig is so considerable that, *a priori*, one might suppose phagocytosis to be the means whereby in these creatures the destruction of erythrocytes is accomplished. But in the cat phagocytosis does not come in for consideration; in normal man, the monkey and the rabbit it cannot be held responsible for the disappearance of any important amount of blood.[45]

The erythrophages apparently attack only injured red blood cells, being particularly abundant after the intravenous injection of distilled water. They serve not alone the purpose of phagocytosis of red blood cells in the spleen but carry these cells to the liver and thereby subserve a function in the process of blood regeneration,[46] or, as Gerlach and Schaffer[47] called it, "endogenous blood production."

It does not seem likely that the normal spleen possesses or produces any hemolysin comparable to the hemolysin *in vitro*. After splenectomy the resistance of the red blood cells to hemolysis increases.[48] Experimentally it reaches its height two months following splenectomy and maintains it for a varying time, even after one year.[49] The erythrocytes of the splenic vein show a lower resistance than those of the splenic artery.[50] This fact is conspicuous in support of the hemolytic power of the spleen.[51 52]

However, nowhere have hemolyzing cells or red blood cell shadows been found. This is evidence that hemolysis in the gross sense does not occur. Instead, another and unsuspected method of blood destruction has been found in the cat, rabbit and dog, namely, disintegration of the cells by fragmentation without loss of hemoglobin while they are still circulating. Extracellular blood destruction produces in the spleen accumulations of microcytes and poikilocytes such as are met with in the circulating blood. The shape of these in the peripheral blood and spleen is to some extent peculiar to the animal species. This constant presence in the spleen of an accumulation of poikilocytes which are subdividing, and of microcytes, and the presence of these elements in the circulating blood indicate that the red cells disappear, in part at least, by fragmentation.[45]

Ehrlich long ago found that the microcytes and poikilocytes of anemia result from fragmentation of the circulating cells while in the blood stream. He based his view on the fragmentation *in vitro* of red cells under the action of various physical and chemical agents. Ehrlich named these true fragmentation forms "schizocytes." Large numbers of the fragments accumulate in the spleen. Many, though, circulate for a greater or less time. In normal and plethoric animals the accumulation of schizocytes in the spleen is striking.

That this organ has some important function in connection with such elements cannot be doubted, and the findings in plethoric animals suggest that the bone-marrow may share the function if blood destruction is great. When human beings are severely burnt many red cells break into hemoglobin-containing fragments. These collect in the spleen so rapidly that within a few minutes practically all are removed from the blood. Not improbably the blood of normal and plethoric animals is kept free of fragments in much the same way. They are not taken so completely from the blood of anemic animals. Perhaps a change in the protoplasm, such as may be thought to accompany normal aging of the cell, is necessary for this. But even in anemia microcytes and poikilocytes accumulate in the spleen to a noteworthy extent.[53]

A constant rapid fragmentation of the effete red cells, one by one, while still circulating, and a prompt utilization of the products of destruction will readily account for the high general standard of cell resistance. Whether, indeed, as the red cells fragment, their resistance lessens, as determined by the ordinary tests, remains to be determined. The fragmentation does not involve a loss of hemoglobin, and, *a priori*, there is no reason why it should be accompanied by a decreased resistance to hemolysins or hypotonic fluids, the ordinary test agents.

Frey[54] reports experiments which show that the blood from the splenic vein contains fewer erythrocytes than the arterial blood or the blood from a vein in the ear. This difference becomes larger after the resistance of the red corpuscles has been reduced by a blood poison, such as during ether anesthesia. The difference grows less and less when the resistance of the red corpuscles is enhanced by substances such as phenylhydrazin. The hemoglobin percentage is alike in both splenic vein and ear vein blood in dogs. As there are fewer erythrocytes in the splenic vein, this finding in regard to the hemoglobin seems to suggest that free hemoglobin is present in the serum of the blood in the splenic vein, an observation also made by Banti[55] and Furno,[56] but not confirmed by Krumbhaar and Musser.[57]

Gilbert[58] believes that a close relationship exists between the loss of splenic function and the appearance of nuclear particles in the blood. These occur in large numbers within a few hours after the removal of the normal spleen, and continue to be present after the blood has become in other respects normal. They occur independent of any primary blood disease. In no other conditions are they found with such constancy and in such large numbers as after splenectomy. There is no definite numerical relationship between the nuclear particles and the presence of the true nucleated red cells or any other quantitative or qualitative changes in the peripheral blood. They originate from otherwise normal nuclei and do not show in themselves a qualitative degenerative process.

Benda[59] described so-called "tingible" bodies in the spleen which he believed to be phagocytosed and degenerated leukocytes. That the leukocytes are destined to undergo changes in the spleen analogous to the erythrocytes is conceivable.

The number of red blood cells per cu. mm. of blood is equivalent to the number of red blood cells produced minus the number destroyed. (Red blood cells in circulation = P.—D.) This, Eppinger[60] calls "Blutmauserung." The same would hold for the hemoglobin production and destruction.

Relation of Spleen Function to Blood Destruction and Jaundice. The natural life of the erythrocytes has been estimated at from ten to fourteen days. This estimate has been made largely on the assumption that biliary pigments are derived entirely from the destruction of erythrocytes. Recent experiments throw considerable doubt on this view. It is therefore quite probable that the life of the red cell is much longer than has been estimated.[61]

Pugliese[62] found a marked lessening of the amount of bile obtained through the biliary fistula following splenectomy, and concluded that the function of the spleen is to gather deteriorating red blood cells and transport them to the liver for destruction. Eppinger[63] believes that the amount of bile produced before and after splenectomy depends upon its original hemolytic functional activity. If the function is prominent in the spleen, the amount of bile pigment after splenectomy will be less.

When hemoglobin is set free in the portal circulation, a larger amount is held by the liver and converted rapidly into bile pigment than is the case when it is set free in the general circulation. Under the former condition, overloading of the liver with bile pigment more readily occurs and jaundice is more apt to develop. This mechanical influence accounts for the lessened tendency after splenectomy to the jaundice which follows blood destruction due to hemolytic agents. Whether the spleen be an active factor in destroying the erythrocytes, or whether it plays merely a passive part as a place for the deposition of the disintegrating cells, there can be no question that in this organ, when it is present, a large number of cells undergo their final disintegration after the action of hemolytic poisons. The hemoglobin there liberated passes by the portal system directly to the liver. When the spleen is removed this disintegration occurs in other organs, notably in the lymph nodes and bone-marrow, and the hemoglobin from these organs passes not into the portal but into the general circulation, from which it reaches the liver more gradually and in a more dilute form.[64]

Animals whose splenic blood supply has been diverted from the liver into the renal vein or inferior vena cava show a lessened tendency to jaundice similar to that exhibited by splenectomized animals receiving hemolytic serum. The lessened tendency to jaundice is, in part at least, due to a mechanical factor dependent on the course of the blood supply to the liver.[65 66]

In hemolytic jaundice there is excessive fragmentation and destruction of blood in the spleen-liver system because the circulating erythrocytes are usually fragile. There is, however, no bile in the urine, but bilirubin is found in the blood, urobilin in large amounts in the stools and the urine, and the bone-marrow shows signs of hyperfunctioning. This disease may in one member of the family cause merely enlargement of the spleen, without jaundice or much anemia; another may have the enlarged spleen, anemia and urobilinogenuria but no jaundice, and a third may have all of these. The enlargement of the spleen may be a work-hypertrophy. The jaundice is no index of the gravity of the condition. The same symptoms characterize the type which develops without any known inherited tendency. The exacerbations may resemble gall-stone trouble, and the anemia may assume the pernicious type during the exacerbations; they are inclined to be more abrupt in the acquired than in the familial type.[67]

In all these hemolytic groups the removal of the spleen has proved the means of curing most, if not all, of both subjective and objective disturbances; only occasionally the red cells may still display a certain fragility.[68]

Hijmans van den Bergh applied the diazo reaction for a fairly exact determination of bilirubin in the blood serum (it is not present in the corpuscles). Among other important results he found that bilirubin reacts in different ways, according to whether its increase is due only to a mechanical obstruction or to other causes. The bilirubin of the mechanical icterus reacts with the diazo reagent in the uncoagulated serum (direct reaction), is largely adsorbed by the coagulated proteins and is oxidized and excreted more readily than bilirubin of the other group. The second group gives the reaction only when the serum proteins have been coagulated by alcohol (indirect reaction). This he calls "dynamic icterus."[69] The question of dissociation between the elimination of bile pigments (bilirubin and urobilin) and of bile salts is of the greatest importance. Both are found in the urine in cases of mechanical obstruction to the outflow of bile. In hemolytic icterus only bile pigment is present (urobilin). In a third—the greatest—group of cases attributed to hepatic insufficiency both bile pigments and bile salts can be present in the urine.[70]

Jaundice in the newborn cannot be attributed to mechanical stasis, for it gives the indirect reaction. The formation of bilirubin in the spleen in pernicious anemia and in some intoxications has been proved directly by comparison of the amount of bilirubin in the vessels. The question whether bilirubin can form outside the liver (also in extravasates) is definitely settled in the affirmative.[71]

Role in Iron Metabolism. In 1834 Johann Müller[72] first showed the existence of iron-containing pigment in the spleen, which von Kölliker[73] and Ecker,[74] in 1847, showed to be present in the pigmented cells.

The spleen is one of the richest iron-containing organs and is a storehouse for the iron which is liberated from the decomposition of the blood tissues. The liver, on the contrary, is the storehouse of the iron ingested, but may partake of the splenic function.[75] Tedeschi[76] found that after splenectomy the liver and bone-marrow become richer in iron and give histological evidence of the increased iron content.

The iron output following experimental splenectomy or roentgen ray of the spleen is much greater than normal. It must therefore be considered that the spleen contains nascent iron, controlling both the exogenous and endogenous iron, since the increased output maintains both in hunger and on meat diet. The increase of output is still found eleven months after the operation.[77]

Experimental plethora can be produced by injecting defibrinated blood in splenectomized animals. The blood picture returns to normal the same as in normal controls. The anemia following poisons is recovered from also the same as in the normal. If the diet is iron-free following splenectomy anemia develops more promptly than on the normal diet; while on iron-rich diet the red blood cells increase.[78] Feeding iron in normal animals increases the iron of the spleen macrophages and of the liver Kupffer cells as well as of the kidney cells. Following splenectomy the preponderance of iron is in the liver cells and also in the epidermis.[79]

Chevalier proposed the following theory of the function of the spleen in relation to iron metabolism. He believes that the source or origin of the iron conditions its distribution in the body and its output. He thus speaks of an excretory tissue and an assimilative tissue. The skin, liver and kidney epithelium he places in the first class as excretory tissues; the macrophages or Kupffer cells of the spleen and liver and the endothelial cells of the skin and interstitial perivascular cells belong to the assimilative group. These he names siderocytes.[80]

On this basis the spleen has the function to: (1) Serve as a storehouse for siderocytes and (2) to st

storehouse for siderocytes and (2) to stimulate the activity of siderocytes in other organs of the body. It thus serves as a controlling organ for the entire siderocyte system. If the spleen fails in the latter function the iron-storing property of these cells is also lost. The spleen removed, the siderocytes partly take on its function, at the same time storing iron for the economy of the organism. If the siderocyte system fails, as it often does after splenectomy, the iron output is increased in the excretory cells.

Blood destruction due to a single injury, as by sodium oleate acting through a short period of time, or by toluylenediamin or hemolytic immune serum, as well as the continuous blood destruction of essentially a chronic experimental anemia, caused by infecting the dog with Trypanosoma equiperdum is not characterized in the absence of hemoglobinuria by an increased elimination of iron in the urine or the feces. This evidence of the power of the body to conserve the iron resulting from erythrocytic disintegration is further emphasized by the increased storage of iron in the liver and spleen.[81]

In view of this definite evidence of the power of the animal body to conserve iron, it is obvious that in the hemolytic anemias in man characterized by excessive elimination of iron in the feces some other factor than mere blood destruction is operative. Theoretically, it may be assumed that it is a disturbance of the mechanism concerned in the retention or conservation of iron.

Regulating Influence on Blood-producing Organs. Krumbhaar, Musser and Pearce[82] believe that the spleen has a stimulating influence on the blood-forming organs, since anemia due to bleeding or hemolytic poisons recovers with much greater difficulty and slowness in the splenectomized than in normal dogs. Eppinger concurs in this belief.

The lipoids and cholesterin in the blood increase with hemolytic anemia as after toluylendiamin and the blood regenerates quicker, possibly because of the presence in the circulation of the material for regeneration by the bone-marrow. The iron, besides, may also stimulate the bone-marrow. This occurs also after injection of erythrocyte lipoids, but not after posthemorrhagic anemia. The spleen possesses these iron-containing lipoids and nucleoproteins, and its function as a stimulant of the bone-marrow may depend upon these. The administration of spleen subcutaneously and intraperitoneally produces an increase in the red blood cell count, perhaps by an organic stimulus to the bone-marrow.

Gilbert[83] found a tremendous bone-marrow stimulation immediately after splenectomy in two patients, as evidenced by the marked leukocytosis, the increased nuclear red forms and increase in the large mononuclear and transitional groups. One year later the differential count was very much the same, except for the increase in the lymphocytes and the marked increase in the number of nucleated red cells. It would seem that the spleen has a very definite relation to bone-marrow cell production and to the maturing of the red cells, especially in the destructive metabolism of their nucleus. After a definite remission in these two patients there was much greater evidence of hemolysis than before. The bone-marrow in both cases showed marked activity, the principal change being the large number of normoblasts and of all stages in the formation of nuclear particles.

Brinchman's[84] experimental work also shows that in some indirect way the spleen exerts a regulating influence on the blood-producing organs, steadying the factors which direct the normal production and destruction.

Freytag and Eppinger[85] have shown an increase of the red blood cells following splenectomy and concluded from that fact that the spleen has a regulating function on the bone-marrow, inhibiting its production of red blood cells. Frank[86] believes that it is a hormone produced by the spleen that stimulates the bone-marrow.

Stradomsky[87] seems to have demonstrated that the spleen has a two-fold hormone action on the bone-marrow, an inhibiting action on the production of red corpuscles in the bone-marrow, and at the same time a stimulating action to increased destruction of these cells. Normally these two influences balance each other, but when the spleen hormone is abnormal or lacking the bone-marrow produces unlimited quantities of red cells; but their quality deteriorates. They die off more readily, and this increased erythrocytosis sets up an automatic vicious circle. Among the facts on which these assumptions are based are the increased numbers of red corpuscles found in the blood stream after splenectomy, the number rising in the course of one, four to six weeks after the removal of the spleen, while almost at once afterward the red corpuscles present Howell-Jolly bodies, showing that these erythrocytes are young immature forms.[88 89]

These findings indicate that the bone-marrow is functioning to excess after having been released from the controlling influence of the spleen hormone. After splenectomy, administration of spleen extract is liable to give results confirming this role of the spleen as a regulator of blood production. Another argument in favor of this assumption is the atrophy of the follicles in the spleen to which Hutchinson[90] and others have called attention in cases of polycythemia. It might be objected that polycythemia would follow in every case of disease of the spleen, but the diversity of pathologic conditions in the spleen may leave some parts of the organ intact, at least enough to produce sufficient of the hormone to prevent excessive production of red blood cells. There is also a possibility that the bone-marrow may not respond in every case in the same way.

The reason for the inconstant results as to the increase of red blood cells following splenectomy is explained by Eppinger[91] by the original condition of the spleen. If it be rich in blood before removal the effect on the erythrocytic blood picture would be different than if the red pulp be deficient in red blood cells.

Following removal of a ruptured normal spleen, Hall[92] found a considerable increase in the total leukocyte count which persisted with much irregularity for over three months. In the early period all types of leukocytes were increased in nearly the same proportion. This period represents the effect of removal of the spleen on the organs of blood formation and destruction. In the second period both total and differential counts showed such marked variation as to render averages valueless, but the total count was usually high. This period, lasting about two months, was one of adjustment of the organism to the new conditions while other tissues were possibly taking over the functions of the absent organ. In the final period a comparative equilibrium was reached, with a moderate increase in the total count, due entirely to lymphocytes and endothelial cells, while the granular leukocytes showed strictly normal figures.

The immediate increase of all cells after operation suggests the removal of some factor that either restricts production of white cells or destroys those that have passed their usefulness. In the Arneth index we have for the neutrophils a means of estimating which factor is mainly concerned. In the first period in this case the index was very slightly increased. As the neutrophils were present in more than double normal numbers it seems probable that the increase was not entirely due to lessened destruction. Moreover, the coincidence of a rise of the index with the first sharp drop of the neutrophils at the beginning of the second period, the fact that during this period high points in the neutrophil curve tended to coincide with high points of the index, and that the index remained high with a normal number of neutrophils in the final period, all suggest that the variations in the cell count are due at least in part to variations in the number of cells produced rather than to changes in the rate of destruction. This point of view would result in the conception of the normal spleen as exercising a resfrictive action on the production of the leukocytes.

It has been proved experimentally on normal animals that the spleen and the lymph nodes are the most sensitive organs in the body to the action of radium and roentgen rays. A few hours after the radiation of a normal animal there is noticed destruction of the cells of the lymphoid tissue and the spleen.

Cases of myeloid leukemia given a brief and mild course of roentgen-ray treatment of the spleen have shown the blood count to return practically to normal. This suggests that the spleen may have a special function in some circumstances, manifested by an inhibiting and impairing of the functioning of the bone-marrow. This special function seems to be set in action by the influence of certain morbid processes in the spleen itself.[93]

Function Concerned with Digestion. The exact role of the spleen in digestion is not known. The theories proposed are that:

1. The spleen gives to the blood stream during digestion a substance which activates or leads to the further elaboration of the gastric enzymes, especially pepsin.
2. The spleen is a storehouse for the temporary reception of the products of protein digestion, much as the liver is for glycogen.
3. The spleen is merely a diverticulum of the portal system to receive the excess blood rushed to the splanchnic area during the digestive period and to act as an abdominal heart for supplying this blood to the stomach and other abdominal organs as needed.

The idea that the spleen must be of some significance in this regard has been prompted by the gland's intimate anatomic connections with the portal system; its blood supply from the celiac axis; its marked congestion and swelling observed during the digestive period, with a gradual resumption of its normal size after several hours; its proportionately excessive atrophy during starvation and inanition; and by references by many experimental investigators, as well as many clinicians, to a state of hunger and voracious appetite after splenectomy.

The pepsinogenic function of the spleen has, indeed, often been mentioned as a possibility of physiologic importance. Tarulli and Pascucci[94] carried out a set of experiments on dogs in which they determined the digestive activity of the gastric juice before and after splenectomy. They concluded that during gastric digestion the spleen elaborates a pepsinogenic substance which is carried to the gastric glands through the blood stream and induces an increased amount of pepsin secretion. Gallenga[95] found increase in activity of the pepsin of the gastric filtrate from a splenectomized patient in artificial digestion by the addition of an extract of lambs' spleen, and concluded that this action of the spleen must depend on a pepsogenic internal secretion.

Trampedach[96] arrived at the conclusion that extirpation of the spleen has no diminishing influence on the digestive power of the stomach.

Recently, Inlow[97] studied the gastric secretion of animals under carefully controlled conditions before and after splenectomy, and concluded that a definite pepsinogenic function of the spleen has not been demonstrated and that the relation of the spleen to gastric secretion is probably merely vascular, the diminution in the amount of the juice secreted after splenectomy being attributable to decreased gastric blood supply from injury to the gastrosplenic circulation.

Cholesterinogenic Function. King,[98] Eppinger[99] and Denis[100] each found that there occurs an increase in the total fats and cholesterin in the blood after splenectomy.

Abelous and Soula,[101] during research on the action of the spleen, have made the new observation that the injection of dilute hydrochloric acid into the duodenum produces increase of cholesterin in the arterial blood. This does not take place in splenectomized animals. From this they concluded that the spleen possesses a cholesterinogenic function and that the liver possesses this function only to the very slightest extent.

Internal Secretion. It has repeatedly been alleged that the spleen is an endocrine organ with the function of influencing, in an obscure manner, some portion of the digestive apparatus by way of the blood stream or of activating one or more of the digestive enzymes by an internal secretion.

The hypothesis that the spleen produces an internal secretion is supported by: (1) The changes in the erythrocytes after splenectomy; (2) the modification of the blood picture in hyperplasia of the spleen, ameliorated in the same cases at least by splenectomy; and (3) the specific effects on the red blood corpuscles of injection of splenic extract. The chief function of the spleen is the removal from the circulation of the disintegrated erythrocytes; the splenic cells elaborate this material, producing from either the stroma or pigment portion an internal secretion. This internal secretion reduces the resistance of all the red blood corpuscles, the effect amounting to actual destruction of the older cells; and, finally, this internal secretion, possibly after modification by the liver, stimulates the erythrogenic function of the bone-marrow and is used up in the manufacture of new corpuscles.[102]

The presence of a spleen hormone to explain the lymphocytosis and the hypertrophy of the lymph glands following splenectomy was also proposed.[103] Krumbhaar[104] and his associates believe that a specific hormone of the spleen is activated by passage through the liver. Their experiments showed that the anemia which develops after splenectomy is more marked in animals on essentially a cooked, mixed diet than on a diet of raw meat. This suggests the possibility that heat alters the substance which, in the absence of the spleen, the body cannot utilize.

Reasoning hypothetically, Mayo[106] surmises that the spleen does not possess an internal secretion of importance, not only because removal of the normal organ does not disturb the body metabolism, but also because of its extremely limited sympathetic nerve supply. It is to be noted that the organs of primary internal secretion usually act through the sympathetic nervous system. The adrenals and the pituitary are so closely connected with the chromophil system that their union amounts almost to a single organ, half sympathetic and half secretory. Other organs, like the thyroid, gonads, pancreas, etc., which have internal secretion acting to a large extent through the blood stream, had at one time or still possess an external secretion as well as an internal.[105] The spleen does not properly fall into either of these categories.

On hypothetical grounds also it seems probable that the spleen develops certain enzymes which are important to its function, but it is equally evident that the function of the spleen is shared by other lymphoid and adenoid structures in the body, and that on the removal of the organ the function is continued by these collaborating structures.[107]

Kaznelson[108] has shown recently that the spleen possesses a thrombolytic function.

Although other investigators have shown that an enzyme or enzymes exist in the spleen capable of hydrolyzing peptone and also fibrin, Morse[109] found that the proteins of the spleen itself autolyze only in neutral or acid, not in alkaline solution. He suggests, therefore, that it is probable that the a-protease of Hedin is not an autolytic enzyme of the spleen but rather a heterolytic one resident in the white blood cells.

Detoxicating Function. The spleen is derived from mesoblastic tissue and is probably concerned largely with filtration of certain substances from the blood and the product of its activities is delivered to the liver through the splenic vein, suggesting at once what clinical experience has shown, a detoxicating function of the spleen.

Bacterial cultures were made of human spleens removed for surgical purposes. These usually remained sterile. In some instances the group of organisms found represented parasitic but nonpathogenic flora of the human body.[110]

Ozaki[111] found that the accumulation of bacteria in the spleen, such as occurs in experimental bacteremia, is principally dependent on the vital activity of the cells, and the mechanical filtration of bacteria by the spleen is not an important factor in their detention. He found that the spleen acts as a close filter for foreign erythrocytes, allowing very few to pass in dogs.

In typhoid fever the spleen becomes enlarged as a result of its straining function. The accumulated bacteria which have been strained out of the blood are sent to the liver for destruction. A failure in elimination of the bacteria from the spleen to the liver may result in multiple or single abscesses containing pure culture of typhoid bacillus.[112]

Enlargements of the spleen from chronic sepsis are not uncommon and may act as secondary distributing centers of infections.[113] Focal infections in various parts of the body may act as the primary source of the bacterial invasion. Septic endocarditis is a notable example.[114]

While tuberculosis of the spleen is considered by some observers as never primary, this condition has occasionally constituted the only known focus in the body.[115]

Spirochetal hibernation in the spleen is not unusual, and failure to eradicate the disease by arsphenamin and prolonged mercurial treatment may result in a syphilitic spleen which permits not only luetic reinfection of the body but also causes a high grade of chronic anemia.[116]

It is probable that some form of chemotaxis attracts to the spleen all of these various agents.

The characteristic change following splenectomy, as Ehrlich has shown, is an increase of eosinophil cells the second year after removal.

The decrease of eosinophils in the peripheral circulation following starvation and the indications of a very close relationship between eosinophils and intestinal secretion suggest that the eosinophils may convey a hormone which is important for proper cellular activity in the intestine.[117] Their relation to anaphylaxis suggests that they are, in some measure, a reaction of the organism against the penetration of foreign proteins.[118] Eosinophils possess important phagocytic properties both for bacteria and cells and are well adapted to the absorption of toxic products and may play an important role in the maintenance of immunity.[119 120 121]

Giffin[3 122 123] reported a case of persistent eosinophilia with hyperleukocytosis and splenomegaly in which the spleen was finally removed. Examination of the organs four and a half years later showed eosinophilic polynuclears and myelocytes abundant in the bone-marrow and the abdominal lymph glands. In this case the permanent increase of the leukocytes following splenectomy for a period of four and a half years considered in connection with the occurrence of more or less constant eosinophilia after splenectomy for various other conditions may be indicative of some special function of the spleen with respect to eosinophilic cells or with respect to the toxins which eosinophilic cells are capable of absorbing.

The results recorded by Hektoen[124] show that splenectomy may diminish the output of antibodies, especially when done about the same time as antigen is injected. Antibodies appear earlier in the spleen than in the blood; antigen is fixed by the spleen and in the presence of antigenic substances cultures of splenic tissue outside the body may produce antibodies. The results of several experiments indicate, however, that after antibody production is well under way splenectomy has little or no effect on the course of the antibodies in the blood. The antibody content of the blood is not diminished markedly by splenectomy or roentgenization at or near the height of the curve. The nature of this so-called resistance remains obscure.

Effects of Splenectomy and Compensation for Spleen Function. We know that the removal of the normal spleen rendered necessary by traumatism, etc., introduces no serious bodily change.

The absence of the spleen has no influence on either the adult or the growing organism, and seems to be without influence on the mother or child if removed during pregnancy.[125] This holds for animals and for man. Henn[126] showed that the spleen is not essential to the life of young rats, rabbits, kittens and puppies and that splenectomy has a negligible influence on their growth.

There seems to be no change in the general metabolic processes following removal of the spleen.[127] This holds for well-fed and poorly nourished animals, for the basal metabolism, carbon dioxide and sugar metabolism.[128] The spleen diminishes in size like the rest of the body with hunger.[129]

The fact, however, that the spleen can be extirpated without causing death or even considerable detriment to the animal organism does not militate against the conclusion that it is an organ of prime importance for the organism. Other organs (hemolymph nodes, bone-marrow and adenoid tissues in general) may assume part of the role of the spleen when this is absent, but only the severity of the blood-destroying agent and the individual resistance can determine whether the body can stand the strain when deprived of the spleen. Cases of death from removal of the malarial spleen indicate this strongly.[130]

After splenectomy the lymph glands of the greater curvature of the stomach and the omentum hypertrophy and become distinctly red, and new ones develop in the neighborhood of the extirpated spleen.[131] Hyperplasia of the lymphatics also gradually develops first in the vicinity of the portal vessels and then inside the liver lobes. This hyperplasia is evidently a compensating process in the lymphatic elements in the depths of the liver; it explains the increase in size of the liver which follows removal of the spleen.[132]

Schmidt[133] found iron-containing cells in the liver similar to the Kupffer cells, reminding him of spleen follicles. In these he found deteriorating red cells which he assumed developed to take on splenic function. The increase of Kupffer cells in the liver and changes in lymph glands and bone-marrow indicate a compensatory function on the part of these tissues in supplying a missing factor in blood formation and destruction.[134]

According to Freytag,[85] spleen function is fully compensated for within five or six weeks.

Physical Diagnosis of the Spleen. Palpation gives the only definite information as to the size of the spleen; if it cannot be felt, percussion is a poor and misleading substitute. We are as yet unable to study the earlier manifestations of associated diseases in relation to the size of the spleen, and its lesions are gross before we can be certain that it is concerned in the production of the symptoms from which the patient suffers.

To estimate more accurately the size of the spleen, Chauffard[135] draws a line from the middle of the axilla to the trochanter region, the arm held above the head. This line serves as the base from which the ovoid spleen is palpated and percussed, and the outline marked also on the skin. A line is then drawn from the base line axially to the farther limit forward of the spleen. This axial line is bisected in the center by a line perpendicular to it. We thus have two lines that can be measured and compared from case to case, giving thus the approximate size of the spleen.

Radiographic examination of the spleen has been of comparatively little assistance in the diagnosis of its function. By means of the roentgen ray the outlines of the spleen may be fairly well determined. The examination is made, moving the patient from side to side so as to change the position of the adjacent hollow organs. The left costophrenic sinus indicates the position of the upper

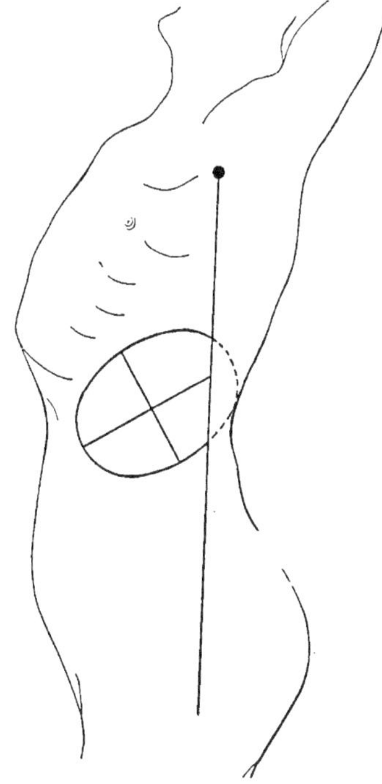

Chauffard's Method of Estimating Size of Spleen.

pole and external surface of the spleen. Gas in the stomach or air introduced by tube may help in outlining the lower surface and right boundary of the spleen. In children who are easily moved about the outlines are more clearly defined. In pathologic spleens manifesting large tumors this method of examination, as well as insufflation of the colon with air, is necessary for differential diagnosis.[136 137]

Puncture of the spleen is attended with danger and is not practised clinically for diagnosis except in cases of suspected abscess.

Here the danger of infection is great and its use as a diagnostic method has been strongly opposed even in localized infections.[138]

Causes of Enlargement of the Spleen.[139]

I. In children.
- (*a*) Disturbances of metabolism, rickets, amyloid disease.
- (*b*) Chronic intestinal affections.
- (*c*) Large but ill-defined group of intestinal disorders, particularly in the tropics.
- (*d*) The pseudoleukemia infantum.

II. In the infections.
- (*a*) Syphilis.
- (*b*) Malaria.
- (*c*) Kala-azar and other forms of tropical splenomegaly.
- (*d*) Hodgkin's disease.
- (*e*) Tuberculosis.

III. In primary disorders of the blood-forming organs.
- (*a*) Leukemia.
- (*b*) Pernicious anemia.
- (*c*) Chlorosis.
- (*d*) Hemachromatosis.
- (*e*) Polycythemic splenomegaly.

IV. In cirrhosis of the liver.
- (*a*) Syphilitic.
- (*b*) Alcoholic.
- (*c*) Hypertrophic of Hanot.

V. Hereditary and family forms of splenomegaly.
- (*a*) Congenital acholuric icterus.
- (*b*) Constitutional disturbances, dwarfing, etc.

VI. Newgrowths and parasites.
- (*a*) Sarcoma.
- (*b*) Primitive endothelioma of Gaucher.
- (*c*) Echinococcus.
- (*d*) Schistosoma of Japan.

VII. Splenomegaly not correlated with any of the above or with any known cause.
- (*a*) Banti's disease with its three stages:
  1. Simple enlargement.
  2. Splenomegaly with anemia.
  3. Splenomegaly with anemia, jaundice and ascites.

REFERENCES AND BIBLIOGRAPHY.

1. Eppinger: Die Hepato-Lienalen Erkrankungen, Berlin, 1920.
2. v. Ebner: Handbuch der Gewebelehre des Menschen, 1902, **3**, 257.
3. Giffin: Am. Jour. Med. Sci., 1919, **158**, 618.
4. Weidenreich: Arch. d. mikr. Anat., 1901, **58**, 247.

5. Socoloff: Virchows Arch., 1888, **112**, 209.
6. Wicklein: Virchows Arch., 1891, **124**, 1.
7. Kalenkiewicz: Diss. Dorpat., 1892.
8. Mall: Am. Jour. Anat., 1903, **2**, 315.
9. Weidenreich: Verhandl. d. anat. Gesellsch., Halle, 1902.
10. Grawitz: Pathologie des Blutes, 1911, **4**, 179.
11. Eppinger: See ref. 1.
12. Naegeli: Fol. Haematol., 1905, **2**, 327.
13. Ehrlich: Charite Annalen, 1878, **5**, 198; Ibid., 1885, **12**, 288; Ibid., 1888, **13**, 300. [Krumbhaar: Jour. Lab. and clin. Med., 1922, **8**, 11.]
14. De Laet: Ann. de l'Inst. Pasteur, 1919, **33**, 807.
15. Rieux: Arch. d. mal. du cœur, 1920, **13**, 254.
16. Normet: Bull. de l'Acad. de méd., Paris, 1920, **83**, 163.
17. Vierordt: Arch. f. physiol. Heilk., 1854, **13**, 259.
18. Weidenreich: Leukocyten u. Verwandte Zellformen, Wiesbaden, 1911.
19. Pappenheim u. Fukushi: Fol. Haematol., 1913, **16**, 177.
20. Kurloff: Ehrlich-Lazarus: Anämien, 1 Abteil, 1898, p. 65.
21. Audibert et Valetti. Compt. rend. Soc. de biol., Paris, 1907, **62**, 536.
22. Port: Arch. f. exper. Path., 1913, **73**, 251.
23. Dubois: Biochem. Ztschr., 1917, **82**, 141.
24. Noguchi· Berl. klin. Wchnschr., 1912, **49**, 1839.
25. Bayer: Grenzgebiete, 1910, **22**, 111 and 532, Ibid., 1913, **27**, 311.
26. Bain: Jour. Physiol., 1903, **29**, 352.
27. Ehrlich: Ztschr. f. klin. Med., 1880, **1**, 553; Farbenanalytische Untersuchungen z. Histol. u. Klinik des Blutes, Berlin, 1891.
28. Dominici: Arch. de Méd. expér. et d'anat. path., 1900, **12**, 563.
29. Elliott and Kanavel: Surg., Gynec., Obst , 1915, **21**, 21.
30. Hartmann and Lang: Jour. Pharmac. and Exper. Therap., 1919, **13**, 417.
31. Frey: Ztschr. f. exper. Med., 1914, **3**, 416.
32. Blumenfeld: Berl. klin. Wchnschr., 1918, **55**, 92.
33. Sanguinetti· Policlinico, 1921, **28**, 97.
34. Freidberg: Monatschr. f. Kinderh., 1920, **18**, 432.
35. Abrams· Med. Rec., 1919, **95**, 96.
36. Scalas: Riforma med., 1920, **36**, 781.
37. Eppinger: See ref. 1.
38. Schmincke: München. med. Wchnschr , 1916, **63**, 1005.
39. v. Kölliker: Mitteil. d. Zürch. Naturforschbreges, 1847, p. 120.
40. Virchow: Virchows Arch., 1852, **4**, 515; Ibid, 1853, **5**, 405; Ibid., 1900, **160**, 247.
41. Perls· Virchows Arch., 1867, **39**, 42.
42. Metchnikoff: Ann. d. l'Inst. Pasteur, 1899, **13**, 737.
43. Gabbi: Ziegler's Beitr., 1893, **14**, 351.
44. Hunter: Lancet, 1892, **2**, 1209.
45. Rous and Robertson: Jour. Exp. Med., 1917, **25**, 651.
46. Lintwarew: Virchows Arch., 1911, **206**, 36.
47. Gerlach: Ztschr. f. rationelle Med., 1949, **7**, 75.
48. Troissier: Rôle des hemolysins, Thèse de Paris, 1910.
49. Pel: Deutsch. Arch. f. klin. Med., 1912, **106**, 592.
50. Botazzi: Arch. Ital. d. biol., 1895, **24**, 1462.
51. Pearce and Minor: Jour. Exp. Med., 1913, **18**, 494; Ibid., 1914, **20**, 19.
52. Charlier et Charlet: Jour. d. physiol. et path. gén., 1911, **42**, 728.
53. See ref. 45.
54. Frey: Deutsch. Arch. f. klin. Med., 1920, **133**, 223.
55. Banti: Klin.-therap. Wchnschr., 1912, **19**, 156.
56. Furno: Arch. de biol. norm. et pathol., September and October, 1913.
57. Krumbhaar and Musser Jour. Exp. Med., 1914, **20**, 108.
58. Morris. Arch. Int. Med., 1915, **15**, 514. Gilbert: Arch. Int. Med., 1917, **19**, 105.
59. Benda: Arch. f. Anat. u. Phys., 1896, 347.
60. Eppinger: See ref. 1.
61. Whipple and Hooper: Jour. Exp. Med., 1913, **17**, 612; Am. Jour. Physiol., 1916, **40**, pp. 332 and 349; Ibid., 1917, **42**, pp. 256, 264 and 544.
62. Pugliese: Arch. f. Anat. u. Physiol., 1899, 60.
63. Eppinger: See. ref. 1.
64. Austin and Pepper: Jour. Exp. Med., 1914, **22**, 675.

65. Krumbhaar and Musser: Jour. Exp. Med., 1916, **23**, 87.
66. Burket: Jour. Exp. Med., 1917, **26**, 849.
67. Biffis: Policlinico, 1919, **26**, 393.
68. Turk Deutsch. med. Wchnschr., 1914, **40**, 371.
69. van den Bergh: Der Gallenfarbstoff, 1916.
70. Brulé: Recherches récentes sur les ictéres, Paris, Masson et Cie., 1919.
71. Lepehne: Deutsch. Arch. f. klin. Med., 1921, **135**, 79.
72. Muller: Müllers Arch., 1834, p. 80.
73. v. Kolliker. See ref. 39.
74. Ecker: Ztschr. f. rationell. Med., 1847.
75. Schmidt: Verhandl. d. pathol. Gesellsch., Jena, 1912, **15**, 91.
76. Tedeschi: Jour. de physiol. et de path. gén., 1899, **1**, 23.
77. Asher and Grossenbacher: Biochem. Ztschr., 1909, **17**, 78.
78. Paton and Goodall: Jour. Physiol., 1903, **29**, 411.
79. Eppinger: See ref. 1.
80. Chevallier: La Rate: Organe de l'assimilation du fer, Thèse de Paris, 1913.
81. Dubin and Pearce: Jour. Exp. Med., 1917, **25**, 675; Ibid., 1918, **27**, 479.
82. Krumbhaar, Musser and Pearce: Jour. Exp. Med., 1913, **18**, 119.
83. Gilbert: Michigan State Med. Soc. Jour., 1917, **16**, 412.
84. Brinchman: Norsk Mag. f. Lægevidensk., 1916, **77**, 1253; Ibid., 1916, **77**, 1451; Acta Med. Scandin., 1920, **52**, 689.
85. Freytag: Pflüger's Arch., 1907, **120**, 501; Ibid., 1908, **122**, 501.
86. Frank: Berl. klin. Wchnschr., 1915, **52**, 490.
87. Stradomsky: Russkiy Vrach, 1916, **15**, 1122.
88. Hirschfeld and Weinert: Verl. klin. Wchnschr., 1914, **51**, 1026.
89. Port: Berl. klin. Wchnschr., 1914, **51**, 546.
90. Hutchinson: Tr. Med. Soc., London, 1908, **31**, 375.
91. Eppinger: See ref. 1.
92. Hall: Am. Jour. Med. Sci., 1920, **160**, 72.
93. Frank: Berl. klin. Wchnschr., 1915, **52**, 1062.
94. Tarulli and Pascucci: Human Physiology, London, Macmillan, 1913, **2**, 175.
95. Gallenga: Policlinico, 1902, **9**, pp. 11 and 105.
96. Trampedach: Arch. f. ges. Physiol., 1911, **141**, 591.
97. Inlow: Am. Jour. Med. Sci., 1921, **162**, 325.
98. King. Arch. Int. Med., 1914, **14**, 145.
99. Eppinger: Biochem. Ztschr., 1914, **59**, 419.
100. Denis: Arch. Int. Med., 1917, **20**, 79.
101. Abelous et Soula: Compt. rend. Acad. d. Sc., Paris, 1920, **83**, 455 and 663. Presse méd., 1920, **170**, 619 and 759.
102. Eddy: Endocrinology, 1921, **5**, 461.
103. Schulze: Cited by Eppinger, see ref. 1.
104. Austin and Pearce: Jour. Exp. Med., 1915, **22**, 682; Krumbhaar, ibid., 1916, **23**, 87.
105. Kendall: Jour. Am. Med. Assn., 1916, **66**, 811.
106. Mayo: Med. Rec., 1917, **92**, 706.
107. Warthin: Am. Jour. Med. Sci., 1901, **121**, 63.
108. Kaznelson: Wien. klin. Wchnschr., 1916, **29**, 1451.
109. Morse: Jour. Biol. Chem., 1917, **31**, 303.
110. Sellards: New Orleans Med. and Surg. Jour., 1917, **69**, 502.
111. Ozaki: Jour. Med. Research, 1917, **36**, 413.
112. Socoloff: Virchows Arch., 1875, **66**, 171.
113. Bardach: Ann. de l'Inst. Pasteur, 1889, **3**, 577.
114. Douglas and Eisenbrey: Am. Jour. Med. Sci., 1914, **147**, 479.
115. Fischer: Wien. med. Wchnschr., 1909, **59**, 2506.
116. Wile and Elliott: Am. Jour. Med. Sci., 1915, **150**, 512.
117. Opie: Am. Jour. Med. Sci., 1904, **127**, 217.
118. Lepsky: Compt. rend. Soc. de biol., 1915, **78**, 629.
119. Mesnil: Ann. de l'Inst. Pasteur, 1895, **9**, 301.
120. Weinberg: Ann. de l'Inst. Pasteur, 1915, **29**, 323.
121. Fiessinger: Arch. de med. exper. et d'anat. path., 1916, **27**, 270.
122. Aubertin and Giroux: Presse méd., 1921, **29**, 314.
123. Stillman: Med. Rec., 1912, **81**, 594.
124. Hektoen: Jour. Infect. Dis., 1920, **27**, 23.
125. Diastre: Compt. rend. de Soc. biol., 1893, **45**, 357.
126. Henn: Am. Jour. Physiol., 1920, **52**, 562.

127. Paton: Jour. Physiol., 1900, **25**, 443.
128. Verzár: Biochem. Ztschr., 1913, **53**, 69.
129. Eppinger: See ref. 1.
130. Morris: Jour. Exp. Med., 1914, **20**, 379.
131. Tizzoni: Arch. ital. de Biol., 1882, **1**, 129.
132. Silvestrini: Riforma medica, 1916, **32**, 266.
133. Schmidt: Ziegler's Beitr., 1892, **11**, 191.
134. Austin and Pearce. Jour. Exp. Med., 1912, **16**, 780.
135. Chauffard: Bull et mém. Soc. méd. d. hôp. de Paris, 1919, **43**, 554.
136. Le Page: La Radioskopie et Radiographie de la Rate, Thèse de Paris, 1912.
137. Rantenberg: Berl. klin. Wchnschr., 1914, **40**, 1205.
138. Stubenrauch: Beitr. z. klin. Chir., 1914, **88**, 712.
139. Osler: British Med. Jour., 1908, **2**, 1151.
140. Held: Med. Clin. North Amer., 1919, **3**, 519.

THE AUTOLYSATE-PRECIPITIN REACTION IN TYPHOID FEVER.

(A PRELIMINARY REPORT.)

By JOHN L. LAIRD, M.D., JOHN R. CONOVER, M.D.,

AND

DONALD C. A. BUTTS,*

PHILADELPHIA.

(From the Division of Laboratories, Pennsylvania Department of Health.)

THE obvious necessity for improvement in the laboratory methods of diagnosis of typhoid infection and the failure of bacteriologic and direct immunologic research studies to accomplish it, has led us to seek a solution of the problem by an entirely new route. Research in typhoid determination has dealt almost entirely with attempts to discover more sensitive culture media for the differentiation of the nonlactose fermenting group as a first step in the diagnosis. Endo, Conradi-Drigalski, Teague's, malachite green, brilliant green and litmus media have been used and advocated by the various workers. All have shown results of about equal efficiency in the hands of their respective advocates. None has shown any appreciable advantage over the others, nor any advance in accuracy of differential diagnosis.

The reason for the failures to determine the typhoid bacillus in the excretions of typhoid cases and carriers by these methods, we believe to be twofold: (1) They depend upon bacterial action on lactose. This presupposes a goodly number of culturally typical typhoid bacilli in the stools and urine, a condition which probably rarely exists; (2) it is beyond reasonable doubt that many of the

* The authors wish to express their indebtedness to the Philadelphia General Hospital for the privilege of their wards, to the H. K. Mulford Company for a supply of antityphoid serum which made possible continued experimentation and to Miss Nora Heffernan, Research Technician in the State Laboratories, for technical aid in this research.

typhoid bacilli infesting the small intestine of the typhoid case are autolyzed during their passage through the intestinal tract, and, therefore, are not culturally demonstrable. Bacteriologic technic, under the most favorable conditions, will average about 25 per cent of positive results upon known typhoid excretions. The typhoid organism, even of the preëminently stable strains, such as Rawling's or Stewart's, so commonly used in the laboratories because of stability for agglutination tests, have been known to undergo mutation, to acquire the ability to ferment lactose. This has occurred several times in this laboratory, and has been verbally corroborated by other bacteriologists; the colonies showing marked fermentation having been identified as pure typhoid by other methods of determination. How much more likely, then, that this change in cultural characteristics should occur in the average unstable strain from the typhoid case. An examination by such method, therefore, fails in its first step.

It should be easily perceptible from the foregoing that one of three methods of attack must be adopted for improvement in typhoid determination.

1. To determine the typhoid bacillus by the other differential methods applied to all organisms present in the original culture of the excretions, regardless of their action upon lactose.

2. To employ a method of treatment to the excretions which will bring about a reclamation of the typhoid bacillus to cultural type before the application of the differential cultural methods.

3. To determine the presence of an autolysate of the typhoid bacilli in the excretions.

The first method is one appropriate to the more purely research laboratory. The second has shown some promise in this laboratory, in the use of the "living-culture tube" devised by Laird, the detailed description of which cannot be given in this article. This publication will deal entirely with the preliminary work upon the third method, the autolysate-precipitin reaction in typhoid stools and urine.

The autolysate-precipitin reaction should not be confused with the precipitin reaction heretofore employed in the diagnosis of typhoid.[1] Our reaction is dependent upon the determination of the existence of the autolysed typhoid bacilli in the excretions of the patient by means of a known specific typhoid rabbit's serum, in direct contrast to the older method which depended upon a precipitin reaction in the serum of the suspected patient by means of a known typhoid solution.

The technic of the autolysate-precipitin reaction was in part suggested by the promising work of Robinson and Meader upon the precipitin reaction in the diagnosis of gonorrhea.[2]

[1] Hiss and Zinsser. Text Book of Bacteriology, p. 424. Norris: Jour Infect. Dis., 1904, **1**, 3.

[2] Robinson and Meader: Jour. Urol., 1920, **3**, 772.

Before entering into the actual procedure of our experiments the technic of preparing the serum and specimens will be described.

PREPARATION OF RABBIT'S SERUM (PRECIPITIN). *Method* 1. A suspension of typhoid bacilli is made, in N/00 NaCl, of two billion organisms per cubic centimeter and placed in the incubator for four days. It is then centrifuged and the clear supernatant solution used and kept at room temperature. One cubic centimeter is injected intravenously into rabbits at intervals of five to seven days for five injections; the rabbits are bled on the fifth day after the last injection.

The agglutination titer should be at least 1 : 1000 and the serum should show a definite precipitate with the original autolysate.

Method 2. One-hundredth of a twenty-four-hour agar slant of typhoid bacilli suspended in 1 cc of N/00 NaCl and killed at 60° for one hour is injected subcutaneously every seven days for five injections. The rabbits are bled on the fifth day after the last administration. The agglutination titer and the specific precipitation should be the same as No. 1.

Method 3. Injections of killed typhoid bacilli are given, first subcutaneously and then intravenously every day for nine days, according to the following table:

1st day	500	million killed bacilli	subcutaneously.
2d “	500	“ “ “	“
3d “	1000	“ “ “	“
4th “	1000	“ “ “	“
5th “	500	“ “ “	intravenously.
6th “	1000	“ “ “	“
7th “	1000	“ “ “	“
8th “	1000	“ “ “	
9th “	1000 / 1500 / or / 2000	“ “ “	“
		depending upon the condition of the animal.	

Allow animals to rest seven days, then make a test bleeding for agglutination titer and autolysate-precipitin reaction. Final bleeding is made upon the ninth day if tests are satisfactory.

All three methods have shown equally good results in the autolysate-precipitin reaction, but method 3 showed the highest agglutination titer, 1 : 6400.

PREPARATION OF THE INFECTED STOOL. Two grams of the stool from the typhoid patient are emulsified in 20 cc of physiologic salt solution (N/00 NaCl)* until a uniform suspension is obtained. A loopful of the suspension is placed upon a hanging-drop slide and examined for suspicious organisms. If any are present a portion is plated upon endo medium and incubated for eighteen to twenty-four hours. Suspicious colonies upon the plate are examined in

* Twenty cc of N/00 NaCl are used for the suspension because smaller amounts, due to absorption during filtration, yield an insufficient amount for the test.

the hanging-drop and transplanted to litmus milk and plain agar and incubated for twenty-four hours. Suspension is made from any growth upon the agar slants and the presence of the Bacillus typhosus verified by hanging-drop and specific agglutination.

While these routine examinations are being conducted the bulk of the original suspension is allowed to stand at room temperature until the insoluble matter has settled to the bottom of the tube, or, if the examinations have shown living organisms suggestive of Bacillus typhosus the suspension is placed in the incubator for twelve hours in order to insure sufficient autolysis. The supernatant liquid is then decanted and centrifuged for thirty minutes at 3000 r.p.m. The supernatant portion is again transferred to another tube and 0.5 gm. of Kieselguhr (diatomaceous earth) is added, agitated and filtered through filtering paper.

It was found that the above method yields a clear filtrate most suitable for our tests.

Preparation of Infected Urine. Before clarification for the tests the urine must be examined qualitatively for albumin, as it has been found that albumin causes precipitation with specific serum which might be falsely interpreted as a positive reaction. The other abnormal constituents of the urine do not influence the precipitin reaction. If albumin is present it is eliminated by adding dilute acetic acid, boiling until the albumin is precipitated and filtering. The resultant acidity interferes in no way with the precipitin test, but it may be neutralized to litmus with dilute sodium hydroxid solution. Moreover, we are led to believe that specimens infected with the Bacillus typhosus have a high degree of acidity which increases with the progressive autolysis. The determination of the actual hydrogen-ion concentration of these specimens has not been performed, but will be taken up in a later publication.

The specimen, free from albumin, is centrifuged for fifteen minutes or longer at 2000 r.p.m. to produce a clear supernatant fluid, to which Kieselguhr is added and filtered. Absolute clarity of the specimen is imperative, otherwise any sediment or cloudiness might be misconstrued as a positive reaction.

The controls for our experiments have been normal feces and urines treated under the same conditions as the infected specimens, together with direct controls of the latter to which no serum has been added and the unmixed serum.

Before performing the autolysate-precipitin test upon actual cases of typhoid, normal urines and stools were infected with Bacillus typhosus. (For this purpose a two-billion per cc suspension of Bacillus typhosus, Rawling's strain, was used.) The infected specimen was incubated for varying periods, six hours, twenty-four hours, four and seven days. Although we received positive reactions at the expiration of the incubation periods in all cases, it was found that with increased autolysis there was increased precipitum. It was also found that the autolysate-precipitin reaction was consistently positive only with the specific serum: Other reagents used were mercuric potassium iodid, ammonium sulphate, ethyl alcohol and heat, but the varying degrees of accuracy eliminated them as possible precipitins.

It was observed, microscopically and culturally, that the Bacillus typhosus was appreciably lessened and the characteristics greatly altered after a long period of incubation, it being impossible to isolate the organism after four to six days. On the other hand, the autolysate-precipitin reaction became more marked.

Technic of Autolysate-precipitin Reaction. Specimens of the stools and urine were collected daily from the cases under our observation and prepared and examined as described under the separate headings.

The precipitin rack is set up, using three tubes for each patient. In the first and second rows place 1 cc of typhoid serum in each tube. To the first row add 1 cc of the specimen to be tested and slightly agitate. To the second row 1 cc of normal urine or extract of feces is added and the tubes agitated. In the third row 2 cc of the corresponding test specimen is placed and agitated. The tubes are allowed to stand at room temperature for one hour and then placed in the ice-box over night. In the morning the rack is again placed at room temperature for several hours.

At the expiration of four or five hours it will be noted that the solutions in the first row of tubes have become turbid or show appreciable precipitation in the positive cases. The second and third rows (controls) should be clear or contain a very small amount of precipitate due to deterioration, the supernatant solution remaining clear in contrast to the turbidity of the positive tests. Of course the specific serum control should accompany each set of tests and should remain clear.

Having observed satisfactory autolysate-precipitin reactions upon one hundred and fifty-two specimens of stool and urine from typhoid cases and convalescents, we deemed it advisable to perform the test upon autolysates of other pathogenic organisms occurring within the intestinal tract. For this purpose we used twenty-four-hour cultures of the following organisms: Bacillus morgani, Bacillus shigæ, Bacillus para coli and five strains of the Bacillus dysenteriæ-flexner (V, W, X, Y and Z),[1] together with Bacillus typhosus, Bacillus paratyphosus A and Bacillus paratyphosus B.

[1] Classification of the Dysentery-Flexner bacillus:
V = Oxford Flexner—Standard Laboratory—Old Flexner.
W = Cable, British Front, 1914 (new variety).
X = Hughes, Carrier, University War Hospital, Southampton (new variety).
Y = Original Hiss-Russell strain.
Z = Whittington, Carrier, University War Hospital, Southampton (new variety).

TABLE I.—AUTOLYSATE-PRECIPITIN EXPERIMENTS. NORMAL STOOLS INFECTED WITH B. TYPHOSUS.

No.	Feces, gm.	Sterilization.	B. typhosus 1 cc = 2 billion.	Incubation.	N/00 NaCl.	Incubation autolysis.	Hanging drop.	3000 r.p.m. centrifuge.	Hanging drop.	Reactions.			
										Typhoid serum.	Autolysate.	Immediate.	Time.
1.	1.02	30 minutes at 250° C.	1 cc	21 hours	10 cc	6 hours	++	30 minutes	±	0.5 cc	0.5 cc	None	Marked.
2.	1.40	30 minutes at 250° C.	1 cc	47 hours	10 cc	24 hours	++	30 minutes	+	0.5 cc	0.5 cc	None	Marked.
3.	1.35	30 minutes at 250° C.	1 cc	95 hours	10 cc	4 days	+	30 minutes	±	0.5 cc	0.5 cc	Slight	Very marked.
4.	1.20	30 minutes at 250° C.	None	21 hours 47 hours 95 hours	10 cc	6 hours 24 hours 4 days	−	30 minutes	−	0.5 cc	0.5 cc	None	None.

++ = Many motile bacilli. + = Some motile bacilli. ± = Few motile bacilli. − = No motile bacilli.
The precipitin used to produce the reactions was undiluted typhoid serum (rabbit), titer 1: 6400.

Suspensions of the cultures were made in N/00 NaCl and diluted to contain approximately two billion organisms per cc. They were placed in the incubator for six, twelve and seventy-two hours and then centrifuged to obtain clear autolysates.

The reactions gave very encouraging results with the specific typhoid serum. The members of the typhoid group (Bacillus typhosus, Bacillus paratyphosus A and Bacillus paratyphosus B) showed clearly positive while the seventy-two hour autolysates of the other intestinal organisms were negative. Here again it was noted that the reaction upon the typhoid group became more pronounced with the increased autolysis. The seventy-two-hour autolysate showed almost immediate precipitation.

Table I shows the results of the increased autolysis upon the autolysate-precipitin reaction.

It can be seen from this table that precipitation becomes more pronounced with increased autolysis; the ninety-five-hour autolysate showing almost instantaneous precipitation, while the twenty-four and seventy-two-hour autolysates required twelve hours for the reaction to occur.

Table II illustrates the reaction carried out with specific typhoid serum upon other potentially pathogenic intestinal organisms in comparison to the typhoid group.

TABLE II.—AUTOLYSATE-PRECIPITIN EXPERIMENTS. SEVENTY-TWO-HOUR AUTOLYSATE.

Organism.	Incubation.	Centrifuged at 3000 r.p.m.	Reactions.	
			Immediate.	Time.
Morgan 1 . . .	72 hours	15 minutes	None	None.
Shiga	72 "	15 "	None	None.
Typhosus . . .	72 "	15 "	Slight turbidity	Marked.
Para A	72	15 "	Marked turbidity	Marked.
Para B	72	15	Marked turbidity	Marked.
Para coli . . .	72	15 "	None	None.
Flexner V . . .	72	15	None	None.
Flexner W . . .	72	15	None	None.
Flexner X . . .	72	15	None	None.
Flexner Y . . .	72	15	None	None.
Flexner Z . . .	72	15	None	None.

Suspension of 2,000,000,000 organisms per cubic centimeter used in the above experiment.

It will be noted that the reaction is markedly positive with the typhoid group, including the paratyphoid bacilli, while it is negative with the other organisms.

Table III shows the results of the autolysate-precipitin reaction upon actual typhoid stools and urine in the progressive stages of the disease and upon carriers and normal specimens.

TABLE III.

Day of fever	Specimens examined, 297.	culture	Widal	Bacteriologic		Autolysate-precipitin reaction.					
						Immediate.		Time.			
				rine	Stool	Urine.	Stool.	Urine.		Stool.	
								+	−	+	−
1st to 7th	9			7			.	7		2	
8th to 14th	9			2				3		6	
15th to 21st				13	5		..	13		5	
22d to 28th	27		1	15	11			16		11	
29th to 40th	24			17	7			17	..	7	
41st to 60th	33			26	7	2 5	2	24	2	5	2
Carriers	32	2	5					19	..	13	
Normal (control)	152			105	17				105	.	47

The blood culture and the idal reactions were, of course, not performed as repeatedly as tl bacteriologic examination and the aut precipitin reaction nor were they performed upon every pecimens represe ed in this table were obtained from ses, 5 convalesce , 2 carriers and 10 normal persons. ight be called to tl fact that the bacteriologic examina- specimens from tl known typhoid cases was positive about 6 per cent, wl e the autolysate-precipitin reaction positive in 100 per cent n to the fifty-sixth day of the disease, ter which the two negative were obtained. The reaction in all instances was clearly perceptble, read and checked by several workers, except during the lte convalescent period as the final negative was approached. Iring convalescence, after two negative bacteriologic examinatios of the stool and urine released the patient from quarantine rtrictions, the autolysate-precipitin reaction remained positive fc many days.

Summary. A brief discussn of the problem of typhoid diagnosis is given with the reasoi leading to the present investigation.

Experimental autolysate-pecipitin reactions and the technic of preparation of the reagets and performance of the test are described.

Autolysate-precipitin reactns upon autolysates of other intestinal organisms with typhoi precipitin showed negative results. The reaction was positive n only to the Bacillus typhosus, but to the paratyphoid A and B ntolysate.

The autolysate-precipitin action showed clearly positive in all cases of typhoid fever and ca riers up to the fifty-sixth day of the disease. The carriers were many years' standing, one dating back eighteen years.

The bacteriologic [illegible]
cent of known typhoid [illegible]

Conclusions. It [illegible]
early stage of experim[illegible]
tion is distinctly m[illegible]
previous methods [illegible]

Inasmuch as th[illegible]
chemical derivative [illegible]
a positive reaction m[illegible]
the patient from w[illegible]
In other words, as lo[illegible]
positive the patient [illegible]
potential menace a[illegible]
depend upon any in[illegible]
presence of the chen[illegible]
the excretions and, th[illegible]
is free from this infe[illegible]

The persistence of t[illegible]
bacteriologic examina[illegible]
from quarantine restr[illegible]
tion as a better meth[illegible]

The result of the [illegible]
stages of the disease [illegible]
diagnosis as well as [illegible]
usefulness in the acute [illegible]
of typhoid which ha[illegible]
because of the eva[illegible]
sequent absence of m[illegible]

It should eliminate [illegible]
logic diagnosis in [illegible]

The distinct specific[illegible]
suggests its possibilitie[illegible]
tions with the use of pro[illegible]

It seems appropriate [illegible]
of time and expen[illegible]
control, if further [illegible]
ability.

It must be under[illegible]
be interpreted as t[illegible]
cases. Many pert[illegible]
only by continued [illegible]
phases and upon the [illegible]

TABLE III.

Day of fever.	No. of specimens examined, 297.	Blood culture		Widal.		Bacteriologic				Autolysate-precipitin reaction							
										Immediate.				Time.			
						Urine		Stool		Urine		Stool		Urine.		Stool	
		+	−	+	−	+	−	+	−	+	−	+	−	+	−	+	−
1st to 7th	9	1	1	4	..	..	7	1	1	..	..	..	..	7	..	2	
8th to 14th	9	..	..	1	..	1	2	1	5	..	..	..	..	3	..	6	
15th to 21st	18	..	1	..	..	..	13	..	5	..	..	..	..	13	..	5	
22d to 28th	27	..	1	..	1	1	15	..	11	..	..	..	..	16	..	11	
29th to 40th	24	..	..	..	..	..	17	..	7	..	..	..	..	17	..	7	
41st to 60th	33	..	..	..	..	..	26	..	7	4	2	5	2	24	2	5	2
Carriers	32	..	2	5	1	..	19	5	8	..	..	..	..	19	..	13	
Normal (control)	152	..	..	..	..	..	105	..	47	..	..	..	..	..	105	..	47

The blood culture and the Widal reactions were, of course, not performed as repeatedly as the bacteriologic examination and the autolysate-precipitin reaction; nor were they performed upon every case. The specimens represented in this table were obtained from 9 typhoid cases, 5 convalescents, 2 carriers and 10 normal persons. Attention might be called to the fact that the bacteriologic examination upon specimens from the known typhoid cases was positive in only about 6 per cent, while the autolysate-precipitin reaction was positive in 100 per cent up to the fifty-sixth day of the disease, after which the two negatives were obtained. The reaction in all instances was clearly perceptible, read and checked by several workers, except during the late convalescent period as the final negative was approached. During convalescence, after two negative bacteriologic examinations of the stool and urine released the patient from quarantine restrictions, the autolysate-precipitin reaction remained positive for many days.

Summary. A brief discussion of the problem of typhoid diagnosis is given with the reasons leading to the present investigation.

Experimental autolysate-precipitin reactions and the technic of preparation of the reagents and performance of the test are described.

Autolysate-precipitin reactions upon autolysates of other intestinal organisms with typhoid precipitin showed negative results. The reaction was positive not only to the Bacillus typhosus, but to the paratyphoid A and B autolysate.

The autolysate-precipitin reaction showed clearly positive in all cases of typhoid fever and carriers up to the fifty-sixth day of the disease. The carriers were of many years' standing, one dating back eighteen years.

The bacteriologic diagnosis was positive in only about 6 per cent of known typhoid cases.

Conclusions. It seems reasonable to conclude even at this early stage of experimentation, that the autolysate-precipitin reaction is distinctly more sensitive and accurate than any of the previous methods of typhoid determination.

Inasmuch as the unknown quantity in the reaction is a direct chemical derivative of the typhoid bacillus (typhoid autolysate) a positive reaction must signify the presence of typhoid bacilli in the patient from whom the test excretions have been obtained. In other words, as long as the autolysate-precipitin reaction remains positive the patient is harboring living typhoid bacilli and is a potential menace as a typhoid carrier. The reaction does not depend upon any immune process in the patient, but upon the presence of the chemical constituents of the typhoid bacillus in the excretions and, therefore, should not persist after the subject is free from this infection.

The persistence of the positive reaction long after the negative bacteriologic examinations, upon which patients have been released from quarantine restrictions, indicates the advantage of its adoption as a better method of control of typhoid cases and carriers.

The result of the autolysate-precipitin reaction in the early stages of the disease gives promise of its usefulness in the field of diagnosis as well as control of typhoid. It also gives promise of usefulness in the accurate diagnosis of abortive and atypical cases of typhoid which have hitherto been so difficult to determine because of the evanescent character of the infection and the consequent absence of immunologic effect.

It should eliminate, also, the confusion encountered in the serologic diagnosis in cases which have received typhoid prophylaxis.

The distinct specificity of the reaction to the typhoid groups suggests its possibilities in the diagnosis of other intestinal infections with the use of precipitins specific to them.

It seems appropriate to make passing mention of the saving of time and expense in this as a routine method of diagnosis and control, if further experimentation prove its promising dependability.

It must be understood that the foregoing conclusions should not be interpreted as final, in consideration of the limited number of cases. Many pertinent questions arise which can be answered only by continued experimentation upon typhoid in all of its phases and upon the other diseases.

THROMBOSIS OF THE CORONARY ARTERIES, WITH INFARCTION OF THE HEART.

By Joseph T. Wearn, M.D.,
BOSTON, MASS.

(From the Medical Service of the Peter Bent Brigham Hospital.)

Introduction. Coronary thrombosis with infarction of the heart as a clinical entity is a condition which is generally classed among the rarities of medicine. Indeed, it is considered so rare and of so little importance that most of the text-books of medicine fail to give it mention or perhaps dismiss it with a brief paragraph, while several of the larger systems of medicine ignore it altogether. It has even been said by a very eminent physician[1] that "there are no characteristic physical signs or symptoms by which thrombosis of the coronary arteries can be diagnosed." So at best it is usually looked upon as a terminal event, impossible to diagnose and therefore of little clinical import. The literature on the subject, moreover, consists for the most part of a very small number of case reports; no attempt has been made to study a large series of cases, confirmed by necropsy, so that a clinical picture might be constructed which would enable one to recognize the condition. It is little wonder then that the diagnosis is generally left for the pathologist to make.

As a matter of fact the condition is not a very rare one; it merely goes unrecognized during life. To account for this failure of recognition, in part at least, one needs only to consider the mode of death of the individuals who die from this cause. As a rule, death is sudden or follows a brief acute illness, so that many of the patients are never seen by a physician at all, or are only examined after death by a coroner. A few, however, survive the attack, and on their account it is of great importance that the condition be recognized and properly treated. Its recognition is of further importance because of the close resemblance of the condition to acute diseases of the chest or abdomen; not infrequently it has been mistaken for pneumonia, pleurisy, acute cholecystitis, pancreatitis or perforated gastric or duodenal ulcer, and undoubtedly some of the so-called "negative laparotomies" could have been prevented had the condition of the coronary arteries been duly considered before the decision to operate was made.

Until comparatively recent years the literature yielded nothing more than a few case reports, and no attempt had been made to correlate these. Indeed, from the time of William Harvey to

[1] Broadbent, Sir William H.: Heart Disease, New York, 4th ed., 1906, p. 324.

the latter part of the nineteenth century little or no progress was made in the recognition of cardiac infarction. Harvey, however, reported a case[2] which was almost certainly one of coronary thrombosis, although he did not interpret it as such. The interest of it makes it worth quoting: "A noble knight, Sir Robert Darcy, an ancestor of that celebrated physician and most learned man, my own dear friend Dr. Argent, when he had reached to about the middle period of life, made frequent complaint of a certain distressing pain in the chest, especially in the night season; so that dreading at one time syncope, at another suffocation in his attacks, he led an unquiet and anxious life. He tried many remedies in vain, having had the advice of almost every medical man. The disease going from bad to worse, he by and by became cachectic and dropsical, and finally, grievously distressed, he died in one of his paroxysms. In the body of this gentleman, at the inspection of which there were present Dr. Argent, then president of the College of Physicians, and Dr. George, a distinguished theologian and preacher, who was pastor of the parish, we found the wall of the left ventricle of the heart ruptured, having a vent in it of the size sufficient to admit any of my fingers, although the wall itself appeared sufficiently thick and strong; this laceration had apparently been caused by an impediment to the passage of the blood from the left ventricle into the arteries."

A number of cases have been reported since Harvey's time, and in many of them some new sign or symptom has been observed and emphasized by the author, so that after a number of years the literature furnishes most of the important facts about the condition, though in a somewhat scattered and noncorrelated form. Morgagni,[3] Heberden,[4] and Caleb Hillier Parry[5] were among the first to associate anginal pain with lesions of the coronary arteries, and, in more recent years, Leyden,[6] Kernig[7] and Pawinski[8] reported pericardial friction rubs following angina, but apparently they did not realize the significance of the sign. Gorham[9] reviewed the literature on this point and reported several cases of cardiac infarction in which a friction rub was heard, and, on account of the constancy of this finding, he emphasized it as one of the most important of the diagnostic signs. Huchard[10] called attention to the persistence of pain or the so-called *status anginosus*, while Krehl[11]

[2] Harvey, William: The Works of William Harvey, Second Disquisition to John Riolan, Junior, p. 127. (Printed for the Sydenham Society, London, 1847.)

[3] Quoted by Osler.[13]

[4] Commentations on the History and Cure of Disease, London, 1816, 4th ed., p. 302.

[5] An Inquiry into the Symptoms and Causes of Syncope Anginosa, Commonly Called Angina Pectoris, London, 1799.

[6] Ztschr. f. klin. Med., 1884, **7**, 459. Quoted by Gorham.[9]

[7] St. Petersburger med. Wchnschr., 1892, **17**, 177. Quoted by Gorham.[9]

[8] Deutsch. Arch. f. klin. Med., 1897, **58**, 565. Quoted by Gorham.[9]

[9] Albany Med. Ann., 1920, **41**, 109.

[10] Tome II, Paris, 1899, p. 128.

[11] Nothnagel's System, **12**, 535, 699.

described cases of coronary obstruction without pain and recognized the compatibility of coronary occlusion with life. In this country Dock[12] was one of the first to emphasize the possibility of diagnosing the condition before death, and, in 1896, he lamented the fact that the profession was so slow in taking up the study of the disease. He also observed that a heart, although extensively necrosed, "may continue to act for some time fairly well," and he was among the first to recognize the true relationship of pericarditis to the syndrome.

It is to Osler,[13] however, that we are indebted for the first real correlation of the clinical and pathologic findings. In his study, the material for which came from his private practice, he gave a very thorough discussion of practically every side of angina pectoris and reported several cases of coronary thrombosis. Allbutt[14] also recognized the condition and discussed at length the origin of the pain and the cause of sudden death in this disease. Herrick and his co-workers [15] [16] [17] [18] have made a very careful study of the clinical aspects of a few cases, and have written an excellent description of the clinical features of the disease which has added much to the present-day knowledge of the condition. Sternberg,[19] Englehart,[20] Obrastzow and Straschesko[21] and others have reported cases in the past few years, some of which will be referred to later.

This paper is based upon a study of 19 cases of cardiac infarction observed at the Peter Bent Brigham Hospital. As each case came to necropsy many of the symptoms and signs observed in the physical examination during life could be correlated with the postmortem findings, and from the data so obtained an effort has been made to construct a clinical picture which might make the diagnosis of the condition less difficult. These cases fall under the general heading of acute cardiac infarction, and for the sake of convenience they have been subdivided into two groups: (*a*) Those cases in which there have been no signs or symptoms of beginning cardiac failure and little or no evidence of an impaired circulation previous to the infarction, and (*b*) those in which there had been organic heart disease with symptoms and signs of long standing, and, previous to the obstruction of the coronary arteries, the clinical evidence of a failing heart muscle.

Etiology. The idea has gained prevalence as a result of the reports of most writers that the disease is almost always limited

[12] Notes on Coronary Arteries, Ann Arbor, 1896.
[13] Lumleian Lectures, Lancet, 1910, No. 1, pp. 697, 839 and 973.
[14] Diseases of the Arteries, Including Angina Pectoris, London, 1915.
[15] Jour. Am. Med. Assn., 1912, **59**, 2015.
[16] Ibid., 1918, **70**, 67.
[17] Ibid., 1918, **70**, 1887.
[18] Ibid., 1919, **72**, 387.
[19] Wien. med. Wchnschr., 1910, **60**, 14.
[20] Deutsch. med. Wchnschr., 1909, **35**, 838.
[21] Ztschr. f. klin. Med., 1910, **71**, 116.

to the upper classes. Osler emphasized this point and others have remarked on the fact that it was a disease rarely seen among hospital ward patients or groups of poorer people. The explanation of this belief is due undoubtedly to the fact that the majority of the cases recorded are from the private practices of the writers; for the same reason it has been called a disease of professional men or men accustomed to large business worries. Osler, for instance, speaks of the high incidence of medical men in his series, and gives a list of well-known names which includes John Hunter, Charcot, Nothnagel and William Pepper, all of whom died of coronary disease. In our small series, however, the disease has not been partial in its selections but has included among its victims clerks, machinists, housewives, and, among others, one man who gave as his occupation "Christian Science healer." Nor has the disease confined itself chiefly to men, as has been noted in most of the previous reports, for 9 of the 19 cases were in women. With one exception all our patients were over forty years of age, being mostly in the sixth or seventh decades.

A thorough search of the records of these patients did not reveal any factors which might play a direct role in the etiology of the condition. Heredity was dismissed at once, for there was only one instance of sudden death in a previous generation. Evidence of syphilis and rheumatic fever was naturally very carefully sought, in view of the close relationship of both these diseases to heart disease and of syphilis to lesions of the bloodvessels. But not one of the 19 patients gave a history of syphilis, and of the 13 whose Wassermann reactions were done, all were negative. Finally, the lack of any evidence of syphilis at the postmortem examinations enables one to say that that disease was not an etiologic factor in this series of cases of cardiac infarction. Rheumatic fever was also unimportant as a causative factor, for in one patient only was there a previous history of this disease, and at necropsy this individual was the only one whose heart showed an old endocarditis. One could likewise rule out other conditions such as diphtheria, pneumonia, scarlet fever, chorea, acute tonsillitis, nephritis and hyperthyroidism as important causative factors, for not one of them occurred in more than two of the patients. There was also no history of excessive use of alcohol, tobacco, tea or coffee.

Attempts to establish vascular hypertension as a factor in the disease met with difficulties. In 3 of our patients hypertension was known to exist before the appearance of any other symptoms referable to the cardiovascular system, while several other patients had an elevated blood-pressure upon entrance to the hospital. But it is evident, of course, that no direct relationship is established, though hypertension as an accompanying factor deserves more consideration in the future than it has received in the past. Every patient in this series showed some degree of arteriosclerosis, and the final cause of the infarction in every case was coronary arteriosclerosis. The factors, therefore, which lead to arteriosclerosis play an indirect part in causing cardiac infarction.

Onset of the Disease; Symptoms. When one considers the end-result and terminal condition of the heart, and especially of the coronary arteries, he is surprised to find in many instances no previous symptoms referable to the heart, and in others only mild symptoms which certainly would not indicate the true state of the coronary arteries. Eight of the patients, for instance, had noticed dyspnea on climbing stairs or walking fast. In three of these the dyspnea was of a paroxysmal type, coming on suddenly after exertion and disappearing after a short rest—in other words, the sign of what McKenzie calls a senile heart. In six instances there were previous anginal attacks which had begun only a few weeks or months before the terminal attack. In contrast to this group, with few signs or symptoms of warning, is the group of four other patients who entered the hospital primarily on account of moderately severe cardiac decompensation or failure resulting entirely, so far as could be determined, from sclerosis of the coronary arteries. Two of this group had also had hemiplegias.

The onset of symptoms of cardiac infarction then is sudden and abrupt and may be the first sign to the patient of any trouble with his cardiovascular system. He may be enjoying practically normal health one minute and in the next be seized with an excruciating pain, or perhaps with extreme dyspnea. Or the onset may occur after a number of anginal attacks which, together with dyspnea, may constitute the only previous warnings of involvement of the coronary arteries. But with this latter type the patient recognizes instantly that his attack (indicative of the infarction) is unlike any that he has ever experienced before. In this group, with few or no previous symptoms, pain is certainly the most prominent symptom of the onset—sudden, sharp, knife-like, excruciating and constant as a rule. The pain may occur in the epigastrium, over the heart, under the lower end of the sternum or in all these and in other regions; it may radiate to the nipples, to the arms or to the abdomen, and to various other places. There are, however, other types of onset, such as sudden severe dyspnea usually associated with extreme weakness. One patient, for instance, who was seated in the house at the time of onset, was seized with a sudden dyspnea which was so extreme that he ran out of doors to get air.

Following closely upon the pain or dyspnea, at times occurring almost simultaneously, there may be nausea, vomiting and diarrhea. Generalized sweating, cough, hemoptysis, cyanosis, aphasia, delirium, collapse and coma were noted in some instances. The skin was usually cold, moist and of a characteristic pale, ashen color. It is very interesting to note the relation of physical activity to the time of onset of cardiac infarction, since some anginal attacks seem to be brought on by exertion and at times by overeating. In 3 of the patients the onset of the symptoms of the infarction followed severe exertion while in 5 other instances the patients were at rest at the time. In only 1 did the signs and symptoms of coronary obstruction begin after eating, so that it seems safe to consider that the onset of cardiac infarction is unrelated to the taking of food and bears little relation to exertion as a causative factor.

The onset in the group of patients with signs and symptoms of antecedent cardiac failure is in marked contrast to the group just described. In the first place 3 of the 4 patients were irrational, so that the occurrence of pain could not be ascertained, and, in addition, dyspnea, edema and other signs of heart disease had been present for some time and in such degree as to mask the onset of the thrombosis of the coronary arteries. One of these patients, however, before becoming irrational had a sudden increase in dyspnea and weakness, and, in a second one, a sudden increase in dyspnea with cyanosis had been noted. In the fourth patient, who was rational until death, no pain was felt, but several days previous to her entrance to the hospital she had noticed a sudden increase in dyspnea and became cyanotic at the same time. It appears then that in those individuals with signs and symptoms of a decompensated heart muscle the onset of coronary infarction is apt to cause a sudden increase in these signs and symptoms. The patients in group 2 did not exhibit the gastrointestinal symptoms or the other signs and symptoms shown by group 1, or else their symptoms were so masked that they were not detected. The skin of these individuals, for instance, was cyanotic and did not show the typical pale, ashen hue which was so characteristic of the other group.

With many cases of infarction of the heart death comes with the onset and is instantaneous; some patients may live a few hours or a few days; a third group of individuals recover, become ambulatory and are able to return to light work.

There are many characteristic features about the pain of cardiac infarction. In the first place it is usually persistent once it has begun, lasting hours or days, and this feature, together with the distribution of the pain, has given rise to the term *status anginosus*. This stands out in contrast to the attacks of simple angina pectoris, where the pain is more apt to last minutes. In some instances there are temporary periods during which the sharp, intense pain may change to a dull ache in the same region, but it is apt to return to its previous state of severity. In other cases the pain may be intermittent with periods of complete absence. The pain may be precordial, referred deeply within the chest (substernal), especially under the lower end of the sternum or in the epigastrium. At times it may cover the whole upper abdomen, but usually when abdominal it is located either in the epigastrium or in the right upper quadrant. When the pain occurs in this region in repeated attacks it may resemble very closely the colicky pain of certain acute abdominal conditions; when tenderness and muscle spasm are associated with the pain in this region the diagnosis is a difficult one. Points of radiation of the pain vary considerably, but in this series there was radiation from the precordial and substernal areas to one or both arms, sometimes to the upper arms only, at others to the finger tips, to the left side of the neck, through to the back, across to the right chest or around both sides of the chest. From the epigastrium the radiation was apt to be upward toward the precordium or to the region of the nipples. In several individuals the taking of food or drink and exertion made the pain definitely worse, while in others eating and moving about caused no discomfort. Quotations from some of the patients' descriptions of their pain are rather vivid in some of the more unusual types. One individual said, "It feels as though someone has a vise on the end of my heart and is gradually tightening it." Another said, "It feels as if a large stick had been forced into my chest (substernal), and it is pressing on everything else in there." Still another complained of a "constriction inside," while those with the epigastric type of pain usually complained of sharp, stabbing pains in that region.

The attitudes of the patients as they lay in bed presented a marked contrast to that of patients with acute abdominal or acute respiratory conditions. In the abdominal type of pain the patients are constantly attempting to protect this part and to lessen the pain by such changes in position as bended knees, flexed thighs or any position which relieves the muscular tension; similarly in acute conditions of the chest, as pleurisy, for instance, the patient is apt to lie upon the affected side or to assume postures which lessen the motion on that side. In patients with cardiac infarction, however, nothing of this sort is seen. They lie in any position or may be propped up in bed, but soon find that no relief is obtained by changes in position. The pain seems to be beyond reach.

In 10 of our patients the so-called *status anginosus* was present, but after several days there was a gradual decrease, and, in some, a disappearance of the pain; in 2 the pain returned after a week in severe form and death followed the same day. Relief was impossible to obtain, in some instances large doses of morphin failing to influence the pain.

Dyspnea was a prominent and almost constant feature, being present in 16 of our cases of cardiac infarction. It was the predominant sign and chief complaint of four of the patients who had no previous signs of cardiac failure, being of such a severe type that it was out of proportion to the other findings in the heart and lungs. One woman, for example, sat up in bed and literally gasped for air, yet on physical examination the condition found in the heart and lungs did not seem to account for the extreme difficulty in breathing. This point alone should suggest the possibility of cardiac infarction. There were other patients in whom dyspnea was not a prominent sign, and, indeed, in some it appeared only after mild exertion, such as lifting themselves in the bed or similar mild exercise. Despite this frequency of dyspnea, however, only 6 of the patients were orthopneic, and 2 of these were in the group with cardiac symptoms of long standing. Observations upon the vital capacity of the lungs of 2 patients were made; in 1 the reading was 900 cc, or 22 per cent normal on two occasions, and 800 cc, or 20 per cent, on another; in the second patient only one observation was made, the reading of which was 700 cc, or 17 per cent. This last result is of doubtful value, as the patient had fluid in the right thoracic cavity. Both results are very low, but it is felt that the first one is of definite value, for the patient was extremely dyspneic.

A slightly productive cough troubled some of the patients; in a few instances this was a troublesome factor, for with the severe dyspnea and weakness it was very exhausting. Hemoptysis was noted in 2 instances, but was not profuse in either, consisting chiefly of blood-streaked sputum. No infarcts were found in the lungs of these patients, but it is probable that the severe grade of congestion which was found would account for the hemoptysis. The postmortem findings of edema and congestion in the lungs of practically every patient accounts for all the respiratory signs and symptoms mentioned. These findings seem significant, as they show that the first sign of failure of the heart, regardless of whether the injury is on the right or left side of the heart, appears in the pulmonary circulation. In later stages of the disease as the myocardium became weaker, 7 of the patients showed the Cheyne-Stokes type of respiration.

In the group of patients with antecedent heart disease the effect of the infarction was to accentuate those signs and symptoms already present, but they were not altered to any extent and did not change the picture from that ordinarily seen in patients with a rapidly failing heart muscle.

General weakness was present in 15 of the 19 patients, and in some it was so extreme that the slightest movement on their part would cause complete exhaustion. One woman, for instance, by merely lifting an arm would become dyspneic and completely exhausted.

The mental state seems to follow no rule. Patients may remain perfectly rational up to the time of death, though they may seem acutely sick and in a critical condition throughout their illness; while others, whose general condition seems much better in comparison and whose myocardium does not seem to be failing, may be irrational from the beginning. Of the patients studied here

11 were rational up to the time of death while 8 became stuporous, irrational or unconscious.

Almost all of the patients showed distress, anxiety or apprehension in their faces, and the expressions in many were those of extreme suffering. The color of the skin has been commented upon by Libman[22] and others, and in many cases it is certainly striking. In some of our patients the skin was pale, while in others it was a "pasty, ashen color," frequently being cold and moist to the touch, so that the individual resembled a person in "shock." In two of the patients of the group with chronic organic heart disease cyanosis was rather marked, but it was not seen in the others. A diffuse red flushing of the skin was noted in three patients, and, in one instance, this was a striking feature; it was only a temporary phenomenon which appeared twice, lasting about six hours each time. In this patient the skin over the head, body and extremities showed a bright red flush, and during this time she complained of severe heat, and requested that she be fanned or have cold sponges. There was profuse sweating with the flushing but no change in temperature. Profuse sweating without the flushing was also observed in four others soon after the onset. Jaundice was observed in two of the patients.

Loss of appetite, nausea and vomiting were disturbing factors in about one-half of the patients, and in one instance food was vomited which had been eaten the day before. These symptoms and the fact that several of the patients refused to take food for fear of increasing the pain made the problem of nourishment a difficult one. Constipation and diarrhea were infrequent. A very distressing complication was abdominal distention; in some patients this symptom was rather marked and embarrassed an already difficult respiration. In view of these gastrointestinal disturbances during the acute illness it may be significant that seven of the patients had for some months noticed discomfort from gaseous distention after meals, some of them stating that the symptoms were accentuated by the acute illness. The group with antecedent chronic heart disease exhibited none of these features.

Physical Examination. A study of the physical examinations of these patients revealed the fact that there are several signs in this condition which occur with remarkable constancy. The type of dyspnea and the color of the skin are helpful points, but it is from the physical findings in the heart and lungs, together with the history of the illness, that one can expect to recognize the occlusion of a coronary artery with the resulting infarct of the heart.

On auscultation of the lungs, and especially of the bases, one is very apt to hear crackling rales. These persist after deep breath-

[22] Med. Record, New York, 1919, **96**, 521.

ing and coughing and represent the earliest evidence of pulmonary edema; which in turn signifies a failing myocardium. The rales may be confined to the bases or to the regions of the axillæ or again may be widely distributed throughout both lungs. They are usually found soon after the onset of symptoms and were present in two patients who were seen and examined within two or three hours after the beginning of their attacks. In one of these individuals the rales were widely distributed, giving the picture of an extensive pulmonary edema, and with this point in mind it is not unreasonable to believe that many cases of cardiac infarction may be diagnosed as acute pulmonary edema without recognition of the true underlying cardiac condition. The rales were present in 17 of the 19 cases, and, as a rule, persisted throughout the illness, generally increasing as the heart muscle grew weaker. In a few instances, however, they disappeared after a few days. Only one individual in the group without antecedent cardiac symptoms developed a hydrothorax, whereas two of those in the group with antecedent chronic heart disease had a hydrothorax, a third had ascites and all of them had rales widely distributed throughout both lungs. The frequency of the occurrence of rales in the lungs makes it a sign of definite value and especially in those cases resembling acute intra-abdominal conditions, where it may serve as an important differential point and lead to the correct diagnosis.

In the physical examination, when one considers all factors in an effort to determine the condition of the heart, one is able to find many points which individually and collectively lead to one conclusion, namely, a weak heart action. The ease with which dyspnea is provoked, exhaustion from the least effort, a weak and feeble pulse, and then in the heart itself an apex impulse that can neither be seen nor felt and scarcely audible heart sounds, all these findings indicate a failing heart. By percussion the heart was found to be enlarged in fourteen instances; in the other five the hearts, while apparently within normal limits on percussion, were found to be enlarged at necropsy. The enlargements, as a rule, were not great but there were exceptions, as shown by the weights given later. On auscultation one could scarcely hear the heart sounds. Those heard in the apical region are described as "weak," "faint," "distant" and frequently of a "tic tac" quality. The same condition was found to be true in listening over the base of the heart, except in 6 individuals in whom the systolic blood-pressure was elevated and in whom there was an accentuation of the aortic second sound. Of the 15 patients in the group with the acute onset of symptoms, 6 had systolic murmurs which were heard best in the apical region, but it was felt by the observers that these did not indicate valvular lesions except in the 1 patient who had had rheumatic fever. In the group of patients with chronic heart disease all were found to have blowing systolic murmurs at the apex. Pericardial friction rubs were heard in only 2 patients, and in 1 of these a definite pericarditis was found after death. In 4 other patients necropsy revealed a fibrinous exudate and other signs of a pericarditis, but no friction rubs had been heard in these individuals during life. No signs of pericarditis were found in the patients in the group with chronic heart disease either before or after death. Pericarditis has been claimed by some to be present in all cases of cardiac infarction, but in this series many of the infarcts were deep within the myocardium, and as a result no inflammation of the pericardium resulted. These findings then give to the pericardial friction rub its true value as a diagnostic sign, namely, that if present it is an additional point in favor of infarction, but its absence is of no diagnostic significance.

Pulsus alternans was looked for in only three of the patients and was found in two of them. Likewise a protodiastolic gallop rhythm was noted in six instances. These are signs which are frequently found when sought for, and it is very probable that they occurred in many others of this series.

Examination of the peripheral arteries revealed little that was of value in a diagnostic sense. One expects to find a certain amount of sclerosis in the bloodvessels of patients the age of these, and all of them showed it, while about two-thirds of them had marked sclerosis of the radial, brachial and temporal arteries. The fact that some had only a slight change in the peripheral vessels merely illustrates the fact that the condition of these vessels is no index of the condition of the vessels elsewhere in the body.

Blood-pressure observations showed a wide variation, but the significance of the readings is not great unless the time at which they were made is considered. In several instances only single readings were made upon entrance to the hospital, while in others numerous records were obtained. One patient, for instance, showed many rapid changes of blood-pressure. It happened that she had temporary tachycardia with a rate of 160 beats per minute, and during this time her systolic blood-pressure was so low that a reading was impossible but a few minutes later her rate changed to 60 beats per minute and at the same time her blood-pressure rose to 150 mm. of mercury. Several other patients also showed fluctuations, so that a single observation is of little value.

The abdominal examination is an important one, for it is here that one is most frequently misled in attempting to make a diagnosis. The pain is frequently localized either in the epigastrium or in the right upper quadrant, rarely below the umbilicus. At times there may be spasm of the muscles or the wall of the abdomen with tenderness on pressure, or less frequently a so-called "board-like" belly, so that when the physical examination is limited to this region surgical treatment certainly seems to be indicated.

Levine and Tranter[23] and other writers have emphasized the resemblance of cardiac infarction to acute abdominal conditions. In addition to the findings just mentioned one frequently finds an enlarged, tender liver. This observation was made in about half of our patients and probably represents another sign of a failing circulation.

Laboratory Findings. There are two other signs in cardiac infarction which are almost constant and tend to confuse one with acute inflammatory conditions, especially if the pain is in the abdomen, namely, fever and leukocytosis. Fever is commonly present and in one patient began within twenty-four hours of the onset. The average height of the temperature was 101° or 102° F., though some temperatures ran as high as 104° F. Other patients had subnormal temperatures with a terminal rise to above normal. Levine and Tranter noted a leukocytosis in their 2 cases, but few other authors have noted this fact or realized the importance of this sign. Its real significance is obvious when one notes that only 3 of the 19 patients did not have a leukocytosis. In these 3 only one count was made. The cause of the fever and the leukocytosis without the presence of an infection is not absolutely clear. It is not unreasonable, however, to consider the necrotic heart muscle as a foreign protein which upon being absorbed into the circulating blood produces fever and leukocytosis, as is known to occur when a foreign protein is injected into the blood stream. Furthermore, histologic study of the heart muscle shows many leukocytes in the infarcted area of the heart. These two points are of great value, especially in the patients with precordial type of pain, for in their presence one can rule out an attack of simple angina pectoris.

The urinary findings in our cases were consistent with a generalized arteriosclerosis in which the kidneys shared. The specific gravity readings showed wide variations—from 1.008 to 1.036—and in most instances albumin was found. The sediment contained hyaline and finely granular casts. In only 4 instances were further studies made, and in 2 of these the blood-urea nitrogen was increased, the amounts being 40 mgm. and 90 mgm. per 100 cc of blood. At necropsy the 2 patients with increased blood-urea nitrogen were found to have a chronic nephritis of the arteriosclerotic type. The 2 others studied showed normal function tests and only slight vascular changes were found in the kidneys at the postmortem examination.

Clinical Course. The clinical course of the condition after the infarction of the heart takes place is a stormy one. There is no doubt that death is instantaneous in many cases of coronary thrombosis. Osler saw deaths of this type, and in his Lumleian Lectures gives a vivid graphic picture of them. When one reads almost

[23] Am. Jour. Med. Sci., 1918, **155**, 57.

daily of sudden deaths from "heart failure," "acute indigestion" or "cerebral hemorrhage," one questions if he is not reading of the result of a thrombus in a coronary artery. The typical course of a cerebral hemorrhage in most cases is certainly not so abrupt, "acute indigestion" is meaningless, and what other type of heart failure could one expect to find in an ambulatory person able to be at work? Then a second group is recognized in which the first shock of the obstruction is survived and the patient lives a few hours or a few weeks. Here the pain, dyspnea and other signs may persist, and later the early signs of a break in compensation may develop, or all signs and symptoms may improve, and death, without warning, may occur. One patient, for instance, who had almost recovered from his pain and seemed to be improving, while sitting up in bed gave a sudden gasp and fell over dead. Another was lying quietly in bed having complained of an increase in her precordial pain a short time previously, when she gasped suddenly and stopped breathing. A nurse who was at the bedside at the time was unable to feel any pulse after the gasp, and when the patient was seen by a physician a minute later the heart had stopped beating.

The type of death just described is characteristic of this condition, and in this series thirteen of the patients with the acute type of onset died very suddenly. Here, again, the group with chronic heart disease differs from the others, for only one of the four patients in this group died suddenly while the deaths of the other three were gradual, not unlike that of any patient with a slowly failing heart. With this type of death in mind the records were studied to determine the relation of rupture of the heart to sudden death, but no definite relation was made out, many having died suddenly in whom no rupture was found at necropsy. It was noted also that rupture of the heart does not depend upon the age of the infarct, for in one instance the rupture occurred within eighteen hours after the onset of symptoms while in another the heart ruptured two weeks after the onset.

Not all patients, however, die from infarct in the heart; many survive and may live for months or even years. Dock, Herrick, Osler and others have recognized this fact, and it is on account of this point that the recognition of the disease is important. Herrick has followed patients after recovery in whom the lesions were finally verified at necropsy. At the present time two patients from this hospital are being followed who survived the attack and have been ambulatory for several months. The activities of both patients are greatly limited, the least exertion producing dyspnea, and one of them complains of a persistent dull ache over the precordium which becomes worse on exertion. Previous to the infarction both of them had anginal attacks from which they had obtained relief by the use of nitroglycerin, but since the occlusion of the coronary artery this drug has no effect upon the pain.

Electrocardiographic Studies. From the clinical observations on our patients it was found that the heart rhythm in 12 of them was regular and remained so throughout their illnesses. The others at some time had an irregular rhythm due, for the most part, to premature beats, but in two instances to heart-block. In only one instance did the auricles fibrillate, and that occurred after digitalis therapy, and was transient. In addition to these routine observations electrocardiographic studies were made upon 10 of the patients, although in most instances only one record was obtained on account of the brief duration of the illness. A summary of the findings in these records is given in Table I, and since few opportunities arise for making electrocardiographic observations on patients with cardiac infarction it seems worth while to review these findings very briefly.

In 6 of the patients the cardiac rhythm was regular, although 1 of this number had complete heart-block at the time records were obtained. Of the individuals with irregular rhythm, in 3 it was due to premature beats, the origin of which was ventricular in 2 instances and auricular in the other. In the remaining 1 the irregularity was due to heart-block with frequent changes in rhythm. As this last patient was studied carefully and frequent electrocardiographic records were obtained (see Fig. 1), it will be of interest, perhaps, to discuss the findings in her case more at length. When the patient was first seen it was noted that the heart rhythm was distinctly irregular, due to very frequent sudden changes in rate, there being three distinct rates of 56, 110 and 160 beats per minute. The rapid changes from one rate to the other were without any special sequence and without any subjective symptoms whatever. Twenty-four hours later, however, this patient began to have frequent fainting spells, and auscultation again showed the three rates with definite pauses at the time of the changes in rhythm. It was also observed that at times during the tachycardia (160) the patient would faint and the rate would then change to 56 per minute. Blood-pressure readings during the tachycardia showed a blood-pressure of 50 mm. of mercury or less, so that accurate reading was impossible; but with the change to the slowest rate (56) the systolic blood-pressure rose to 150 mm. and the diastolic to 105 mm. Electrocardiographic tracings were obtained of the two slower rates, but unfortunately only a pulse tracing was obtained of the rate of 160 per minute. When at the rate of 56 per minute the record showed complete heart-block, and several records of a change from this rate to a normal rhythm at 110 per minute were obtained. On the third day there was a marked lengthening of the *QRS* interval and the

TABLE I.

Medical No. and initials.	Rhythm.	Conduction time (P–R interval).	Q.R.S. complex.	Amplitude of curves.	T-waves.	Time relation of electrocardiographic record to onset and death.	Digitalis.	Miscellaneous.
[illegible]	[illegible]egular; prema- [illegible] auricular	Normal	Normal	Diminished	Slightly inverted in leads 2 and 3	Record obtained 4 days after onset, 2 days before death	Small amount given	
[illegible]	[illegible]	Complete heart-[illegible]	Definite spread	Normal	Inverted in lead 1; low but upright in leads 2 and 3	Two days after onset, on day of death	None given	Left ventricular preponderance
[illegible]	[illegible]	[illegible]	Normal	Diminished greatly in all leads	Practically isoelectric in all leads	Nine days after onset, on day of death	Given.	
[illegible]	[illegible]	[illegible]	[illegible]	Normal	Isoelectric in leads 1 and 2	14 days after onset, 10 days before death	None given before record obtained	
[illegible]	[illegible] dropped	Delayed [illegible] later complete heart-block	[illegible] 4th, 14th days; marked lengthening on 6th and 7th days; typical of intraventricular defective conduction	Normal on 4th, 12th and 14th days; diminished on 6th and 7th days	4th day diphasic in lead 1, isoelectric in 2, inverted in 3. 7th day diphasic in lead 1; 14th day diphasic in leads 1 and 3, isoelectric in 3	Died on 14th day	Small amount after 1st tracing but not enough to influence the curves, [illegible] given.	[illegible]
[illegible]	[illegible]	[illegible]	Normal	Slightly diminished	Isoelectric [illegible] 3	[illegible] days after onset, [illegible]	None given	
[illegible]	[illegible]	Normal	Normal	Slightly diminished	[illegible]	[illegible]	None	
[illegible]	[illegible]	[illegible]	[illegible]	Normal	[illegible]	[illegible]		
[illegible]	[illegible]	[illegible]	Normal	[illegible]	[illegible]	[illegible]	[illegible]	

form of the e trocardiogram was entirely different from that of the first day. Again on the fifth day there was delayed auriculoventricular co uction with changes in the rate from 110 per minute to about 55 p minute with complete heart-block. Later records showed a dis cated pacemaker with a return of the electrocardiogram to ts original form with a prolonged *QRS* complex. In another pat nt three distinct rates were noted and records were obtained of tl two slower ones; these showed complete heart-block with a r e of 28 per minute and a normal rhythm of about 60 per minute It seems most probable that the tachycardia in these instances was of the ventricular type, as reported by Herman.[24] The two insta es just mentioned are the only ones in which the auriculoventric lar conduction time was delayed, for in the other eight patients t was normal. This seems rather remarkable in view of the n ure and location of the lesion in the heart, for in many insta c there was extensive damage to the septum.

Abnormaliti of the *QRS* complex were noted in three of the records, and each instance there was a lengthening typical of the so-called traventricular defective conduction. Fortunately several record were obtained upon two of these patients, and it was found tha the lengthening of the *QRS* complex was not permanent. In e of them the lengthening occurred on the sixth day after the set of symptoms of infarction and disappeared on the eighth day The other patient was irrational, so that the time relation of the ate of the electrocardiographic records to the onset of the disease ould not be determined. The amplitude of the *QRS* complex r initial ventricular deflection was regarded as diminished in ne-half of the patients observed, and in some instances it s so markedly diminished that the curves were almost isoelect .

It will be se from Table I that in all of the ten patients there was some alter ion of the *T*-waves in at least one of the leads, and frequently n ads I and II, so that these changes, while not abnormal in s e of the individual curves, may be significant when taken as a grou. Many were inverted while others were isoelectric or diphasic, bu in one record only was the *T*-wave found to come off the *R*-wav as described by Parde his occurred in lead II, but in a re rd obtained the next this patient the type of cu e had changed, and ave no longer came fr m the down stroke of es of two other pat nts were practically not n of the isoelectric rves which were noted in the third lead of th (Fig. 2). l findings are no d in

Jour. Mi Med. Assn.,
Arch. Int . 26, 244.

TABLE I.

Medical No. and initials.	Rhythm.	Conduction time (P–R interval).	Q.R.S. complex.	Amplitude of of curves.	T-waves.	Time relation of electrocardiographic record to onset and death.	Digitalis.	Miscellaneous.
2741 H. C.	Irregular; premature auricular beats	Normal	Normal	Diminished	Slightly inverted in leads 2 and 3	Record obtained 4 days after onset, 2 days before death	Small amount given.	
4784 J. T.	Regular; complete heart-block	Complete heart-block	Definite spread	Normal	Inverted in lead 1; low but upright in leads 2 and 3	Two days after onset, on day of death	None given	Left ventricular preponderance.
7223 W. S.	Irregular, trigeminy; premature ventricular beats	Normal	Normal	Diminished greatly in all leads	Practically isoelectric in all leads	Nine days after onset, on day of death	Given.	
14600 C. C.	Regular	Normal	Normal	Normal	Isoelectric in leads 1 and 2	14 days after onset 10 days before death	None given before record obtained	
15301 M. H.	Irregular; dropped beats	Delayed and later complete heart-block	Normal on 4th, 12th and 14th days; marked lengthening on 6th and 7th days, typical of intraventricular defective conduction	Normal on 4th, 12th and 14th days; diminished on 6th and 7th days	4th day diaphasic in lead 1, isoelectric in 2, inverted in 3, 7th day diphasic in lead 1; 14th day diphasic in leads 1 and 3, isoelectric in 3	Died on 14th day	Small amount after 1st tracing but not enough to influence the curves; disturbances in rhythm all present before digitalis was given	Dislocation of pacemaker on 13th and 14th days; pulse tracing shows tachycardia of 160 per minute.
14652 A. D.	Regular	Normal	Normal	Slightly diminished	Isoelectric in lead 3	Three days after onset, day before death	None given.	
16216 I. M.	Irregular; rare premature ventricular beat	Normal	Normal	Slightly diminished	Diphasic in lead 3	One day after onset, on day of death	None given	Left ventricular preponderance
15989 M. N.	Regular	Normal	Normal	Normal	Diphasic in 1; comes off the down stroke of R wave in lead 2; 2d day normal	1st and 2d days after onset; 5th and 6th days before death	After first record	Left ventricular preponderance; second day different form of complex with disturbed pacemaker.
8681 J. J. H.	Irregular; premature ventricular beats	Normal	Normal	Normal	Flat in all leads	Onset indefinite	Given after first record	Left ventricular preponderance.
13063 C. Y.	Regular	Normal	Normal	Normal	Diphasic in 1; inverted in 2 and 3	29 days before death	None given	Left ventricular preponderance; notching of R wave in all leads.

form of the electrocardiogram was entirely different from that of the first day. Again on the fifth day there was delayed auriculoventricular conduction with changes in the rate from 110 per minute to about 55 per minute with complete heart-block. Later records showed a dislocated pacemaker with a return of the electrocardiogram to its original form with a prolonged *QRS* complex. In another patient three distinct rates were noted and records were obtained of the two slower ones; these showed complete heart-block with a rate of 28 per minute and a normal rhythm of about 60 per minute. It seems most probable that the tachycardia in these instances was of the ventricular type, as reported by Herman.[24] The two instances just mentioned are the only ones in which the auriculoventricular conduction time was delayed, for in the other eight patients it was normal. This seems rather remarkable in view of the nature and location of the lesion in the heart, for in many instances there was extensive damage to the septum.

Abnormalities of the *QRS* complex were noted in three of the records, and in each instance there was a lengthening typical of the so-called intraventricular defective conduction. Fortunately several records were obtained upon two of these patients, and it was found that the lengthening of the *QRS* complex was not permanent. In one of them the lengthening occurred on the sixth day after the onset of symptoms of infarction and disappeared on the eighth day. The other patient was irrational, so that the time relation of the date of the electrocardiographic records to the onset of the disease could not be determined. The amplitude of the *QRS* complex or initial ventricular deflection was regarded as diminished in one-half of the patients observed, and in some instances it was so markedly diminished that the curves were almost isoelectric.

It will be seen from Table I that in all of the ten patients there was some alteration of the *T*-waves in at least one of the leads, and frequently in leads I and II, so that these changes, while not abnormal in some of the individual curves, may be significant when taken as a group. Many were inverted while others were isoelectric or diphasic, but in one record only was the *T*-wave found to come off the *R*-wave as described by Pardee.[25] This occurred in lead II, but in a record obtained the next day from this same patient the type of curve had changed, and, along with it, the *T*-wave no longer came from the down stroke of the *R*-wave. The curves of two other patients were practically normal, with the exception of the isoelectric curves which were noted in two leads of one and in the third lead of the other (Fig. 2). A few other incidental findings are noted in Table I.

[24] Jour. Missouri State Med. Assn., 1920, **17**, 406.
[25] Arch. Int. Med., 1920, **26**, 244.

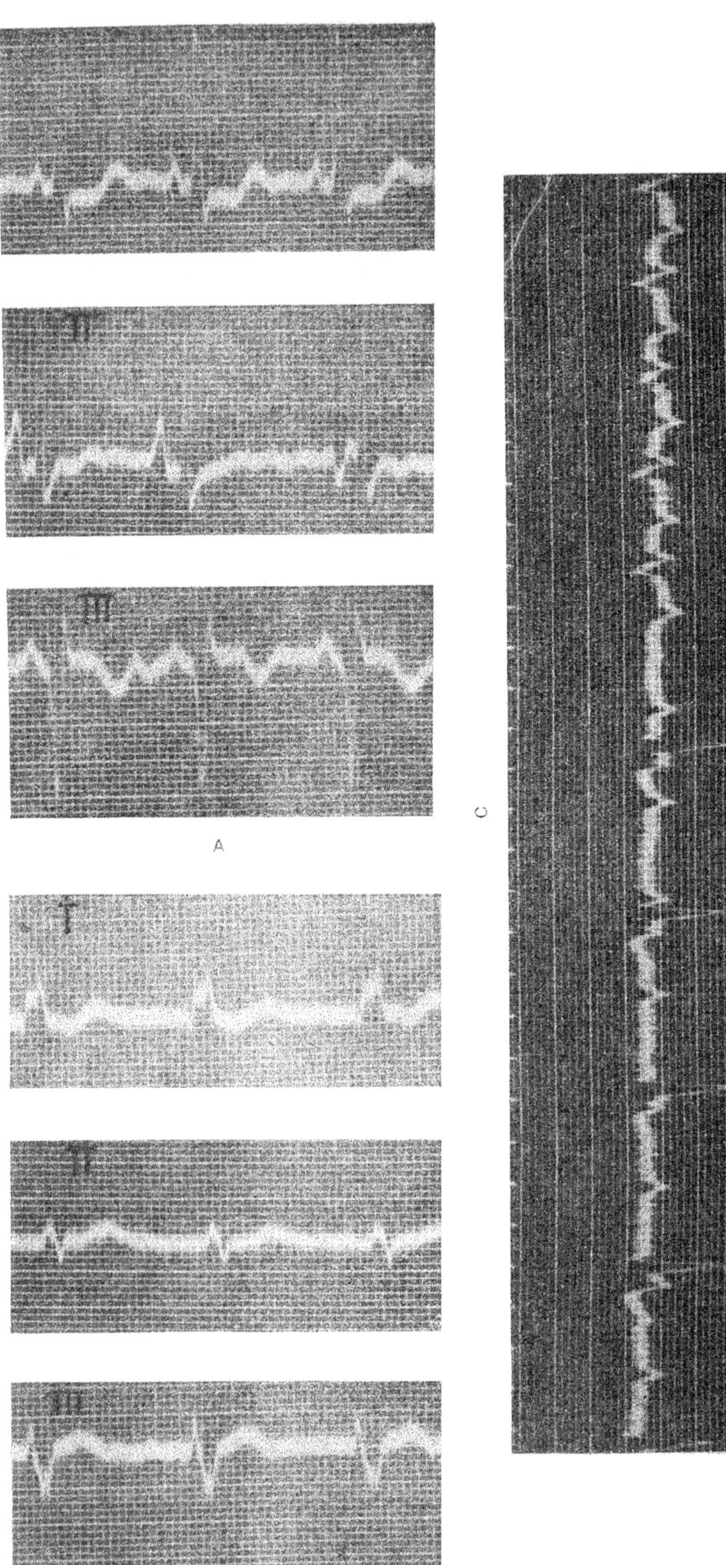
A
C

Owing to the variations in the relation of the onset of the attacks to the time that these records were made, and owing to the small number of patients, no definite conclusions can be drawn, but it is obvious that no one form of electrocardiogram is characteristic of this condition. The location of the lesion and the amount of

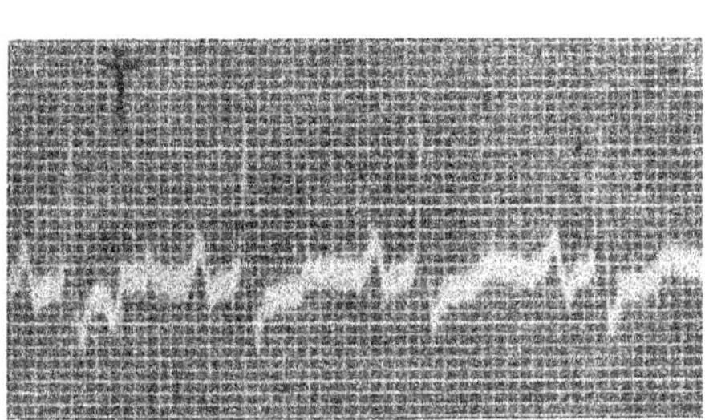

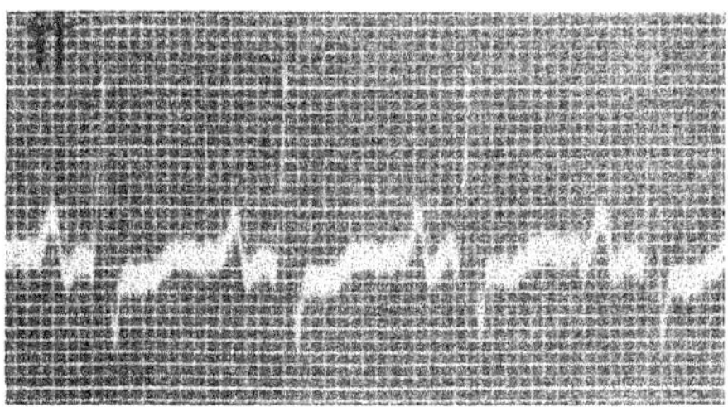

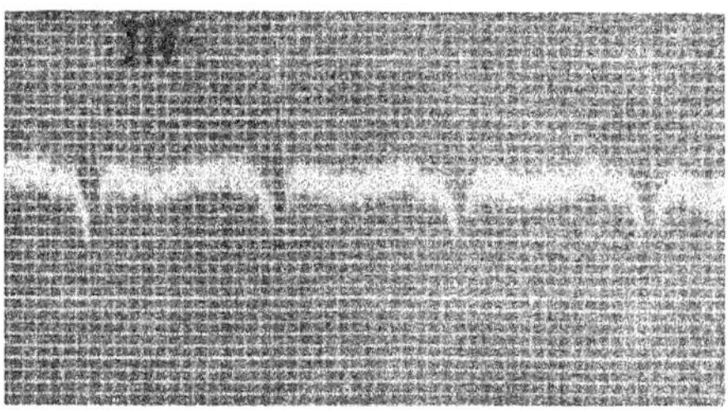

D

Fig. 1.—Records from Case No. 15301. Frequent changes are shown in the records of the different days. Those of the fourth day are labelled *A*, sixth day *B*, eighth day *C*, and the thirteenth day after the onset or the day of death, *D*. Note the change in the form of the electrocardiogram in *A* and *B* with the return to the original form in *D*. *C* shows the change from a regular rhythm to complete heart-block.

damage to the conduction system probably influence the type of curve, although in this series many of the pathologic lesions appeared almost identical while the curves differed a great deal. Disturbances of the *T*-wave and a diminished amplitude were the most constant findings, but disturbance of the pacemaker, complete heart-block, delayed auriculoventricular conduction, lengthening of the *QRS* complex and the occurrence of tachycardia and other changes in rate illustrate the great variety of possible alterations in the cardiac mechanism that may be found in patients with cardiac infarction.

Treatment. It seems most probable that the eventual outcome of the individual patient depends upon the amount of damage caused by the infarct in the heart and in the conduction system of the particular patient. Treatment was directed toward absolute

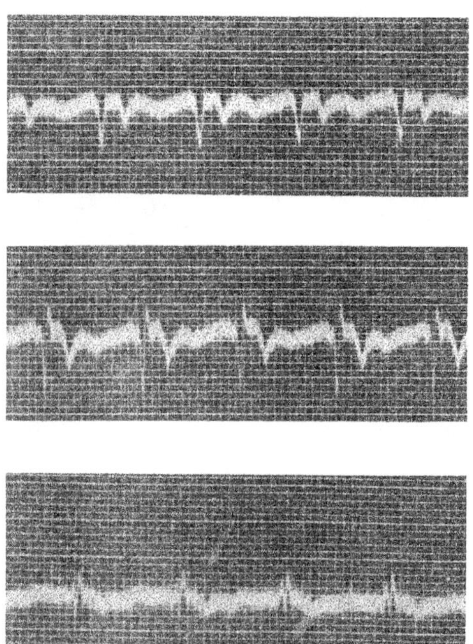

Fig. 2.—Record from Case No. 14652, which shows a practically normal electrocardiogram. This tracing was taken on the third day after the onset of the infarction and on the day before the death of the patient. The interventricular septum was included in the area of infarction in this individual.

rest, and every effort was made to spare the patient any bodily exertion. The fluid intake was limited and in eight of the patients digitalis was employed, the usual result being that the patient felt better and that the circulation improved, as shown by a diuresis and disappearance of the rales in the lungs. These signs of improvement did not occur in every patient who was given digitalis nor can the improvement be credited wholly to this drug; but it was the feeling of the observers that digitalis was beneficial and that it is indicated in this condition. In no instance did the nitrites relieve the severe pain; frequently large doses of morphin were required and these failed to control the pain in some instances. There were very critical times with some of the patients when the blood-pressure dropped and they showed other signs of collapse, and during these times stimulants were employed freely. Caffein and camphor were used with almost immediate relief, and in one patient who was having frequent changes of heart-rate, with numerous fainting attacks and Cheyne-Stokes respiration, caffein and camphor were used, with the result that the heart-rate became regular in complete block, the blood-pressure rose and the respiration became regular. The effect usually lasted about two hours and was obtained again by repetition of the drugs. No instances of ruptured hearts followed the use of stimulants.

Necropsy Findings An analysis of the postmortem findings in these 19 patients shows several points of interest and explains many of the signs and symptoms observed during life. The one finding which serves as a basis for the whole picture is arteriosclerosis; in practically every one of the patients there was found a generalized sclerosis of the vessels. In some instances the aorta was markedly involved, showing varying grades of the sclerotic process from mere fatty plaques to extensive atheromatous ulcerations with calcification, but in several instances the condition of the aorta was surprisingly good, showing an elasticity normal for the age and with little or no sclerosis, especially in the ascending portion of the arch. These findings in the aorta are interesting because of their relation to Allbutt's views on the cause of anginal pain. In several of the patients with pain resembling the anginal type the pathologist found little in the aorta that would account for it, while in one patient in whom dyspnea was the predominating sign, and there was no pain, the aorta showed an extreme degree of ulceration and even calcification. The degree of sclerosis frequently varied in different groups of vessels, with the exception of the coronary arteries, which in every instance were markedly sclerosed. Their finer branches were frequently closed because of this process and in many of the larger branches the lumen was contracted so that only a very small opening remained. The lack of elasticity of the bloodvessels of the heart could limit the supply of blood to the heart muscle and could most probably account for some of the clinical symptoms.

Rene Marie[26] and Le Count[27] have reported interesting studies of the pathologic findings in the hearts. In view of the finding of enlarged hearts by clinical methods it is of interest to note that the heart was moderately enlarged in practically every one of the 19 cases in our series, varying in weight from 365 gm. to 670 gm., the average weight of fourteen of the hearts being 471 gm., and

[26] L'infarctus du myocarde et ses consequences, Paris, 1897.
[27] Jour. Am. Med. Assn., 1918, **70**, 974.

while the weights of the other five hearts were not given, the pathologist noted the hearts as enlarged in most of those instances. The number showing pericarditis was surprisingly small in view of the nature of the main lesion, but this was most probably due to the position of the infarct and to the fact that many of the patients died before the inflammatory changes became widespread. Only four of the total number showed exudate or injection of the pericardium, a much lower percentage incidence than in the cases reported by Gorham.[28]

The frequence of the occurrence of the thrombus in one particular branch of the coronary arteries was striking. In 16 of the 19 instances the occlusion occurred in the anterior descending branch of the left coronary artery, and in 15 of these the thrombus was situated on the site of a contracture in the lumen due to an atheromatous change in the vessel wall. In one instance the thrombus was not found but the artery was practically closed at one point by an atheromatous constriction of the lumen. As would be expected from the distribution of this branch of the coronary artery the infarction was usually in the anterior wall of the left ventricle. At times the thrombus was so high in the course of the vessel that the interventricular septum and the papillary muscles of the left ventricle were included in the infarction. The posterior descending branch of the left coronary artery was thrombosed in one instance, the infarct being in the posterior wall of the left ventricle. The two other instances in which vessels other than the anterior descending branch of the left coronary artery were involved were in the patients with chronic heart disease. In one the thrombus was found in the descending branch of the right coronary artery, with the infarct in the anterior wall of the right ventricle; in the other the thrombus was located in the posterior circumflex branch of the left coronary with infarction of the posterior wall of the left ventricle. No essential difference was noted in the clinical findings between occlusion of the right and of the left coronary artery. It does not appear, therefore, that a prediction can be made from the clinical findings as to which artery or branch is occluded, but there is a statistical preponderance in favor of the anterior descending branch of the left coronary artery.

Gross examination of the heart outside of the area of the infarct revealed many small fibrous scars. These were verified as such microscopically, and, in addition, many of the small branches of the coronary arteries were found to be closed as a result of an old atheromatous process. In other words, aside from the acute infarction there was, in general, a so-called chronic fibrous myocarditis in a heart with a moderate degree of hypertrophy. In view of these findings it is not surprising that dyspnea occurred

[28] Loc. cit.

when any increased strain was thrown upon the heart, even before the occlusion of the coronary artery. Indeed, it is difficult to understand why these patients did not show more severe signs and symptoms referable to the heart before the onset of the infarction.

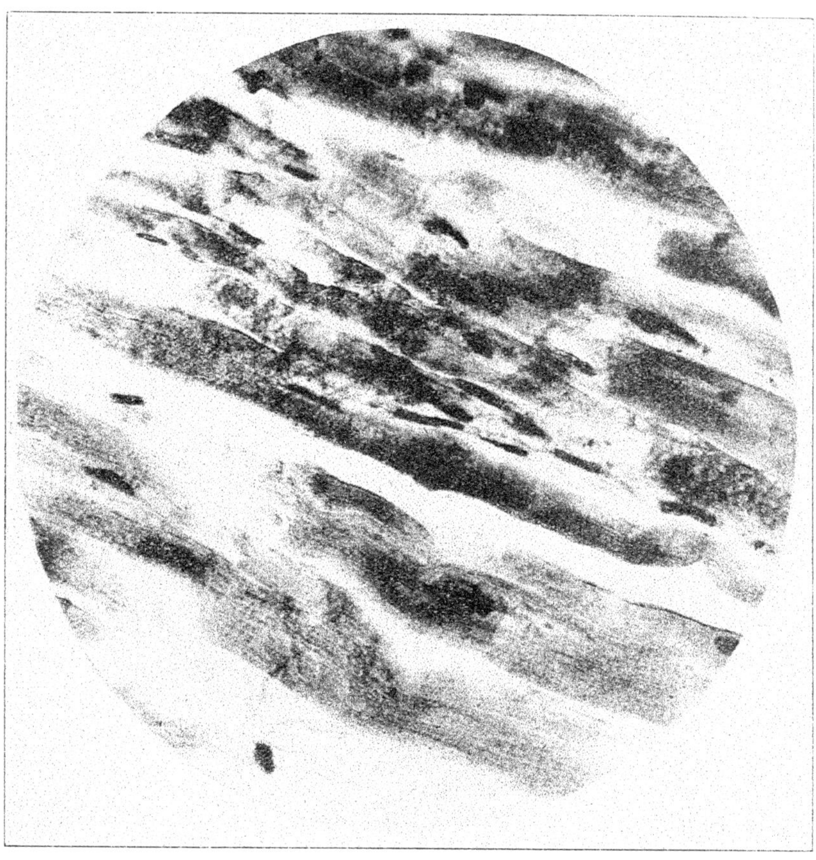

Fig. 3.—Acute degeneration of the myocardium in a patient who died about twenty-four hours after the occlusion of the coronary artery. The muscle fibers show swelling, granulation and loss of striations, and there is marked shrinking of the nuclei. (High power.)

Sections through the area of the infarct were practically identical in every case. Acute necrosis with rupture and fragmentation of the muscle fibers was practically always found, except in the patients in whom death resulted almost immediately after the infarction. In these there was a coarse granular appearance within the muscle fibers, the nuclei of these fibers being small and piknotic (Fig. 3). Edema of the heart muscle was also a frequent finding and a moderate amount of fatty degeneration was present in a few instances.

In later stages or in patients who died weeks after the infarction fibrous changes had begun to appear at the site of the infarct. Following the acute stage of the infarct in a case of coronary thrombosis, repair begins, the area of infarction being replaced by granulation tissue, and, finally, if the patient survives long enough a fibrous cicatrix is formed. Very small scars of this type are frequently found distributed throughout the heart muscle in individuals

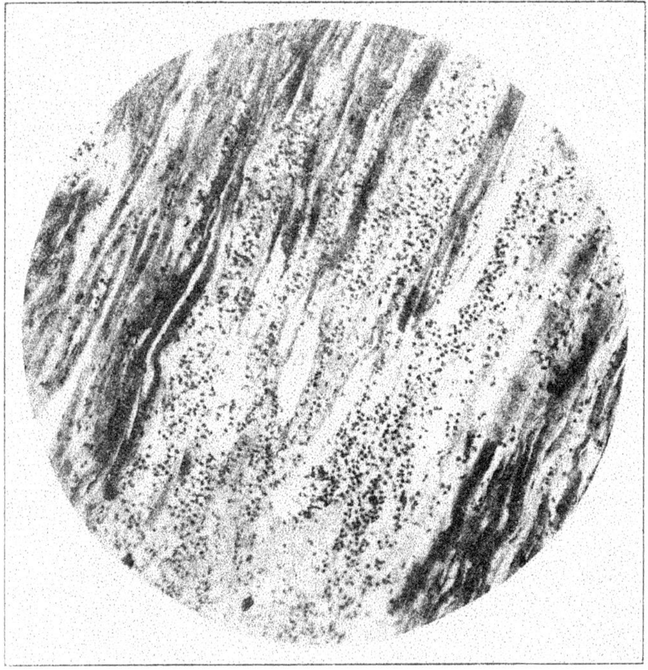

Fig. 4.—This section through the area of infarction shows necrosis of the myocardium and the exudate of polymorphonuclear leukocytes. (Low power.)

with marked sclerosis of the coronary vessels, and they are possibly the result of closure from sclerosis of the very small branches of the coronary arteries. When a main branch is obstructed and the patient lives a large fibrous scar is formed; it is possible that these scars may result in the small aneurysms not infrequently found at the apex of the heart. It certainly seems significant that the majority of infarcts occur near the apex in the left venticle and that aneurysms frequently occur at the same point.

Another observation which was made in every case in this series was the presence of polymorphonuclear leukocytes in the infarcted area (Fig. 4). They were found invading the necrotic tissue and at times in such great numbers that the process resembled an abscess. This probably accounts for the leukocytosis which was found during life. In a few instances there was also a round-cell or lymphocytic infiltration.

With the numerous systolic murmurs heard during life in mind it is interesting to find that in only one instance did the heart show an endocarditis with a valve lesion, and this was in the patient with a history of rheumatic fever. In another instance a very

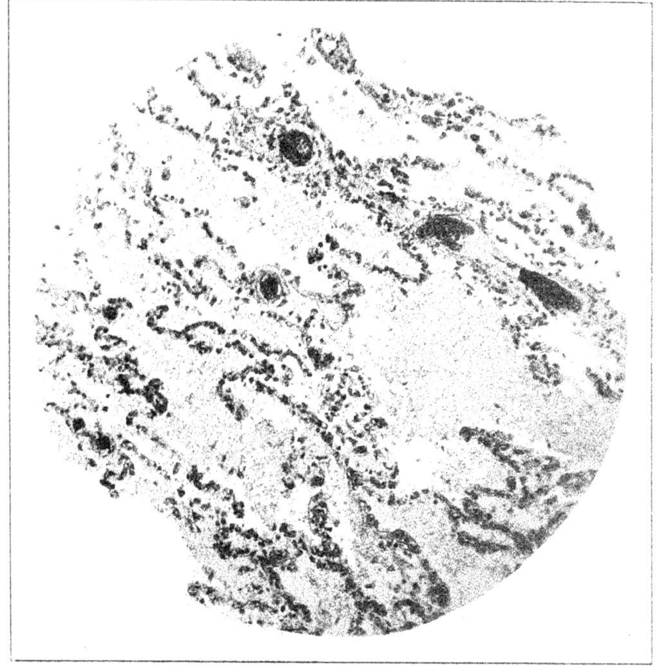

Fig. 5.—Section of the lung of a patient who died twenty-four hours after the occlusion of the coronary artery, showing the marked pulmonary edema. (Low power.)

small vegetation was found upon the mitral valve, but it was calcified, and in the smears made from it no organisms were found. A frequent occurrence, however, was the formation of numerous small mural thrombi which were generally found over the endocardial surface of the infarcted area.

The interventricular septum was included in the infarcted area a number of times, and, on some occasions, quite extensively. A serial section study of the septum has not been made, but the gross appearance and the amount and extent of the necrosis of the septum bore no relation to the form of the electrocardiographic curve.

The pathologic changes in the lungs were practically the same in every case. With one exception either edema or congestion was found, and in most cases both were present. This held true for the early as well as the late cases, one patient who died twenty-four hours after the onset of symptoms showing an extensive edema (Fig. 5). This patient was in the hospital at the time the infarction occurred, and although previous to the onset he had not been dyspneic, he became markedly so almost immediately afterward. The heart muscle of this patient is shown in Fig. 3. The degree of edema and congestion varied, of course; in some of the lungs only the bases were edematous while in others the edema and congestion extended throughout. Such an extensive filling of the lungs as is shown in Fig. 5 would readily account for severe dyspnea, a lowered vital capacity and the rales so frequently noted. In several of the patients small amounts of fluid were found in the thoracic cavities, but the quantity was rarely above 200 cc except in the group with antecedent chronic heart disease. In most instances all the abdominal viscera were found to be congested, this being especially true of the liver and spleen. As a result these organs were enlarged to such an extent that the enlargement of the liver was frequently discovered during life. The kidneys were generally congested, and, in addition, the renal vessels were sclerotic. This sclerosis in some instances had reached the stage of a vascular nephritis, a condition discovered in several of the cases during life. Infarcts were also found in the kidney, spleen, lung and brain, but only infrequently.

Briefly the necropsy findings in cases of coronary thrombosis reveal arteriosclerosis, usually generalized, and especially marked in the coronary arteries. Because of this arteriosclerosis a thrombus forms in one or more of the arteries, with a resulting infarct of the heart. Usually the anterior descending branch of the left coronary artery is occluded and the infarct involves the left ventricle and part of the septum. In the necrotic tissue polymorphonuclear leukocytes are found in great numbers. The heart is generally enlarged, and outside of the area of infarction a so-called chronic fibrous myocarditis is usually found. From the cardiac lesion, in turn, result edema and congestion of the lungs and congestion of the abdominal viscera.

Summary. If then the data from the clinical studies of nineteen patients with a diagnosis, confirmed by necropsy, of infarct of the heart be summarized and a typical case be constructed therefrom we will obtain a picture much as follows: We will find a patient, usually a man, possibly less frequently a woman, beyond the age of forty, probably over fifty, complaining of severe pain over the heart or under the lower end of the sternum, or almost as frequently of pain in the epigastrium. Less frequently the complaint may be of a sudden attack of extreme shortness of breath, persistent and uurelieved by rest. A glance at the patient gives the warning that the nature of the illness is very serious and the condition of the patient correspondingly so. From the presenting signs and symptoms and from the complaint attention is usually directed to the heart and a few questions soon establish the fact the patient had not had the usual forerunners of heart disease, such as rheumatic fever. Furthermore, in view of the severity of the dyspnea and other symptoms referable to the heart, one is surprised to find either little or no evidence of heart disease in the past history. Dyspnea on exertion, such as climbing stairs, may have been noticed for a few months, or some patients may have experienced a few attacks of anginal pain; but the exceptional person only has been incapacitated or prevented from carrying out his daily routine.

The onset of symptoms with the infarction is very sudden and without warning. The patient may have been in good or fairly good health the minute before being seized by an excruciating pain either in the region of the precordium or in the epigastrium, a pain which in most instances radiates into the shoulders and down one or both arms. Unlike anginal attacks, which may have been experienced previously, it persists, and relief at times seems impossible. With the pain may be an extreme type of dyspnea, or, in some instances, the dyspnea may occur alone. The attack may have begun after exertion or, as frequently happens, the individual may have been asleep at the time of the onset. If the patient has experienced attacks of anginal pain or dyspnea previously he needs no one to tell him that this attack is of an entirely different nature; most patients make this observation for themselves. While the pain of angina pectoris lasts minutes the pain of cardiac infarction lasts for hours or days, the same holding true for the shortness of breath. Closely following the pain and dyspnea may be nausea, vomiting, weakness or even collapse, so that the condition may actually resemble shock. In a few patients the heart may have begun to fail before the onset of the infarction, so that they may have been dyspneic, edematous and bedridden. In these people the occlusion of the coronary artery either accentuates the signs and symptoms already present, or, as is possible, the onset of the infarction may be masked by the severity of the previous illness.

When one examines the patient he is impressed by the severity of the symptoms and by the fact that they seem out of all proportion to the physical findings. A careful search, however, is rewarded by finding enough points to enable one to recognize the true condition in the heart. The skin, a pale ashen color, is moist and cold; the expression of anxiety and suffering suggests the severity of the condition. In the lungs signs of edema, either a few crackling rales at the bases or scattered extensively through both lungs, give the first clue of the failing circulation. Percussion reveals a moderately enlarged heart, and then, on further examination of it, one is struck by its weak action. The apex impulse can neither be seen nor felt, and on auscultation the weak, distant and scarcely audible sounds indicate also the weakness of the heart. Occasionally a pericardial friction rub is heard, and, if present, is an additional point in favor of infarction. Unfortunately a friction rub does not occur very frequently. One may find a regular rhythm or irregularities due to premature beats or less often to heart-block, and not infrequently one finds a tachycardia with a rate as high as 150 per minute. Electrocardiographic tracings may be helpful, but one cannot expect to make a diagnosis from them alone, as there is no typical or characteristic curve in the condition.

On palpation of the abdomen one is apt to find an enlarged liver which may or may not be tender. In patients with the epigastric type of pain, tenderness and even spasm may be found in this region. Finally the presence of a fever and a polymorphonuclear leukocytosis adds to the number of findings which occur with sufficient constancy to make them of definite value in recognizing the condition. A careful search for and consideration of the points which have been mentioned make the diagnosis of cardiac infarction much less difficult and enables one to treat more intelligently those patients who survive the first stage of occlusion of the coronary artery.

The writer wishes to thank Drs. H. A. Christian and S. A. Levine for many helpful criticisms and suggestions during the preparation of this paper.

HEMATEMESIS IN NEPHRITIS.

By Howard F. Shattuck, M.D.,

Associate Attending Physician, Postgraduate Hospital, New York.

The determination of the cause of hematemesis is often a matter of considerable difficulty. This symptom has become almost inseparably associated with peptic ulcer. And yet the number of cases of gastric hemorrhage due to other causes is considerable.

One of these causes is chronic nephritis or its allied states of arteriosclerosis and vascular hypertension. Massive hematemesis in these conditions is comparatively rare. But it occurs often enough to make us bear it in mind when dealing with an obscure case of this dramatic symptom. In this connection I wish to report the following case:

Case History. Mrs. M., a white American housewife, aged thirty-one years, was admitted to the medical service of the Post-graduate Hospital on March 20, 1920, complaining of having vomited a "cupful" of blood five hours previously. Her family history is of no interest. She married at seventeen and her husband and two children are in good health. At fourteen she had typhoid fever with complete recovery. Her appendix, both ovaries and uterus were removed when she was twenty-eight. Following the operation she had good health for two years. The morning of the day of her admission to the hospital she had a severe headache and vomited "a cupful" of bright red blood. Further questioning showed that for the past year she had suffered with severe headaches, becoming increasingly severe in the last three months. During the same period her appetite had been poor; she had been troubled with nausea, and frequently vomited small amounts of clear mucus (rarely any food). She had gradually lost weight (twenty pounds) and had become so weak she could no longer do her housework. For several months she had noticed that any unusual exertion caused moderate dyspnea. Urination had averaged six times during the day and two or three times at night for eight months. During the last month she noticed numbness and formication in her hands and legs. There had been no abdominal pain or other symptoms referable to the gastrointestinal tract except the anorexia, nausea and vomiting noted above.

Physical Examination. The patient was a poorly nourished woman in early adult life. Her skin and mucous membranes were rather blanched. Ears, nose, throat and teeth were all negative. There was no general lymphadenopathy. The lungs were clear except for a few fine, moist rales in the left axilla. The apex of the heart was in the fifth left interspace, 11.5 cm. from the mid-sternal line; the right border at the sternal margin. The second aortic sound was loud and ringing; there were no murmurs; the action was regular and rate 102. The blood-pressure was 194 systolic and 124 diastolic. On admission the abdomen was not examined because of the recent hemorrhage. Later examination showed no tenderness, palpable viscera, masses or free-fluid. There was no edema. The reflexes were normal.

Ophthalmoscopic Examination. Right fundus: Margin of disk completely obliterated; veins dilated; arteries contracted; numerous stellate hemorrhages scattered over the peripapillary area; large whitish spots here and there in equatorial zone. Left fundus: Similar changes though less marked. (Two days after admission.)

Laboratory Findings. Blood count; red blood cells, 3,488,000; white blood cells, 10,600; hemoglobin (Sahli), 60 per cent; differential, 65 per cent polymorphonuclear leukocytes and 35 per cent large and small lymphocytes. Red blood cells showed slight central pallor.

Urine: Specific gravity, 1010 to 1016; persistent faint trace of albumin; no sugar; few hyaline casts.

Gastric analysis (made three weeks after hemorrhage): Fasting contents, 10 cc; faintly greenish fluid; lactic acid, 0; occult blood, 0 (benzidin and guaiac); Boas-Oppler bacilli, 0; free HCl, 10; combined, 12; total acidity, 22. No food remnants.

Ewald test meal: 60 cc yellowish fluid; mucus, +; bile, 0; lactic acid, 0; occult blood, 0 (benzidin); Boas-Oppler bacilli, 0; free HCl, 16; combined, 14; total 30.

Stool: Examination made three weeks after hemorrhage; bile, ++; no ova or parasites; blood, 0 (benzidin and guaiac).

Roentgen-ray report (Dr. W. H. Meyer): Lungs show no pathology; heart shows left-sided enlargement. Gastrointestinal tract: Stomach hypotonic; diminished peristalsis; no defect seen in stomach or duodenum; stomach empty in six hours; examination suggests only gastroenteroptosis.

Blood chemistry: Urea, 11.4 mg. per 100 cc of blood; creatinin, 2.14 mg. per 100 cc of blood; uric acid, 3.5 mg. per 100 cc of blood; sugar, 0.124 per cent; chlorides as NaCl, 0.419 per cent. (Patient had been on low protein diet several days preceding this examination.)

Phenolsulphonephthalein elimination: 130 cc urine with 30.4 per cent in two hours.

Response to nephritic test meal: Total day urine, 794 cc; specific gravity range, 1008 to 1013; total night urine, 1385 cc; specific gravity, 1007; day urine (sodium chloride), 0.36 per cent; total, 2.85 gm.; night urine, 0.16 per cent; total, 5.06 gm.; day urine (nitrogen), 0.21 per cent; total, 1.69 gm.; night urine, 0.097 per cent; total, 1.34 gm.

Progress Notes. During the first twenty-four hours the patient vomited fresh blood, once about four ounces, once about two ounces and once about six ounces. The vomiting ceased after the first twenty-four hours. She was given the routine treatment for hematemesis, followed by salt-poor diet, forced fluids, sodium nitrite, luminal, chloral and rest. She rapidly improved and was discharged on April 3, having only an occasional headache and gaining in weight and strength. Blood-pressure on discharge was 210 systolic and 118 diastolic. She returned to the hospital on July 25, 1920, saying she had been getting worse for the past month, losing weight and strength and suffering with severe headaches. She was quite dyspneic on slight exertion and vomited several times, but no more blood. Physical examination was the same as during her previous stay in the hospital, except that the retinal hemorrhages were more numerous and extensive. Blood-pressure was 250 systolic, blood chemistry showed no essential change, phenolsulphonephthalein excretion was 28 per cent in two hours. After leaving the hospital August 5, 1920, she became gradually worse and died in uremic coma October 20, 1920. Autopsy was refused.

Discussion. It is difficult to learn the frequency of hematemesis in chronic nephritis, arteriosclerosis or vascular hypertension. However, since Richard Bright gave us his description of the disease that bears his name, there have appeared from time to time scattered through the literature, chiefly in France, reports of gastrointestinal hemorrhages including hematemesis occurring in these diseases. Bright[1] himself, in 1829, spoke of gastric and intestinal hemorrhages in some cases of nephritis, but he saw only a clinical coincidence in the occurrence and did not suspect the relationship that might exist between them. Even before this Latour, in 1815 (quoted by Riesman[15]), described epistaxis and other forms of bleeding in dropsy; and still earlier Morgagni reported the case of a woman with the odor of urine in her breath, who vomited blood and had epistaxis with beneficial results. Later the association of various forms of hemorrhage, including gastro-intestinal hemorrhage in nephritis and uremia was noted and reported by a number of observers. Among these were Rayer,[2] Malmsten,[3] Johnson,[4] Treitz,[5] Fournier,[6] Moxon,[7] Bartels,[8] Dodet,[9] Mathieu and Roux,[10] Monpeurt[11] and Lancereaux.[12] Most of these observers described chiefly the intestinal hemorrhages and their lesions which occur more often than those in the stomach.

In a group of 68 cases of uremia collected by Dickinson,[13] however, there were 3 with hematemesis, and Bonifas[14] reported a severe gastric hemorrhage in a case of nephritis, aged thirty years, with recovery. In reviewing the hemorrhagic manifestations occurring in nephritis, Riesman[15] discusses hematemesis among others. He believed that renal disease was a cause of hemorrhagic diathesis, the factors being hypertension, arterial disease and toxemia, and, further, that there was some toxin in the blood acting on the capillary endothelium and impairing the integrity of the blood. Decreton[16] described a case of gastric hemorrhage and tarry stools in a man showing Cheyne-Stokes breathing, uremia and a high blood urea, 79 mg. per 100 cc of blood becoming 11.7 mg. per 100 cc of blood six weeks later. He then discusses the differential diagnosis of gastric carcinoma and ulcer in patients with hematemesis showing evidence of nephritis, arteriosclerosis and hypertension, pointing out the importance of determining the blood urea before deciding. It is very interesting in this connection to note the low figures for blood urea in the case reported by the writer. The blood chemistry was determined in both instances, however, after the patient had been taking a low-protein diet for several days. Uric acid was increased in the writer's case. Crispin,[17] in a general discussion of gastric hemorrhage, mentions nephritis and vascular hypertension as causes and urges a careful search for them in unexplained cases of gastric hemorrhage. He reports a case of hematemesis in which a gastroenterostomy was done in 1914 for supposed peptic ulcer. Because of repeated gastric hemorrhages the patient was explored at the Mayo Clinic in 1915, but no ulcer was found. He had a blood-pressure of 185 systolic, slight left-sided cardiac hypertrophy, phthalein excretion of 43 per cent and a negative gastrointestinal roentgen-ray, except for a normal functioning gastroenterostomy. Three months after leaving the Mayo Clinic he had another severe gastric hemorrhage and a blood-pressure of 250 systolic.

Pathology. No uniform pathologic findings have been reported by those who have had the opportunity of studying these cases. Monpeurt,[11] reviewing the work previously appearing on the subject, found that nephritis most often gives rise to intestinal ulcerations, and that in the aged gastric ulcerations do not occur without intestinal lesions. Ulcers in the stomach and ileum in uremia were classified as follows by Gandy[18]: (*a*) Hemorrhagic infiltration; (*b*) simple erosion; (*c*) true ulcer. Treitz[5] described uremic lesions in the stomach and intestines as thinning of the mucous membrane, hyperemia and finally ulcerations; while Lancereaux,[12] in a case of gastric hemorrhage in nephritis, was unable to find any gastrointestinal ulceration. Pineau[19] believed that both hematemesis and melena in nephritis are due to increased blood-pressure, increased permeability of the bloodvessels and minor alterations of the mucosa. A man aged thirty-eight years, dying of hematemesis, is reported by Hirschfeld,[20] who showed at autopsy only marked lesions of sclerosis of the gastric arteries, of which one was the seat of a small aneurysmal dilatation. Widal and Boidin[21] described a patient dying in hematemesis and showing no ulcer or cancer. They found only endarteritis of the gastric vessels. In four cases of pronounced hematemesis Fisher[22] found only small white kidneys.

Summary. 1. A case of severe hematemesis is reported due, as far as could be ascertained, to chronic nephritis with hypertension.

2. A review of the literature shows several reports of this rather unusual complication, but gives no uniform conclusions about the cause or pathology of this symptom.

BIBLIOGRAPHY.

1. Bright, Richard: Reports of Medical Cases, London, 1827.
2. Rayer, P.: Traité des maladies et des reins, Paris, 1839.
3. Malmsten, P. H.: Ueber die Brightische Nierenkrankheit, Bremen, 1846.
4. Johnson, George: Diseases of the Kidney, London, 1852.
5. Treitz: Monographie sur les maladies des reins, 1859.
6. Fournier: De l'urémie, Thèse d'agrégation, Paris, 1863.
7. Wilks, S., and Moxon, W.: Lectures on Pathologic Anatomy, London, 1875.
8. Bartels, C.: Maladies des reins, Paris, 1884.
9. Dodet, L. E.: Des hemorrhagies dans l'urémie, Paris Thesis, 1901.
10. Mathieu, A., and Roux, J. C.: Arch. gén. de méd., 1902, **1**, 14.

11. Monpeurt, H. C. V.: Ulcerations gastriques d'origine cardiorenal chez le vieillard, Paris Thesis, 1910.
12. Lancereaux, E.: Texte d'atlas d'anatomie pathologique, Paris, 1871.
13. Dickinson, W. H.: On the Pathology and Treatment of Albuminuria, London, 1868.
14. Bonifas, J.: La normandie médicale, 1898, **13**, 102.
15. Riesman, David: Tr. Assn. Am. Phys., 1907, **22**, 498
16. Decreton: Rev. gén. de clin. et de thérap., 1916, **30**, 646.
17. Crispin, E. L.: California State Jour. Med., 1917, **15**, 308.
18. Gandy, C.: L'ulcère simple et la nécrose hémorrhagique des toxémies, Paris Thesis, 1899.
19. Pineau, M.: Des hémorrhagies gastro-intestinales d'origine uremique, Paris Thesis, 1899.
20. Hirschfeld, H.: Berl. klin. Wchnschr., 1904, **41**, 584.
21. Widal and Boidin: Bull. et mém. Soc. méd. d. hôp. de Paris, 1905, **22**, 696.
22. Fisher: Bristol Med.-Chir. Jour., 1904, **22**, 234.

REVIEWS.

The Defective Delinquent and Insane. By Henry A. Cotton, M.D. Pp. 201; 32 illustrations. Trenton, N. J.: Princeton University Press.

This remarkable book presents the widely known views of its author on the relation of infection to mental diseases. An illustration of the many reactions which it can rouse is found in its preface where Dr. Meyer regards the book as a stimulant to the production of well-endowed research centers which will afford "a certain surplus of opportunity instead of the deplorable and disgraceful halfway measures with which the study of mental diseases has had to skimp along."

The reader can well become interested in the writer's positive views: "Psychoses arise from a combination of factors, some of which may be absent, but the most constant one is an intracerebral, biochemical, cellular disturbance arising from circulating toxins, originating in chronic focal infections situated anywhere in the body and probably to some extent in disturbances of the endocrine system." This is a proposition that can be studied without prejudice. The chapter about the pathology of the mouth can be left for bacteriologists and dental surgeons to judge, after they have had plenty of time to satisfy themselves by their own work. The general clinical statement, that in the impacted molars and other infected teeth of children lies the explanation for such abnormal characters as the shut-in personality, cannot be controlled so definitely. In fact in the clinical statements and data which the author gives, the most astonishing feature is the number of interpretations that are possible. The following case will serve as an example. A boy, aged nineteen years, in a profound depression, showed by roentgen-ray studies four impacted third molars, a serious gastrointestinal infection and had badly infected tonsils. He was taken home improved, became maniacal and has been confined in various institutions where no attention has been paid to the gastrointestinal tract.

Many clinical cases are given in some detail to show that recovery and improvement have followed surgical and other procedures directed to the detoxication of the patient. The records of other hospitals, where other methods are practised, will show parallels of these individual cases. We quote from a reprint which by chance was received in the same mail as the author's book: "I recollect one instance of an inmate who had been four years regarded as a hopeless dement, and for whom an early death was anticipated . . . and yet, a twenty-minute interview showed that this man was merely a profoundly timorous psychasthenic, who had completely lost heart, overburdened with the psychologic puzzles he had been endeavoring to solve before his incarceration. He returned to normal life after four months' careful body and mental nursing.' The careful physician will want time enough to see the results of any new therapy demonstrated in some cases which he himself knows pretty well. Many physicians have a group of cases in mind who have gone to Trenton and have not apparently been benefited; it is possible that some of these have not submitted to all the procedures which the author thought necessary. Among other unsettled points there is the question of how much psychic effect is produced by the intense enthusiasm and activity which the new patient meets at Trenton, and as the author suggests, a patient must be glad to believe that his trouble is a physical one from which he can be relieved without much effort on his own part.

It is embarrassing to criticise the author's conclusions as to the value of certain detoxicating procedures when one sympathizes with his position on the restraint of patients, with his optimism, his determination to leave no stone unturned to send a patient home well, and the way in which he has brought into his psychopathic wards the atmosphere of the general hospital. One does not need to turn his back upon these good things to urge slowness in accepting a certain technic which deals with very complicated and varying organisms.

We think the author would agree with the following way of stating his position. There are not many persons who acquire mental disease because their ancestors had it, nor are there many, who, hereditarily tainted, are tipped over by the mental distresses they meet. Most psychotics have been riding in flat-bottomed boats, not in canoes, and it has taken an infection from outside to tip them over. Those people who have infections and do not capsize are veritable rafts in their stability. It is a hopeful view, especially since even the canoe may be kept right side up if the essential disturber, infection, be eliminated. We can hope that in time it will turn out to be a correct view. O.

MEDICAL RECORD VISITING LIST, OR PHYSICIANS DIARY. Revised. New York: William Wood & Co., 1922.

THIS annual visiting list is made up for the year 1923 in the usual attractive form. In addition to the spaces for recording professional services there are many tables of drugs, doses, and condensed information of value for quick reference. W.

Diseases of the Skin. By Henry H. Hazen, A.B., M.D., Professor of Dermatology in the Medical Department of Georgetown University. Second edition. Pp. 608; 241 illustrations, including 2 color plates. St. Louis: C. V. Mosby Company, 1922.

The present volume contains about seventy more pages than the first edition, published seven years ago. The entire work shows signs of careful revision. Changes have been made in classification and several new subdivisions have been formed. There are a number of new illustrations and some of the old ones have been omitted. The technic of superficial roentgentherapy has been brought up to date and a brief consideration of radium and phototherapy added. Almost every chapter has been improved by some addition or suppression. The discussion of the etiology of eczema shows accordance with the modern viewpoint. The author has previously indicated his interest in skin diseases in the negro race and references to this phase of the subject occur more often than in other manuals. His key to diagnosis is rather novel and decidedly practical. In therapy the writer frequently diverges from the worn path, but he is not at all radical. The entire subject is handled in a direct, common-sense manner. Owing to the lack of a confusing variety of treatment for each disease, the book should be especially useful to the student. Briefly, an excellent medium-sized work on dermatology has been improved and modernized. C.

Clinical and Operative Gynecology. By J. M. Munro Kerr, Professor of Obstetrics and Gynecology, Glasgow University (Muirhead Chair); Gynecological Surgeon, Royal Infirmary, Glasgow. Pp. 832; 225 illustrations and colored plates. London: Henry Frowde, Hodder & Stoughton, 1922.

Dr. Kerr emphasizes the clinical aspects of gynecology in this excellent book, and this attitude toward the clinical side is strengthened by the inclusion in the text of a large number of abridged case histories illustrative of a certain point under discussion. The sections on Anatomy, Nervous Disorders of Women and Venereal Diseases have been ably handled by colleagues. The very sane discussion of the endorine glands is to be commended. Radium does not seem to be regarded in as wide a therapeutic range as in this country, and its possibilities as a cure in cancer are rather questioned. The operative details incident to the surgical side of this specialty are clearly and briefly described, the line drawings of the stages of operations accompanying the text are well executed. The reviewer notes the omission of the consecutive numbering of the illustrations after a certain point, thus rendering correlation between them and the foregoing text rather difficult. Personal preference or objection to various operative measures are frankly stated. The color plates by Maxwell are unusually good, as indeed are most of the illustrations. Chapter XX gives a *resume* of the conditions in nearby organs which may simulate pelvic disease. There is little to criticize and much to commend in this well-balanced treatise. W.

A Manual of Pharmacology and Its Applications to Therapeutics and Toxicology. By Torald Sollmann, M.D., Professor of Pharmacology and Materia Medica in the School of Medicine of Western Reserve University, Cleveland. Second edition. Pp. 1066. Philadelphia and London: W. B. Saunders Company, 1922.

If a man may be told by the company he keeps, still more should be revealed by the book he writes. The author's comprehensive presentation within the limits of an octavo volume is, we believe, a demonstration of this axiom. Aiming to combine the broad conceptions of a text-book with the mass of minute details of a reference book, he has had to make liberal use of large and small print, side headings, black face, italics, footnotes and similar devices. Although this often entails as many as six forms of type on one page, we feel that the resultant loss of ease and continuity is more than compensated for by the saving of space and reader's time. Appendix A—a tabulation of average doses in four groups according to their practical importance—should be a useful aid to the undergraduate student; while the bibliography of over six thousand titles should be of great value to students of all grades. K.

Protein Therapy and Nonspecific Resistance. By William F. Peterson, M.D., Associate in Pathology, University of Illinois; College of Medicine, Chicago, Ill. With an introduction by Joseph L. Miller, M.D., Professor of Medicine, Rush Medical College, University of Chicago, Chicago, Ill. Pp. 314. New York: The Macmillan Company, 1922.

This book is a pioneer in its field. It is not a text-book or a dogmatic statement of the subject—the time is not yet ripe for that—but a careful compilation, review and analysis of all the evidence that has accumulated in a voluminous literature. The task has been well performed by a man particularly fitted for it by his knowledge of the problems of immunity and by his large clinical experience with protein therapy, a man who combines enthusiasm with a sound and usually conservative judgment.

Diseases of the Skin. By H... ...describes the various
fessor of Dermatology in ... proceed, and the theories
town University. Second ... of the reaction. He next
including 2 color plates ... manner his own conception of
1922. ... of the book is taken up with
... result obtained in a variety
The present vol... ...s with indications and contra-
first edition, ...ntly alluded to throughout
signs of care... ...been a trifle fuller, or perhaps
and sever... ...ll bibliography with over 1200
numbe... ...erapy is finding an increasing
omitt... ...is that of the clinician as well
b... ...atologist. book should have and deserves a
...ingly wide appeal. K.

...'s Handbook of Physiology. Revised by ... Greene. Tenth American edition. Pp. 820; 524 illustrations. New York: William Wood & Company, 1922.

This well-known text-book has been considerably revised for this new edition. It has certain advantages over most of the other text-books for anyone commencing the study of the subject who needs a comprehensive knowledge of the more elementary facts. These advantages depend partly upon the fact that details of histology and of fundamental biochemistry are given as well as the physiologic deductions that can be made from them, and partly because definite statements are made, while less stress is laid on the evidence on which these statements are based.

Such a statement of the main facts of physiology, without dealing too much in theory, should make the book useful for certain types of students, but this method of teaching is doomed to failure unless the facts are absolutely accurate. Unfortunately, this is not the case in this edition, for there appear to be some serious mistakes, presumably misprints, which greatly diminish the value of the book, and some of which the reviewer mentions in a spirit of friendly criticism in the hope that they will be modified.

Thus, in dealing with the gases found in the lungs and tissues, excellent reproductions of some of Barcroft's curves are included; but further on the oxygen tension of the arterial blood is repeatedly given as 29 mm. of mercury, which is entirely inconsistent both with the curves and figures given previously and with our modern knowledge. In the same place wrong figures for the carbon-dioxide tension in expired air are given.

Another part of the book which ... revision in order to make the physiologic basis agree ... clinical findings is that describing the passage of sensory ... spinal cord.

her criticims which might be made are that, while in places of the bok has been brought up to date, including even the ork of Iacleod on insulin, in other places old methods are ribed, nd even at times old conclusions are drawn. On a such mportance as hemoglobin estimations it is a pity er th Sahli nor the Haldane method, the two most oder clinical methods, are included; and that in a mpotant as heart sounds, graphic records should still ed otained by Einthoven, using an obsolete method me f the records that have been obtained recently in this coi by Viggers.

If a few of these errors could be corrected, particularly in the misprints of figues dealing with gases, the book would have a real value as an elemntary text-book which covered the whole subject very thoroughly B.

OTO-RHINOLARYNOLOGY FOR THE STUDENT AND PRACTITIONER. By GEORGE LURENS, M.D.; authorized English translation of the fourth revi-d French edition by H. CLAYTON FOX, F.R.C.S. (IRELAND), wit a foreword contributed by SIR J. DUNDAS-GRANT, M.A., M.D., F.R.C.S. Second English edition. 589 illustrations. New York: William Wood & Company, 1922.

THIS translatio of the fourth French edition of George Laurens' treatise on disease of the nose, throat and ear is of special value to the student an general practitioner. The author has endeavored to give to th general practitioner the necessary data which would enable him to diagnose and treat the more common ailments of the nose, throatand ear, making it clear, however, that certain diseases cannot b successfully handled, except by a specialist. Methods of treatmet and the more simple operations are described in sufficient detail to enable the general practitioner, with a certain amount of practiceto take care of the common diseases. Operations and other tecnics demanding special training are only mentioned and not desribed in detail, as the author rightly believes such cases should b referred to a specialist. One of the valuable parts of the book i contained in the "What to Avoid" remarks. Though in a few dtails we cannot agree with the author, on the whole, the book is very reliable one and a safe guide for those beginning the study of otolaryngology. It is well illustrated with numerous and clear though not elaborate, illustrations, and the text is very easily readable. In this edition particular mention has been made of Vicent's angina, hay-fever, rhinometry, pseudohemoptysis of laryngeal origin and vaccine therapy. Also aural vertigo and the intitracheal injections of medicated liquids is given special attentio. W.

Beginning with a historical review, the author describes the various nonspecific agents, the typical reactions produced, and the theories hitherto advanced as to the mechanism of the reaction. He next states in a clear and convincing manner his own conception of this mechanism. The second half of the book is taken up with a review and discussion of the clinical results obtained in a variety of diseases. The final chapter deals with indications and contra-indications. While these are frequently alluded to throughout the book, this chapter might have been a trifle fuller, or perhaps more advantageously placed. A full bibliography with over 1200 references is appended. Protein therapy is finding an increasing application in infections. Its field is that of the clinician as well as the immunologist. This book should have and deserves a correspondingly wide appeal. K.

KIRKES'S HANDBOOK OF PHYSIOLOGY. Revised by C. W. GREENE. Tenth American edition. Pp. 820; 524 illustrations. New York: William Wood & Company, 1922.

THIS well-known text-book has been considerably revised for this new edition. It has certain advantages over most of the other text-books for anyone commencing the study of the subject who needs a comprehensive knowledge of the more elementary facts. These advantages depend partly upon the fact that details of histology and of fundamental biochemistry are given as well as the physiologic deductions that can be made from them, and partly because definite statements are made, while less stress is laid on the evidence on which these statements are based.

Such a statement of the main facts of physiology, without dealing too much in theory, should make the book useful for certain types of students, but this method of teaching is doomed to failure unless the facts are absolutely accurate. Unfortunately, this is not the case in this edition, for there appear to be some serious mistakes, presumably misprints, which greatly diminish the value of the book, and some of which the reviewer mentions in a spirit of friendly criticism in the hope that they will be modified.

Thus, in dealing with the gases found in the lungs and tissues, excellent reproductions of some of Barcroft's curves are included; but further on the oxygen tension of the arterial blood is repeatedly given as 29 mm. of mercury, which is entirely inconsistent both with the curves and figures given previously and with our modern knowledge. In the same place wrong figures for the carbon-dioxide tension in expired air are given.

Another part of the book which requires revision in order to make the physiologic basis agree with the clinical findings is that describing the passage of sensory impulses up the spinal cord.

Other criticisms which might be made are that, while in places much of the book has been brought up to date, including even the latest work of Macleod on insulin, in other places old methods are still described, and even at times old conclusions are drawn. On a subject of such importance as hemoglobin estimations it is a pity that neither the Sahli nor the Haldane method, the two most accurate modern clinical methods, are included; and that in a subject so important as heart sounds, graphic records should still be reproduced obtained by Einthoven, using an obsolete method instead of some of the records that have been obtained recently in this country by Wiggers.

If a few of these errors could be corrected, particularly in the misprints of figures dealing with gases, the book would have a real value as an elementary text-book which covered the whole subject very thoroughly. B.

OTO-RHINOLARYNGOLOGY FOR THE STUDENT AND PRACTITIONER. By GEORGE LAURENS, M.D.; authorized English translation of the fourth revised French edition by H. CLAYTON FOX, F.R.C.S. (IRELAND), with a foreword contributed by SIR J. DUNDAS-GRANT, M.A., M.D., F.R.C.S. Second English edition. 589 illustrations. New York: William Wood & Company, 1922.

THIS translation of the fourth French edition of George Laurens' treatise on diseases of the nose, throat and ear is of special value to the student and general practitioner. The author has endeavored to give to the general practitioner the necessary data which would enable him to diagnose and treat the more common ailments of the nose, throat and ear, making it clear, however, that certain diseases cannot be successfully handled, except by a specialist. Methods of treatment and the more simple operations are described in sufficient detail to enable the general practitioner, with a certain amount of practice to take care of the common diseases. Operations and other technics demanding special training are only mentioned and not described in detail, as the author rightly believes such cases should be referred to a specialist. One of the valuable parts of the book is contained in the "What to Avoid" remarks. Though in a few details we cannot agree with the author, on the whole, the book is a very reliable one and a safe guide for those beginning the study of otolaryngology. It is well illustrated with numerous and clear, though not elaborate, illustrations, and the text is very easily readable. In this edition particular mention has been made of Vincent's angina, hay-fever, rhinometry, pseudohemoptysis of laryngeal origin and vaccine therapy. Also aural vertigo and the intratracheal injections of medicated liquids is given special attention. W.

THE ORIGIN AND EVOLUTION OF THE HUMAN DENTITION. By WILLIAM K. GREGORY, PH.D., Associate Professor of Vertebrate Paleontology, Columbia University; Curator of the Department of Comparative Anatomy, American Museum of Natural History, New York. Pp. 548; 353 illustrations. Baltimore: Williams & Wilkins Company, 1922.

IN this very exhaustive treatise is traced the gradual development of the teeth from the earliest times and from the lowest vertebrates up to those of modern man. A detailed review could only be undertaken by a paleontologist. Those seeking the reasons for the present formation of the human dental organs will find here many points elucidated. It is through the labors of such purely scientific workers as the author, that true principles for the modern practice of medicine and dentistry are established. I.

DISEASES OF THE SKIN AND THE ERUPTIVE FEVERS. BY JAY F. SCHAMBERG, A.B., M.D., Professor of Dermatology and Syphilis, Graduate School of Medicine, University of Pennsylvania; Dermatologist to the Philadelphia General Hospital and the Jewish Hospital; Fellow of the College of Physicians of Philadelphia; ex-President of the American Dermatological Association. Fourth edition. Pp 625; 228 illustrations. Philadelphia and London: W. B. Saunders Company, 1922.

THE author's excellent book on *Diseases of the Skin* has forty-one additional pages more than in the last edition. The volume has been brought up to date by the following additions: Eczematoid Ringworm or Tinea of the Extremities; Copra Itch; Larva Migrans; Brown-tail Moth Dermatitis; Trichoptilosis; Granuloma Annulare; Purpura Annularis Telangiectodes; Sarcoid; Gangosa; Espundia; Paraffinoma; Leukemia Cutis.

The chapter on Roentgen-ray Therapy has been rewritten, giving the MacKee-unit method for the treatment of various cutaneous diseases. Syphilis has been much amplified, as the third edition of this book contained but twenty-five pages, and in the present volume this subject is covered in fifty-four pages. New pictures have been added under the following headings: Eczema, Pemphigus Vegetans, Herpes Zoster, Lichen Planus, Acne Necrotica, Pityriasis Rosea, Larva Migrans, Xeroderma Pigmentosum, Sarcoid, Syphilis, Yaws, Gangosa, Espundia (Leishmaniasis).

The volume is extremely readable and well edited. K.

PROGRESS

OF

MEDICAL SCIENCE

MEDICINE

UNDER THE CHARGE OF

W. S. THAYER, M.D.

PROFESSOR OF MEDICINE, JOHNS HOPKINS UNIVERSITY, BALTIMORE, MARYLAND,

AND

ROGER S. MORRIS, M.D.,

FREDERICK FORCHHEIMER PROFESSOR OF MEDICINE IN THE UNIVERSITY OF CINCINNATI, CINCINNATI, OHIO.

Prevention of Goiter.—McCLENDEN (*Science*, 1922, **56**, 269) emphasizes that the goiter belt seems to be a low iodide belt. Practically all the world's supply of iodin is now in the sea, where there is a calculated total of sixty billion metric tons. The writer, therefore, suggests the prevention of goiter by the use of table salt, made from sea-water. A less attractive possibility is the addition of powdered kelp for food.

Arteriosclerosis and Diet.—NEWBURGH and CLARKSON (*Jour. Am. Med. Assn.*, 1922, **79**, 1106) studied the bloodvessels of rabbits, which had been fed on diets containing various percentages of protein. Diets containing 27 and 36 per cent of protein were followed by internal changes which resembled true arteriosclerosis. Large groups of rabbits fed on normal vegetable diets failed to show such changes. The time of appearance and the severity of the vascular change were roughly proportional to the amount of protein fed and the duration of the feeding. All rabbits who ate high protein diets for six months or more showed extensive changes. It is not claimed that human arteriosclerosis is caused by a high protein diet. It is pointed out, however, that carnivorous animals show a higher incidence of arterial disease than do herbivorous.

Phthisiogenesis and Latent Tuberculous Infection.—OPIE (*Am. Rev. Tuberc.*, 1922, **6**, 525) states that pulmonary tuberculosis in early childhood is not selective; it affects any portion of the lung. It is progressive with almost no tendency to heal or to form fibrous tissue. The miliary form is common; 16 per cent of fatal cases die of meningitis. The incidence of pulmonary tuberculosis at autopsy on children (dead of other cause) agrees substantially with the incidence of infection as indicated by the von Pirquet skin test. Children sick with "masked" tuberculosis—"frequent coughs and colds, attacks of unexplained fever, loss of weight, anorexia and asthenia"—show a very high percentage of positive skin tests and complement-fixation tests. An absolute differentiation between latent tuberculous infection and clinical tuberculosis in children cannot be made. Primary intestinal tuberculosis is well recognized, but the bacillus leaves local lesions along its path of entry in Peyer's patches, mesenteric nodes, cervical nodes, etc. After the seventh or eighth year of life, lung lesion tends to become localized at the apex and the lesion is more fibrotic and more chronic, and is without the caseation of the bronchial lymph nodes, which is common in children. This type of lesion—latent apical infection—is easily differentiated from phthisis (chronic, fibrotic tuberculosis) and is "transformed into phthisis only when the tuberculous lesion becomes active and progressive." At autopsy this type of latent lesion occurs in one-sixth of the people dying from whatever cause. Adult phthisis may be and probably is occasionally acquired in childhood, as is strenuously maintained by von Behring, but by far the most of the children infected under one year of age soon die. The lesion in chronic lung tuberculosis is predominantly fibrotic rather than caseous or pneumonic, and it is probable that the ordinary case is one which has been infected, probably repeatedly, prior to the development of clinical phthisis. Many workers have reported fibrotic lesions (phthisis-like) in experimental animals which have been reinfected, but not in animals with primary infection. The primary infection in animals has more the appearance of the tuberculosis of infants and young children. Adults may become repeatedly infected, even though sources of infection are at times difficult or impossible to find. Most adult tuberculosis comes at a period when the childhood infections are healed. In adults the course is chronic and the disease fibrotic because the adult has a relative immunity from a former infection. Adult phthisis seems to come usually from infection through the air passages. The extensive experiments of Calmette do not convince one that phthisis necessarily arises from infection through the intestinal tract. It has been found that from 350 to more than 500 times the number of tubercle bacilli are required for infecting an animal by ingestion as by inhalation. Sputum from phthisis remains a great source of danger, as does also contaminated milk.

Pernicious Anemia and Protein Sensitization.—Faber (*La presse méd.*, 1922, **81**, 873) for several years had good results in the treatment of pernicious anemia from the administration of fermented milk (kefir). It was thought that the action of this kefir might be due to its protein effect. Therefore a case of pernicious anemia which failed to respond to the ordinary methods of treatment was when almost moribund given an intramuscular injection of 5 cc of sterilized milk. There was an intense immediate reaction with a high fever, which was followed shortly by a very marked subjective and objective improvement. Subsequent cases similarly treated have shown various results but some have been definitely improved. These observations led Faber to some very interesting speculations concerning the pathogenesis of pernicious anemia. He summarizes the familiar arguments for the origin of pernicious anemia in an intestinal intoxication. He points out that the achylia, which is known frequently to precede the onset of the anemia, will permit an abnormally abundant bacterial flora in the part of the intestine in which absorption is most rapid and will also permit the proteins of the food to reach the small intestine practically unchanged. Thus he thinks proteins may be absorbed as such and sensitization result. He suggests then that pernicious anemia may be a "sort of chronic alimentary anaphylaxis" and that the relapses and remissions may be due to variations in the immunity of the organism.

Reticulated Erythrocytes.—KRUMBHAAR (*Jour. Lab. and Clin. Med.*, 1922, **8**, 11) suggests the word "Reticulocyte" to designate red blood cells revealing a reticulum by methods of vital staining and that when the normal percentage of those cells in the peripheral blood is exceeded the condition be designated "Reticulosis." He reports that in experimental plethora in dogs the reticulated cells are greatly diminished. The normal variation in reticulated cells in the human adult is from 0.1 to 1 per cent. Infants show an increased percentage during the first week of life. By the end of the first week the picture should resemble that of the adult. It is pointed out that the degree of reticulosis is a better index of the functional activity of the bone marrow than the study of polychromatophilia or nucleated forms.

Erythropoietic Action of Germanium Dioxide.—KAST, CROLL and SCHMITZ (*Jour. Lab. and Clin. Med.*, 1922, **7**, 643) treated 16 cases of anemia with germanium dioxide. They gave 100 to 200 mg. daily or every two or three days until about 1 gm. had been given. An apparent erythropoietic action was observed in several of these cases. The most marked changes in red count and hemoglobin occurred in anemia secondary to hemorrhage. Total solids in the blood were increased, but not sufficiently to explain the increase in red cells on the ground of decrease in plasma volume. No deleterious effects of the drug were noted.

Intravitam Bone Marrow Studies.—MORRIS and FALCONER (*Arch. Int. Med.*, 1922, **30**, 485) have devised a drill for trephining long bones to secure living bone marrow for histological and cultural study. They have obtained marrow specimens from numerous animals without untoward results. The marrow obtained by this method showed the same characteristics as were visible in sections of the marrow made after killing the animal. The authors feel that this method of examination can be used safely in human beings and that it might throw much light on early phases of obscure blood diseases.

Etiology of Scarlet Fever.—BLISS (*Jour. Exper. Med.*, 1922, **36**, 575) reports further studies of scarlet fever strains of streptococcus. Contrary to the traditional idea that this organism is present in many but not in all cases of scarlet fever, Bliss reports its occurrence in 100 per cent of scarlatina patients during the first week of the disease. While these organisms had no special morphological or cultural criteria, and in fact varied in their growth characteristics, 80 per cent of them were identical as regards their reaction to specific agglutinating sera. Of special interest was a strain recovered from a mastoid infection with a scarlet rash, which serologically fell into the scarlatinal group of strains. The writer is very conservative in interpreting his findings, but implies that a special group of hemolytic streptococci is at least an invariable concomitant of scarlet fever.

Thyroid Function. — Marine (*Phys. Reviews*, 1922, 2) reviews our present knowledge of the functions of the thyroid gland. He points out that the thyroid has been shown to develop from a single ventral tubular down-growth of pharyngeal endoderm. The so-called "lateral thyroid anlagen," formerly believed to form the lateral thyroid lobes, are accidental inclusions which later undergo atrophy. A review of the literature shows that the relation between the number of mitochondrial granules and the pharmacological activity of the gland is not generally accepted in view of the abundance of these granules in the thyroid in myxedema. Thyroid adenomata are believed to develop from cell rests which atrophy under normal conditions but which form adenomata under certain conditions calling for increased thyroid activity. Thyroidectomy in animals has resulted in an average maximum reduction in total metabolism of 35 to 40 per cent, which figure "corresponds closely to that observed in the severest forms of human cretinism and myxedema and may be designated as the myxedema level." A close interrelationship of suprarenal cortex and thyroid has been observed, and Marine believes that exophthalmic goiter is intimately involved with cortical exhaustion and epinephrin stimulation. The review includes a survey of our present knowledge of the bearing of iodine metabolism upon the physiology of the thyroid gland and of the interrelationship of the thyroid and the other glands of internal secretion. The paper is brief and the clinician will find it well worth the reading in detail.

THERAPEUTICS

UNDER THE CHARGE OF

SAMUEL W. LAMBERT, M.D.,

NEW YORK,

AND

CHARLES C. LIEB, M.D.,

ASSISTANT PROFESSOR OF PHARMACOLOGY, COLUMBIA UNIVERSITY.

Report on Artificial Pneumothorax.—Burrell and MacNalty (*Medical Research Council.* Special Report No. 67, abstracted as one of the leading articles in the *British Medical Journal*, September 30, 1922, p. 606) in the first part of the report discuss pneumothorax from all aspects and give a summary of Burrell's first 150 cases. It is found that patients with a low resistance and in whom the disease is progressing rapidly are but little benefited by the operation; patients with high power of resistance usually do well with sanitorium or other medical treatment. It is in the intermediate cases (those in whom the disease is subacute and in whom the healthier lung is not too seriously involved) that artificial pneumothorax offers the greatest hope of permanent benefit. The risks of the operation are so slight and the danger of the disease spreading so great, that all patients of this class are entitled to the probable benefit afforded by the operation. Burrell's 150 cases may be divided into three classes: in the first group, an efficient pneumothorax was produced; in the second, only a partial pneumothorax was induced and in the third, none was obtained because of the pleural adhesions. There were 107 cases in the first group; in 40 the disease was arrested and in 22 there was improvement. The result in the other groups was not nearly so good. The second part of the report consists of the answers to a questionnaire sent to sixteen British physicians. The replies indicate that these physicians are unanimous in their approval of pneumothorax as a therapeutic measure, and their approval gains weight when it is learned that these sixteen physicians have induced pneumothorax in 14,000 to 15,000 patients. There is a difference of opinion as to which patients are most suited for the collapse treatment; but the general consensus of opinion appears to be that after institutional treatment has been given a fair trial, as soon as it is noted that the disease is not responding, pneumothorax should be induced. The collapse treatment shows that the first essential to the arrest of active pulmonary tuberculosis is immobilization and the more complete the rest given the tuberculous lung, the better the healing. Thus the same principle is applicable to surgical and pulmonary tuberculosis, and that is, rest.

The Intratracheal Injection of Oils for Diagnostic and Therapeutic Purposes.—Corper and Freed (*Jour. Am. Med. Assn.*, 1922, **79**, 1739) studied the effects produced by the intratracheal injection of small quantities (0.05 to 1 cc) of some oils that have been highly recommended in the treatment of tuberculosis. Some of these substances have hitherto been regarded as quite harmless to the pulmonary tissue and of considerable bactericidal power; others were thought to be sufficiently irritant to elicit a mild fibrosis which promoted the healing of the diseased area (lung abscess, bronchiectasis, etc.). Corper and Freed found that the injection of so-called "bland" oils is accompanied by grave danger. Chaulmoogra oil and the mixed esters of chaulmoogra oil are, when injected into rabbits, intensely irritant and cause profound pathological changes in the lung which may range from acute pneumonic consolidation with abscess formation to a proliferative bronchopneumonia, depending on the localization of these oils in the lung and on their concentration. Even so dilute a solution as 10 per cent chaulmoogra oil in olive oil or liquid petrolatum produces a distinct proliferative bronchopneumonia. Olive oil or liquid petrolatum injected intratracheally is aspirated into the pulmonary alveoli and may remain there unabsorbed for months causing a mild type of localized pneumonia. It is probable that the local application of one of these oils to the larynx or to a bronchus through the use of the bronchoscope, is followed by the aspiration of the oil from the site of application and by its distribution throughout the adjacent alveoli. The conclusion that seems obvious is that even "inert" oils are dangerous when aspirated, and that the greatest care must be used in introducing any foreign body into the normal or diseased lung.

Temporary Disturbances of the Circulation and Respiration Due to Local Anesthetics.—The object of the studies reported by Ross (*Jour. Lab. and Clin. Med.*, 1922, **8**, 1) was the determination of the changes occurring in the respiratory and circulatory systems when the commonly used local anesthetics were applied to animals by the same methods that are used in medical practice. The local anesthestics (cocain and procain) were injected into the tonsillar tissue or painted on the pharynx; the epinephrin was injected submucously into the tonsils. The submucous injection of epinephrin (adrenalin) elicited practically no effects, raising blood-pressure only 8 per cent and accelerating breathing by 16 per cent. Cocain injections had a more marked effect, elevating arterial blood-pressure by 83 per cent and venous pressure by 100 per cent; the heart rate was increased only 3 per cent and respiration 9 per cent. When both epinephrin and cocain were injected into the same tonsil, profound circulatory and respiratory changes ensued; arterial pressure rose 233 per cent, and venous pressure 467 per cent; the heart rate declined 18 per cent and respiratory rate was doubled. The preliminary injection of atropin and morphin lessened these striking changes to a slight degree only. In another series of experiments cocain (20 per cent) was painted on the pharynx and subsequently epinephrin was injected into the tonsils. The effects on circulation and respiration were greater than when epinephrin alone was injected but much less than when both the epinephrin and cocain were injected together. Procain (20 per cent) when swabbed on the tonsils and pharynx caused no definite reduction in the effects of cocain-epinephrin injection. Ross draws the following conclusions: The submucous injection of epinephrin and cocain into the tonsillar tissue brings on systemic reactions similar to those that follow the intravenous injection of these drugs, and causes an enormous increase in arterial and venous pressures. The latter is increased more than twice as much as the former, and the great rise in venous pressure may cause cerebral asphyxia and thus explain all the temporary disturbances that occur in medical practice after the use of local anesthetics. Cocain and epinephrin injected submucously are powerful synergists. Sufficient cocain is absorbed from sponging the pharynx with a 20 per cent solution to increase markedly the sensitiveness to epinephrin. Novocain and epinephrin are not synergists and novocain does not materially neutralize the extent of the synergistic action of cocain and epinephrin.

PEDIATRICS

UNDER THE CHARGE OF

THOMPSON S. WESTCOTT, M.D., AND ALVIN E. SIEGEL, M.D.,
OF PHILADELPHIA.

The Rate of Secretion of Breast Milk.—SMITH and MERRITT (*Am. Jour. Dis. Children*, 1922, **24**, 413) from their observations noted that nursing infants obtain the greater part of their feeding of breast milk in the first few minutes, from 40 to 60 per cent in the first two minutes and from 60 to 85 per cent in the first four minutes. This holds true whether the supply is abundant, moderate or scanty. After eight minutes very few babies get any milk whatever. Only 17 of their observations showed any increase in weight after eight minutes. Fourteen of these were from good feedings and only 3 of them obtained milk after ten minutes. A few large vigorous infants nursing from an abundant supply, may get small amounts of milk up to sixteen minutes. The babies who needed both breasts usually got less from the second breast than from the first, except where one breast regularly yielded a better supply. The rate at which a baby gets milk from the second breast is similar to that of the first breast. After that time very little is obtained. The time after which a baby gets no more milk from the second breast is usually shorter than on the first breast. The poor feedings are usually completed in a shorter time than the good ones. When the breast supply is evidently failing, the baby gets all that he will get in from three to five minutes as a rule. It does no good to leave a baby a longer time at breast in hopes that by so doing an additional amount will be ingested. If a baby empties the breast in from five to eight minutes and shows no evidence of discomfort from an adequate feeding obtained in that time, there seems to be no good reason why he should not take his bottle in the same time. If the nipple holes are of good size so that the milk flows freely, nearly all strong infants will finish the bottle in less than ten minutes. They evidence less distress than the nurse does over the rapid feeding. On the other hand a slow nipple either discourages the infant so that he will give up in disgust before he has finished, or else make him swallow so much air that he vomits or has colic.

Faulty Diet and Its Relation to the Structure of Bone.—SHIPLEY (*Jour. Am. Med. Assn.*, 1922, **79**, 1563) says that there are several dietetic principles concerned in the growth of bone. First there is an uncharacterized organic substance which is distinct from fat soluble A. This is found in certain oils principally those of the cod, burbot and shark livers in large amounts. It is present in very small quantities in butter fat and in cocoanut oil. Fat soluble A is missing from the latter of these. It may belong to the group of the vitamins, and is known to be much more resistant to heat and oxidation than fat soluble A. Other essential principles are calcium, phosphorus, water soluble B and fat soluble A. Water soluble C was found to influence the structure of the bone of the guinea-pig, but the rat either does not need this substance or is able to synthesize it. The writer was able to show that the lack of fat soluble A was not responsible for the developing of rickets. Bones of animals whose diet is adequate except for fat soluble A are perfectly calcified, but a high degree of osteoporosis develops. The same result follows the administration of diets having a deficiency only in water soluble B. When this factor is deficient there is also an aplasia of the marrow, such as follows complete starvation, and later there is hemorrhage into the medullary cavity. If a guinea-pig is deprived of water soluble C, his bones are identical with those of a rat which has been given an insufficient supply of water soluble B. When the organic factor mentioned before is absent from the diet or only present in small quantities, all other factors being so far as can be ascertained in optimal concentration, any variation in the ratio between calcium and phosphorus results in a profound disturbance in the structure and functional capacity of the skeleton. A disease of the osseous system which has the clinical and pathological characteristics of rickets may be induced in rats by diet. It may be induced by diets which are within certain limits low either in phosphorus or in calcium, all other dietary factors being maintained at the optimal level for growth and function. If the organic factor which is so abundantly present in fish oils is supplied freely, rickets will not develop in spite of a faulty ratio of calcium to phosphorus in the food. Cod-liver oil will protect against rickets, or cause the healing of the lesion even if the salt content of the diet is such that rickets will invariably develop without the oil. It was found that animals were enabled to compensate for faulty calcium-phosphorus ratiosin the diet if they were exposed to the rays of the sun or to the iron-chromium or cadmium arcs or to the light of the mercury vapor quartz lamp. The same changes are induced under the influence of the rays as by cod-liver oil.

Immunization Against Measles.—HERMANN (*Arch. Pediat.*, 1922, **39**, 607) claims that 75 per cent of the deaths from measles occur in infants under two years of age, and 90 per cent under five years. He feels that any method of immunization which aims to control or eradicate this disease must be employed in early infancy on all or nearly all children. Infants, whose mothers have had measles are relatively immune during the first five months of life. This immunity gradually disappears, but in many it persists to the sixth or eighth month. The immune bodies in the mother's blood are probably conveyed to the fetus through the placental circulation. Artificially fed, as well as breast fed babies enjoy this relative immunity. It is not conveyed to any great extent through the breast milk, for infants of six or more months, who are still nursed are just as susceptible as bottle fed babies. In measles the infectious material is regularly present in an active form in the nasal discharge from twenty-four to forty-eight hours before the eruption begins. It is not necessary to isolate and identify the infectious material, or to obtain its growth in pure culture, in order to immunize against the infection. In measles the infectious material is conveyed usually from the nasal mucous membrane of the patient to the nasal mucous membrane of the child infected. Immunization follows the same path. The nasal mucous discharge of patients, free from other diseases, is taken from twenty-four to forty-eight hours before the appearance of the eruption. It is mixed with a small amount of normal saline solution, and bacteria and other extraneous material separated by centrifugalization. If passed through a Berkfeld filter, the organisms are eliminated but the virus loses some of its potency and cannot be depended upon for the purpose of immunization. A little tricresol is added as a preservative. A few drops of this solution is applied to the nasal mucous membrane of the child to be immunized. Only healthy infants between four and five months are immunized. The method attempts to convert the temporary relative immunity into an immunity which persists during the first few years when the disease is the most dangerous. The best results are obtained in those cases in which a rise in temperature follows on the eighth to the sixteenth day.

Congenital Hypertrophic Pyloric Stenosis and Its Treatment by Atropin.—HAAS (*Jour. Am. Med. Assn.*, 1922, **79**, 1314).says that uncertainty of etiology is the cause of the differences of opinion in treatment. Medical treatment was formerly practised until the Rammstedt operation caused surgery to be advocated exclusively. To see and to feel a pyloric tumor, he thinks, and to observe the histologic appearance makes faith in any other view difficult. He thinks, nevertheless, that the problem is a medical one, and that atropin is practically a specific. He holds that pyloric stenosis is only an advanced degree of pylorospasm. It is only a single manifestation of a general hypertonic state, whose etiologic factor is an overaction of the vagus portion of the autonomic nervous system. There is usually an excitability of severe degree of all motor functions. This condition has been described variously as the hypertonic infant, myotonia, myotonia spastica perstans, arthrogryposis, essential contractures, pseudotetanus, tetanoid conditions, infantile tetany, spasmophilia and vagotonia. Experimental work supports this view. Further support is found in the reports of cure by other than surgical methods. Differential diagnosis between pylorospasm and pyloric stenosis is practically impossible. The symptoms of pyloric stenosis are projectile vomiting, visible peristalsis, constipation, starvation stools, rapid loss of weight and pyloric tumor. Closer observation will reveal pallor, lividity, loss of turgor, circumoral cyanosis, cold, clammy, cyanotic hands and feet, subnormal temperature unless obscured by starvation elevation, and spasm not only of the pylorus but often of the larynx, pharynx, esophagus, cardia and various portions of the intestines. There is also hypertonicity of the skeletal muscles. Irritation of the infant nervous system produces an effect predominantly stimulating. An inhibiting effect is virtually absent. In the treatment certain points should be observed. Errors in diet or hygiene must be corrected. In advanced cases saline must be given subcutaneously at frequent intervals, until enough fluid is taken by mouth to supply body needs. Atropin, like digitalis, must be active. In the milder cases the drug may be given by mouth or in the bottle, and in breast-fed babies in a teaspoonful of water, before feeding. In the severe cases the drug must be administered hypodermically until vomiting is controlled. The dose is variable, from $\frac{1}{1000}$ grain at each feeding up to a maximum which either controls symptoms or produces physiologic reaction. Treatment may be required only for a few weeks or it may be necessary for the most of the first year. Few cases require a smaller dose to begin with. Occasionally constipation with severe tenesmus occurs. This is relieved by the omission of a few doses of atropin. The author bases this report upon more than forty cases.

Toxin-antitoxin Immunization Against Diphtheria.—PARK (*Jour. Am. Med. Assn.*, 1922, **79**, 1584) has had twenty-five years of experimental and practical experience in the immunizing effect of toxin-antitoxin injections, and has made many Schick tests. He has found that three injections of a suitable toxin-antitoxin, 1 cc each, at intervals of one or two weeks, will cause about 85 per cent of susceptible children or older persons to develop sufficient antitoxin to give the negative Schick reaction and produce marked if not absolute protection against diphtheria. The development of the immunity is slow. The amount of antitoxin sufficient to prevent the positive Schick reaction develops in the different children in from one to six months after receiving the injections. Antitoxin as heretofore must continue to be used to produce immunity immediately. The duration of the immunity in at least 90 per cent of the children is for more than six years and probably for the remainder of life. There seems to be no difference between these and those who develop antitoxin naturally. Toxin-antitoxin injections should not be given without an interval of two weeks having elapsed since the administration of antitoxin. Otherwise the toxin is slightly overneutralized and the resulting development of antitoxin is lessened. Mixtures made from old toxin and antitoxin are fairly stable and may be used for a period of one year. Even such preparations are at their best when first sent out, as the mixtures slowly tend to become at first neutralized and then slightly antitoxic. This change gradually lessens the immunizing power of the toxin. The toxin-antitoxin should be kept cool and in a dark place. It is best to use the mixtures within three months of final preparation. A toxin-antitoxin mixture of stabilized materials which is safe when it leaves the laboratory cannot become toxic on being kept. The Schick test is an extremely reliable means of separating the individuals who have antitoxic immunity from those that have none. Although it is a simple test, it must be carried out with extreme care. The toxin must be retained intracutaneously, and the toxin must be neither 25 per cent more or less than the desired amount. It is extremely important to choose a glass of suitable chemical composition for the containers in which the toxin is to be placed, as rapid deterioration may ensue from improper containers. The preliminary Schick test is usually omitted in children under three years of age. Two-thirds of these require the toxin-antitoxin anyway. It is not certain that those who give negative reactions are immune. In school work the Schick test is usually omitted up to the sixth year, because it is easier to inject the children than to wait for the test. After the sixth year the preliminary Schick test should be made whenever possible. No child should be pronounced immune upon receiving three injections of toxin-antitoxin. A negative Schick test is absolutely necessary before one can be certain. The toxin-antitoxin injections are inadvisable before six months of age. During this time most infants retain the antitoxin received from their mothers. Up to the age of three months immunizing injections are usually ineffective. During the first three years there is almost no annoyance from the injections.

DERMATOLOGY AND SYPHILIS

UNDER THE CHARGE OF

JOHN H. STOKES, M.D.,

MAYO CLINIC, ROCHESTER, MINN.

Agglutination of Red Blood Cells by Arsphenamin.—OLIVER, DOUGLASS and YAMADA (*Jour. Pharm. and Exper. Therap.*, 1922, **19**, 187, 199 and 393) have been conducting important studies on the effect of arsphenamin solutions upon the blood stream, which illuminate the mechanism of reaction to this drug under therapeutic conditions. They find, following the work of Karsner and Hanslick, that arsphenamin as a chemical substance in colloid suspension produces an agglutination of red blood cells. This property is shared by other colloids, such as acacia and gelatin, and may explain the anaphalactoid reactions which follow their use in intravenous injection. Oliver and Douglas succeeded in showing that the agglutinative power of arsphenamin solution is markedly increased by the presence of an electrolyte, such as sodium chloride, and the agglutinative power can be inhibited by colloids such as are present in blood serum. The agglutinative titer of arsphenamin seems to be fairly constant for red blood cells. The reaction is most marked in human cells and least marked in chicken cells. The arsphenamin is absorbed by the red blood cells, but no agglutination occurs except in the presence of an electrolyte. There is a drop in the tier of salt dilutions of arsphenamin if they stand in the open air. It is furthermore demonstrable that a physical change in the degree of dispersion of arsphenamin results when an electrolyte is added to the drug in solution. These authors, therefore, suggest that the action of the electrolyte, in producing an agglutination of red blood cells is primarily upon the absorbed arsphenamin of sensitized cells. In a subsequent article Oliver and Yamada demonstrated a protective effect of many hydrophilic colloids.

Cause of Early Arsphenamin Reactions.—In a subsequent article (*Jour. Pharm. and Exper. Therap.*, 1922, **19**, 393) OLIVER and YAMADA take up experimental studies into the relation of this peculiarity of arsphenamin solutions to the clinical reactions produced by the drug. They differentiate arsphenamin reactions into early and late types, a distinction which has long been clinically recognized, and point out that the early reactions partake distinctly of the so-called anaphylactoid characteristics; while the late reactions exhibit the ill-effects incident upon the chemical base of the drug (arsenic). In a study of a series of rabbits following acute arsphenamin death, they succeeded in showing that even after use of the disodium arsphenamin salt, now so widely advocated for intravenous administration, agglutination of red blood cells occurs. They succeeded in showing that the characteristic pathologic picture of acute arsphenamin death is that of wholesale agglutination of red blood cells with the formation of multiple emboli in the terminal capillaries. Where the agglutination is minimal death does not occur immediately and the development of secondary reaction phenomena following embolism can be observed. The paper contains a series of very beautiful photographic demonstrations of the accuracy of the authors' work. Controlled studies of the effect of intravenous injection of red blood cells previously agglutinated *in vitro* by arsphenamin yielded the same clinical pictures and similar pathologic findings. The authors point out that acute arsphenamin death is identical with the clinical picture of multiple embolism as produced by the intravenous injection of oils and liquid fat, the emboli in the case of arsphenamin being composed of agglutinated red blood cells. This agglutination of red blood cells is in accord with that observed in the studies above mentioned and arises from the physical characteristics of the arsphenamin solution rather than its chemical composition. This work unites in a comprehensive study of arsphenamin reaction the observations of a number of observers. The increased pulmonary pressure noted as a feature of arsphenamin administration by Jackson and Smith, and Bissell's observations on the pulmonary pressure in fat embolism are shown to be comparable, and due to the formation of multiple emboli in the pulmonary capillaries. It has been shown that the physical properties of the arsphenamin solution are markedly influenced by the presence and efficiency of protective colloids, the character and concentration of electrolytes present and the hydrogen-ion concentration. The authors are extending their study to the late reactions to arsphenamin in the hope of ascertaining whether the physical properties of the drug have any bearing upon these reactions and of confirming the observation of observers such as Kolmer and Lucke. The authors are convinced from their observations that there is a purely chemical as distinguished from a physical factor in the late reactions to arsphenamin.

[Editor's Note.—In studies of the histologic changes produced experimentally in rabbits by arsphenamin and neoarsphenamin, Kolmer and Lucke (*Arch. Dermatol. and Syph.*, 1921, **3**, 483) found agglutination thrombi similar to those here described, but marked focal necroses as well.]

Arsenic Distribution following Arsphenamin Treatment of Children.—Clausen and Jeans (*Am. Jour. Syph.*, 1922, **6**, 567) report the result of a series of determinations of the distribution and excretion of arsenic following arsphenamin administration in children, using the analytical method of Gutzeit (modified). "Arsphenamin rapidly disappears from the blood, but 10 per cent remaining in one hour. In the blood it is present exclusively in the plasma. The organs taking up the largest amounts are the liver and the small and large intestine. The excretion begins immediately, is very rapid at first, gradually diminishing until at the end of two weeks only traces are found. However, at the end of two or even three weeks 50 per cent is still stored in the tissues. It is excreted five times as rapidly in the stools as in the urine. The curve of excretion *via* the urine is a peculiar one and is evidently a composite of two curves. It seems likely that the curve of excretion *via* the stools would be of the same type, if the stools could be collected accurately at stated intervals. The amount of arsenic found in the cerebrospinal fluid is greater in the first hour (in some cases two hours) after the intravenous administration. The amount of arsenic found in the cerebrospinal fluid seems to depend upon the amount of inflammation present. In some children with no evidence of neurosyphilis no arsenic was found. The greatest amounts were found in those cases with evidence of the most active inflammation. Much more was found in infants with neurosyphilis than in older children similarly affected, which may explain the occasional need for intraspinal therapy (Swift-Ellis) in older children. In all patients was noted a diminishing amount of arsenic in the cerebrospinal fluid at succeeding injections and for the same time intervals. The arsenic content of the spinal fluid is at least as great in cases of cerebrospinal syphilis after intravenous administration of arsphenamin as would result from the intrathecal injection of arsphenamin serum according to the Swift-Ellis technic." It was also noted that no arsphenamin was present in the skeletal muscles, but that the drug was present in the heart muscle of the kitten.

Cause of Hutchinson's Teeth.—NICHOLAS, MASSIA and DUPASQUIER (*Ann. de dermat. et syphil.*, 1922, **3**, 321), in an extensive and interesting review, have endeavored to collect and correlate facts and observations tending to relate a group of clinical manifestations of osseous syphilis with one of the embryonal anlagen of the bones of the face, the "incisor bud" which as part of the frontal prominence, has an origin different from the lateral parts of the upper jaw; the latter originate according to some authorities from the first branchial arch. This conception is of particular interest as applied to the origin of Hutchinson's teeth. These the authors regard as the products of a dystrophic influence upon the embryonal anlagen, and not as either a syphilid in the strict sense or as the result of damage to the developing teeth. They suggest that the dystrophic injury is to the "incisor bud" and not to the tooth germ as such. This accounts for the appearance of Hutchinsonian lateral incisors as well as central incisors, and explains also the existence of aplasias. The authors further suggest that future studies may suggest a relationship between the dysplasias of this region in heredosyphilis and cite Hutinel's observations on their possible relation to endocrine dysfunction. The authors collected 19 cases, including 3 of their own, in which late gummatous changes were so exactly limited to the region developed from the "incisor bud" (intermaxillary bone) as to support strongly the belief that this part of the jaw and face preserves even in the adult a certain amount of autonomy in its reaction to the Spirocheta pallida, and justifies the term "syndrome of the incisor bud." They emphasize that treatment is primarily medical treatment for syphilis, and not surgical intervention. The possibility of confusion of the gummatous process with alveolar abscess and maxillary cyst is pointed out.

OBSTETRICS

UNDER THE CHARGE OF

EDWARD P. DAVIS, A.M., M.D.,

PROFESSOR OF OBSTETRICS IN THE JEFFERSON MEDICAL COLLEGE, PHILADELPHIA.

The Coagulability of the Blood During Pregnancy and in the New Born.—Falls (*Jour. Am. Med. Assn.*, 1922, **79**, 1816) divides hemorrhage complicating parturition into maternal and that of the new born. The mother loses a quantity of blood in labor which varies greatly. In 3 per cent of all cases the bleeding is serious. The amount of loss varies from 500 cc to 2 liters or more. The effect of hemorrhage in the parturient woman cannot be foretold and is not dependent upon the quantity of blood loss. We recognize that hemorrhage in both mother and child occurs from mechanical or chemical causes. The latter, the writer thinks, is confined to the new born. In this he apparently neglects the toxemia of pregnancy which produces important chemical changes in the mother's blood. He cites hemophilia as very rare in the female members of a family, but transmitted through them to the male members. Postpartum hemorrhages have been observed clinically much more frequently in patients who were delivered under ether anesthesia than in patients who had no anesthesia. A study of the blood was made to determine whether anesthesia by ether changed the coagulability of the blood. The results of these studies show that the coagulability of the blood in women before, during and after labor, when estimated by the coagulation, calcium and prothrombin tests, is within the limits of normal blood coagulability. There is the same coagulation time for the blood of mother and child. There is no evidence from these studies that pregnancy predisposes to a condition of the blood favorable for hemorrhage and certainly not to hemophilia. Postpartum hemorrhage can very rarely be ascribed to such a cause. In the normal fetus at birth the blood clots with normal rapidity and firmness. Subsequent tendencies to hemorrhage cannot be detected by coagulation tests made soon after birth. Patients who took ether had the same coagulation time as those who did not, and hence postpartum hemorrhage must depend upon something else than alteration in the coagulability of the blood occasioned by ether.

Infectious Abortion and the Human Subject.—In the *Lancet*, November 4, 1922, **2**, 979, the reports of various observers upon infectious abortion in cows and the possibility of its communication to the human subject are discussed. It will be remembered that an organism known as B. abortus was isolated in 1890 by Bang, and thought to be the cause of infectious abortion in cattle. This germ can be cultivated with difficulty and compared with other well-known bacteria is remarkably inert. Another similar germ was discovered in mares. Both of these are thought to produce infectious abortion. As regards the human subject, the organism found in bovine cases is also present in many instances in milk; and such milk injected into guinea-pigs produces disease. The question whether this germ can produce pathological conditions in the human subject has been raised by Moore, because the organism has been found in the throat and tonsils of children. Larsen and Sedgwick, in examining 425 children, found this germ in 6 per cent. Antibodies were found in the blood in these cases, thus demonstrating the pathological character of the germ. It has further been shown by Evans that the bacillus of infectious abortion in cattle is closely related to the germ of Malta fever. The bacillus producing Malta fever can and not infrequently does infect the human body. The study of these cases suggest a very practical point, namely—that there are many causes of abortion in the human subject not clearly defined, and that some obscure cases may be caused by the bacilli described in this paper, conveyed through milk or drinking water.

The Use of Salvarsan During Pregnancy with a Fatal Result.—In the *Zentralblatt für Gynäkologie*, 1922, No. 41, p. 1634, Kirstein describes an unusual case as follows: The patient was in her second pregnancy at eight months and had a contracted and rachitic pelvis. She came to the clinic evidently syphilitic. There was slight edema of the under portion of the thighs and abdomen; the urine contained no albumin. She was sent to a clinic for the treatment of venereal disease. In twenty days she was given 3 cc of a preparation known as cyarsal-Riedel, 2 cc kontraluisin and 1.35 cc neosalvarsan. About six weeks later there was an eruption over both breasts and the urine contained a trace of albumin. The eruption speedily disappeared and the patient was twice given injections of kontraluisin and 0.45 cc of neosalvarsan; in all 1.8 cc of neosalvarsan. Four days after the giving of the last dose the urine was evidently albuminous, and an exanthem developed over the entire body, beginning with irritation in the region of the breasts and occasioning a great deal of itching and annoyance. The patient became very cold, had violent cough and nasal catarrh. A few days later the whole body was covered with small reddish blotches, followed by moderate fever. Labor pains developed and the patient was brought to the obstetric clinic. In addition to the eruption of the skin there was edema of the face, but the urine was free from albumin. Labor slowly developed, the membranes ruptured and there were evidences of birth pressure in the feeble heart sounds and the escape of meconium. Dilatation of the cervix was but partially accomplished, and after a tedious labor a normally developed living child was born, in spontaneous labor. The placenta was naturally expelled about an hour afterward, and twenty minutes later the patient had a chill followed by fever of 104.5° F. An illness of fourteen days followed with fever without chills and the presence in the vaginal discharge on the

second day of hemolytic staphylococci in great abundance. Blood cultures on the second, nineth and fourteenth days were sterile. The patient died on the fourteenth day, having developed symptoms of catarrhal pneumonia, double femoral thrombosis and septic infection. Autopsy showed influenza-pneumonia and also an infection of the genital tract. In the right wall of the uterus there were two small abscesses connecting with the venous channels of the uterus. On closer study of the case, there was no evidence that the pneumonia was metastatic. There could be no question but that the results of the salvarsan treatment contributed greatly to the fatal issue. The writer has collected 9 deaths in parturient women following the use of salvarsan. In these cases, hemorrhagic encephalitis was the cause. Meirowski reports 20 deaths from salvarsan, where in 12 there was no doubt concerning the cause; in 5 a possible question, and in 3 the salvarsan had only an indirect effect. In the writer's clinic 39 syphilitic pregnant women have been treated, and neosalvarsan has been used in a total quantity amounting to 3.15 G. In only 1 case was there fever, and that patient received inunctions of mercury in addition.

GYNECOLOGY

UNDER THE CHARGE OF

JOHN G. CLARK, M.D.,

PROFESSOR OF GYNECOLOGY IN THE UNIVERSITY OF PENNSYLVANIA, PHILADELPHIA,

AND

FRANK B. BLOCK, M.D.,

INSTRUCTOR IN GYNECOLOGY, MEDICAL SCHOOL, UNIVERSITY OF PENNSYLVANIA, PHILADELPHIA.

Myomectomy.—For the past several years the operation of myomectomy, as opposed to hysterectomy, seems to have been regaining some of its lost popularity and perhaps the foremost advocate of this operation has been MAYO (*Minnesota Med.*, 1922, **21**, 235). He prefaces his argument by stating that the menstrual cycle, aside from its function in reproduction, has a marked effect on the female during the period between puberty and menopause. All surgeons have seen the shrinkage of the uterus and shortening of the vagina accompanied by trophic changes which follow ovariectomy. The nervous and psychic changes of the normal menopause are aggravated in young women by operations which check the menstrual flow. The effect on the patient is essentially the same, whether menstruation is stopped by removing the ovaries and leaving the uterus, or removing the uterus and leaving the ovaries, according to Mayo's observations. It is probable, he thinks, that menstruation itself has some important endocrine function. Conservation of the reproductive function is of first importance, but conservation of the ovary for the continuance of its internal secretion and its effect on the production of menstruation is second only to the generative function. Even if reproduction is impossible, conservation of the ovary or some portion of it for the sole purpose of continuing menstruation is of the greatest importance. The technic of hysterectomy has been so thoroughly organized and perfected that there is a tendency to perform the operation so readily that many patients are deprived not only of the right to motherhood; but also of the function of menstruation, which is so important to the endocrine system. Hysterectomy is seldom necessary for benign myoma in a woman under thirty-five years, and demands an excellent reason in a woman under thirty. It has been argued against myomectomy that it is a more dangerous operation than hysterectomy, but the mortality in the series of the Mayo Clinic of 909 cases with 7 deaths was a trifle under 1 per cent (0.7 per cent). In cases of abdominal myomectomy the mortality was 0.5 per cent. Vaginal myomectomy gave a death rate of 2.7 per cent on account of the infection present. The statement has been made that often myomas develop after myomectomy. Only 2.56 per cent required secondary operations. In more than half of these the second operation was performed five or more years after the myomectomy, and in 1, thirteen years afterward. More than half the secondary operations were performed for inflammatory disease and in no case was a malignant condition found. In the cases in which a second operation was performed for recurrence of the myomas, the use of radium would probably be considered now. In none of the cases reported were the recurrent tumors large, because the patients, knowing their former condition, were on the alert. Hysterectomy was usually performed at the second operation, but the patient had been carried along by the myomectomy to an age in which a radical operation is of less consequence. While considering this report from the Mayo Clinic, it will be of interest to review a series of 100 consecutive myomectomies which have been reported by BONNEY (*Lancet*, 1922, **2**, 745), a well known British gynecologist. He states that neither the number nor the position of the tumors within the uterus, nor the presence of degeneration, nor the accompaniment of menorrhagia or pregnancy are a bar to the successful performance of the operation. He believes, however, that patients suffering from profound anemia due to fibroids should not be treated by myomectomy, because in them the continuance of even normal periods is undesirable, so much is their blood content depleted. Moderate menorrhagic anemia however, does not contraindicate myomectomy, provided the operation is carried out so that all the tumors are removed and the uterus left behind is not too big for the involution that occurs after myomectomy to restore it to normality. One of the risks urged against myomectomy is that of menorrhagia continuing after operation, but where this occurs it is nearly always due to the surgeon's failure to achieve these two desiderata. In all cases of fibroids with menorrhagia where myomectomy is performed, Bonney believes that the uterine cavity should be opened in order to make certain that no small fibroid on the mucous surface, or mucous polypus, or great thickening of the endometrium is missed. The chief risk of an extensive myomectomy is hemorrhage during and after the operation. It can be guarded against by temporarily securing the main vessels going to the uterus, by properly placing the sutures and by cutting away sufficient tissue to leave an organ of manageable size to suture. The incision should be a single anterior incision in the uterus with extraction of all the tumors through that incision. An anterior incision has these great advantages: if postoperative bleeding occurs, the blood accumulates in the utero-vesical space and the intestine is least likely to adhere in consequence of it; if the operator doubts that the incision is blood-tight he can suture it to the anterior abdominal wall or the back of the bladder and render it safe, while the single incision reduces the area of possible blood leakage and intestinal adhesion to a minimum. The fibroid most easily accessible through the anterior incision should be removed first and the incision should be carried right into the substance of the tumor so that there is no difficulty in finding the plane of cleavage between the tumor and capsule. This fibroid having been enucleated, the next most accessible should be reached by a secondary incision starting in the wall of the cavity left by the first tumor. In this way tumors of the posterior wall can be reached by a track which skirts around the uterine cavity but does not open it. One of the most important parts of a myomectomy is the suturing of the enucleation cavities, which usually consists of deep mattress sutures supplemented by superficial approximation sutures. The number of tumors removed by Bonney varied from 1 tumor in 49 cases to as high as 30 tumors in 1 case and the mortality of the entire series was 2 per cent.

Pneumopyelography.—Since the introduction of the method of injecting oxygen and later carbon dioxid and even air, into the various body cavities as an aid in roentgen-ray diagnosis, its use has become comparatively common and varied; however, the injection of gas into the renal pelvis has not been popularized to the extent which it deserves according to THOMPSON (*Jour. Urology*, 1922, **7**, 285). When the ureter or pelvis has been filled with an opaque solution and a roentgenogram obtained, it causes a white shadow on the plate bringing into relief only the pelvis and calices and not the kidney tissue itself, as the shadow is so dense that it obscures the tissues causing lighter shadows directly in front or behind the opaque media. For instance, the shadow of a stone in the ureter or pelvis is obscured by the heavier shadow of the opaque solution. The injection of oxygen into the ureter or renal pelvis causes no shadow at all, but creates a space which shows up black on the roentgen-ray plate, and brings into relief not only the pelvis and calices, but also the kidney tissue, as it does not obscure the shadows caused by the tissues either in front or behind. For example, the shadow of a stone will not be obscured by the oxygen and the size, shape and position of the stone can be easily determined. The black of the oxygen against the lighter shadow of the kidney substance makes a better contrast for the study of the kidney substance than does the white shadow of the opaque solution against the surrounding lighter shadow of the kidney. The apparatus required for the oxygen injections includes an oxygen tank, about 3 feet of rubber tubing in the center of which is a tube connected to a manometer, 2 cc Luer syringe barrel, a hypodermic needle large enough to fit snugly in the end of a No. 6 F. ureteral catheter, and a non-opaque ureteral catheter. The patient must be prepared in such a manner as to exclude all gas from the intestine so that no confusing shadows will be on the plate. For this purpose two ounces of castor oil should be given the night before, a soap-sud enema is given six hours before and repeated two hours before the roentgen-ray examination. The ureters are catheterized in the usual manner, a number 6 French ureteral catheter is preferable. The oxygen is then allowed to flow into the catheter until the patient complains of a fulness in the kidney region. The pressure in the manometer is noted at this point and then oxygen is allowed to flow until the pressure has reached 20 mm. above this point and then the roentgenogram is made.

PATHOLOGY AND BACTERIOLOGY

UNDER THE CHARGE OF

OSKAR KLOTZ, M.D., C.M.,

DIRECTOR OF THE PATHOLOGICAL LABORATORIES, SAO PAULO, BRAZIL,

AND

DE WAYNE G. RICHEY, B.S., M.D.,

ASSISTANT PROFESSOR OF PATHOLOGY, UNIVERSITY OF PITTSBURGH, PITTSBURGH, PA.

The Experimental Production of Periarteritis Nodosa in the Rabbit with a Consideration of the Specific Causal Excitant.—The various describers of the 54 cases of periarteritis nodosa on record have discussed, at length, whether or not the vascular lesions constitute a disease entity or represent a peculiar invasion of the vascular structures by the "virus of syphilis" or by certain known microörganisms. Because of the rarity of the disease and its infrequent recognition during life, and inasmuch as search for an etiological agent was attempted in less than one-fourth of the reported cases and, among these, attempts at transmission of disease to animals in only three, periarteritis nodosa has afforded a small field for experimental study. Recently, HARRIS and FRIEDRICHS (*Jour. Exp. Med.*, 1922, **36**, 219) reported the clinical and autopsy findings of a negro, aged thirty-two years, in whom characteristic lesions were found in the gastroepiploic, renal and coronary arteries and to a lesser degree in the hepatic and mesenteric lymph node arteries. Macroscopically, these lesions consisted of aneurysmal dilatations which were most marked in the right kidney, where rupture of capsule had occurred, resulting in a hemoperitoneum. The lesions could be divided into three groups: (1) the inflammatory reaction in the vessel walls; (2) the resultant vascular lesions arising from those of the first group, namely, aneurysms both true and false, thrombosis and vascular rupture with extravasation of blood; and (3) retrograde lesions in the structures involved through impairment of blood supply, chiefly because of the lesions of the second group. Microscopically, the adventitia and media were especially affected. In either or both of these layers, polymorphonuclear neutrophils and fibrin with or without a zone of necrosis in the media and fragmentation of the elastic membrane were seen. In some instances, an acute cellular and fibrinous exudate extended through the media to the subendothelial layer and at times a lymphoid or plasma cell and eosinophilic infiltration were noted in the outer vessel area. Cultures of several kidney lesions on various media remained sterile. By inoculating emulsions of the affected human organs or tissue emulsions and filtrates from rabbits previously injected with emulsions of human nodules, into the ear vein of full-grown rabbits, gross lesions consisting of aneurysms and hemorrhages in the liver and lungs of many of the rabbits were produced. In all the rabbits microscopic changes of some degree of intensity, resembling those occurring in periarteritis nodosa of man, existed. These changes consisted of infiltrations of the arterial adventitia, media and even the intima with neutrophils, eosinophiles, lymphocytes and plasma cells. Degeneration and necrosis of the media, dilatation of the vascular lumen and thrombosis were encountered. The veins were only exceptionally affected. The authors believe that the results of their experiments afford additional evidence for eliminating Treponema pallidum as the inciting cause of periarteritis nodosa, noting that the pathological character of the gross and microscopic lesions suggests a specific inciting agent, which is transmissible to rabbits and belongs to "the group of so-called filter passers."

Experimental Studies on the Etiology of Typhus Fever.—Having "shown *Jour. Exp. Med.*, 1921, **34**, 525) that the typhus virus, in inducing the typical experimental disease in guinea-pigs, readily invites invasion in the bodies of these animals of a number of bacteria, which complicate the typhus infection but, on the other hand, have no etiological relationship to the disease," OLITSKY (*Jour. Exp. Med.*, 1922, **35**, 115) has continued his investigations by means of a deductive method, so as to study the nature of any inciting agent which might reside in the virus. Accordingly, 4 cc of active citrated blood obtained from the guinea-pigs during the height of the experimental reaction was added to an equal quantity of various media, as normal rabbit plasma, normal horse serum (diluted), veal infusion broth, human ascitic fluid, under aërobic and anaërobic conditions at 37° C. After varying intervals of time, the lower 5 cc were injected intraperitoneally into a guinea-pig, the criteria of the experimental disease being the transmissibility from animal to animal, the presence of the characteristic vascular lesions particularly in brain, the absence of secondary invasions with ordinary bacteria and the development in recovered animals of immunity to subsequent injections of typhus virus. In those media from which oxygen was excluded by a petrolatum seal, the typhus virus tended to die rapidly, the viability period being twenty-four to forty-eight hours, whereas the virus survived as long as five days under aërobic conditions. In another communication (*Jour. Exp. Med.*, 1922, **35**, 121) additional observations, relating to that supposed intracellular nature and filtrability of the virus, as it exists in the organs of guinea-pigs during the height of the typhus reaction to inoculation, are presented. Fourteen experiments were made with infected spleen and brain, including three with the frozen infected tissue, two with the desiccated tissue, three with the crushed tissue and six with the ground tissue. The results of the different procedures were practically identical. Those guinea-pigs which were inoculated, intraperitoneally, with 2 cc of the infected tissue which was not disintegrated showed, after an incubation period of from five to ten days, typical experimental typhus fever, as did those animals receiving, similarly, infected tissue which had been repeatedly frozen and thawed, desiccated, crushed or ground. However, guinea-pigs injected with 5 cc of filtrates through Berkefeld V and N candles of suspensions of the frozen, desiccated, crushed or ground infected tissues, failed to exhibit the typical experimental disease and all of those animals reinjected with active typhus virus failed to show any immunity. The author indicates the possibility of an extracellular condition of the typhus virus as shown by his experiments. Later (*Jour. Exp. Med.*, 1922, **35**, 469), OLITSKY described experiments "to show that these filtrates, which are free, so far as we can ascertain from a living multiplying agent, can occasionally induce in guinea-pigs not only the typical lesions of the disease, but also an immunity to later injections of the active virus." Of the twenty guinea-pigs, injected intraperitoneally with 5 to 10 cc of Berkefeld V and N candle filtrates of typhus infected and subsequently disintegrated spleen and brain, five showed a rise in temperature (above 104° F.) for one to three days, first noticed from two to five days after inoculation. On the nine guinea-pigs similarly inoculated with filtrates and reinjected after ten to sixteen days with active typhus virus, six showed no immunity, two showed a partial and one a complete immunity. In four of ten guinea-pigs inoculated with the filtrates and sacrificed seven days after injection, histopathological lesions characteristic of experimental typhus fever were found. The author believes that the general indications are that the substance which causes these occasional reactions is not a living organism.

———

Experimental Studies of the Nasopharyngeal Secretions from Influenza Patients. VI. Immunity Reactions. — Having identified "the active material pathogenic for rabbits and guinea-pigs found in the nasopharyngeal secretions of patients in the early hours of uncomplicated influenza" in the anaërobic organism (Bacterium pneumosintes) OLITSKY and GATES (*Jour. Exper. Med.*, 1922, **35**, 1) conducted a series of immunity experiments on rabbits which had recovered after the inoculation of various materials, including nasopharyngeal washings from influenza patients, suspensions of lungs of affected rabbits, and washed mass cultures of Bacterium pneumosintes. In order to arrive at the presence of protection or cross-protection, similar material was injected at varying periods after recovery. It was found that the experiments gave additional evidence of the "pathogenic character and the virtual identity of the various strains of the active agent derived from the nasopharyngeal secretions of influenzal patients with which the transmission experiments in rabbits" had been carried out. As the active material had been demonstrated to be of antigenic nature, the rabbits were protected from the effects of a second inoculation. The authors state that their experiments indicate the antigenic identity of the various strains of the active agent with each other and with Bacterium pneumosintes, and that the protection may persist for fourteen months, which was the longest period yet tested.

HYGIENE AND PUBLIC HEALTH

UNDER THE CHARGE OF

MILTON J. ROSENAU, M.D.,

PROFESSOR OF PREVENTIVE MEDICINE AND HYGIENE, HARVARD MEDICAL SCHOOL, BOSTON, MASSACHUSETTS,

AND

GEORGE W. McCOY, M.D.,

DIRECTOR OF HYGIENIC LABORATORY, UNITED STATES PUBLIC HEALTH SERVICE, WASHINGTON, D. C.

Physiological Effects of Exposure to Low Concentrations of Carbon Monoxide.—SAYERS and MERIWETHER (*Public Health Reports,* 1922, **37,** 1127) summarize their work as follows: (1) The exposure for six hours to 2 parts of CO in 10,000 of air caused: (*a*) Saturation of 16 to 20 per cent of the hemoglobin of the blood with CO; (*b*) very mild subjective symptoms of CO poisoning at the end of the test; (*c*) no noticeable effects after the test. (2) The exposure to 3 parts of CO caused: (*a*) Saturation of 22 to 24 per cent of the hemoglobin with CO after four hours, and 26 to 27 per cent after five hours; (*b*) symptoms at the end of two hours absent; after four hours, mild effects attributed to CO poisoning; and after five hours, moderate effects; (*c*) after-effects of four hours' exposure mild; of five hours' exposure moderate. (3) The exposure to 4 parts of CO in 10,000 caused: (*a*) Saturation of 15 to 19 per cent of the hemoglobin with CO at the end of one hour and 21 to 28 per cent at the end of two hours; (*b*) after-effects, moderate to marked. *With the subject exercising strenuously:* (1) The exposure for one hour to 2½ parts of CO in 10,000 caused: (*a*) Saturation of 14 to 16 per cent of the hemoglobin with CO; (*b*) moderate symptoms of CO poisoning at the end of the test; (*c*) after-effects mild to moderate. (2) The exposure for one hour to 3.3 parts of CO in 10,000 caused: (*a*) Saturation of 17 per cent of the hemoglobin with CO; (*b*) mild to moderate symptoms of CO poisoning; (*c*) after-effects mild to moderate (3) The exposure for one hour to 4 parts of CO in 10,000 caused: (*a*) Saturation of 23 per cent of the hemoglobin with CO; (*b*) moderate symptoms of CO poisoning; (*c*) moderate after-effects. *With the subject at rest. Temperature and humidity high.* (1) The exposure for one hour to 3.1 parts of CO in 10,000 caused—(*a*) Saturation of 16 per cent of the hemoglobin with CO; (*c*) mild symptoms of CO poisoning; (*c*) mild moderate after-effects. *Conclusion.* (1) The combination of CO with hemoglobin takes place slowly when the subject is exposed to low concentrations and remains at rest, many hours being required before equilibrium is reached. (2) The rate of combination of CO with hemoglobin takes place much more rapidly during the first hour of exposure than during any succeeding hour, with the subject remaining at rest. (3) Strenuous exercise causes much more rapid combination of CO with hemoglobin than when the subject remains at rest. The symptoms of CO poisoning are emphasized by exercise. (4) High temperature and humidity, with a given concentration of CO cause more rapid combination of CO with hemoglobin than do normal conditions of temperature and humidity. All symptoms and effects described in this paper are called acute in character. None of the subjects has shown any permanent deleterious effects from the exposure to CO.

The Decline in the Death Rate, 1901-1910 and 1910-1920.—Data from the Statistical Office, U. S. Public Health Service (*Public Health Reports*, 1922, **37**, 1625), show that the gross death-rate from all causes in the original registration state declined from 17.2 per 1000 in 1900 to 15.6 in 1910 and 13.9 in 1920, a decrease of 9.3 per cent in the first decade and 10.9 per cent in the second decade. Taking into consideration the fact that a secondary but severe epidemic of influenza-pneumonia occurred in the early part of 1920, the indicated decline from 1910 to 1920 is less than it would have been had 1920 been a normal year. In forty-two cities in the United States, having a population of over 100,000, the excess death-rate during the 1920 epidemic period from influenza-pneumonia alone was about 1.13 per 1000. If the same excess may be presumed to have occurred in these original registration states, the death-rate in 1920 would have been approximately 12.8 per 1000, and the decline from 1910 would have been about 18 per cent. A comparison of the specific death-rates and the expectation of life at various ages for the three periods suggests that, in addition to the accelerated decline in the mortality-rate during the decade 1910–1920, some extremely interesting and highly significant changes have taken place. Such a comparison has been made possible in a table recently published by the statistical bureau of the Metropolitan Life Insurance Company in its *Statistical Bulletin* for May, 1922. The changes in the death-rates have altered materially the complete expectation of life in 1920 as compared with 1910 and 1901. From the figures prepared by the Bureau of the Census and the Metropolitan Life Insurance Company, have been computed the decreases or increases in the expectation of life in 1910 over 1901 and 1920 over 1910. The "expectation of life" tells the story in a better way than do the mortality-rates. In 1910, at the ages of forty to eighty, the expectation of life had actually decreased over what it was in 1901. But in 1920, in spite of abnormally high mortality, especially in certain age groups, from the influenza epidemic, there was a gain in the expectation of life over 1910 in practically every age shown.

Development of Paratyphoid-enteritidis Group in Various Foodstuffs.—Koser (*Jour. Infect. Dis.*, 1922, **31**, 79) investigated several type strains of the paratyphoid-enteritidis group to gain some idea of their ability to develop in miscellaneous foodstuffs, such as various vegetables, fruits, meats and evaporated milk. The effects of different conditions, such as temperature of incubation and the hydrogen-ion concentration and the texture of the food were considered in relation to multiplication and the ability to spread throughout the foodstuff. Koser found that all the strains of the Gärtner-group multiplied readily in the liquor of several common cooked vegetables, with the exception of the highly acid sauerkraut. In the fruit juices a rapid destruction of the organisms occurred. In several meat products Gärtner-group organisms exhibited a marked ability to spread from one original point of inoculation throughout the foodstuff, although this occurred only under optimum temperature conditions. The author states that the development of the Gärtner-group in foodstuffs is usually not accompanied by visible alteration or spoilage, which observations are in accord with the reports of previous outbreaks of "food poisoning" caused by this group of organisms.

Clostridium Botulinum.—TANNER and DACK (*Jour. Infect. Dis.*, 1922, **31**, 92) found that the different strains of Clostridium botulinum studied in their investigation showed different resistance to dry heat. This, they state, was probably due to inherent characteristics and, in a large measure, to the age of the cultures used. At 110° C. the time of survival averaged beyond one hundred and twenty minutes. At 140° C. the variation was between sixty minutes and fifteen minutes, a rather wide variation. At higher temperatures of 160° C. and 180° C. the times of survival were short, between five and fifteen minutes. The modern methods of dry-heat sterilization seem, then, to be adequate for sterilizing apparatus which has been used for cultivating Clostridium botulinum. Young spores of Clostridium botulinum are more resistant to dry heat than old ones. Clostridium botulinum, like other pathogenic anaërobes, is commonly present in nature. In this investigation 11 of 73 of the samples of soil contained it. Three specimens of hog feces contained it, but it was not isolated from 3 specimens of cow feces. It was isolated from 1 sample of sewage. Clostridium botulinum is probably a common saprophyte widespread in nature. The results of this investigation do not conflict with those of Meyer and Geiger, who propose a regional distribution of the organism. It may be that it is more common in recently manured soils. Further investigation must be carried out before a better understanding of the characteristics of Clostridium botulinum is attained. The occurrence of the organism in stools of healthy individuals is one phase of the subject which is being investigated. In a later study TANNER and DACK (*Jour. Am. Med. Assn.*, 1922, **79**, 132–133) state that 2 of 10 specimens of feces from healthy persons were found to contain Clostridium botulinum. Five other specimens gave strong evidence of its presence. The two strains absolutely identified as Type B strains formed powerful toxins in sheep-brain medium.

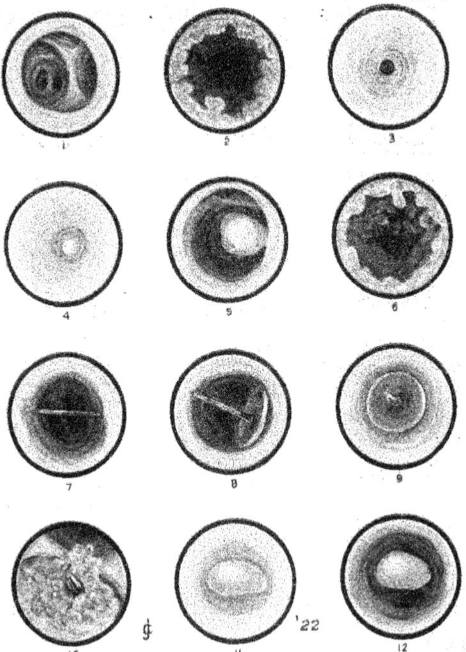

Bronchoscopic views.
(See page 317.)

THE

AMERICAN JOURNAL

OF THE MEDICAL SCIENCES

MARCH, 1923

ORIGINAL ARTICLES.

THE MECHANISM OF PHYSICAL SIGNS, WITH ESPECIAL REFERENCE TO FOREIGN BODIES IN THE BRONCHI *.

By Chevalier Jackson, M.D.,

PROFESSOR OF LARYNGOLOGY, JEFFERSON MEDICAL COLLEGE; PROFESSOR OF BRONCHOSCOPY AND ESOPHAGOSCOPY, UNIVERSITY OF PENNSYLVANIA, GRADUATE SCHOOL OF MEDICINE.

It would seem interesting for me to illustrate for the internists present the bronchoscopic views of the most frequently seen departures from the normal in the interior of the bronchi. In other words to consider the changes in physical forms that must necessarily influence, according to the laws of physics, the physical signs as elicited by the internist examining through the barrier of the thoracic wall. At the outset it should be said that I am incompetent to elicit physical signs partly because while I have been endeavoring to train my eyes and fingers to the requirements of endoscopic technic, the training of my ears to the niceties of auscultation and percussion have been neglected. Fortunately, however, my patients and I have had the advantage of a number of the most skilled internists. Since roentgen-ray diagnosis of non-opaque foreign bodies in the lung by the discovery of Iglauer and its development to a high degree of perfection by my colleague, Willis F. Manges, it may be said that the roentgen ray is our most valuable means of diagnosis in all cases of suspected foreign body in the lung; but this does not lessen the necessity for the study of the physical signs. It would be a great misfortune if careful physical examination were neglected in any case. Every foreign

* Report of a "chalk talk" given at the meeting of the Section on General Medicine of the College of Physicians, February 27, 1922.

body case should be gone over as carefully as if the roentgen-ray had not been discovered and the signs should be recorded and interpreted *before* the roentgen-ray examination so the examiner will not be biased, or, as is often the case, hindered by his efforts not to be biased. It is so much easier simply to record "in cold blood" and interpret the findings as elicited with no knowledge of the ray-findings, that all of the internists with whom I have collaborated preferred to work that way.

Changeability of Physical Signs. One of the outstanding features of the physical signs, especially in foreign body cases, is their changeability, as pointed out by McCrae.[1] This changeability is well illustrated in all the bronchoscopic views except 1 and 7. The bronchial movements and the shifting of the secretions, the granulations and the foreign body all contribute to the changeability of the physical signs. The outstanding feature of all bronchoscopic endobronchial pictures is also the incessant change. The bronchoscopist without moving his bronchoscope from one location sees a never-ending panoramic series of changes from one image to another. The image is modified by:

(*a*) The bronchial movements.

(*b*) The presence, absence or shifting of secretions.

(*c*) The presence and movements of foreign bodies.

Necessarily in obedience to physical laws, the physical signs must in some degree change also. That they do thus change is abundantly evidenced by the clinical observations of the Bronchoscopic Clinic, a few of which are herewith illustrated.

The normal bronchial movements are probably not fully realized by anyone who has never looked through a bronchoscope into the normal living lung. It is an awe-inspiring sight. The bronchi are not rigid tubes like gas-pipes. They expand, contract, elongate, shorten; they bulge out, dinge in; bend and twist to an astonishing degree. Often the lumen of a normal bronchus proximal to a foreign body is noticed to be obliterated so as completely to hide a foreign body from view, simply by the momentary contraction of the normal walls of the bronchus. The same thing occurs from momentary bending and dinging in of the bronchial wall. These movements follow each other in rapid succession. They are rhythmically evident during respiration. Expansion and lengthening of a bronchus occurs during inspiration, contraction and shortening during expiration. These movements change the picture at the rate of 18 or more times per minute. They are enormously exaggerated during the expiratory blast of cough and the deep inspiration that immediately follows cough. The transmitted movements of the heart and great vessels change the picture at the pulsatory rate of seventy or more times per minute.

[1] Am. Jour. Med. Sci., 1920, **159**, 313.

The Shifting of Secretions. Secretions, unless the bronchus is completely occluded (by a foreign body itself or by secretions, granulations, swollen mucosa, etc.) are constantly shifting. They go upward under the influence of the cilia, the "squeezing" of the contractile lung, the expiratory current, or the tussive blast. They may have a retrograde tendency, usually less marked, under the influence of gravity and of the inspiratory current. Speaking broadly, there is a tidal effect in the alternate accumulation of secretions and their tussive expulsion. They may be partially expelled and aspirated into the other lung, giving marked signs in the univaded side for a time at least.

Foreign Bodies in the Air Passages. Symptomatology and Diagnosis. *Initial symptoms* are choking, gagging, coughing, and wheezing, often followed by a symptomless interval. Foreign body may be in the larynx, trachea, bronchi, nasal chambers, nasopharynx, fauces, tonsil, pharynx, hypopharynx, esophagus, stomach, intestinal canal, or may have been passed by bowel, coughed out or spat out, with or without knowledge of patient. Initial choking may have escaped notice, or may have been forgotten.

Laryngeal Foreign Body. One or more of the following laryngeal symptoms may be present: Hoarseness, croupy cough, aphonia, odynphagia, hemoptysis, wheezing, dyspnea, cyanosis, apnea, subjective sensation of foreign body. Croupiness usually means subglottic swelling. Obstructive foreign body may be quickly fatal by laryngeal impaction on aspiration, or on abortive bechic expulsion. Lodgement of a non-obstructive foreign body may be followed by a symptomless interval. Direct laryngoscopy for diagnosis is indicated in every child having laryngeal diphtheria without faucial membrane. (No anesthetic, general or local, is required.) In the presence of laryngeal symptoms we should, I think, consider the following possibilities:

1. A foreign body in the larynx.
2. A foreign body loose or fixed on the trachea.
3. Digital efforts at removal.
4. Instrumentation.
5. Overflow of food into the larynx from esophageal obstruction due to foreign body.
6. Esophagotracheal fistula from ulceration set up by a foreign body in the esophagus, followed by leakage of food into the air-passages.
7. Laryngeal symptoms may persist from the trauma of a foreign body that has passed on into the deeper air or food passages or that has been coughed or spat out.
8. Laryngeal symptoms (hoarseness, croupiness, etc.) may be due to digital or instrumental efforts at removal of a foreign body that never was present.
9. Laryngeal symptoms may be due to acute or chronic laryn-

gitis, diphtheria, pertussis, infective laryngotracheitis, and many other diseases.

10. Deductive decisions are dangerous.

11. If the roentgen-ray is negative, laryngoscopy (direct in children, indirect in adults) without anesthesia, general or local, is the only way to make a laryngeal diagnosis.

12. Before doing a diagnostic laryngoscopy, preparations should be made for taking a swab-specimen and for bronchoscopy and esophagoscopy.

Tracheal Foreign Body. (1) "Audible slap;" (2) "palpatory thud," and (3) "asthmatoid wheeze" are pathognomonic. The "tracheal flutter" has been observed by McCrae. Cough, hoarseness, dyspnea and cyanosis are often present. Diagnosis is established by roentgen ray, auscultation, palpation, bronchoscopy. Listen long for "audible slap," best heard at open mouth during cough. The "asthmatoid wheeze" is heard with the ear or stethoscope bell (McCrae) at the patient's open mouth. History of initial choking, gagging, and wheezing is important if elicited, but is valueless negatively.

Bronchial Foreign Body. Initial symptoms are coughing, choking, asthmatoid wheeze, etc., noted above. There may be a history of these or of tooth extraction. At once, or after symptomless interval, cough, blood-streaked sputum, metallic taste, or special odor of foreign body may be noted. Non-obstructive metallic foreign bodies afford few symptoms and few signs for weeks or months. Obstructive foreign bodies cause atelectasis, drowned lung and eventually pulmonary abscess. Lobar pneumonia is an exceedingly rare sequel. Vegetable organic foreign bodies, such as peanut-kernels, beans, watermelon seeds, and the like cause at once violent laryngotracheobronchitis, with toxemia, cough and irregular fever, the gravity and severity being inversely to age of child. Bones and metallic bodies after months or years produce changes which cause chills, cough, foul expectoration, hemoptysis, in fact, all the symptoms of chronic pulmonary sepsis, abscess or bronchiectasis, and many signs which may suggest pulmonary tuberculosis. The apices, however, are normal and bacilli are absent from the sputum.

Physical Signs. The following is a brief *resume* of the results of the work of the various eminent internists who have collaborated with me: The physical signs vary in different cases and at different times in the same case. The results of my endoscopic studies of the mechanism of the production of the physical signs throw much light, I think, on the subject, as I shall now endeavor to show by a few drawings.* Secretions, normal and pathologic, may shift from one location to another; the foreign body may

* Reproduced in the color plate.

change position admitting more, less, or no air, or it may shift to a new location in the same lung or even in the other lung. A recently aspirated pin may produce no signs at all. The signs of diagnostic importance are chiefly those of partial or complete bronchial obstruction, though a nonobstructive foreign body, a pin for instance, may cause limited expansion (McCrae) or, rarely, a peculiar rale or a peculiar auscultatory sound. The most nearly characteristic physical signs are: (1) Limited expansion; (2) decreased vocal fremitus; (3) impaired percussion note; (4) diminished intensity of breath sounds distal to the foreign body. Complete obstruction of a bronchus followed by drowned lung adds absence of vocal resonance and vocal fremitus, thus often leading to an erroneous diagnosis of empyema. Varying grades of tympany are obtained over areas of obstructive or compensatory emphysema. With complete obstruction there may be tympany from collapsed lung for a time. Rales in case of complete obstruction are usually most intense on the uninvaded side. In partial obstruction they are most often found on the invaded side distal to the foreign body, especially posteriorly, and are often most intense at the site corresponding to that of the foreign body. A foreign body at the bifurcation of the trachea may give signs in both lungs. Early in a foreign body case, diminished expansion of one side, with dulness, may suggest pneumonia in the affected side; but the decreased vocal fremitus and the diminished breath-sounds with absence of, or decreased, vocal resonance, and absence of typical tubular breathing, should soon exclude this diagnosis. Bronchial obstruction in pneumonia is exceedingly rare.

Description of the Color Plate. Reference to the color plate reproduction of the chalk drawings along with the following notes of the outstanding features of the physical signs in the corresponding cases will doubtless be of interest. To avoid confusion all signs that seemed without special significance will be omitted. By this, however, it is not meant that the signs are due to the conditions illustrated, as, of course, it is impossible to say. The clinical facts are recorded for what they may be worth. Unless otherwise mentioned the physical signs noted corresponded to the tributary area of lung.

1. Bronchoscopic view looking down the right main bronchus of the living patient. The bronchoscopic tube-mouth is at the orifice of the main bronchus. The author's belief is that the normal breath sounds are largely produced by the impinging of the air-blast on the thin sharp edges of the spurs between the branch orifices. The view is somewhat composite, inasmuch as the bechic, respiratory, pulsatory and bronchial movements prevent a simultaneous view of all the branch-bronchial orifices shown, as mentioned in the paragraph on bronchial movements.

2. View looking down the right main bronchus in a case of post-

pneumonic pulmonary abscess. The walls of the bronchus are lined with exuberant granulations which have also obliterated the normal thin, sharp dividing spurs seen in illustration 1. Obviously, by the laws of physics, air rushing through such a tube must give an auscultatory sound different from the passage of air through a normally lined tube and impinging on sharp dividing spurs, as shown in the preceding illustration. A brass horn lined with obstructing masses of grease and incrustations would give a note perceptibly different to sensitive ears, from that obtained from a clean, polished, unobstructed horn. The difficulties encountered at the Bronchoscopic Clinic in designating a peculiar sound as characteristic of this state of a bronchial tube is due to the almost invariable association with pus produced by the granulations. The granulations shown at 2 are often seen to flap to and fro in the respiratory current or bechic blast. They are quite often associated with the conditions shown at 5 and 6, though the latter represent other cases. Coughing up the purulent secretions may in a few moments restore the condition shown at 2. Dr. O. H. Perry Pepper elicited the following signs: Limited expansion; dulness at base; expiration prolonged and of bronchial quality; breath sounds absent at base; vocal resonance unaltered; no whispered pectoriloquy.

3. Arachidic bronchitis, due to aspiration of a peanut-kernel which does not show. The bronchial mucosa has swollen until only a small lumen remains. For convenience this is called a pin-hole lumen, though it may be considerably larger than a pin-hole. The outstanding physical signs in this case before bronchoscopy were: Limited expansion on the invaded side, diminished, sometimes absent, breath sounds, impaired percussion note and occasionally a long, wheezing expiratory rale, alternating with absence of rales.

4. Same case as shown at 3, a few moments later. The pin-hole lumen has been occluded with a thick, firm clot of pus which was removed with forceps. Although no physical examination was made at the moment this bronchoscopic image was seen, the inference is logical that the intermittent disappearance of all breath sounds corresponded with an intermittent occlusion of the lumen similar to that noted at bronchoscopy and shown in this and the preceding illustration.

5. Pus coming into the right main bronchus from the upper-lobe bronchus (recumbent patient); partial occlusion of the right main bronchus. A few moments later the pus was aspirated into the orifice of the middle-lobe bronchus which is here shown anteriorly (above and beyond the pus in the drawing). Physical signs: Limited expansion and coarse rales all over right side; intermittent diminution of breath sounds over middle lobe; impaired percussion note right upper lobe.

7. A slender bit of steel (shaft of a dental instrument) transfixed across the lumen of the left stem bronchus. The logical hope would

be that some peculiar eolian note might be heard from the air-blast rushing past the slender wire. Nothing of the kind could be made out. Instead a most illogical and so far unexplained phenomenon was observed in this case by Dr. McCrae; namely, a limitation of expansion on the invaded side. In consideration of the fact that there was, as clearly shown at bronchoscopy and illustrated here, no obstruction to the airway, this curious, phenomenon is difficult to explain. Since this case the same thing has been noted in a great many similar cases. The only other sign of note was the presence of fine "tissue-paper" rales. Both these and the limitation of expansion disappeared after bronchoscopic removal of the foreign body.

8. A tack in the right stem bronchus. In this position there is a partial by-passage of air. Physical signs were limitation of expansion, impaired percussion note, diminished breath sounds and coarse rales. In the case of a piece of bone in this same location, Dr. Stengel localized the bone by exaggerated harsh breath sounds having their maximum intensity posteriorly corresponding to the endobronchial location from which I subsequently removed the foreign body with the bronchoscope.

9. This tack, because of the position of its head, completely occludes the bronchus. Physical signs: Limitation of expansion, absence of breath sounds, flat percussion note, absence of rales on the invaded side, loud rales in great variety in the other lung. Illustrations 8 and 9 show different cases of the same kind of tack, of which nearly two dozen have come to the Bronchoscopic Clinic. In a number of these cases I have noticed at bronchoscopy the tack shifting from a position similar to that shown at 8 to a position similar to that shown at 9. It is logical to suppose that a similar shifting occurs to account for the changeability of the signs so often noted in this kind of foreign body and, in fact, in almost all kinds of foreign bodies.

10. A tack in the lower-lobe bronchus, embedded, because of its prolonged sojourn, in a mass of soft, flabby, exuberant granulations which are partially occluding the orifice of the middle-lobe bronchus. Before the bronchoscopy Dr. McCrae had noticed intermittently a diminution of breath sounds over the middle lobe. The natural inference is that there were intermittent and varying degrees of obstruction of the middle-lobe bronchus because of the location of the tack, the granulations and the pus at its orifice. The physical signs were: Limitation of expansion, a flat percussion note and absence of rales and breath sounds over the right lower lobe; a flat percussion note and absence of rales and breath sounds over the right lower lobe; a variety of rales and, intermittently, diminished breath sounds over the middle lobe; coarse rales at times in the other lung. In a number of similar cases a rib resection has been done under a mistaken diagnosis of empyema.

11. A peanut-kernel in the right bronchial orifice almost completely occluding the bronchus *during expiration only.*

12. The same patient as in illustration 11; view a moment later, at the *beginning of inspiration.* The "forceps spaces" have opened up for the inspiratory by-passage of air, the exit of which is impeded by the collapse of the bronchial wall shown in the preceding illustration. This is the explanation, afforded by bronchoscopy, of the most important diagnostic phenomenon of obstructive emphysema, discovered by Iglauer and developed to a high degree of certainty by Manges.

THE NATURE OF THE COMPLEMENT FIXATION REACTION IN SYPHILIS IN RELATION TO THE STANDARDIZATION OF TECHNIC.*

By John A. Kolmer, M.D.,

PROFESSOR OF PATHOLOGY IN THE GRADUATE SCHOOL OF MEDICINE OF THE UNIVERSITY OF PENNSYLVANIA.

(From the Dermatological Research Institute of Philadelphia and the Department of Pathology and Bacteriology of the Graduate School of Medicine of the University of Pennsylvania.)

The literature upon the Wassermann and other serum reactions in syphilis has become so voluminous and the subject has been discussed so frequently and with such detail, that it would appear almost superfluous to devote more time to it. On the other hand, syphilis is so widespread and of such high economic importance, is so likely to be encountered in every specialty of medical practice, and may so easily escape clinical detection in certain stages, that the subject is one of universal interest and great importance, and improvements in our aids to diagnosis are to be welcomed. No other strictly laboratory test has been more used and abused, lauded and condemned and frequently misunderstood than the Wassermann test; yet its intrinsic worth has enabled it to weather all storms so that it probably stands today, potentially at least, the most important single laboratory procedure, full of possibilities for great good when properly conducted and interpreted, but of even greater possibilities of harm when technically incorrect and misunderstood.

The Proper Function of the Complement Fixation Reaction in Syphilis. Syphilis in its first and especially in its later manifestations may so readily engage attention in every specialty in medicine that all physicians must expect to encounter it in their practice. Specialists are usually highly skilled in detecting the disease when it involves

* Read by invitation before the New York Academy of Medicine, December 20, 1921.

their particular domain of work, but in its later stages with varied clinical manifestations the disease may easily escape detection by the general practitioner. In its latent stages it may escape diagnosis by even the most skilled physician, as likewise the atypical case with a negative or indefinite history. The complement fixation test in order properly to fulfill its function must prove of most aid under these conditions—not to replace clinical acumen and judgment, but to furnish an additional and accurate means of diagnosis of the clinically difficult, doubtful or unsuspected case. When and where clinical skill is least, reliability of the serum test should be greatest, and for this reason the technic is deserving of more attention as part of the nation-wide movement for the diagnosis and thorough treatment of syphilis.

Probably with the majority of physicians the Wassermann test is acceptable only as confirmatory evidence of syphilis. Many are unwilling to ascribe any significance to the reaction in either a positive or negative way unless the result meets with their clinical expectancy. Doubtless not a few have been forced into this attitude by actual experience. I believe, however, that it is possible to avoid technical errors and greatly improve the diagnostic status of the test, and that it should be the aim and purpose of serologists to evolve a test capable of correctly detecting the disease when this is not possible by clinical means; to me the complement fixation tests fails in its ultimate mission and purpose if it fails to do so. I believe that falsely positive reactions are most likely to be caused by technical errors, and that, as in other branches of medicine, skill and experience are required to reduce their incidence to a minimum. I believe that with improved technic the incidence of falsely positive reactions will be negligible because there is no biological reason for their occurrence in any nonsyphilitic disease other than frambesia tropica. Falsely negative reactions, however, will probably always occur for biological reasons, because no matter how sensitive a test may be made it cannot detect in the serum or spinal fluid something that is practically absent, and it would appear that in some cases of latent syphilis the activity of spirochetes is so slight or their numbers and virulence so reduced, that demonstrable amounts of "reagin" are not produced.

I trust that this high ideal of the complement fixation test in syphilis is justifiable. According to my own observations and experiences I believe it is, although I admit that the full possibilities of the test are realized only by close coöperation between clinician and serologist or by him who possesses training and experience in both branches.

Nature of the Complement Fixation Reaction in Syphilis. The complement fixation reaction occupies a very unique position among immunological phenomena. At first regarded as a specific reaction, it is now known to be biologically non-specific, but in most parts of the world this does not seriously reduce its diagnostic value in syphilis because the peculiar antibody-like substance to be found in the blood or spinal fluid or both, and responsible for the reaction, is known definitely to occur only in syphilis and frambesia tropica, or yaws.

Infection with spirochetes of these two diseases results in the elaboration of a substance aptly called "reagin" by Neisser, which has the property of uniting or reacting with certain lipoidal substances, the resulting complex regarded as a precipitate by some investigators, being able to absorb or fix hemolytic complement in the test tube. This "reagin" is probably produced by the cells directly in contact with and stimulated by the spirochetes; it is first found therefore in the tissue juices of the chancre, as recently shown by Klauder and myself. As the spirochetes are disseminated through the body the tissues of various internal organs, including those of the brain and spinal cord, very probably participate in the production of this Wassermann substance or "reagin." Even the cells of the cardiovascular system may participate in the process as likewise the lymphocytes and other cells of inflammatory stimulation surrounding the nests of spirochetes. It may be that the lipoids of spirochetes are antigenic and induce the production of the "reagin," but so far all attempts to produce antibodies with pure lipoids have failed, and even if it were true, one would expect a certain degree of specificity on the part of these lipoids which has not been demonstrated. This view does not coincide with our present conception of the tissues usually concerned in antibody production in infectious diseases, but there are no valid reasons for regarding this cellular "reagin" as a true antibody. In the first place the amount to be found in the body fluids bears a more or less direct relation to the severity of infection, although this relation may not be clinically apparent if the spirochetes are active in tissues of minor physiological importance. In the second place it may be present during the latent or resting stages of the disease in such small amounts as to escape detection, whereas if it were a true antibody capable of forcing the spirochetes into these periods of latency, it should be demonstrable in large amounts. For these and other reasons the complement fixation reaction is to be regarded as an index of the degree of infection rather than of immunity, and if this is true the phenomenon is unique, not only for this reason but likewise because of the peculiar nature of the "reagin."

This "reagin" has the power of fixing complement in the presence of a suitable suspension of lipoids. It is probably not itself a lipoid or identified with the lipoid content of serum or spinal fluid, although this phase of the subject is by no means a closed chapter and requires further investigation.

The Practical Specificity of the Complement Fixation Reaction in Syphilis. The important practical question is—May similar cellular "reagins" be produced in diseases other than syphilis and frambesia, capable of bringing about the physico-chemical phenomenon of complement fixation in the presence of extracts of lipoids? Do the positive Wassermann reactions which have been recorded as occurring in leprosy, diabetes mellitus, during the febrile stages of malaria, typhoid fever, pneumonia, late pregnancy, and so on, answer the question affirmatively? When one remembers the many chances of technical error capable of involving every important element and phase of the test, the answer must be given with great caution. Furthermore, may not pregnancy, an intercurrent infection, a metabolic disease and so on, stimulate latent foci of syphilitic spirochetes into activity with the production of "reagin," just as trauma may possibly be provocative or stimulating?[1] I am sure that this question of non-specific reactions cannot be answered by a mere review of the literature upon the Wassermann reaction in nonsyphilitic diseases because too much of it has been built upon obvious technical errors. Neither do I disclaim the possibility of observing positive complement fixation reactions with a correct and acceptable technic in nonsyphilitic diseases, but I do know that the clinician is not always infallible in his judgment that syphilis can escape clinical detection and that these unexpected positive reactions are not always due to laboratory error. My question remains—Is a "reagin" similar to that produced in syphilis and frambesia, or a physico-chemical alteration of the blood and spinal fluid similar to that occurring in these diseases, to be found in other infectious and non-infectious diseases? A final answer cannot be given, as the subject requires further investigation; but if I may be permitted to express a prediction, I believe that the answer will be negative and that as clinical and pathological knowledge of syphilis is developed and more especially as our complement fixation technic is perfected, more and more emphasis will be placed upon what may be called the "syphilitic significance" of these unexpected and weakly positive reactions with the sera of individuals regarded tentatively as nonsyphilitic.

A source of clinical error worthy of keeping in mind is that a positive Wassermann reaction does not necessarily mean that a particular lesion is syphilitic; for example, a tuberculous ulcer may occur in the larynx of an individual with latent syphilis and fail to improve with antiluetic treatment. On the other hand the complement fixation reaction may yield falsely negative reactions, and not a few physicians regard the test as insufficiently sensitive.

Biologically Falsely Negative Reactions and the Necessity for a Sensitive Test. These false reactions may be due to the presence of insufficient amounts of "reagin" in the blood or spinal fluid or

[1] A recent paper by Klauder on Syphilis and Trauma (Jour. Am. Med. Assn., 1922, **78**, 1029) is very instructive in this connection and answers this question affirmatively.

to technical errors. The mere fact that a person is known to have contracted syphilis does not necessarily mean that the "reagin" is present in detectable amounts. There must be a certain degree of spirochetic activity and doubtless numbers of spirochetes, their virulence and location in the body are important modifying factors. Warthin has shown that spirochetes may exist in the tissues with practically no inflammatory reaction and under these conditions "reagin" production must be very slight.

Therefore the technic of the complement fixation reaction in syphilis should be as sensitive *as is possible with specificity*. Every serologist knows that the test may be rendered so delicate as to incur the risk of non-specific reactions, but the harmfulness of these is so apparent that they are not included in the present discussion. Whether or not cases of latent syphilis unexpectedly detected by the complement fixation reaction are subjects for mild, moderate or intensive treatment is likewise aside from the present discussion. There ought to be, however, no difference of opinion of the desirability of having a complement fixation test as sensitive as is possible with practical specificity in order to avoid falsely negative reactions and especially when the test is employed as a guide to treatment to avoid the regrettable error of undertreating the disease. Even under these conditions we will continue to secure falsely negative reactions for the very good biological reason that where "reagin" is practically absent from the serum and spinal fluid it cannot be detected in the test tube. In connection with this subject of biologically falsely negative Wassermann reactions it is worthy of remembering that while "reagin" may not be present in detectable amounts in the blood, sufficient may be present in the spinal fluid for yielding positive reactions. The reason is unknown. It may be that in these cases the spirochetes are mainly located in the tissues of the brain and spinal cord and that the "reagin" produced by these tissues finds its way into the spinal fluid where it may be detected in smaller amounts than is possible in the serum because five to ten times more spinal fluid may be employed in the Wassermann test than is permissible with serum. I believe this to be the principal reason, but in addition it may be that some of the "reagin" is filtered out of the spinal fluid during its reabsorption into the lymphatic and vascular systems.

Studies in the Standardization of Technic. During the past six years my colleagues and myself[2] have been actively interested and engaged in a series of investigations aiming to study every phase of complement fixation in syphilis for the purpose of building up a test possessing a maximum degree of sensitiveness with the minimum possibility for yielding non-specific reactions. I realized

[2] Series of thirty-two papers being published in the Am. Jour Syph., beginning 1919, 3, 1.

that the task was big before a start was made, but did not conceive that it would require the very large amount of work that has been done. As our investigations proceeded it became evident that every detail, regardless of how trivial it may at first appear, was worthy of careful study. My associates and myself have striven always to conduct the work without preconceived ideas and without bias. It can scarcely be hoped or expected that we have escaped technical errors and erroneous conclusions, but we have faithfully described what we have done and what we have observed. These investigations have finally enabled us to build up a new complement fixation test for syphilis which I hope others will find as satisfactory as ourselves and that clinicians and serologists will at least consent to give it a fair trial alongside of their own technic.

Standardization of the complement fixation reaction has been discussed and if accomplished may yield certain advantages. For example, it would enable a closer analysis and evaluation of different kinds and methods of treatment and greatly increase the confidence of the medical profession as a whole in the test as an aid in the diagnosis of syphilis.

Doubtless many physicians have had the unhappy experience of securing varying reports on the Wassermann reaction with portions of the same blood sent to different laboratories. This is regrettable but not altogether unexpected, when one remembers the great influence of technic upon the reactions and the numerous modifications being practised. Standardization of technic would aim to correct this situation, but it is easy to fall into the error of making the "remedy worse than the disease." For example, if it were desired to simply unify the results insofar as positive or negative reactions were concerned, a simple modification of the original Wassermann reaction could be made to fulfill the requirement. In other words by adopting a technic capable of detecting only relatively large amounts of "reagin" the weakly positive or doubtful cases which constitute those giving varying results would be weeded out by giving negative reactions. Only gross technical errors would interfere with uniform results under these conditions, but is such a reaction worth while? Are not the truly syphilitic cases in the latent stages worthy of detection even though antiluetic treatment may not be given? Should not a reasonable attempt be made to make treatment as thorough as possible? When treatment is being guided by the complement fixation reaction, should not the test be made as sensitive as is possible with practical specificity in order that a truly positive reaction may be the last symptom to disappear and the first to return if complete sterilization has not been accomplished?

I have not called our new test a standardized test because it must earn that designation by common consent. But experience with it has been favorable, and I am hoping that it may, at least, high degree of sensitiveness as is permissible with practical specificity; (2) technical accuracy and uniformity in results insofar at least as positive or negative reactions are concerned. Slight variation in the degree of positiveness will occur, but these do no harm as long as the primary question of whether a serum does or does not yield a positive or negative reaction is answered; (3) to yield a truly quantitative reaction in order to give an index of spirochetic activity and the influence of treatment; (4) to be technically simple in order to reduce the minimum of error, and (5) economical of time and materials insofar as this is consistent with the best work. Simplicity is but a relative term; for the inexperienced any technic is apt to be complicated, but for the experienced my new test is simple. It is not a short-cut method and has never aimed to be, because too many sources of error require attention and correction to fulfil the primary aim of sensitiveness and specificity.

The new complement fixation test for syphilis has aimed to meet these requirements as follows, a fuller discussion and all technical details being given elsewhere:[3]

I. *The requirement of sensitiveness* by the following procedures:

(*a*) By using a highly sensitive antigen.

(*b*) By using relatively large amounts of antigen.

(*c*) By using relatively large amounts of serum and spinal fluid.

(*d*) By heating sera for only fifteen minutes at 55° C. instead of for thirty minutes.

(*e*) By using a mixture of guinea-pig complements prepared in a manner tending to increase sensitiveness to fixation.

(*f*) By mixing serum and antigen for a brief period before the addition of complement.

(*g*) By using a primary incubation of fifteen to eighteen hours in a refrigerator at 6° to 8° C. plus ten minutes in a water-bath.

(*h*) By close adjustment of the hemolytic system.

(*i*) By using an antisheep or antiox hemolytic system, although the test can be conducted with an antihuman system.

(*j*) By reading the reactions within three hours after the conclusion of the secondary incubation.

[3] Kolmer, J. A.: Am. Jour. Syph., 1922, **6**, 82.

II. *The requirement of practical specificity by:*
   (*a*) Close adjustment of the hemolytic system to a primary incubation of fifteen to eighteen hours at 6° to 8° C.
   (*b*) Careful titration of antigen under conditions rendering the dose employed suitable for this kind of primary incubation.
   (*c*) Including numerous and adequate controls.

III. *The requirement of technical accuracy and uniformity in results by:*
   (*a*) Adopting the principle that pipetting relatively large amounts of fluid (0.2 to 1 cc) tends to greater accuracy than measuring smaller amounts (less than 0.2 cc).
   (*b*) Using a total volume of 3 cc with sufficient corpuscles and test-tubes of suitable size to yield clear, sharp, and easily read reactions.
   (*c*) By using a reading scale prepared each time the tests are conducted and with the same reagents.

IV. *The requirement of a true quantitative reaction*, so important in connection with the use of the complement fixation test as a guide and control in treatment, has been met by working out a series of five dilutions of patient's serum and spinal fluid which may be set up rapidly and accurately.

V. *The requirement of simplicity* has been met insofar as experienced serologists are concerned. Simplicity is but a relative term, inasmuch as the simplest technic is a complicated problem for the inexperienced and insufficiently trained worker, whereas a more complicated technic is perfectly simple to the experienced serologist. I am quite sure that my new test can be satisfactorily conducted by any person possessing a working knowledge of the technic of complement fixation.

VI. *The requirement of economy* has been met insofar as materials are concerned; in regard to time the new test is not a short-cut method and is not shorter than other methods in general use.

A few lines may be added on the subject of uniformity in results: It must be emphasized that the anticomplementary activity of serum or spinal fluid is very important in relation to reactions, and for this reason tests conducted with portions of the same specimen of blood in different cities cannot be expected to yield absolutely similar results, nor even in the same city, if serologists vary in their methods of preserving blood until the tests are conducted.

Two or more serologists working in the same or different laboratories testing portions of a sample of blood or spinal fluid from one person should agree at least upon the question of positive or negative reactions; in my experience most variation occurs with sera yielding weakly positive or borderline reactions. Slight discrepancies in the reports on the degree of complement fixation must be expected, inasmuch as the personal equation plays an important part in reading the degree of hemolysis, as it does in matching colors in other lines of work. Slight discrepancies of this kind do no harm as long as the primary and fundamental question of whether a serum does or does not yield a positive or negative reaction is untouched, and particularly with sera yielding borderline results.

Is Standardization Advisable and Possible? Standardization is desirable if these aims are served and satisfied: The first purpose should be to secure as good a technic as is possible to evolve in the light of our present knowledge. Mere unification of results in Wassermann tests in different laboratories means little or nothing unless the test is technically correct and as sensitive as is possible with practical specificity. Even under these conditions individual variation in the scientific attainments and accuracy of different serologists will ever be modifying factors, if the test aims to be a sensitive one; but I believe standardization is possible under these conditions, and my own efforts have been and will continue to be dedicated to that end.

THE PRODUCTION OF HEART MURMURS.*

By William D. Reid, M.D.,
BOSTON, MASS.

The detection and study of murmurs if present form perhaps the most important feature of cardiac auscultation. That not all murmurs indicate disease of the heart has long been recognized, but it is often difficult to decide as to the interpretation to be placed on a given murmur. The recent emphasis laid on the relative unimportance of a systolic murmur heard over the cardiac apex has given the matter a renewed interest. To interpret correctly heart murmurs an understanding of the chief facts pertaining to the production of murmurs would seem to be essential. It is the purpose of this paper, therefore, to discuss in part the literature on the subject and then to present the results of a few simple experiments and clinico-pathologic observations.

Literature. Laennec,[1] the father of auscultation, explained murmurs as due to a spasmodic contraction of the heart or arteries.

* Read in part before the Harvard Medical School Research Club, February 24, 1922.

[1] Traité de l'auscultation mediate, 1826, 2, 441.

His main proof of this conception was that postmortem examination failed to disclose any constant findings and that often the heart was found to be structurally normal. That spasm could not be the cause of heart murmurs was clearly shown by Corrigan, the Dublin physician whose name is still linked with the collapsing or water-hammer pulse of aortic regurgitation. Corrigan subjected the matter to experiment, using a length of small intestine attached to a water pipe from which a stream of water was allowed to pass through the piece of bowel. As a result of his observations he attributed the causation of murmurs to the formation of a jet. Thus he wrote: "When an artery is pressed upon . . . the action of blood in the artery immediately beyond the constricted part (looking from the heart) is no longer as before. A small stream is now rushing from a narrow orifice into a wider tube and continuing its way through the surrounding fluid."[2] And in a later paper appeared his conception of the action of this jet as follows: ". . . its particles tending to leave vacuums between them throw the sides of the tube into vibration, which can be very distinctly felt by the finger and which gives to the ear the peculiar sound *bruit de soufflet* and to the touch *fremmissement*."[3]

Corrigan's ideas were the subject of much controversy, and it was not until 1858 that Chauveau, of Lyons, placed the question of murmurs on a sound basis. This French physiologist and veterinarian carried out a large series of observations, mostly on horses, in which a considerable length of the carotid artery or jugular vein was easily exposed by surgical means and subjected to experiment. Chauveau's work was so carefully done, and so many of his conclusions appear correct even today, that it seems worth while to repeat the latter here. The details of the experiments on which he based his statements may, for the most, part be omitted, as to include them would unduly lengthen this paper. The observations of this clear-headed scientist[4] are, then:

1. Vascular murmurs do not depend directly upon the quantity or the quality of the blood which is circulating in the vessels.
2. The asperities which roughen the internal surface of the circulatory tubes, without modifying the caliber of the latter, cannot be a cause of a murmur.
3. When a dilatation exists in the course of a vessel, the blood, on arriving at this dilated part may produce a murmur.
4. Narrowing of the vessels may cause a murmur, but the latter is not due to the entry of the blood into the narrowed part or through it. . . . The murmur occurs just beyond.
5. A dilatation is necessary, but also (*a*) sufficient dilatation and (*b*) a certain force to the blood stream.

[2] Corrigan, D. J.: Lancet, 1828, **2**, 4.
[3] Corrigan, D. J.: Edin. Med. and Surg. Jour., 1832, **37**, 225.
[4] Chauveau, M. A.: Gaz. méd. de Paris, 3me Série, 1858, **13**, 247. The translation adheres to the author's words as far as is consistent with good English.

6. Although it is true that there is necessary a certain difference in diameter between the dilatation where the murmur takes place and the narrowing, real or relative, which precedes this, so that the murmur is manifest, it does not follow that the more pronounced the difference the greater the intensity of the sound produced. When the entrance to the dilated part becomes very small and permits the passage of only a very small thread of blood, the murmur though remaining distinct, rough even, loses much of its intensity, the more so as the thread of blood is the less voluminous. It is when the blood arrives as a large wave in a large cavity that one is more likely to observe a strong murmur.

7. The pressure must be at least one-quarter of that in the left ventricle (in the horse 5 cm. column of mercury). If this pressure is increased the intensity of the murmur increases proportionately.

8. The murmur is propagated along the vessel beyond and on the near side of the point of production (farther if more intense) but always farther with the blood stream. On the near side it has the sound of a file cutting on iron, and beyond, with the stream, that of the rasp of wood being sawn.

9. Like all possible sounds the immediate cause of murmurs are molecular vibrations.

10. In anemia the lessening of the number of cells is accompanied by a lessening of the blood volume. This diminution, while lowering the pressure exerted during diastole on the semilunar valves, greatly increases the force of the impulsion which animates the blood when it is driven into the arterial system. This force of impulsion is further increased, often, by the greater energy which the heart-beats acquire in anemia.

11. The essential stethoscopic sign of anemia is a cardiac murmur synchronous with ventricular systole.

12. Anemia does not cause arterial murmurs, but one can produce them by pressure, perhaps, a little easier than in healthy adults.

13. In anemia murmurs may be heard in the veins of the neck, as here only does one find the conditions which cause a *veine fluide*,[5] the cause of a murmur.

It will be noted that Chauveau is quoted as asserting that "the asperities which roughen the internal surface of the circulatory tubes, without modifying the caliber of the latter, cannot be a cause of a murmur." This is a contradiction of the observation of Theodor Weber,[6] who, in 1854, reported that roughness of the internal surface of the vessel caused a murmur.

About ten years later, in 1868, appeared an important monograph

[5] This term, originating in the French, is now freely used by English writers. Perhaps the word jet is a good translation.

[6] De Causis Strepituum in Vasis Sanguiferis, Leipzig, 1854, p. 8.

by Bergeon[7] on the production of murmurs. This author accepts the principles established by his predecessor, Chauveau, to whom he courteously gives full credit, and adds some further points. Of these there are two which take preëminence.

1. The *veine fluide* is a secondary phenomenon, just as are the rings in a mill pond into which a stone has been dropped. The phenomena of compression and reaction, which take place as a fluid under pressure passes by a spot where there is a sudden change in the caliber of the vessel, constitute the primary disturbance or shock (*l'ébranlement*). Perhaps this will be a little clearer if I quote a few sentences: "As all the molecules cannot pass the constriction at the same time, some will be crowded back and compressed. These latter, as a result, acquire a greater tension and in their turn go out, at the same time compressing and crowding back others, etc. From this results a series of alternating motions of equal intervals and in close succession."[8] This is Bergeon's explanation of the vibrations in the *veine fluide,* and it is these vibrations, he asserts, which produce the murmur.

2. The phenomena of compression and reaction also occur when there exists a cul-de-sac against the current and the murmur occurring under this condition is propagated up stream. Bergeon finds the occurrence of the cul-de-sac analogous to the bevel which is found in the mouthpiece of a flute.

Some lesser points concerning the production of murmurs are described by the same author. Thus the murmur was unaffected by the composition of the narrow area. Tests were made with copper, glass, porcelain, gutta-percha and rubber. Also the thickness of the wall at the constricted area was without influence. As regards the viscosity of the fluid flowing through the tubes, Bergeon agreed with Potain[9] that it modifies the murmur by its effect on the speed of the current; but he also satisfied himself by experiment that it influences the manner of vibration of the liquid. A musical quality of the murmur was found to result from impinging of a thin piece of membrane in the trajectory of the *veine fluide.* Bergeon quotes instances in which postmortem examination had disclosed some fibrous pathological formation[10] which had so influenced the character of the murmur. The jet, or *veine fluide,* it is to be remembered, had already been produced by a sudden narrowing of the lumen of the vascular tube. Murmurs are modified in transmission at times. Thus a metallic quality has been found to be associated with the resonating effect of some cavity, as the stomach distended by gas, a suitably located cavity in the lung, and in pneumothorax.

[7] Des causes et du mechanism du bruit de souffle, Adrien Delahaye, Libraire-Editeur, Paris, 1868.

[8] Idem, p. 79.

[9] Compt. rend. de la Gazette d. hôp., May 28, 1867, p. 252.

[10] Not mere roughening.

The conditions attending the presence of murmurs are again considered in 1881 by the French physiologist Marey. In a rather tiresome chapter[11] this author advances the theory that a sudden change in the blood-pressure is the essential condition in the production of a murmur. Of course that is just what occurs, according to physical laws,[7] on either side of a narrowing sufficient to cause some obstruction to the passage of the blood stream. A little thought makes it evident that Marey's experiment in raising and lowering the pressure in a tube just beyond a constricted area may more properly be considered as merely influencing the speed of the flow past the narrowing. It seems like putting the cart before the horse to attribute to the alteration in the blood-pressure on either side of a narrowing of the lumen the primary cause of a murmur. Marey, with his attention centered on alterations in blood-pressure as the real cause of murmurs, helps us, however, by pointing out that where the arterial tension is lowered by peripheral dilatation (relaxation of the arterioles) the occurrence of murmurs is favored. Fever is cited as an example. Perhaps this is one of the factors influencing the frequent occurrence at the aortic area of a systolic murmur along with the diastolic in those cases of aortic regurgitation in which there is a well-marked Corrigan pulse (a lowering of the diastolic pressure is characteristic).

Davison calls attention to the sound produced if the *veine fluide* strikes the surface of the bloodvessel. He writes: "When a membrane enclosing a liquid receives on its internal surface a stream which impinges on it, at any angle whatever, it will be thrown into sonorous vibrations, these vibrations giving rise to a sound when the stream impinges with rapidity and force, the pitch of which sound will depend upon the relative thinness of the membrane (the thinner the membrane the higher the pitch) and the intensity will depend upon the force of the stream, the vibrations giving rise to a soft blowing murmur when the stream impinges with little rapidity and force, and to a rough murmur when the rapidity and force are increased."[12] This, of course, is but an enlargement of certain observations previously made by Bergeon. It may be of help in explaining the greater transmission of murmurs with the course of the blood stream.

Geigel,[13] in 1893, concluded that murmurs are due solely to lateral vibrations of the vessel walls and sometimes of the valves. He admitted, however, that eddies, etc., occur at such places where murmurs are present; Heynsius made them visible by mixing powdered amber with the fluid. Geigel approved Weber's apt comparison of the blood with the bow of the violin and the vessel wall with the string.

[11] Marey, E. J.: Le Circulation du sang, Paris, 1881, p. 647.
[12] Davison, J. T. R.: Lancet, 1895, **1**, 1597.
[13] S. Virchow. Arch., 1895, **140**, 385.

Henri Soulier,[14] of Lyons, believes in the *veine fluide* but would add the murmur of the solid bodies (*souffles solidiens*), or, in other words, the murmur produced by the vibration of the valve involved. Soulier writes of the murmur down stream and up stream from the site of the narrowing, but these were both mentioned by Chauveau and Bergeon, while the latter described conditions (the cul-de-sac up stream) in which the murmur would both originate and be propagated up stream. Soulier points out that in mitral insufficiency the murmur heard in the back (especially if the transmission of that at the apex ceases in the axilla) may well be the murmur travelling down stream, *i. e.*, transmitted from the left auricle.

The explanation of the apex being the point of maximum audibility of the systolic murmur occurring in regurgitation through the mitral valve is commonly accepted as due to the fact that the apex is the part of the left ventricle which most closely approaches the chest wall. But, as Graham Steele points out, "the incompetent valves project backward into the blood stream, exactly like the lip or rim employed by Bergeon."[15] Thus the cul-de-sac against the stream exists (in addition to the narrowing through which the blood passes back to the left auricle) and if Bergeon's conclusions are sound there should be a murmur here and its transmission is up stream.

Thayer and MacCallum, in 1907, published an excellent paper[16] on the experimental production of murmurs in dogs. Their work and that of others demonstrate the ease with which murmurs may be produced artificially in animals.

Experimental. In the hope of obtaining a better understanding of the nature of murmurs detected in the physical examination of the patient, I have made some study of the murmurs which may be produced in rubber tubes through which a stream of water is passing. At first the work was done alone and consisted largely in the repetition of some of the simpler experiments of Gannet, Austin Flint and others, but finally realizing my ignorance of physics and the close connection of the latter with the problem of heart murmurs, I went to Prof. E. L. Chaffee, of Harvard University, for advice. Prof. Chaffee not only answered my questions but insisted on making some apparatus which enabled me to conduct experiments of greater reliability. It seems sufficient to merely summarize some of the tests and the results:

Rubber tubes, of pure rubber and of the caliber of 13 mm. and 7 mm. respectively, were connected with a number of appliances made of brass and representing various alterations in the caliber and contour of the vessel wall. The tube was auscultated above and below the appliance for the presence of a murmur as the water

[14] Lyon méd., 1899, **91**, 289.

[15] Med. Chronicle, Manchester, 1888, **8**, 105.

[16] Thayer, W. S., and MacCallum, W. G.: Am. Jour. Med. Sci., 1907, **133**, 256.

flowed through it. The fitting of the stethoscope with a short piece of rubber tubing, which had been burned to fit the curve of the tube through which the water was flowing, enabled one to auscult accurately without causing a stenosis by pressure of the end of the stethoscope in the effort to make an air-tight contact.

When the rubber tube is compressed with the fingers a murmur is readily produced. This is loudest just below the compressed area and is transmitted farther with the current than against. It varies in intensity with the velocity of the stream and the amount of the stenosis, but if the narrowing is progressively increased there is a point beyond which the maximum murmur is no longer audible. The accompanying diagrams (Diagram 1) show some of the conditions tested.

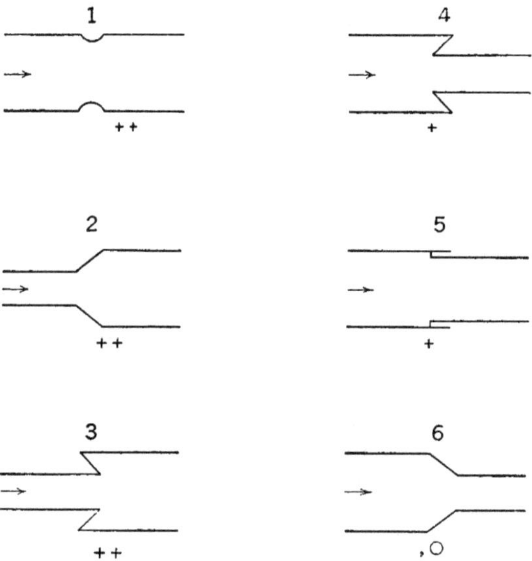

DIAGRAM I.—Cross-section of some of the conditions tested. The arrows indicate the direction of flow. ++ equals a good murmur. + is for a less intense murmur, O is used to signify an absence of murmur.

Figs. 1, 2 and 3 represent conditions favorable for the formation of a *veine fluide* or jet, and readily produced a murmur. Figs. 4 and 5 are examples of the cul-de-sac against the current, whose importance was emphasized by Bergeon. In the condition indicated by Fig. 5 there is merely a sharp lip where the rubber tube was passed over the end of a glass tube; there resulted a sharply localized murmur. In Fig. 6 there was essentially no murmur. The murmur was distinctly louder when associated with a condition which produces a *veine fluide*, as in Figs. 1, 2 and 3, and was heard better and transmitted farther down stream. The audibility and transmission of the murmur in Figs. 4 and 5 was greater up stream. In all cases, as noted in the experiment of digital compression of the tube, a certain degree of velocity of the fluid was necessary and, within limits, the intensity of the murmur was proportional to the velocity of the circulating fluid.

Contrary to the observation of Bergeon it was found that the character of the murmur was influenced by the composition of the wall at the point where the murmur was produced. Thus there was a murmur where the stream of water from the faucet entered the rubber tube and the pitch of this became progressively higher as the auscultation was carried back to the faucet. In another instance the brass tube was connected to a glass tube with almost complete exclusion of the usual rubber tubing, and it was found that the murmur was weaker and of a different pitch.

The rubber tube was opened and for a distance of about two inches fine sand was stuck to its inner aspect by rubber cement. The slit in the vessel wall was then closed by rubber cement. When the water was turned on no murmur could be auscultated save one of very faint character when the stream was flowing at a high velocity. The tube was reopened and it was proved that the sand had not been washed away. In another experiment bits of the inner surface of the tube were cut out, leaving a surface definitely roughened by little pits with sharp edges averaging 1 to 2 mm. in depth and 3 to 4 mm. in greatest diameter. Result: no murmur could be detected.

It was found that when much sand or other material was made adherent to the inner wall of the tube a murmur was readily produced, but it is obvious that this was not a satisfactory test of the influence of roughness, as some degree of stenosis was then also present. It should be recalled that Chauveau cautioned against this error.

An experiment originally performed by Richard Geigel, to show the origin of the actual sound in the vessel wall, was repeated. A pail (Diagram II), was substituted for the glass beaker used by Geigel. In this experiment a murmur was present when the tube delivering the water practically impinged upon the bottom of the pail. A faint sound was detected when the tube was withdrawn so that the eddy around its mouth was made to play upon the bell of the stethoscope.

Clinico-pathologic. I have compared the clinical records and pathologic findings of the last 80 autopsies, all in 1921, at the Boston City Hospital. The group includes only cases which had been on one of the medical services; as there alone would one expect a careful record of the auscultatory findings. It is admitted that the records were written by interns who, of course, vary in skill, but it seems fair to believe that in the majority of instances the results of the physical examination were confirmed by the visiting physician. In any case these records represent examinations of at least equal skill if not better than those of the average physician, and are confidently believed to be suitable for my purpose.

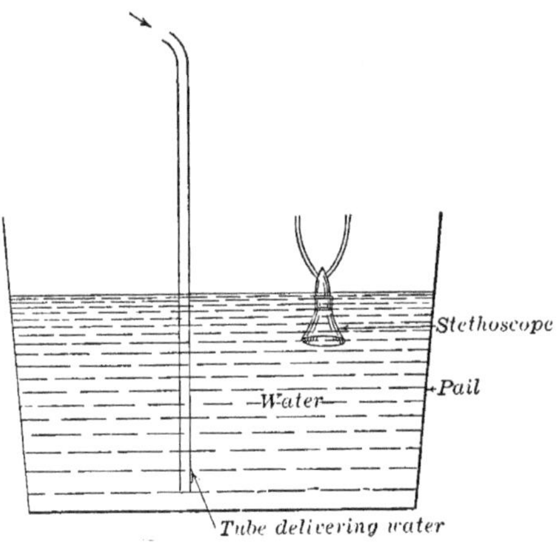

DIAGRAM II.

The comparison is limited to the aortic valve at which the conditions are seemingly simpler. In 56 of the 80 cases the valve was normal and no murmur was recorded. In 6 instances a systolic murmur was present; the postmortem findings were: 4 cases of organic stenosis, a fifth in which a much enlarged heart was associated with hypertension and arteriosclerosis, and in the sixth the valve was normal and the murmur not explained.

In the 18 cases remaining the aortic valve was disclosed to be definitely roughened from various sclerotic changes, in most of which calcification was present, and yet no systolic murmur at the base was recorded. It might be thought that in some of these cases the presence of a systolic murmur over the lower precordia might have caused one at the base to be overlooked. On this point it was found that of the 18 cases, without a systolic murmur at the base in spite of a roughened aortic valve, 5 did have a systolic murmur at the apex; in 3 of these organic changes of the mitral valve were evident and in the remaining 2 none.

In brief then, of 23 cases in which at autopsy the aortic valve found to be definitely roughened, in only 5 was a systolic murmur detected in life. In these latter sufficient cause other than roughness existed.

Comment. A review of the literature pertaining to the mechanism of the production of vascular murmurs appears to disclose that the most common and effective condition giving rise to a murmur is the *veine fluide*. This results from a true stenosis of the vessel or an abrupt widening of its lumen. A sufficient degree of pressure and velocity of blood flow are necessary.

The second condition which favors the production of a murmur is that of a cul-de-sac against the current, as described by Bergeon. This factor is operative apparently when there is merely a sharp edge or lip opposed to the stream. It would seem that the structure of the mitral valve is such that a cul-de-sac against the stream is often present in addition to the conditions that produce a *veine fluide*.

There is a lack of agreement as to the importance of roughening of the inner aspect of the vessel. The difference of opinion is probably due to a difference in the experimental procedure used to determine the effect of roughness. Thus, as already mentioned, Theodor Weber's experiment, in which he stuck bits of cork to the inner aspect of a tube, would appear unsound. In his original report[6] Weber makes no statement as to the exact size of the small pieces of cork or of the amount introduced; in fact he has nothing to say as to what precautions he took to avoid introducing some degree of stenosis. The details of this observer's experiment are seldom referred to, but, if I am correct, his conclusions are often quoted and have exerted much influence in establishing the belief that roughness of the inner aspect of a vessel is an adequate cause for the production of a murmur.

Let us see what methods Chauveau used in getting the evidence on which he based the assertion that the asperities that roughen the internal surface of the circulatory tubes, without modifying the calibre of the latter, cannot be a cause of a murmur. He reports two experiments:

1. Ten to 15 cm. of the carotid artery in a horse were exposed surgically. When with a coarse string tightly drawn around the vessel he cut the lateral and median coats at four or five points rather near together. The coats of the artery torn by this constriction form, producing, to follow closely Chauveau's words,[4] rugosities on the inner aspect of the vessel. These rugosities can be made still more numerous and prominent by pinching the artery with forceps and thereby crushing irregularly the friable layers of the vessel wall. No murmur resulted from this experiment.

2. A metal tube of about the caliber of the artery in diastole was made rough in the interior by powdered gritstone blown in on collodion or varnish. The tube was then introduced into the course of the carotid artery. Result: no murmur.

Chauveau warned that great care must be used not to alter the caliber of the vessel in these experiments. He also pointed out that the clinical study of senile ossification of the arteries agrees with the above experiments in that roughness does not produce a murmur.

My experiments would tend to confirm those of this distinguished

Frenchman. I realize, however, the difficulty in satisfactorily testing the effect of roughness alone, but may say that this work has led to a conviction that if roughness is any factor in the production of vascular murmurs it is very slight and in no sense comparable with the cul-de-sac against the current or the conditions which produce a *veine fluide.* The clinico-pathologic findings reported above are in agreement with this view.

That the composition of the walls at the point at which the murmur is produced has an influence on the murmur would seem to be a logical conclusion from the experiments which I have described. An analogy is found in the alteration in the character of the aortic second sound which is observed when arteriosclerotic changes have occurred in the valve and adjacent aortic wall.

One of the best books on physical diagnosis states, "If the mitral curtains are fixed or made rigid by calcification, so that the vibration with the mitral direct current of blood does not take place, either the murmur may be wanting or its usual characteristic quality may be absent."[17] Another explanation for the absence of the murmur is suggested by certain observations of John Tyndall. The latter, in studying the sounds produced by the flame from gas burners, noted that a certain flame, that made a clear singing sound when surrounded by a long tube was silent when a shorter tube was substituted. He writes: "This large flame, in fact, is not able to accommodate itself to the vibrating period of the shorter tube. . . . But on lowering the flame it soon bursts into vigorous song, its note being the octave of that yielded by the longer tube."[18] Thus the physics of sound are such that certain relations must be present between the surrounding tube and the jet of gas or of fluid, which acts similarly, according to Tyndall, who exhaustively studied the subject, in order that a sound may be produced. It would seem probable, therefore, that the absence of a murmur in the type of mitral valve described by Flint is due to the phenomena observed by Tyndall, *i. e.*, a nonexistence of the relations between the jet and the surrounding tube that are necessary for production of a sound. The same laws must apply to the other cardiac orifices.

The experiment similar to that of Richard Geigel, with the stream of water flowing into the pail of water, is said to demonstrate that the sound is due to vibrations of the vessel walls. Eddies occur in the fluid, but unless they set the walls in vibration no sound is heard. The apt comparison by Theodor Weber of the *veine fluide,* eddy, and so on, to the bow and the vessel wall or valve to the string of a violin has already been mentioned. Apparently also the sound varies in accordance with what is set in vibration; an

[17] Flint's Physical Diagnosis, revised by H. C. Thatcher, Lea & Febiger, 1920, p. 283.
[18] Tyndall, John: "Sound," D. Appleton & Co., 1867, p. 225.

analogy to this are the sounds produced by a stream of water from a hose played upon a window pane and then upon the piazza floor.

In eddies and whirlpools the molecules of water or other fluid continue to move from the spot from which they started. This is a different phenomenon from sound which travels by waves transmitted from one molecule to another similar to the impact transmitted through a row of billiard balls.[18] A wave[19] is a disturbance which travels through any medium without permanently displacing the parts of that medium. Since fluids are practically incompressible, and certainly not so at any such pressure as exists in the human body, Bergeon's conception of alternate compression and reaction of the fluid at the point of murmur production does not seem satisfactory. The literature dealing with the question as to whether the sound originates in the fluid or in the vessel wall is extensive. It does not seem profitable for me to attempt further discussion of the point.

Vascular murmurs, being but one form of sounds, are subject to all the laws of the latter. Thus in their transmission to the surface of the chest considerable alteration may occur due to reflection and refraction as the sound waves from one medium to another of a different density. The sound may be increased by resonance, just as the hollow part of the violin acts with the sound produced by the vibrating string. Further discussion on these aspects of vascular murmurs is beyond the scope of this paper.

Conclusions. 1. A murmur is most readily produced where the conditions exist for the formation of a *veine fluide* or jet. Such conditions are:

(*a*) A stenosis or narrowing of the vessel.

(*b*) A sudden increase in the caliber of the tube.

2. A certain velocity of the stream is necessary.

3. Within certain limits the loudness or intensity of the murmur is proportional to the velocity of the stream.

4. The murmur is propagated both up stream and down, but better in the latter direction.

5. A second condition, easily giving rise to a murmur, is the cul-de-sac against the current. A mere sharp edge or lip is sufficient to cause a murmur.

6. The murmur produced by the cul-de-sac against the current is less intense than that associated with the *veine fluide,* and it is better transmitted up than down stream.

7. Roughness of the inner surface of a vessel appears not to be a cause of a murmur, or if this be not literally true then a murmur due to roughness of the vessel wall is very slight and in no sense comparable to those produced when a *veine fluide* or a cul-de-sac against the stream are present.

[19] Hall and Bergen: A Text-book of Physics, Henry Holt & Co., 1899, p. 443.

Earlier observers are not in agreement as to the influence of roughness of the vessel wall in the production of a murmur. In testing this experimentally great care is necessary to avoid the presence of stenosis also. This error appears to destroy the value if certain experiments, as a result of which some observers have concluded that roughness is a sufficient cause for the production of a murmur.

8. The conditions suitable for the formation of a *veine fluide*, a cul-de-sac against the stream and roughness of the vessel wall may be and often are present together in the human heart.

9. The quality of the murmur is influenced by the character of the vessel wall at the point of production.

10. In their transmission murmurs may be altered by the effect of resonance and of the reflection and refraction of sounds.

11. Murmurs are not mysterious phenomena incapable of explanation, but are one kind of sounds and are subject to the laws that the science of physics has shown pertain to sounds.

THE VALUE OF THE ROENTGEN RAY IN CARDIAC DIAGNOSIS.*

By Frank N. Wilson, M.D.,

ASSOCIATE PROFESSOR OF INTERNAL MEDICINE, UNIVERSITY OF MICHIGAN,

AND

E. Forrest Merrill, M.D.,

SENIOR INTERN IN ROENTGENOLOGY, UNIVERSITY HOSPITAL, ANN ARBOR.

According to an old adage, "Seeing is believing." The roentgenray has a greater appeal than the older methods of physical diagnosis in that it brings the living human heart within the range of that special sense upon which we place greatest dependence. Nevertheless, like many of the special methods of examination that have been introduced into clinical medicine in recent years, the roentgenologic examination of the heart has suffered in reputation from two causes; many not familiar with the type of evidence furnished by the method have expected too much of it; others, specializing in its use, have exaggerated its importance, making extravagant claims which have tended to bring it into disrepute. When it was first employed cases were reported in which sclerotic coronary arteries or an open foramen ovale could be visualized, and it was used by the advocates of special "cures" to demonstrate that certain systems of calisthenics or courses of baths had a definite and favorable effect upon the cardiac silhouette.[1] Looked upon

* Read by Dr. F. N. Wilson at a meeting of the New York Association of Cardiac Clinics, February 8, 1922.

as an ultrascientific method it is still considered by many a veritable *autopsia in vivo*. In its proper sphere, where it is used as an adjunct to our older clinical methods and not as a substitute for them, the roentgen-ray examination of the heart is an invaluable method; it has not failed and it cannot fail in the future to bring us more complete and accurate knowledge, but it is a method which we should be careful not to misuse.

A thorough and systematic study of the normal must always precede the investigation of the abnormal; the experience of the world war has recently emphasized the fact that many errors in diagnosis arise from an insufficient appreciation of the variability of the normal. In the case of the roentgen-ray our knowledge of the normal cardiac silhouette, in spite of the large amount of work that has been done, is still insufficiently comprehensive.

Appearance of the Heart on Fluoroscopic Examination. From the standpoint of the roentgenologist no other organ is so favorably situated as the heart. On ordinary dorsoventral fluoroscopic examination it stands out clearly as a deep shadow against the brightly illuminated lung fields to the right and left. This shadow is continuous above with that of the sternum, the vertebral column and the great vessels, and below with the shadow of the diaphragm and the structures that lie beneath it. The normal cardiac silhonette is bounded on the right and on the left by well-defined arcs corresponding to the lateral borders of the individual cardiac chambers and the great vessels. On the right there are two arcs: The lower is formed by the right auricle and the upper by the superior vena cava or by the more dense ascending aorta. On the left border three and sometimes four subdivisions can be made out; the uppermost arc is formed by the arch and descending aorta; the lowermost arc by the left ventricle; and the middle arc by the pulmonary artery; between the lowest and the middle arcs a fourth, formed by the left auricular appendage, may sometimes be seen. The cardiac apex is frequently lost in the shadow of the dome of the diaphragm which lies behind it; it is best seen when the cardiac end of the stomach contains a bubble of gas or during deep inspiration.

The position and shape of the normal heart varies greatly; in tall, slender individuals (asthenic habitus) with long, narrow chests the cardiac silhouette is also long and narrow and its longest diameter may be nearly vertical; in short, stout subjects (hypersthenic habitus) it may, on the other hand, be nearly horizontal. In persons of average build the longest diameter makes an angle of between 30 and 40 degrees with the horizontal.

The density of the shadow cast by the heart and the great vessels is not uniform. The shadow of the superior vena cava is very faint, so that the more dense aorta can be seen through it; the descending aorta is also visible in many instances through the structures which lie in front of it. The shadow of the left auricular appendage and that of the apex are relatively faint. In some individuals with cardiac disease an indistinct shadow is seen running upward and to the right from the border of the left ventricle; it corresponds fairly well in position to the interventricular septum, which it was believed by Moritz to represent. Groedel[1] has observed it only in cases in which the left auricle was thought to be greatly enlarged and believes it is the shadow of the lower border of this chamber seen through the shadow of the ventricles.

By rotating the subject through an angle of 45 degrees, so that the rays pass through the chest obliquely or by lateral illumination, in which the rays pass through the chest from right to left, other views of the heart may be obtained. With these procedures the distance of the heart from the screen is considerably greater than with dorsoventral illumination and the depth of tissue which the rays must penetrate is much increased; the result is a greater exaggeration of the heart shadow and a marked reduction of contrast. The configuration of the cardiac silhouette in these positions and the identity of the chambers which form various parts of its outline vary according to the exact position of the subject with reference to the direction of the rays, and have been worked out much less fully than in the case of dorsoventral illumination.

With the subject in the right anterior oblique position, in which the rays enter the left back and emerge on the right side anteriorly, the posterior mediastinum appears as a clear band of uniform but variable width.[2] It is bounded on the posterior side by the vertebral column and anteriorly by the aorta in its upper third, the left auricle in its middle third and the right auricle in its lower third.[2] No definite arcs can, however, be made out. The anterior border of the cardiac silhouette is bounded below by the right or left ventricle according to the angle of view and above by the pulmonary artery. The aorta appears as a narrow band at the top of the shadow. The width of the clear posterior mediastinum increases with inspiration and decreases with expiration.

With the subject in the left lateral position we get some idea of the anteroposterior diameter of the heart. In the average normal subject it makes up about 0.7 of the total sternovertebral distance.[3] The posterior margin of the cardiac silhouette is formed by the left ventricle below, the left auricle in its middle portion and the aorta above; the anterior margin by the right ventricle and the pulmonary artery. The lack of contrast makes it very difficult, however, to distinguish details.

As Groedel[1] has pointed out, the lateral and oblique positions show that the longest diameter of the heart is not parallel to the anterior surface of the chest; it makes an acute angle with the vertical axis of the body; the heart is therefore foreshortened by projection upon a plate or screen in contact with the ventral surface of the chest.

The Cardiac Pulsations. With dorsoventral illumination the pulsations of the heart can be seen plainly, but the amplitude of the movement varies greatly in different normal individuals. The movement of the right auricular border is usually so small as to be hardly measurable; the superior vena cava may be motionless or may show slight movement alternating with that of the auricle. The systolic pulsation of the aorta is easily seen though not of large amplitude; the pulsation of the pulmonary artery is less conspicuous. The greatest movement is shown by the border of the left ventricle; it differs in character from that of the right auricle and that of the great vessels, in that it is more deliberate and gives the impression of being more forceful. At the junction of the left auricle and the left ventricle there is a sort of walking-beam effect with a node of no motion which moves up and down with each cardiac cycle.

Our knowledge of these pulsation phenomena is as yet very imperfect and will remain so until some adequate method of recording them has been devised. Some progress in this direction has recently been made. Crane[4] has a method for taking what he calls "roentgenocardiograms." A lead sheet with a transverse slit about 2 cm. wide is placed between the patient and the plate in such a way that the slit overlaps the heart borders of which the movements are to be recorded. The plate is moved in front of the slit at a uniform speed. By this method tracings somewhat resembling pulse tracings may be made; those so far published have been rather poor from a technical standpoint, but this defect may perhaps be overcome. Flohil[5] and Eyster and Meek[6] have devised methods for taking instantaneous (exposure of 0.04 second) roentgenograms at chosen points in the cardiac cycle; an electrocardiogram is taken simultaneously, and this, through induction, records the time of the exposure with reference to the electrocardiographic deflections. Eyster and Meek have been able by using a special plate-changing device to take plates at the beginning and at the end of the same systole. From such plates they compute, using the tables worked out by Bardeen,[7] the systolic output of the heart. They find that "usually the maximum change is at or near the apex and decreases upward, but the reverse may be seen. The movement of any one point on the left border may give an entirely erroneous idea as to the extent of the contraction of the heart." They describe a typical cardiac contraction as follows: "When the auricles contract the right auricular border decreases slightly and there is a corresponding enlargement along the lower border of the left and right ventricles. The apex moves about 1 mm. to the left and the heart becomes slightly more elongated from base to apex. . . . As the ventricles contract the right auricular border enlarges slightly and extends outward slightly more than immediately before the auricular systole. The bases of the ventricles descend a few millimeters and the whole heart becomes more globular in outline. The apex moves upward and to the right, the right ventricular border moves toward the base and the left ventricular border to the right." These observations are very interesting; it is to be hoped that they will be continued and that they will be extended to include instances of heart disease.

It is rather difficult to see, however, how it is possible to measure the movements of the right ventricular border and of the ventricular base accurately, for these borders are not clearly visible in the roentgenogram. It is also difficult to see the value of computing the systolic output by the method mentioned, for changes in auricular volume cannot be distinguished with certainty from changes in ventricular volume, since the position of the *A-V* junction cannot be accurately determined. It is quite within the range of possibility that in some instances the chief alterations in auricular and in ventricular volume are accomplished by changes in the position of the auriculoventricular septum. According to Van Zwaluwenburg,[2] hearts of the pendulous type often show more movement of the apex than hearts of the sessile type. He believes that in the former, which are in a way suspended from the great vessels, the *A-V* septum moves less and the apex consequently more.

Effects of Respiration and Change in Posture. The cardiac silhouette is altered in position and in form by the respiratory movements and by changes in the posture of the body. With forced inspiration the heart follows the diaphragm downward and the long diameter rotates in a clockwise direction.[5] The long diameter of the heart increases slightly while the transverse diameter decreases considerably.[1] There is probably also some torsion of the heart. Whether these changes in the position and shape of the heart are accompanied by changes in its volume has been much disputed; quiet breathing seems to cause comparatively little change in the size of the cardiac shadow. Cohn,[8] who has recently investigated this subject, found that in the majority of individuals both the long and the transverse diameters as well as the area of the cardaic silhouette were slightly greater in inspiration than in expiration. It has been shown that the Valsalva experiment causes a definite decrease in the size of the heart shadow while the Müller experiment causes a definite increase. Forced expiration and forced inspiration probably have similar though less marked effects. Forced expiration causes a greater shift in the position of the heart than forced inspiration when the subject is in the erect position; the opposite is true when the subject is in the supine position.

The changes in the cardiac silhouette which accompany a change from the horizontal to the vertical posture are in part due to the change in the level of the diaphragm and the tendency of the heart to drop down of its own weight when the subject stands. There is, however, a definite decrease in the area of the heart shadow on assuming the vertical posture. The heart volume is said to be about 25 per cent less with the subject standing,[1] and the area of the cardiac outline to be about 13 per cent less.[8] The cause of these variations is not altogether clear; they have been attributed to traction on the cavæ and the pericardium in the standing position, to hydrostatic factors and to pressure of the dome of the diaphragm on that part of the heart which lies between it and the anterior chest wall in the lying position.

Of the changes in the cardiac silhouette which accompany other changes in posture nothing need be said; they are for the most part such as might be anticipated. It should be noted, however, that the pendulous heart is much more mobile than the more sessile organ, which is firmly held in the angle between the dome of the diaphragm and the anterior chest wall. On one occasion a tall, thin student consulted one of us because he found that when he lay on his right side the cardiac impulse was best felt to the right of the sternum; his heart was normal but of the pendulous type.

The Roentgen-Ray in the Diagnosis of Cardiac Enlargement. Upon few subjects that have received an equal amount of attention are there greater differences of opinion than upon the roentgenologic estimation of the size of the heart. In preroentgenologic days the clinician depended for this purpose upon the position and character of the apex-beat and upon the percussion outline of the deep cardiac dulness. How inadequate these methods are we all realize. Before the days of the orthodiagram there was, even among the masters of percussion, no general agreement as to the usual limits of the deep cardiac dulness in the normal subject. It is only within recent years that the percussion outline has been made to correspond with the orthogonal projection of the heart upon the anterior chest wall. But inaccurate though they be, inspection, palpation and percussion are very useful in judging the heart's size; they rarely lead to gross errors because we are familiar with their limitations. With the roentgen-ray with which they cannot compete in accuracy we are not altogether satisfied because we have, without reason, expected it to enable us to distinguish infallibly between a heart which is just beginning to enlarge as a result of disease and one which is normal. This is manifestly impossible; no sharp line can be drawn between health and disease; a zone of uncertainty is inevitable.

In the roentgenologic examination of the heart two methods

are available: orthodiagraphy and teleroentgenography. As a general method the former is certainly preferable; it is much less expensive and it allows us to mark the junction of the left auricular and the left auricular border and the junction of the right auricular border and that of the great vessels, and to follow the left ventricular border below the dome of the diaphragm. It gives us a view of the cardiac pulsations. Its chief disadvantages are that it requires more skill and is more subjective. When possible a combination of the two methods should be used.

Before the roentgen-ray could be used successfully in the diagnosis of cardiac enlargement it was necessary to establish normal standards. In establishing such standards it is desirable, in order to make the normal range as small as possible, to take into consideration all of the factors which are known to affect the size of the normal cardiac silhouette. It is known that the heart shadow varies in size with the body weight, the height, the posture, the heart-rate, the sex, the phase of respiration, the position of the heart and the amount of physical exertion to which the subject is accustomed. It must be remembered that the heart is an elastic organ; its size varies with the volume of its contents; the venous pressure, the intrathoracic pressure, the tension of the pericardium, the elasticity of the heart muscle probably play a part in determining the volume of the heart. It is true that the influence of many of these factors is probably so slight that no great error is made in neglecting them, but the normal standards at present in use take into consideration only the posture, the body weight and the phase of the cardiac cycle. The subjects are usually examined in the erect posture. the diastolic size of the heart shadow is determined and the subjects are classified according to weight.

As to the best method of measuring the size of the heart shadow there is no general agreement. The most popular method is to measure the area of the silhouette by means of the planimeter or to compute the approximate area by some formula such as that for the ellipse. One difficulty with this method arises from the continuity of the heart shadow with that of the great vessels above and that of the liver below; the upper and lower borders must be drawn in more or less arbitrarily before its area can be measured. The error is probably not great in dealing with the normal heart; it is certainly much greater in dealing with the abnormal heart, of which the shape varies greatly. Another difficulty, one which is common to all the roentgenologic methods of determining the presence of cardiac enlargement that have so far been proposed, arises from the width of the normal range. As Cohn[8] has recently pointed out, individual normal subjects may show silhouette areas larger by 30 per cent or more than the average area for normal subjects of the same weight. Similar deviations from the normal average have been found by all observers except

Smith;[9] they are therefore probably not to be avoided by any refinement or variation in technic.

The method in use in Ann Arbor was introduced by Van Zwaluwenburg. He found that by treating the cardiac silhouette as an ellipse and computing the area by multiplying the product of the long and short diameters by 0.7854, he obtained figures which showed an average deviation from the planimeter values of only 3 or 4 per cent; the greatest deviation amounted to 8 per cent.[2] He also found it convenient to express the area of the cardiac shadow of individual cases in percentages of the average area of normal subjects of the same weight. Since the area computed by this method is a constant fraction of the *product of the diameters* (*POD*), the latter may be utilized instead of the former as a measure of the heart's size. The average *POD* (in square centimeters) of normal subjects, expressed as a function of the weight, is approximately equal, according to Van Zwaluwenburg, to $3.72\sqrt[3]{\text{weight in pounds}}$.[2] This standard falls considerably below that of Bardeen.[7] A variation of 10 per cent in either direction is considered to be within normal limits. The subjects are examined in the erect posture and the cardiac silhouette is recorded by means of the orthodiagraph.

The smallest values observed have been in the neighborhood of 85 per cent, the largest in the neighborhood of 280 per cent. The great majority of abnormal hearts show values in excess of 130 per cent, but occasionally cases of mitral stenosis and of cardiosclerosis show values within 10 per cent of the standard figures. We frequently see, on the other hand, values as high as 140 per cent in cases in which no abnormality of the heart can be discovered by other methods and in which there are no clinical findings that would lead us to anticipate cardiac enlargement. It is possible that in such cases we are dealing with slight idiopathic cardiac enlargement, but we very much doubt that this is often the case. We believe that in most of these instances the heart is normal; the patients are usually asked to return in six months for a second examination.

Several other methods of diagnosing cardiac enlargement from the cardiac silhouette have been advocated. One that has recently received considerable attention is the determination of the ratio of the total transverse diameter of the heart (the total transverse diameter of the heart is the sum of the greatest perpendicular distance from the midline to the right border (*MR*) and the greatest perpendicular distance from the midline to the left border (*ML*)) to the internal diameter of the chest.[10] When this ratio exceeds a value of 0.50 the heart is considered to be abnormally large. In order to get a better idea of this very simple method we went over 60 orthodiagrams, selected at random, and compared this ratio with the *POD* expressed in the percentage of the standard. In 28 cases both methods indicated cardiac enlargement; the *POD* varied between 116 per cent and 272 per cent, the ratio between 0.50 and 0.75. In 16 cases both methods indicated no cardiac enlargement; the *POD* varied between 85 per cent and 110 per cent while the ratio varied between 0.37 and 0.50. In 10 cases the *POD* indicated enlargement while the ratio did not; in one of these cases the *POD* reached a value of 150 per cent. In 6 cases the ratio indicated enlargement and the *POD* did not; in one of these cases a *POD* of 93 per cent was associated with a ratio of 0.63. We got the impression that the ratio varies greatly with the shape of the chest and the position of the heart. In individuals of asthenic build it may fall as low as 0.35, while in individuals of hypersthenic habitus it may exceed 0.50 even though the heart is normal. It tends to give high values in cases of arteriosclerosis of the aorta in which the heart is transversely placed. It would also seem that it must undergo considerable variations with the phases of respiration, for inspiration tends to increase the transverse diameter of the chest while it tends to decrease the transverse diameter of the heart. It has the additional disadvantage that great variations in the size of the heart produce only slight variations in the ratio.

In a third method of determining the presence of cardiac enlargement the total transverse diameter of the heart shadow is compared with the average value of this measurement in normal subjects of the same weight. The total transverse diameter has the advantage that it can be measured with a high degree of accuracy; the right and left margins of the heart stand out clearly against the lung fields so that there is no uncertainty in locating them as there is in locating the apex, which is necessary to the measurement of the long diameter, or the upper and lower borders of the cardiac silhouette, which are necessary to the measurement of the silhouette area. The chief objection to this method is that the transverse diameter varies with the angle of inclination of the long axis of the heart; when the heart is of the pendulous type the transverse diameter is very small; when the heart is horizontally placed the transverse diameter is relatively large. In Cohn's tables[8] the range of the transverse diameter for normal subjects of 74 kilos is 5 cm. In these tables the angle made by the long diameter with the horizontal is given for each subject; if we consider only those subjects (weighing 74 kilos) in which this angle varies between 40 and 45 degrees the range of the transverse diameter is reduced to 3 cm. If we had standards which took into consideration the inclination of the long axis of the heart the usefulness of the transverse diameter in determining the heart's size would be greatly increased.

In this connection it should be pointed out that the long diameter and the area are influenced in a similar fashion by the inclination of the long diameter of the heart to the axis of the body.[1] How variable this may be we do not at present know, but the possibility that it may have an important influence upon the measurements mentioned must be borne in mind.

We must conclude that with the standards at present in use it is impossible for the roentgenologist to diagnose with certainty grades of cardiac enlargement that are not recognized or suspected by the clinician. This fact should be emphasized; failure to realize it is sure to do harm. There is need for a much more comprehensive study of the normal cardiac silhouette than has yet been attempted. In such a study all of the factors which are known to influence the size of the heart shadow should be included. Not only height and weight, but the body surface, the sitting height the heart rate, the age, the diameters of the chest, the angle of inclination of the long axis of the heart and the amount of physical exertion to which the subject is accustomed should be recorded so that the influence of each may be determined. The anterior-posterior diameter of the heart and the inclination of its long diameter with reference to the axis of the body should be measured. And finally the subjects should be selected with great care and should be reëxamined after from two to four years so that incipient cases of heart disease might be excluded; this could easily be done in any medical school where freshmen could be chosen as subjects and could be kept under observation until graduation. In this way the width of the normal range could probably be reduced considerably and the roentgen ray could be made much more serviceable in the diagnosis of cardiac enlargement than it is at present.

But even if all of the variables mentioned were included in the standard tables the normal range would probably still be relatively wide. The weight of the heart is probably much more constant than its volume, and certainly the weight of the heart can be determined with much greater accuracy than we shall ever be able to determine its volume by means of the roentgen ray. Nevertheless it is almost as difficult to diagnose cardiac hypertrophy after death as it is to diagnose cardiac enlargement during life. The figures of Müller[11] and of Lewis[12] show that the ratio ventricular weight body weight varies in controls within wide limits. Thus in Lewis's series of cancer controls, in which no cardiovascular abnormality could be discovered at autopsy, this ratio varies between 0.00200 and 0.00421, and has an average value of 0.00301. The individual variations are as great as those found by Cohn for the cardiac silhouette area. It is clear, therefore, that the normal range is not likely to be brought within narrow limits. Neither in clinical medicine nor in pathology is it possible to recognize the slighter grades of cardiac enlargement.

Variations in the Size of the Heart. In following the variations in the size of the heart in individual patients with cardiac disease the roentgen-ray is vastly superior to any other method. For this purpose it is much better to superimpose successive teleroentgenograms or orthodiagrams than to compare measurements of these; errors due to changes in the position of the heart may thus be more easily avoided. The constancy of the heart's size in many cases of chronic heart disease is, as Grodel has pointed out, surprising. Such patients may go for long periods of time without measurable change in the cardiac shadow. A rapid increase in the size of the heart is usually of evil omen. We have recently seen, however, a case in which considerable variations in the size of the heart shadow took place without any appreciable change in the clinical condition. The patient was a young man with rheumatic aortic insufficiency and mitral stenosis; he had no cardiac symptoms whatever. The first orthodiagram showed a greatly enlarged cardiac shadow with a transverse diameter of 145 mm. The second orthodiagram, taken two months later, showed, when superimposed upon the first, a general increase in the size of the heart shadow; the transverse diameter was 172 mm. The third orthodiagram showed, when compared with the second, a slight decrease in the silhouette area; the transverse diameter remained about the same. The patient's clinical condition was unchanged.

The various therapeutic procedures, rest and digitalis, which bring about striking changes in the degree of heart failure, only occasionally give rise to a conspicuous decrease in the size of the heart. Patients are not usually examined by the roentgenologist, however, when the cardiac weakness is at its maximum, because of the technical difficulties involved. Most observers agree that a striking decrease in the size of the chronically enlarged heart is uncommon, and one observer states that when a conspicuous decrease takes place in such cases a pericardial effusion should be suspected.[1]

The case is quite difficult when the increase in size is not of long standing. Transient enlargement of the heart shadow has been noted frequently in various infectious diseases, including rheumatic fever, diphtheria, pneumonia and scarlet fever[1] and during attacks of paroxysmal tachycardia.[13] As to the exact factors involved in the infectious diseases we have no accurate knowledge. An increase in the size of the cardiac silhouette cannot, so it seems to us, be safely attributed to cardiac weakness unless it is accompanied by signs of venous engorgement or diminished blood flow. In paroxysmal tachycardia with increase in the size of the heart such signs have been observed.

The Recognition of Enlargement of Individual Cardiac Chambers. Most of the older text-books on physical diagnosis, and many of the newer ones, describe signs which are supposed to differentiate between hypertrophy and dilatation of the ventricles and between enlargement of the right and enlargement of the left ventricle.

Enlargement of the left ventricle is said to displace the cardiac impulse to the left and downward; enlargement of the right ventricle to displace the apex to the left. Left ventricular hypertrophy is said to cause a heaving apex-beat; right ventricular hypertrophy, to cause systolic retraction at the apex or in the epigastrium. Most of these signs, in so far as they have been tested by comparison with postmortem findings, have proved thoroughly unreliable. The electrocardiographic indications are likewise not to be depended upon.[14] It is, of course, possible to diagnose preponderant enlargement of the right or left ventricle correctly in many cases from a knowledge of the type of heart lesion present; we know that aortic insufficiency and chronic hypertension usually produce preponderant enlargement of the left ventricle and that mitral stenosis and pulmonary stenosis usually produce preponderant enlargement of the right ventricle. Such inferential diagnoses have little value. The roentgen-ray furnishes some real evidence of the size of the individual cardiac chambers, but here also caution is necessary in drawing conclusions.

The roentgen-ray signs of enlargement of individual cardiac chambers have been worked out by studying the shape of the cardiac silhouettes that have been shown to be characteristic of various valve lesions. It is difficult to check the roentgen-ray picture against the autopsy findings because of the changes in the heart which take place during the agonal period and after death through the occurrence of rigor mortis; nevertheless too little work along this line has been attempted. The relation of the component arcs of the normal cardiac shadow to the different cardiac chambers is no longer a subject of dispute; in the case of the abnormal heart, however, considerable difference of opinion exists. Much stress is often laid upon the character and time of the pulsations of a given border of the heart shadow in identifying the chamber which forms it; but since these pulsations have, heretofore, been studied by simple inspection only, and since the movements of a given arc are not solely due to the activities of the chamber of which it forms the margin, conclusions based upon such data must be looked upon with some skepticism.

There is also a tendency invariably to attribute increased saliency of a given margin of the cardiac silhouette to enlargement of the chamber which normally forms that margin, and to assume that increase in the size of a given chamber must invariably give the same picture. When we consider the great variability of the normal heart in size, shape and position it is hard to believe that this assumption is justified. It is to be expected that the picture of enlargement of a given chamber will vary greatly in individuals of different build. It must also be remembered that the heart is a mobile organ and its mobility differs in different individuals. When the enlargement of one of its cavities causes a shift in its center of gravity it must readjust its position, and the new position like the old will depend upon a great many factors which vary from person to person. That auricular enlargement may be distinguished from ventricular enlargement in the majority of cases and that enlargement of the left auricle may be distinguished from enlargement of the right is hardly to be doubted. That the roentgenologist can say in every case of ventricular enlargement which of the two ventricles is chiefly affected remains to be proved. To show that certain signs held to indicate enlargement of the left ventricle only are present in aortic insufficiency and absent in pulmonary stenosis is not sufficient justification for considering these signs pathognomonic of left ventricular enlargement under all manner of conditions.

Hypertrophy and Dilatation; Cardiac Weakness. The roentgenologist can, in some measure, distinguish between hypertrophy and dilatation. Hypertrophy alone can, of course, cause comparatively little enlargement of the heart; the increase in the thickness of the heart wall which takes place when the heart hypertrophies rarely amounts to more than a few millimeters, and can hardly cause a recognizab[illegible] diameters of the cardiac shadow. Recognizable [illegible]ent means dilatation; if the enlargement has [illegible] space of a few hours it means dilatation [illegible]alone. All chronically enlarged hearts are hypertrophied as well as dilated; the increase in size is due almost entirely to dilatation, but the shape may depend upon the amount of hypertrophy present. Viewed with the fluoroscope many enlarged hearts show well-defined arcs corresponding to the various cardiac chambers and a shape characteristic of the valve lesion present. Others appear shapeless; they are enlarged in all diameters and no distinct arcs are seen; the heart appears flaccid in that the shadow rests upon a broad base and is narrow above, so that it looks somewhat like a leather bottle filled with water; in such cases the pulsations are usually of small amplitude. The roentgenologist is prone to speak of hearts of the first type as hypertrophied and to describe hearts of the second type as dilated. Which of these forms the heart assumes when it becomes much enlarged may depend in part upon the chambers affected or it may depend upon the thickness of the ventricular walls.

The roentgenologist sometimes makes such diagnosis as "myocardial insufficiency" or "cardiac decompensation." In such cases he bases his opinion upon the presence of "dilatation" and upon the character of the cardiac pulsations. In describing the latter such terms as "feeble," "vigorous," "weak" or "strong" are used; we believe that such words should usually be avoided; they are apt to be considered descriptive of the condition of the heart muscle. The character of the pulsations seen on fluoroscopic examination is greatly influenced by the size of the heart, the heart-rate and the position of the heart, and bears no close relation to the efficiency of the heart as a pump. Large hearts are usually bad hearts, but the terms *dilatation* and *cardiac weakness* are not synonymous. That there is a relation between the two conditions is not to be doubted; it is not, however, a close one. Very large hearts, more especially large shapeless hearts, are seen chiefly in patients who suffer or who have suffered from advanced cardiac failure; but a relatively large heart is compatible with fair cardiac function and a relatively small heart with poor function. The efficiency of the heart must be measured in terms of blood-flow; cardiac weakness must be diagnosed largely by the presence of signs and symptoms produced by a slowed circulation of the blood; for this purpose the examination of the heart itself is of quite secondary importance. In heart failure of the type associated with venous engorgement the right auricle is usually greatly dilated, so that there is a wide extension of the heart shadow to the right; this sign belongs in the same class with congestion of the liver and distention of the veins of the neck. Except in so far as this sign is of value in the diagnosis of cardiac weakness this diagnosis does not lie within the province of the roentgenologist.

The Diagnosis of Valve Lesions. Valve lesions can be diagnosed by roentgen-ray only in so far as they produce characteristic changes in the size and shape of the cardiac chambers affected, and thus alter the configuration of the cardiac silhouette and the saliency and pulsation of its component arcs. The roentgenologist is prone to regard these changes as a quantitative measure of the valve defect and to look upon valve lesions which are not associated with more or less characteristic alterations of the cardiac silhouette as comparatively unimportant. But the importance of a valve lesion does not depend solely upon the magnitude of the disturbance of cardiac mechanics which it produces; it depends even more upon the nature of the disease process to which it is due. In aortic insufficiency the clinician is, on the whole, less anxious to know the amount of blood which regurgitates than he is to know whether the lesion is a sign of arteriosclerosis, of syphilitic aortitis or of an old rheumatic carditis, or to know the nature and extent of the inflammatory and degenerative changes that have taken place in the ventricular muscle. In answering these questions the roentgen-ray, though less important than the history and physical examination, is often of service. The changes in the size and shape of the heart in chronic heart disease are not due solely to changes in the fluid pressures within its chambers, but in part to the associated myocardial changes. The roentgen-ray picture is often more significant in cases in which the cardiac silhouette is not characteristic of the valve lesion present than in cases in which it is.

In typical cases of mitral stenosis the cardiac outline is characterized chiefly by an abnormal saliency of that arc which forms the margin of the left auricular appendage. This encroaches upon the left ventricular arc, which in the absence of left ventricular enlargement is shorter than in the normal. There is sometimes an abnormal extension of the shadow to the right of the midline; whether this is rightly attributed to enlargement of the right ventricle by Vaquet and Bordet[15] is questionable; it is by no means always present. The enlarged left auricle may also be seen by oblique illumination, in which it causes a constriction of the posterior mediastinum in its middle third (right anterior oblique illumination). When this picture is modified by rounding of the apex, by an increase in the length of the lower left arc, by an increase in the distance of the left border from the midline and by an increase in the anterior posterior diameter of the ventricular shadow the roentgenologist makes a diagnosis of mitral stenosis plus mitral insufficiency. Whether in such instances the ventricular enlargement is due entirely to the regurgitation of blood through the mitral orifice or whether the diagnosis of mitral insufficiency, mitral stenosis being present, has any particular value is, it seems to us, questionable. In some cases of mitral stenosis the pulmonary arc is prominent. Vaquet and Bordet[15] have described a case in which this was a conspicuous feature and in which there was a soft blowing diastolic murmur along the left border of the sternum which they took to be a Graham Steele murmur. Whether the Graham Steele murmur is a frequent phenomenon is still uncertain; we regard it as rare, believing that most of the basal diastolic murmurs which are so common in mitral stenosis are due to slight damage to the aortic valve. The origin of such murmurs, no changes in the pulse being present, is not of great practical interest.

In typical cases of aortic insufficiency the cardiac silhouette extends far to the left, whereas the width of the ventricular shadow (that is the diameter perpendicular to the long diameter) is not greatly increased. The apex is blunt and the arc of the left ventricle is lengthened and more sharply curved near the apex, so that the upper left margin of the ventricular shadow is sometimes described as "round-shouldered." According to Groedel[1] the apex is elevated, according to Vaquet and Bordet[15] it is depressed; its actual position probably depends upon the shape and position of the heart before the lesion developed and upon the presence or absence of changes in the aorta. The pulsations of the aorta are usually exaggerated; in rheumatic aortic insufficiency the aorta is of normal caliber while in syphilitic aortic insufficiency it is usually diffusely dilated. In the former mitral stenosis is often associated and a salient left auricle is added to the picture. Oblique examination shows an increase in the thickness of the ventricular shadow. The pulsations of the left border are deliberate and give the same impression of power that is gained from the heaving apex-beat.

Aortic stenosis is said to give a similar picture except that there is less enlargement and the aortic throbbing is absent. Chronic hypertension may give a picture closely resembling that of aortic insufficiency; the increased movement of the aorta is absent; the aorta is dense, lengthened and often diffusely dilated.

Open ductus arteriosus gives a cardiac silhouette characterized chiefly by abnormally salient and violently pulsating pulmonary arc. In pulmonary stenosis, which is very often associated with other congenital lesions, the apex according to Vaquet and Bordet[15] is often much elevated, so that the ventricular shadow resembles a "sabot" in appearance. We have not seen such a picture. Recently we have seen a patient with congenital heart disease and a loud systolic murmur with a pronounced thrill in the pulmonic area in whom the cardiac shadow was normal in every respect. An open ventricular septum is also said to give a characteristic cardiac shadow. In the cases which have been observed the silhouette was globular and extended far to the right and systolic pulsations of wide excursion were present at both right and left margins.[1 15]

Many roentgenologists believe that tricuspid insufficiency can be recognized by roentgen-ray examination. It is indicated when in addition to a greatly increased extension of the cardiac shadow to the right of the midline, produced by enlargement of the right auricle, the auricular arc and the vena cava show well-marked systolic pulsations. Whether this sign is more reliable than systolic distention of the liver and the positive venous pulse which were formerly much in favor is to be doubted. We cannot refrain from pointing out here to those who believe that tricuspid insufficiency causes recognizable expansile pulsation of the liver, that an increase of 30 cc, one-half the systolic output of the normal right ventricle, in the volume of a much congested liver with a volume of let us say 2000 cc, will cause an increase of less than 1 mm. in any one of its linear dimensions. Can a systolic distention of this magnitude be recognized through the abdominal wall and distinguished from mere nonexpansile movement? The case of the enlarged right auricle is similar; when one remembers that the movements of the margin of the normal right auricle are often barely visible he doubts the possibility of recognizing such systolic distention of a much enlarged auricle as could be produced by any amount of blood that is likely to regurgitate through the tricuspid orifice.

In *the diagnosis of diseases of the aorta,* arteriosclerosis, dilatation, syphilitic aortitis and aneurysm the roentgen-ray is exceedingly useful, but lack of space prevents us from considering this subject here.

Fibrinous pericarditis produces no roentgen-ray signs. Large *pericardial effusions* give large, roughly, triangular "water-bottle" like shadows which extend far to the right and rest upon a broad base. The contour changes with changes in posture.[16] The silhouette borders are practically motionless. The cardiohepatic angle is maintained. It is sometimes difficult on a single examination to distinguish between a pericardial effusion and a very large heart; in such instances the clinical picture usually aids in reaching a decision. Small effusions are recognized with difficulty. The roentgen-ray has also proved useful in the *diagnosis of adherent pericardium* either through the visibility of extrapericardial adhesions or through the effect of the adhesions upon the mobility of the heart. The roentgen-ray diagnosis of adherent pericardium is, however, scarcely less difficult than the clinical diagnosis.

Conclusion. The roentgen-ray appears to us an indispensable instrument in the diagnosis of cardiac disease, but we must not allow the roentgenologist to make our diagnoses for us. We should ourselves be able to interpret his findings and to allot to them their proper place. We should be especially careful in the diagnosis of cardiac enlargement from the roentgen-ray picture alone, particularly in cases in which no cause for such enlargement can be found. Finally the exaggeration of the importance of the roentgen-ray examination of the heart, at the expense of other methods, which is to be seen in some of the recent French literature, is to be deplored. Special aspects of a subject are not to be neglected, but they must be subordinated to the subject as a whole.

REFERENCES.

1. Groedel, F. M.: Atlas und Grundriss der Röntgendiagnostik in der inneren Medizin, Munich, 1909 (J. F. Lehmann).
2. Van Zwaluwenburg, J. G.: Am. Jour. Roentgenol., 1920, **7**, 1.
3. Laubry, Ch., Mallet, L., and Hirschberg, F.: Arch. d. mal. d. cœur, 1921, **14**, 394.
4. Crane, A. W.: Am. Jour. Roentgenol., 1916, **3**, 513.
5. Flohil, A.: Arch. Neerland. d. Physiol., 1918, **2**, 562.
6. Eyster, J. A. E., and Meek, W. J.: Am. Jour. Roentgenol., 1920, **7**, 471.
7. Bardeen, C. R.: Am. Jour. Roentgenol., 1917, **4**, 604.
8. Cohn, A. E.: Arch. Int. Med., 1920, **25**, 499.
9. Smith, B.: Arch. Int. Med., 1920, **25**, 522.
10. Martin, C. L.: Am. Jour. Roentgenol., 1921, **8**, 295.
11. Müller: Die Massenverhältnisse des menschlichen Herzens, Hamburg and Leipzig, 1883.
12. Lewis, T.: Heart, 1914, **5**, 367.
13. Wilson, D. C.: Heart, 1921, **8**, 303.
14. Herrmann, G. R., and Wilson, F. N.: Unpublished observations which will appeart in Heart.
15. Vaquet, H., and Bordet, E.: The Heart and the Aorta (translated by Honeij and Macy), Yale University Press, 1920.
16. Holmes, G. W.: Am. Jour. Roentgenol., 1920, **7**, 7.

SUDDEN DEATH FOLLOWING THORACENTESIS.

By Ernest S. du Bray, A.B., M.D.,
INSTRUCTOR OF MEDICINE, UNIVERSITY OF CALIFORNIA MEDICAL SCHOOL, SAN FRANCISCO, CAL.

Clinicians of wide experience can usually recall in their own memories accidents and fatalities attending or following simple puncture of the thorax for either exploratory purposes, the drainage of fluid and more recently for the institution of an artificial pneumothorax in the treatment of certain cases of pulmonary tuberculosis. Notwithstanding the fact that these mishaps are comparatively uncommon and that the practice of thoracentesis is now considered a harmless and simple procedure, the well-known possibility of syncope, collapse and even death during or shortly following it should be sufficient grounds for regarding this procedure more seriously and inducing us to take any known precautions that may prevent the occurrence of untoward symptoms.

Physiologic Mechanisms. The physiologic mechanisms through which syncope, collapse and death are brought about have been the subjects of several signal investigations, and although it cannot be said that the mechanism is understood in every case, nevertheless certain facts have been demonstrated which rationally explains the mechanism in most cases. Russell[1] studied this subject in 1899, and he came to the conclusion that the syncope which sometimes attends or shortly follows simple thoracentesis is based upon direct injury to the vagus nerve fibers in the lung tissue with secondary reflex impulses conveyed to the heart. This explanation does not take into consideration any reflex which might arise and be propagated through the pleura itself, and is, in consequence, not in accord with the results of the splendid experimental investigations afterward performed by Capps[2] and his associates.

The Pleural Reflex. Capps's[3] interest in this subject was aroused by a fatal case of collapse which came under his observation in a patient with a pleural effusion. The collapse immediately followed the puncture of the pleural cavity after only a few cubic centimeters of fluid had been removed. The autopsy failed to reveal anatomic evidence for the cause of the unfortunate accident, although lesions such as laceration, hemorrhage and edema of the lung were sought as well as an investigation of the brain. It was to the careful experimental work of this investigator that clinical medicine owed the neurogenic conception of the mechanism of collapse in these cases. Capps proved the existence of a true pleural reflex, and any one interested in this subject cannot do better than review his original papers.[4 5 6 7]

By ingenious and convincing animal experimentation he showed that the healthy pleura is tolerant to irritation, whereas the inflamed pleura may react to irritation, whether mechanical or chemical, by marked reflex circulatory disturbances. To use his own words he says, "The pleural reflex may act on the cardioinhibitory fibers of the heart through the vagus nerve-endings or on the vasomotor centers through the sympathetic nerves."

Capps's conclusions, based on his experiments, are as follows:

"1. Syncope during aspiration is the result of direct cardiac inhibitiou.

"2· Syncope during aspiration results from irritation of the pleural or pulmonary nerves either by the trocar or by congestion. It is most common toward the end of the operation when the instrument is most likely to scratch the pleura and when the lung is most congested.

"3· Syncope occurring within forty-eight hours after aspiration is probably due to the circulatory reflexes arising from congestion of the lungs.

"4. Syncope during irrigation of the pleural cavity is the result of a reflex arising from the chemical irritation of the pleura."

Pulmonary Lesions Produced by Thoracentesis (Injury and Congestion). Besides the foregoing fairly clear-cut type of collapse now believed to be due to the pleural reflex (often called pleural shock) there is another rather mixed group of cases which are seen but which have a varied pathogenesis. The cases referred to are, however, constant in one particular—in that they are practically always associated with demonstrable anatomic lesion of the lung parenchyma, either in the form of lacerations or puncture wounds caused by the trocar accidentally in the course of the thoracentesis or definite pulmonary congestion of an extreme grade.

Air Embolism. In 1912 Brauer[8] directed attention to the question of air embolism of the cerebral vessels. Stivelman,[9] in a recent paper, has been inclined not only to minimize the importance of this occurrence but to question its existence. More recently Spencer[10] has reviewed the literature on the subject of air embolism following thoracentesis and advances considerable evidence that the phenomenon is a physiologic-pathologic entity. Schlaepfer[11] quoted the case by Saugman of a young woman with pulmonary tuberculosis who was being treated by the artificial pneumothorax method. The trocar in this case was connected with a manometer and inserted 5.5 cm., when the manometer showed only small excursions, so a stylet was passed and on drawing this out a little blood followed. Immediately the patient felt giddy and the trocar was withdrawn. She turned pale and was laid on her back; she was unconscious and the head and eyes, with contracted pupils, turned to the left. Then the respiration became irregular and failed, the pupils dilated and she died. In this case it was found that the trocar had penetrated a vein in the lung and gas bubbles were found in the bloodvessels at the base of the brain, including the sylvian artery. This instance, quoted by Schlaepfer, together with his review of the literature, afford clinical evidence of the existence and consequent results of air embolism involving especially the cerebral vessels.

Pulmonary Edema. In this mixed group of cases there occur those which present the well-recognized clinical picture of acute pulmonary edema. The phenomenon usually supervenes after the drainage of the pleural cavity, though it is known to occur after simple exploration. The exact mechanism of acute pulmonary edema has long been a moot question among pathologists, and in spite of the tremendous impetus of the late war to solve once and for all this perplexing problem it remains in dispute.

Schlomovitz[12] concludes his long paper, which is a critical review of the important work done on experimental pulmonary edema, with the statement that the mechanism of its causation must be sought beyond the immediately obvious causes, such as intravenous emboli, intravenous injection of drugs, injury to the chambers of the left heart, particularly the ventricle, electrical stimulation of the lung tissue directly, alterations in the content or the amount of blood, or any of the many other causes which have been advanced. It is conceivable that acute pulmonary edema may be the resultant of a group of causes.

Other Pulmonary Lesions. Pulmonary thrombosis, following lung puncture, with blood-clot embolism to the heart or brain, may also cause untoward symptoms. Pulmonary hemorrhage and congestion, with or without hemoptysis,[15] is at times the chief causative factor in the production of the disagreeable and dangerous sequelæ of thoracentesis. Albuminous expectoration is one of the well-recognized but less common results of pleural tapping.

In this mixed group, which has just been reviewed, it is more than likely that several of these factors combined account for the collapse in most instances.

Pneumothorax. Besides the mechanisms mentioned above, namely, the pleural reflex of Capps and this second group of cases with mixed pathogenesis, in which there are always demonstrable lung parenchyma lesions, there is one other condition of lesser importance that must be mentioned as a cause of untoward symptoms and even death. Numerous cases of spontaneous pneumothorax have occurred following exploratory thoracentesis, as pointed out years ago by Sears;[15] but since the institution of the treatment of pulmonary tuberculosis by the artificially induced pneumothorax method[16 17] the wealth of clinical experience offered by this procedure has shown that this sequel is not of serious import and is rarely the cause for untoward symptoms.[18] Doubtless many of the fatal cases reported in the older literature which were accredited to the accidental production of a pneumothorax following exploratory thoracentesis, or the treatment of empyemas, or the withdrawal of pleural effusions, would in the light of our present ideas be better explained on the basis of the pleural reflex or pulmonary injury and congestion.

The following case stimulated my interest in this subject, and is presented rather completely both from the clinical and pathologic standpoint because it exemplifies an instance of a fatal accident following therapeutic thoracentesis.

Case Report. *Clinical History.* The patient was a married woman, aged twenty-three years, who was admitted to the Urological Service of the San Francisco City and County Hospital on July 27, 1921, with the complaint of continuous sharp pain over the right side of the abdomen. The family history was essentially negative, she being the mother of three healthy children and with no history of miscarriages. The anamnesis disclosed the fact that she had had the usual children's diseases without known complications and also malaria at eight years of age and influenza at twenty. She had lost ten pounds during the three months previous to admission.

The present illness dated from November, 1920, with the onset of frequency of urination and incontinence of urine. The patient consulted a physician in April, 1921, who told her that she had "bladder trouble." During the last few months before admission she has been disturbed by some dyspnea, night-sweats and dull abdominal pain following her bowel movements.

The important findings made out in the physical examination at this time pertained to the chest, abdomen and the urine. There was slight bulging of the chest at the right base, and over this area expansion was poor, the percussion note was definitely impaired and both tactile fremitus and the breath sounds were absent. The right flank was bulging and there was an increased muscular resistance over the entire right abdominal wall. The pelvic examination was negative. A catheterized specimen of urine was reddish brown in color, contained many pus cells, with the polymorphonuclear type predominating; there were many bacteria present, but no tubercle bacilli could be demonstrated at this time in the centrifugalized specimen. The usual morphologic study of the blood showed: erythrocytes, 4,600,000; leukocytes, 17,000; a differential count with an increase of the mononuclear elements. The blood Wassermann was negative and the ordinary phthalein kidney function test showed a normal output for the two-hour period. Ureteral catheterization of the right kidney showed marked reduction of function on this side and a urine which contained much pus and some tubercle bacilli. A diagnosis of pyonephrosis of tuberculous origin was made and a surgical operation decided upon.

On August 5 a right nephrectomy was performed and a large

pyonephrotic kidney was removed. For several weeks following the operation the patient's condition was fairly satisfactory; however, the pulse, temperature and respiration remained elevated, which simulated the preoperative picture. The condition at the base of the right lung was thought to be due to a pleurisy with effusion, and this was concurred in by the fluoroscopic examination. Cystoscopic examination of the bladder showed a marked chronic, diffuse cystitis with secondary contraction.

On August 22, at 4 P.M., it was decided to perform an exploratory thoracentesis. The patient was elevated to the usual sitting position and the skin over the seventh interspace in the posterior maxillary line was anesthetized with a 1 per cent novocain solution. The exploratory trocar was attached to the usual 20 cc Luer syringe and the puncture was made at the above-mentioned point. The trocar was sharp and no undue resistance was observed by the operator. On an attempt to aspirate the pleural cavity nothing was recovered, and consequently the trocar was partially removed and then thrust forward in several directions. In the course of these explorations it was suddenly noted that an abrupt change had occurred in the patient. The first striking symptoms observed were the presence of cyanosis of the face and neck and a general stiffness of the body. This was followed rapidly by a loss of consciousness. Immediately after this condition was noted the aspirating trocar was withdrawn and measures were taken to relieve the apparent collapse. The head was lowered, adrenalin and atropin were administered subcutaneously and an ice-bag applied to the precordium. Within a few minutes after the onset of the symptoms the respirations became labored, tracheal rales were heard and considerable pinkish fluid was regurgitated by the mouth. Thereupon the breathing slowed and artificial respiration was begun, and this was followed by the administration of oxygen. The pulse had elevated and varied between 150 and 200. Unfortunately no blood-pressure determinations were made during the twelve-hour period of collapse before death. Within a half-hour after the mishap the reflexes were investigated and it was found that there was a definite jaw clonus present, the pupils were dilated and did not react to light, a bilateral ankle clonus was present and a positive Babinski was found on the right side, whereas it was doubtful on the left. During the next twelve hours the patient remained in this state of shock and at no time regained consciousness. The reflexes varied from time to time but the picture in general was constant. The patient died at 4 A.M. on the morning of August 23, just twelve hours after the thoracentesis and onset of the disastrous accident. A few moments before death a large amount of grumous, blood-stained material was regurgitated from the mouth. There were no involuntary movements of the bowels or bladder during the comatose state immediately preceding death. Although there were various reflex disturbances, indicating cerebral irritation, there were no definite paralyses or convulsions.

AUTOPSY. The chief findings of the postmortem examination, five hours after death, were the following: General survey showed the body of a well-developed and fairly well-nourished woman of about her stated age. In the right posterior-axillary line, at the level of the sixth interspace, there was a small puncture wound. In the right lumbar region there was a long, recently healed, surgical scar, extending from the eleventh rib about 4 cm. from the spine downward and obliquely forward for about 16 cm. to the crest of the ilium, reaching a point 5 cm. posterior to the anterior-superior spine of the ilium. The lower angle of the wound presented a draining sinus and at the upper angle there was a small fluctuant area.

Abdomen. The abdomen was opened by the usual midline incision. The peritoneum appeared normal except in the region of the hepatic flexure, where there were fibrous adhesions binding this flexure and the posterior-inferior surface of the liver high up to the posterior abdominal wall and the diaphragm. There were numerous fibrous adhesions about the spleen. The mesenteries of the ascending and descending colons were unusually long. The stomach was tremendously dilated and was filled with a black liquid.

Pleural Cavities. The diaphragm was in the normal position. The left pleural cavity was practically obliterated by dense fibrous adhesions, whereas the right cavity also showed the same general condition, except that the adhesions were less numerous and dense. There was no free fluid in either pleural cavity.

Pericardial Cavity. The pericardium was normal and there was no fluid in the pericardial sac.

Heart. The heart appeared about normal in size and weighed 220 gm. The epicardium was smooth and glistening and the myocardium was of good color and consistency and showed no scars or areas of necrosis. The endocardium and the valves were normal throughout. The valve measurements were normal and the coronary arteries were negative.

Aorta. The aorta was normal in position. The intima was smooth and delicate.

Lungs. The surfaces of both lungs were extensively roughened by the thick, dense, pleural adhesions mentioned above. The lungs were moderately voluminous, hypercrepitant, and on section appeared to be markedly edematous; scattered throughout there were noted numerous moderate-sized, irregular, hyperemic areas. From the cut surfaces of both lungs considerable frothy, pinkish fluid exuded, which, however, did not appear blood-stained. In some areas there was also a certain small amount of pus which could be pressed from the bisected bronchioles. In the posterior portion of the left lower lobe there was seen a depressed, dark-colored, irregular area which measured 2 x 3 cm. in diameter. On section through this area there appeared a poorly defined, dark, bluish-red area slightly firmer than the surrounding tissue and extending for about 2 cm. into the cut surface of the lung. In the upper lobe near the apex on the left there was a firm, grayish-yellow, opaque, raised area about 1 cm. in diameter which was surrounded by a narrow, pale, translucent zone. Considerable interest centered around the right middle lobe, which on section presented several moderate-sized, dark-bluish, slightly raised areas. In the center of one of these dark areas there was a definite puncture wound. The entire lung parenchyma in this region disclosed the fact that the mid-lobe was the seat of extensive hemorrhage. This hemorrhage extended down to the region of one of the large branches of the pulmonary vein, but actual rupture of the wall of this vein could not be demonstrated. No clots were found in the bronchioles supplying this portion of the midlobe. The larger bronchial branches in both lungs contained a considerable amount of frothy fluid.

Liver. The liver was slightly enlarged and over the cut surface there were scattered irregularly a few small, round, yellowish-brown, opaque areas which were less than 1 mm. in diameter. The gall-bladder and ducts appeared normal.

Spleen. The spleen was large and the capsule was attached to the inferior, left, diaphragmatic surface by diffuse adhesions. On section the spleen showed nothing remarkable.

Intestines and Pancreas. These structures were normal.

Mesentery. The mesentery was normal except for the adhesions mentioned above.

Lymph Nodes. The posterior mediastinal lymph nodes appeared somewhat enlarged. There was no definite involvement of either the mediastinal or the retroperitoneal nodes.

Kidneys. The right kidney was absent (nephrectomy six weeks before death). The left kidney was slightly enlarged, weighed 200 gm., and the capsule stripped readily, leaving a brownish-red surface. The cut surface of the bisected kidney showed normal markings, however; the cortex was somewhat increased in thickness, measuring 7 to 8 mm. in diameter. The glomeruli were readily visible as white points. The medulla was also moderately increased in thickness and was sharply separated from the cortex. The renal pelvis, ureter and vessels appeared normal. In the right lumbar region, at the site of the nephrectomy, the tissues were diffusely thickened and scarred, involving the psoas muscle as well as the fascia and the adjacent fibro-fatty tissues. The region lying immediately below the skin under the operative scar presented a surface covered with necrotic tissue, in the midst of which were seen numerous small, opaque granules, while section through the upper portion of this tissue mass disclosed the right adrenal buried within the dense tissue. The gland, however, showed no evidence of tuberculous involvement. The left adrenal was normal.

Bladder. The urinary bladder was small. The mucosa showed an extensive, irregular, rather superficial, ulcerative process scattered over its surface, together with numerous small, semitranslucent nodules. The ureteral orifices were situated at some distance from the urethra. The one on the left was readily found and was more or less surrounded by definite tubercles, whereas the right orifice presented a funnel-shaped depression while the tissue surrounding it was extensively involved in the tuberculous ulcerative process. The distal bladder portion of the left ureter appeared normal; on the other hand the right ureter showed a marked thickening of the wall throughout, with small, scattered ulcerations over the mucosa.

Brain. Permission was not obtained to remove the brain.

COMPLETE ANATOMIC DIAGNOSIS. Right nephrectomy; marked tuberculous ulcerative cystitis; marked tuberculous involvement of the right ureter; extensive tuberculous inflammatory reaction in the tissues of the right lumbar region with burial of the left adrenal in the fibrous tissue; fibrous adhesions about the hepatic flexure and the posterior-inferior surface of the right lobe of the liver; small focus of pulmonary gelatinous and caseous pneumonia in the left upper lobe; extensive pulmonary edema; disseminated hyperemic foci in both lungs; slight purulent bronchitis; puncture wound of the midlobe of the right lung with moderate hemorrhage into the pulmonary tissue; recent hemorrhagic infarct in the lower lobe of the left lung; diffuse pleural adhesions bilateral; acute gray splenic tumor; perisplenic fibrous adhesions; parenchymatous degeneration of the viscera; moderate endothelial hyperplasia in the retroperitoneal and mediastinal lymph nodes; marked dilatation of the stomach with "coffee-ground" contents; moderate compensatory hypertrophy of the left kidney.

Conclusion. In the foregoing case, it is obvious from the autopsy findings, outlined above, that the collapse during exploratory thoracentesis and the subsequent death of the patient within twelve hours of the puncture were not produced primarily by the pleural reflex, or, on the other hand, by the production of an accidental, rapidly formed, spontaneous pneumothorax. The puncture wound in the middle lobe of the right lung, which was surrounded by hemorrhage and congestion, in association with the presence of extensive pulmonary edema, justify the supposition that this accident was caused by the combined physiologic-pathologic mechanism discussed as our second group, namely, injury and congestion of the lung parenchyma plus acute pulmonary edema with secondary circulatory reflexes, appear to have been responsible for the fatal outcome. Nothing was observed either in the clinical picture or the autopsy findings to suggest that air embolism was a factor.

BIBLIOGRAPHY.

1. Russell, A. E.: Death Occurring during or after Exploratory Puncture of the Lung, St. Thomas's Hosp. Reports, 1899, **28**, 465.

2. Capps, J. A.: Oxford Medicine, 1920, **2**, 163.

3. Capps, J. A.: Forchheimer's Therapeusis of Internal Medicine, Appleton & Co., New York and London, 1916, **3**, 455.

4. Capps, J. A.: Some Observations on the Effect on Blood-pressure of the Withdrawal of Fluid from the Thorax, Jour. Am. Med. Assn., January, 1907, **48**, 22.

5. Capps, J. A., and Lewis, D. D.: Observations upon Certain Blood-pressure Lowering Reflexes that Arise from Irritation of the Inflamed Pleura, AM. JOUR. MED. SCI., 1907, **134**, 868.

6. Capps, J. A., and Lewis, D. D.: Blood-pressure Lowering Reflexes from Irritation of the Chest in Empyema, Arch. Int. Med., 1908, **2**, 166.

7. Capps, J. A.: An Experimental Study of the Pain Sense in the Pleural Membranes, Arch. Int. Med., 1911, **7**, 717.

8. Brauer, L.: Ueber Arterielle Luftembolie, Ztschr. f. Nervenh., 1912, **45**, 276.

9. Stivelman, B. P.: The Dangers of Artificial Pneumothorax, New York Med. Jour., 1919, **109**, 187.

10. Spencer, W. G.: Air Embolism Following Thoracentesis, Med. Sci , Abstracts and Reviews, Oxford University Press, 1921, **3**, 521.

11. Schlaepfer, K.: Ein Fall von Dreitägigen Erblindung nach Probepunktion der Lunge. Ueber Arterielle Luftembolie nach Luftaspiration in Lungenvenen, Deutsch. Ztschr. f. Chir., 1920, **159**, 152.

12. Schlomovitz, B. H.: Experimental Pulmonary Edema, Arch. Int. Med., 1920, **25**, 472.

13. Caillé, A.: Fatal Hemoptysis Following Exploratory Puncture of the Chest in Young Children. Contributions to Medical and Biological Research, P. Hoeber, New York, 1919, **1**, 373.

14. Riesman, D.: Albuminous Expectoration Following Thoracentesis, AM. JOUR. MED. SCI., 1902, **123**, 620.

15. Sears, G. G.: Accidents Following Thoracentesis; Pneumothorax; Sudden Death from Exploratory Puncture, Tr. Assn. Am. Phys., 1906, **21**, 177 (with a bibliography).

16. Riviere, C.: The Pneumothorax Treatment of Pulmonary Tuberculosis, Oxford University Press, 1917, Chapter VIII, p. 151.

17. Sachs, T. B.: Artificial Pneumothorax in the Treatment of Pulmonary Tuberculosis, Jour. Am. Med. Assn., 1915, **65**, 1861.

18. Lemon, W. S., and Barnes, A. R.: Clinical and Surgical Experience in Diseases of the Chest with Special Reference to Pneumothorax, Med. Clinics North America, 1921, **5**, 295.

SUPPLEMENTARY BIBLIOGRAPHY.

Cordier, V.: Recherches complémentaires sur les troubles nerveux d'origine pleurale, Rev. de méd., 1911, **31**, 213.

Cordier, V.: Reactions nerveuses de la plèvre expérimentalement infectée, Lyon méd., 1911, **117**, 1446.

Dayton, H.: Accidents and Death from Exploratory Puncture of the Pleura, Surg., Gynec., Obstet., 1911, **13**, 607.

Ewart, W.: The Dangers of Artificial Pneumothorax, Prog. Med., 1919, **3**, 36.

Hamilton: Accidents in Thoracentesis, Montreal Med Jour., 1907, **36**, 749.

Jeanselme, E.: Des Accidents nerveux consécutifs à la thoracentésis en à empyèma, Rev. de méd., 1892, **12**, 502.

Mollard, J., Favre, M., Cordier, V.: Mort par ponction exploratrice du thorax (crises epileptiformes), Lyon Méd., 1920, **119**, 883.

Vallery-Radot, P., and Apert, E.: Sudden Death during Puncture of the Pleura, Bull. et mém. Soc. méd. d. hôp. de Paris, 1920, **44**, 935.

Zesas, D. G.: Zur Frage der Pleurogenen Reflexe, Zentralb. f. Chirurg., 1914, **41**, 371.

DIFFUSE GLOMERULO-NEPHRITIS.

By Herman Elwyn, M.D.,
Assistant Visiting Physician Gouverneur Hospital, and Clinical Assistant, Out-Patient Department of the Mt. Sinai Hospital, New York.

With the increasing knowledge of kidney disease our viewpoint has gradually undergone transformation. We have learned to separate the various forms of tubular nephritis or nephrosis as definite entities. We have learned to separate the purely arterio-sclerotic kidney. In the realm of glomerulo-nephritis or nephritis proper, we have learned to separate the focal and embolic forms from the diffuse forms. In the diffuse forms the conceptions are still much confused, and in spite of the immense amount of work on the pathology of the kidney and on the blood chemistry there is still little proper understanding of the processes involved. This paper is written with the object of giving a clear view of this disease and especially to give due prominence to Volhard's theory of the pathogenesis of diffuse nephritis, which has not been sufficiently appreciated.

To understand the disease processes involved one must continually realize that diffuse glomerulo-nephritis is in point of time an extremely variable process. It always has its origin in an acute form, often in early childhood. When it passes into a chronic form it may only last a few months or may stretch over years, and may even find its terminal stage more than twenty years later. The pathologist who studies such kidneys sees the changes at the time of death only, and these are often complicated by the addition of recent and acute changes to the old and chronic ones, as well as by the secondary changes in the arteries and arterioles.

The pathology of diffuse glomerulo-nephritis has been definitely placed on a firm footing by the work of Nauwerck[1] and of Langhans[2] among the older writers, and the recent investigators especially by Loehlein,[3] Fahr,[4] Herxheimer,[5] Jungman[6] and others.

The following description of the pathologic histology of the kidney is from the work of the above-named authors.

Acute Diffuse Glomerulo-nephritis. The earliest pictures are characterized by a more or less equal involvement of all the glomeruli. The glomeruli are enlarged, entirely filling the capsular space and often protruding into the neck of the tubule. The individual capillaries are enlarged, swollen and there is an increased number of nuclei partly belonging to endothelial cells but mostly to a greatly increased number of leukocytes which can be demonstrated, as Graff[7] has shown, by the oxydase method. The loops of the capillaries are especially characterized by their bloodlessness while the intertubular capillaries are filled with blood. The walls of the glomerular capillaries are thickened, and the lumen is empty of blood but contains a granular protoplasm in which the proliferated endothelial cells and the leukocytes are embedded. Here and there the glomeruli are sprinkled with fat droplets.

The capsular epithelium shows at this stage cloudy swelling, fatty degeneration with beginning proliferation of cells. In the capsular space here and there where the glomerulus does not quite fill it some red cells and coagulated albumin may be seen.

The convoluted tubules show cloudy and fatty degeneration and in some areas desquamation of cells. These are secondary to the changes in the glomeruli especially to the bloodlessness. It is the bloodlessness of the glomeruli which dominates the pathologic picture of acute diffuse glomerulo-nephritis, and it is the intensity and duration of the bloodlessness which dominates the further progress of the disease.

There are four possibilities in the further developments of this disease.

1. The capillaries of the glomeruli are again filled with blood, the swelling lessens and the glomeruli gradually return to normal. Of course, kidneys showing such a return to normal of the glomeruli are rarely seen post mortem and are only obtained when death is due to some complication occurring just at this time. Volhard and Fahr[8] describe such a case. Herxheimer's[9] cases X and XI are such cases.

2. The bloodlessness persists in its intensity and the changes in the glomeruli are rapidly progressive. The capillaries of the glomeruli are now shrunken and partly hyalinized and contain an increased amount of cellular elements. The proliferation of the capsular epithelium increases and forms concentric and semilunar masses of cell layers, which also become partly hyalinized and contain fat droplets. They fill the capsular space and are often larger than the glomerulus.

The tubules are dilated, atrophied, the cells are flattened, degenerated and the lumen is filled with casts. The interstitial tissue is here and there infiltrated with round cells and young connective tissue. The vessels show a proliferation of the intima.

This is the severest form. It corresponds to the extracapillary form of Volhard and Fahr and has been termed subacute nephritis by Volhard.

3. In this form the bloodlessness is not quite complete and here and there in the first divisions of the vasa afferentia blood may be seen. The glomeruli show a variety of pictures. The capillaries are broad, their walls thickened and partly hyalinized, some glomeruli are entirely hyalinized. The capsular epithelium is not proliferated but is surrounded by concentric layers of connective tissue. The tubules are dilated, regeneration of tubular cells is found here and there, but fatty and lipoid degeneration predominates throughout.

The interstitial tissue is markedly increased and also contains fats and lipoids. The vessels, especially the small ones, show definite proliferation of the intima. This form, which may last for a long time, has been termed by Volhard the subchronic form and corresponds to the intracapillary form of Volhard and Fahr.

4. This forms the secondary contracted kidney. The markedly increased connective tissue dominates the picture. It is irregularly distributed and in places infiltrated with round cells. Embedded in the connective tissue are masses of hyalinized glomeruli and atrophied tubules. Scattered among these are areas containing enlarged glomeruli of normal appearance and of normal blood content. The tubules belonging to these glomeruli are dilated, their epithelium is low, and fatty degeneration may be seen. Some of the glomeruli may be seen to be partly hyalinized and surrounded by concentric formations of connective tissue. The vessels, the large as well as the small ones, show marked arteriosclerosis with proliferation of the intima and splitting of the internal elastic membrane, and fatty degeneration, while some vessels are completely occluded. This is the chronic form or endarteritic form of Volhard.

In viewing the histological pictures one important fact stands out clearly, namely, the bloodlessness of the glomeruli and the reaction to this bloodlessness. This is the prime factor and its importance is insisted upon by Loehlein and more so by Volhard and Fahr. The changes in the tubules are secondary to it. In the acute diffuse glomerulo-nephritis it is the bloodlessness of the glomeruli which causes the infiltration of leukocytes and proliferation of the endothelial cells. It is the intensity of the bloodlessness which determines the severity of the acute form, and it is the duration of the bloodlessness which determines whether the changes in the glomeruli will retrogress and their capillaries again become permeable to the entrance of blood or whether the glomerular changes will become progressive, resulting in the subacute and subchronic forms. If the intensity or completeness of the bloodlessness of the glomeruli is marked and the duration sufficiently prolonged, the capillaries of the swollen glomeruli gradually begin to shrink, and the capsular space which is now functionless becomes filled with the proliferated capsular epithelium and at times with a leukocytic and hemorrhagic exudate which also becomes hyalinized. The permanent marked diminution of the blood supply results also in the changes in the tubules previously mentioned. These changes and their variations, resulting from the bloodlessness of the glomeruli which form the characteristics of the subacute form, determine the duration of the disease. As these changes, once established, are not retrogressive a fatal outcome is necessarily the result in the subacute form.

The subchronic form results when the duration of the bloodlessness is sufficiently prolonged, but is much lessened in intensity and completeness. The glomeruli are really not bloodless but blood-poor, and although some capillaries contain blood, most of them do not, and have undergone permanent changes with shrinkage, and resulting increase in the interstitial tissue. The duration of this form, whether months or years, depends upon how much the capillaries again become permeable to the entrance of blood; and also whether the pressure necessary to force the blood through the capillaries is available.

All the variations in the histological pictures, as well as in the clinical forms, depend, therefore, upon these factors. (1) The duration and intensity of the bloodlessness. (2) The extent of the proliferative and infiltrative reaction as a consequence of this bloodlessness. (3) The extent to which, in spite of these reactions, the capillaries of the glomeruli can again become filled with blood.

The very chronic form, in which the glomeruli remain normal for many years after the subsidence of the acute stage, and which however, eventually results in the histological pictures described above, is more complex and we shall return to this form later.

The essential element and the starting point is the bloodlessness of the glomeruli. All the recent investigators in this field insist on this point. It has been assumed that this bloodlessness is secondary to the changes in the glomeruli. Volhard,[10] who has brought to the study of the nephritides a greater understanding and insight than any other worker in this field, has proposed a new explanation for this bloodlessness of the glomeruli, which gives a new viewpoint to the whole pathogenesis of the disease. Volhard comes to the conclusion that the starting point of all forms of diffuse glomerulo-nephritis and the cause of the bloodlessness of the glomeruli is a spastic contraction of the arteries above the afferent artery to the glomerulus; and that everything we have said above as resulting from the bloodlessness of the glomeruli is in the last instance the result of the intensity and duration of the spastic contraction. The arterial narrowing is at first functional and not the result of organic changes in the vessel wall, but with the duration of this spastic contraction organic changes result in the vessel below the choking, as well as in the glomeruli. The changes in the vessel wall below the point of choking have the character of a proliferating endarteritis with a consequent permanent narrowing of the lumen. As long as the choking of the blood stream is due to a functional spastic contraction the vessels may again become permeable when the choking is released. Once the organic changes have developed it depends upon their extent whether the vessels become permeable and to what degree. In the acute diffuse form the blood-vessels may always become permeable, but with the organic changes in the blood-vessels definitely developed it depends upon the intensity and extent of these organic changes, whether the disease passes into the rapidly fatal subacute form, or into the slowly progressive and fatal subchronic form.

This theory of acute ischemia of the glomeruli, at first functional and due in the progressive cases to organic changes in the vessels and glomeruli, is of very great importance. Volhard observes, in the support of this theory, that he has found in kidney sections obtained at operation for decapsulation of the kidney, that the proliferative changes in the glomeruli were minimal, although the glomerular capillaries were bloodless. In support of the functional origin of the ischemia, he observes that he has been able in some cases in the early acute stage to relax the choking of the vessels by the single administration of a large quantity of water. This release would not have been obtained if the choking were of organic origin. He also observes, in support of this theory, that the acute form may heal without leaving any changes in the vessels or glomeruli.

Huelse,[11] in discussing Volhard's theory, remarks that while there are some objections to the theory that have not been overcome, no critic of this theory has been able to supply anything more plausible.

With the assumption of an angiospastic ischemia of the glomeruli as the beginning of diffuse nephritis, we enter the field of functional processes and changes. Our problems here are as follows:

1. What is the normal control of the flow of blood to the glomeruli, and what effect have the normal variations of this control on the function of the kidney?

2. How is the excessively increased control which results in an angiospastic ischemia of the glomeruli brought about?

3. What is the effect of this ischemia on the function of the kidney, and how is this effect compensated?

4. How can the clinical phenomena be explained on the basis of this ischemia?

The function of the kidney is to eliminate the nitrogenous waste products of body metabolism, to eliminate promptly any excess of water in the body, and to help maintain the constancy of the blood volume and blood composition. An excess of fluid intake is at once eliminated by the kidney in a urine of low specific gravity. Diminution of the fluid intake causes the kidney to produce a highly concentrated urine so as to save the water and certain salts for the body economy. It is not necessary here to enter into the age-old controversy between secretion on the one hand and filtration and reabsorption on the other. A mediating view has been put forward by Metzner[12], who assumes filtration by the glomeruli and reabsorption as well as secretion by the tubules. Recently Cushny[13] has most thoroughly presented the case for the filtration and reabsorption theory. Glomerular filtration is practically assumed by all leading physiologists, and recently Richards[14] has added some new evidence, especially as to the role that the blood-pressure plays in the urine formation. Filtration and reabsorption can be said to be definitely proven, and we must discuss our first problem on this basis.

We know that the kidney can eliminate an added intake of more than 12 liters in twenty-four hours. We know that in diabetes insipidus 10 to 12 liters of urine can be eliminated daily. We know that to produce such quantities of urine enormous quantities of blood must pass through the glomeruli. What is the control that prevents, normally, in everyday life, such quantities of blood plasma from being filtered through the glomeruli? The answer is, in the extensive vasomotor control of the small vessels of the kidney and in the normal shutting off of a great number of glomeruli from active function. Richards, in the Harvey lecture mentioned above, quotes Hermann to the effect that one part of the excreting surface of the kidney may rest or be active, while another part is held in reserve. Richards and his co-workers have been able to observe the active glomeruli in the lateral border of the ventral surface of a frog's kidney by focussing the light of an arc lamp on the kidney. They have observed that the number of glomeruli that could be seen in a field varied and could be made to vary with the introduction into the blood of various substances. This led them to conclude that all the glomeruli of the kidney of the frog do not receive blood simultaneously. Injection of saline increases the number of the glomeruli; adrenalin lessens the number seen. When we realize that the effect of adrenalin is on the sympathetic nerve endings of the small vessels, and consider the experimental evidence of diminution of urine production by the stimulation of the renal nerves, and the increased flow of urine from cutting these nerves, it is evident that we have in the vasomotor mechanism of the kidney an extremely sensitive control of the blood supply to the glomeruli. The sensitiveness of this control can be judged from the easy reflex response to various distant stimuli, such as catheterization, cerebral injury, chilling of the body surface and others. It is this extremely sensitive control which regulates the amount of blood which passes through the glomeruli and in consequence the amount of urine formed. So sensitive is this mechanism that it responds with a diluted urine to a fluid intake which dilutes the blood so slightly that it cannot be detected by ordinary methods (Cushny).

What is the effect of the variations of this vasomotor mechanism on the function of normal kidney to eliminate water and nitrogenous waste products, and to keep the blood volume and composition constant?

We understand the function of the glomeruli to be that of filtration of a deproteinized plasma from the blood, which is then concentrated in the tubules by the reabsorption of the water and those salts which the body needs for its economy, in a solution comparable to that of Locke's fluid, while the rest appears as urine. The quantity reabsorbed and therefore the concentration of the urine depends upon the length of time the glomerular filtrate remains in the tubules, and this again upon the flood coming from the glomeruli. It is obvious that with the sensitive mechanism which opens and shuts the vascular gates to the glomeruli in response to varying amounts of blood dilution, we have the explanation of the ability on the part of the kidney to produce a highly concentrated urine on water starvation, or to produce an extremely diluted one after a debauch on immense quantities of liquids and liquors.

When the vasomotor control is so stimulated as to shut off all the blood to the glomeruli, kidney function ceases and anuria results, and in this we have the explanation of the various reflex anurias. These are usually temporary. It is the sufficiently long duration of this angiospastic shutting off of the blood to the glomeruli, which forms, according to Volhard, the ischemia of the glomeruli, which is the beginning of diffuse glomerulo-nephritis. What produces this excessive vasomotor shutting off of the vessels to the glomeruli? This question, of course, coincides with that of the etiology of diffuse glomerulo-nephritis.

The etiology is unknown. Despite all possible speculation concerning the cause of glomerulo-nephritis, we are still no nearer the solution. That it is of an entirely different variety than the causes of the focal glomerulo-nephritides is at once obvious. In the latter we have local inflammatory reactions at the seat of the invading organism, a true defensive reaction involving only a portion of the glomerulus and only that portion where the invading organism happened to lodge. The rest of the glomerulus is free to carry on its function and there is usually enough of it left to do it. In acute diffuse glomerulo-nephritis there is no chance involvement of a glomerulus, but all the glomeruli of the kidney and with the exception of the very rare cases of unilateral glomerulo-nephritis, all the glomeruli of both kidneys are equally involved and to a more or less equal degree at the beginning. Whatever the cause, it must naturally have a central point of attack, and with the assumption of an angiospastic ischemia as a starting point, it must be something that will attack either all the vessels supplying the glomeruli or the vasomotor control of these vessels. This is perhaps comparable to the phenomena of anaphylaxis such as the contraction of the bronchial musculature in the guinea-pig, or the contraction of the pulmonary arterioles in the rabbit. For both of these possibilities, that is, for a reflex angiospastic contraction, and for the possibility of its being an anaphylactic phenomenon, there are suggestions in the literature.

The vasomotor supply of the kidney has its origin, according to Gaskell,[15] in the renal ganglion, and the connector fibres are to be found in the thoracico-lumbar outflow of the sympathetic nervous system, in the roots of the spinal nerves from the fourth dorsal to the fourth lumbar, while the skin and the blood-vessels are supplied with nerve fibers from the same thoracico-lumbar outflow. Exposure to cold causes afferent impulses to travel by way of the somatic nerves with reflex vasoconstriction resulting in blanching of the skin, increase in blood-pressure due to constriction of the splanchnic vessels, and diminution of the urine due to constriction of the renal vessels.

Exposure to cold is often given in the literature as a causative factor in nephritis. The tendency has been to discredit this factor and ascribe the nephritis to an accompanying affection. Krehl[16] says that "it is the experience of our best physicians that inflammations of the kidney are produced by the influence of intensive cold on the skin," and speaks of a "mysterious connection between the skin and the kidney." That a history of recent exposure to cold is often obtained in cases of acute nephritis is everyday knowledge. Classical cases have been reported. Horn[17] reports the case of a stoker on a steamboat who fell into the Rhine and on the next day had pains in the kidney region followed by acute nephritis with edema and hematuria. Experimentally, Siegel[18] produced a parenchymatous nephritis in dogs by the application of ice to the exposed kidney and by chilling of the hind legs and lumbar region. Others who repeated his experiments were not so successful.

In the etiology of war nephritis especially, exposure to cold and wet played a great role. Ameuille[19] quotes Chiari and Bruns who "maintain in no uncertain terms that it is almost always the chief cause." Bruns says that "in 70 per cent of the patients there is a clear history of a chill or exposure to dampness and cold." Ameuille himself does not agree with this. Fahr[20] quotes a number of writers who report cases of nephritis with chilling of the body as the causative factor.

For the second suggestion, that the angiospastic glomerular ischemia may be an allergic or anaphylactic phenomenon, there are several points in its favor. We know that nephritis often begins after an infection and especially a streptococcus infection, such as tonsillitis. We know that usually a week or more intervenes between the onset of the tonsillitis and the beginning of the nephritis. We know that the nephritis following scarlet fever always occurs nineteen to twenty-one days after the onset of the scarlet fever. All of these facts suggest resemblance to allergic reactions. Volhard also remarks that he has observed a true hydropic nephritis following vaccination for typhoid fever. Longcope[21] produced changes in the glomeruli and tubules by the injection of foreign protein. Wells,[22] in reviewing anaphylaxis in Physiological Reviews, observes that in anaphylaxis, "presumably, stimulation of unstriped muscle tissue is universal," and "the symptoms observed depend upon the degree of development of these muscles, or their strategic location, in different organs of different species." Disse[23] says that "in the interlobular arteries of the kidney, the walls are very thick. The medium has very little elastic tissue, but has a large amount of muscle fibers." Perhaps the increased development of the muscular coat of these vessels in the kidney, and which may be still more developed in certain individuals as a result of hereditary tendencies, may play a role in the anaphylactic phenomena of the human being.

All these may be very suggestive and still we must repeat that we do not know as yet the cause of the angiospastic renal ischemia.

What is the effect of the angiospastic glomerular ischemia on the function of the kidney and how is this effect compensated?

In discussing the bloodlessness of the glomeruli, we have spoken of its intensity and duration. We mean by its intensity, the degree or completeness of vascular contraction. If this is extreme, and if it is not overcome, as we shall see later that it can be, no blood enters the glomeruli and anuria is the result. Anuria often ushers in an acute diffuse nephritis, and those cases which succumb in the early stages of acute nephritis show practically the absence of red cells in the glomeruli before any exudative or proliferative changes have taken place. The effect on the kidney function is obvious. There is no glomerular filtration, no filtrate for the tubules to concentrate and there are changes in the composition and volume of the blood due to the accumulation of water and nitrogenous waste products in the blood. The total non-protein nitrogen, the urea, uric acid and creatinin which can be determined are found to be increased, the blood is diluted by the water which is not excreted, which can be easily determined by the proportionate fall of the red cells and hemoglobin. If the angiospastic contraction is less intense and if it is overcome to a varying extent, the glomeruli receive some of the blood plasma even though the red cells are not able to enter the capillaries and filtration occurs just to that extent. Concentration by the tubules is effected insofar as they are functionally capable in spite of the degenerative changes in them. Water and nitrogenous waste retention varies with the degree of glomerular permeability to the inflow of plasma and is practically a function of this and of the mechanism which attempts to overcome the angiospastic contraction.

What is this mechanism? Reflex vasoconstriction carries with it an attempt to remedy the vasoconstriction. One would naturally conclude that to overcome obstruction to blood flow, increased pressure above the seat of the obstruction would be the remedy. We mentioned that afferent vasomotor impulses from exposure of the skin to cold will cause diminution of the urine due to constriction of the renal vessels and at the same time an increase in blood-pressure due to constriction of the splanchnic vessels. It is this increase in blood-pressure which is produced by the mechanism concerned in the production of the angiospastic ischemia, which is the means of overcoming the obstruction to the inflow of the blood into the glomeruli. The ability on the part of the body to maintain this increase in blood-pressure may be little or much at the beginning of the angiospastic contraction, according to the reserve of pressor substances at its command, but as the disease progresses the body evidently acquires the means of maintaining the blood-pressure. Langhans[24] was able to inject the glomeruli in kidneys of acute nephritis with Prussian blue, but with a much increased pressure. Huelse[25] was able to inject the glomeruli of three cases of nephritis with practically the same pressure which these cases presented during their illness. That the increase in blood-pressure in diffuse glomerulo-nephritis, which may be maximal, is just for the purpose of overcoming this resistance to filtration is apparent when we consider that without this increase in pressure filtration by the glomeruli becomes impossible.

We do not know the entire mechanism for the maintenance of the increased blood-pressure. Volhard[26] assumes, and with reason, that the reflex stimulation of the splanchnic nerves, which causes increase in blood-pressure by constriction of the splanchnic vessels, causes at the same time an increase in the production of adrenalin. He also assumes that the afferent impulses from the nerves of the renal vessels stimulate the vasomotor center or the splanchnic nerves direct with an increased output of adrenalin. The inability to find an increased amount of adrenalin in the blood is not against this, as the adrenalin is continuously used up at the seat of its activity.

How can we explain the clinical phenomena on the basis of the glomerular ischemia?

It is not the purpose of this paper to discuss every possible symptom of nephritis, but the essential clinical phenomena of the various forms of diffuse glomerulo-nephritis. This disease, as we have said before, has always its origin in an acute form, and, according to Volhard's theory, in an acute angiospastic ischemia. It may also appear without the obvious symptoms and so remain unnoticed by the patient who has, therefore, at a later stage, no recollection of the acute beginning.

The essential clinical phenomena of the acute stage of diffuse glomerulo-nephritis are: (1) The urinary changes, of which hematuria is the distinctive feature, with albumin and casts; (2) the edema; (3) the increase in blood-pressure; (4) the changes in the blood; (5) as a complication, the phenomena, especially of the nervous system, which go by the name of uremia.

The angiospastic obstruction to the inflow of blood into the glomeruli carries with it, as we have discussed above, the immediate consequence of oliguria, compensatory increase in blood-pressure and changes in the composition of the blood. These three phenomena are always functional variables of the intensity and duration of the bloodlessness. The *hematuria* has probably several sources. Owing to the bloodlessness of the glomeruli there is an increased filling and back pressure in the venous system of the kidney with engorged intertubular capillaries with rupture. A second source is the rupture of the first divisions of the vasa afferentia of those glomeruli which have already become permeable to the entrance of blood. A third source is the exudation of blood through the capillaries around the glomerular capsule. The albuminuria is not a distinctive feature, as it is common to all forms of nephropathies. Undoubtedly some of it is due to the increased permeability of the glomerular membrane as a result of the ischemia; some may also come by way of the tubules. We have no definite knowledge about this.

The *edema* of acute diffuse glomerulo-nephritis is general and the edema fluid differs in composition from the edema of cardiac failure as well as from the edema of nephrosis. It is characterized by relatively high protein content and is practically a filtered plasma. Beckman[27] in examining fluids of all the three varieties of edema found the highest protein content in the edema fluid of acute glomerulo-nephritis. The production of this form of edema is best explained by filtration through the capillaries. The factors which cause the acute angiospastic contraction in the kidney is also responsible for the angiospastic contraction of the small vessels and capillaries in the skin. Weiss[28] observed, with his new method, the skin capillaries in a case of nephritis following a cold. He found the capillaries tortuous, the blood flow slow and granular. We must assume that there is an increased pressure in the capillaries with filtration or possibly a lessened nutrition of the capillaries with a consequent increased permeability of their walls.

The *increase in blood-pressure* we have attempted to explain. In the acute cases an increase of 30 to 50 mm. of mercury is usual. It rarely goes above 180, and the dropping of the previously increased blood-pressure in acute nephritis is one of the first indications that the glomeruli are returning to normal.

The *changes in the blood*, namely the increase in the blood of water and nitrogenous waste products, are purely a function of the glomerular ischemia and vary with it, and vary inversely with the blood-pressure insofar as the blood-pressure is able to overcome the ischemia and cause filtration.

The uremia we shall discuss later.

In discussing the pathologic histology we have spoken of four directions in which the process of acute diffuse nephritis may proceed. We have said that the first possibility is that the glomeruli again become permeable to the entrance of blood and return to normal. Clinically, this means that the acute nephritis is cured. That acute diffuse glomerulo-nephritis is curable forms a part of our understanding of the disease, and it is curable as long as the changes in the glomeruli have not advanced beyond those which we have described under the heading of the acute form.

The clinical phenomena of the subacute, subchronic and chronic forms have this in common, in that they all show the phenomena of renal insufficiency, with an increase in blood-pressure to overcome the resistance to the entrance of blood into the glomeruli.

The subacute form is characterized by a subsidence of the acute symptoms, especially the hematuria, and often by the subsidence of the edema. The increase in blood-pressure persists and is dependent upon the ability of the body to produce pressor substances, especially adrenalin. Whatever filtration is possible is dependent upon the increase in pressure, and with the fall in pressure the renal insufficiency increases to a maximum. The waste substances in the blood increase proportionately, and death is due to renal insufficiency or at times to an acute convulsive seizure.

The subchronic form is characterized clinically by the persistence of the hypertension after the disappearance of the acute symptoms. The kidney at first assumes more of its function with the increase in the pressure, but gradually renal insufficiency develops. This form may run without edema, but it is just in this form that there is often marked fatty and lipoid degeneration in the tubules with a corresponding edema and marked albuminuria. These cases of the subchronic form Volhard calls "nephritis mit nephrotischem Einschlag." They are the mixed cases in which Epstein[29] found, in addition to the hypertension, the phenomena of nephrosis, an increase in the cholesterol of the blood, reduction of the blood protein, and an inversion of the albumin-globulin ratio. As a result of the hypertension there is cardiac hypertrophy. Termination of these cases is usually from renal insufficiency which results from the inability of the hypertension to overcome resistance to the entrance of blood into the glomeruli. Renal insufficiency may also result from the fall in blood-pressure due either to the failure on the part of the body to supply sufficient pressor substances, or to cardiac failure as a result of excessive demand on the heart by the increase in blood-pressure.

The very chronic or endarteritic form presents phenomena which are more complex. The duration is many years. The acute stage may have been severe or so mild that the patient does not remember it. The acute stage subsides, the blood-pressure returns to normal and only the continual presence of albumin in the urine may remain. The angiospastic renal ischemia has been relieved and the glomeruli again obtain the full supply of blood.

But here as a result of the ischemia changes in the smaller vessels have developed with thickening of the intima which shows in places degenerative changes. These changes are permanent and are of the character of an obliterating endarteritis. The lumen gradually becomes narrowed, and here and there some vessel becomes obliterated. This results again in an ischemia of some glomeruli, but as these changes in the vessels are organic and permanent, the glomeruli which are supplied by these vessels become entirely obliterated. The process is a slow one, and for many years the gradual reduction in the number of the glomeruli, although it affects the kidney reserve, does not produce any clinical phenomena. That the reserve is reduced often becomes manifest when the patient notices that after drinking heavily elimination of water is not so prompt and he has to get up at night, although this is not necessary on his ordinary fluid intake. Transient rises of blood-pressure occur at such times with an increased water content of the blood.

With the gradual reduction in the number of the glomeruli as a result of the obliterating endarteritis, the lumen of the smaller vessels which supply the rest of the glomeruli becomes narrowed to a degree that threatens the maintainence of normal blood-pressure of these glomeruli. A certain height of blood-pressure must be maintained in the glomeruli if filtration is to occur. Experimentally, it has been shown that urine production ceases at a blood-pressure of about 40 to 45 mm. of mercury. For normal filtration a much higher pressure is necessary, and the pressure in the glomeruli normally is probably very little lower than that of the aortic pressure. We know that in Addison's disease when the blood-pressure sinks permanently to 75 or 80 mm. of mercury, functional renal insufficiency becomes evident from the increase in the blood of the waste products of metabolism.

The result of the narrowing of the arterioles is an increase in blood-pressure, which gradually increases as the lumen of these vessels becomes more and more narrowed by the changes in their walls, and as more of the glomeruli are destroyed as a result of the obliteration of these vessels. The hypertension is compensatory with the object of maintaining filtration pressure in the glomeruli. It is effected here by reflex vasoconstriction of the entire peripheral vascular system. Reflex impulses from the diseased arteries cause the vasoconstriction, and with the reflex stimulation of the splanchnic nerves, an increased output of adrenalin which persistently maintains the vasoconstriction. The evidence for the generalized peripheral vascular constriction can be found by observing the skin capillaries according to modern methods, and better still, by observing the vessels of the retina with the ophthalmoscope. These show at this stage constriction of the arteries and after a time, as a result of the ischemia, areas of degeneration with lipoid deposits.

We have then as the clinical expression of the very chronic form, at first a period of complete absence of any indication of renal disease with the exception, possibly, of a persistent albuminuria. This is followed by a second period characterized by a gradually increasing hypertension with a gradual diminution in the kidney reserve. The hypertension is often very high and the whole second period, which may last for many years, may present nothing else but this hypertension. As a result of the high blood-pressure, there is cardiac hypertrophy, and at times headache is complained of. Kidney reserve is diminished. This may be tested by giving a single large quantity of water, when it will be found that elimination is not prompt and is prolonged over a longer period of time than normal. The intake of a measured quantity of protein, or of urea, will cause a greater than normal increase of urea in the blood, and the increase will remain longer, indicating that elimination is prolonged. With the reduction in the number of the glomeruli there is also a loss of the corresponding tubules, and therefore, a lessening of concentration which is evident from the lower specific gravity of the urine. As absorption in the tubules is diminished, larger quantities of urine must be eliminated, but the urine is dilute and more nearly approaches the glomerular filtrate.

This second period of chronic glomerulo-nephritis so commonly presents only hypertension that it is often indistinguishable from the essential or benign hypertension of renal arteriosclerosis, the nephrocirrhosis arteriolosclerotica (Ashoff). In the benign sclerosis there is also a gradual narrowing of the smaller vessels, but this is due, not to an obliterating endarteritis following an acute ischemia, but to a true arteriosclerosis of the smaller vessels. The process is much slower, the patient usually older, there is no history of a previous acute nephritis, and, as this is the main point, the functional reserve of the kidney is much less, or not at all, disturbed. The symptoms are mainly cardiac and arterial, and not renal. In some cases occurring in younger individuals differentiation may be difficult.

Both diseases, the benign arteriosclerosis of the kidney and the second period of chronic glomerulo-nephritis, are often spoken of together as focal nephrosclerosis. This name only expresses the histological picture and lays emphasis on the areas of connective tissue growth which are really only the burial grounds of the glomeruli. It does not express what is really the main thing, that it is the changes in the vessel wall and the narrowing of the lumen which are responsible for the compensatory increase of blood-pressure, and that it is the ability of the rest of the glomeruli to filter or not, and of the tubules to concentrate or not, which is responsible for the variations in the kidney reserve function. Nor does this name express whether the clinical picture is that of the benign arteriosclerosis or of the progressive second stage of chronic nephritis.

During the second period of the chronic form there occur attacks of acute ischemia, such as are responsible for the beginning of the disease. These attacks have the same pathogenesis and probably the same ultimate cause. The kidney, once the seat of an acute ischemia, seems predisposed to its recurrence. The acute ischemia adds its symptoms to the chronic symptoms, and as far as the symptoms are due to the acute process they are retrogressive. It often happens that a patient with a history of an acute beginning, and in whom the gradual development of hypertension has been followed, is taken sick with edema, an enormous increase in the blood nitrogenous waste products, with hematuria and albuminuria. This subsides under rest and treatment, and credit is then claimed for the form of treatment employed in curing a supposedly chronic nephritis. When we realize that only the acute forms are retrogressive, and that the clinical phenomena of chronic glomerulo-nephritis is due to permanent organic changes in the vessels and the glomeruli, which cannot, by their very nature, retrogress, we must also realize how little we can claim for any treatment from which we expect to widen the narrowed lumen of vessels or bring to life obliterated glomeruli.

The third stage of the chronic form of glomerulo-nephritis appears when the changes in the vessels of the glomeruli have progressed to a stage where, despite increased pressure, and despite maximal efficiency of the remaining glomeruli, kidney function cannot be maintained. The "kidney rest," as some express it, is unable to maintain normal function even on a low food and water intake, and kidney reserve has entirely disappeared. Clinically, this expresses itself in the phenomena of renal insufficiency. Blood-pressure is very high, usually above 200. When this sinks and remains low, the degree of renal insufficiency is increased. The evidence for a prolonged contraction of the peripheral vessels is found in the eye grounds. Especially the radiating star-shaped white lines around the macula represent degenerated areas where the vessels have become obliterated.

The renal insufficiency manifests itself in the changes of the composition of the blood, in diminished glomerular filtration and diminished concentration by the tubules. The glomeruli are enlarged, but small in number, and are working with maximum efficiency. In spite of this they are unable to filter the excess of waste products from the blood, and we have, therefore, a gradual accumulation of water and these waste substances in the blood. The water increase in the blood can best be determined by counting the red corpuscles and by determining the hemoglobin. Both are found to be reduced in proportion. The anemia which is thus found does not represent the real loss of blood elements, but represents a dilution of the blood; a true hydremia. The color index is usually around one, and there is no evidence of either blood regeneration or blood destruction. Occasionally bleeding from the mucous membranes adds to the degree of the anemia. The anemia occurring in nephritis has been recently investigated by B. N. Berg in the wards of the Mt. Sinai Hospital.

The following figures represent the blood composition of a man aged thirty-six years who had an acute glomerulo-nephritis at the age of twelve, several recurrent attacks, the last one at the age of twenty-six, with a gradual increasing hypertension. A week before his death his systolic blood-pressure was 230 mm. of mercury, and his diastolic 140. At that time his blood figures were as follows:

Hemoglobin	54
Red corpuscles	2,500,000
Platelets	110,000
White blood cells	16,000
Polymorphonuclears	91 per cent
Incoagulable nitrogen	151.2 mgm. per 100 cc
Urea nitrogen	270 0 " " "
Uric acid	6.5 " " "
Creatinine	21.0 " " "

The figures of the blood elements represent practically a dilution to half, with a marked leukocytosis. The figures for the nitrogenous waste products are exceedingly high.

As the remaining normal glomeruli filter with maximal efficiency in response to the diluted blood, and as the tubules concentrate maximally, a practically constant quantity of urine is produced which does not vary with the fluid intake. In the case mentioned there was a constant production of urine of about 30 cc per hour or about 720 cc in twenty-four hours. The urine was of a fixed specific gravity of 1010, of light color and containing a small amount of albumin. It is often said that the water elimination in these cases is normal, and the fact that the patient can pass three-fourths of a liter of urine in twenty-four hours, would seem to indicate that such is the case. This is misleading. We have to consider that normally many liters of the glomerular filtrate must pass through the tubules to be concentrated to produce one liter of normal urine (Cushny). In a case like the one above, the urine is only very slightly concentrated above that of the glomerular filtrate. Yet, instead of the many liters that should be passed because of this lack of concentration, granted water filtration were really normal and concentration alone impaired, we have only 720 cc of a dilute urine, probably very closely resembling the glomerular filtrate.

The course of this third or final period is dependent upon the rapidity with which the glomeruli become obliterated, upon the maintenence of the hypertension, upon the cardiac sufficiency. Edema is not an essential part, but occurs at times with the fall in blood-pressure, and also from myocardial insufficiency.

Death is due to uremia. In this, the chronic form, we mean that it is due to poisoning of the system by the retained waste products, especially urea. We have said before that uremia also occurs as a complication in the acute diffuse glomerulo-nephritis. What then is meant by uremia? Definition is difficult, and we shall not attempt it. We mean by it certain phenomena which occur in the course of the various forms of nephritis, which are especially the results of cerebral involvement. We accept Volhard's division of uremia into, (1) true chronic uremia; (2) chronic pseudouremia; (3) acute convulsive or eclamptic uremia.

True chronic uremia is due to the prolonged retention of the nitrogenous waste products, and always expresses the clinical end stage of chronic nephritis. It is characterized by a gradually increasing fatigue and drowsiness combined with irritation phenomena. There is tremor of the extremities, sudden contraction of muscles, tendon jumping, the normal reflexes are increased, but there are no abnormal reflexes, such as a Babinski. There is a loss of flesh which was thought by Senator to be due to a toxic destruction of protein, and was produced experimentally by Bradford, by the reduction of the kidney tissue to one-fourth its volume. This loss of flesh is probably due to the increased metabolism as a result of the dynamic action of the amino acids of the blood, which are also increased. There are also disturbances of the gastro-intestinal tract, such as loss of appetite, singultus, vomiting, diarrhea, stomatitis, gastritis, and enteritis, with urinary fetor *ex ore*. Due to the retained acid phosphate salts there is diminution of the alkali reserve in the blood, resulting in a slow and deep breathing sometimes periodic in character, and which is characteristic of states of acidosis. Pericarditis is a common occurrence. Before death there is usually a fall in temperature. Convulsive seizures are not part of the essential picture of true uremia, and although occasionally convulsions do occur, more often they do not.

The symptoms of pseudouremia occur in the course of prolonged hypertension. They are not due to retained waste products and occur in the second period of chronic nephritis, but more often with the hypertension of the benign kidney ateriosclerosis or arteriolosclerosis. They are arterial in character, and due to sudden temporary angiospastic ischemia in the different organs, especially in the brain. Depending upon the location there occur transitory paralyses, aphasia, epileptoid phenomena, bulbar symptoms, Cheyne-Stokes breathing, and others. Osler[39] describes such classical cases.

The acute convulsive or eclamptic uremia occurs occasionally in the end stage of chronic nephritis, but its typical occurrence is more commonly a complication in the course of acute diffuse glomerulo-nephritis. It is not an essential part of the clinical picture, and the course of an acute diffuse nephritis may run entirely without any convulsions. It is characterized by the classical epileptiform attack with coma, or some equivalent form such as headache, restlessness, vomiting, unconsciousness, blindness. The convulsions are sometimes tonic, more often clonic, occasionally only on one side and with or without an aura. There are psychic equivalents ranging from fits of depression to maniacal conditions. The headache, vomiting, slowing of the pulse and choked disk may simulate a brain tumor. Lumbar puncture relieves and often stops the convulsions.

In explaining the pathogenesis of convulsive uremia occurring as a complication in acute diffuse glomerulo-nephritis, Volhard assumes that the angiospastic contraction, which is general, occurs also in the brain. The angiospastic contraction of the peripheral blood vessels results in edema due to filtration through the capillaries or to increased permeability of the capillaries, as a result of disturbances in their nutrition. The same process occurs also in the brain, resulting in an edema of the brain. The brain swells and is compressed in the rigid cranium with consequent irritation of the cortex. This is aided by the added increase in blood-pressure which always precedes the convulsive attack. He quotes Loeschke as showing that when death results from convulsive uremia, the brain when properly cut *in situ* snugly fits the walls of the skull, and the ventricles of the brain show themselves as linear slits. This explanation leans on the old Traube theory of swelling of the brain. It is more reasonable and more in accord with the pathogenesis of diffuse nephritis than the hypothetical poisonous irritant assumed by many investigators.

Conclusions. Volhard's theory of acute angiospastic renal ischemia as the starting point of diffused glomerulo-nephritis is the best explanation so far offered for the pathogenesis of this disease. We have attempted to follow the consequences of such an ischemia on the kidney function of filtration and concentration and on its function in helping to maintain the constancy of the volume and composition of the blood. We have also attempted to follow the changes occurring in the kidney following the angiospastic ischemia, and to explain the clinical phenomena on the basis of such changes. The theory is also of value in the treatment of this disease. We must realize that our efforts can only be directed toward those changes which are still retrogressive. When these changes have passed on to a stage where they are no longer retrogressive, treatment can only be directed toward lessening the functional load of the kidney. At all times where the functional reserve of the kidney is lessened or has entirely disappeared, either by acute ischemic or by chronic changes, treatment should be directed toward limiting the intake of those substances which in their normal quantities cannot be eliminated by the kidney which has become limited in its function. These substances are protein food and water, and their reduction is always indicated when the blood shows an increase in the nitrogenous waste substances.

BIBLIOGRAPHY.

1. Nauwerck, C.: Beitr. z. path. Anat., 1886, **1**, 1.
2. Langhans, Th.: Virchows Arch., 1879, **76**, 85, and 1888, **112**, 1.
3. Loehlein, M.: Arb. a. d. pathol. Inst. z. Leipzig, 1907, 1.
4. Volhard and Fahr: Die Brightsche Nierenkrankheit, Berlin, 1914.
5. Herxheimer, G.: Deutsch. med. Wchnschr., 1916, **42**, 869.
6. Jungman, P.: Ztschr. f. klin. Med., 1917, **84**, 1.
7. Graff, S.: Deutsch. med. Wchnschr., 1916, **36**, 1092.
8. Volhard and Fahr: L. c., p. 142, case 18.
9. Herxheimer, G.: L. c.
10. Volhard, F.: Die Doppelseitigen Haematogenen Nierenerkrankungen, Berlin, 1918.
11. Huelse, W.: Deutsch. med. Wchnschr., 1920, **46**, 1244.
12. Metzner, R.: Nagel's Handbuch d. Physiologie, 1907, **2**, 207.
13. Cushny, A. R.: The Secretion of Urine, London, 1917.
14. Richards, A. N.: Am. Jour. Med. Sci., 1922, **163**, 1.
15. Gaskell, W. H.: The Involuntary Nervous System, London, 1916, p. 36.
16. Krehl, L.: Pathologische Physiologie, Seventh Edition, Leipzig, 1912, p. 585.
17. Horn, P.: Med. Klin., 1916, **12**, 685.
18. Siegel, W.: Deutsch. med. Wchnschr., 1908, **34**, 454.
19. Ameuille, P.: Jour. Urol., 1918, **2**, 51.
20. Fahr, Th.: Ergebnisse d. Allg. Pathol., 1919, **19**, 1.
21. Longcope, W. T.: Jour. Exper. Med., 1913, **18**, 678.
22. Wells, H. S.: Physiological Reviews, 1921, **1**, 44.
23. Disse, J.: Von Bardeleben's Handb. d. Anat. d. Menschen, Jena, 1902, **7** (Part I), 75.
24. Langhans, Th.: L. c.
25. Huelse, W.: L. c.
26. Volhard, F.: L. c., p. 153.
27. Beckman, K.: Deutsch. Arch. f. klin. Med., 1921, **135**, 173.
28. Weiss, E.: München. med. Wchnschr., 1916, **63**, 925.
29. Epstein, A. A.: Med. Clinics North Amer., 1920, **4**, 145; Am. Jour. Med. Sci., 1922, **163**, 167.
30. Osler, Wm.: Canad. Med. Assn. Jour., 1911, **1**, 919.

STUDIES OF GRAVES' SYNDROME AND THE INVOLUNTARY NERVOUS SYSTEM.*

By Leo Kessel, M.D., Charles C. Lieb, M.D.,

AND

Harold Thomas Hyman, M.D.,

NEW YORK.

General Introduction. These studies result from an attempt to promulgate a definite policy for the management of individuals

* These studies were carried on in the Medical Department of the Mt. Sinai Hospital and in the Department of Pharmacology of the College of Physicians and Surgeons, Columbia University. The work has been made possible by a fund established for the purpose by the New York Foundation and by Mr. Felix Warburg. The basal metabolism readings throughout were made by Dr. Herman Lande to whom we are indebted for his painstaking, accurate and conscientious work.

suffering from Graves' syndrome. In our hospital this condition has been handled by the surgeons, internists and radiotherapists. Each group has reported successful results, not only in those patients who had received no previous treatment, but also where other treatments had proved a failure. For two reasons it was impossible to compare or estimate therapeutic reports: (1) There has been no concordance as to just what constituted Graves' syndrome, and (2) data as to end-results have been meager and subject to individual interpretation.

A survey of the literature failed to clarify the situation. The diagnostic criteria varied; case reports were frequently not supplied; personal opinion and interpretations rather than actual facts were presented; end-results were either obscurely reported in massed statistics or were not given at all. Satisfactory individual records, however, are to be found in the papers of Du Bois[1] and Means and Aub.[2]

One of us (H) visited the leading goiter clinics in 1920 to determine whether more could not be learned from personal observation. While each clinic had its definite plan as to diagnosis and therapy, no two clinics were found with policies that were similar; even in the same institution the widest possible variation obtained among different services.

We decided, therefore, that a small group of patients with fully developed Graves' syndrome† be studied carefully from every angle. In order to eliminate the personal factor it was determined not to include in this group a patient in whom the clinical diagnosis was not confirmed by a distinct and continuous elevation of the basal metabolism. The course of the basal metabolism was accepted as the best available objective[1] criterion of the severity and progress of the disease. The complete data of this group of definite Graves' syndrome are compiled in paper III.[7]

A large number of patients were referred to us who, while they presented many of the cardinal clinical symptoms, *i. e.*, tachycardia, exophthalmos, goiter and tremor, associated with some of the minor symptoms (diarrhea, sweating, palpitation, etc.), nevertheless showed no constant elevation of the basal metabolism, and gave no histories suggestive of a previous crisis. They were studied separately for classification and for the purpose of establishing the differential diagnosis from Graves' syndrome. Of these the first subgroup was composed of patients who had an enlargement of the neck. They had no other manifestations of Graves' syndrome, and no elevation of the basal metabolism. It became apparent that these patients were suffering: (1) From an existing hyperplasia

† For its historical interest we have retained the term "Graves' Syndrome." The introduction of basal metabolic studies has thrown new light on the syndrome, and we have altered our conception in accordance, as will be seen from the text.

of the thyroid gland; (2) from the results of a previous hyperplasia, (3) from adenoma. A review of the etiology, physiology and clinical associations of hyperplasia and adenoma, with the case reports in this subgroup, form the basis for paper I. In a second subgroup were patients, who, with or without goiter, exhibited many of the classical manifestations of Graves' syndrome. In these there was no significant elevation of the basal metabolism and no reason to believe that an elevation had ever existed. Their manifestations were clinically divisible into three groups: (1) The registration in consciousness of somatic activities which normally proceed unconsciously, as palpitation; (2) objective functional disorders in organs which themselves were apparently healthy (tachycardia, diarrhea); (3) symptoms of obscure origin which were accentuated by the administration of adrenalin (tremor, asthenia). With the possible exception of thyroid enlargement, all of these symptoms and signs were sympathomimetic.‡ To these clinical disturbances of the involuntary nervous system we have applied the term *Autonomic Imbalance.* The clinical study of patients with autonomic imbalance is presented in paper II.[8]

Because the symptoms of Graves' syndrome and autonomic imbalance were found to be due to disturbance in the realm of the involuntary innervation we studied the physiology and pharmacology of the involuntary nervous system.

We do not claim that either Graves' syndrome or autonomic Imbalance is necessarily an inherent derangement of the involuntary nervous system, but that whatever the ultimate cause it must operate either primarily or secondarily through the involuntary nervous system. The attempt to find an index for the activity of the involuntary nervous system is described in paper IV.[4] By means of this index, the role of alleged etiologic and therapeutic influences, as well as factors which maintain the tonicity of this system, were investigated. These results are presented in papers V, VI and VII.[4]

Finally, a definite therapeutic policy for Graves' syndrome was sought. In a disease where "specific" results have been claimed for general medical treatment; for tonsillectomy; for roentgen-ray exposures of thyroid or thymus, or both; for mechanotherapy; for spondylotherapy; for surgery, from injections to ligations, and from partial to subtotal thyroidectomy; for endocrinology,—the suspicion was aroused that there was a "nonspecific" factor common to all these "cures" and that the course of the disease was toward spontaneous arrest. Accordingly we studied fifty patients (Paper III) with Graves' syndrome without employing "specific" measures, in

‡ Adopting the term of Barger and Dale[3] to denote manifestations that are tantamount to electrical stimulation of the thoracico-lumbar division of the involuntary nervous system, or to stimulation of the same system by adrenalin.

order to determine its natural history as an index for the evaluation of therapeutic procedures.[6]

A general summary of the clinical and laboratory work on the involuntary nervous system constitutes paper VIII[5], and a discussion of the pathogenesis and an evaluation of popular therapeutic procedures constitutes paper IX.[6]

BIBLIOGRAPHY.

1. Du Bois: Arch. Int. Med., 1916, **17**, 915.
2. Means and Aub: Arch. Int. Med., 1919, **29**, 645.
3. Barger and Dale: Jour. Physiol., 1910, **41**, 19.
4. Lieb and Hyman: Jour. Exp. Pharm. and Therap., 1922, **63**, 60, 68, 83, 88.
5. Lieb, Hyman and Kessel: Jour. Am. Med. Assn., 1922, **79**, 1099.
6. Kessel and Hyman: Jour. Am. Med. Assn., 1922, **79**, 1213.
7. Kessel, Hyman and Lande: Arch. Int. Med. (to be published).
8. Kessel and Hyman, Am. Jour. Med. Sci., 1923, **165**.

STUDIES OF GRAVES' SYNDROME AND THE INVOLUNTARY NERVOUS SYSTEM.

I. Thyroid Enlargement in Individuals Without Sympathomimetic Manifestations.

By Leo Kessel, M.D.,

and

Harold Thomas Hyman, M.D.,

New York.

Studies on the condition of thyroid enlargement are usually made in lake districts where goiter is endemic, and consist of massed statistical reports.[1] The great frequency of endemic goiter has obscured the study of thyroid enlargements due to other causes.

Our work was done at a seaport where thyroid enlargement is relatively infrequent. An out-patient department was organized and an attempt made to determine the etiological factor in the individual patient. The conditions associated with and resulting from the thyroid enlargement were studied with the object of investigating the possible relationship between goiter and Graves' syndrome.

Of over 200 patients investigated, 55 furnished material for this paper. Of these, 32 patients (Table I) presented as their sole symptoms the "lump in the neck." The other 23 patients (Table II) had, beside thyroid enlargement, some other unrelated disease which was responsible for the presenting symptoms.

TABLE I.—THYROID ENLARGEMENT IN INDIVIDUALS FREE FROM SYMPATHOMIMETIC SYMPTOMS AND WITH NORMAL BASAL METABOLISM.

No.	Sex.	Age.	Age onset goiter.	Duration of goiter.	Previous treatment.	Tonsils.	Miscellaneous.	Effect of iodide.
8673	F.	43	?	?	None	Infected	Calcification	
8545	F.	36	?	?	25 roentgen-ray	.....	Small adenoma referred as exop. goiter	
8543	F.	56	44	12	Roentgen-ray	.....	Referred as exop. goiter	
5066	M.	33	21	12	Roentgen-ray	Infected		
9234	F.	14	12	2	Chiropractor	.....	Puberty hyperplasia	
9080	F.	50	26	24	.....	.....	Regarded as exop. goiter (?)	
8651	F.	50	?	?	.....	Infected	Referred as exop. goiter	
9220	F.	33	?	?	.....	.....	Discrete tumor	
9198	F.	34	19	15	.....	.....	Referred as exop. goiter	
8718	F.	30	30	5 wks.	.....	.....	Discrete tumor	3 cm. 5 mos.
8803	F.	26	?	?	.....	.....	Discrete tumor; removed for relief of cough. Still coughs	
9215	F.	37	34	3	.....	.....	Referred as exop. goiter	
9125	F.	18	15	3	Ops. 2 yrs ago	.....	Gland still enlarged	
8891	F.	36	36	1 mo.	.....	.....	Discrete tumor	8 cm. 6 mos.
8766	F.	29	?	?	Injections into gland	.....	Referred as exop. goiter	
8517	F.	26	?	?	.....	.....	Referred as exop. goiter	
8581	F.	30	?	?	.....	.....	Referred as exop. goiter	3 cm. 10 mos.
8748	F.	29	25	4	.....	Infected	Puberty hyperplasia	
8681	F.	14	11	3	.....	.....	Puberty and starvation	
8963	F.	30	?	?	.....	Infected	Referred as exop. goiter	2 cm. 4 mos.
8760	F.	18	8	10	.....	.....	Referred as exop. goiter	3 cm. 8 mos.
8869	F.	23	?	?	.....	Infected		
9157	F.	18	16	2	.....	Infected		
8863	F.	38	34	4	.....	Infected	Thyroid exhaustion (?)	7 cm. 6 mos.
9193	F.	28	11	7	Ops.	.....	Post-partum; increased after ops.	
8734	F.	47	44	3	.....	.....	....	5 cm. 6 mos.
8882	F.	19	19	2 mos.	.....	.....	....	2.5 cm. 3 mos.
8674	F.	19	15	4	30 roentgen-ray	.....	....	3 cm. 9 mos.
9194	F.	30	?	?	.....	.....	....	3 cm. 1 mo.
8606	F.	50	?	?	.....	.....	Referred as exop. goiter	
8599	F.	43	?	?	.....	.....	Referred as exop. goiter	
8832	F.	42	?	?	.....	.....	Referred as exop. goiter	

CHART 1.—Note wide variation in age at time of admission; variation in age of onset of goiter and in duration of goiter; roentgen-ray fails to shrink goiter; compensatory hyperplasia after operation; 8 have infected tonsils; character of goiter varies some diffuse and others discreter preponderance of females; shrinkage with iodide; 14 referred as exophthalmic goiter.

Clinical Data. *Sex and Age.* Fifty-two of the 55 patients were females. The ages of the patients were between fourteen and fifty-six. The two extremes at which the goiter was first noted were also at fourteen and fifty-six years, and the duration up to the time of admission varied between one month and twenty-four years.

TABLE II.—THYROID ENLARGEMENT IN INDIVIDUALS WHO ARE SUFFERING FROM ANOTHER BUT UNRELATED DISEASE AND WHO HAVE NEITHER SYMPATHOMIMETIC SYMPTOMS NOR ELEVATION OF BASAL METABOLISM.

No.	Sex.	Age.	Thyroid.	Associated condition.	Miscellaneous
5144	M.	32	Cyst	Tuberculosis (healed); anxiety neurosis	Referred as exop goiter.
9219	F.	25	Removed in 2 ops.	Manic-depressive psychosis	Ops as exop goiter.
8515	F.	50	Diffuse	Diabetes mellitus	
8535	F.	42	Cyst	Anxiety neurosis	Referred as exop goiter.
8679	F.	59	Diffuse	Diabetes mellitus	
5619	M.	70	Substernal	Myocarditis, emphysema; chr. bronchitis	Cough supposed to be due to thyroid.
8854	F.	33	Diffuse	Anxiety neurosis	Referred as exop. goiter.
8501	F.	47	Diffuse	Chronic hypertensive nephritis, prominent eyes	" " "
9214	F.	?	Diffuse	Fainting spells	Referred as exop. goiter.
8650	F.	29	"	Asthenia after flu	" " "
8600	F.	14	"	Myositis, infected tonsils	" " "
8585	F.	20	"	Sinusitis	" " "
8580	F.	37	"	Pregnancy	" " "
8542	F.	46	"	Gastric symptoms	" " "
				Infected tonsils and sinusitis	Had roentgen-ray therapy.
8548	F.	34	"	Polyarthritis	Referred as exop. goiter.
8925	F.	29	"	Cystorectocele	" " "
8660	F.	24	"	Psychoneurosis	" " "
8661	F.	16	"	Dysmenorrhea	" " "
8743	F.	43	"	Cholelithiasis	" " "
8922	F.	26	"	Sterility, infantile uterus	" " "
8824	F.	34	"	Mitral stenosis	" " "
8560	F.	40	"	Diabetes mellitus	" " "
8532	F.	38	"	Cancer of uterus	" " "

Note tendency to attribute to thyroid rather than other obvious associated condition the presenting symptoms.

Etiology. In many of the patients the etiological factor could not be determined, because they were not at all sure as to the time of appearance of the goiter. The relationship to puberty and to the child-bearing period was definite in 13. Infected tonsils were present in 8. In one girl the goiter was apparently congenital.

Symptoms. In the first group (Table I) the only symptom was the thyroid enlargement. In the second group (Table II) presenting symptoms were due to a great variety of associated conditions, one each; cancer of the uterus, cholelithiasis, mitral stenosis, cystorectocele, pansinusitis, diabetes mellitus, arthritis, pregnancy, chronic nephritis, generalized atherosclerosis and infantile uterus and neuroses in 6. One woman suffered from a manic-depressive psychosis.

Diagnosis. Of the 32 patients listed in Table I at least 17 were referred with the diagnosis of exophthalmic goiter. In many others the presumption is strong that this diagnosis had been made by the attending physician. Four had received frequent roentgen-ray exposures and 3 had been subjected to operations on the thyroid gland. Of these 1 suffered a compensatory hyperplasia, so that the gland is now larger than prior to operation.

Of the patients recorded in Table II, practically all were referred to us as examples of exophthalmic goiter and in almost all there was supposed to be a definite connection between the associated conditions already mentioned and the thyroid enlargement. The patient with the manic-depressive psychosis had had thyroidectomy twice without any effect upon her condition. Three had had unsuccessful treatment of the thyroid gland with frequent roentgen-ray exposures. Except for the goiter none of the individuals in either group had had at any time evidences of any of the manifestations of Graves' syndrome. None presented metabolic disturbances as measured by the basal metabolism.

The Type of Gland. From clinical examination it was impossible to determine the pathological type of thyroid enlargement. In no instance was opportunity for histological examination afforded. This, however, is of little importance, because in those glands that were uniformly enlarged a colloidal or hyperplastic picture must have been present at the time of examination. In either instance it may be assumed that the patient had passed through a stage of hyperplasia [3 4] without sympathomimetic manifestations.

In 6 individuals the enlargement was due to the presence of a discrete nodule, presumably an adenoma. No symptoms accompanied this enlargement. In 2 patients the goiter was substernal.

Treatment. All these patients received small doses of syrup of the iodide of iron,[5] 10 to 30 drops twice a day. The majority of these patients were referred to us merely for diagnosis and no attempt was made to follow them. Of the 11 who were followed not one failed to show a definite softening and decrease in the size of the gland as a result of the iodine administration. On the average the shrinkage in the circumference of the neck was 1 cm. a month. Seven had had treatment by roentgen-ray before being referred to us, and none of these patients reported diminution in the size of the goiter as the result of the exposures. Four had had thyroidectomy. Of these, 2 still had thyroid enlargement; 1 had such a marked compensatory hyperplasia that the gland was actually larger than it had been before operation. In the remaining 2 the gland was definitely smaller; however, in both of these latter patients the operation had been done not for the cosmetic effect but for the relief of cough in the one and manic-depressive psychosis in the other. Neither of these conditions was affected.

Discussion. 1. ARCHITECTURE OF THE THYROID GLAND. There are two special pathological conditions that give rise to uniform enlargement of the thyroid gland. These have been described by Marine[6] in his classical article in which he recognized as ground types; the normal, the hyperplastic, and the colloid gland. The histology of the normal gland is familiar. The hyperplastic gland differs in that the epithelium is higher, the colloid is less, the walls of the alveoli may be thrown up into plications, the intercellular substance and the vascularity are increased, and there may be round cell infiltration of the stroma. The colloid gland presents large amounts of colloid material, distending alveolar spaces, a flattened epithelium and relatively enormous thickening of the walls of the bloodvessels. In each type variations in intensity may be present. Transitional forms are also observed, in which there is evidence of hyperplasia in a colloid gland, and *vice versa*. There may be present, particularly in the colloid type, secondary changes such as cyst formation, hemorrhage and calcification, which are accidental.

Discrete enlargements of the thyroid gland are due to cysts or adenomata. The latter may present the same alterations as the non-tumor tissue, so that the adenoma may resemble normal, colloid or hyperplastic thyroid tissue. The non-tumor tissue of the gland is not necessarily of the same architecture[7] as the adenomata.

2. The Chemistry of the Thyroid Gland. Investigation of the chemistry, particularly of the iodine metabolism, clarifies the otherwise inexplicable mechanism of the ground types.

Of all the tissues of the body, the thyroid gland alone contains iodine in appreciable quantity. Given by any route or in any form, iodine is quickly bound by the thyroid.[8 9] The iodine content of the normal gland is 1 mg. per gram of dried tissue.[10] The potency of a thyroid extract is directly proportionate to its iodine content. Because of its increased weight the total iodine content of colloid glands either equals or exceeds that of the normal gland. The hyperplastic gland always contains less than 1 mg. of iodine per gram of dried tissue. The total quantity of iodine is always less than in the normal or the colloid gland, and the iodine content is inversely proportional to the degree of the hyperplasia.

The problem of determining whether the architecture depends upon the chemistry or the chemistry upon the architecture, has been definitely solved by the work of Marine.[3] In animals whose glands are rendered hyperplastic, the administration of iodides invariably produces an involution to colloid, but never a resumption of the normal architecture. If iodides are now withheld and the factors producing the hyperplasia remain operative, hyperplasia is reinduced. The resumption of iodides again changes the hyperplastic to the colloid form. From this it must be quite clear that the architecture of the thyroid gland is bound up with the iodine content; that the hyperplastic gland presents a low iodine content, and that the colloid gland has a relative and absolute iodine content that is at least normal: that the colloid gland has passed through a stage of diminished iodine storage. The histological appearance and exposures and 3 had been subjected to operations on the thyroid gland. Of these 1 suffered a compensatory hyperplasia, so that the gland is now larger than prior to operation.

Of the patients recorded in Table II, practically all were referred to us as examples of exophthalmic goiter and in almost all there was supposed to be a definite connection between the associated conditions already mentioned and the thyroid enlargement. The patient with the manic-depressive psychosis had had thyroidectomy twice without any effect upon her condition. Three had had unsuccessful treatment of the thyroid gland with frequent roentgen-ray exposures. Except for the goiter none of the individuals in either group had had at any time evidences of any of the manifestations of Graves' syndrome. None presented metabolic disturbances as measured by the basal metabolism.

The Type of Gland. From clinical examination it was impossible to determine the pathological type of thyroid enlargement. In no instance was opportunity for histological examination afforded. This, however, is of little importance, because in those glands that were uniformly enlarged a colloidal or hyperplastic picture must have been present at the time of examination. In either instance it may be assumed that the patient had passed through a stage of hyperplasia [3, 4] without sympathomimetic manifestations.

In 6 individuals the enlargement was due to the presence of a discrete nodule, presumably an adenoma. No symptoms accompanied this enlargement. In 2 patients the goiter was substernal.

Treatment. All these patients received small doses of syrup of the iodide of iron,[5] 10 to 30 drops twice a day. The majority of these patients were referred to us merely for diagnosis and no attempt was made to follow them. Of the 1 who were followed not one failed to show a definite softening and decrease in the size of the gland as a result of the iodine administration. On the average the shrinkage in the circumference of the neck was 1 cm. a month. Seven had had treatment by roentgen-ray before being referred to

types; the normal, th hyperpla
histology of the norm gland is
differs in that the epitelium is higher. The hyp
of the alveoli may be thrown up into the colloid is
substance and the vasclarity are increased, the
cell infiltration of the stroma. The colloid
amounts of colloid ma rial, distending alveolar
epithelium and relativ y enormous thickening of the
bloodvessels. In each ype variations in intensity may
Transitional forms are lso observed, in which there is
hyperplasia in a collo l gland, and *vice versa.* The
present, particularly in he colloid type, secondary chan
cyst formation, hemorrage and calcification, which ar

Discrete enlargemen of the thyroid gland are
adenomata. The latte may present the same alte
non-tumor tissue, so at the adenoma may resem
colloid or hyperplastic tyroid tissue. The non-tumor t
gland is not necessarily f the same architecture[7] as the ad

2. The Chemistry c the Thyroid Gland. Investi
the chemistry, particulrly of the iodine metabolism, cla
otherwise inexplicable mchanism of the ground types.

Of all the tissues of te body, the thyroid gland alone
iodine in appreciable quatity. Given by any route or in a
iodine is quickly bound by the thyroid.[8 9] The iodine co
the normal gland is 1 m. per gram of dried tissue.[10] The
of a thyroid extract is dectly proportionate to its iodine
Because of its increased veight the total iodine content o
glands either equals or xceeds that of the normal glan
hyperplastic gland alwa contains less than 1 mg. of iod
gram of dried tissue. Te total quantity of iodine is alwa
than in the normal or tl colloid gland, and the iodine cont
inversely proportional to he degree of the hyperplasia.

The problem of deternining whether the architecture dep
upon the chemistry or the hemistry upon the architecture, has b
definitely solved by the wrk of Marine.[3] In animals whose glan
are rendered hyperplastic the administration of iodides invariabl
produces an involution t colloid, but never a resumption of the
normal architecture. If iodides are now withheld and the factors producing the hyperplasia reain operative, hyperplasia is reinduced.
The resumption of iodide again changes the hyperplastic to the
colloid form. From this it must be quite clear that the architecture
of the thyroid gland is bond up with the iodine content; that the
hyperplastic gland presers a low iodine content, and that the
colloid gland has a relativ and absolute iodine content that is at
least normal: that the cloid gland has passed through a stage
of diminished iodine storge. The histological appearance and

chemical examination of the gland merely give information regarding the question of the storage of iodine. Whether the lowered content in the hyperplastic gland is due to: (1) An increased demand for iodine by the body; (2) a decreased supply; (3) an inability on the part of the gland to store iodine, or (4) a modification of the circulating iodine itself, cannot be determined from these examinations. Functionally and in its iodine content the colloid gland departs in in no way from the normal. A gland that is colloid must at one time have gone through a period of hyperplasia. No gland that has undergone any degree of hyperplasia can ever resume its normal appearance.

The hyperplastic gland is therefore the only important structural variation. Until the secretion of the thyroid gland can be accurately measured, no statement regarding the relationship between function and morphology can rise beyond the realm of speculation.

The adenomatous tissue has always less avidity for iodine than the non-tumor tissue of the same gland.[11] In other words, iodine will be bound by the non-tumor tissue before the tumor grasps it, and alterations in the morphology of the tumor are not affected by the iodine until the non-tumor tissue has responded. This suggests that while the iodine metabolism of tumor tissue is qualitatively the same as that of non-tumor tissue, quantitatively it is less active.

3. THE ETIOLOGY OF THYROID HYPERPLASIA. Hyperplasia of the thyroid gland occurs as the result of many dissimilar conditions: low iodine intake, the ingestion of polluted water,[12] alterations in the activity of the sex apparatus,[17] after partial thyroidectomy, after the ingestion of large quantities of fat,[13] vitamine insufficiency,[13] the drinking of water from glacial strata, hyperplasia of the thyroid of the gravid mother; and it occurs in congenital cretinism, the hairless pig malady,[14, 15] and in Graves'[16] syndrome. Whatever the cause, the use of iodine in any form will result in involution to the colloid type. This strongly suggests that alteration in the iodine metabolism is either a primary or an essential secondary step in the production of hyperplasia by the dissimilar conditions mentioned above.

The architecture of the thyroid gland, in both health and disease, depends therefore upon the iodine economy.

4. THE ETIOLOGY OF THYROID ADENOMATA. Thyroid adenomata are seen in congenital cretinism and in many otherwise normal glands. They may show any of the ground types seen in non-tumor thyroid tissue. The fetal adenomata[7] present the most marked degrees of hyperplasia, and the relationship between the histological appearance of the adenoma and the iodine content differs in no way from the relationship in non-tumor tissue. There is no evidence to support a view that the adenomata arise *de novo* in response to an injury, and there is no evidence to show that alterations in the function of an adenoma can occur without altera-

tions in the non-tumor tissue. From the response of the tumor to iodine and from the results of feeding tumor, it is much more likely that in the same gland the tumor is less active than the non-tumor[11] tissue.

5. The Nervous Mechanism of the Thyroid Gland. The nerve supply to the thyroid gland has been demonstrated anatomically. The innervation of the bloodvessels is so abundant that the vascularity of the gland may be most delicately regulated.

The influence of the nerve supply upon the specific secretion of the thyroid gland has not been definitely settled, and about this point has arisen considerable academic controversy. In support of the nervous regulation of secretion the following have been offered: (1) Electrical stimulation[18] of the vago-sympathetic nerves decreases the iodine[19] content; (2) stimulating the vago-sympathetic nerves increases the thyroid secretion as measured by the vascular response to adrenalin;[20] (3) the subcutaneous injection of adrenalin causes an induction current in the gland;[21] (4) continuous stimulation[22] of the nerves, as by phrenico-sympathetic anastomosis, produces a condition resembling Graves' syndrome, which in turn is supposed to be due to hyperthyroidism. In opposition to these there may be offered: (1) Experiments using alteration of iodine content as an index of secretion are complicated by two technical factors (*a*) the iodine distribution in a gland is not uniform[23] and (*b*) the iodine-containing substance may be mechanically squeezed[24] out as a result of the powerful vasoconstriction following nerve stimulation. Again the interpretation of these results is open to the objection that the decrease in the iodine content does not necessarily connote increased secretion, but merely a diminution in the iodine store; (2) we have shown that after stimulating the thoracico-lumbar system with adrenalin[25] the augmented pressor response is due, not to alterations in the thyroid secretion, but to changes in the involuntary nervous system; (3) the production of the induction current may well be due to alterations in the vascular bed rather then in the secretory activity; (4) despite perfect nerve union no changes occur after phrenico-sympathetic anastomosis.[26 27 28]

While the chemical influence on thyroid secretion is so clearly demonstrable and so subtly adjusted it seems quite unnecessary to assign, in the presence of such inconclusive experimental data, more than a minor role to the influences of nervous impulses. Those who hold that the nervous influences control the secretion regard as the augmentor nerve to the thyroid gland the thoracico-lumbar division. If the theory of Gaskell[29] as to the double segmentation of the vertebrate ancestor is correct, then we should expect the augmentor nerve to the endodermal thyroid gland to be bulbo-sacral in origin.

6. Thyroid Hyperplasia and its Effects. In the majority of individuals and in animals in whom thyroid hyperplasia exists,

no extra-thyroidal alterations are constant.[2] In brook-trout[30] and many other animals in which thyroid hyperplasia has been studied, there are evidences in some of increase in weight, diminution in activity, susceptibility to infection, and in mammals a shedding of the hair; in other words, many of the symptoms of myxedema. In the "hairless pig malady,"[14 15] the highest degree of hyperplasia is present and the clinical condition is identical with myxedema. There is little doubt, therefore, that the functional activity of the thyroid may be apparently normal or greatly diminished in the presence of a hyperplasia. The frequency with which hyperplasia occurs in Graves' syndrome has led to the supposition that hyperplasia is an indication of hyperfunction, *i. e.*, a true hyperthyroidism.[31 32] Four facts make this hyperplasia-hyperthyroid theory difficult to maintain: (1) The definite cause and effect relation between the hyperplasia and the marked myxedema in the "hairless pigs;" (2) the association of hyperplasia with almost complete absence of iodine content in human congenital cretinism (myxedema); (3) the low iodine content of hyperplased glands; (4) failure to demonstrate the hormone in the blood from a hyperplased gland even after electrical stimulation of the nerves.

7. Specific Secretion of the Thyroid. The specific secretion of the thyroid is an iodine-containing substance that has been isolated by Kendall[33] and has been named thyroxin.[34] Many other gland extracts have been prepared, most of which are potent, but the compound of Kendall has the advantage of being crystalline, having an exact dosage, a constant chemical composition and it is fit for intravenous injection. As yet no potent compound has been obtained that is free from iodine and the potency of a preparation varies directly with the iodine content. Iodine-poor compounds cannot be made potent by treatment with iodine after or during extraction. Thyroxin is built up by the thyroid cells and stored in the colloid. The synthesis probably takes at least[35] eight to twenty hours. It is secreted into the thyroid veins rather than the lymphatics. Elimination is slow, probably taking forty-eight hours to ten days. Plummer[36] has estimated that the amount circulating is 12 to 14 mgm., or about 1 mgm per 10 pounds of body weight. Allowing the high figure for blood of 10 per cent of body weight, the amount in the blood is 1 mgm. to the pound or a concentration of 1 : 2,200,000. This amount is not detectable by chemical methods and the biological method of Gudersnatch[37] is utilized for the qualitative detection of small amounts. This test relies upon the increase in the rate of metamorphosis in the tadpole when thyroid extract is fed. The iodine content of the thyroid colloid is ordinarily sufficient to be estimated chemically. As has been stated, this varies as the histological appearance of the gland and is normal in normal or colloid glands and adenomata and greatly decreased in general or

local hyperplasia (gland and adenoma). The secretion has been detected in the thyroid veins[38] after electrical stimulation of the vago-sympathetic trunk to a normal gland. Similar stimulation of a hyperplastic gland produced no such effect. This meagre information is all we possess of the estimation of the output from the thyroid and would indicate that the output from a hyperplastic gland, like the storage, is less than the normal and confirms the clinical findings of myxedema associated with hyperplasia. Those who regard hyperplasia as indicating hypersecretion (hyperthyroidism) have difficulty correlating their theory with these findings.

Of the factors that control secretion three have been mentioned: iodine, nervous influences and the circulating epinephrine. Of these the first is potent and delicately adjusted, the second remains unconfirmed and the third is dubious in view of the fact that[38a] we were unable to confirm the data on which the supposition rests even with large amounts of adrenalin. This theory is also opposed by the phylogenetic evidence[23] which would lead one to expect that the stimulation of the thoracico-lumbar division and hence epinephrine would inhibit thyroid secretion.

Reports of feeding experiments with large amounts of thyroid are at variance. At the one extreme are those who claim that all the symptoms of Graves' syndrome including exophthalmos can be reproduced. At the other extreme is Carlson[39] who in an elaborate investigation on various animals and man found loss of weight, gastro-enteritis, and diarrhea as the only symptoms constantly produced. He concludes "It would require considerable imagination or an undue influence of one's wish or of one's judgment to identify the symptom complex of excessive thyroid feeding in experimental animals with exophthalmic goiter." Certain it is that in concentration comparable to that in the circulating blood thyroid extract cannot produce these symptoms. Indeed the effects of small doses indicates a metabolic reversal so that the thyroid is anabolic, and not catabolic. This remarkable finding of Janney[40] emphasizes the need for quantitative studies with thyroid extract. The status of this problem is not unlike that of the question of the function of epinephrin before the quantitative work of Hoskins.[41] It will be remembered that after it was shown that adrenalin elevated blood-pressure it was immediately assumed that epinephrin maintained the vascular tonus. When it was found that the action of adrenalin was reversible[42] and that with small doses vaso-dilatation occurred, Hoskins made quantitative study and found that the concentration of adrenalin necessary to give a pressor effect was also sufficient to cause intestinal inhibition. This experience with adrenalin indicates the fallacy of concluding that the same effects must necessarily be produced by thyroid secretion in the amounts circulating in the normal economy as are produced by the administration of this substance in large quantities.

The most definite information regarding thyroid effects has been obtained from metabolic studies. On the one hand thyroid feeding increases the heat production in myxedema and on the other hand diminished heat production results from diminution in the thyroid function (ablation, fibrosis or extreme hyperplasia). That the thyroid is not the sole regulator of the heat mechanism is obvious from (1) the fact that the elevation of the basal metabolism caused by adrenalin (stimulation of the thoracico-lumbar division of the involuntary nervous system) is not altered appreciably by thyroidectomy[43] and (2) destruction of the adrenal cortex causes a prolonged and sustained elevation of the basal metabolism in the presence of the thyroid gland.[43] It is clear, therefore, that the basal heat production may be altered by at least three factors—the thyroid, the adrenal cortex and the involuntary nervous system.

Summary and Conclusions. 1. A study made at a seaport of 55 individuals with thyroid enlargement is presented.

2. None of these patients presented sympathomimetic manifestations or alterations of their basal metabolism.

3. The efficacy of iodides in reducing neck circumference is again demonstrated.

4. The thyroid enlargement where uniform is due to existing hyperplasia or the results of a previous hyperplasia.

5. The mechanism of the production of hyperplasia is through diminution in the iodine store.

6. We are unaware of the mechanism that produces the deficiency in the iodine store.

7. Alterations in the iodine store throw no light on the function of the gland.

8. Hyperplasia of the thyroid gland is compatible with normal economy, and it may be present in cretinism.

9. That hyperplasia of the thyroid gland indicates hypersecretion is based on inferences which are not compatible with the available data.

10. Discrete enlargements of the thyroid gland are due to cysts or adenomata. Cysts are of no functional importance. Adenomata function apparently in no way different from non-tumor tissue, except that they are less active in their avidity and response to iodine.

11. There is no evidence to support the theory of the toxicity of adenomata.

12. The influence of nervous impulses upon the secretion of the thyroid gland has not been demonstrated, and in view of the subtle chemical reaction the nervous influences probably play a minor role, if any.

13. While the active principle of the thyroid gland has been isolated, we are as yet unable to make any determinations upon the rate of secretion.

14. Feeding thyroid extract in toxic amounts does not reproduce Graves' syndrome.

15. The role of the thyroid in the production of clinical symptoms is greatly overemphasized. Of the 55 patients recorded, in 41 attention had been specifically directed to the thyroid gland. Either the symptoms were attributed to a disturbance of the function of the gland, while the true pathological condition that was operative was overlooked, or else specific therapy was directed toward the thyroid gland without any relief of symptoms which could not possibly have been caused by thyroid disturbance.

16. Roentgen-ray exposures of the thyroid gland do not cause an appreciable reduction in size.

17. Operations upon the thyroid gland may be followed by compensatory hyperplasia.

18. Thyroid enlargement can be present for many years without in any way altering the bodily economy.

BIBLIOGRAPHY.

1. Marine: Jour. Lab. and Clin. Med., 1917, **3**, 40.
2. Jour. Am. Med. Assn., 1919, **73**, 1873.
3. Arch. Int. Med., 1909, **3**, 66.
4. Idem, 1908, **1**, 349.
5. Jour. Exp. Med., 1910, **12**, 311; 1911, **13**, 455.
6. Arch. Int. Med., 1911, **7**, 506.
7. Jour. Med. Res., 1910, **27**, 229.
8. Jour. Biol. Chem., 1915, **22**, 547.
9. Jour. Pharm. and Exp. Therap., 1916, **8**, 437.
10. Arch. Int. Med., 1908, **1**, 349.
11. Graham: Jour. Exp. Med., 1916, **24**, 345.
12. Marine: Bull. Johns Hopkins Hosp., 1911, **21**, 95.
13. McCarrison: Jour. Am. Med. Assn., 1922, **78**, 686.
14. Hart and Steenbock: Jour. Biol. Chem., 1917, **33**, 313.
15. Smith: Jour. Biol. Chem., 1916, **29**, 215.
16. Wilson: Am. Jour. Med. Sci., 1914, **147**, 344.
17. McCarrison: Proc. N. Y. Path. Soc., 1921, **21**, 154.
18. Rahe, Rogers, Fawcett and Beebe: Am. Jour. Phys., 1914, **34**, 72.
19. Watts: Am. Jour. Phys., 1915, **38**, 356.
20. Asher and Flack: Zentr. f. Phys., 1910, **24**, 211; Arch. f. Phys., 1911, **139**, 562.
21. Cannon and Levy: Am. Jour. Phys., 1918, **41**, 392.
22. Cannon and Cattell: Am. Jour. Phys., 1918, **41**, 58.
23. Vandyke: Am. Jour. Phys., 1921, **56**, 168.
24. Watts: Am. Jour. Phys., 1915, **38**, 356.
25. Lieb and Hyman: Jour. Pharm. and Exp. Therap. 1922, **63**, 60, 68, 83, 88.
26. Marine, Rogoff and Stewart: Am. Jour. Physiol., 1918, **45**, 368.
27. Burget: Am. Jour. Phys., 1917, **44**, 492.
28. Troell: Arch. Int. Med., 1916, **17**, 582.
29. Gaskell: The Involuntary Nervous System, Monograph, 1916.
30. Marine: Jour. Exp. Med., 1914, **19**, 70.
31. Plummer: Tr. Assn. Am. Phys., 1916, 138.
32. Plummer: Am. Jour. Med. Sci., 1913, **146**, 790.
33. Kendall: Jour. Biol. Chem., 1919, **40**, 264.

34. Kendall: Jour. Am. Med. Assn., 1918, **71**, 871.
35. Plummer and Boothby: Proc. Am. Phys. Soc., 1920.
36. Plummer: Jour. Am. Med. Assn., 1921, **77**, 243.
37. Marine: Jour. Pharm. and Exp. Therap., 1917, **9**, 57.
38. Rogoff: Jour. Pharm. and Exp. Therap., 1918, **12**, 193.
38 a. Lieb and Hyman: Jour. Pharm. and Exp. Therap. 1922, **63**, 60, 68, 83, 88.
39. Carlson: Am. Jour. Phys., 1911, **30**, 128.
40. Janney: Arch Int. Med., 1920, **26**, 392.
41. Hoskins and McClure: Am. Jour. Phys., 1911, **31**, 59.
42. Cannon and Lyman: Am. Jour. Phys., 1911, **31**, 376.
43. Marine and Lenhart: Am. Jour. Phys., 1920, **54**, 248.

ON THE SIGNIFICANCE OF THE SEQUENCE AND MODE OF DEVELOPMENT OF SYMPTOMS AS AN AID TO THE DIAGNOSIS OF MULTIPLE SCLEROSIS IN THE EARLY STAGES.*

By Williams B. Cadwalader, M.D.,

Assistant Professor of Neurology at the University of Pennsylvania; Neurologist to the Presbyterian Hospital, Philadelphia; Consulting Neurologist to the Bryn Mawr Hospital,

and

J. W. McConnell, M.D.,

Associate in Neurology at the University of Pennsylvania; Neurologist to the Philadelphia General Hospital and to the Howard Hospital, Consulting Neurologist to the West Philadelphia Hospital for Women.

Multiple sclerosis is regarded by European authors as one of the most frequent conditions that affect the central nervous system. The number of cases of multiple sclerosis, however, in which the clinical diagnosis can be made with certainty by no means exceeds the number of cases in which the differential diagnosis is perplexing. Spiller, as well as Taylor, has drawn attention to the infrequency with which cases of multiple sclerosis with necropsy are recorded in this country, an apparent rarity that is probably due to the great difficulty with which the clinical diagnosis is made.

Considerable difference of opinion seems to exist regarding the symptom-complex that would justify a diagnosis of multiple sclerosis, particularly during the early stages of the disease. When Charcot, in his earlier descriptions, emphasized the importance of such symptoms as intention tremor, nystagmus, and scanning speech, he did not wish to imply that these manifestations were an invariable accompaniment of the disease, and most neurologists now agree that a positive diagnosis of multiple sclerosis may be

* Read at the second meeting of the Association for Research in Nervous and Mental Diseases, held in New York, December 27, 1921.

justifiable even in those cases in which the three classic signs of Charcot are not present at the same time. Great stress must, however, be laid upon all the points in the history, to show the sequence in the development of subjective and objective signs arising during the course in a given case. This view is of great importance in diagnosis, since it brings about a broader conception of the disease and tends to create a unanimity of opinion, as well as to help toward an appreciation of the mildest types of the disease that might lead to the realization that abortive cases or spontaneous cures do occur. Thus far this theory has not been confirmed.

For purposes of logical discussion it is necessary to state briefly that the clinical and histologic evidences that have been recorded up to date[1] seem to us to be strongly in favor of the view that the disease possesses a distinct entity, and that it is essentially infectious in origin and inflammatory in character, notwithstanding the fact that there is considerable evidence to show that the symptoms of multiple sclerosis may be produced by other diseases. Thus, for example, Spiller and Camp[2] reported a case of malarial fever that presented symptoms similar to those of multiple sclerosis. These authors[3] also found a form of multiple sclerosis that was syphilitic in origin. Other investigators have made similar observations. In another case reported by Mills and Spiller[4] the symptoms were found to be due to arteriosclerosis. We are convinced that in one of our cases (Case I) the disease was directly related to a previous attack of "influenza" and epidemic encephalitis. The relation of multiple sclerosis, both clinically and histologically, to epidemic (lethargic) encephalitis is a subject of great importance, and merits careful individual consideration.

During this meeting Dr. Spiller will demonstrate the microscopic lesions of the central nervous system in cases of epidemic encephalitis which very closely resemble those observed in certain cases of multiple sclerosis.[5] Years ago, Marie, Oppenheim, and others commented upon the relation of influenza to multiple sclerosis. The relation of influenza to epidemic encephalitis, although not proved, is admitted by many. These unsettled problems are referred to here more particularly to emphasize the fact that the knowledge that an infectious process had existed before the earliest symptoms of multiple sclerosis developed may be of importance in forming the diagnosis.

In the earliest stages of multiple sclerosis many of the symptoms

[1] Dawson: Review of Neurology and Psychiatry, 1917, **15**, 47; 1918, **16**, 287.

[2] Am. Jour. Med. Sci., 1900, **120**, 629.

[3] Spiller and Camp: Jour. Nerv. and Ment. Dis., 1907, **34**, 760.

[4] Jour. Nerv. and Ment. Dis., 1909, **36**, 747.

[5] Since the preparation of this manuscript, Dr. Spiller presented before the Philadelphia Neurological Society, at the meeting of February 27, 1922, a report on a form of epidemic encephalitis that resembled, both clinically and histologically, multiple sclerosis.

are so mild as to escape detection. It must be remembered, however, that these symptoms may subside without leaving any trace, and yet recur later and become progressively more intense. The most minute cross-examination on the part of the physician is, therefore, necessary in order to determine the mode of succession of the objective signs in a given case; this requires so much time and patience that it is not at all surprising that but little can be gained for this particular purpose from a study of many of the histories that are recorded in routine hospital practice.

If, in a given case, spastic paraplegia, intention tremor, scanning speech, optic atrophy, and nystagmus are present, the diagnosis presents but little difficulty, since these symptoms point to an advanced stage of the disease. But in the earliest stages of multiple sclerosis, before any of these signs have developed fully, the diagnosis is exceedingly difficult. The point that we wish to emphasize and discuss at this time is that a knowledge of the mode of succession of the symptoms may constitute sufficient evidence on which to base a positive diagnosis in the early and undeveloped stages. When accurate information is obtainable, a careful analysis of all the circumstances leading up to the development of the very earliest forms of disability is of as much value for diagnostic purposes as are the individual symptoms. Isolated objective signs, such as impairment of vision, ocular paralyses, weakness of one or more of the extremities, associated with paresthesia, are exceedingly common. These phenomena are, however, transitory, and are frequently so fleeting as to be overlooked.

Remission of the onset symptoms is far more common than is generally believed, and is prone to occur in the majority of cases. Birley and Dudgeon[6] have shown that most cases run an intermittent course, accompanied by a haphazard series of relatively acute disturbances due to focal lesions.

In one of the cases (II) studied at the University Hospital the earliest evidence of the disease, dating back to 1907, was a paralysis of the left leg that lasted one month, disappeared, and returned within two months. It was absent again for a prolonged period, but in 1909 it recurred, and remained as an intermittent feature up to and for some time after the full development of marked bilateral spastic paraplegia and other symptoms of multiple sclerosis about eight years later.

This case shows that transitory paralyses may constitute the only objective sign of disease, and may recur and subside at irregular intervals, covering a period of time varying in duration from months to years, and gradually becoming fixed and permanent, and later associated with other manifestations characteristic of the late stages of multiple sclerosis.

[6] Brain, London, 1921, **44**, 150.

In one of our cases (III) the only complaint was of intermittent diplopia over a period of three years before other characteristic signs developed. In another case (IV) there were irregular attacks of sudden but transient blindness preceding the development of optic atrophy; and in still another case (V) there developed very rapidly bilateral oculomotor paralysis that persisted for eighteen months, no other symptoms, either objective or subjective, being present. Tremor, scanning speech, and weakness of the extremities developed later. Case VI presented the signs typical of hemiplegia of rapid onset, which had been mistaken for the results of an apoplectic attack from vascular occlusion; these persisted for a number of months without the development of other symptoms. Numerous similar examples could easily be collected, since they appear to be quite common, and tend to show the difficulties in diagnosis in the earliest stage in the absence of other phenomena.

For diagnostic purposes isolated symptoms of the disease under consideration are of little value, but the knowledge that paralytic phenomena were at first isolated and later became permanent and were combined with nystagmus, scanning speech, tremor, or other manifestations may be of considerable importance.

It has been our experience that the classic symptoms, *i. e.*, nystagmus, scanning speech, and intention tremor, differ from the other signs of this disease in that they are not so frequently remittent in character, although occasionally they appear as isolated signs. Once established, they tend to become permanent and to progress. Each of these symptoms seems to point to a more or less widespread distribution of the inflammatory lesions, and for this reason they are of far greater importance than almost any other single sign of the disease. Scanning speech or other dysarthria indicates disturbance in the combined motor function of the respiratory, laryngeal, palatal, lingual, and lip muscles that are supplied by different cranial nerves; and each one of these cranial nerves has its origin at a different level within the brain-stem. One lesion sufficiently severe to have destroyed all of these must, therefore, be very diffuse.

A purely spinal type of multiple sclerosis is exceedingly uncommon. It is not unusual, however, to find that a diagnosis of multiple sclerosis has been made when the symptoms of spastic paraplegia and loss of abdominal reflexes are present without any involvement of the structure of the brain. In our opinion this is not always justified, although we do not deny that the disease may present this picture. A case of this kind was reported in 1900 by Burr and McCarthy,[7] the diagnosis having been confirmed by autopsy, but which presented only the signs of combined sclerosis of the spinal cord. When, however, these symptoms are followed by

[7] Jour. Nerv. and Ment. Dis., 1900, **207**, 634.

nystagmus, intention tremor, or scanning speech, the diagnosis is, we believe, clear. Such a case recently came to our notice, in which spastic paraplegia had existed for two years, after which nystagmus, scanning speech, and tremor of the upper limbs rapidly developed. Other cases have been reported in which symptoms attributable to the spinal cord were entirely lacking. Here, again, in the absence of the classic trio, scanning speech, nystagmus, and intention tremor, the diagnosis may be uncertain. Thus in Case V bilateral oculomotor paralysis developed very rapidly in the spring of 1919, and persisted for eighteen months, although no cause for it could be found. Months later, however, the patient began to complain of difficulty in writing with his right hand, due to tremulousness. This tremor gradually extended, until now it involves the four extremities and is associated with moderate weakness in the right lower limb, increased tendon reflexes, and the Babinski sign, ankle clonus, and scanning speech. At the beginning a diagnosis of multiple sclerosis was impossible, but now that the other symptoms have developed, together with the involvement of the lower limbs, the diagnosis seems quite clear.

Conclusion. We would emphasize that the sequence, mode of development, and the combination of signs are more important than the individual symptoms themselves. In addition, the occurrence of cerebral symptoms, most particularly scanning speech and nystagmus, either alone or after spinal symptoms have developed, or the reverse, spinal symptoms following the cerebral manifestations, is strongly indicative of the dissemination of the pathologic process. If there is a history of earlier remissions or of a discontinuance of the process in the early stages, followed by a progressive course, the nature of the disease can be determined with considerable accuracy. With the exception of syphilis, no subacute or chronic disease other than multiple sclerosis presents this remittent picture so constantly.

Case Reports. CASE I.—J. K., aged eighteen years.

Chief Complaint. Tremulousness.

Family History. Negative.

Personal History. Was well until October, 1918, when he was very ill with "flu." Was confined to bed for two weeks; fever and delirium were present and patient was extremely weak. He gradually recovered from his acute symptoms, and was out of bed in about four weeks. Although believed to have fully recovered, he states that he has never regained his strength, particularly in his lower limbs. About January, 1919, while driving a motor car at night and looking at the headlights of another car approaching, he first noticed diplopia. This has been irregular and inconstant, but most annoying. During this time he has developed very gradually weakness of the lower limbs, associated with marked tremor and uncertainty in gait. General health remained fairly good.

Examination showed weakness of the right sixth and of the left third nerve; marked intention tremor of all four limbs; adiadokokinesia on each side; dysmetria in both upper limbs; marked ataxia and spasticity of both lower extremities; increase of all the tendon reflexes; ankle clonus on the right and Babinski sign present; speech is slurring.

Diagnosis. Multiple sclerosis developing after an attack of "flu."

CASE II.—E. Z. D. White male, aged thirty-three years. First examined April 20, 1911.

Chief Complaint. Weakness of the left leg.

Family History. Negative.

Personal History. The patient is a highly educated man. He has been partially blind since 1908, the impairment being due to unilateral optic atrophy, considered by the ophthalmologist to be the result of a sphenoidal sinusitis. There was some difficulty in convergence at this time, believed to have been due to weakness of the internal rectus muscle of the left eye. About a year preceding the difficulty with his eye (1907) he noticed a weakness of the left leg which lasted about one month, disappeared for two months, then recurred for about a month, disappeared again, and recurred in 1909. Shortly after the last recurrence he experienced difficulty in writing and in shaving, which he attributed to weakness and stiffness of the right hand and arm.

Following the appearance of these symptoms he gradually developed a spastic paraplegia, scanning speech, and intention tremor—a typical picture of *disseminated sclerosis,* from which condition he is suffering at the present time.

Blood Wassermann was negative.

CASE III.—K. N., white female, aged eighteen years. First examined in 1905.

Chief Complaint. Nervousness.

Personal History. For about a year she has had attacks of double vision lasting for varying periods of time, the longest being seven weeks. After several attacks of double vision during a period of three years she gradually developed a marked tremulousness of the hands and noticed disturbances of speech. Following this her symptoms progressed quite rapidly, and she died two years after first coming under observation. This was a typical advanced case of *disseminated sclerosis.*

CASE IV.—W. W. P. White male, aged twenty-four years. First examined February 2, 1916.

Chief Complaint. Nervousness.

Personal History. The patient states that he was perfectly well up to December, 1915, at which time he suffered a severe nervous shock, and immediately after noticed that his vision was blurred. Within a few days be became blind and had some trembling of the hands and a slight difficulty in walking. All these symptoms disappeared completely. About two weeks previous to his admission to the hospital he again developed tremulousness of the hands, and had considerable difficulty in using his legs for locomotion. He gave no history of excesses of any kind, and was a man of unusual education and of splendid physique.

Physical examination at the time of his admission to the hospital presented the neurologic features of a fairly well-advanced case of *disseminated sclerosis*, namely, intention tremor, scanning speech, spastic paraplegia, and optic atrophy.

He remained in the hospital for a short time, and was under observation for about two years. Within six months after leaving the hospital he improved so greatly that he was regarded as almost completely recovered. This remission in the symptomatology was of very short duration, however, and the symptoms that followed progressed with tremendous rapidity. At this time he presents a picture of a well-marked case of *disseminated sclerosis*, and is almost helpless.

Wassermann reaction, both of the blood and of the spinal fluid, was negative.

CASE V.—J. W., aged seventeen years.

Chief Complaint. Headache and inability to look upward.

Personal History. In May, 1919, following an acute attack that was diagnosed as "flu," and that had confined him to bed for two weeks, the patient found that he was unable to look upward or downward, and had frequent severe frontal headaches. On examination in June, 1919, there was inability to rotate either eyeball upward or downward, although the external and internal rotations were performed normally. No cause for the condition could be determined, and no other objective sign could be discovered. The patient continued under observation at the Presbyterian Hospital, and about October, 1919, he complained of an inability to write because of tremor of the right hand. This condition progressed, and weakness of the right lower limb also developed. About 1920 his speech became indistinct, and in 1921 examination showed partial bilateral third nerve paralysis, with marked scanning speech, intention tremor, dysmetria, and adiadokokinesia on both sides, but most marked on the right, weakness of the right lower limb, with ankle clonus and increased tendon reflexes.

Diagnosis. Multiple sclerosis.

Case VI.—M. S. White male. First examined at the Philadelphia General Hospital.

Personal History. Patient was almost completely blind. The right half of his body was practically powerless, and he had considerable difficulty in using the left side of his body. Nevertheless, he was able to move about. The history of his present illness was to the effect that about a year before coming to the hospital he had a sudden attack of what was believed to have been "an apoplectic stroke, which resulted in paralysis of the right arm and right leg." This was soon followed by failure of vision, which gradually grew worse.

On admission to the hospital he presented weakness of all four limbs, but greater on the right side; a partial blindness, due to optic atrophy; slurring speech; marked nystagmus; tremor of the left upper extremity following use of the limb; marked increase of all the reflexes, and bilateral Babinski sign.

Wassermann, both of the blood and of the spinal fluid, was negative, as was also the general physical examination.

The disease pursued a continued progressive and typical course up to the time of death, which occurred in 1921.

Diagnosis. Disseminated sclerosis.

OBSERVATIONS REGARDING THE CONDITION OF TRAUMATIC CEREBRAL EDEMA.

By William Sharpe, M.D.,

PROFESSOR OF NEUROLOGIC SURGERY, NEW YORK POLYCLINIC MEDICAL SCHOOL AND HOSPITAL, NEW YORK CITY.

Within recent years the presence or not of a linear fracture of the vault or of the base of the skull in conditions of brain injury has become of comparative unimportance, whereas the degree of associated cerebral edema has become more and more a significant factor to be considered in the diagnosis and in the treatment of these patients, not only during the acute condition but for a period of months and even of years following the cranial injury. Varying degrees of cerebral edema undoubtedly accompany all severe cranial injuries, whether there is a fracture of the skull or not and whether there is an associated intracranial hemorrhage or not, and it is difficult to conceive that a traumatic intracranial hemorrhage can occur without there being associated with it a cerebral edema of more or less severity and especially of the localized type.

By the term cerebral edema is understood a "wet" edematous condition of the cerebral tissues. Most probably it is merely an excess amount of normal cerebrospinal fluid; in this regard the condition of cerebral edema differs from the edema of other body tissues following a bruise or injury and it is, therefore, not simply a transudation of lymph. The excess amount of cerebrospinal fluid in the acute traumatic cerebral conditions may be due to hypersecretion of the fluid from the blood stream on the part of the choroid plexus in the third ventricle, or, and most probably, in my opinion, it is due to a lessened absorption (hypoexcretion) of the cerebrospinal fluid through the normal excretory channels, chiefly in the walls of the supracortical veins, sinuses and Pacchionian bodies, and thus a partial blockage of the excretion of the cerebrospinal fluid is temporarily produced. It is not known whether or not this lessened excretion of the cerebrospinal fluid through the little stomata of exit in the walls of the supracortical veins and sinuses in these acute traumatic conditions, is due to the associated vasomotor disturbance—in effect, a paralytic retardation of the excretory function of the supracortical veins. It is an interesting observation, however, that, during the period of severe initial shock so frequently following the cranial injury, the condition of cerebral edema is rarely present; this may be due to the associated lowered blood-pressure, both general and intracranial, and, therefore, resulting in possibly a diminished secretion of the cerebrospinal fluid by the choroid plexus, so that the condition of cerebral edema does not occur during this period of shock, even though at the same time the excretory function is also lessened as a result of the condition of shock and its accompanying vasomotor disturbances.

Cerebral edema of toxic origin, such as occurs in nephritic and diabetic disease and in alcoholic and arteriosclerotic patients, is most probably due to an increased secretion of the cerebrospinal fluid rather than to a partial blockage of its excretion through the little stomata of exit in the walls of the supracortical veins lying in the sulci between the convolutions of the cerebral cortex—the chief channels of the normal excretion of the cerebrospinal fluid, and, to a lesser degree, through the walls of the Pacchionian bodies and of the large dural sinuses into the blood stream. Cerebral edema, resulting from toxic conditions, is, therefore, most probably due to a hypersecretion rather than to a lessened absorption or partial blockage of the excretion of the cerebrospinal fluid, and yet in acute traumatic cranial conditions associated with cerebral edema of varying degree, it is not definitely known whether the "wet" edematous brain of an excess amount of cerebrospinal fluid is due to a temporary increase of the secretion or, and more probably, to a decrease in the amount of absorption or excretion of the cerebrospinal fluid.

In reviewing the literature upon cerebral edema of traumatic origin, it has indeed been most surprising to realize the apparently slight interest in this serious complication of cranial injuries; the literature itself is most meagre and with the exception of papers by Jones,[1] Baehr,[2] Preston,[3] Hollander,[4] Reichardt[5] and two or three others, and brief mention of the condition in various general surgical treatises and text-books, such as Rawling, Keen, Mills, Stewart and Herrick, little or no attention has been directed toward a better clinical understanding of the condition and its treatment. It is only within recent years that the factor of cerebral edema in conditions of brain injuries has been recognized as being a most important one, not only from the standpoint of the diagnosis, but of the treatment and of the prognosis. Traumatic localized cerebral edema, however, has frequently been diagnosed as a possibility in producing various neurologic signs, such as the alteration of the reflexes, paralyses of varying degree and occasionally aphasia in its various forms, and the diagnosis itself has been confirmed, in selected cases at operation, immediately upon opening the dura and thus permitting a careful exposure of the involved cerebral cortex.[6]

In those cases of localized cerebral edema developing from the associated operative traumatism of opening the bone and the dura, and of the effect of cold air upon the cortex, producing a dilatation of the supracortical veins and thus a temporary partial blockage of the excretion of the cerebrospinal fluid, a localized cerebral edema can develop within a few minutes to the extent that the involved cerebral cortex may bulge and tend to protrude through the dural opening; a lumbar puncture with spinal drainage, however, will usually permit the protrusion to recede so that no cortical damage results.

Until several years ago, patients dying within twelve to forty-eight hours following a cranial injury, were usually diagnosed as conditions of "shock," "fracture of the skull," "hemorrhage of the brain," and yet when an autopsy was performed (and only too frequently the importance of autopsy findings has been overlooked)[7]

[1] Jour. Am. Med. Assn., 1918, **11**, 1265.

[2] Lancet-Clinic, 1914, **111**, 696.

[3] Jour. Nerv. and Ment. Dis., 1894, **21**, 494.

[4] Jahrb. f. Psychiat., Wien, 1882, **3**, 176.

[5] Allg. Ztschr. f. Psychiat., Berlin, 1918, **12**, 622.

[6] Vide report of case of localized cerebral edema by my associate, Dr. G. E. Espejo, Jour. Am. Med. Assn., 1918, **70**, 1278.

[7] During the past seven years I have insisted, before performing an operation upon any patient having a chronic neurologic condition, that the nearest relatives give me, in writing, permission to make a postmortem examination in case the patient should die (and naturally one does not expect the patient to die), in order to ascertain the real cause of death rather than accept the common report of "shock," "cerebral or pulmonary embolus" and "thrombus formation." If death is due to an operative error or to some avoidable complication, then it is for the surgeon to realize it so that its repetition can, if possible, be prevented in future patients; moreover, the accuracy of the diagnosis is thus confirmed or disproved and the pathologic lesion is carefully examined. The coöperation of the nearest relative in permitting these examinations has been the rule; in only two instances in a series of over 1000 patients operated upon was a flat refusal maintained, and no operation was performed.

the report was often characterized as being "merely a wet brain," thus apparently confirming the diagnosis of "shock," but not always that of "fracture of the skull" or of "cerebral hemorrhage." If, however, a fracture of the vault and particularly of the base of the skull was disclosed, and, especially, if an area of subdural hemorrhage could be demonstrated, then the diagnosis was considered complete—the cause of death ascertained. This was, and is, so often the case in the large municipal hospitals, where many nephritic and arteriosclerotic patients associated with the condition of chronic alcoholism are admitted following cranial injuries of even an apparently trivial nature and yet, upon autopsy within several days, merely a wet edematous condition of the brain is disclosed; shock is a definite factor in the high mortality in many of these patients, but the condition of acute cerebral edema producing a marked increase in the intracranial pressure is a far more serious and important complication in the diagnosis and treatment of these patients. The presence or absence of a fracture of the skull, either of the vault or of the base, and the presence or absence of a small amount of intracranial hemorrhage, even though the cerebrospinal fluid may be termed bloody at lumbar puncture, is of little significance in the treatment and prognosis of the condition. The most important point to be considered is the presence or not of a marked increase of the pressure of the cerebrospinal fluid, whether due to hemorrhage or to cerebral edema or to both; it is this factor of increased intracranial pressure which has been overlooked so frequently in the past, unless it was of such a height as to produce the definite and, unfortunately, the late signs of medullary compression—increased blood-pressure, retarded pulse and respiration-rates with the irregular Cheyne-Stokes rhythm—a most serious condition for the patient, as the chances of recovery of even life, not to mention normality, are not favorable.

No doubt the condition of severe initial shock is a frequent cause of death in cranial injuries, and in these extreme cases the diagnosis can usually be made from the clinical charts alone: subnormal temperature, pulse- and respiration-rates increased to 140 plus and 40 plus, respectively, and the blood-pressure 90 and lower, and yet this diagnosis of shock as being the cause of death has been frequently asserted in the presence of a temperature of 100 plus, pulse and respiration rates of 70 and 16 and lower, respectively, and a blood-pressure of 140 plus. At autopsy upon a number of these patients, who finally succumbed from the more advanced signs of medullary compression and, finally, of medullary edema—rapidly rising temperature to 106 plus, pulse and respiration rates of 160 plus and 50 plus, respectively, and a falling blood-pressure of 80 and lower, only too frequently in these cases was "merely" a cerebral edema ascertained and no fracture or even intracranial hemorrhage disclosed; the condition of shock might have been an initial factor in precipitating the acute medullary edema, but surely the cause of death and the diagnosis should not be labelled as one of "shock." In a recent work upon the diagnosis and treatment of brain injuries,[8] I realize now that I did not emphasize sufficiently the relative unimportance, in my opinion, of a definite increase of the blood-pressure, except as indicating the lateness of the time for operative interference, since this increase of the blood-pressure is a sign of medullary compression, and the patient should be given an opportunity to recover by an earlier lowering of the increased intracranial pressure, either by the expectant palliative or by the operative method. If we wait in the treatment until the blood-pressure is definitely increased above normal, then we are letting the patient reach a very serious condition of medullary compression and it is then frequently too late to aid him even with an operation of decompression and drainage. In my opinion, the ophthalmoscopic and spinal mercurial manometric findings are much more valuable than the status of the blood-pressure, as definite and delicate tests in ascertaining *early* the intracranial condition of an increase of the intracranial pressure, whether due to hemorrhage or to an excess cerebrospinal fluid. The presence of shock is characterized by a lowered blood-pressure together with a subnormal temperature and an increased pulse-rate, whereas the stage of medullary edema presents a rising temperature, pulse- and respiration-rates, and also a falling blood-pressure, so that clinically these two periods can usually be differentiated. It is the general neglect in the recognition of the importance of the factor of cerebral edema in the diagnosis and treatment of brain injuries that will be discussed in this paper.

The significance of cerebral edema as being the most important factor in the statistics of the high mortality following cranial injuries in patients of the large municipal hospitals, is just being recognized, and their high mortality-rate cannot be compared, with justice, to the much lower rate in private patients or in the patients of the smaller private hospitals; this natural difference is due to the lessened general resistance of the majority of patients admitted to the municipal hospitals with severe cerebral injuries, a lessened resistance to the onset of acute cerebral edema following even apparently trivial cranial injuries and due to chronic alcoholism associated with varying degrees of nephritis and arteriosclerosis. These patients are poor risks and their prognosis is always much more grave than in patients of good habits and especially in the absence of nephritis and arteriosclerosis, because in the latter selected patients a dangerous degree of cerebral edema is only to be feared as the result of *severe* cerebral injuries and not

[8] The Diagnosis and Treatment of Brain Injuries, with and without a Fracture of the Skull, J. B. Lippincott Company, Philadelphia, 1921.

following the milder type of cranial injuries. This is true also of children, in whom traumatic cerebral edema is a rare complication unless the cerebral injury is of the greatest severity. Therefore, the mortality-rate of brain injuries in children and adolescents is much lower than in adults of either sex; and in a rather large series of acute brain injuries, the mortality-rate in the female patients has been definitely lower than that of the male patients, most probably due to the greater resistance of women to the onset and development of cerebral edema, owing to their better habits of life in regard to alcohol and to the strain and stress of modern life, and thus a greater freedom from arteriosclerotic disease. In this connection, it may be of interest to note that the increased intracranial pressure developing in children of either sex and in adult female patients, following cranial injuries with or without a fracture of the skull, less frequently reaches a height necessitating the operative treatment of decompression and drainage than in adult male patients, because in the former patients (women and children) the condition of extensive cerebral edema is only associated with the severe types of cerebral injuries, and, therefore, the expectant palliative treatment of absolute rest, quiet, ice helmet, liquid diet and catharsis usually suffices to obtain an excellent recovery of life and of normal function; while in the adult male patients, the greater frequency of the development of extensive cerebral edema necessitates in a larger proportion of these patients the operation of subtemporal decompression and drainage in order to obtain the best results by an early lowering of the resulting increased intracranial pressure.

Acute Cerebral Edema. The onset of acute cerebral edema with and without an intracranial hemorrhage may occur so rapidly following the cranial injury that the initial period of shock is obscured and overshadowed by the signs of high intracranial pressure, due to the excess amount of cerebrospinal fluid associated or not with varying degrees of hemorrhage. In these severe cases the signs of medullary edema resulting from the extreme condition of cerebral edema may be evident upon the patient's admission to the hospital—rapidly rising temperature of 104° plus, pulse and respiration rates increasing to 140 plus and 40 plus, respectively, while the blood-pressure falls steadily; naturally in these extreme cases the condition is a hopeless one, the patients being moribund. They all die, operation or no operation. In this regard it may be stated that no patient should be operated upon during the terminal period of medullary edema, cerebral surgery being thereby merely discredited, and this moribund period together with that of the initial stage of extreme shock immediately following the injury form the two periods of brain injuries when no operation should be performed, and if a patient should recover following an operation during the period of severe initial shock, then he recovers in spite of the operation. It has been the neglect in observing and in recognizing in the past the danger as well as the futility of operating during these two periods that has discouraged the operative treatment of brain injuries during *any* period, and thus the rational treatment of these acute patients has lagged behind the great advances of modern surgery.

In a much larger percentage of the patients developing an extensive cerebral edema, the onset of the condition is by no means such a rapid and overwhelming one; the condition of the patient upon admission to the hospital and even for several days may be considered as "fair" or indeed "good;" a normal temperature or a slightly elevated one, pulse and respiration rates normal or mildly increased respectively, and a blood-pressure within physiologic limits; then gradually the pulse and respiration rates descend slowly during a period of hours to 70 and 18 and then to 60 and 16, respectively, and even lower, and the blood-pressure possibly (but by no means always) rises to 140 and occasionally higher, and yet the temperature remains the same. It is during this period of mild medullary compression that it is most important to ascertain the presence or not of a high intracranial pressure, as indicated in the fundi ophthalmoscopically and by means of the spinal mercurial manometer at lumbar puncture.[9] If the mercurial manometer should register the pressure of the cerebrospinal fluid less than twice the normal pressure, which is 6 to 8 mm., then, whether the cerebrospinal fluid is bloody or not, the expectant palliative treatment, with or without the repeated lumbar punctures of spinal drainage, will usually suffice to obtain excellent recovery of both life and apparent normality in slightly over two-thirds of the patients, whereas if the pressure of the cerebrospinal fluid at lumbar puncture is greater than twice the normal pressure (that is, over 16 mm.), then in my opinion, these selected patients should receive the benefits of an early subtemporal decompression and drainage—both to assure a recovery of life and, more especially, to permit the greatest return of normal

[9] The condition of measurable papilledema to the degree of "choked disks" (2 D+) is rarely to be observed with the ophthalmoscope in those patients having acute brain injuries; a measurable papilledema does occur when the intracranial pressure is extreme and of slow formation, as in cases of large middle meningeal extradural hemorrhage and thus producing a tumor pressure, but the usual fundal picture in the acute patients having a definite increase of the intracranial pressure is that of dilated retinal veins associated with an edematous blurring of the nasal and temporal margins and of the nasal halves of the optic disks. During the period of initial shock following the cranial injury, it is most uncommon for ophthalmoscopic examinations to disclose the fundal signs of an increased intracranial pressure—the general blood-pressure being lowered and, therefore, it is physiologically impossible for a high intracranial pressure to develop even if a large vessel or sinus is torn; in this manner, the condition of initial shock within moderate limits may be a most valuable aid of Nature in affording the organism a period of time to readjust itself to changed intracranial conditions—by the thrombosis of torn vessels and thus avoiding or at least lessening the later intracranial hemorrhage.

function physically, mentally and emotionally. These patients with high intracranial pressure, even to the degree of medullary compression, may recover with life without an operation, and a large number of the milder ones do, but the percentage of recovery of normal function, let alone life itself, is very low indeed in this class of patients and when recovery of life does occur, then it is most rare to obtain as normal an individual as before the injury. These are the patients forming a large class of chronic brain injuries and their condition will be discussed under the heading of chronic cerebral edema. The technic of cerebral surgery has so advanced during the past two decades, and especially the operation of subtemporal decompression as devised by Cushing, that these operations should no longer be deferred until the patient reaches the most serious stage of extreme medullary compression, but rather an early operative lowering of the high intracranial pressure will permit not only a higher percentage of recovery of life, but in some cases of even greater importance, the maximum degree of normality. In this series of over 1000 patients, upon whom the subtemporal decompression was performed, the mortality was only slightly over 10 per cent.

In adults, and especially in alcoholic males, the onset of acute cerebral edema following even apparently trivial injuries of the head may develop so rapidly and to such a degree that upon admission to the hospital the condition has become one of medullary edema—rising temperature, pulse and respiration rates with a falling blood-pressure; the period of initial shock in these patients may be of very short duration and at times it would seem that the condition of shock merges directly into that of medullary edema without there having been evident the clinical signs of medullary compression—moderate temperature, lowered pulse and respiration rates and a possible increase of the blood-pressure. The condition in these extreme cases may have been so overwhelming that the signs of medullary compression were only obscured rather than being absent. At autopsy, however, the usual findings are a very "wet" edematous brain under high tension, associated or not with hemorrhage of varying degree with or without a fracture of the skull. These acute and extreme cases occur only too frequently in active hospital practice, and they are the moribund patients for whom little if anything can be done; and most assuredly, *no* operation. On the other hand, those patients eventually developing the condition of acute cerebral edema after a period of twelve to forty-eight hours, and especially after several days to even two weeks following the injury, they are the ones whose clinical charts are typical—the usual period of initial shock of varying degree and of several hours' duration, then the general condition of the patient so improves that an excellent prognosis may be stated; with the exception of headache, the patient may have no complaints. After a period of hours or even days, the pulse rate may descend slightly to 74 and to 70 and the respirations register 20 and later 18, yet "the temperature is slightly increased and the blood-pressure is normal," and the excellent prognosis is reassured with the expectant palliative treatment. The condition seems favorable and fortunately in many patients the recovery is uneventful; on the contrary, however, the pulse- and respiration-rates may continue to descend to 62 and to 16 respectively, and may even remain in this relative position for a period of hours and of several days, and the temperature only slightly increased and the blood-pressure possibly raised a few points; "still the patient is perfectly conscious, a little drowsy and the headache is only natural." Even from this condition of evident mild medullary compression, the patient may recover with life after a period of days and weeks and with the expectant palliative treatment alone, but it is this type of patient who so frequently never regains his former normality, especially in the mental processes and the emotional reactions. But should this condition of mild medullary compression remain apparently stationary for a period of days and should then, either suddenly (within two to six hours) or gradually (twelve to forty-eight hours), progress to the degree that the pulse- and respiration-rates descend to 54 and 16, and lower, respectively, then this mild condition of medullary compression becomes the most serious one of severe medullary compression, which may rapidly change into that of medullary edema in spite of any known treatment, operative or otherwise; and once the temperature rises rapidly to a 104 plus, the pulse rate to 70, 80, 100, 120, 140 plus and the respiration rate to 18, 22, 28, 34, 40 plus and the blood-pressure to fall steadily—the typical onset of medullary edema—then all treatment is futile and these patients all die within twelve to forty-eight hours. To permit patients to reach this degree of extreme intracranial pressure during a period of hours and even of days, and sufficient to produce the signs of medullary compression, without ascertaining accurately and frequently the intracranial pressure, by means of routine examination of the fundi with the ophthalmoscope, and especially by the repeated daily use of the spinal mercurial manometer, medical treatment of this careless character is typical of the period of at least twenty years ago, when it was considered remarkable for a patient to recover with life "and a fracture of the base of the skull was present." The rational treatment of brain injuries depends chiefly upon the presence or not of a marked increase of the intracranial pressure, whether due to hemorrhage or to cerebral edema or to both, and the clinical signs of medullary compression should not be awaited before the patient is given an opportunity to recover not only life but the former normality. If an operation is advised, then the operation of choice is the subtemporal decompression and drainage, removing an area of bone two to three inches in diameter beneath the temporal muscle and opening the dura widely and permitting it to remain open. These apparent elementals in the operative treatment of brain injuries are mentioned because only recently, in the year 1921 in New York City at a large active hospital, the leading surgeon operated "to relieve a brain pressure following a fracture of the skull with hemorrhage" by turning down a large bone flap over the motor area with a hammer and chisel and then pricked the dura to permit the underlying hemorrhage to escape (several drops); the bone flap was then replaced and the relief of intradural pressure was practically nil; this procedure may be called an operation, but by no means a useful one.

It has long been recognized that children and young adults withstand the effects of cranial injuries much better than patients over forty years of age, and unless there are present in these young patients definite contusions and lacerations of cerebral tissues, then the associated cerebral edema is only of moderate degree; as gross lesions of the cerebral tissues in these traumatic cases of peacetimes are unusual (only occurring in 12 per cent of the acute cases in this series of 582 patients), their much lower mortality-rate is explained by the comparative absence of the extreme condition of cerebral edema and thus a relatively lower intracranial pressure, usually insufficient to produce the signs of medullary compression and the subsequent medullary edema. It is for this reason—the comparative rarity of extensive traumatic cerebral edema in children and young adults—that makes possible in the large majority of cases their successful treatment with the expectant palliative method alone, whereas in the older patients the greater frequency of the development of an extreme degree of cerebral edema with the resulting high intracranial pressure necessitates in a large percentage the operative method of treatment; however, even in the adult cases of this series the operative treatment was considered advisable in only 31 per cent, the expectant palliative method being sufficient in slightly over two-thirds of the patients.

In this connection, I should like to report briefly the case history of a child developing an extreme condition of acute cerebral edema several days following the cranial injury; unless the cerebral tissues are badly contused or lacerated, not only is it uncommon for a child to develop such a marked condition of acute traumatic cerebral edema as to make obligatory a cranial decompression and drainage, but that the onset of the resulting high intracranial pressure should be delayed until four and a half days after the cranial injury and the edematous condition should then persist in a mild degree (in spite of the drainage operation) for a period of several weeks—these are the unusual features of this case history.

No. 1741. Edward, aged seven years; white; school; United Sates. Admitted, October 9, 1921, to the Swiney Sanitarium, hyonne, N. J. Operation, October 14, 1921 (3 A.M.), four and a half days after the injury. Left subtemporal decompression ad drainage. Discharged, November 23, 1921, forty-three days ater injury. Family and past medical histories were negative. Lual diseases of childhood.

Present Illness. While playing at home, the patient fell headlog down the stairway, striking upon the top and left side of had; stunned but no complete loss of consciousness. No bleeding frm nose or ears. Immediately carried to the sanitarium and D. M. A. Swiney made the following notes: Temperature, 98°; plse rate, 94; respiration rate, 22. Mild condition of shock. Dowsy and restless at times; vomited twice within the first eight hors after admission. No paralyses nor sensory impairments. Pnils were equal and reacted normally. Reflexes were negative. Lcally, over the upper left parietal area the scalp was contused, bcgy and distinctly tender upon palpation. Treatment: For shck and the expectant palliative, quiet, external warmth (heated blnkets, hot-water bottles), ice helmet, etc.

xamination. October 10, 1921, twenty-four hours after injury an admission. Consultation with Dr. Swiney. Temperature, 99 °; pulse rate, 100; respiration rate, 22; blood-pressure, 118. Petectly conscious, but rather confused and irritable; complains of eadache. No signs of shock. Over the left parietal area the scal is ecchymosed and edematous, associated with marked tenderness. No bleeding from nose or ears; no mastoid ecchymos; otoscopic examination, negative. No paralyses nor sensor impairments. Pupils, negative. Reflexes, superficial: right epiastric and abdominal skin reflexes less active than left; deep: patllar increased, but equal; no ankle clonus nor definite Babinski. Furli, negative except for a slight dilatation of the retinal veins; no dematous blurring of either optic disk. Roentgen-ray report: "Vrtical linear fracture of left parietal bone extending downward int squamous portion of left temporal bone."

N lumbar puncture was advised as the condition appeared to be mply one of fracture of the skull, with a mild associated cerebral oncussion and no signs of a definite increase of the intracranial pre ure or of any intracranial lesion. (It is usually better judgmen to perform a lumbar puncture upon these traumatic cases afte the signs of initial shock have disappeared in order to obtain the most accurate information regarding the intracranial condition the presence or absence of a definite increase of the intracranial presure, whether of hemorrhage or of cerebral edema, so that if a secod test becomes advisable the results may be compared and thus the progress of the intracranial condition may be the more ready understood.) Treatment: The expectant palliative method

was continued and the prognosis was considered excellent in the absence of a high intracranial pressure, and especially in view of the fact that the patient was a child. The pulse and respiration rates to be noted every thirty minutes.

Upon the following afternoon (October 11, and forty-eight hours after the injury) the pulse and respiration rates became 88 and 20 respectively, the restlessness subsided and there were no complaints with the exception of a slight headache. This favorable condition continued until late in the afternoon of October 13, four days after the injury, when the pulse- and respiration-rates gradually descended within three hours to 72 and to 18, and four hours later to 60 and to 16 respectively; more drowsy, with complaints of headache and of dizziness of an objective character; the temperature and the blood-pressure remained normal. An examination at this time did not disclose any gross change in the physical condition. The child was conscious, with no paralyses nor sensory impairments, but the retinal veins of each fundus were observed ophthalmoscopically to be dilated and the nasal halves and temporal margins of both optic disks were obscured and blurred by edema; the physiologic cups were both shallow. A lumbar puncture, using the spinal mercurial manometer to estimate the pressure of the cerebrospinal fluid, recorded a marked increase—22 mm. For fear of the acute onset of the signs of medullary compression—the rhythmical Cheyne-Stokes respiration—and pulse-rates, with an increased blood-pressure of varying degree (late signs of high intracranial pressure, whether of hemorrhage or of cerebral edema alone), an immediate left subtemporal decompression and drainage were advised as being not only of much less risk of life to the patient than a continuance of the high intracranial pressure, but as offering to the patient a much greater chance of future normality—physically, mentally and emotionally.

Operation. October 14, 1921, four and a half days after injury. Left subtemporal decompression and drainage: usual vertical incision and bone removed; linear fracture passed downward to the base through this area of bone, and thus permitting an ecchymosis and edema of the muscle fibers beneath the temporal fascia (a very reliable sign of fracture of the underlying bone). Several small extradural clots. Dura bulging, tense and non-pulsating; upon incising it, slightly straw-colored cerebrospinal fluid spurted to a height of several inches and upon enlarging the dural opening, a very "wet" edematous cortex tended to protrude but did not rupture; owing to the rapid escape of a large amount of cerebrospinal fluid, the cerebral cortex began to pulsate, and soon its bulging lessened so that normal pulsation occurred. No hemorrhage nor any gross cortical lesion ascertained, only a marked condition of "cerebral edema." Usual closure with a small drain of rubber tissue at the upper and lower angles of the incision;

duration, forty minutes. Postoperative notes: Excellent operative recovery; temperature never exceeded 102°, while the pulse and respiration rates within six hours after operation became 96 and 20, and eighteen hours after operation reached and remained around 84 and 20, respectively, during the operative convalescence. There were no complaints of headache nor of dizziness. Incision healed per primam, all sutures being removed on the seventh day and the bandage on the tenth day postoperative. The operative area, however, bulged beyond the flush of the surrounding scalp, and although the pulsation was normal, yet it was considered advisable to keep the patient quietly in bed in the hope that the persisting cerebral edema would gradually lessen so that the intracranial pressure would descend to normal, and thus the operative area become depressed and sunken in—a process usually requiring about three weeks postoperative. The absorption of the excess cerebrospinal fluid, traumatic cerebral edema, did progress, but much more slowly than is usual and especially in children, so that at the delayed discharge of the patient from the hospital (forty-three days after injury) the decompression area was only slightly depressed, but with normal pulsation; the general physical and neurologic examination was otherwise negative. *Treatment:* Parents were advised to continue the patient's hospital treatment at home to lessen the condition of cerebral edema until the operative area became depressed—a quiet inactive life with no exciting games, and at least twelve hours of sleep each night and six other hours to be spent in bed; vegetable, fruit and cereal diet, with no meat and meat soup and naturally no tea or coffee; fresh fish and the white of chicken not more than twice a week; daily warm bath; bowels to move freely. (In selected cases thyroid and thymus gland may be used to diminish the secretion of the cerebrospinal fluid.) Last examination: September 6, 1922, eleven months after operation. No complaints. Operative area definitely depressed and pulsates normally; pupils, negative; reflexes, negative; fundi, negative.

Remarks. Delayed traumatic cerebral edema in a child and of degree sufficient to necessitate an operative decompression and drainage is most unusual, and especially in the absence of severe cerebral lesions, extensive subdural hemorrhage, cerebral contusions or lacerations; this case history is common in adults, particnlarly in the alcoholic and arteriosclerotic types of patients with or without intracranial hemorrhage, but in children it is indeed rare. The general character of the cerebral edema, without localizing signs pointing to a definite area of the brain as being involved, is also the rule in adults.

In less severe cases having a lower intracranial pressure (not above 16 mm.) repeated lumbar punctures of spinal drainage may be used, but this method of decompression is distinctly dangerous when the intracranial pressure is high, and especially in the presence of signs of medullary compression, for fear of an acute choking of the medulla in the foramen magnum.

The comparative unimportance of the fracture of the skull is also illustrated in this case history; its presence rather aided the patient to decompress himself by permitting the escape of any hemorrhage and cerebral edema from the otherwise closed cranial cavity into the tissues of the scalp (and in other patients externally through the ears and nose), and this lessening of the intracranial pressure, together with the other means of natural absorption, frequently suffices to permit the milder cases of intracranial pressure to recover with the expectant palliative treatment alone, whereas, if no fracture of the skull were present, then repeated lumbar punctures and even a cranial decompression might be indicated to obtain not only a recovery of life but the maximum of future normality.

Rarely is the measurement of the blood-pressure of value in the early diagnosis and in the early treatment of these traumatic intracranial conditions. Naturally, the diagnosis of initial shock is confirmed by subnormal temperature and blood-pressure, associated with increased pulse and respiration rates, but to delay the rational treatment of these patients with and without a fracture of the skull until the pulse and respiration rates are markedly retarded below 60 and 26 respectively, and in the presence of edematous fundal changes, and especially with the spinal mercurial manometer registering the pressure of the cerebrospinal fluid above 16 mm. merely because the blood-pressure is not definitely increased (this is a dangerous sign of advanced medullary compression),—it has been this method of "watchful waiting" that has permitted many of these patients to pass from this preliminary stage of increased intracranial pressure into that of pronounced medullary compression, where the blood-pressure is always increased and at the great risk to the patient's life, operation or no operation.

Chronic Cerebral Edema. Within the past few years the profession has been more and more impressed with the end-results in these patients. To be sure, the preservation of life is essential, and yet the treatment of the acute condition should be not only to preserve life, but also to restore a condition of approximate normality, both mentally and physically. The attitude of the profession has largely been one of surprise if a patient with a "fracture of the skull," and particularly of the base, recovered; and if the mental, emotional or physical condition was not so normal as before the injury, "Well, he had a fracture of the skull and should consider himself fortunate to be alive." It has been this feeling of comparative helplessness that has permitted these patients to be very much neglected, it being considered that the mental and physical impairment was due to a definite gross primary brain lesion at the time of the injury and, therefore, an irreparable condition. Fortunately, however, this is a fact in only a small percentage of the patients having had severe cranial injuries with or without a fracture of the skull, and these are the selected patients having the so-called "chronic brain injuries" that I wish to discuss here.

During the past eight years I have had the opportunity to examine and to treat a large series of patients having acute brain injuries, and it has been very impressive to note, either at autopsy or at operation, the comparative rarity of extensive cerebral laceration in these patients. It is conceded that in large compound, depressed fractures of the vault and in the occasional gunshot injuries of civil life, extensive cerebral laceration does occur and, therefore, if the patient should survive then an irreparable brain injury presents its symptoms and signs. Yet it is indeed most infrequent for gross tears in the cerebral cortex to occur in the usual cranial injuries, with or without a fracture of the vault or of the base of the skull. At autopsy upon those patients, who have died from the extreme initial shock or from an infective meningoencephalitis or from a terminal medullary edema resulting from high intracranial pressure of hemorrhage and of excess cerebrospinal fluid, the most common of cerebral lesions was a contusion of the superficial layers of the cortex of the anterior and inferior surfaces of either frontal lobe and of the tip of either temporosphenoidal lobe, but no extensive laceration, merely a bruising of these areas covered by a thin layer of localized supracortical hemorrhage. Even these findings, however, were not frequent. The most common postmortem condition was a large amount of free bloody cerebrospinal fluid associated with a layer of supracortical hemorrhagic clot of varying thickness, the brain itself being swollen and edematous, and of the so-called "wet" and "water-logged' type. This condition of supracortical hemorrhage and excess cerebrospinal fluid is also the usual operative finding, and rarely is a gross cerebral laceration exposed. The relative infrequency of large cerebral lacerations is also demonstrated clinically in those patients who make such excellent recovery of function from hemiplegia, following most severe cranial traumata with and without an operative decompression, and thus confirming the opinion that the immediate paralysis was due to local compression of hemorrhage and of cerebral edema rather than to a gross cerebral laceration. It is in those patients having high intracranial pressure, especially when it is due chiefly to hemorrhage, that the subtemporal decompression and drainage is the treatment of choice, from the standpoint not only of recovery of life, but also of the ultimate recovery of function.

We are now concerned with those patients who have recovered from the immediate effects of the acute cranial injury and yet remain with symptoms and signs of definite impairment—severe persistent headaches, early fatigue, inability to work throughout the day as formerly, dizzy spells, a definite change of personality of the depressed or of the excitable and irritable type, and even epilepsy in its various manifestations. These are cases that form a most interesting group for study.

It is an opinion rather common among the laity and, to a less extent, in the medical profession that once an individual has had a fracture of the skull he is never the same again, if not mentally and physically, then at least in the emotional reactions; that he is more irritable, with periods of depression or of excitement, frequently complains of persistent headache, has a sense of early fatigue so that the former day's work is impossible or at least difficult, occasional spells of vertigo and at times even epileptiform seizures. Definite changes of the personality have been very frequently observed, as manifested by less interest in surroundings and ambitions for the future, and unreliability to such a degree that he is termed "a loafer and a good-for-nothing." The condition of a large percentage of those patients was called that of "post-traumatic neurosis"—a functional disturbance resulting from the "shock" of the injury, "concussion" of the brain, etc., while the condition of the smaller number of these impaired patients was considered as being due to a gross organic injury of the brain at the time of the accident, such as cerebral contusions and lacerations associated with hemorrhage of varying degree. In the absence of macroscopic lesions to be observed with the naked eye, then the condition was believed to be due to minute and possibly microscopic changes, not only in the cortical nerve cells themselves, but also in their interrelationship and associated nerve tracts, and thus an irreparable condition.

With this post-traumatic condition in mind, in 1912, I attempted to ascertain the status of those patients at three of the large hospitals in New York City, who had had a "fracture of the skull" during the preceding decade of 1900–1910. The mortality of the acute condition was 46 to 64 per cent, while the operative mortality itself was 87 per cent; this latter was due chiefly to the type of operation performed, usually an extensive osteoplastic flap exposure, and the frequent performance of the operation during the initial stage of extreme shock or during the terminal stage of medullary edema. Under these conditions, Pearce Bailey was undoubtedly correct in the belief then, that these patients "get along just as well without as with operation." Of the total patients who were discharged from those three hospitals as "well," "cured" or "improved," I was successful in locating only 34 per cent, but of this number 67 per cent were still suffering from the effects of the former injury, the chief complaints being headache, early fatigue, change of personality and, in a very small number, convulsive seizures. The records of these impaired patients were very instructive, in that their hospital residence was usually longer than that of the other cranial injury cases by a number of days and even of weeks, while frequent notes were found of prolonged stupor and even of unconsciousness, of severe headache and of retarded pulse rate—symptoms and signs indicative of an increased intracranial pressure; rarely was an ophthalmoscopic examination made and even more rarely had a lumbar puncture been performed. In examining these chronic cases, I was very much surprised to find in a large number of them the definite evidence of an increase of intracranial pressure, as observed with the ophthalmoscope and particularly with the estimation of the pressure of the cerebrospinal fluid at lumbar puncture. Upon 9 of these selected patients the operation of subtemporal decompression and drainage was performed, even at this late date following the injury, and the operative findings were all similar, no gross cortical lesions exposed, but a "wet," swollen edematous brain under varying degrees of increased pressure; along the supracortical veins in the sulci, however, was a cloudy induration of new tissue formation surrounding the vessel walls, which were also thickened. Microscopic sections have now been made of this condition occurring in similar patients and also in children who have had a supracortical hemorrhage at the time of birth; this tissue formation is now recognized as the organization residue of connective tissue of a former layer of supracortical blood, which had collected chiefly in the sulci about these veins and thus had blocked the little stomata of exit of the cerebrospinal fluid through the walls of these vessels—the main channels of excretion of the cerebrospinal fluid into the blood stream. In this manner, a mild condition of external hydrocephalus had been produced by this partial blockage of the excretion of the cerebrospinal fluid.

Microscopic sections of the cortical cells and their normal arrangement have only rarely disclosed a definite change of structure, although this added complication cannot be excluded in any case. It is the pathologic condition, however, about the supracortical veins that has been overlooked in the past; and it has only been since we have learned that over 80 per cent of the excretion of the cerebrospinal fluid occurs through the supracortical veins lying in the sulci, that it was recognized that this condition of new tissue formation following the hemorrhage was the main lesion in causing the edematous brain, due to the partial blockage of the excretion of the cerebrospinal fluid with the resulting varying degrees of intracranial pressure. Those patients making excellent recoveries with the expectant palliative treatment alone, and over 50 per cent do, undoubtedly are the ones in whom the natural means of absorption have been sufficient to take care of the free supracortical blood, so that no real residue or new tissue formation results, since practically all of the hemorrhage has been absorbed. I have had the opportunity to demonstrate the confirmation of this opinion in 3 patients who had had cranial injuries with a resulting intracranial hemorrhage, as indicated by the bloody cerebrospinal fluid at lumbar puncture, which was not sufficient, however, to produce a marked increase of the intracranial pressure, so that the expectant palliative treatment alone was indicated in order to obtain an excellent recovery. Later, upon death from other causes, autopsy in these 3 cases disclosed little, if any, new tissue formation about the supracortical veins in the sulci, the hemorrhage having been entirely absorbed. The brain was not edematous, there being no blockage of the excretion of the cerebrospinal fluid.

These chronic patients having had an intracranial injury, and most probably a supracortical hemorrhage, with or without a fracture of the skull, who have not recovered their former normality and in whom headache, early fatigue, change of personality or even convulsive seizures persist, should be most carefully examined from the standpoint of the presence or absence of an increased intracranial pressure, as found in the fundi with the ophthalmoscope and, more accurately still, by the spinal mercurial manometer at lumbar puncture. If no increase of the intracranial pressure is present, then the treatment can be only of the expectant palliative type because the intracranial damage has already occurred, whether due to a primary gross or to a minute microscopic lesion of the cortical cells or to a prolonged high intracranial pressure, which has gradually become lowered as a result of the atrophy of the cerebral cells—a permanent impairment, being a compensatory lowering of intracranial pressure at the expense of the brain itself. But if a definite increase of the intracranial pressure persists in spite of the usual medical expectant palliative treatment, then the patient can be greatly benefited and improved by means of an early subtemporal decompression and permanent drainage of the blocked cerebrospinal fluid. The dura should naturally be opened widely and permitted to remain open and not resutured, otherwise the decompression and drainage is of only temporary value. Excellent results have been obtained in this class of patients and the earlier the condition of increased intracranial pressure can be lowered to normal, just so much more of an improvement can be expected from the operation; naturally, in those chronic sclerotic patients, greatly deteriorated during a period of years, even to the degree of dementia, little, if anything, can be expected at this late date.

In closing, let me merely mention the similar chronic condition occurring in children as the result of an intracranial hemorrhage at the time of birth, most frequently in difficult labor, with or without instruments. They are usually first children, and unless convulsive twitchings occur within several days after birth, or the child is abnormally excitable or stuporous, the condition is commonly overlooked and the baby may be considered a normal child until the seventh or eighth month, and even later. Then it is observed that the child is not holding up its head, and later does not sit up or attempt to stand until months after the normal time; convulsive twitchings may or may not be present; speech is usually retarded,—in fact, the entire physical and mental activities are delayed and retarded in varying degree. If examinations now show a marked increase of the intracranial pressure, these are the selected patients who can be greatly benefited by subtemporal decompression and permanent drainage of the blocked cerebrospinal fluid, even at the late date of several years following the injury, just as in the chronic brain injuries occurring in adults. However, the ideal treatment of these conditions of intracranial hemorrhage is at the time of the acute condition—within the first few days following birth in the baby, and within a period of hours following the injury in adults. In these new-born babies, if repeated lumbar punctures with removal of large amounts of blood cerebrospinal fluid do not suffice to lower permanently the increased intracranial pressure, then a modified subtemporal decompression and drainage operation is immediately indicated, just as in the acute brain injuries of adults having the symptoms and signs of high intracranial pressure. Infants surviving a birth hemorrhage, whose increased intracranial pressure has not been lowered to normal, cannot develop as they should, either mentally or physically; as a result of this condition, these patients are eventually added to that large group of spastic and defective children—the bane of the pediatrist, orthopedist and neurologist. After a lapse of years, however, the selected children having an increased intracranial pressure can be only improved by the operative lowering of the pressure. I have now operated upon 572 of these children out of 5000 cases personally examined, of ages varying from five hours to twenty-three years, and I may state that the lesion is practically the same as occurs in adults from cranial injuries with a supracortical hemorrhage; the persistent increase of intracranial pressure is due to the partial blockage of the excretion of the cerebrospinal fluid by the connective-tissue formation resulting from the supracortical hemorrhage about the veins in the sulci, producing the characteristic "wet," edematous condition of the brain.

Conclusion. It is only in those patients having a definite increase of the intracranial pressure that any improvement can be afforded by means of the cranial decompression and drainage. Naturally, if minute sclerotic changes have taken place in the cortical cells themselves, then an irreparable damage has occurred, and even if the increased intracranial pressure is lowered to normal by operation, these advanced patients cannot make a complete recovery of function, although the relief of the pressure should improve their condition.

It is, however, in those early patients in whom the increased pressure, resulting from a partial blockage of the excretion of the cerebrospinal fluid, is the main pathologic condition, and especially in those who have no organic cellular changes, that the operation of subtemporal decompression and permanent drainage affords the greatest ultimate improvement and, in the more fortunate ones, even an apparent recovery of function.

THE PROGNOSIS IN CANCER OF THE BREAST.*

By Harry C. Saltzstein, M.D.

DETROIT, MICHIGAN.

The prognosis in cancer of the breast may be said to depend upon four factors: (1) The surgical removal; (2) the variety of the cancer; (3) the immunity of the patient; (4) the duration of the disease before operation. This paper is concerned with an evaluation of these factors, especially what variations in each are possible or to be expected, and what influence there will then be upon the prospect of cure.

The Surgical Removal. The beginning of the surgical cure of breast cancer can be said to date from 1867, when Moore asserted that cancer was a purely local disease, curable by local eradication. From 1870 to 1880 Danish, German and Austrian surgeons were the only ones to grasp this principle, and they alone reported cures, 9 per cent.

From 1880 to 1894 various isolated surgical principles for malignancy of the breast were formulated. Volkman advised removal of the axillary glands; Gerster advised wide excision, and gentleness in handling, stating that pulling on retractors, hooks, and so on, forced cancer cells into the lymphatics. Heidenhain traced lymphatic spread underneath the pectoralis major and advised removal of this muscle. The pectoralis major was sometimes removed, both muscles only rarely, the axilla only partially cleaned out, and the operation was frequently done in two stages. With these procedures various operators reported 20 to 25 per cent of cures, but some with wide experience stated that they had "seen cartloads of breasts removed without a single cure."

In 1894 Halsted and Willy Meyer described the present-day radical removal and advocated this technic in all cases: the extirpation of the entire contents of the axilla, removal of both pectoral muscles and the breast in one complete block; the excision

* From the Surgical Service of Dr. Max Ballin, Harper Hospital. Dr. Carl Gaines assisted in part of this work.

of all suspected tissues with the widest possible margin, in one unentered and little manipulated mass. Cures jumped to 40 to 45 per cent. Since this milestone in technical progress there have been only slight modifications in methods (the Rodman incision, the Jackson flap, Handley's wide excision of fascia), and, as a general statement, the limit of improvement in operative technic has been said to have been reached. This is reflected in the fact that Halsted's and Willy Meyer's results published in 1904-5 are essentially those of the present day, 40 to 45 per cent cures is still the average figure. Radium and the roentgen-ray have won definite places as adjuncts to surgery. In some series they have increased the percentage of cures and they uniformly inhibit local metastases. How much more cancer we will cure by perfected ray and radium methods is problematical; certainly there will be some increase, but probably there will be no radical change.

The operation then has been quite well standardized, and as a factor in prognosis will probably not be found to vary markedly in the future. The extensive cautery excision recently described by Percy[1] may prove to be another exception. No results were published, however, and the procedure has not, as yet, become generally adopted.

The Variety of the Cancer. The importance of the variety or type of the cancer when determining the prognosis, has been emphasized repeatedly. (Halsted,[2] Bloodgood,[3] and Ewing,[4]) "Scirrhous cancer represents only a part of what has existed. The struggle against cancer cells, resulting in fibrous tissue production, is not always futile, and when minute foci of cancer epithelium have been destroyed, the new fibrous tissue may, in part, be absorbed also. Thus scirrhous disease may be active and metastases take place a long time before the visible, or palpable tumor is developed." (Halsted).[2] Cases such as these may show only neuritis, paraplegia, then paralysis, in spite of careful examinations. Finally a small scirrhus of the breast will be felt and the roentgen ray show spinal metastases.

Medullary, encephaloid, or simplex, are clinical terms designating the average soft cellular tumor with very little stroma and small active cell nuclei. There is rapid progress, early skin invasion, extensive dissemination, and early cachexia.

Certain rare forms, colloid cancer, for example, tend toward encapsulation and may grow to enormous size without invading the axilla. Other types, as acute carcinosis, cancer cysts, may be rapidly fatal, occasionally in less than two months.

[1] Surg., Gynec. and Obst., 1921, **33**, 417.

[2] Tr. Am. Surg. Assn., 1907, **25**, 61.

[3] Diagnosis and Treatment of Borderline Pathological Lesions, Ann. Surg. 1913, **58**, p. 282.

[4] Neoplastic Diseases, Ed. 2, 1922.

Adenocarcinoma has been credited with a very high percentage of cures. A recent study by Bloodgood[5] raises the question of whether many of these cases are cancer at all. Seventeen cases diagnosed adenocarcinoma were in reality benign non-encapsulated adenomata, and, of course, if added to total cured cases markedly increased the percentage.

The Immunity of the Patient. As the lymphatics are invaded, especially the axillary glands, there is a tendency for previously slowly growing tumors to approach the cell type of the rapidly growing forms with correspondingly increased virulence.

An immune mechanism against cancer undoubtedly exists in the lymphatic elements of the blood. In experimental cancer a failing cancer graft is absorbed by mononuclear cells, and a lymphocytosis, a "lymphocytic crisis," marks the triumph of the body defence and the death of the graft. If the lymphoid tissue is destroyed by roentgen-ray, the animal's susceptibility to cancer is increased. If the lymphoid tissue, instead of being destroyed, is stimulated by a smaller roentgen-ray exposure, the immunity of the animal is markedly increased. (Murphy and Norton.[6])

Similarly J. W. Vaughan[7] states that early malignancy shows an increase in the large mononuclear blood cells. When these cells decrease, and the polynuclear elements increase, the tumor is growing rapidly. Then, and only then will metastases take place. He has used this differential blood count as an index of operability. However, the disturbance causing polymorphonuclear leukocytosis can be brought about by so many other factors than the spreading of cancer, that it is difficult to gauge operability from relative leucocyte percentages.

McCarty[8] has shown in his studies that the prognosis in cancer of the breast is dependent on factors analogous to the variety of the tumor and immunity of the patient. The more closely the tumor type resembles the embryonic cell, the more virulent is the growth. Vice versa, if the cell shows marked differentiation from the primitive, the growth is much more benign. Breast cancers showing cellular differentiation had 57 per cent greater postoperative length of life than the normal average of the group studied. He also measured the prognostic value of the defense pictures seen about the tumor, lymphocytic reaction, fibrosis, and hyalinization. Patients showing all of these reactions had 37 per cent greater expectancy than the normal average, and 42 per cent greater expectancy than if none of these factors were present.

What relative importance the patient's immunity is in determining the ultimate outlook, as contrasted with the type or variety

[5] Arch. Surg., 1921, **3**, 527.
[6] Science, 1915, **42**, 842.
[7] Jour. Am. Med. Assn., 1917, **49**, 1952.
[8] Ann. Surg., 1922, **75**, 61.

of the tumor, is problematical. If the cell type changes as the tumor progresses, is this simply an index of lowered resistance, or is the cell metamorphosis primary? Does a cancer begin as a scirrhus rather than a medullary form because one patient has a greater immunity, with more tendency to fibrous tissue formation, or does the type of growth determine the tissue reaction? It is apparently the same enigma met with in infection and resistance, the pneumococcus strain against the body defence.

Practically, however, these considerations are important as follows: a rapidly growing type, unless treated almost as an emergency disease, and with extensive radical removal, is hopeless (Fig. 1). Secondary operations are of no avail. The patient lives longer without them. Another type may be cured by incom-

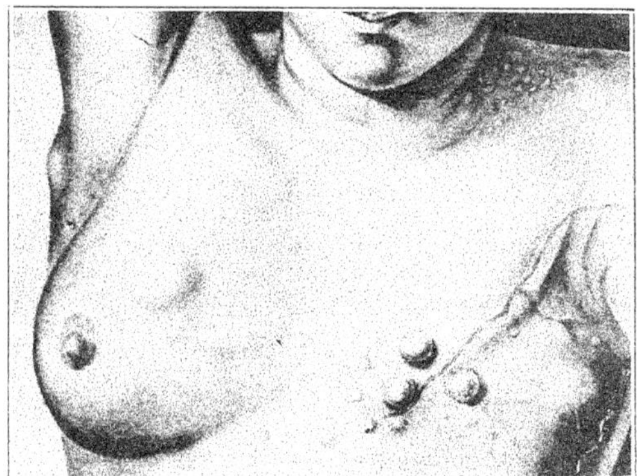

Fig. 1.—Case I. Advanced medullary carcinoma. Appearance five months after radical amputation of left breast. Operation was performed five months after tumor was noted. Axillary glands were badly infected at that time. Three months after operation metastases appeared in left side of neck and in the region of the scar. Soon there was edema of the arm, numerous skin metastases, and symptoms of abdominal metastases with death six months after operation. To offer any prospect of cure such a case must almost be considered as an emergency disease.

plete removal. Metastases may be resected, sometimes repeatedly and with good result. (Fig. 2—an extensive local metastasis was removed by a cancer fakir by means of arsenic paste). Willy Meyer has stated that statistics of cures in cancer of the breast are worthless as regards the prognoses in an individual case, because the cure depends so much on the virulence of the tumor.

The Duration of the Disease before Operation. Cancer radiates in a sphere; on the surface, growth is expressed in square dimensions, not as linear increase. Consequently, doubling the time increases the risk of recurrence not twice but two to the square dimension or four times. (E. Wyllis Andrews[9].) If a tumor has grown to a certain size in two months, after two more months have elapsed,

[9] Ann. Surg., 1905, 42, 903.

the probability of a cure is not one-half, but one-fourth. When the axilla is free from disease, the prognosis is generally stated to be about 80 per cent cures (Crile 80 per cent; Johns Hopkins 85 per cent). When the axilla is involved, the prognosis for cure ranges from 25 per cent (Halsted, Rodman) to 12 to 14 per cent (Massachusetts General and Crile) and in some cases as low as 4 per cent.

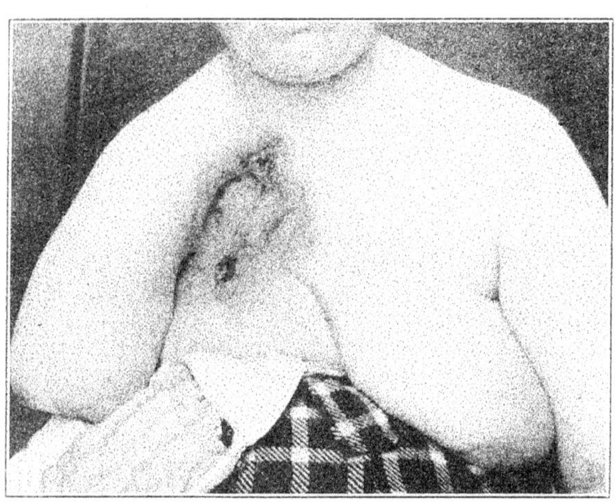

FIG. 2 —Case II. Extension locally only. Repeated removal indicated. April, 1919, radical removal of right breast. A lump 2 cm. in diameter in the outer upper quadrant, had been present four months. Three months after operation a tumor was noted in the neighborhood of the right second and third ribs anteriorly. May, 1920 there was a two-fist size local recurrence, attached to the clavicle and thorax, and firmly fixed in Mohrenheim's fossa. Three surgeons independently pronounced it inoperable. Not satisfied, the patient consulted a cancer quack (June, 1920), who made daily applications of arsenic paste, each day clipping off the dead eschar before reapplying the caustic. After five months of this treatment, the anterior thoracic wall, the right clavicle and apparently the growth were destroyed. In October, 1920, there was sudden profuse hemorrhage from the axillary vessels, which stopped spontaneously in thirty minutes. One week later the forearm was gangrenous and had to be amputated above the elbow. November, 1920 the necrotic remnants of the right clavicle, right second and third ribs were removed, and skin grafts placed directly over the lung tissue. There was no evidence of recurrence. April, 1921, a local recurrence was excised from the region of the fourth costochondral junction. This was followed by a severe attack of erysipelas. July, 1921, a similar local recurrence was excised, roentgen-ray still showing the thorax clear of metastases. (The photograph was taken the day before the operation). Thus, two and a half years after its initial appearance, a carcinoma showed no thoracic involvement in spite of continuous local growth. Repeated removal was certainly indicated.

Of the cases coming to Harper Hospital from 1914 to 1920, 80 per cent already had metastases in the axilla: in only 20 per cent was the axilla clinically free. That is, when adequate treatment was first instituted, four-fifths of the patients had three in four chances of succumbing; one-fifth had three in four chances of cure.

What is early? This question perplexed no less a student of cancer than the late J. B. Murphy. The small circumscribed carcinoma, or the microscopic cancer metamorphosis may have 100 per cent chance of cure, and may even have that prognosis with incomplete removal; the fully developed carcinoma may within the space of a very few weeks become hopeless. If one accepts Handley's view that cancer spreads along the fascial lymphatics as a gigantic ringworm, far in advance of any demonstrable deposits, how early must surgical intervention take place to regularly establish a cure?

We may never have an answer to this question, chiefly because different cancers progress with different degrees of rapidity depending on the patient's immunity and the type of the tumor. One is encapsulated for months and then suddenly bursts forth into a very malignant tumor; a scirrhus may grow very slowly, but the defence of the organism may hold the primary as well as multiple secondary growths in check for months or years. There have been well authenticated cases of spontaneous disappearance. On the other hand patients with certain virulent cellular growths (so-called acute carcinosis) may be doomed almost from the start. (Fig. 1.)

The axillary glands are uniformly involved within twelve months, and then the prognosis is 25 per cent to 12 per cent cures, as above stated, whereas a few months before the same case had 80 per cent chance of cure.

If we cannot exactly define early, we can continue exhorting earlier diagnosis and operation. The probability is that cancer must in a certain percentage of cases be treated as an emergency disease if the surgical intervention is to take place soon enough to allow of radical removal beyond the involved area.

Women are surely coming sooner for operation than formerly, and this decrease in the time factor is a most hopeful and promising sign. Where increasing percentages of cures have been reported in recent series, the increase has often been ascribed to the inclusion of a greater number of early cases rather than to improvements in technic. Bloodgood's[10] data show the following interesting facts: At Johns Hopkins, from 1890 to 1915, the proportion of benign lesions of the breast has risen from 32 to 59 per cent of the total number of breast tumors coming to operation. The percentages of borderline cases, where the surgeon is in doubt regarding the gross nature of the lesion has risen; whereas formerly there was 10 per cent error in these cases, now the error is 15 per cent. Fully developed carcinoma of the breast has decreased from 90 per cent of the total in 1890 to 78 per cent in 1913.

The following table compiled from admissions to Harper Hospital during the years 1914 to 1920, likewise shows a slow but significant steady decrease in the time factor.

[10] Jour. Am. Med. Assn., 1916, **66**, 552.

AVERAGE DURATION OF TUMOR BEFORE OPERATION. (PATIENT'S STATEMENT.)

1914	16.5 months
1915	13.4 months
1916	17 months
1917	15 months
1918	14 months
1919	13 months
1920	10 months

Of the factors upon which the prognosis of a given case of carcinoma of the breast depends (the surgical removal, the immunity of the patient, the variety of the tumor, and the duration of the disease before operation), the last, the duration of the disease before operation, is the only one capable of any wide variation at our hands.

The ever widening realization of this fact, the popular spread of Bloodgood's doctrine that "the cure of cancer is its early recognition," will do more to change the percentage columns of cancer statistics than anything known to medicine today.

Conclusions. 1. Radically different methods of surgical removal of breast cancers are not to be expected. Improved operative proceedures will play little role in increasing the percentage of cures. 2. The clinical variety of the tumor, or the variety divided by the patient's immunity, is of profound importance in determining the prognosis. 3. Operations upon recurrent carcinoma of the breast are distinctly indicated in certain cases, when the type is favorable. If the type is not favorable, operation hastens death. 4. Eighty per cent of admissions to Harper Hospital already had axillary involvement. When the axilla is involved the prognosis is 4 to 25 per cent cure; uninvolved the prognosis is 80 per cent cure. 5. There is substantial evidence that in breast cancer women are seeking advice and operation earlier than formerly, but in this matter it may be said that the surface only has been scratched. 6. Since the time factor is capable of such wide variation at our hands and is capable of such influence upon the ultimate prognosis, our best efforts should be directed toward reducing the interval between appearance and eradication, toward transposing "80 per cent with axillary involvement" to "80 per cent clinically benign." This will be realized only when popular information is so widespread that every woman regards a lump in her breast with dread suspicion as soon as, and not six months after, she first perceived it.

MAGNESIUM SULPHATE AS A SEDATIVE.

By Paul G. Weston, M.D.

and

M. Q. Howard, M.D.

Warren, Penna.

In a series of papers in the *American Journal of Physiology* beginning in 1904, Meltzer and Auer reported the action of magnesium sulphate when injected subcutaneously or intravenously. They found that the "primary effect of magnesium upon the nerve cells is that of paralysis without any preceding excitation. The effect seemed to be exclusively of an inhibitory character." They also noted that calcium antagonizes the abnormal activity of its three inorganic associates in the animal body, sodium, potassium and magnesium, be the activity an over-inhibition or an over-excitation. In one of their experiments a rabbit was given sufficient magnesium sulphate solution to cause complete muscular paralysis. The intravenous injection of a very small amount of calcium chloride caused this paralysis to disappear at once. Based on the fatal dose for rabbit, the fatal dose for a man weighing 75 kg. (165 lbs.) would be approximately 120 gm. (4 ounces) given hypodermically.

It occurred to us that since magnesium sulphate has such a paralyzing action on the nerve cell, it should be of use as a sedative in excited states, inasmuch as the toxic dose is very high and the antidote prompt in its action. We have therefore been using the salt as a sedative for a little over two years and our results are here recorded.

Preparation of the Salt. The crude magnesium sulphate of the apothecary shops is recrystallized three times and a perfectly pure product obtained. It was found that C. P., U. S. P. and "reagent" magnesium sulphate were quite impure and none would give a clear, colorless solution. It cannot be stated whether these impurities are toxic or not, for only pure salt was used in our cases.

A 50 per cent solution of the salt with its water of crystallization was made in distilled water and sterilized in the autoclave. The solution was dispensed in 50 or 100 cc bottles closed with a rubber stopper having a thin rubber diaphragm in its center, such a stopper as is used in bacterin bottles.

The usual dose was 2 cc of the 50 per cent solution. It was injected subcutaneously or intramuscularly, the usual aseptic technic being employed. No local pain and no sloughing followed the injections. The dose was repeated at half-hour intervals when necessary. At first a 25 per cent solution of the salt was used and the results with mildly excited patients were very satisfactory; but it was so often necessary to repeat this dose for more excited patients that we changed to a 50 per cent solution and have used this strength regularly.

For convenience we have placed the patients in the following arbitrary groups:

Group 1. Patients who remained in bed talking quietly to themselves in response to hallucinations. They did not awaken or annoy other patients in the same ward and did not sleep.

Group 2. Patients who remained in bed talking loudly and frequently shouting or screaming. They annoyed the other patients and awakened the sleeping ones.

Group 3. Patients who persisted in getting out of bed and annoying other patients who were sleeping. They were excited, walked up and down the floor and shouted. They could not be persuaded to remain in bed.

Group 4. Patients who showed the same general reaction as those of Group 3 but were more excited and noisy.

Effects of Magnesium Sulphate. Group 1. Nine patients; all responded readily and slept from five to seven hours.

Group 2. Twelve patients; 11 responded readily; 1 patient showed no effect after the injection of three doses.

Group 3. One hundred and fifty-eight patients; 128 of these responded to one dose of 2 cc and 10 after two doses. Twenty patients, 12.6 per cent, failed to respond to three or more doses.

Group 4. Twenty-four patients; 20 of these responded after one dose and 2 after two doses. Two patients were unaffected by three or more doses.

Most of the patients went to sleep in from fifteen to thirty minutes after the salt had been injected. A small number did not sleep but remained quietly in bed. One of these was an old morphin addict. She was well aware that she had been given some drug that she had never had before but a good description of her subjective sensations was not obtainable. Many of the patients required a sedative each night for varying periods of time. Of those who reacted to the salt the first time it was injected, all but one reacted to subsequent injections. This one received an injection of 2 cc on each of two succeeding nights and slept six hours each time. Six months later when she had a second attack of excitement, the salt had no effect whatever. Within two and a half hours she was given 15 cc of the solution, representing $7\frac{1}{2}$ gm. of the salt but no effect was observed. The excitement of the second attack was apparently of the same degree as the first. In two other instances 15 cc of the solution were injected during two and a half hours with no apparent effect.

The pulse rate was determined before and every half hour after the injection for a period of three hours. In no case in which the pulse rate before the injection was not over 72 was there a diminution of more than 5 beats per minute. In those cases in which the pulse rate was over 80, the decrease was more marked, 8 to 12 beats, but the decrease was only that which occurs physiologically when a person is asleep or resting quietly in bed. In short, there was no change in pulse rate due to the magnesium. Meltzer and Auer emphasized this point in their papers. The duration of the sedative action was from five to ten hours.

We have used the salt in a number of persons, not insane, who were suffering from severe pain. The results were very gratifying. The anesthetic effect was quite marked and in 2 cases the pain was so severe and protracted that the continuous use of morphin would almost surely have led to the formation of a habit. In both these cases salicylates and morphin had previously been used.

After we had been using magnesium sulphate for some time, the paper of Gwathmey[1] appeared in which he recommended giving morphin in a 25 per cent solution of magnesium sulphate to prolong the action of the morphin. We had found that in cases not quieted by 6 to 10 cc of 50 per cent magnesium sulphate solution, morphin also was of no value except in heroic doses, and that when the magnesium sulphate alone failed to give relief, it was of no effect when used in combination with $\frac{1}{4}$ gr. of morphin.

Summary. Pure, recrystallized magnesium sulphate with its water of crystallization was made into a 50 per cent solution with distilled water and sterilized. The solution was injected subcutaneously and intramuscularly more than a thousand times. No local pain or sloughing occurred when proper aseptic technic was used. In 82.7 per cent of the cases the sedative action was prompt, the patient becoming quiet after fifteen or thirty minutes and sleeping from five to seven hours. In a few instances the patient became quiet but did not sleep. The effect persisted for from five to ten hours. The salt was found to be a very excellent substitute for morphin and hyoscin in many cases. It was found necessary to repeat the dose of 2 cc in 6 per cent of the cases before sedation was obtained. In 11 per cent of the cases no effect at all was noticed after the injection of three or more doses. The salt is quite harmless in the dose necessary to produce sedative effect and can be given liberally when necessary. No opportunity has presented itself for using the salt in preoperative or postoperative cases or in acute thyrotoxicosis.

[1] Jour. Am. Med. Assn., 1921, **76**, 22.

NEPHRITIS: AUTOPSIED CASES AND RECENT VIEWS.

By Rolfe Floyd, M.D.,
New York.

The French school believe in a dissociation of function in renal diseases—difficulty in eliminating salt in one type; difficulty in eliminating nitrogenous waste in another. While this dissociation is probably frequent in early stages, the cases as we meet them in the hospital wards usually show a failure of both salt and urea elimination; that is, they have retention both of salt and nitrogen.

That fatal azotemia may occur in pure type is shown by the following case which died on my service at Roosevelt Hospital and on which I performed the autopsy.

Case I.—*Fatal Azotemia*. Woman, aged thirty-six years. General health said to have been good; no renal symptoms. Miscarried at six weeks, on July 13, 1921. Curetted at Roosevelt Hospital on July 16. After operation she became jaundiced and vomited; the jaundice cleared but the vomiting persisted until, on July 21, she was transferred to the medical service. She was much prostrated. Her heart, lungs and abdomen were normal. Her tongue was dry; reflexes normal; no edema. Blood-pressure: 118 systolic, 80 diastolic. Hemoglobin, 70 per cent; red cells, 4,920,000; white cells, which had been 44,000 with 94 per cent polynuclears on July 16, had fallen to 8400 with 68 per cent polynuclears on July 21, but later rose to 21,400 with 87 per cent polynuclears on July 29. A spinal puncture resulted in a dry tap.

Five examinations of her urine were made on the gynecological service. The specific gravity varied between 1015 and 1025; a trace of albumin was always present, but no casts. One examination after her transfer to my service showed specific gravity 1020; no albumin or sugar; no casts.

She was put on a Murphy drip and teaspoon doses of milk by mouth. The vomiting diminished; the rectum, however, became intolerant and the drip was discontinued.

An acute and painful parotitis developed the day after the transfer and lasted a week, interfering with taking fluid or food by mouth and retarding her progress.

An intense general erythematous eruption, simulating that of severe measles, appeared on July 27, just as the parotitis was subsiding. This faded in three days. By this time she was taking and retaining a fair amount of fluid and some nourishment by mouth.

Her blood chemistry was reported on July 30 to be nonprotein nitrogen 539, urea nitrogen 293, creatinin 12, uric acid 14.3, sugar 18. All these figures and those appearing later in this paper indicate milligrams in 100 cc of blood serum.

On July 31, she became stuporous and sank into coma. On August 2, she died.

Autopsy. The autopsy was done eight hours after death and included examination of the brain.

The heart was not enlarged, weighing 330 gm.; its valves and wall were normal.

There was no significant lesion anywhere except in the kidneys.

The kidneys were slightly large, weighing 330 gm. Their surfaces were smooth, capsules free, their color decidedly lighter than normal. Cortex of normal thickness but with obscure markings.

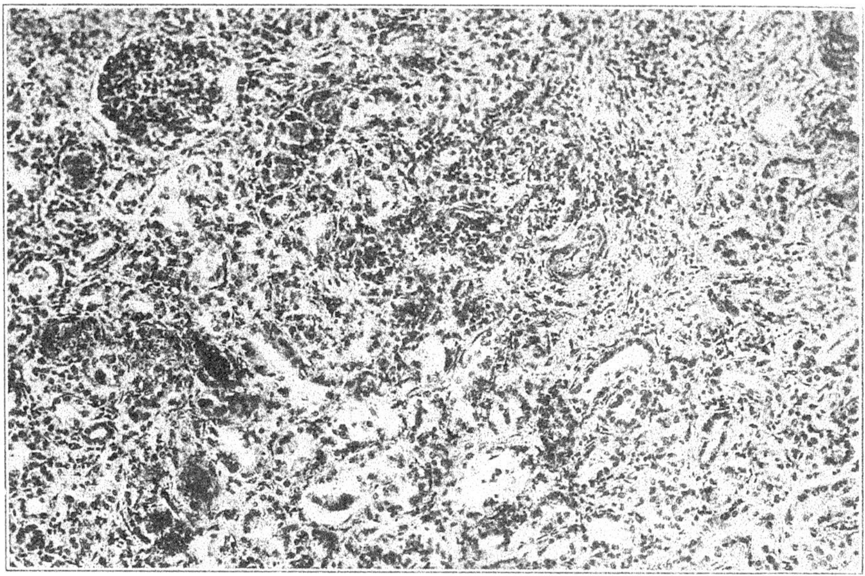

FIG. 1.—Kidney in pure azotemia. The dark bodies in some of the tubes are blood casts. × 133 and reduced.

Under the microscope there is a decided and general increase of the connective tissue in the cortex. There is a marked swelling of the tubular epithelium. The lumina of the tubes, which are narrowed by this swelling, contain red cells and some hyaline and blood casts. The glomeruli show much less pathological change than the tubes and stroma. Many of them are normal, but many others show a definite increase of tuft cells, obscuring the outline of individual loops. There are a few round-cell foci at the junction of cortex and medulla. There is no sclerosis of the arteries (Fig. 1).

Comment. Volhard and Fahr[1] consider hypertension an "obligatory" result of nitrogenous retention except in advanced tuberculosis or pronounced alcoholism. Tension they say may fail with failure of

[1] Die Brightsche Nierenkrankheit, Mannheim, 1914.

heart power, but then a cardiac hypertrophy will be found at autopsy. This case is entirely at variance with their view and they evidently had not seen one like it when they wrote (1914).

On the other hand the case demonstrates the correctness of the view held by Widal and Ambard[2] that in disease one of the renal functions may fail without the others.

So far as my own experience goes the case is unique. The sudden development of uremia in this woman without premonitory renal symptoms was probably due to the low urinary volume incident to reduced fluid intake. Normal kidneys can concentrate the urine to the point where about 500 cc a day can carry off the urea that must be excreted during the 24-hour period in order to prevent retention. Damaged kidneys cannot concentrate urea so much and, depending on how weak this power, 1000 cc, 1500 cc, even more will be the smallest urinary volume that can prevent urea retention. This woman probably did not pass over 600 cc, and a resulting residue of urea retained each day in her blood thus rapidly raised the total. Ambard has especially insisted on this cause of retention.

Had I adequately realized this danger I might have obviated it by introducing fluid beneath her skin or in her veins. If, however, the kidneys had reached the point where they were incapable of excreting enough urea to keep the blood concentration below the fatal point, no matter what the urinary volume, no such plan of treatment would have been effective.

Nephrosis as a disease entity is especially insisted on by Volhard and Fahr, who define it as follows:

We have found with the same "parenchymatous picture" two types, one with increased blood-pressure and one without, and this distinction has been found to correspond to an anatomical difference. In the gross, "large white kidneys" are found both without and with increased blood-pressure, and this has led to the false conclusion that large white kidneys were all the same lesion, and the blood pressure an unessential complication. When the blood-pressure fails, so do the evidences of inflammation, viz., hyperemia, stasis, exudation and proliferation. In this group degeneration of the epithelium is the essential change, the stroma and bloodvessel changes sinking far into the background, though when fully established, they do show leukocyte infiltration as well as stroma increase. Unquestionably these inflammatory changes, because of their meagreness and their absence in fresh cases, are to be regarded as secondary and stimulated, as Weigert interprets them, by the products of cell degeneration and as a replacement fibrosis that finally reaches a large diffuse development and may lead to contraction.

If now we turn to inflammation and its primary vascular changes

[2] Physiologie normale et pathologique des reins, Paris, 1920.

it is evident that these must be present in and characterize any true nephritis. The degeneration cases in which inflammatory changes fail can then be called nephrosis in contradistinction to the inflammatory ones.

The evidences of nephritis are increased blood-pressure and blood in the urine, and, under the microscope, an inflammation of the glomeruli as well as extensive epithelial degeneration, which is common to both types of large white kidney and on which extensive dropsy chiefly depends.

The waxy kidney has been described as a separate type of disease, but it has been noted how often it gives the clinical picture of nephrosis without cardiac hypertrophy, retinitis or uremia. We do not believe that a typical amyloid kidney can be differentiated from nephrosis without amyloid. We therefore regard it as an unessential complication of nephrosis and regard both epithelial and vascular changes as due to the same cause. The same conclusion holds for the contracted nephrotic kidney with and without amyloid. Amyloid changes in no way alter the symptoms. For these reasons the amyloid kidney as a separate entity is omitted from the classification."[3]

I have always questioned the validity of this conception of Volhard and Fahr, and have expressed my doubts in an article[4] comparing their classification of Bright's disease with that of Delafield.[5] The following case has helped to confirm my skepticism.

Case II.—*Symptoms of Nephrosis; Lesions of Nephritis.* Man, aged thirty-seven years; a cook. First came to Roosevelt Hospital in July, 1919. He had been a drinker. For one year he had been short of breath following a pleurisy; for two months there had been dropsy of the legs; for three weeks vomiting. There were physical signs at both apices confirmed by roentgen ray, and tubercle bacilli were found in the sputum. His urine varied in gravity from 1010 to 1024; it contained large amounts of albumin and many casts. His nonprotein nitrogen was 26.9. His Wassermann was positive.

He was much improved by hospital care and went to work on a farm for six months. He then considered himself cured and resumed his work in this city as a cook. He has been short of breath ever since 1919.

His second admission to the hospital occurred March 28, 1921. Three weeks prior to admission he caught cold and began to cough and expectorate. For ten days there had been rapidly increasing dropsy of the legs and swelling of the abdomen. He was having two or three liquid stools a day.

[3] This quotation is not a *verbatim* translation. It is both abbreviated and free, but an accurate statement of the authors' views so far as I comprehend them.

[4] Floyd, R.: Two Classifications of Bright's Disease, Med. Rec., April 2, 1921.

[5] Lectures on Practice of Medicine with Cases and Charts, New York, 1903.

His face was waxy white and much swollen; there was extensive subcutaneous dropsy and fluid in the abdomen. There were signs of tuberculosis at the right apex, of general bronchitis and of fluid at the right base. Three examinations showed no tubercle bacilli in the sputum.

The heart was not enlarged. Blood-pressure: 120 systolic and 62 diastolic. Wassermann negative. Hemoglobin, 80 per cent; red cells 4,600,000; white cells 15,200, with 77 per cent polynuclears. Five urine examinations resulted as follows:

Specific gravity.	Albumin.	Sugar.	Microscope.
1050	Boiled solid	None	Many hyaline and granular casts.
1038	" "	"	" " " "
1031	" "	"	" " " "
1030			" " " "
1028			" " " "

The blood chemistry showed nonprotein nitrogen, 29.8; urea nitrogen, 13.5; creatinin, 0.98; uric acid, 2.4; sugar, 0.1; chlorides, 6. In the plasma there were 3.79 per cent of albumin and 5.61 per cent of globulin.

The phenolsulphonephthalein test, done twice, resulted as follows:

1st hour.	2d hour.	Total.
36	23	59
20	15	35

The nephritic test-meal gave a total day urine of 2295 cc and a total night urine of 200 cc. The specific gravities of the various specimens varied from 1020 to 1028.

About 1000 cc of serum was drawn from the right chest on each of four occasions. He grew progressively weaker and died on April 22.

I performed the autopsy four hours after death. There was an extensive old and largely healed tuberculosis in the right upper lobe with much fibrosis and some bronchiectasis. There were a few large tubercles scattered through the rest of the lungs. There were extensive pleural adhesions, a large amount of serum in the right chest, much less in the left.

The heart was entirely normal, weighing 290 gms. There were no other significant lesions except in the kidneys.

The kidneys were very large, 660 gm. together. Capsules free, color light buff mottled with red. Cortical markings gone. Pyramids red in sharp contrast to cortex.

Under the microscope there are patches of new connective tissue all through the cortex, in which the tubes are compressed and the tubular epithelium flat. Outside of these patches the tubular epithelium is swollen and distorted, but rarely desquamated, its cytoplasm takes a universally faint stain and sometimes contains large faintly purplish granules. There is a very extensive exudate of pus cells throughout the cortex, both in the new connective tissue and in the tubes. There is also an exudate of red cells into the tubes, but these are much fewer in number than the pus cells. Casts and coagulated matter also occur in the tubular lumina. The glomeruli are all profoundly waxy; not only is there not a single normal one, but not one in which the permeability of the loops is not greatly reduced. Most of the glomeruli are of normal size or a trifle large. It is hard to judge of the tuft cells because of the enormous development of amyloid; there is no increase of the capsule cells and no thickening of Bowman's capsule. The arterioles show no sclerosis (Fig. 2).

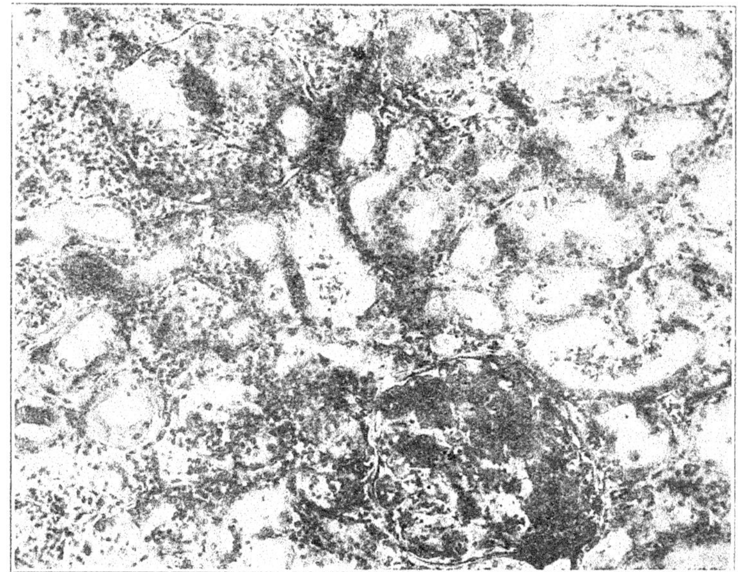

Fig. 2.—Kidney in nephrosis. Note the intense glomerular lesion, the pus in the tubes, the growth of new connective tissue and in some tubes the swollen and faintly staining epithelium. × 133 and reduced.

Here, then, is a case with all the typical symptoms of nephrosis: Anasarca, excessive albuminuria, high specific gravity, no nitrogenous retention, no hypertension, no cardiac hypertrophy, practically normal dye test and test-meal, pallor out of proportion to anemia and watery stools.

The lesions, on the other hand, are definitely inflammatory, for even if one chooses to call the connective tissue a replacement fibrosis, which it does not look like in the sections, the pus exudate is altogether too great to be regarded as incidental, and red cells, which Volhard and Fahr regard as the especial indicators of inflammation, are also exuded. As to the glomeruli, it is all very well to say that amyloid makes no difference in the symptoms. It is perfectly obvious that such an amyloid change as occurs in these glomeruli must seriously compromise their function by the structural occlusion of their loops alone.

In this case dropsy and albuminuria go hand in hand with extensive degeneration of the tubular epithelium, just as Volhard and Fahr claim, but in all other features the findings run counter to their conception of nephrosis.

Volhard and Fahr believe that sclerosis of the renal arterioles may exist for long periods without any other changes in the kidney, and that hypertension almost invariably accompanies this lesion.

They believe this lesion leads to inflammation of other kidney structures and that then a fatal termination presently results. They do not report cases in which death results from hypertension with renal sclerosis the only significant lesion. It is such a case that I have, in conclusion, to report.

Case III.—*Death with Cardiac Hypertrophy and a Renal Lesion Confined to the Arterioles.* Colored man, aged forty-two years, brought to Roosevelt Hospital moribund January 9, 1922. His wife stated that he had never been sick until four months ago, when he began to have trouble with his heart. This was relieved by digitalis. Three days before admission he was taken with sudden, severe dyspnea and went to bed. He has grown steadily worse.

A huge negro, powerful but not fat; skin moist and cold; marked pulmonary edema. Heart could not be heard; apex in anterior axillary line; pulse too weak to count. Temperature 101.8°, respirations 32. No edema. Blood-pressure 110 systolic. Neither blood nor urine examined. He died a few hours after admission.

The autopsy I did fifteen hours after death. The lungs show marked edema and congestion but no pneumonia. Thyroid gland normal. The heart is enormous, 900 gm. There is massive hypertrophy with enlargement of all chambers. The valves are all normal. Coronaries show a little sclerosis but no stenosis. The heart muscle is normal. Pericardium is normal. The aorta shows very slight atheroma. The kidneys weigh 360 gm. and are about in normal proportion to the size of the body. Their capsules are somewhat adherent; surfaces smooth; cortex and medulla normal on section.

Under the microscope the only striking change is an enormous thickening of nearly every arteriole by the process of ordinary arteritis. The glomeruli all show the dilated loops of chronic congestion and many of them show a little increase of the tuft cells obscuring the individual loop outlines. Rarely the divisions of the tuft are matted or Bowman's capsule a little thickened. These glomerular lesions are secondary or very minor.

There is no formation of new connective tissue. The tubules

are normal in size and contents; their epithelium is somewhat swollen and a little desquamated but shows nothing that may not be easily accounted for by fifteen hours of postmortem deterioration (Fig. 3).

This man, then, apparently died of the failure of an enormously hypertrophied heart. Both the hypertrophy and the failure were presumably caused by a prolonged hypertension, for I believe it is accepted that, when there is no valvular or myocardial lesion, no adherent pericardium and no goiter, cardiac hypertrophy is to be ascribed to hypertension. A blood-pressure of 110 in a patient dying of heart failure with an uncountable pulse, of course, gives no basis for judging his antecedent tension. In such cases every-

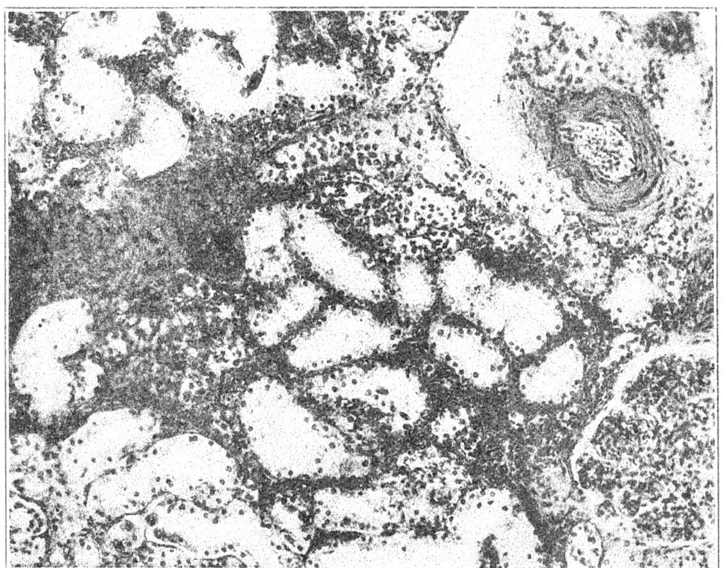

Fig. 3.—Kidney in hypertension. Note the greatly thickened arteriole without other lesions. (× 133 and reduced.)

one looks to a renal lesion for an explanation, and here we find a pronounced renal lesion of peculiar type with no significant pathological changes anywhere else in the body.

It is obvious that, as no one knows what causes increased blood-pressure, any generalizations from such a case are unwarranted. However, as I find myself opposed to Volhard and Fahr's views on nephrosis, so I am much convinced that their work on renal sclerosis is a brilliant contribution and am glad to report a case that strongly supports their contention that there is a close relation between hypertension and vascular renal lesions.

These cases are reported in the belief that as our knowledge of renal function grows it must be correlated as far as possible with changes in structure.

REVIEWS.

Thyroid and Thymus. By André Crotti, M.D., F.A.C.S., formerly Professor of Clinical Surgery and Associate Professor of Anatomy, Ohio State University; Surgeon to Grant and Children's Hospitals, Columbus. Imperial octavo. Pp. 774; 105 engravings and 39 colored plates. Half Morocco *de lux*. Philadelphia: Lea & Febiger, 1922.

This is the most beautiful example of medical bookmaking which has come from the press in recent years. Binding, paper, type, illustrations and arrangement are all superlative. Opinions may differ as to propriety of issuing in expensive *de lux* form such contributions to medical literature, which are necessarily somewhat ephemeral because of continued progress and knowledge concerning the subject. In defence, it may be said that the book is a joy to the bibliophile, and its comprehensiveness gains for it an expectation of more than ordinary duration of life and usefulness. The book is a happy combination of compilation from the literature and the author's personal views. Whether or not one agrees with the author's opinions, as, for instance, that Graves's disease is a toxic thyroiditis, it is of interest to follow his line of thought, set forth not too dogmatically. The work and opinions of the great masters in this field are freely drawn upon, and due credit given. An excellent balance is maintained between the fundamental, scientific and literary aspects, and the strictly practical considerations. Altogether, this work is the most comprehensive and satisfactory which has yet been issued in single volume on the subject. P.

Text-book on Minor Surgery. By John C. Vaughan and Athel C. Burnham, Director and Visiting Surgeon, Beekman Street Hospital, and Colonel in the United States Army, respectively. Pp. 605; 459 illustrations. Philadelphia and New York: Lea & Febiger, 1922.

In this work the authors have very clearly portrayed many valuable diagnostic points with their well-chosen illustrations and their descriptions of conditions are also well given. Their outlines of treatment are very good for those who have repeatedly had to deal with like conditions, and from this standpoint it is not a book for students so much as it is for the dispensary surgeon, industrial surgeon or busy general practitioner.

Many of the subjects are really within the realm of major surgery, but their inclusion makes it a more complete and useful reference book, especially for those coming in contact with emergency surgery.

B.

PREMATURE AND CONGENITALLY DISEASED INFANTS. By JULIUS H. HESS, M.D., Professor and Head of the Division of Pediatrics, University of Illinois, College of Medicine; Chief of Pediatric Staff, Cook County Hospital. Pp. 388; 189 illustrations. Philadelphia and New York: Lea & Febiger, 1922.

THIS book should be of inestimable value to all those concerned with the care of the newborn, for it deals in a capable and comprehensive manner with those two most difficult problems, the bringing to maturity of a premature baby and the diagnosis and proper treatment of the congenitally diseased infant.

The section on the etiology of the premature child should be of much interest to the obstetrician, even though he early delegates the care of infants to the pediatrician, for it is in more thorough prenatal care that the percentage of prematurity will be lowered. The subject of the diet of the premature is considered in accord with the physiology of the immature digestive tract. Wet nursing, maternal feeding and artificial diets are fully discussed. The subject of incubators is handled in detail.

There is nothing to criticize and much to praise in the handling of the subject of general diseases of the newborn, and of the diseases to which the premature infant is particularly prone. Respiratory diseases and syphilis are gone into in detail, with reference to treatment especially. The book closes with a very pertinent chapter on the treatment and care of the premature infant after it has reached extrauterine maturity.

W.

SURGICAL CLINICS OF NORTH AMERICA. Vol. II, No. 5. Southern number. Pp. 326; 126 illustrations. Philadelphia: W. B. Saunders Company, 1922.

IT is an exceedingly difficult undertaking to write a real review of the Surgical Clinics. The multiplicity of writers and subjects makes it almost impossible to touch upon them all. Suffice it to say, however, for the benefit of those who know the magazine, that this number is up to standard. Among the contributing authors we find representative men from all over the South, men whose names signed to an article guarantee the reader valuable information and enjoyable reading. E.

DIE PHYSIOLOGIE DES KREISLAUFES. Vol III. By ROBERT TIGERSTEDT, Helsingfors, Finland. Second edition. Pp. 320; 134 illustrations. Berlin and Leipzig: Vereinigung Wissenschaftlicher Verleger, 1922.

THE third volume, devoted to the flow of blood in the general circulation, discusses in eight chapters such topics as Torricelli's and Poiseuille's laws, blood viscosity, elasticity of vessel walls, factors changing the flow of blood and blood-pressure in arteries, veins and capillaries. The first two volumes on the movements and the innervation of the heart appeared in 1921, and a fourth volume on the innervation of bloodvessels is expected before the end of 1922. But little comment is needed on the value of this volume as a book of reference—as a text-book for American students it will not have much vogue for obvious reasons. K.

DISEASES OF CHILDREN, MEDICAL AND SURGICAL. By H. T. ASHBY AND C. ROBERTS. Originally by H. ASHBY AND G. A. WRIGHT. Sixth edition. Pp. 769; 202 illustrations. London: Henry Frowde, Hodder & Stoughton.

To the reviewer's knowledge this is the only book which deals both with the medical and surgical diseases of children. Like so many volumes from the pens of our English colleagues, it is well written and does not partake of a too dry or stereotyped style. The subject of pediatrics seems thoroughly covered with thirty-six chapters devoted to physiology, hygiene and diet, diseases of the various systems, scurvy, rickets, metabolisn, radiography and similar topics. In addition there is an appendix describing various diagnostic and therapeutic procedures and formulæ. Without the desire to be unduly critical, several noticeable omissions in the text should be mentioned, especially as the preface contains the usual statement that the book has been brought up to date. In the first place the chapter on feeding is very short and lacking in detail; top milk mixtures are recommended, but one can gain little idea of just how to proceed in feeding the individual infant. Again in the discussion of rickets and spasmophilia no mention is made of the recent studies of the mineral metabolism, nor is the therapeutic action of light in rickets noted. American pediatrists have become so dependent upon the intraperitoneal administration of fluids in dehydrated conditions, that it is surprising to find that it does not receive recognition in a pediatric text-book. In other respects the text seems as full as the size of the volume warrants. The amount of space allotted to the subjects is well balanced and the important pediatric problems receive due consideration. Taken all in all the book is interesting and useful in a library containing other standard works on pediatrics. M.

TREATMENT OF FRACTURES. By CHARLES L. SCUDDER, M.D., Assistant Professor of Surgery at the Harvard Medical School. Ninth edition, revised, octavo. Pp. 749; 1252 illustrations. Philadelphia: W. B. Saunders Company, 1922.

THIS, the ninth edition, gives to its readers the last word in fractures. The World War gave an enormous impulse to the study of fracture treatment and as a result, many of the old standard ideas have been discarded. The author presents these improvements in the fullest manner possible. Every fracture that the human frame is heir to is discussed fully, and its treatment minutely outlined not only in the written text but by numerous photographs of the deformities as shown on the surface anatomy and by roentgen-ray. An entire chapter is given over to the operative treatment, and other chapters take up the questions of gunshot fractures ambulatory treatment, the roentgen-ray and its relation to fractures, the anatomy of the epiphyses and the use and abuse of plaster-of-Paris dressings. The last chapter deals with a number of dislocations.

The author, in the preface of his work shows clearly that he has aimed at the very latest and best in this line of work. He voices arguments that will make for better and more speedy results in the fracture. E.

ATLAS OF SYPHILIS. By PROF. LEO V. ZUMBUSCH, Munich. Pp. 34; 64 illustrations. New York: William Wood & Co., 1922.

THIS "Atlas of Syphilis" represents a new departure in medical illustration and consists of 64 colored photographs taken direct from patients by color photography. The pictures are true to life, the accuracy of coloration being a remarkable achievement, and form a valuable collection of realistic clinical pictures of the more common forms of the disease. The 4 illustrations of the spirochæta pallida were taken from water-color drawings and are excellently done. The translation of the work has been prepared by Dr. J. Snowman. The publishers particularly wish to draw the attention to the desirability of using this Atlas in conjunction with a text-book dealing systematically with venereal disease, such as "The Venereal Clinic," by Dr. Clarkson. B.

An Essay on the Physiology of Mind. By Francis X. Dercum, A.M., Ph.D., Professor of Nervous and Mental Diseases, Jefferson Medical College. Pp. 142. Philadelphia: W. B. Saunders Company, 1922.

The author considers the development of the mind from a biological and biochemical standpoint. He clearly reviews the evolution of the nervous system from the lowest to the highest levels, dealing only with well established facts. With such a basis, he undertakes an explanation of the transmission of impulses in the nerve pathways, leading up to the field of consciousness. Consciousness is defined as from necessity, an ever changing process. The "unconscious mind" he holds to be a contradiction in terms and substitutes "unconscious field" for it. He reiterates his theory expounded in 1895 that hysterical attacks are a result of the retraction of the processes of the neurones, producing in effect an interruption at the synaptic junctions. A brief consideration as an Addendum is given to certain pathological mental states, viewing them from the same biochemical and biological viewpoints. The book is entertainingly written, clear in diction, and easily read. It is of particular value to the neuropsychiatrist for review, and sufficiently free of technicalities to be easily understood by the general practitioner. Even though nothing really new is added to the subject, old concepts and present-day facts are so logically arranged that the sequence is easily followed. It is highly recommended by the reviewer. P.

Ten Postgraduate Lectures. Pp. 216. New York: William Wood & Co., 1922.

This little book contains ten lectures delivered before the Fellowship of Medicine of London. There is a short preface written by Sir Clifford Allbutt in his characteristic delightful style. Among the contributors, one finds such well known authorities as Savage, Hale-White and Rolleston. The lectures deal with divers topics including Morbid Mental Growths (Savage), Prognosis of Exophthalmic Goiter (Hale-White), After-effects of Anesthetics (Mortimer) and Disabilities of the Feet Due to Static or Mechanical

Causes (Trethowan). The lectures are apparently designed to interest general practitioners rather than specialists, and the subjects are discussed in a practical manner. It is hinted that this volume is the first of a series of Fellowship lectures to be issued. If the others conform to the high standard set in the first volume, the project deserves success. W.

A TEXT-BOOK ON GONORRHEA AND ITS COMPLICATIONS. By GEORGES LUYS, M.D., Late Assistant to the Urological Clinique, Hôpital Lariboisière, Paris; Prizeman of the Faculté de Médecine, Paris; Chief Medical Officer of the Urological Center at the Military Hospital, Versailles. Translated and edited by ARTHUS FOERSTER, Capt., R.A.M.C., (C.T.), M.R.C.S., L.R.C.P. (Lond.), Late Resident Medical Officer, London Lock Hospital. Third revised edition. Pp. 400; 212 illustrations and 5 colored plates. New York: William Wood & Company, 1922.

THE general character of this text-book has not been changed from the first edition which appeared in 1913, the chief features being new chapters which deal with the technic of urethroscopy and urethroscopic treatment. The colored plates of the normal urethra and those depicting the pathological conditions of the urethra due to gonorrhea are particularly good. This book contains twelve chapters. The history of gonorrhea, its etiology, a full description of the gonococcus, the clinical picture of gonorrhea and the symptomatology of this disease are fully described in the early chapters. The numerous complications of gonorrhea are then reviewed and there is a special chapter devoted to gonorrhea in women and children. In the last two chapters there is given a full description of the treatment of acute and of chronic gonorrhea; the methods which have stood the tests and if properly applied, lead to a "certain cure." The book has been illustrated with special care. B.

DIATHERMIE ET DIATHERMOTHERAPIE. By H. BORDIER. Pp. 490. Paris: Baillière.

THIS book of about 500 pages presents the subject agreeably and logically. The usual details of currents, their nature and uses, as well as the physiological and chemical effects, are clearly set forth. The mathematics contained can be understood by others than the physicist. In therapeutics the work is the best since Nagelschmidt. The subjects are well worked out from the standpoint of a physician, but would be better for more detailed clinical histories. Some surgeons will surely criticize the claims to benefit chronic appendicitis, salpingitis and anterior poliomyelitis, but the enthusiasm of authorship may surely claim some allowance.

PROGRESS

OF

MEDICAL SCIENCE

MEDICINE

UNDER THE CHARGE OF

W. S. THAYER, M.D.

PROFESSOR OF MEDICINE, JOHNS HOPKINS UNIVERSITY, BALTIMORE, MARYLAND,

AND

ROGER S. MORRIS, M.D.,

FREDERICK FORCHHEIMER PROFESSOR OF MEDICINE IN THE UNIVERSITY OF CINCINNATI, CINCINNATI, OHIO.

Congenital Porphyrinuria Associated with Hydroæstivale and Pink Teeth.—L. Mackey and A. E. Garrod (*Quart. Jour. Med.*, 1922, **15**, 319) report a remarkable case of congenital porphyrinuria with hydroæstivale, with pink coloration of the milk teeth. The authors have reviewed the literature and find that not more than 15 cases of congenital hematoporphyrinuria have been reported, 10 of which were in males. Hydroæstivale may or may not be associated. The authors' case is unique, in that the teeth of the patient were colored pink. From birth, the patient's mother had noted that the urine had a ruby red color. The first tooth cut had a pink color, and this has been noted in all the teeth of the first dentition. During the period of observation, none of the permanent teeth had been cut. Since it has been shown that there are at least three porphyrins in man, *i. e.*, hematoporphyrin, uroporphyrin and stercoporphyrin, all differing in chemical formula, the author's suggest that the term, hematoporphyrinuria, is a misnomer, as it is not hematoporphyrin which is found in the urine but uroporphyrin. They, therefore, propose that the designation, porphyrinuria, is a more accurate one and should be preferred.

Planorbis Metidjensis as Intermediate Host of Schistosoma Hematobium.—A. Bettencourt and I. Borges (*Compt. rend. Soc. de biol.*, Paris, 1922, **87**, 1039) have made an experimental study, the result of which demonstrates that *Planorbis metidjensis* may serve as an intermediate host for *Schistosoma hematobium.* Mice and guinea-pigs were used as the experimental animals. The hair of the abdomen was shaved, and the animals were then placed in vessels containing water, in which there were many cercariæ derived from *Planorbis metidjensis.* The shape of the vessels was such that the animals had to remain immersed in the water to their necks, thus offering a large surface for the cercariæ to penetrate. The animals were subjected to infestation during several consecutive or alternate days, and remained in the water each time forty to fifty minutes. Of the mice exposed to infestation, three died. The first had had seven exposures to infestation between May 18 and 25 and died August 2. The second and third were infested after four exposures and died August 16 and 25 respectively. The remaining mice and all the guinea-pigs have survived. Autopsies on the three mice showed adults of *Schistosoma hematobium* in the portal vein, the parasites being already coupled. The ova found were also typical of *S. hematobium*.

SURGERY

UNDER THE CHARGE OF

T. TURNER THOMAS, M.D.

ASSOCIATE PROFESSOR OF APPLIED ANATOMY IN THE MEDICAL SCHOOL AND ASSOCIATE PROFESSOR OF SURGERY IN THE SCHOOL FOR GRADUATES IN MEDICINE IN THE UNIVERSITY OF PENNSYLVANIA; SURGEON TO THE PHILADELPHIA GENERAL AND NORTHEASTERN HOSPITALS.

Urinary Lithiasis in Children.—THOMAS and TANNER (*Jour. Urol.*, 1922, 8, 171) says that urinary lithiasis is frequent in childhood and infancy, the average occurrence in the three large series reported being 43 per cent; the average age is seven years. The youngest patient was ten months old. The authors were unable to determine the etiology of urinary stones in infants, although in their opinion infection is one of the factors (21 per cent of the cases). The frequency of involvement of the right kidney to the left is as 21 is to 8. Only 8 per cent were arrested in the ureter. Assuming that the majority of urinary stones in infants (except in the presence of urethral obstruction or malformation) originate in the kidney, 69 per cent will pass into the bladder. The symptomatology in the order of occurrence is as follows: Pain and colic, hematuria, frequency, pyuria, dysuria, nausea and vomiting. The infant ureter is capable of great distention or in some other manner facilitates the easy passage of ureteral stones. Diagnosis depends upon the following positive findings: Roentgen ray, cystoscopy, urinalysis and clinical findings alone (in a minor portion of the cases). Surgery is indicated when stones do not progress through the urinary tract. When stones are bilateral surgery should be carefully considered. Urinary stones in children may remain symptomless for many years.

Tumors of the Testicles.—TARNER (*Surg. Gyn. Obstet.*, 1922, 25, 565) says that new growths of the testicle occur about once in 2000 male hospital admissions. The disease is practically unilateral, involving both sides only as a metastatic growth from the skin or seminal vesicles. Trauma as an etiological factor in these tumors evidently has some foundation. Practically all cases occur between the ages of eighteen and fifty years, the period of greatest sexual activity, while either testicle is involved with about equal frequency. Undescended testicles within the canal are more apt to become malignant than normally placed organs. Undescended testicles within the abdomen are relatively immune to malignant changes. In this series, the mortality was about 70 per cent. The so-called mixed type of tumor gives a much higher mortality than the carcinomatous type. Tumors containing cartilage and squamous epithelium seem to have a decidedly unfavorable prognosis.

Treatment of Chronic Empyema Where the Recognized Surgical Procedures Have Failed to Produce Obliteration.—Keller (*Ann. Surg.*, 1922, **76**, 549) says that the chronic type of empyema, especially those with large cavities should occur but seldom if early aspiration followed by negative pressure treatment is promptly instituted. Empyema cavities can be obliterated by discission and chemical decortication plus implantation of certain muscle bodies. Chemical decortication if used injudiciously may result in rupture of the visceral pleura, dangerous herniation of the lung and hemorrhage. Subperiosteal resection of ribs at the point of division should be discarded and rib section flush with peristeum adopted. Obliteration by expansion of lung which means increased vital capacity should be practised, rather than cavity diminution by collapse of the chest wall. Sterilization of the cavity can often be accomplished, even in long standing cases, but reinfection will invariably occur if the parietal pleura is not removed in a case of over one year's duration, especially if it is of the hemolytic streptococcus variety. Moreover, daily cultures of the wound are necessary to check the progress and to determine the amount of Dakin's solution to be used. The many-step, open or fractional operation, has the following advantages; it permits direct inspection and Dakinization of the entire cavity; it permits the detection and eradication of diverticulæ which are often missed on roentgen-ray examination. It aids in the detection of osteomyelitis and foreign bodies; it insures such immediate improvement in profoundly septic cases that they will permit further operative procedure being carried out with low mortality; it allows the detection and direct closure of bronchial fistulæ; finally the operation can be discontinued at any stage only to be finished later when the patient's condition permits with a mortality far below that of the standard radical operation.

The Pathology and Mechanism of Prostatic Hypertrophy.—Tenenbaum (*Jour. Urol.*, 1922, **8**, 431) says that the progress made in prostatic pathology leads to the conclusion that the so-called prostatic hypertrophy is really a hyperplasia of the periurethral glands. The prostate itself undergoes atrophy through compression, by growth intruding upon it, or primarily as a physiological presenile process occurring in advanced life. Moreover, it cannot be considered a disease. It is with the secondary changes in the urinary tract caused by proliferation of the periurethral glands that the true pathological process develops. The changes in the urethra in regard to size, lumen and curve are the result of various coöperating and antagonistic forces of which the direct pressure of the intruding glands, the indirect influence of the changes in the bladder upon the urethra and the anatomical peculiarities of the latter are the most important factors. The part of the urethra which is directly subjected to moulding by the growth is the supramontane part of the prostatic urethra. There are two types of intrusion of the growth into the bladder. The direct invasion occurring on or near the sphincter of the bladder which is associated with alterations in the symmetry of the bladder. The indirect raises the floor of the bladder *in toto*, without affecting its symmetry directly. The early stage of bladder involvement is marked by its increased muscular activity while the later stage shows distension and atony combined with impaired muscular activity. The early stages of renal involvement in prostatics are marked by congestion of kidneys with nocturnal polyuria.

Fracture of Tibial Spine.—BLAISDELL (*Arch. of Surg.*, 1922, **5**, 560) says that variation in the anatomical constituents of a part must be considered. These affect size, strength and length and are often a part of a peculiar body habitus. Injuries to the knee-joint which may appear slight or trivial, are occasionally accompanied by a crucial triad involvement. Sprain-fracture of knee may be present without giving objective signs. Experiments on the cadaver have demonstrated that force applied over the distal and anterior surface of the thigh driving the femur backward on the tibia when the leg is fixed, will produce rupture of the anterior crucial ligaments and fracture of the tibial spine anteriorly. Inward or outward rotation of the leg may involve an element of the crucial triad, especially when they are accomplished by direct muscular action or mechanical violence.

THERAPEUTICS

UNDER THE CHARGE OF

SAMUEL W. LAMBERT, M.D.,

NEW YORK,

AND

CHARLES C. LIEB, M.D.,

ASSISTANT PROFESSOR OF PHARMACOLOGY, COLUMBIA UNIVERSITY.

Insulin and Diabetes.—J. J. R. MACLEOD, (*Brit. Med. Jour.* November 4, 1922) in this "General Statement of the Physiological and Therapeutic Effects of Insulin" summarizes the work that has been going on in his laboratories for some time. As he points out, the diabetes following pancreatectomy has been long ascribed to the absence of a hormone essential for the complete metabolism of sugar. Attempts to isolate this hormone have heretofore been fruitless because the hormone, which has been named insulin (or isletin), is destroyed by the proteolytic ferments also present in the pancreas. Recently the destruction has been circumvented by tying off the pancreatic duct so that the cells that secrete the digestive enzymes degenerate completely; whereas the isles of Langerhans, which apparently secrete the antidiabetic hormone, remain more or less intact. When extracts of such degenerated glands are injected into dogs rendered diabetic by pancreatectomy, they decrease the hyperglycemia and the glycosuria and cause a great improvement in the general condition of the animal and prolong its life. Active extracts can also be prepared from fetal pancreas, in which proteolytic enzymes have not yet appeared, and from adult ox pancreas by fractional precipitation by alcohol. Insulin preparations are so potent that they must be carefully standardized. For the unit of activity has been selected the amount of insulin which, on subcutaneous injection, lowers the percentage of blood sugar to 0.045 within four hours in a rabbit weighing about 2 kg. and from which food has been withheld for sixteen to twenty-four hours previously. The solution is then concentrated so that 1 cc contains one unit. If the sugar is lowered below 0.045 per cent the animal develops characteristic symptoms consisting of violent convulsions with intervals of coma. These symptoms usually terminate fatally but if the animal is injected subcutaneously with dextrose (1 gm. per kilo), it immediately recovers and usually remains free from symptoms; should the symptoms recur, another injection of dextrose is a successful antidote. The respiratory quotient is a reliable qualitative index of the type of metabolism, having a value of 1 if carbohydrates are the chief foods undergoing katabolism; 0.7 for fats and 0.8 for protein. In diabetes of the severest type, in depancreatized dogs, for example, the respiratory quotient often falls below 0.7 and is not raised by feeding carbohydrates. When diabetic dogs are given insulin along with carbohydrate food, the respiratory quotient immediately rises, showing a restoration of the power to metabolize this class of food; the acetone bodies disappear from the urine and remain absent so long as the administration is continued. In depancreatized dogs, the glycogen content of the liver is very low whereas that of the heart is abnormally high; after insulin and sugar, the per cent of glycogen in the liver rises (to 12 per cent) while that of the heart falls. The fat content of the liver decreases from the abnormally high figure of 12 per cent in untreated animals to below 5 per cent in those treated with insulin and there is, simultaneously, a marked fall in the fat of the blood. These observations indicate that insulin, possibly through its influence on carbohydrate metabolism, also affects that of fat. The hyperglycemia of diabetes disappears and insulin restores the blood sugar to a normal or even subnormal level. All these facts indicate that this new hormone is an essential factor in the regulation of carbohydrate metabolism. Not only does insulin remove the symptoms of diabetes due to the absence of this hormone, but it prevents the development of hyperglycemia (and presumably of glucosuria) which usually follows such procedures as puncture of the floor of the fourth ventricle, the subcutaneous injection of epinephrin, and the various forms of asphyxia, including ether anesthesia. The mode of action of insulin is not yet known. From the fact that insulin causes an increased consumption of sugar by the heart, it appears probable that the site of action is the muscle cell itself, and that it either increases the rate of combustion of the sugar or hastens its conversion into glycogen. Possessed of all these facts learned from animal experiments, it seemed fair to the author and his co-workers to select cases of human diabetes and try the curative effects of insulin. From all the cases treated the following conclusions seem justified: When insulin is administered subcutaneously in adequate doses, it is capable, within a remarkably short time, of removing the cardinal symptoms of diabetes for a period of several hours. To suppress the symptoms permanently, the injections must be repeated and the practise at present is to give two injections daily. So long as the administration is continued, the patient is able to assimilate much more carbohydrate than previously; he gains in weight and in mental and physical vigor, and the despondency and apathy that are so prominent in these cases disappear. It is in the adolescent forms of the disease that the results have been most marked but there can be little doubt that when insulin comes to be more available, its exhibition, along with intelligent control of diet, will have the same beneficial results in all serious forms of the disease. In cases of threatened coma, insulin is invaluable and the same is true for its use as a precautionary against postoperative risk in surgical practice. Insulin will be put on the market only by licensed manufacturers and not until its usefulness has been fully determined.

Carbon Tetrachloride in the Treatment of Hookworm Disease.—S. M. Lambert (*Jour. Am. Med. Assn.*, 1922, **79**, 2055) concludes from his study on more than twenty thousand inhabitants of the Fiji Islands, that carbon tetrachloride is a potent vermifuge and vermicide and is especially effective in the treatment of hookworm disease and less valuable in infection with ascaris, bothriocephalus dispar and oxyuris. Carbon tetrachloride is administered in doses of 0.2 cc per year of age up to fifteen years; the maximal dose thereafter is 3 to 4 cc according to the weight of the patient. After some preliminary tests, the following routine procedure was adopted: the carbon tetrachloride was administered on an empty stomach in the morning and three hours later a dose of magnesium sulphate was given. The carbon tetrachloride is itself a purge but there is less danger of absorption and of systemic action if a saline cathartic is administered after it. No food should be taken for several hours before nor for several hours after the vermifuge. Systemic symptoms include headache, sleepiness, nausea and vomiting and all are prevented or alleviated by the saline purge. The danger of absorption is greatly enhanced if alcohol is taken within several hours of the vermifuge or if the patient is naturally constipated. Reëxamination of the feces of 823 patients indicated that one treatment lowered the infection rate from 100 per cent to less than 9 per cent. Lambert concludes that carbon tetrachloride is well adapted to mass treatment since it is effective, its administration is simple and the cost low (four pence halfpenny per patient).

Respiratory Paralysis Following Quinidine Therapy.—W. D. Reid, (*Jour. Am. Med. Assn.*, 1922, **79**, 1974). The author's case of respiratory paralysis is the fifth to be reported in the literature and is the only one which resulted fatally.

PEDIATRICS

UNDER THE CHARGE OF

THOMPSON S. WESTCOTT, M.D., AND ALVIN E. SIEGEL, M.D.,
OF PHILADELPHIA.

The Early Diagnosis of Intussusception.—Zschau (*München. Med. Wchnschr.*, 1922, **69**, 1408) found that intussusception as affecting children particularly was too little appreciated or understood by general practitioners. In a Children's Hospital in Nurnberg there were 19 cases in the period between 1906 and 1921, which was less than 0.1 of 1 per cent of the total admissions. Strong healthy children, many of them breast fed, were suddenly seized with vomiting and severe abdominal pain in paroxysms. After a time diarrhea would develop, and the stools would become bloody. The child would grow continually worse and the facies abdominalis would become marked. The attacks of colic are especially significant. A child that has been quiet will suddenly cry out and writhe in pain. The abdomen becomes flatulent and the intestines become hard. Finally a roller like, only slightly movable, swelling usually above the umbilicus and extending in an oblique direction, can be felt. The temperature is only slightly elevated, the pulse is small and accelerated. Conservative treatment may be tried but Zschau claims that as a rule no result will be experienced. In only 1 of his 19 cases was disinvagination brought about without operation. In 12 of the cases the invagination was ileocolic; in 4 in the colon, and in 2 in the ileum. In 2 cases resection of the intestines was necessary. The earlier the operation was undertaken the less difficult it was. Recovery took place in all but 1 case when the operation was performed within thirty-six hours. The mortality was 30 per cent. The most frequent false diagnosis was dysentery or hemorrhagic enteritis. The false diagnoses were confined mainly to infants in whom there were 4 deaths in 11 cases. Zschau feels convinced that in infants the invagination often is unrecognized, and the cause of death is given as intestinal catarrh. In older children the diagnosis is more accurate probably due to the fact that they can indicate the location of the pain.

Artificial Pneumothorax in Children.—Babonneix and Denoyelle (*Arch. d. med. d. enf.*, 1922, **25**, 599) found in 28 children with progressive pulmonary tuberculosis that the disease was strictly unilateral in 12. Of this number 7 were treated with artificial pneumothorax. In 5 others, pleural adhesions interfered, but in only 2 of these cases had the adhesions been diagnosed. They conclude from their observations that shrinking of the wall on the side of the penumothorax and scoliosis occur early. In 3 cases out of 6, the pneumothorax was followed rapidly by the appearance of a localized pneumonic focus on the opposite side which retrogressed fairly quickly and completely. It seemed to be due to the contamination of the healthy lung by expectoration of bacilli from the diseased lung. To prevent such accidents, compression should always be slow and progressive so as not to force into the bronchi the contents of the cavity. In 1 case the general condition improved but the bacilli persisted in the sputum. In 3 other cases the local and general results were excellent and seemed possible of being permanent.

A Scarlet Fever Epidemic in an Agricultural School.—Diehl and Shepard (*Jour. Am. Med. Assn.*, 1922, **79**, 2079) describe the observations made by them during this epidemic. This school admits as regular students boys and girls who have completed the eighth grade of public school, and as special students mature men and women. Exclusive of a number of service men who are taking vocational training, most of the students came from rural districts, 59 per cent of them living in places of less than 100 inhabitants. The age period represented was from sixteen to twenty-five, and the individuals had presumably very little immunity to the usual diseases of childhood. At the school 36 per cent of these students lived in dormitories, and 40 per cent took their meals in a common dining room. Most of the others roomed near the campus and took their meals at restaurants or boarding houses. In all 59 cases developed between January 25 and March 26. Of the patients 93.3 per cent were boys and 6.7 per cent were girls; 55.9 per cent lived in rural communities; 33.9 per cent lived in towns of less than 5,000 inhabitants, and 10.2 per cent in cities of more than 5,000 inhabitants. New cases developed at the rate of from 1 in three days to 4 in one day during the epidemic. By means of daily throat inspection with isolation of all suspicious contacts and cases, the epidemic was kept under partial control. It was not until all students with even slightly reddened throats were isolated that new cases failed to develop. From the study of the epidemic, it seems probable that students showing no symptoms other than a moderately reddened throat were responsible for the transmission of much of the infection. A review of the clinical notes in the cases shows a great diversity of symptoms and complications. There were no deaths.

A New Eruptive Fever Associated with Stomatitis and Ophthalmia.—Steven and Johnson (*Am. Jour. Dis. Child.*, 1922, **24**, 526) have observed 2 cases of a generalized cutaneous eruption not conforming to any recognized dermatological condition. Both cases occurred in boys, one being seven years of age, and the other eight, coming from widely separated sections of New York City with no possibility of contact. Both cases manifested a purulent conjunctivitis, one going on the panophthalmia and total loss of vision, the other responding to treatment, but leaving a severe corneal scar. The pus showed pyogenic organisms, but no gonococci. A high and continuous fever was present in both cases. In the case with loss of vision there was a lobar pneumonia, which may explain the fever. In the other cases the fever was present without other cause than the skin condition. The eruption showed certain characteristics identical in both cases. The onset was with fever, the rash appearing on the back of the neck and chest, spreading to the face, arms and legs during a period of about eighteen days, the last lesions to appear being on the soles of the feet and the palms of the hands. At this time resolution of the first lesions began. The eruption consisted of oval, dark red to purplish macules, separated by areas of normal skin. These became in a few days raised firm papules of brownish-purple from 0.5 to 2 cm. in diameter, without areola, and without subjective symptoms of pain or itching at any time. A few of the largest spots showed a yellow, dry, necrotic center. The lesions on the forearms and shins were smaller and more thickly together. No pustules or vesicles were to be seen. The scalp was at all times free of lesions, but the mouth and lips were intensely sore and inflamed. In one case bullæ were present in the mouth. After the third week resolution began in the order of the appearance of the lesions. This consisted of the shrinking of the macule to a horny oval of dark brown color with raised papery edges. From the fourth week these scales dropped off, leaving a faint pigmented area; there was no pitting or scarring. By the fifth week the chest, face and back were clear except for the pigmentation, while resolution and crusting were still going on in the arms and legs. Fall of temperature coincided with the period of resolution of the skin lesions. Investigation rules out the possibility of drug rash. In the entire absence of gastro-intestinal symptoms it was not thought to be the rash of food idiosyncrasy. Syphilis was excluded clinically and by laboratory tests. Hemorrhagic measles was the primary diagnosis, but the later course ruled out this possibility. Sepsis with generalized eruption was considered but the superficial nature of the lesions, their character and progressive appearance over three weeks and the leukopenia were the reasons for excluding this diagnosis. Erythema multiforme was also eliminated. The authors feel that this represents a distinct disease which has not been previously recognized.

DERMATOLOGY AND SYPHILIS

UNDER THE CHARGE OF

JOHN H. STOKES, M.D.,
MAYO CLINIC, ROCHESTER, MINN.

Precipitation Tests for Syphilis.—The development of precipitation tests for syphilis has resulted in a group of reactions whose clinical standing is, on the whole, distinctly inferior to that of the Wassermann test. The procedures thus far described have in general involved complexities almost as great as those attached to the Wassermann reaction, without a corresponding gain in reliability or sensitiveness. Recently, however, Kahn (*Arch. Dermat. and Syphil.*, 1922, **5**, 570; ibid., 1922, **5**, 734; ibid., 1922, **6**, 332) has devised a precipitation test for syphilis applicable to the blood serum, which is so simple that it may have wide application in the clinical consulting room and the small private laboratory. The method is described in detail in the articles mentioned. The antigen consists of extract of fresh beef heart, one test being performed with a cholesterinized and the other with a noncholesterinized antigen. The antigen is diluted with physiologic sodium chloride solution and is best used freshly diluted. The blood serum is obtained by centrifugation and inactivated for one-half hour in the water-bath at 56° C. The diluted antigen and the serum are shaken together and the test read for the spontaneous or strongly positive reactions which take place immediately, the flocculation being visible to the naked eye. The remaining serums are incubated over night at 37.5° C. and read the next morning without shaking. KEIM and WILE (*Jour. Am. Med. Assn.*, 1922, **79**, 870) report the results of a comparison of this test with the Wassermann reaction as carried out in two different standard laboratories in a total of 350 cases. In primary syphilis fifty spontaneous reactions were obtained with agreement between the three tests in 66⅔ per cent. In 33⅓ per cent positive tests were shown by the Kahn reaction, which were negative by the Wassermann. In a treated case the Kahn reaction showed positive in the face of a negative Wassermann. In secondary syphilis the two tests compared favorably in sensitiveness. In osseous late syphilis the Kahn test proved to be less sensitive than the Wassermann with ice-box fixation. In visceral involvement the Kahn test was slightly the more sensitive of the two. In neurosyphilis the two tests compared favorably. In congenital syphilis the Kahn reaction had a slight advantage, and in latent syphilis the Kahn test has a very definite advantage. In the control serums of nonsyphilitic patients, 154 to 157 cases were uniformly negative. The Kahn test showed partial positives as against negative Wassermann reactions in 3 patients with acne, variola and diabetes respectively. Keim and Wile point out the great simplicity of the test, the rapid reading and the visibility of the precipitates and the greater possibilities for standardization in the simplified precipitation test. HERROLD (*Jour. Am. Med. Assn.*, 1922, **79**, 957) has proposed a ring modification of the Kahn test.

Studies in Asymptomatic Neurosyphilis.—J. E. MOORE, (*Johns Hopkins Hosp. Bull.*, 1922, **33**, 231). The author's article is a comprehensive and valuable summary of the experience of the Syphilis Clinic of the Johns Hopkins Hospital in this particular field and gives tangible form to many current clinical impressions. In 352 cases of primary and secondary syphilis, 26.4 per cent were found to have neurosyphilis as detected by neurological examination plus routine spinal puncture after one or two courses of treatment. It is recognized that this probably reduces the percentage of original incidence of this type of involvement. Three groups are recognized, the first presenting only slight pleocytosis, and slight increase in globulin, the second marked pleocytosis and a negative or only mildly positive Wassermann and the third a strongly positive Wassermann with a marked pleocytosis and marked globulin increase. The first group responds to routine continuous treatment; the second to a slight intensification of treatment, and the third requires intraspinal therapy to secure any response. Of the 94 cases presenting neurosyphilitic involvement, 76.6 per cent were asymptomatic and detected only by routine puncture. Of the primary syphilis cases, 29.9 per cent had abnormal fluids, and of the patients with secondary syphilis, 22 per cent. 25 per cent of the cases fell into the first group; 53.1 per cent into the second group, and 23.6 per cent into the third group. The author emphasizes the fact that the constancy of the percentage of neurosyphilis in early and late cases argues that the fate of a patient with reference to neurosyphilis is decided early in the infection. The optimum time to detect its presence would appear to be by spinal puncture between the twelfth and eighteenth month. An interesting justification of the idea of continuous treatment as compared with lapsing or irregular treatment was found in the fact that three times as many patients who had been irregular in treatment developed neurosyphilis as compared with those whose treatment was regular or continuous. By regular or continuous treatment is meant overlapping courses of arsphenamine and mercury without rest intervals. The author notes that his cases in group two, continue to increase in number with the duration of the infection even during treatment. After reaching 17 per cent it begins to decline again. Patients with strongly positive spinal fluid Wassermanns and high cell counts early in the disease prove resistant and probably constitute the recruiting ground for late neurosyphilis. Negroes were found to present a markedly lower percentage of neurosyphilis than whites. There appears to be some evidence that neurosyphilis tends to appear in an increasing proportion in patients who have mild early cutaneous manifestations. If the blood Wassermann reaction is still positive after a second course of arsphenamine plus all interim mercurialization, a particularly careful search should be made of the osseous, cardiovascular and nervous systems. Of the cases of early neurosyphilis, 21.4 per cent had a resistant blood Wassermann as compared with 8.4 per cent of patients with negative spinal fluids. The author estimates that a systematic intensive continuous treatment should reduce the ultimate incidence of neurosyphilis from between 20 and 30 per cent to approximately 5 per cent. He wisely opposes too much individualization of treatment in early cases urging that it is preferable to treat to a standard which cures the majority rather than to undertreat by an overasymptomatic plan. He suggests that treatment be continued for a full year after the patient has reached complete serological negativity on both the blood and fluid.

The Non-specificity of "Luetin."—Another aspect of the ubiquitous question of non-specificity in the reactions of the body to the *Spirochæta pallida* is the recent demonstration by Kolmer and Greenbaum (*Jour. Am. Med. Assn.*, 1922, **79**, 2063) of the complete non-specificity of the luetin reaction, and the danger of proceeding to the interpretation of cutaneous tests without properly controlling the non-specific elements and ingredients employed. These authors confirmed the observations of Stokes on the instrumentality of agar in the production of the luetin reaction, and removed the last trace of specificity from the test by showing that the killed *Spirochæta pallida* from pure culture did not produce any reaction when injected into the skins of syphilitics. The reaction is therefore dependent upon secondary factors, such as the medium (ascites agar) upon which the organisms were grown. The worthlessness of much commercial luetin at the present time was recently demonstrated by Alderson (*Arch. of Dermat. and Syph.*, 1922, **5**, 610). The great importance of using as controls in cutaneous tests, especially on syphilitics, substances which are capable of engendering the same non-specific reactions as the testing substance, is emphasized.

OBSTETRICS

UNDER THE CHARGE OF

EDWARD P. DAVIS, A.M., M.D.,

PROFESSOR OF OBSTETRICS IN THE JEFFERSON MEDICAL COLLEGE, PHILADELPHIA.

Tubal Gestation Treated by Salpingotomy. — As a result of careful dissections and study, WHITEHOUSE (*Jour. Obstet. and Gynec. of the Brit. Emp.*, 1922, **29**, 93) has concluded that tubal mole is the direct result of intratubal rupture, and the mole invariably retains a very narrow basis of attachment to the tubal wall, usually on the floor of the tube and always at the proximal end of the mole. When tubal abortion takes place the pedicle of a mole is torn through by peristaltic action of the tube endeavoring to expel the foreign body. Clots may be expelled from the tube through the ostium abdominale without separation of the mole occurring, such clots being frequently ovoid in shape. The conformation of a tubal mole or tubal abortion is the result of pressure of the tubal wall upon the clot, the impression of the normal rugæ being frequently observed. The deciding factor as to whether intra- or extratubal rupture shall occur is the direct outcome of the combination of tissue erosion and tissue tension. This is influenced by the site of the implantation of the ovum in the ampullary, isthmic or interstitial portions of the tube. Evidence, either macroscopic or microscopic, of preëxisting inflammation of the tube appears to be the exception rather than the rule in cases of tubal mole and abortion. The two points upon which the writer would lay special emphasis are: (1) The existence of a pedicle or narrow basis of attachment in all cases, and (2) the ease with which the rest of the mole can, in the case of fresh specimens, be detached from the tubal mucosa. These two points suggested to him the possibility of removing a mole from the tube *in situ* and raised the question as to whether we are justified in sacrificing the tube on all occasions. In a small series of ten cases therefore, previous to removing the tube, he performed salpingotomy and extracted the gestation, which was done without difficulty or hemorrhage either from the pedicle or the tubal wall which was not readily controlled by suture. The tube in these ten cases was then removed and examined in detail for evidence of inflammatory change and in all the specimens the tissues appeared to be normal, and the abnormal implantation of the gestation to be purely accidental in origin. There seemed, therefore, to be quite a good case for salpingotomy and on five subsequent occasions he adopted this method in the treatment of tubal gestation, all of the patients making a normal recovery. Although the writer seems to be quite enthusiastic over this procedure, nevertheless he states that salpingectomy is probably the better procedure, because in the presence of severe hemorrhage life is more important than conservatism, and the interests of the patient are possibly better served by excising rather than suturing a badly lacerated tube. Salpingotomy appears to be worthy of a trial as an alternative procedure, but time alone will prove whether its adoption is followed by other complications, such as recurrence of the accident, the subsequent development of hydrosalpinx, or the incidence of a tubal chorion-epithelioma.

What is the Present Death Rate in Parturient Women?—This question which is of considerable interest medically and economically receives answer from J. P. Greenhill (*Surg. Gyn. and Obst.*, 1922, **35**, 614). His statistical material was 10,000 parturient women, among whom occurred 39 deaths, mortality 0.39 per cent. As to the relative mortality of the mother in hospital, among the 39 deaths were 5 delivered by the outpatient service of the hospital in their homes; 1 gave birth before the outpatient physicians could arrive; 1 was delivered by a general practitioner, and 1 by a midwife. There remained 31 deaths in hospital of whom 7 were hospital-ward cases, and 24 were in hospital before under the care of private physicians. This may be understood from the fact that the obstetrical hospital furnishing these statistics is open to the practice of over 300 different physicians. It may represent the practice of the average general physician, but conducted in hospital. In the 39 deaths, what is called general sepsis is charged with 6; peritonitis with 6; shock with 6, the latter divided equally between hemorrhage and rupture of the uterus. There were 5 eclampsias; 4 embolisms; 4 pneumonias; 3 cardiac deaths; 3 toxemic; 3 thrombosis of the vessels of the heart proved by autopsy; 1 status lymphaticus proved by autopsy. The fact that the deaths in hospital are divided among such a number of causes, illustrates the average and probably unavoidable mortality of parturition at the present time. Eight autopsies were obtained, and among the septic cases there were 3 who died before admission to hospital in outpatient service. It is interesting to note that 1 woman died four days after spontaneous birth from a ruptured and infected appendix. Another died after a spontaneous birth from perforation of the small intestine. The 3 deaths from hemorrhage were equally divided among premature separation of the placenta, postpartum hemorrhage and rupture of the uterus. There were 46 cases of eclampsia in the 10,000 with a mortality of 10.9 per cent; 3 patients were said to have toxemia probably without eclampsia; 1 had vaginal hysterotomy, dying on the nineteenth day from embolism; 2 had classic Cæsarean section. The unusual circumstances pertaining in this hospital where over 300 physicians attend patients with hospital advantages make these statistics of unusual interest. The fact that hospital advantages afforded to men of average skill and ability give a low mortality, suggests that further improvement is to be sought in two ways. First by prenatal care, concerning which nothing is said in this report, and second, in making obstetrics a specialty and allotting obstetric cases to obstetricians only.

The Diet Required During Lactation.—Hartwell (*Lancet*, 1922, **2**, 963) has studied the effects of diet upon warm-blooded animals while nursing their young, to determine the relative quantity of protein and non-protein material needed. If protein matter be given in excess (about 46 per cent of the total solids), the results are bad, and in some of the lower animals spasms and ultimate death ensue. Fresh cow's milk acts as an antidote to some other proteins, and upon examining milk to determine what it contained which produced this result, there was evidence that vitamin B was the efficient substance. Accordingly, experiments were made with 19 substances commonly used in food. The animals studied were given protein in excess together with butter, lemon juice and salt. To neutralize food of excessive protein content, fruit and vegetable juices were found amply efficient. Best of these were the tomato, potato, carrot and artichoke. Next in efficiency were apple, orange, beet root and vegetable marrow. The juice of cucumbers and juice of grapes had practically no value in the chemistry of food metabolism. Preparations of wheat foods containing yeast and the yolks of eggs were useful. Of all substances fed to nursing animals the yolks of eggs produced the best results upon the offspring. The extracts of beef muscle, cod and herring were useful, and the watery extract of wheat, when it was used in large quantities gave the desired result. Apparently the best of all these substances for neutralizing excess protein in the nursing mothers was the tomato, the active principles of wheat, the yolks of eggs and preparations containing yeast.

GYNECOLOGY

UNDER THE CHARGE OF

JOHN G. CLARK, M.D.,

PROFESSOR OF GYNECOLOGY IN THE UNIVERSITY OF PENNSYLVANIA, PHILADELPHIA,

AND

FRANK B. BLOCK, M.D.,

INSTRUCTOR IN GYNECOLOGY, MEDICAL SCHOOL, UNIVERSITY OF PENNSYLVANIA, PHILADELPHIA.

Complications of Double Kidney.—It is almost an axiom, in reviewing surgical literature, that when one desires to know something about uncommon surgical conditions a reference to the work of the Mayo Clinic will show, as a rule, that the condition is not so uncommon as thought, and, furthermore, the latest thoughts on the subject will usually be presented. For example, BRAASCH and SCHOLL (*Surg., Gynec. and Obst.*, 1922, **35**, 401) state that anomalies in the urinary tract, of themselves, are of no clinical significance. It is only when some pathological complication occurs that their recognition becomes of clinical, as well as of surgical, importance. Pathological, and particularly surgical, complications are prone to develop in the presence of such anomalies, and their clinical discovery is, therefore, comparatively frequent. The most common anomaly in the urinary tract is duplication of the renal pelvis and ureter; such duplication may be unilateral or bilateral, complete or incomplete. When it occurs in a solitary kidney, it is usually termed fused or horseshoe kidney. That duplication is comparatively common is evident from the literature, although it is doubtful if any other clinic has carefully observed 144 cases of this type, as has been done at the Mayo Clinic. The incidence of aberrant and bilateral duplications of ureters and pelves reported in the literature is too high, owing to the tendency to report the more unusual cases. Of the patients in this series, the duplication was unilateral in 135 (94 per cent) and bilateral in 9 (6 per cent). Of the 135 patients with unilateral duplication, 36 (25 per cent) had complete duplication and 99 (68.7 per cent) had incomplete duplication. Of the 9 patients with bilateral duplications, 8 had complete duplication and 1 had incomplete. Duplication may vary from duplication confined to the renal pelvis to duplicate pelves, with separate ureters opening into the bladder. The pelves are generally unequal in size, the upper being the smaller, and are separated by a bridge of normal renal cortex of variable extent. When an unusually small renal pelvis is outlined in the pyelogram, the possibility of duplication should be suspected. Complete duplication will be discovered more often if a careful search is made routinely for anomaly at the time of cystoscopic inspection. In cases of partial duplication, the diagnosis is made only by means of a pyelo-ureterogram. Hydronephrosis is the most common pathological complication, and is due to ureteral obstruction, generally in the region of the junction of the two ureters in cases of incomplete duplication. In tuberculosis of double kidneys, gross evidence of the disease is generally confined to one segment, usually the lower; but in all cases histological examination reveals tubercles in the intervening renal tissue and extending into the remaining segment. Occasionally, when only one pelvis is outlined by the pyelogram, its unusual shape and contour may be misconstrued with pathological changes occurring in single kidneys, such as atrophic pyelonephritis. Only 61 (42 per cent) of the patients in this series were without pathological complications, and the anomaly was discovered in the examination for other conditions. Fifteen of the 30 patients operated on submitted to primary nephrectomies and 4 to heminephrectomies; 2 of these later required complete nephrectomy. Six pyelolithotomies and 3 ureterolithotomies were performed. In 1 patient hydronephrosis was relieved by the cutting of an aberrant vessel, and in another symptoms were relieved by the ligation of an aberrant ureter from the upper pole of a double kidney. In the treatment of pathological complications in a double kidney, the indication for heminephrectomy is limited to but a few favorable cases, since the remaining half of the resected kidney may become infected and require subsequent removal.

End-results of Surgical Treatment of Cancer of the Cervix.—The enthusiastic acclaim which has greeted the use of radium in the treatment of cancer of the cervix has well nigh put a stop to the operative treatment of this disease in many of the large clinics of this country. DAVIS (*Ann. Surg.*, 1922, **76**, 395), however, is unwilling to abandon the operative treatment in appropriate cases until more evidence of lasting cures by radium is at hand. The operation which he performs consists of a total abdominal hysterectomy, including a liberal cuff of vaginal wall and wide removal of parametrial tissue. Systematic dissection of the pelvic lymph nodes has not been attempted, while ligation of the internal iliacs has not proved to be of material advantage, and has been given up since his early cases. In cases presenting a bulky cauliflower outgrowth from the cervix, filling the vault of the vagina, preliminary curettage and cauterization, followed ten days later by radical hysterectomy, have been done. In his series of 32 cases, there have been three operative deaths, an operative mortality of 9.3 per cent, while there has been no mortality in the last 12 cases. These 32 cases were selected out of a series of 85 cases of carcinoma of the cervix applying for treatment, so that his operability rate is 37.6 per cent, although in the latter part of the series the operability rate fell to 33 per cent, in spite of an active publicity campaign carried on in his community. Hysterectomy was undertaken in all cases in which the disease was apparently confined to the cervix, or had invaded the vaginal walls to a limited extent. Mere bulk of the cervical outgrowth into the vagina has not been considered a contraindication, nor has limited parametrial invasion. Actual involvement of the rectal or vesical walls is now considered a contraindication, also massive infiltration of the broad ligaments, as determined by rectal palpation. Mere fixation of the growth in the pelvis has not been found to be a contraindication, as in several cases this has been proved by laparotomy to be due to inflammatory exudate and adhesions. It cannot be denied that there have been distressing complications in those patients who survived the operation. Of the 17 patients who have lived more than five years, there were 4 afflicted with urinary fistulas, although 1 of these closed spontaneously. Postoperative shock was noted in 3 cases, while pyelitis, phlebitis, cystitis and wound sepsis were recorded once each as complications. There were 20 cases operated upon more than five years ago, all of whom have been traced. In 3 cases death occurred as an immediate result of the operation, giving an operative mortality of 15 per cent. In 7 cases the patients are now living and well, while in 1 case the patient died of intercurrent disease without recurrence, seven years after operation. This gives a total of eight five-year cures, or 40 per cent. Recurrence of disease was noted in 9 cases, taking place within one year in 7 cases. The prevalence of urinary fistulas in these cases can be ascribed largely to errors of technic and judgment as the operator was acquiring his early experience. A more conservative selection of cases with substitution of rubber for gauze drainage, avoidance of stripping bare the ureter for considerable distances, and gentleness in its handling, have reduced the incidence of this most distressing sequel in later cases, and yet with all care, ureteral fistula the result of necrosis, remains the great bugbear of the operation, an inherent risk of thorough removal of parametrium.

Ovarian Transplantation.—For many years MARTIN (*Surg., Gynec. and Obst.*, 1922, **35**, 573) has been greatly interested in the subject of ovarian transplantation, and we have quoted him on several previous occasions. His latest contribution to this subject consists of a collective review of the literature, with an extensive bibliography, which will be of great use to those especially interested in this fascinating branch of gynecology. He summarizes his impression of the whole subject by saying that, as more evidence is accumulated from the literature, the claims of the earlier enthusiasts seem to become less and less substantial. The one most hopeful feature that he is able to glean from the mass of more or less loosely recorded evidence is that the clinical records dealing with transplantation in the human show that, while autotransplants give some evidence of success, homotransplants and heterotransplants give practically none at all. On the other hand, definite evidence of success is recorded as the result of carefully conducted experiments on animals, in which matters of selection of appropriate material and proper technic are more controllable than in dealing with the human. The present status of the question, as may be gleaned from the more recent opinions expressed, is that clinically there is very little to encourage one to believe that transplantation of ovaries, as practised up to the present time, has more than speculative value as a surgical procedure. There is some evidence that autotransplants are of some value in deferring the symptoms of the menopause and delaying the cessation of menstruation. It is difficult, however, not to attribute some of this evidence to suggestive therapeutics or to unattached ovarian tissue left *in situ*. There is practically no convincing evidence that homotransplants or heterotransplants have been successful where the human female has been the recipient, although there is some encouraging evidence recorded in experimental animal surgery that not only autotransplants, but homotransplants and even heterotransplants have been successful, and the sexual function of the castrated animal maintained. The technic followed by the various operators on the human females, in too many instances, seems unsurgical and too often is incompletely and loosely recorded, leaving the impression that the conclusions derived from such work must be unreliable. There is, however, encouraging evidence in all this endeavor to lead one to hope that the subject will be pursued experimentally, especially for the purpose of devising a rational and simple technic, based upon the work of serologists, endocrinologists, hematologists and practical clinical surgeons.

PATHOLOGY AND BACTERIOLOGY

UNDER THE CHARGE OF

OSKAR KLOTZ, M.D., C.M.,

DIRECTOR OF THE PATHOLOGICAL LABORATORIES, SAO PAULO, BRAZIL.

AND

DE WAYNE G. RICHEY, B.S., M.D.,

ASSISTANT PROFESSOR OF PATHOLOGY, UNIVERSITY OF PITTSBURGH, PITTSBURGH, PA.

A Ten Year Old Strain of Fibroblasts.—EBELING (*Jour. Exp. Med.*, 1922, **35**, 755) described the actual condition of a strain of fibroblasts, obtained from the heart of a chick embryo which had completed the tenth year of its life *in vitro*. At that time the cultures represented the 1860th generation of the connective-tissue cells. The growth of the tissue fragments was as rapid as during the past years, each fragment generally doubling its volume in forty-eight hours. The cultures had not modified their appearance, many cells dividing mitotically. Although other experimenters believe that cells cultivated *in vitro* did not use the substances contained in the medium and that the masses of tissue did not increase, Ebeling indicated that this was not the case, when the tissues are grown in a medium containing embryonic tissue juices, pointing out that in ten years more than 30,000 cultures had been derived from this fragment of heart less than 1 c.mm. in size and that "If it had been feasible to multiply the tissue to their greatest possible extent, today their mass would be very much larger than the sun," and further, "That the existence of the ten year old strain demonstrates also that the cells are potentially immortal." These experiments have aided in the study of certain biological problems. Pure cultures of cells were found to be as necessary in physiology as pure cultures of bacteria in bacteriology. The cells remained indefinitely young or grew old according to the food material they were given and the extent of the elimination of their catabolic substances. Since it has become possible to obtain strains of lymphyocytes and of epithelial cells living *in vitro* by practically the same procedure that was employed for fibroblasts, the author states that the scope of these studies will be increased.

The Tetanus Bacillus as an Intestinal Saprophyte in Man.—While it is recognized that *B. tetani* is widely distributed in Nature, the role of man as a carrier of this organism has received little attention. It is often stated in the literature that the tetanus bacillus is present in the digestive tract of man, the statement being based, apparently, on the work of Pizzini and also on the fact that this offers the best explanation for some idiopathic cases of tetanus and for those following typhoid fever, dysentery and hemorrhoid operations. TENBROECK and BAUER (*Jour. Exp. Med.*, 1922, **36**, 261) found that 34.7 per cent of 78 male Chinese, save 1, harbored tetanus bacilli in their stools. The organisms were isolated by heating impure cultures to 80° C. for twenty minutes, transferring to sterile bouillon plus tissue in a fermentation tube and plating when the tetanus-like forms predominated. Virtually all the film examinations were made after the tubes had been inoculated four days but latterly it was learned that the tetanus bacilli were more abundant after incubation of five or six days. Field or white mice were inoculated subcutaneously with the centrifugalized branch fluid of the culture tube after incubation of ten days, two receiving 0.001 cc, two 0.01 cc, two 0.01 cc plus approximately 1 unit of tetanus antitoxin, and two 0.1 cc plus the same amount of antitoxin. Only those cultures were called *B. tetani* which produced characteristic spasms and death in mice receiving 0.001 cc and in those mice injected with 0.1 cc plus about 1 unit of tetanus antitoxin in which there were no spasms and the mice survived at least five days. The authors are convinced that tetanus bacillus was growing in the digestive tract, inasmuch as it was present in persons receiving a practically sterile diet for a month or more and because one individual may eliminate several million spores of *B. tetani* in a single stool.

Changes in the Number of Small Lymphocytes of the Blood Following Ligation of the Thoracic Duct.—The extent of appearance of the lymphocyte in the thoracic duct under ordinary conditions or its appearance in the blood stream after splenectomy has been studied by Biedl and von Decastello, after extirpation of important glands by Ehrlich and Rembach, after administration of pilocarpine by Rous and following ligation of the thoracic duct by Davis and Carlson, and Bunting and Huston. During the progress of work on intrathoracic ligation of the thoracic duct in five young adult male cats, LEE (*Jour. Exp. Med.*, 1922, **36**, 247) had an opportunity to observe the effect of ligation of that vessel on the number of small lymphocytes in the blood. The blood for counting was procured from the ear. Differential counts were made by applying Wright's stain to the smears and counting 300 or more cells. It was found that the thoracic duct ligation "produced an immediate decrease in the number of small lymphocytes to the extent of 56 per cent." The preoperative level was again reached at about the end of three weeks. The author believes "that the gradual return of the number of small lymphocytes to the preligation level took place *pari passu* with the establishment of the collateral circulation of the thoracic duct, although," he says "there is no absolute proof of this." It is evident from these observations that the thoracic duct is an avenue for the entrance of at least half of the small lymphocytes to the circulating blood in the cat.

HYGIENE AND PUBLIC HEALTH

UNDER THE CHARGE OF

MILTON J. ROSENAU, M.D.,

PROFESSOR OF PREVENTIVE MEDICINE AND HYGIENE, HARVARD MEDICAL SCHOOL, BOSTON, MASSACHUSETTS,

AND

GEORGE W. McCOY, M.D.,

DIRECTOR OF HYGIENIC LABORATORY, UNITED STATES PUBLIC HEALTH SERVICE, WASHINGTON, D. C.

Dermatosis Following the Use of Cutting Oils and Lubricating Compounds.—MCCONNELL (*Public Health Reports*, vol. **37**, No. 29, p. 1773) summarizes a rather exhaustive study of the subject as follows: "In this report attention has been particularly directed toward the practical method of preventing the dermatosis, but it is realized that only a minimum reduction in the number of cases is effected by merely recommending preventives to the workmen without providing adequate sanitary arrangements and employing responsible supervision. The weight of the evidence collected in this investigation incriminates oils and lubricating compounds of all types carrying extraneous matter in suspension as the primary cause in producing the initial dermatosis by mechanical obstruction of the sebaceous orifices, the underlying or basic cause being a deficiency of the natural oiliness of the skin. Infecting organisms, which usually inhabit the body surface, but which may be carried by cutting liquids, frequently find ingress to the skin through the primary dermatic lesions by reason of the sufferer's scratching the affected surface or by reason of other irritation, and thereby produce a secondary infection of the dermatosis as a complication. In other cases the abrasions produced by particles of the metal become infected and complicate the dermatosis. The condition so arising is not, however, allied to the primary dermatosis, but is similar to conditions, which would be classified under the head of abrasions and infections, such as are commonly found wherever bacteria are present. Prevention depends, first, upon thorough cleanliness, and, second, upon the application of lanolin or lanolin and castor oil to the skin at the beginning of the work period. Cure is accomplished by rest of the affected parts and by constant use of the preventive measures."

Influenza: Framingham Epidemic and Postepidemic Observations.—Studies conducted under the FRAMINGHAM COMMUNITY HEALTH AND TUBERCULOSIS DEMONSTRATION (*Framingham Monograph*, 1922, No. 9) led to the following conclusions: (1) A very small percentage (1 per cent) of the group have had a recurrent attack of influenza subsequent to the primary epidemic. (2) A fairly large percentage seemed to have acquired the practice of going to their own physician for an examination, either as a result of the general medical examination propaganda, or partly as a result of the emphasis given to this idea in connection with the postepidemic activities. Twenty-nine per cent of the individuals canvassed in the second follow-up stated that they had been to their own physician at least once during the preceding six months for medical advice, other than for specific medical treatment. (3) Cardiac signs seem to have been moderately stirred up by the epidemic, the percentage of cases, as compared with preëpidemic examinations, increasing from 5 to 8 per cent in the first follow-up. However, the disappearance of these symptoms in the second follow-up seems to have been substantial, and the general wave of cardiac symptoms seems to have subsided to a figure approximately the same as the preëpidemic finding. (4) Persistent, vague and undiagnosed respiratory findings were increased by the epidemic, this increase apparently persisting during the second and third follow-ups. (5) While the number of active cases of tuberculosis discovered in the group after the epidemic in the first follow-up was increased by 1 per cent over the preëpidemic findings, this apparent lighting up of the disease seems to have been more than compensated for by the rearrest of the active process in this group, as indicated both by the findings in the second and third follow-ups (0.3 per cent in the second follow-up) and by the general observations of the medical staff, leading to the conclusion that the epidemic has not been a conspicuous, responsible factor in increasing the prevalence of active tuberculosis. The conclusion is further substantiated by the mortality-rates in Framingham and, indeed, throughout the United States.

Analysis of 123 Cases of Anthrax in the Pennsylvania Leather Industry.—SMYTH and BRICKER (*Jour. Indust. Hyg.*, 1922, **4**, 53) report

123 cases of anthrax connected with the tanning industry in the twelve years from 1910 to 1921, inclusive. This number represents almost 12 per cent of the directly exposed employees. The mortality among these 123 cases was over 21 per cent. The authors state that in the five-year period for which accurate statistics were made, there was a yearly morbidity rate of almost 2 per cent of the directly exposed employees. The directly exposed employees include those handling raw stock and those soaking and liming this stock. Anthrax has been contracted from the handling of non-packer cattle hides from Texas, Mexico, China, India and South America, and from goat skins from many regions. Anthrax has been contracted from the handling of both dry and wet salted hides and skins, and from both certified and uncertified stock, and anthrax bacilli have been isolated from both. The present practice of certification offers little or no protection to the tanner. The mortality of cases treated in hospitals has been considerably less than one-half that of unhospitalized cases. In Pennsylvania apparently the best results of treatment have been obtained by the injection of strong phenol solutions (25 to 50 per cent) locally around the area of the initial lesion, with or without excision of the lesion. The use of antianthrax serum with excision of the local lesion has also given excellent results, and the authors do not desire to create the impression that it should not be used. They state they would be inclined, from a consideration of the Pennsylvania experience, to advocate the continued intensive use of a reliable serum subcutaneously or intravenously, combined with excision of the local lesion and the injection of concentrated phenol solution around the wound. Early diagnosis, prompt hospitalization if possible, and absolute rest are essential for success in any form of treatment. Anthrax continues to be a decided menace to both the cattle hide and goat skin tanner and will continue to be so until some method is developed whereby tanneries cease to receive anthrax infested raw stock. Seymour-Jones advocates for England the prohibition of the importation of any raw stock not previously converted to the wet salt state by means of his formic acid and mercuric chloride method. Whatever method may be finally adopted the authors feel strongly that all undisinfected imported stock should be disinfected at one or more centrally located government disinfecting stations before being shipped to the tanners, as the English government is doing at present with wool and hair.

Notice to Contributors.—All communications intended for insertion in the Original Department of this JOURNAL are received only *with the distinct understanding that they are contributed exclusively to this* JOURNAL.

Contributions from abroad written in a foreign language, if on examination they are found desirable for this JOURNAL, will be translated at its expense.

A limited number of reprints in pamphlet form, if desired, will be furnished to authors, *providing the request for them be written on the manuscript.*

All communications should be addressed to—

DR. JOHN H. MUSSER, JR., 262 S. 21st Street, Philadelphia, Pa., U. S. A.

THE

AMERICAN JOURNAL

OF THE MEDICAL SCIENCES

APRIL, 1923

ORIGINAL ARTICLES.

SOME OBSERVATIONS UPON THE HISTOLOGICAL CHANGES IN LYMPHATIC GLANDS FOLLOWING EXPOSURE TO RADIUM.

By J. C. Mottram, M.D.,

(From the Research Department, Radium Institute, London.)

The following observations were made with reference to certain problems of cancer immunity, although here they are published largely divorced from the cancer problem. They are concerned with the histological changes in the iliac lymphatic gland of the rat which follow exposure of the whole animal to radiations from radium. In this very difficult and controversial field conclusions have only been drawn with great diffidence, and perhaps more especially with a view to encourage other workers to take up what appears to be a profitable line of investigation.

A brief description of the histological structure of the normal iliac lymph gland of the rat is a necessary preliminary. The gland is enclosed in a fine connective tissue capsule, which sends fine processes throughout the gland, dividing it into a sponge-like meshwork. At one or more places a hilum is seen where a thicker band of connective tissue enters the gland, carrying with it bloodvessels and lymphatic vessels. The whole gland is composed of a spongework of lymphatic channels and reticular cells; the afferent lymphatic vessels open into this system at the surface of the gland, the efferent leave it centrally via the hilum. Between these channels lie the various cell masses shown diagrammatically in Fig. 1.

(*a*) Irregular islands of plasmoidocytes occupy the center of the gland; they usually extend to the margin in a few places (X and

Y in Fig. 1). They are grouped around the bloodvessels, and separated by lymphocytic channels, The exact nature of these cells is in doubt; some observers describe them as plasma cells, other consider that they are lymphoid myeloblasts. They closely resemble cells which give rise to red cells in the spleen, and very occasionally have been seen having the same function in the iliac

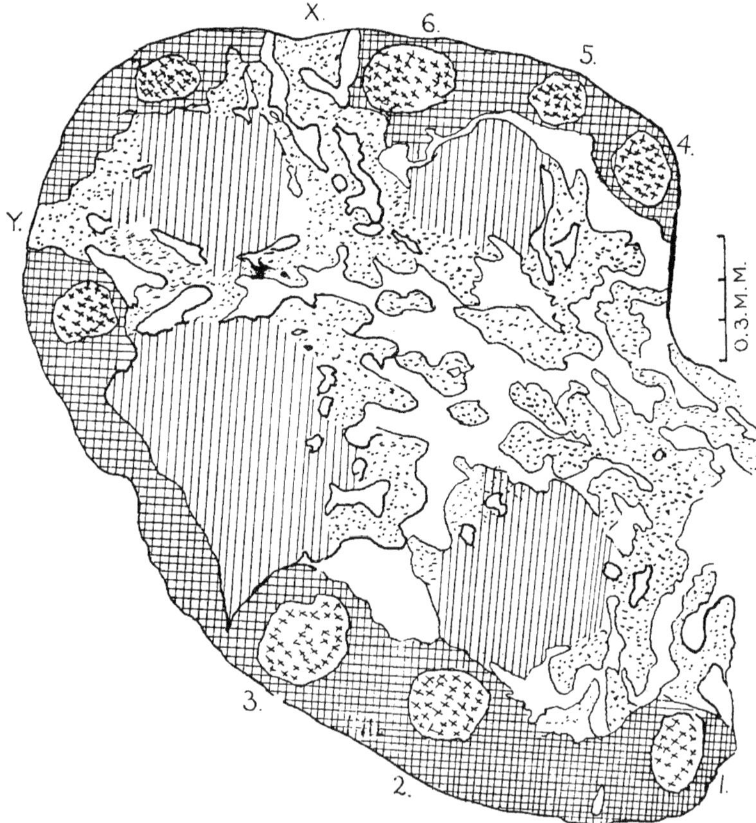

FIG. 1.—Projection drawing of a normal iliac lymphatic gland. Dotted areas, plasmoidocytes; plain areas, lymphatic channels; lined areas, central group of lymphocytes; cross-hatched areas, marginal ring of lymphocytes; areas with crosses, follicles.

lymph gland. As they have not quite typical plasma cell characters, Maximow called them plasmoidocytes, and this term is used throughout this communication.

(*b*) More or less circular masses of lymphocytes are also centrally placed, and grouped around the bloodvessels. They are directly continuous with the plasmoidocyte masses, as shown in Fig. 1

(lined areas). When they occur the lymphatic channels are collapsed, or filled with lymphocytes.

(*c*) Just within the capsule of the gland there is a ring of lymphocytes (cross hatched areas), quite distinct from the central group of lymphocytes, and not continuous with the plasma cell groups. This ring, as already mentioned, may not be complete; it is absent where the plasma cells reach the margin. It varies considerably in thickness.

(*d*) Round the margin and lying among the marginal lymphocytes are follicles consisting of circular collections of macrophages (clasmatocytes or phagocytic endothelial cells). (Areas with crosses.) Around the outer half of these corpuscles the marginal lymphocytes are especially accumulated, whereas on their inner side they are scanty or absent.

With this general description attention may now be directed to more detailed histological findings. Dividing cells are only to be seen in two situations, among the cells forming the follicles, and among the plasma cells. Mitotic figures, though specially stained for, have never been seen on either the marginal or central groups of lymphocytes.

As regards the follicles, the generally accepted view is that they are the mother cells of the lymphocytes found more or less surrounding them. The following facts are, however, against this conclusion:

1. As before mentioned, the surrounding lymphocytes are numerous toward the outer side, and few or absent on the inner of the follicles: whereas the distribution of the mitotic figures is exactly the reverse (Fig. 2). It follows that cell division is confined to the side where few or no lymphocytes are found.

2. Mitotic figures are not especially confined to the outlying cells of the follicles, and yet lymphocytes are never seen scattered among these cells either in the center of the follicle or toward its inner margin. They are, however, to be seen among the cells forming the outer margin of the follicle, where, however, mitotic figures are very rarely seen.

3. The lymphocytes surrounding the follicles have not the characters of young cells recently divided off. Their protoplasm is not scanty, and the nucleus is irregular in shape, pyknotic, and stains palely. They have, in fact, the characters of old partly degenerated cells rather than young (Fig. 3, *b*).

4. These degenerated appearances are especially marked among the lymphocytes directly abutting on the follicles, and especially among these found scattered among the follicle cells along the outer margin (Fig. 3, *c*).

5. There is evidence that these margin lymphocytes are carried on to the gland by means of the afferent lymphatics. The afferent lymphatics enter the gland all along its outer margin, opening directly into the lymphatic space immediately within the capsule,

and it is clear that any lymphocytes carried in the afferent lymph will be deposited here.

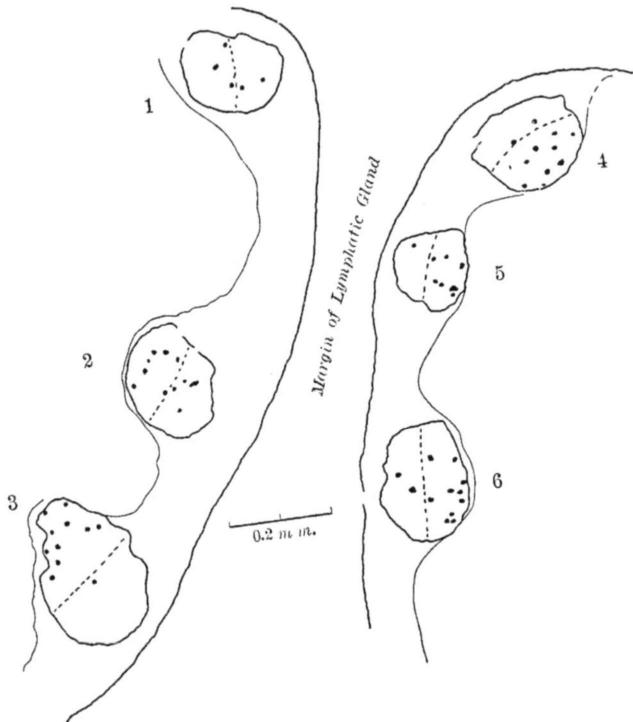

FIG. 2.—The six follicles of Fig. 1, showing the distribution of the mitotic figures. Note that the mitoses are for the most part internal to the middle line (dotted).

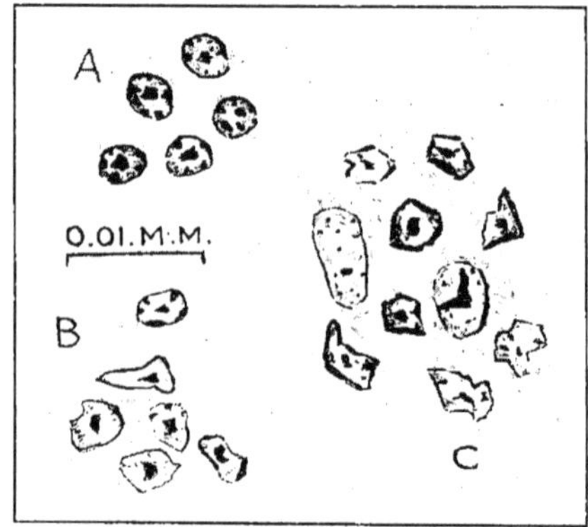

FIG. 3.—Lymphocytes, *a*, from the central group; *b*, from the marginal group; and *c*, lying among the outer cells of the follicles.

To test this the following experiment was carried out. The right iliac glands of six rats were removed. During the succeeding night the animals were subjected to β and γ radiation (unscreened) sufficient to produce a marked disappearance of lymphocytes from the circulation; the left iliac glands were removed the next day, in some cases immediately, and in other cases, a few hours after the radiation was stopped. A histological comparison on the two sets of glands was then made, and it was found that in each case a very great increase in the number of marginal lymphocytes had occurred, without any increase in the number of mitoses in the follicles, and further, that these lymphocytes presented degenerative changes. Control experiments carried out without radiation, using six animals, showed no such change.

If the cells of the follicles do not produce lymphocytes by mitosis they must be converted into some other cells, for their accumulation in the lymphatic gland is limited, and yet their rate of division is rapid, judging from the great number of dividing cells seen. Evidence will be brought forward later as regards their destination.

Nevertheless, they have some relation to the lymphocytes, which accumulate around them in this characteristic manner. The clue to this relationship is given by the numerous cell inclusions to be seen within vacuoles in their protoplasm. They were first described by Flemming, who called them "stainable particles," and concluded that they were particles of chromatin. They stain very deeply with basic dyes, as do dividing and some forms of degenerating chromatin. It is now certain that they represent the phagocytosis of lymphocytes.

The drawing shown in Fig. 4 represents all the stages from the first inclusion of a lymphocyte within the vacuole to its final disintegration into fine granules. The first change is a loss of the structural detail of the nucleus, accompanied by a tendency to stain more darkly than the nuclei of the surrounding, but not yet ingested, lymphocytes. The next change is a fragmentation of the darkened nucleus into at first large, and subsequently small dark granules. Finally these granules gradually change their staining qualities. For instance if stained with pyronin-methyl-green after fixation with acetic alcohol, they first stain purple, but finally the fine granules take only the pyronin, or if stained with eosinate of methylene blue and eosin after fixation with formol-potassium-bichromate, they first stain dark blue, then purple, and finally red. Thus the basic nuclear staining quality gradually changes to a more protoplasmic acid type.

The last stage consists of the disappearance of the vacuole and the disposition of the red granules in the protoplasm chiefly around the surface, away from the nucleus. It is possible that the vacuole may be to some extent due to shrinkage during fixation, as it varies much in size in different specimens.

It may be here mentioned that the amount of this phagocytosis is directly proportional to the number of lymphocytes around the follicles, and it is not seen in the absence of marginal lymphocytes, whereas it is especially abundant with the great marginal accumulation following radiation.

It is doubtful whether all of the marginal lymphocytes are in this way destroyed, or only the more degenerated forms, the others passing through the gland by means of the lymphatic channels and efferent lymphatics.

Turning now to the plasmoidocytes (or myeloblasts) occupying the central areas of the gland, they, like the cells of the follicles, are to be seen undergoing mitosis. It is possible that this division to some extent results in an increase in the number of plasmoidocytes; but such an increase must soon reach a limit, as there is no evidence that these cells leave the gland either in the blood or lymph, or by

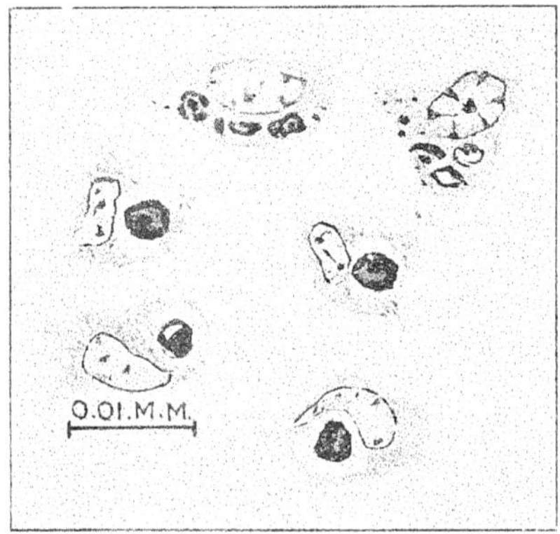

FIG. 4.—Follicle cells containing lymphocytes in various stages of phagocytosis.

other means. From the following observations it is concluded that they by their division give rise to lymphocytes:

1. The central groups of lymphocytes occupy similar positions to the plasmoidocyte groups (Fig. 1).

2. At the margins these groups of lymphocytes are directly continuous with the plasmoidocyte groups (Fig. 1.)

3. At this junction of lymphocytes and plasmoidocytes, dividing plasmoidocytes are especially to be seen, as if the change by division was occurring here.

4. There is a correlation between these two groups; when central "lymphocytes are abundant" plasmoidocyte groups are scanty and *vice versa*.

5. The lymphocytes of the central group have the characters of young cells. They have a scanty protoplasm, a small round darkly stained nucleus, and often show the kataphase condition of mitosis.

6. The return of lymphocytes to the circulation is associated with division of the plasmoidocytes in the gland, as is shown by the following experiment.

The prolonged exposure of an animal to radium irradiation or roentgen-rays results in a great destruction of lymphocytes through-

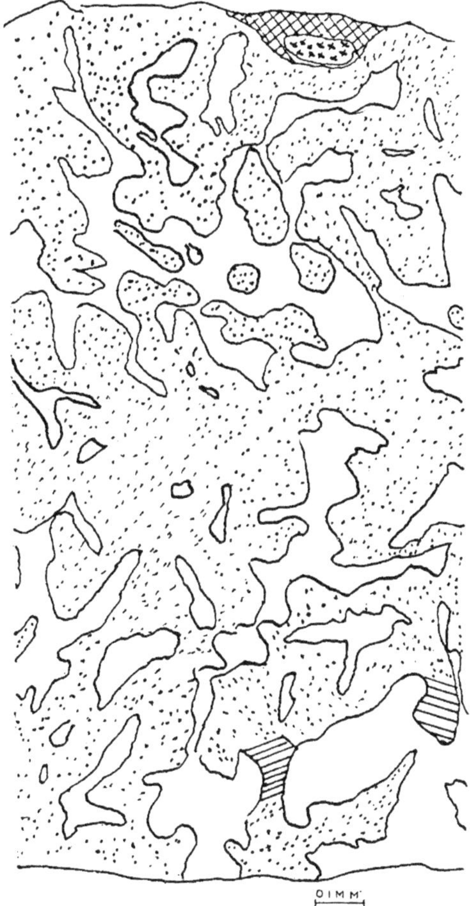

FIG. 5.—Projection of an iliac lymphatic gland after an exposure of the animal to 0.22 rads; the various cell groups are indicated as in Fig. 1.

out the body, so much so that sections of lymphoid tissues such as the spleen or lymphatic gland may fail to show a single lymphocyte (Fig. 5). It is evident that not only must existing lymphocytes have been destroyed, but also the production of fresh lymphocytes must have been inhibited. If lymphocytes are derived from the division of plasmoidocytes in the lymphatic gland of the rat, then prolonged exposure to radium by inhibiting this division should result in the accumulation of these plasmoidocytes.

This expectation was found to be the case. After exposure to γ radiation for twelve days (0.22 rads), the inguinal lymph glands in the case of five animals were found to consist almost solely of plasmoidocytes, in some cases entirely.

It has already been mentioned that there is evidence that the cells of the follicles do not by division form lymphocytes, but have some other relation. The following facts suggest that they may become converted into plasmoidocytes:

1. It is possible to trace every intermediate stage between a macrophage cell of the follicle and a plasmoidocyte.

2. The macrophages gradually accumulate, by the digestion of lymphocytes, red granules in their protoplasm which have exactly similar staining qualities as the red granules of plasmoidocytes, and these granules tend from their first appearance to be deposited not near the nucleus, but toward the outside of the cell, as is the case with the plasmoidocytes.

3. It often occurs that the plasmoidocyte group extend right to the margin of the gland, and where this occurs neither marginal lymphocytes nor follicles are seen. In the absence of marginal lymphocytes, the follicle cells cease to divide, and their place is taken by plasmoidocytes.

4. The follicle cells are arranged around bloodvessels on exactly the same way as the plasmoidocytes are.

The functions, origin, and fate of the plasmoidocytes in the lymphatic gland have now been dealt with, and as regards the follicle cells, their function and fate have also been considered, only their origin remains to be discussed.

If a rat be given sufficient γ radiation to produce a profound lymphopenia, it has been seen that a few hours later a considerable accumulation of marginal lymphocytes occurs. If a further interval of time be allowed to elapse before the examination of the gland is made, then numerous young follicles will be seen. The following exposure was found to give good results: 100 mg. $RaBr_2 2H_2O$, screen 2 mm. lead, distance eight inches, time five days, animal killed at end of exposure.

Under these conditions, along the inner edge of the marginal lymphocytes will be seen numerous small bloodvessels and capillaries, lying among a network of lymphatic spaces, lined by endothelial cells. Detailed examination will show, that in many cases, lying in vacuoles of these endothelial cells are the nuclei of lymphocytes in the various stages of digestion shown in Fig. 6. It is here, in fact, that the early stages of this digestion are especially to be seen. Not only do these lymphatic endothelial cells (reticular cells) show this digestion, but also the endothelial cells lining the small bloodvessels.

As further evidence, that there is a close relation between a typical endothelial cell and the cells of the follicles, is the fact that every gradation from one to the other can easily be found, as shown in Fig. 7.

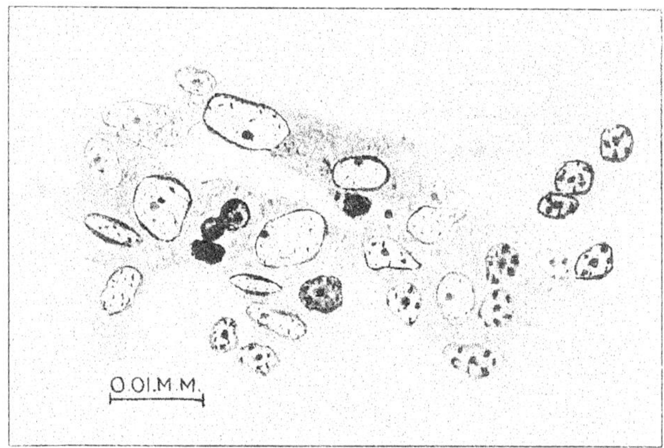

Fig. 6.—Endothelial cells lining a lymphatic channel, showing phagocytosis of lymphocytes.

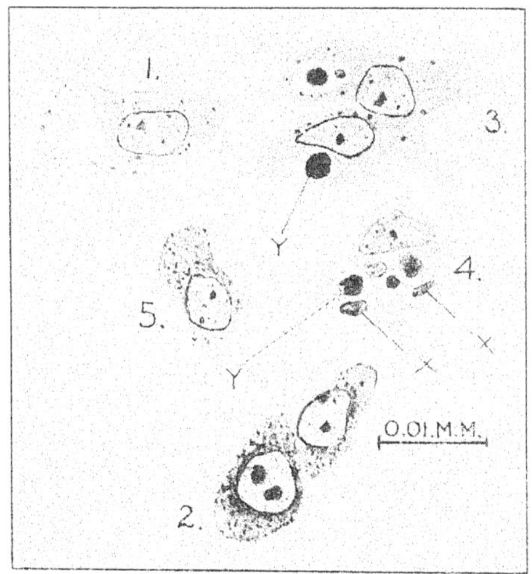

Fig. 7.—Shows transition from endothelial cell, 1, to follicle cell, 2, 3 and 4, endothelial cells phagocytosing lymphocytes; 5, endothelial cell intermediate in respect of granules between endothelial and follicle cell.

The follicle cell differs from the endothelial cell only qualitatively, the pale staining nucleus is common to both; both have one or two nucleoli, large in the follicle cells, small in the endothelial cell. In both the protoplasm is moderate in quantity and finely reticular, it contains fine red granules when stained with eosinate of methylene blue, numerous in the follicle cell, and scanty in the endothelial cell. Other staining methods do not differentiate any qualitative difference.

The way in which the lymphocytes arising from division of the plasmoidocytes leave the lymphatic gland and find their way into the blood stream remains to be considered. The finding of many young lymphocytes in the efferent lymphatic vessels is strong evidence that this is a way of exit. Nevertheless examination of the bloodvessels running among the central groups of lymphocytes often reveals lymphocytes lying between the lining endothelial cells, as shown in Fig. 8. Thus this direct migration into the blood stream appears to be an alternative way.

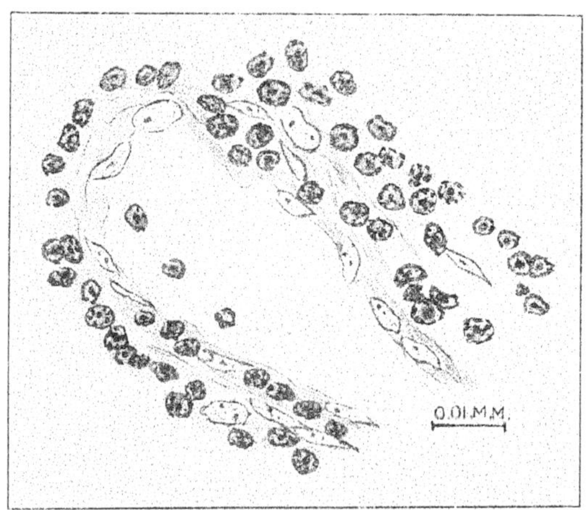

Fig. 8.—Portion of a small bloodvessel traversing a central group of lymphocytes, showing lymphocytes lying between the endothelial cells.

As before mentioned plasmoidocytes are not seen in either of these situations.

The accompanying diagram (Fig. 9) gives a concise view of the conclusions which have been drawn, the arrow denoting the direction of the changes. Some conclusions have been drawn with confidence, such as the phagocytosis of lymphocytes by follicle cells, others with doubt, such as the conversion of follicle cells into plasmoidocytes.

Lymphocytes, *L*, enter the gland by the afferent lymphatics, and are devoured by endothelial cells, *E*. These cells then gradually change into follicle cells, *M*; increasing in numbers by cell division, they next become converted into plasmoidocytes or myelocytes, *P*. The plasmoidocytes divide into lymphocytes, which leave the gland by the efferent lymphocytes, or possibly by the bloodvessels.

These observations have an important bearing upon the work being carried out at the Middlesex Hospital[2 3 4], and the Rockefeller Institute[5 6 7] upon the relation between lymphocytes and cancer immunity. For instance, at the Rockefeller Institute numerous communications have appeared showing that an exposure of animals to small doses of roentgen-rays and dry heat is followed by an increase in the number of mitotic figures in the corpuscles of the spleen and lymph glands, and this has been taken as evidence of a stimulation of lymphocytic formation, whereas according to the views here laid down, it is due to the accumulation of degenerated lymphocytes as a result of the treatment.

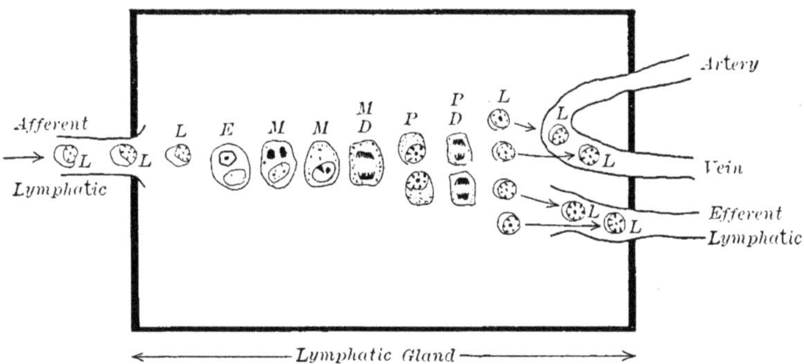

Fig. 9.—Diagram of the conclusions which have been arrived at. *L*, lymphocyte; *E*, endothelial cell; *M*, macrophage of follicle; *M D*, macrophage, dividing; *P*, plasmoidocyte; *P D*, plasmoidocyte dividing. The sequence of changes reads from left to right.

It may be mentioned that Murphy and his associates noted the degenerated and pyknotic lymphocytes surrounding the corpuscles. Further reference to their communication will reveal the fact that the lymphocytosis which follows exposure to roentgen-rays and dry heat does not correspond in point of time with the increased number of mitoses in the follicles. This occurs often many days before the lymphocytosis appears in the circulation, and they make special note of this discrepancy, namely the finding of increased mitosis, but without lymphocytosis.

It may be mentioned that two observers, Latta[8] and Maximow[9] have both recently concluded that the follicle cells phagocyte lymphocytes.

REFERENCES.

1. Cleland, Trares: Path. Soc., London, 1905, **56**, 381.
2. Mottram, J. C., and Russ, C.: Proc. Roy. Soc., 1917, **90**, 1.
3. Russ, C., Chambers, H., Scott, G. M., and Mottram, J. C.: Lancet, 1919, **1**, 692.
4. Mottram, J. C., and Russ, C.: Jour. Exper. Med., 1921, **34**, 271.
5. Nakahara, W.: Jour. Exper. Med., 1919, **29**, 17, 83.
6. Murphy, J. B., and Nakahara, W.: Jour. Exper. Med., 1920, **31**, 1, 13.
7. Murphy, J. B., and Nakahara, W.: Anat. Record, 1921, **22**, 107.
8. Latta, J. S.: Am. Jour. Anat., 1921, **29**, 159.
9. Maximow, A.: Compt. rend. Soc. de biol., 1917, **80**, 222.

THE PERMEABILITY OF THE INTESTINAL MUCOSA TO CERTAIN TYPES OF BACTERIA, DETERMINED BY CULTURES FROM THE THORACIC DUCT.

By Carl S. Williamson, M.D.,
Division of Experimental Surgery and Pathology,

and

Rollo O. Brown, M.D.,
Fellow in Surgery, Mayo Foundation, Rochester, Minn.

In many cases of pneumonia developing soon after operations in the abdominal cavity the cause is obscure. In view of the fact that bacteria producing chronic pulmonary lesions often gain access to the respiratory tract by way of the digestive tract and lymphatics, it occurred to us that the same route might be available to bacteria producing postoperative pneumonia. We, therefore, made the investigation which is described here.

An attempt was made to learn if bacteria introduced into the intestinal canal under normal conditions, and conditions comparable to operative procedures could be recovered from the lymph stream. The observations were made on dogs with thoracic duct fistulas. Sterile technic was used in all the operative procedures. The technic for making the thoracic duct fistula was modified from that employed by Biedl and will be described briefly.

Technic of Operation. The animal was fasted for from twelve to sixteen hours, and four to six hours before operation, it was fed a mixture consisting of 300 cc of milk and 200 cc of melted lard. In most instances the animal ate the meal readily, although it was necessary to give the mixture with a stomach tube to some. The meal of fat was given to stimulate the flow of lymph, to distend the lymphatic channels, and to make it easier to identify the thoracic duct. After sufficient time had elapsed, the animal was placed in an etherizing cabinet and anesthetized quickly in order to prevent vomiting; afterward it was placed on the operating table and ether was given by an anesthetometer. The maintenance of artificial respiration was necessary in case of accidental puncture of the pleura during the course of the operation. The purpose of this operation was to make the external jugular vein a conduit for the discharge of lymph, unmixed with blood, to the outside.

A straight incision was made over the left jugular vein extending from the middle of the clavicle upward to the level of the cricoid cartilage. The vein was then dissected free and all tributaries were ligated and sectioned. After the external jugular vein had been freed its junction with the internal was sought and the point of entrance of the thoracic duct located (see illustration). A ligature was then placed around the venous trunk on the cardiac side of the entrance of the duct and another around the internal jugular vein about 1 cm. from its junction with the external. After all veins entering into the common jugular had been ligated, a ligature was placed around the external jugular near the upper border of the thyroid cartilage and the vein was sectioned below. The clotted blood was expressed from the vein and a flow of lymph was established. A soft rubber catheter was inserted into the vein, and

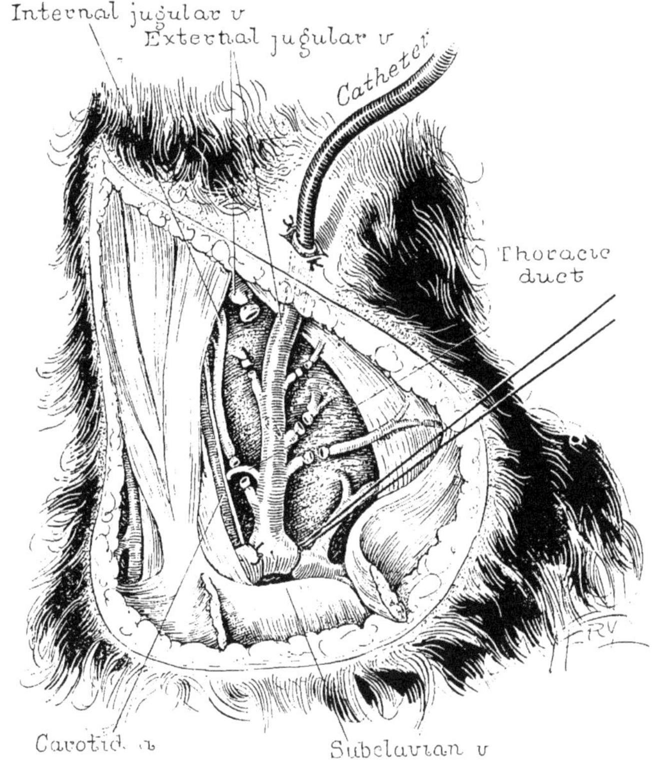

Diagrammatic sketch showing duct fistula.

the vein with its catheter was brought out through a stab wound in the skin and sutured in place with one or two silk sutures. In a few days the catheter came away, leaving a patent fistula.

It was possible, with careful handling, to maintain a flow of lymph for from two to four weeks, but in the majority of instances the fistula closed in about two weeks. Collateral circulation of lymph develops very rapidly in the presence of obstruction, hindering free discharge to the outside.

After the fistula was established, it was necessary to select an organism. It must be easily cultivated, not commonly found in the laboratory, nonpathogenic, and readily identified. Bacillus *prodigiosus* was chosen as the organism most nearly meeting all these requirements. The bacteria were grown either on dextrose-agar plates or in dextrose-bouillon. Cultures forty-eight hours old usually were used for injection. Bouillon cultures were employed in a few experiments only; they were fed or administered by stomach tube. The agar cultures were removed from the plates with as little agar as possible and placed in normal salt solution. This was well shaken to insure even distribution and administered by stomach tube. Attempt to estimate the number of bacteria for each unit of solution was not made. Control cultures were always taken before administration to insure the use of a viable organism. In the case of the salt suspension, the solution used contained enough organisms to make a definite pink color. The amount of suspension given varied from 20 to 30 cc for each dose. Before the bacteria were administered control cultures of lymph from the thoracic duct fistula were always made in order to rule out the possibility of contamination from the animal's cage. After feeding, cultures of lymph were made at hourly intervals during a period of from six to eight hours; in most cases cultures were made twenty-four and forty-eight hours after ingestion. All cultures were taken on sterile cotton swabs and plated on dextrose-agar plates. These were then incubated at room temperature for from twenty-four to forty-eight hours. Suspicious appearing colonies were subcultured and the organisms identified microscopically.

Experiments. Our experiments were divided into eight groups, each group comprising a minimum of five experiments and several groups containing from fifteen to twenty. The standard technic for culturing referred to was used in all experiments with the exception of the group in which the feces were cultures. The technic of this experiment is explained in the summary of Group 7.

Group 1. The animals were fasted for from twelve to twenty-four hours and then bacteria were administered with a small amount of food or, as in some instances, by stomach tube. The condition of the gastrointestinal tract in fasting animals is comparable to that obtained in man by preoperative fasting. All cultures in this group of experiments were negative.

Group 2. In many preoperative cases a purge of castor oil or magnesium sulphate is given. This causes some irritation of the intestinal tract, and might be a factor in allowing the passage of bacteria from the intestinal canal into the lymph stream. In this group of experiments 45 to 60 cc castor oil, or 15 to 20 gm. magnesium sulphate were given twelve to fifteen hours prior to feeding. The technic of feeding and culturing was the same as that employed in Group 1, and the same negative results were obtained.

Group 3. Certain observers have found that the permeability of the intestinal tract to bacteria is increased by certain types of food, particularly fat. By the technic used in the experiments in Groups 1 and 2, we attempted to determine the influence of diet on absorption of bacteria. Besides the bacteria, the animals were given diets rich in protein, fat, and carbohydrates, and some experiments were run in which the animals were on mixed diets. Cultures taken from animals on the various diets were negative for the ingested bacteria.

Group 4. Since we believed that the bacteria might be killed by the gastric juice during their passage through the stomach, it was desirable to obviate this possibility and at the same time, to introduce them near the beginning of the jejunum. This, besides lessening the concentration of the hydrochloric acid, would provide for maximal absorption. A loop of the jejunum, 15 to 30 cm. below the ligament of Treitz, was sutured beneath the skin ten to twelve days before the experiment was performed. A middle line incision was made under sterile technic, and the jejunum was brought up the desired distance from the ligament of Treitz. The recti muscles were sutured together beneath the loop of intestine with interrupted sutures of No. 2 catgut. Care must be taken to insure a sufficient opening at the point of exit from and entrance into the abdominal cavity. If caution is not used the points of exit and entry are apt to be too small and result in obstruction. It is also important, in drawing the edges of the recti muscles together, not to place the sutures too close together or to pull them too firmly else they are apt to obstruct the flow of blood to the transposed loop of intestine. We usually transpose a loop 12 to 15 cm. long and use four sutures to hold the recti together beneath it. After the edges of the recti were sutured together the subcutaneous fascia was closed with a continuous layer of catgut sutures. The skin was then closed with a continuous suture of linen. The wound healed in a few days and a thoracic duct fistula was made as in previous experiments. With a syringe and needle 20 to 30 cc of a salt solution suspension of bacteria were injected directly into the jejunum, which was readily felt beneath the skin. Cultures from these animals were entirely negative, showing that the gastric juice is not a factor in the negative cultures obtained from the lymph of the thoracic duct, and from the feces.

Group 5. In the experiments in Groups 1 to 5, the permeability of the normal intestinal tract to bacteria, exclusively, has been tested. In experiments of Group 5 we introduced a traumatic factor. Dogs with freely discharging duct fistulas were anesthetized and placed on the operating table, and the abdomen was opened. The viscera were brought out of the peritoneal cavity and exposed to the air for from fifteen to twenty minutes. In some instances, also, the viscera were rubbed with a dry gauze sponge until gentle oozing occurred. At the end of the traumatic period, fifteen to twenty minutes, the bacteria, 20 to 30 cc of a pink solution, were injected by a hypodermic syringe directly into the stomach or, as in some instances, into the jejunum, and the abdomen was closed. The animal was then allowed to recover from the ether and cultures were taken as in the preceding experiments. Several cultures were positive, but in each instance the animal had vomited while recovering from the anesthetic and these positive cultures were regarded as contaminations. Cultures of the vomitus were positive. Trauma, then, did not make the intestinal tract more permeable to bacteria, as shown by cultures of the lymph from the thoracic duct.

Group 6. Realizing that the preceding experiments, while similar, are not comparable to operative procedures on the intestinal tract, we performed standard intestinal operations on dogs with fistulas as of the thoracic duct, for example, gastroenterostomies and end-to-end anastomoses. At the completion of operation bacteria were injected into the stomachs of the dogs with gastroenterostomies and into the intestines above the anastomosis in dogs with end-to-end anastomoses. Routine cultures taken following operation in this group of experiments were negative.

Group 7. Since absorption from the colon occurs, as demonstrated by rectal feeding and so forth, we decided to determine whether bacteria injected into the rectum could be recovered from the thoracic duct by culture. From 90 to 100 cc of the standard bacterial suspension was slowly injected into the rectum by means of a rubber tube, and in most instances the animals retained practically all of the injected fluid. However, routine cultures from the thoracic duct were uniformly negative for *Bacillus prodigiosus.*

We wished to learn if bacteria ingested as in the preceding experiments could be recovered from the feces, and, therefore, the feces of a few animals, two or three in each series, were cultured twelve, twenty-four, forty-eight, and seventy-two hours after ingestion. These cultures were always negative, showing that the ingested bacteria disappeared somewhere along the digestive tract.

Group 8. In this series of experiments eight animals with freely discharging ducts were used. From 20 to 30 cc of the standard bacterial suspension were injected with a needle and syringe directly into the peritoneal cavity, and routine cultures from the discharging duct were made. Positive cultures were obtained from four of the eight animals in from two to four hours after injection. This is the only group of experiments in the entire, comparatively large, series in which the results were positive.

Discussion. Much work has been done to show that bacteria pass from the intestinal tract into the blood stream, especially bacteria that produce chronic diseases. Ravenel, working with the bacillus of tuberculosis, recovered the organism from the blood after ingestion in a high percentage of instances. Diet was a factor in the success of these experiments, that is, an animal fed on fat before or simultaneously with the bacteria always showed a greater number of positive blood cultures than did the fasting animal. Nicolas and Descas have also shown the influence of diet on the permeability of the intestine to bacteria as shown by culture of the blood.

In our experiments cultures of the lymph from the thoracic duct following ingestion of *Bacillus prodigiosus*, regardless of the diet of the animal, were always negative, as were cultures of the feces. Somewhere along the digestive tract the bacteria were destroyed or absorbed. We consider that, to a large extent, the germicidal action of the acid gastric juice was ruled out in the experiments of Group 4, but even these cultures were negative. However, it was not possible to rule out the destroying power of the digestive juices for the bacteria. The intestinal tract is host to many types of bacteria, but *Bacillus prodigiosus* is not among them, and it is entirely possible that a new organism in the intestinal tract is promptly destroyed by the action of the digestive fluids. On this point we can offer no direct evidence except to call attention to the countless varieties of bacteria that are constantly being taken into the body with the food, only a small number of which survive unless they are especially resistant, as is the bacillus of tuberculosis.

On the other hand, two other possibilities must be considered in accounting for the disappearance of the ingested organisms. These bacteria may pass through the intestinal villæ directly into the blood stream; but since our problem has to do only with the recovery of the ingested bacteria from a discharging thoracic duct, we have made no observations on this point. The other possibility is that the bacteria did pass through the intestinal wall with the chyle, but were destroyed, or came through in such small numbers by our method of culturing that they were not recovered.

Hess has shown that, if bacteria are injected into the colon and blood cultures made, it is necessary to use a large amount of blood in order to recover the bacteria. We believe that if bacteria come through the thoracic duct in such a small number as not to be detected by our method of culture, they could not be a factor in the production of postoperative pneumonia. Hess also determined that *Bacillus prodigiosus* injected into the rectums and colons of rabbits could be recovered from the upper digestive tract within a few hours after injection and also from the blood stream, if large amounts of blood were cultured. Ravenel and Hammer, in attempting to confirm the work of Hess, concluded, from a small series of experiments, that passage of bacteria from the rectum and colon into the blood stream is problematic. From observations on the possible passage of bacteria from the rectum and colon into the lymph stream we have reached the same conclusion as regards the lymph as Ravenel and Hammer reached in regard to the blood.

The experiments of Group 8 were made as control experiments on the passage of bacteria from the intestinal tract into the lymph. We, at present, are not prepared to discuss the significance of the passage of bacteria from the peritoneal cavity into the lymph; this will be dealt with in a future paper.

Conclusions. 1. It is not possible to recover *Bacillus prodigiosus* from a fistula of the thoracic duct by culture of the lymph after ingestion of the organisms.

2. The negative results were not influenced by diet or by trauma due to exposure of the viscera or to standard operative procedures.

3. Cultures of the feces for the ingested organisms were negative.

4. Cultures obtained from the thoracic duct following injection of the bacteria into the peritoneal cavity were positive in 50 per cent of the experiments of Group 8.

BIBLIOGRAPHY.

1. Hess, A. F.: Antiperistalsis in its Relation to Tubercle Bacilli and Other Bacteria in the Alimentary Tract. Jour. Med. Res., 1910, **22**, 129–144.
2. Nicolas and Descas: Quoted by Ravenel.
3. Ravenel, M. P.: The Etiology of Tuberculosis. Am. Jour. Med. Sci., 1907, **134**, 469–482.
4. Ravenel, M. P., and Hammer, B. W.: Passage of Bacteria through the Intestinal Wall. Jour. Med. Res., 1911, **24**, 513–515.

A STUDY OF THE BILE OBTAINED BY NONSURGICAL BILIARY DRAINAGE, WITH ESPECIAL REFERENCE TO ITS BACTERIOLOGY.*

By George Morris Piersol, M.D.,

and

H. L. Bockus, M.D.,

PHILADELPHIA.

It is our purpose in this paper to point out the information of practical clinical importance that may be obtained from a study of the bile collected by means of duodenal drainage. In 1919, B. B. Vincent Lyon[1] published a paper in which he showed how fresh bile may be obtained through duodenal drainage, basing this work of practical value upon a suggestion made by Meltzer[2] two years before in an article entitled "Disturbances of the Law of Contrary Innervation as a Pathogenetic Factor in the Diseases of the Bile Duct and Gall-bladder." Until recently, such a procedure would

* Read before the American Climatological and Clinical Association, May 3, 1922, at Washington, D. C.

1 Jour. Am. Med. Assn., 1919, **73**, 980.

2 Am. Jour. Med. Sci., 1917, **153**, 469.

have been out of the question, for up to 1919 practically all studies upon the composition and bacteriology of the bile were made entirely upon bile obtained from the gall-bladder at operations or at autopsy, or through postoperative biliary fistulæ, with the exception of studies made on the fasting bile by Einhorn.

It will be recalled that in this connection Meltzer suggested the possibility of causing, through "crossed innervation," the paradoxical situation of relaxation of the sphincter of the common duct and at the same time contraction of the gall-bladder by the local application to the duodenum, by means of the duodenal tube, of a 25 per cent solution of magnesium sulphate. In making this suggestion, Meltzer but elaborated upon the well-proved physiologic observations made over twenty years before by Doyon and Oddi. To Lyon, however, belongs the credit of first making practical use of these physiologic and pharmacologic facts in diagnosis. He showed that when through a duodenal tube hyperisotonic solutions of magnesium sulphate are brought in contact with the duodenal mucous membrane and are withdrawn before absorption takes place, fresh bile may be obtained from the gall-bladder and bile ducts, and further that this bile may be separated into three definite fractions, *i. e.*, "A" bile which comes from the common duct, "B" bile which is of a different character and is derived from the gall-bladder, and "C" bile which is obtained from the hepatic ducts and bile capillaries and canaliculæ.

Abundant confirmation of his earlier work has been obtained by Lyon upon an enormous series of cases, and has been further confirmed by a large number of other observers. Thus there has been established a comparatively simple technic, by which with reasonable certainty fresh bile from various portions of the biliary tract may be collected through the duodenal tube. It is not too much to say that the method has become firmly established, and must be looked upon as a well-recognized and necessary additional method of gastrointestinal examination.

In passing it is perhaps fair to point out that the hypothesis advanced by Meltzer, and its further application by Lyon, have not been accorded uniform approval. There are those who question the validity of applying the law of "crossed innervation" to the gall-bladder and the muscle of Oddi. There are others who question whether the sphincteric action of the muscle of Oddi is definitely established and whether there is a specific action of magnesium sulphate in bringing about this relaxation and stimulation through intraduodenal excitation. Much stress is laid upon the fact that Meltzer's hypothesis is purely theoretical and has never been proved. The careful experimental work of Doyon and Oddi, in 1894 and 1895, seems to refute this latter contention. A thorough discussion of these moot points would here be out of place, but it is our belief, based upon personal observation and experience with the method, in conjunction with increasing clinical and experimental evidence, that the principle enunciated by Meltzer and put to practical use by Lyon is in the main entirely reliable. An admirable critical discussion of the entire question has been furnished by Smithies, Karshner and Oleson.[3]

During the past year transduodenal lavage and stimulation of the flow of bile, by the introduction of hyperisotonic magnesium sulphate solution, has become almost a routine practice in the Gastrointestinal Clinic at the Graduate School of the University of Pennsylvania. In the course of this work we have met with the difficulties and disappointments from time to time that have been common to all workers in this field. On the whole our results have been encouraging and rarely has serious difficulty been experienced in introducing a duodenal tube into the duodenum. As a rule, not over an hour and a half has been required to get the tube in place. We have not had the difficulties claimed by some in determining the position of the duodenal tube. Without resorting to fluoroscopic examination we believe that the presence of the tube in the duodenum can usually be determined: (1) By the presence of the "duodenal tug," that is, when the tube is in the duodenum the plunger of the syringe attached to the free end of the tube will return to its position when traction is made upon it. Such is not the case, as a rule, when the tip is still in the stomach. (2) The appearance of pure yellow alkaline bile on aspiration or a lemon-yellow froth. (3) Failure to obtain water in the syringe after half a glass of water has been taken by mouth. (4) When the tube is in the duodenum, if 30 cc of warm water are allowed to run in and are then siphoned off by gravity the water will return definitely bile-stained. The latter method is particularly efficacious in those cases in which nothing can be obtained by aspiration due to a closed sphincter.

We have experienced but little difficulty in recognizing the three bile fractions referred to by Lyon, namely, the "A," "B" and "C" bile. Doubt has been entertained by some as to whether the dark bile alleged to come from the gall-bladder is actually derived from this source. In this connection observations, which are being carried out by one of us in conjunction with Dr. Eimann, of the Bacteriological Laboratories of the Presbyterian Hospital of Philadelphia, and which await later publication, are suggestive. Estimation of the cholesterin content of the various specimens of bile conclusively shows that in the dark gall-bladder bile the amount of cholesterin is approximately four and a half times greater than that obtained from either the common duct or hepatic duct specimens. This increased cholesterin content results from the concentration and stagnation of the bile which takes place in

[3] Jour. Am. Med. Assn., 1921, 77, 2036.

the gall-bladder. The remarkable ability of the gall-bladder to concentrate the bile, and the restriction of this concentrating ability to the gall-bladder, has been admirably shown by the work of Rous and McMaster.[4] These authors have shown that bile is actually diluted in the bile ducts, whereas the gall-bladder is able to reduce the bulk of bile delivered to it as much as ten and two-fifths times in twenty-two and a half hours.

Five cases of cystic duct obstruction recently observed are interesting from this standpoint. The diagnosis in 3 of them was definitely confirmed, 1 by operation and 2 by roentgen-ray. There was no reasonable doubt about the diagnosis in the other 2. It was not possible to separate the bile into definite "A," "B" and "C" fractions, as there was no color change. In each case, however, the bile was collected in three separate bottles, the bottles being changed at the time when the color change usually occurs in normal cases. Each case was restimulated several times to be sure that no "B" bile was obtainable. In each case the amount of cholesterin in the three collected samples was practically identical. Compare these cholesterin readings with that for normal cases. In the latter the "B" fraction is always about four and one-half times as rich in cholesterin as the "A" and "C" bile. Its ratio is the same as that given by Hawk[5] in his table comparing the composition of liver bile and gall-bladder bile obtained directly from these organs. The "C" fraction usually contains about 10 mg. more cholesterin than the "A" bile, probably due to its being slightly mixed with the "B" bile. All of these cases had patent common ducts. An ample quantity of bile was drained from each. If this "B" fraction is due to liver stimulation or to magnesium sulphate, as has been claimed by some observers, why was it not possible to drain dark bile from these cases of cystic duct obstruction, there being no interference with the drainage of bile from the liver? If the "B" fraction is due to liver activity and not to concentration of bile in the gall-bladder, why was not the cholesterin content of the bile in the middle of the drainage four and one-half times greater than that obtained early and late in the drainage as it was in normal cases without cystic duct obstruction? Cases of this nature, which are constantly found in routine work, are decidedly convincing and seem to indicate that bile can be definitely separated into fractions, and that these fractions represent the bile from the common duct, gall-bladder and the hepatic duct system in that order. Whether or not the gall-bladder is emptied completely is not definitely known. We do not believe it is as a rule, for upon restimulating after having obtained the three fractions a small amount of gall-bladder bile will frequently be obtained the second time.

[4] Jour. Exper. Med., 1921, **34**, 7.
[5] Practical Physiological Chemistry, Seventh Edition.

The technic employed by us for obtaining samples of bile for ordinary study is essentially the same as that advocated by Lyon and now widely employed. The method is so well known that detailed discussion seems unnecessary.

The accumulated observations of many workers during the last couple of years leave no doubt but that valuable data are obtainable from bile collected by the transduodenal route, from which, with a fair degree of accuracy, may be determined the state of the biliary tract. In order to be of value, it is generally conceded that the study of the bile must be carried out when the specimens are fresh. These studies may be grouped under three headings: (1) The gross appearance of the bile; (2) its microscopic appearance; and (3) its bacteriology.

When such examinations are carried out the following conclusions are justified as to the state of the biliary passages.

If the "A" bile obtained from the common duct is turbid and more viscid than normal and shows the presence of a considerable number of bile-stained epithelial cells of the tall columnar variety, less tall than gall-bladder epithelium, mucus, leukocytes and bacteria, it is suggestive of chronic common bile-duct infection.

The study of the "B" fraction is of the greatest significance. Grossly the normal "B" bile is clear, transparent, light amber to dark brown in color. It is free from shreds and gross detritus. The color change between the "A" and "B" fractions is usually sharp. The "B" bile is viscid and averages about 35 to 45 cc. Microscopically it may show an occasional cholesterin crystal or fatty acid crystal, particularly if allowed to stand. A slight amount of amorphous bile salt is frequently seen or an occasional epithelial element. It is not unusual to see elements, the identity of which cannot be determined. Any addition to this picture means, as a rule, some biliary tract pathology. Chronic cholecystitis, the most common condition encountered, causes alteration in the gross appearance of the "B" fraction. The bile is static, deep brown or black color, turbid and very viscid. It frequently contains gross detritus and flakes of mucus. For the microscopic examination one of these flakes should be selected. Microscopy will usually reveal the true condition of the viscus. The presence of clumps of degenerated bile-stained epithelial cells of the tall columnar variety associated with colonies of bacteria is diagnostic of cholecystitis. Frequently mucus, considerable unidentified detritus, leukocytes and pigment crystals add themselves to the picture. We have noticed frequently a considerable quantity of small rectangular prisms vary slightly bile-stained. Whether these are pigment crystals or bile salts we are not prepared to say. An abnormal amount of cholesterin crystals when *en masse* or in clumps is very suggestive of stones.

If the "C" bile shows the more marked departure from the

normal we should infer that the focus is either in the hepatic duct radicles or the liver. We have drained three cases of jaundice following arsphenamin injections and found the most marked change in the liver bile. After several drainings this was very noticeable, the freshly secreted bile coming last being very turbid and full of detritus and degenerated epithelial cells; no organisms were seen.

It must be borne in mind that frequently toward the end of the drainage a milky turbidity will develop, due to an ejection of gastric juice into the duodenum. Hydrochloric acid renders bile turbid. We have been unable to determine the cause.

If one is positive that the tube is in the duodenum and bile cannot be obtained following the stimulation, a hasty conclusion must not be drawn that common bile duct obstruction is present even when jaundice exists. Stimulate at least three times. Usually the sphincter of Oddi, for some reason, does not open until the second or third stimulation. We have noticed this particularly in two types of individuals, patients suffering from vagotonia and those with chronic cholecystitis. If after two or three drainages and the administration of belladonna bile cannot be obtained, a diagnosis of common duct obstruction may be made.

The repeated absence of the "B" fraction means cystic duct obstruction in the presence of a gall-bladder.

A careful study of the bile fractions as to their manner of appearing, the macroscopic and microscopic examination of the bile, all yield important information relative to the condition of the biliary tract.

From a diagnostic, prognostic and therapeutic standpoint, obviously great interest centers about the bacteriologic examination of the bile. A satisfactory technic for carrying out such an examination is obviously difficult, and many factors must be overcome before the result obtained can be regarded as reliable. In numerous instances we have attempted bacteriologic studies of the bile. In an effort to have these observations as reliable as possible the following technic, after the method advocated by Lyon, has been adopted.

The night before the examination is to be made the patient must brush the teeth thoroughly; the mouth and throat are carefully washed by lavoris (weak astringent solution of ZnCl and formalin), followed by liquor antisepticus. From then on no further food or fluid is ingested and the tube is passed the following morning on a fasting stomach. Prior to the passage of the tube the throat and mouth are thoroughly disinfected by lavoris followed by liquor antisepticus. The duodenal tube, having been rendered sterile by careful surgical sterilization, is then passed by an operator wearing sterile gloves and a sterile gown. As soon as the duodenal tube has reached the stomach the stomach is carefully washed with distilled water until the return is entirely clear. It is next washed with a solution of lavoris, 60 cc being diluted with 200 cc of sterile water. This lavage is followed by another lavage of sterile water. Then 250 cc of a 1 to 1000 silvol solution are introduced into the stomach and removed. This is followed by another lavage with sterile water, which is continued until the return flow is entirely clear. Such fluid or contents as is then remaining in the stomach is cultured and the duodenal tube allowed to pass into the duodenum. Before stimulation with magnesium sulphate a culture is made from the duodenal contents. Then stimulation of the duodenum is carried out as usual, with 75 cc of a 25 per cent solution of sterile magnesium sulphate. The bile is then obtained in the usual way, being segregated in the three fractions "A," "B" and "C," from all of which separate cultures are made.

By following this method it is generally possible to render the upper alimentary tract sterile for all practical purposes. By taking cultures from the stomach and duodenum, and possibly the mouth and throat, before stimulation is made, one is enabled to know which, if any, organisms are present in these structures before the flow of bile begins. Exceptionally the only organisms obtained from the bile are the same as those obtained from the stomach or duodenum before the bile has entered it. Under such conditions the organisms found cannot be regarded as in any way peculiar to the bile, and the cultures should be repeated. If the cultures obtained from the bile contain only the commoner mouth saprophytes such as the Streptococcus salivarius, Micrococcus catarrhalis or the Bacillus subtilis, no significance can be attached to the findings, which must be looked upon as due to contamination. The organisms, which, however, are of importance and which have been repeatedly isolated by numerous observers, include streptococci, especially the hemolyticus, the Staphylococcus aureus and albus, the Bacillus typhosus and the colon bacillus. From the somewhat meagre published results of bacteriologic examination of the bile thus obtained it is surprising to note the frequency with which some observers have found hemolytic streptococci. It is also interesting to note that pneumococci have been reported by some, which seems somewhat incomprehensible in view of the well-known bile-soluble property of pneumococci.

It must be admitted that the technical difficulties, as well as the rather meagre knowledge at present available as to the bacteriology of the stomach, duodenum and biliary passages, often make the bacteriologic study of the bile distinctly unsatisfactory.

Elaborate and careful experimental studies on the bacteria, and the static and germicidal properties of the bile have been carried out by Neilson and Meyer.[6] Their experiments were largely done with

[6] Jour. Infect. Dis., 1921, **28**, 542.

test-tubes and included a variety of biles from different animals, such as cats, goats, rats, dogs, oxen, sheep, pigs, and a few observations on bile obtained from man. The human specimens were obtained wholly from cholecystectomized bladders or by aspiration during a laparotomy. These observations were made largely upon organisms of the typhoid-dysentery-paratyphoid group and the vibrio of cholera. In the specimens of bile obtained from man they found that the typhoid bacilli grew well and remained viable for more than ten days, whereas with the cholera bacillus it required eight days before the sterilization was complete. They concluded that the vigor of bacterial growth in average human cystic bile is noteworthy. They further discovered that proliferation is somewhat influenced by artificially reducing hydrogen-ion concentration, but that complete suspension of growth only occurs at a pH_4, which in all probability never occurs in a human body. The importance of their paper, so far as man is concerned, has largely to do with the influence of cystic bile on the human typhoid carrier state.

It was originally our intention to discuss the bacteriologic findings in a series of cases that exhibited disease of the biliary tract or gall-bladder, but in the earlier portion of our work so much difficulty was experienced with the bacteriologic technic that the results obtained were regarded as too unreliable for permanent record. We have, however, had an opportunity of carrying out some successful and interesting bacteriologic observations on a limited number of cases, and in order to demonstrate the importance of the bacteriologic findings in the bile these cases will be reported briefly.

Case I.—C. P., Jr., aged sixty years. On January 1, this man suffered from a gastrointestinal disturbance associated with marked jaundice. A diagnosis was made by his physician of acute catarrhal jaundice. In the course of two weeks the jaundice entirely cleared up. The patient first came under observation by us three weeks after the onset of his jaundice. At that time there was no evidence of jaundice on physical examination. Stools contained bile and the urine was free of it. He exhibited, however, considerable pallor. There was some elevation of blood-pressure; he suffered from a distinct asthenia, coated tongue and loss of appetite. Examination of the urine showed the presence of considerable quantities of albumin, numerous hyaline and granular casts and red blood cells. He was admitted to the hospital apparently suffering from an acute exacerbation of a chronic nephritis. Hematuria became more marked and the anemia progressed, Careful search was made for a focus of infection that might be held responsible for the acute renal manifestations. All possible foci of infection were eliminated except the gall-bladder, over which there was a slight persistent tenderness. With the history of a recent attack of jaundice it was decided that the gall-bladder was in all probability the focus of infection responsible for his progressive anemia and his renal symptoms. Three weeks after coming under observation his hemoglobin was 55 per cent; his red cells 2,860,000 and his leukocytes 17,100. At this juncture duodenal drainage was instituted. A considerable quantity of dark gall-bladder bile was obtained. In this bile were found numerous flakes of mucus, much sediment and epithelial cells. In 3 of the specimens of gall-bladder bile pus was present. On culture on two separate occasions Staphylococcus aureus and albus were found in pure culture in the "A," "B" and "C" bile, and these organisms were not present in the cultures taken from the stomach or from the duodenum before stimulation was resorted to. It was also interesting to note that specimens of urine collected under sterile conditions at about the same time and examined at a different laboratory also gave pure cultures of the same organisms. There seemed, therefore, to be some justification for the assumption that the gall-bladder and renal infections were the result of the same organism. Owing to a steadily falling blood count the patient was given a transfusion of 500 cc of blood. Some slight improvement followed this procedure, although the blood count did not noticeably increase. The most marked subjective improvement followed biliary drainage, which was practised once a week. A vaccine was prepared from the strains of Staphylococcus aureus and albus isolated from the bile. During the past month the patient has been receiving the vaccine every four days. The hematuria has cleared up, the renal symptoms have subsided, the blood count has shown marked improvement and subjectively the patient presents every indication of recovery.

Case II.—E. D., aged fifty-two years, in whom a diagnosis of duodenal ulcer and cholecystitis was made. The condition of the gall-bladder was discovered by a biliary drainage during a course of two weeks' treatment with duodenal feeding. In this patient the microscopic study of the bile showed a considerable number of pus cells, bile-stained epithelial cells, many short motile bacilli, a few pigment crystals and quantities of amorphous bile salts. Bile from the gall-bladder was obtained by the aseptic technic of Lyon. Cultures showed a luxurious growth of colon bacilli. An autogenons vaccine of colon bacilli was prepared and injections were given at intervals of four days up to 1,000,000,000 bacilli. At the same time weekly biliary drainage was practised. The original culture was obtained on January 13. On March 23, a second culture, obtained by the same technic, was sterile. At this time the patient was symptomatically greatly improved. Gastrointestinal symptoms had disappeared.

Case III.—A woman, aged thirty-five years, was suffering from chronic arthritis of eleven years' duration. After exhaustive search for the foci of infection, in the course of which the tonsils were removed and some teeth extracted without improvement, nonsurgical drainage of the biliary tract was instituted. The "B" bile was a deep brown black, very viscid, contained many shreds and particles and on culture showed Streptococcus hemolyticus and Staphylococcus albus in luxurious growths. In view of these findings the gall-bladder, regarded as the probable focus of infection, was removed. At operation no stones were found but a definite chronic cholecystitis existed. Cultures taken from the gall-bladder at operation showed hemolytic streptococcus and Staphylococcus albus. Confirmation by surgical means of the findings obtained by the transduodenal drainage are interesting and significant of the value of the latter method. Biweekly biliary drainage was instituted in this case. Two months after the original culture was obtained from the bile, bile cultures were again made following the Lyon antiseptic technic. This time the Staphylococcus albus alone was present; the streptococcus had disappeared. An autogenous vaccine was prepared and given. A month later the biliary drainage was discontinued and the patient at that time was showing marked improvement; her temperature was practically normal and she was able to be up and to walk about. It is interesting to note in this case that after the cholecystectomy no "B" bile was obtained and absolutely no color change in the bile. We have never observed dark bile sooner than six months after cholecystectomy.

Case IV.—K., aged sixty years. This patient was suffering from a chronic arthritis. Her tonsils had been removed without results. Biliary drainage was instituted and cultures were obtained according to the Lyon technic. A nonhemolytic streptococcus was isolated from the "B" bile. Stomach cultures were sterile. A vaccine was made and is being administered. The patient is still under observation, and although improving it is too early to know the ultimate result.

Case V.—M., aged fifty-three years. The patient gave a history of recurring attacks of slight jaundice and so-called "biliousness." These latter attacks he had since his youth. Biliary drainage was instituted and cultures made from the bile. In this instance, although the bile showed Staphylococcus albus, nonhemolytic streptococci and unidentified micrococci were also found in the stomach cultures. The results obtained from the biliary culture were too uncertain to justify any therapeutic procedure based upon these findings without further checking the results. This case is cited to emphasize the importance of culturing the stomach, even though it is believed to be sterile. Even though a different organism had been isolated from the bile it could not be regarded as significant, since the stomach was not sterile.

These cases have been reviewed in order to point out the possibility of accurate bacteriologic study of the bile by means of biliary drainage and also to again emphasize the frequently forgotten role that the gall-bladder plays in producing focal infection.

The checking by operative findings of the results of biliary drainage in Case II is a gratifying evidence of the reliability of bacteriologic studies made by this technic. A much more impressive example, however, of the value of preoperative duodenal findings in comparison with the lesion found at operation is furnished by Whipple,[7] who, in a series of 27 cases on whom careful studies of the biliary tract were made by means of duodenal drainage before operation, found a striking coincidence in the operative findings with those obtained by a study of the bile before operation.

In carrying out our bacteriologic studies of the bile a caution which has been rightly emphasized by Lyon should be pointed out. Lyon insists upon the importance of replanting from the original broth culture, if one is used, in six hours. If this is not done a rapidly growing colon bacillus may render it extremely difficult to isolate the slower growing streptococcus, should such an organism be present. In order to render the bacteriologic examination doubly safe, bile is planted on broth cultures during the biliary drainage and is transplanted within twelve hours. In addition to this all the bile withdrawn is collected in bottles, separated into "A," "B" and "C" fractions, and streak cultures are made from these fractions on solid media at once. By following this method the isolation of these organisms will be facilitated.

CONCLUSIONS. 1. We believe that the method of biliary drainage instituted by Lyon and based upon the hypothesis of Meltzer is a useful and practical procedure, and that there is every reason for the belief that the bile obtained in this way is derived from the common bile duct, the gall-bladder, the hepatic duct and the biliary capillaries in the order given.

2. In our experience the diseased condition of the gall-bladder and the bile ducts can be recognized in this way by a microscopic and bacteriologic study of the bile, which under pathologic conditions shows alterations which are significant.

3. The bacteriologic study of the bile derived in this way is feasible and is of importance, but in order to be successful a rather elaborate, time-consuming technic is essential.

4. If such a technic is carried out the bacteriologic findings are useful and serve as a guide to therapeutic procedure.

Finally, however, it should be emphasized that it is our feeling

[7] Ann. Surg., 1921, **73**, 556.

that the information obtained by nonsurgical biliary drainage is only a diagnostic adjunct, and in no sense should take the place of a careful history and complete physical examination. It is only when the findings derived from biliary drainage are taken in conjunction with a complete clinical study of the case that accurate conclusions can be drawn. Our knowledge of the bacteriology of the biliary and upper gastrointestinal tract is still so meagre that a great deal of work and much careful observation will be required before this phase of the subject is placed upon an entirely satisfactory basis.

EXPERIENCES WITH NONSURGICAL BILIARY DRAINAGE.

(Meltzer-Lyon Test.)

By Edward Hollander, B.S., M.D.
NEW YORK.

(From the Medical Department, Mt. Sinai Hospital, N. Y.)

In 1917, Meltzer published a theoretical discussion of his views regarding the interrelation between the gall-bladder musculature and the sphincter of Oddi. He invoked the general physiological "law of contrary innervation" (which applies to other neuromuscular reflexes of the alimentary tract), to explain their interplay as antagonists in the normal storage and discharge of gall-bladder bile. He drew an analogy between the action of the gall-bladder and that of the urinary bladder, in that, when the bladder contracts the sphincter relaxes, and when the sphincter contracts the bladder relaxes. To substantiate his contention, he cited the experiments of Doyon,[2] showing the crossed innervation of the gall-bladder and Oddi's sphincter within the splanchnic and vagus nerves.* In a small footnote appended to his paper (which bears repetition because of its frequent misquotation), Meltzer[1] stated: "In experiments with $MgSO_4$, I observed that the local application of a 25 per cent solution of that salt on the mucosa causes a completely local relaxation of the intestinal wall. . . The duodenal tube, however, apparently has reached an efficient, practical stage. I make, therefore, the suggestion, to test in

* Because of the technic employed, Doyon could not demonstrate a contraction of the gall-bladder and a relaxation of the sphincter in the same experiment. He believed that normally they must be practically simultaneous. A consideration of the pressures involved, substantiates this view. Freese[30] found the maximum force of gall-bladder contraction to be 313 mm. of water, whereas Archibald[31] found the resistance of the sphincter to vary between 500 to 650 mm. of water and McWhorter[32] found its maximal value to be 580 mm. of water.

jaundice and biliary colic the local application of a 25 per cent solution of $MgSO_4$ by means of the duodenal tube. It may relax the sphincter of the common duct and permit the ejection of bile, and, perhaps, even permit the removal of a calculus of moderate size, wedged in the duct in front of the papilla of Vater."

It should be noted that Meltzer made no mention of observations on gall-bladder contraction in response to magnesium sulphate. Frequent statements and misquotations that he did, have constantly appeared in the literature.

The Work of Lyon. B. B. Vincent Lyon, correlating the above pregnant suggestion with the "law of contrary innervation," studied the effects of douching the duodenal mucosa with magnesium sulphate solutions injected through a duodenal tube. In a practical communication,[3] he concluded that Meltzer was correct in his application of this law and that it was possible, in normal people, to obtain a fractional separation of the bile from the various portions of the biliary tract. Thus, he stated, it was possible to segregate the gall-bladder, or "B" bile, from the common duct, or "A" bile, and the hepatic duct, or "C" bile. By careful examination (physical, chemical, microscopical and bacteriological), a definite diagnosis could be made of pathological conditions in these portions of the biliary system. In a series of articles,[4, 5, 6, 7, 8, 9] Lyon elaborated a method of diagnosis and treatment of the gall-bladder and ducts heretofore undreamed of.

Criticisms. The subject was immediately taken up by various workers and dissenting opinions were soon expressed. Thus, Einhorn[10, 11] studied the return following the injection of various salts through the duodenal tube, and plotted the values of the color intensity, alkalinity and specific gravity of the bile. He concluded that increases in these values represented liver stimulation through portal absorption and liver excretion of the injected salts. He also claimed that aqueous solutions of 25 per cent magnesium sulphate, 25 per cent sodium sulphate, 25 per cent glucose and 5 per cent peptone possessed the property of marked liver stimulation, whereas 25 per cent sodium phosphate, 13 per cent magnesium citrate, 15 per cent magnesium sulphate, 0.5 per cent sodium chloride, and many other substances, stimulated the liver to lesser degrees. He disagreed with Lyon that these values represented gall-bladder admixtures. It is proper to state that Einhorn's theory is contrary to the evidence of experimental studies of the excretion of magnesium salts,[12] and that he formulated it from clinical data only.

Bassler,[13] failing to observe definite contractions of the exposed gall-bladder after laparotomy under ether anesthesia, came to practically the same conclusions. Both authors also observed a return of dark bile following magnesium sulphate in some cholecystectomized patients, and used this fact as a further argument against the gall-bladder origin of the "B" bile in the non-operated case.

Crohn,[14] failing to obtain gall-bladder contraction in narcotized dogs, doubted the gall-bladder origin of the "B" bile.

Dunn and Connell,[15] in a case of hepatoduodenostomy, injected magnesium sulphate solution through a duodenal fistula into the duodenum and also into the jejunum, and obtained a dark bile fraction with an increased magnesium content. They concluded that portal absorption and hepatic excretion of the salt were the most plausible explanation of their findings.

Discussion of Criticisms. These "criticisms" when correlated with the known facts of experimental physiology are incorrect deductions from observations, rather than true objections to the fundamental principles of the reaction. To explain the source of dark bile which is occasionally obtained in cholecystectomized patients, Doyon[2] demonstrated that the bile ducts, as well as the gall-bladder, can contract. Rost[16] showed, in cholecystectomized dogs, that those developing continence of Oddi's sphincter (with concomitant dilation of the ducts), reacted to injections of peptone in a manner somewhat similar to dogs with intact gall-bladders. He proved, by comparison with the failure of response in dogs with incontinent sphincters, that the bile ducts were stimulated reflexly to discharge their pent up bile. He further showed that after several months, these continent dogs exhibited organic dilatation of the bile ducts, even to the formation of new gall-bladders. These findings have been corroborated by other observers.[17, 18] Since stasis of bile with moderate increase in its color concentration can occur in the ducts, their contraction will result in the discharge of bile of darker color than bile direct from the liver.

The case of Dunn and Connell appears convincing only on superficial examination. It may be interpreted as a reflex discharge of static bile from the hepatic ducts. It must be remembered that this was a case of severe biliary infection of several months' duration, in which damage to the biliary ducts had undoubtedly occurred. As to the increased values of the magnesium content of their so-called "B" bile, which they assume was absorbed and excreted by the liver, sufficient evidence was not adduced, first, that there was no reflux into the duodenum of the magnesium sulphate injected, and second, that the gram-molecular increase of Mg over that of SO_4, in the proportion of $MgSO_4$, was not due to the increased magnesium content of the static duct bile itself. This could have been done by the comparison of the findings following peptone injection.

That magnesium sulphate solution introduced into the duodenum does not proceed directly onward as is usually assumed, can be demonstrated by coloring the injected fluid. In 10 cases, I introduced 75 cc of 33 per cent magnesium sulphate, colored with

2 cc of 2 per cent methylene blue, and syphoned out the fluid immediately. Throughout the discharge of "B" and "C" biles, lasting from one-half to three-quarter hours, irregular jets of bluish to greenish watery bile were obtained, and the bile between these jets showed less or no coloration by the dye. It is also the admixture of such small amounts of the original magnesium sulphate solution throughout the reaction, that can account for the markedly increased specific gravity of the "B" bile, as compared with the actual specific gravity of the gall-bladder content at operation. Thus, as small an amount as a 5 per cent solution of magnesium sulphate in bile will increase its specific gravity from 1013 to 1055.[10]

Regarding the failure to observe actual gall-bladder contraction during operation under anesthesia, it should not be forgotten that we are dealing here with a delicate neuromuscular reflex, which, analogous to the pupillary and conjunctival reflexes, can be abolished according to the depth of the anesthesia. Bainbridge and Dale[19] appreciated this fact and refrained from drawing conclusions from their failure to elicit reflex gall-bladder contractions in their anesthetized animals. Doyon, however, succeeded in registering such reflex contractions following irritation with vinegar and ammonia in curarized (non-anesthetized) dogs. This fact has been overlooked recently by several experimenters.

Gall-bladder Response to Duodenal Irritation. Doyon found that irritation of the gastric and duodenal mucosa caused a relaxation of the common duct sphincter and a contraction of the gall-bladder. This fact can explain the varying colored bile responses following the injection of various chemicals into the duodenum. In studying this phase of the subject, I selected cases in which the "B" return was distinctly atypical, affording a sharp contrast to the "A" and "C" biles, *viz.*, "B" biles of a very dark or tarry appearance, or with special microscopical characteristics. Nine such patients were operated on. Successive injections (from 2 to 4) of various solutions during the same intubation were given, 60 cc being injected and immediately syphoned off. It was found that besides 25 to 33 per cent magnesium sulphate (which acted most energetically, probably because of its peculiar property of relaxation), 5 to 10 per cent peptone, 25 per cent glucose (and occasionally and much more feebly, 25 per cent sodium sulphate), produced similar "B" biles, which were similar to the gall-bladder contents at operation. These are the substances that Einhorn claims possess the property of marked stimulation of the liver. After injection of 15 per cent magnesium sulphate, 13 per cent magnesium citrate, 25 per cent sodium phosphate, and 0.5 per cent sodium chloride, biles which were slightly darker than the fasting liver bile control were usually obtained; but *the same result* was also occasionally observed *after plain water* injected at a temperature slightly above that of the body. Also following successive injections (2 to 3) of these weaker solutions during the same intubation, a distinct "B' return was sometimes obtained, similar to that following 25 to 33 per cent magnesium sulphate or 5 to 10 per cent peptone. In tests made *in vitro* all of these colors could be simulated by mixing various amounts of gall-bladder contents with "C" bile. Furthermore, 7 of the cases which showed a distinctly atypical "B" bile, were studied six to sixteen weeks after cholecystectomy, and *then not one showed a "B" bile.* The inference is forced upon us, that in accordance with the findings of Doyon, these darker specimens are due to varying amounts of gall-bladder bile, dependent upon the strength of gall-bladder contraction coincident with sphincteric relaxation in response to the injected irritant.*

Although Meltzer failed to observe intestinal relaxation if magnesium sulphate solution passed through the stomach, yet with the duodenal tube *in situ*, after swallowing 75 cc of 33 per cent magnesium sulphate, the sequential flow of "A," "B," and "C" bile is usually obtained, though it is not as forceful as when the magnesium sulphate is injected through the tube. Its action is similar to that following the injection of a less hypertonic solution.

To test Lyon's suggestion of the hormonic action of magnesium sulphate, 10 patients were given intramuscular injections in the amount advised in the treatment of tetanus.[10] Intravenous injections were considered too hazardous. Fifteen cc of 25 per cent magnesium sulphate (and in 1 case, 15 cc of 50 per cent solution, due to nurse's error) were injected deep into the gluteal region. No gall-bladder response was observed in any case from one-half to three-quarters hours (at which time in the rabbit full systemic effects occur[21]). Some patients complained of feeling heavy and tired. Otherwise, no effects were noted.

Lyon described "B" bile as bile from the gall-bladder admixed with bile from the liver. That "B" bile is not a uniform fluid, as it should be if it were excreted by the liver, is readily demonstrated in cases with gall-bladder stasis by viewing it in a test tube against a ground-glass background immediately after its return. Whirls of dark colored and viscid bile in a lighter and more limpid bile can be distinguished. In a few minutes, however, the mixture becomes uniform and is of a lighter color than the gall-bladder bile found at operation. In normal cases there is not sufficient color contrast between the gall-bladder bile and the liver bile to bring out such a reaction so distinctly.

Because of this admixture, comparison of the "alkalinity" of the "B" bile with that of the gall-bladder bile, always gives a higher value for the latter. A static gall-bladder bile has an increased nucleoprotein content, which combines with HCl, result-

* Spasm of the sphincter may be brought about by *strong* irritation, mechanical or chemical. According to McWhorter,[31] hyperacidity will produce a spasm of the sphincter. Similar observations are recorded by Archibald.[32]

ing in very high titrations for the "alkalinity." As high as 200 cc $\frac{N}{10}$ HCl (calculated for 100 cc of bile, methyl orange indicator), was obtained in 1 case.

Disadvantages of Magnesium Sulphate in Diagnosis. In studying the effects of different substances injected into the duodenum, it was found, that while magnesium sulphate proved to be the most energetic in causing a gall-bladder response, it has serious diagnostic disadvantages. If after the completion of the reaction to 5 per cent peptone, 25 to 33 per cent magnesium sulphate be injected and a comparison of both samples of "B" and "C" biles be made, it will be found that those specimens obtained after the use of the hypertonic magnesium sulphate are usually contaminated with numerous duodenal flocculi. This occurs even if the duodenum was previously douched with astringent solutions (0.2 per cent zinc chloride or Lavoris). Microscopical examinations (stained and unstained) of these flocculi show very numerous short columnar and cuboidal cells, varying numbers of polymorphonuclears, and rare red blood cells, frequently together with many organisms enmeshed in strands of mucus. It is most likely an osmotic reaction of the mucous membrane to the hypertonic salt, for similar response can be obtained by any strongly hypertonic salt. It is interesting to note that the tall columnar cells, which line the villi, are very few in number, and that the cytological picture is that of exfoliated cells from the deeper portions of the crypts of Lieberkühn. This is not surprising if we bear in mind the fact that inflammatory reaction is most marked in regions where drainage is poor and bacterial nests can form. As the epithelial lining of the biliary tract is histologically similar to that of the duodenal mucosa, and as disease of the gall-bladder is usually associated with an exfoliative duodenitis, to avoid confusion it *is essential to recognize the cellular contamination from this region.* Furthermore, since these duodenal flocculi contaminate the aspirated bile specimens, the bacteriological studies of them must be very misleading regarding the true status of biliary infection. While cultural studies were not made, the microscopical comparison of the specimens of "B" and "C" biles after 5 per cent peptone, with those obtained after the strongly hypertonic salt (consecutive injections during the same intubation), substantiates this criticism. *A priori*, I would suggest, that cultural studies on specimens after 5 per cent peptone injection will give more exact data regarding biliary infection.

Technic. In the early cases, the original plan of Lyon was followed, but after becoming familiar with the details of the test, and with the appearance of extra-hepatic contaminations, the preliminary washings and sterilizations of the stomach were omitted, simplifying the method to meet the demands of outpatient practice. The patient presents himself with a twelve-hour fasting stomach. The relation of the test to previous feeding is important and has not been sufficiently emphasized, for, as Rous and McMaster[12] have shown, the concentration of gall-bladder bile is continuous and dependent on the duration of its sojourn in that organ. After obtaining a specimen of fasting gastric juice, the tube is swallowed slowly, as suggested by Lyon, until the bulb is in the duodenum, which usually takes from one-half to two hours. To determine whether entrance into the duodenum has been effected, roentgenological examination is the best method, but for obvious reasons, it is not practicable for routine work. The litmus test is not entirely reliable, for regurgitation of duodenal contents into the stomach may cause a bluish tinge, and again, the tube may have entered the duodenum and yet an acid reaction is not infrequent. Of the various tests suggested, I have found the most reliable to be the failure to recover swallowed water, or to recover less than half of 90 cc injected through the tube. But in cases of gastroptosis in which the fluid may gravitate beyond the bucket, this too might be misleading. However, when once familiar with the appearance and reaction of the bile, together with the manner of return of swallowed or injected fluid, one can, in most cases, form an accurate judgment regarding the position of the tube.

The duodenal fluid is permitted to syphon into a series of 20 cc test tubes, a separate tube being used for every change in the character of the fluid. As many as 25 tubes may be required during a test, thus obtaining a veritable cinema of the bile discharge. A specimen of the fasting duodenal contents is examined for comparison with later specimens. It has been my experience that bile can be obtained from the fasting duodenum in most cases, even in normal persons. Schneider[23] reports similar findings. Lyon, however, interprets bile in the fasting duodenum as indicating "a lesion of group organs physiologically related to this intestinal zone." Bruno[24] stated that, in animal experiments, no bile appears in the fasting duodenum. However, it is probable that with the tube, the irritation of the metallic bulb causes sufficient relaxation of even a normal sphincter to permit bile to flow from the ducts. Ordinarily, the stimulus is too weak to cause gall-bladder contraction. However, in a small percentage of cases, spontaneous discharge of small amounts of deeper colored gall-bladder mixtures may occur. (Einhorn,[25] attempted to diagnose the condition of the gall-bladder from such specimens.) It is important to recognize that in the same individual, bile samples from the fasting duodenum are of varying color (from light straw to golden yellow), depending on varying dilutions, chiefly by duodenal fluid and gastric juice. One should not designate as "B" bile, the darker samples of "C" bile.

After securing a sample of the fasting duodenal contents, the duodenum is lavaged with 90 cc water at body temperature for the purpose of washing away any superficial mucus, etc. For reasons already given, the gall-bladder response is stimulated by the injection of 60 cc of 5 per cent peptone.* Because of its bland action on the duodenal mucosa, peptone affords a more exact analysis of the various components of the bile tract. We can, with more certainty than after magnesium sulphate, venture an opinion regarding the origin of muco-flakes appearing in the "A," "B," and "C" biles. Thus, the attempt to locate the source of disease is made more practicable. Occasionally, the gall-bladder response to peptone is slow, sometimes not appearing until a half hour after the injection. Occasionally, 10 per cent peptone is effective when 5 per cent fails. Following the reaction to peptone, I always inject 75 cc of 33 per cent magnesium sulphate in order to determine the degree of duodenitis present, and to restimulate gall-bladder discharge. A second or even third injection of 25 cc of 33 per cent magnesium sulphate is given if no gall-bladder response occurred after the previous injections. It is remarkable to what degree exfoliative duodenitis is usually associated with gall-bladder disease. The duodenal flocculi frequently sediment to one-quarter the volume of bile in some of the test tubes. This reaction to the strongly hypertonic salt usually manifests itself quickly, but sometimes, it may not develop fully until after twenty to thirty minutes. Occasionally, no gall-bladder discharge occurs after either 5 or 10 per cent peptone, but following the relaxing effect of magnesium sulphate on the intestinal wall, a forceful flow is obtained. Following the reaction to magnesium sulphate, no further injection or lavage is given, and no ill effects have been noted from the absorption of toxic material. This is not surprising, since most of the bile is syphoned out of the tube.

The entire reaction must be closely watched, as the tube may be dislodged by a cough, sneeze, etc.. and thus vitiate the findings; or small amounts of gastric juice may appear, which must be segregated. Furthermore, the examinations must be made immediately, since oxidation takes place quickly with clouding of the bile. Since only a few minutes are required for serious alterations or even complete destruction of the important cellular elements by the pancreatic ferments, there should be as little delay as possible in the microscopical examinations.

Diagnosis. The practicability of making a diagnosis depends upon one's familiarity with the reaction in normals, and revolves about the careful examinations and *comparisons* of the fasting gastric, and duodenal fluids, and the "A," "B," and "C" biles. The examinations include the following: (1) *Physical*, quantity, color, transparency or turbidity, viscosity, manner of discharge,

* An unrefined peptone is not effective. While Witte peptone is the best preparation, it is too expensive for routine use. I have found that a good preparation by any reliable firm, such as Armour or Eimer and Amend, is equally effective as Witte peptone in stimulating gall-bladder response.

flocculi, presence of sand; (2) *microscopical* (oil immersion on stained and unstained specimens essential for the study of the cellular and bacterial content), epithelium, leukocytes, red blood cells, mucus, bacteria, inflammatory débris, and crystals; (3) *chemical,* alkalinity (methyl orange indicator).

In normal subjects (if the sphincter is closed), 10 to 20 cc of clear light golden-yellow bile, "A" bile, is followed, after one to three minutes, by 1 to 3 ounces of syrupy darker transparent amber bile, "B" bile, and then a varying quantity of light clear golden-yellow bile, "C" bile. Microscopically, there are present occasional epithelial cells, leukocytes, bacteria, scattered bile crystals and traces of mucus from the duodenum or bile. Changes from the *normal* findings indicate *malfunction* or *disease.*

The diagnosis may be made by the correlation of the following observations:

1. Failure to obtain bile after successive stimulations indicates occlusion of the common duct.

2. The volume of "A" bile is dependent on the time interval between the injection and the gall-bladder response, as well as on the degree of dilatation of the common duct.

3. Failure to obtain "B" bile in *repeated* tests is indicative of an organic condition which is interfering with the function of the gall-bladder. This finding, in conjunction with the clinical picture, is a distinct indication for surgical intervention.

4. Sand or agminated crystals, is evidence of a tendency toward or of the actual presence of stones.

5. Swarming or colonizing bacteria indicate active infection.

6. Increased number of or massed leukocytes is indicative of an acute or subacute inflammatory reaction. The use of 2 per cent acetic acid brings out the nuclei more clearly.

7. Darker colors of "B" bile, clear to slightly turbid, (deeper shades of amber to tarry black), with sluggish or intermittent discharge, yielding more than 90 cc or less than 20 cc, are indicative of various degrees of gall-bladder stasis. Lyon interprets this finding as evidence of gall-bladder atony. However, occasionally cases are encountered in which no gall-bladder discharge occurs after peptone, but following the relaxing effect of magnesium sulphate on the intestinal wall, a *forceful* flow occurs. Such a reaction suggests that the primary condition present is not one of atony of the gall-bladder musculature, but rather one of increased tone or spasm at the ampulla with consequent (contrary) relaxation of the gall-bladder as originally suggested by Meltzer. It is frequently associated with varying degrees of duodenitis. Such a condition might well be termed "ampullospasm," analogous to spasms at other sphincters, *viz.*, pylorospasm, cardiospasm, etc. The gall-bladder stasis in relation to this spasm is analogous to the gastric retention in relation to pylorospasm.

It must be pointed out that in cases with sluggish gall-bladder discharge, the resulting "B" specimen will consist chiefly of liver bile and only a small proportion of gall-bladder bile. It is evident that the resulting mixture will be much lighter than the gall-bladder content.

In many cases of gall-bladder stasis, repeated gall-bladder responses to successive injections of peptone were obtained (as many as 6 injections and responses in 1 case). In these, a definite interrelation between the gall-bladder and pylorus was evident. During each discharge of "B" bile, the pylorus remained closed, and cloudy precipitation of the bile by acid gastric juice appeared only after "C" bile was obtained. In relation to this observation, it is interesting to note the frequency after cholecystectomy of regurgitation of bile into the stomach. This gastric bile (if retching was not present), is an indication of disturbed physiology about the pylorus.

8. Columnar cells, especially tall columnar cells, usually degenerating, deeply bile stained, and in fan or rosette formation, when present *only* in the "*B*" *fraction*, represent catarrhal desquamation from the gall-bladder. Frequently intensively bile-stained detritus is also present.

To designate a particular group of cells as derived specifically from the gall-bladder is a difficult task, especially since all recent evidence, clinical and pathological, tends toward the view that chronic cholecystitis is usually associated with inflammatory reactions in the liver and pancreas. However, with increasing experience and care in the technic as described above (careful segregation and comparison of specimens), it can be done.

It should be pointed out that the depth of bile stain bears no constant relation to the origin of a cell from the gall-bladder. Examination of gall-bladder contents frequently shows varying degrees of bile staining of the cells, whereas in reflux bile into an acid stomach, cells become deeply stained. This can be reproduced by adding 2 per cent acetic acid or strongly acid gastric juice to colorless duodenal cells in bile.

9. Mild gall-bladder colic soon (and in some cases a few hours later), after the injections, indicates an inflammatory condition of the gall-bladder.

10. Regarding cultural studies, Whipple's[26] results show that contaminations from the mouth and stomach are unavoidable in many cases, even with the most careful technic. There were conflicting findings in about 50 per cent of his cases. From his results, I conclude, that when gross infection (direct microscopical evidence) is absent, cultural methods are not reliable.

It is necessary to emphasize that a light-colored bile may show marked microscopical evidence of disease, whereas a dark bile may show nothing more than its increased color concentration. The gall-bladder, in disease, may even lose its property of concentrating bile.

It is also necessary to emphasize that this method of investigation enables us to make a diagnosis of early gall-bladder disease when the clinical signs and symptoms are slight and vague. At exploration the surgeon fails to detect this type, for he cannot judge the normality of the organ by sight or touch. I have observed 3 cases in which the surgeon pronounced the gall-bladder normal, but changed his opinion on further examination of the aspirated bile or after the removal of innocent looking adhesions. Judd,[27] in 1916, was suspicious of this fact, and recently Einhorn and Meyer,[28] reported a series of 18 cases of recurrent cholecystitis without stones, from which they concluded that it is not the appearance or softness of the gall-bladder, but rather the examination of the aspirated bile, that is the true criterion of its condition.

Clinical Experience. During the past two years, 415 successful intubations were performed in 128 patients, chiefly gall-bladder suspects. Most of these tests were performed in the outpatient service devoted to the study of gastrointestinal diseases conducted by Dr. Edward A. Aronson, to whom I am indebted for many courtesies.

Normal reactions were obtained in 45 cases, of which 20 were normal persons selected for the study of normal findings; in the remaining 25 cases, roentgen-ray examination proved the presence of calculi in 2, and in 5 others the history and clinical studies were highly suggestive of a chronic cholecystitis. The finding of a normal reaction in chronic cholecystitis has also been reported by Brown.[29] It is a question for future experience to decide, whether with our better understanding of the pathogenesis of gall-bladder disease (removal of foci of infection and relief of biliary stasis), these cases with normally functioning gall-bladders may not carry their evidences of past dysfunction safely without surgical intervention.

The other 83 cases were classified as follows:

I. Repeated absence of "B" bile—22 cases.

This finding is interpreted as evidence of advanced organic disease as discussed above.

II. Abnormal microscopical findings ("B" bile)—19 cases.

On this evidence these cases were classed as cholecystitis or cholelithiasis. In cholelithiasis the examination frequently shows only the findings of the associated cholecystitis. The direct indication of the presence of or tendency toward calculi (sand or agminated crystals) is frequently lacking. In these cases the correlation of the bile examination with a carefully taken history, roentgen-ray examination and other clinical findings is essential to the diagnosis of stones.

III. Static "B" bile (without abnormal microscopical findings) —37 cases.

On the basis of the test, these cases could be classed only as functional (?) atony of the gall-bladder or "ampullospasm." Many cases of enteroptosis were included in this group. Many cases presented the clinical picture of the functional type of relative atony described by Lyon: Vague dyspepsias, so-called "biliousness," often associated with attacks of migraine. Also included in this group, were 7 cases in which the clinical diagnosis of chronic cholecystitis was considered certain. In 2 cases, gall-stones were definitely present and in 1 case stones were found at operation. The differentiation between these clinical types could be made only by the correlation of the test with other clinical data (history, roentgen-ray findings, etc.). The finding of static "B" bile without definitely abnormal microscopical elements, while indicating gall-bladder dysfunction, cannot be interpreted as evidence of definite gall-bladder disease. The elucidation of this large group requires further study, especially of the chemistry of the bile (cholesterin, nucleoprotein content, etc.).

Operation was performed on 17 patients. This group in which our findings were corroborated is most instructive. Operation was advised in 11 patients solely on the evidence of the fractional bile examinations. In these 11 patients either the gall-bladder condition was merely suspected, or an incorrect clinical diagnosis had been made. In 8 of the patients, "B" bile was not obtainable after several attempts, and the operative findings disclosed sufficient gall-bladder disease to account for the failure of the gall-bladder response. In the remaining 9 patients, the *"B" bile* and the *gall-bladder contents at operation* corresponded both in color and microscopical findings. In 7 cases of this group, I had the opportunity to repeat the test six to sixteen weeks after the cholecystectomy, and *then "B" bile could no longer be obtained.*

Besides these, 5 other cholecystectomy cases were studied, and in only 1 (operated on two and a half years previously) was a "B"-type of bile discharged. In this case I obtained 45 cc of light brown bile. However, its manner of discharge was different from that of static bile from the gall-bladder, in that it did not present the whirls of dark bile within a lighter bile as described before. Although stasis of bile in the hepatic ducts is not frequent, it must be borne in mind that it can occur. To differentiate it from gall-bladder bile, its manner of discharge must be closely observed, and here, as in other cases, the findings must be correlated with the history (previous operations), physical examination (presence of icterus), and other clinical data. If such precautions are not taken, errors in interpretation will be made.

Discussion of Cases. (See Table I). Cases I, III, IV, V, VIII, and XIV were clear-cut clinical cases of cholelithiasis. In Case V the only explanation for the failure to obtain "B" bile was the presence of very viscid tarry bile in a thickened gall-bladder. In

TABLE I.

Patient.	Clinical diagnosis.	Meltzer-Lyon test.	Findings at operation.	Repetition of test 6 to 16 weeks later.
1. Mrs. M. S.	Gall-stones	No "B" bile; G. B. colic; exfoliative duodenitis	G. B. full of stones	
2. Mrs. B. R.	Chr. cholecystitis?	No "B" bile; G. B. colic; increased leukocytes after injection	Cystic duct stone; G. B. content mucopurulent	
3. Mrs. S. P.	Gall-stones	No "B" bile; exfoliative duodenitis	Cystic duct stone; G. B. many stones	
4. Mr. H. W.	Gall-stones	No "B" bile	G. B. full of stones	
5. Mrs. F. F.	Gall-stones	No "B" bile	Thickened G. B.; viscid tarry bile; 3 stones	
6. Mrs. R. H.	Suspicious G. B. 1 yr. later obstructive jaundice	No "B" bile; no bile in duodenum	Infiltrating Ca. involving G. B., stomach and pancreas	
7. Mr. H. M.	Duodenal ulcer	No "B" bile; severe G. B. colic	Stone in cystic duct; G. B. content mucopurulent	
8. Mrs. Y. K.	Gall-stones	No "B" bile; exfoliative duodenitis	G. B. full of stones; G. B. content mucopurulent	
9. Mrs. D. R.	Gall-stones	2 tests: No "B" bile 2 tests: Greenish-black "B" bile with agminated cholesterin crystals. Flocculi of degenerating tall columnar cells. Exfoliative duodenitis	G. B. appeared normal. Few small stones in cystic duct and many small stones in G. B. contents similar to "B"	No "B" bile.
10. Mrs. B. F	Chr. cholecystitis?	Greenish-black "B" bile. Flocculi of deeply-stained columnar cells and scattered cocci and leukocytes enmeshed in mucus. Agminated cholesterin crystals. Marked exfoliative duodenitis	Many small stones in G. B.; contents similar to "B"	No "B" bile.
11. Mrs. C. K.	Postop. adhesions; recurrent chr. cholecystitis?	3 tests: No "B" bile 2 tests: Black bile with swarming bacteria, clumps of leukocytes and intensively stained detritus; G. B. colic	Acute cholecystitis; adhesions between G. B. and anterior abdominal wall; contents similar to "B"	No "B" bile.
12. Mrs. R. G.	Appendectomy 12 wks. before, G. B disease not suspected	Tarry black bile; macroscopical sand; marked exfoliative duodenitis	Many small stones in G. B. contents similar to "B"	No "B" bile.
13. Mrs. E. L.	Duodenal ulcer; G. B. (?)	Deep amber clear bile; many agminated cholesterin crystals; small flocculi of columnar cells and deeply-stained detritus; G. B. colic; exfoliative duodenitis	Normal G. B. to sight and touch; small adhesion at fundus; later more small adhesions found; strained bile, 8 small stones; G. B. contents deep amber, clear. Microscopical examination not made	No "B" bile.
14. Mrs. M. B.	Gall-stones	Clear, static (deep brown) "B" bile; no microscopical findings. Marked exfoliative duodenitis	Many small stones in G. B.; contents similar to "B"	Not done.
15. Mrs. C. S.	Hyperthyroidism; gastroptosis	Turbid amber bile; many scattered degenerating columnar cells; many bacilli; scattered leukocytes; agminated cholesterin crystals; detritus	Thickened G. B.; no stones; contents similar to "B"	No "B" bile.
16. Mr. J. R.	1, Luetic crises? 2, Gastric ulcer? 3, G. B.?	Greenish-black bile; small flocculi of degenerating deeply stained columnar cells; exfoliative duodenitis	Three stones in G. B.; contents similar to "B"	No "B" bile.
17. Mrs. A. H.	Appendectomy 4 mos. before	Static (greenish-black) viscid "B" bile; no microscopical findings; marked exfoliative duodenitis	No evidence of disease by sight or touch; aspirated bile similar to "B"	Not done.

Case XIV, clinically cholelithiasis, only the evidence of marked stasis was found in the examination of the "B" bile. In Case II, in several tests, a definite increase in clumped leukocytes was found in the bile following the injection of peptone. These cells were interpreted as evidence of inflammatory reaction in the ducts.

In Cases II, IX, and X the diagnosis of probable chronic cholecystitis had been made clinically. The marked anomalous bile fractions that were obtained made the diagnosis of gall-bladder disease certain. In Case IX, at operation, the gall-bladder appeared and at first felt perfectly normal. However, on careful palpation a few small stones were felt low down in the cystic duct. After extirpation, the gall-bladder was found to contain numerous small stones practically suspended in the bile. It is interesting to note that in two tests no "B" bile was obtained in this case.

Case VI, a very obese woman, complained only of belching after meals, and disease of the gall-bladder could only be suspected. As "B" bile was absent in several tests, the diagnosis of definite organic disease of the gall-bladder was made and operation was urged. Because of her slight symptoms, this was refused. One year later she developed persistent jaundice with complete absence of bile in the duodenum. On exploration, a huge infiltrating carcinoma involving the gall-bladder and invading the stomach and pancreas was found. This case is instructive in that the definite diagnosis of organic disease of the gall-bladder, demanding operation was made one year before the clinical evidence manifested itself. It is a question whether the operation, when first advised (solely on the basis of the repeated absence of "B" bile), might not have saved this woman.

Case VII presented the three cardinal symptoms of duodenal ulcer: Pain two hours after meals, night pains and an "interval history" of several years duration. This diagnosis had been made by three well known gastroenterologists, and the patient had been subjected to a regimen of duodenal alimentation for cure of his ulcer without relief. On duodenal stimulation of the gall-bladder, no "B" bile could be obtained. The injection was followed by severe colic in the gall-bladder region requiring injections of morphine for its control. The patient was then referred for operation with a definite diagnosis of gall-bladder disease, and a subacute empyema with a calculus occluding the cystic duct was found.

In Case XI, a cholecystostomy had been performed four years before coming under observation. Interpretation of the patient's symptoms was difficult because of her markedly neurotic condition, and also because they might have been simply and readily explained by postoperative adhesions. Duodenal examination revealed a "B" bile with swarming bacteria, an increased number of leukocytes, and inflammatory débris. Gall-bladder colic followed the test.

Reoperation was advised. While under observation prior to the operation acute cholecystitis developed, the temperature rose to 104° and immediate operation became imperative. At operation acute cholecystitis was found with adhesions between the gall-bladder and the anterior abdominal wall. These adhesions could account for the failure to obtain "B" bile in three of the tests.

In Case XII, an appendectomy had been performed twelve weeks previously without relief of symptoms. Gall-bladder disease had not even been suspected, as the complaints were referred to the right lower quadrant of the abdomen.

Case XIII, clinically, was considered most probably one of duodenal ulcer. From the "B" bile examination, the diagnosis of cholecystitis with the probable presence of stones was made. At operation, the gall-bladder appeared and felt perfectly normal, but after dividing an innocent looking adhesion at the fundus many more small adhesions became evident. After removing the gall-bladder and straining the bile, 8 small stones were found.

Case XV was one of hyperthyroidism and gastroptosis. With this diagnosis her abdominal symptoms had been explained for many years. The "B" bile showed definite microscopical evidence of disease. At operation chronic cholecystitis was found.

Case XVI was a man with a luetic history and a positive Wassermann reaction. The differential diagnosis lay between luetic crises, gastric ulcer, and possibly, gall-bladder disease. The tubal findings indicated the last. At operation only cholelithiasis was found.

Case XVII, a woman, aged thirty-four years, complained of midepigastric "burning" for two years. Appendectomy was performed four months previously without relief of symptoms. The tubal findings showed a clear, but very static greenish-black viscid "B" fraction without special microscopical features. This was associated with a very marked exfoliative duodenitis. Because of the markedly static bile and the persistence of symptoms, it was believed that gall-bladder disease was present. Because of the patient's objection to medical treatment, reoperation was advised. At operation the gall-bladder showed no external evidence of disease, but the aspirated bile proved to be of a static, greenish-black color similar to the "B" specimen. A cholecystostomy was done, and after surgical drainage for three weeks, the symptoms were completely relieved. It is now three months since the operation. The pathology of the gall-bladder of this case is, of course, undetermined. As far as our data go, the case was one of marked gall-bladder stasis and exfoliative duodenitis. It is probable that as much could have been accomplished with medical drainage.

Summary and Conclusions. 1. Criticisms of the fundamental principles of the Meltzer-Lyon test can be answered, and do not bear strict analysis.

2. Because of its bland action on the duodenal mucosa, 5 per cent peptone is suggested for diagnosis in preference to strongly hypertonic magnesium sulphate solutions.

3. Attention is drawn to the condition of "ampullospasm" in relation to gall-bladder stasis.

4. A normal reaction may be present in chronic cholecystitis. However, in most cases of gall-bladder disease we observe either failure of gall-bladder response, or microscopical abnormalities, or evidence of stasis. The correlation of these findings with other clinical data is essential to a correct diagnosis.

5. The practicability of the test is presented in 17 operated cases. In many cases, the definite diagnosis of gall-bladder disease cannot be made by any other method.

6. Since gall-bladder disease, with its protean clinical manifestations, is a frequent cause of intra-abdominal symptoms (second only to disease of the appendix), this test should be included as a routine in the study of gastro-intestinal cases.

BIBLIOGRAPHY.

1. Meltzer, S. J.: The Disturbance of the Law of Contrary Innervation as a Pathogenic Factor in the Diseases of the Bile Ducts and the Gall-bladder, Am. Jour. Med. Sci., 1917, **153**, 469.

2. Doyon, M.: De l'action exergée par le système nerveux sur l'appareil excreteur de la bile, Arch. de physiol., 1894, **6**, 19.

3. Lyon, B. B. V.: Diagnosis and Treatment of Diseases of the Gall-bladder and Biliary Ducts, Jour. Am. Med. Assn., 1919, **73**, 980.

4. Lyon, B. B. V.: Some Aspects of the Diagnosis and Treatment of Cholecystitis and Cholelithiasis, Med. Clin., No. Am. 1920, **3**, 1253.

5 and 6. Lyon, B. B. V.: Choledochitis, Cholecystitis and Cholelithiasis, New York Med. Jour., 1920, **112**, 1 and 45.

7. Lyon, B. B. V.: Diagnosis and Treatment of Cholecystitis and Choledochitis by a Method of Physiological Drainage, Am. Jour. Med. Sci., 1920, **160**, 515.

8. Lyon, B. B. V: The Treatment of Catarrhal Jaundice by a Rational Direct and Effective Method, Am. Jour. Med. Sci., 1920, **159**, 503.

9. Lyon, B. B. V.: Discussion of the Treatment of a Case of Chronic Arthritis, with Lambliasis, by Duodenal Biliary Drainage, Med. Clinics No. Am., 1921, **4**, 1153.

10. Einhorn, M.: Studies on the Action of Various Salts on the Liver after their Introduction into the Duodenum, New York Med. Jour., 1921, **113**, 313.

11. Einhorn, M.: Action of Various Salts and other Substances on Liver after their Introduction into Duodenum, New York Med. Jour., 1921, **114**, 262.

12. Mendel, Lafayette, B. and Benedict, Stanley, R.: The Paths of Excretion for Inorganic Compounds: IV. The Excretion of Magnesium, Am. Jour. Physiol., 1909, **25**, 1.

13. Bassler, Anthony, Luckett, W. H., and Lutz, J. R.: Some Experiences with the Meltzer-Lyon Method of Draining the Biliary System, Am. Jour. Med. Sci., 1921, **162**, 674.

14. Crohn, B. B., Reiss, J., and Radin, M. J.: Experiences with the Lyon Test, Jour. Am. Med, Assn., 1921, **76**, 1567.

15. Dunn, A. D., and Connell, Karl: Hepatoduodenostomy, with Observations on the Lyon-Meltzer Method of Biliary Drainage, Jour. Am. Med. Assn., 1921, **77**, 1093.

16. Rost, Franz: Die funktionelle Bedeutung der Gallenblase, Experimentelle und anatomische Untersuchungen nach Cholecystektomie; Mitth. a. d. Grenzg. der Med. u. Chir., 1913, **26**, 710.

17. Klee, Ph., and Klupfel, O.: Experimenteller Beitrag zur Funktion der Gallenblase, Mitth. a. d. Grenz. d. med. u. chir., 1915, **27**, 785.

18. Judd, Edward Starr, and Mann, Frank C.: The Effect of Removal of the Gall-bladder: An Experimental Study, Mayo Clinics, 1916, **8**, 253.
19. Bainbridge, F. A. and Dale, H. H.: The Contractile Mechanism of the Gall-bladder and its Extrinsic Nervous Control, Jour. Physiol., 1905, **33**, 138.
20. Handbook of Therapy, Am. Med. Assn., 1918, p. 176.
21. Meltzer, S. J. and Auer, John: Physiological and Pharmacological Studies of Magnesium Salts, Am. Jour. Physiol., 1905, **14**, 366.
22. Rous, P. and McMaster, P. D.: The Concentrating Activity of the Gall-bladder, Jour. Exper. Med., 1921, **34**, 47.
23. Schneider, J. T.: A Study of the Bile Pigments in Pernicious Anemia, Jour. Am. Med. Assn., 1920, **74**, 1759.
24. Bruno, G. G.: L'excitabilité specifique de la magnèse du tube digestif, Arch. des sci. biol., 1899, **7**, 87.
25. Einhorn, Max: Further Experiences with the Direct Examination of the Duodenal Contents in Affections of the Gall-bladder and Allied Organs, Med. Rec., 1918, **93**, 881.
26. Whipple, Allen O.: The Use of the Duodenal Tube in the Preoperative Study of the Bacteriology and Pathology of the Biliary Tract and Pancreas, Ann. Surg., 1921, **83**, 556.
27. Judd, Edward Starr; Cholecystitis; Changes Produced by Removal of the Gall-bladder, Boston Med. and Surg. Jour., 1916, **174**, 815.
28. Einhorn, Max and Meyer, Willy: Diagnosis and Treatment of Recurrent Cholecystitis without Stones, Med. Rec., 1920, **98**, 211.
29. Brown, George E.: The Meltzer-Lyon Method in the Diagnosis of Infections of the Biliary Tract, Jour. Am. Med. Assn., 1920, **75**, 1414.
30. Freese, J. A.: The Force of Contraction of the Gall-bladder and the Course of its Motor and Inhibitory Nerve Fibers, Johns Hopkins Hosp. Bull., 1905, **16**, 235.
31 Archibald, E.: A New Factor in the Causation of Pancreatitis, Trans. Internat. Cong. Med., 1914, **8**, 21.
32. McWhorter, Golden L.: The Surgical Significance of the Common Duct Sphincter, Surg., Gynec. and Obst., 1921, **32**, 134.
33. Archibald, E.: The Experimental Production of Pancreatitis in Animals as the Result of the Resistance of the Common Duct Sphincter, Surg., Gynec. and Obst., 1919, **28**, 529.

STUDIES OF GRAVES' SYNDROME AND THE INVOLUNTARY NERVOUS SYSTEM.

II. The Clinical Manifestations of Disturbances of the Involuntary Nervous System (Autonomic Imbalance).

By Leo Kessel, M.D.,

AND

Harold Thomas Hyman, M.D.

NEW YORK.

Introduction. Comprehensive understanding of the involuntary nervous system requires a study of the phylogeny, embryology and physiology of vertebrates. These arduous and important tasks have been performed mainly by Gaskell's[1 2 3] and Barger and Dale.[4] Gaskell has compiled the literature in his monograph on the "Involuntary Nervous System," and the following review is a coudensation and rearrangement of his data. The rearrangement was necessitated by the fact that Gaskell wrote not with a view to the clinical study of the involuntary nervous system, but to establish the origin of the vertebrate ancestor.

PHYLOGENY AND EMBRYOLOGY OF THE INVOLUNTARY NERVOUS SYSTEM. The cells of the involuntary nervous system arise from those of the cerebrospinal axis. Phylogenetically the involuntary nervous system makes its first appearance in the annelid and it is noteworthy that this is the first phylum in which a vascular system is developed. Of the cells of the primitive involuntary nervous system one group retains as its function the transmission of nerve impulses; the other develops into the chromaffin tissue and acquires secretory activity. In the higher vertebrates the chromaffin cells collect in the adrenal medulla while the nervous cells retain for the most part their segmental arrangement.

ANATOMICAL AND PHYSIOLOGICAL DIFFERENCES BETWEEN THE INVOLUNTARY AND VOLUNTARY NERVOUS SYSTEM. In the voluntary nervous system the motor cell is in the anterior horn and the nerve that emerges in the anterior root is a medullated effector fiber.

In the involuntary nervous system the motor cell occupies a position outside the cord and the medullated fiber that connects it with the central nervous system is a connector and not an effector fiber. The migrated cell gives origin to the true effector fiber, which is non-medullated and is called postganglionic. Whereas the impulse in the voluntary nervous system passes from the cerebrospinal axis to the end-organ without interruption, in the involuntary nervous system it is relayed at the peripheral ganglion. Physiologically the systems differ in that the involuntary nervous system usually functions without entering consciousness and is uninfluenced by the will. "The more the concentrated voluntary nervous system (brain) is freed from the insubordinate involuntary nervous system consistently with the harmonious interaction between the systems, the greater the advantage to the animal." (Gaskell, page 23.)

THORACICO-LUMBAR AND BULBO-SACRAL SUBDIVISIONS OF THE INVOLUNTARY NERVOUS SYSTEM. The involuntary outflow takes place from the midbrain, medulla and thoracico-lumbar and sacral cords. The thoracico-lumbar forms one subdivision and is separated from the others by the plexuses for the limbs. The other three outflows are grouped as the bulbo-sacral division.

It is Gaskell's theory that the ancestor of the vertebrate presented a double segmentation, appendiceal and branchial. The branchial segmentation has given rise to the structures of primitive endoderm and the appendiceal to the structures of primitive ectoderm and mesoderm. The appendiceal segmentation has given rise (1) to the appendages of the skin and the subdermal layer of musculature, (2) the vascular system, including the heart, and (3) the derivatives of the segmental duct from which arise the organs of excretion and reproduction. These structures function for individual and race preservation. They receive excitatory impulses via the thoracico-lumbar and are stimulated by adrenalin. The bulbo-sacral innervation is antagonistic. The branchial segmentation has to do with the metabolic functions in the organism inasmuch as its important derivatives are (1) the gastro-intestinal tract and its accessory glands, and (2) the respiratory tract and such appendages as the thyroid, parathyroid and thymus. Most of these structures receive augmentor impulses over the bulbo-sacral and are accordingly stimulated by acetylcholin. The thoracico-lumbar sends inhibitory impulses to many of these same structures and adrenalin suppresses their functional activity.

Factors that Maintain the Tonicity of the Involuntary Nervous System. With the discovery of the specific action of adrenalin on the thoracico-lumbar division of the involuntary nervous system, nothing was simpler than to assume that its tonic activity was regulated by the epinephrin circulating in the blood. The quantitative work of Hoskins[5] demonstrated quite clearly that adrenalin in amounts sufficient to cause a rise of blood-pressure, inhibits intestinal movement. Hence, the tonicity theory was generally abandoned and for it was substituted the emergency theory of Cannon.[6] This postulates that in times of stress epinephrin is poured forth to stimulate the thoracico-lumbar division. The experimental work of Cannon and his colleagues, however, has not been confirmed by other workers, notably Stewart and Rogoff.[7] For the present Cannon's[8] ingenious theory may be regarded as interesting and stimulating, but not proved.

It has been assumed that some metabolite, possibly a cholin derivative, in an analogous manner regulates the tonicity of the bulbo-sacral division.

Our own[9] work fails to show the factors concerned with the maintainance of the tonus of the thoracico-lumbar; the tonus is quite independent of the adrenals, and we think that the amount of epinephrin necessary to produce an emergency effect is beyond the secretory capacity of the adrenal glands.[10] We have also been unable to confirm the reported stimulating effect of thyroxin[11, 12] on the involuntary nervous system, and we have shown that in acute experiments, at least, thyroxin is quite without effect on the involuntary nervous system.

Autonomic Imbalance. The following report deals with patients whose symptoms can be ascribed to disturbance in the realm of the involuntary nervous system. The symptoms may be divided into three groups. In the first of these the symptoms are objective, and due to disturbed function of an organ in which no lesion can be demonstrated by the most painstaking clinical examination. The second group differs only in that the manifestations are subjective. The third group is composed of such symptoms as asthenia and tremor. Their constant association with the above groups and their accentuation by adrenalin administration has led us to regard them as of similar origin.

To the syndrome presented by the association of these symptoms we have applied the term *autonomic imbalance*. In it we include the conditions ordinarily called larval hyperthyroidism, forme fruste of hyperthyroidism, Basedowoid, suprarenal insufficiency, etc. These terms are discarded because they are either misleading, or are dependent on an erroneous or doubtful hypothesis.

Material Studied. The 86 patients reported, (Table I) were studied in the Outpatient Department of Mount Sinai Hospital.* None had definite or constant elevation of their basal metabolism but all had autonomic imbalance as we have defined it.

Etiology. 1. *Predisposing Causes.* The factors that predispose to this syndrome are at present unknown. Manifestations of the disturbance have been present in most of these patients as far back as they can remember. Whether the predisposition is inherited or whether it is due to some early environmental factor remains to be decided.

2. *Exciting Causes.* As exciting causes may be mentioned: (*a*) sex epochs; (*b*) focal infection; (*c*) psychic insult.

(*a*) In 23 of the 86 patients the symptoms were greatly accentuated at the time of puberty. In 11, pregnancy aggravated the symptoms. Hence in 40 per cent of these patients exacerbation was associated with a sex epoch.

(*b*) In 2 patients infection was the most probable etiological factor. In nearly one-half of the patients focal infection was present and may have been an exciting factor. Forty-one of the patients had tonsils from which we expressed secretion, and 7 had sinus infections.

(*c*) Psychic insult played an essential role in 8 patients and a minor role in at least 12 others.

Symptoms. A. SUBJECTIVE SYMPTOMS. 1. *Palpitation.* Thirty-nine patients complained of palpitation. There was no relationship between this symptom and the pulse rate: for example, No. 8613, a woman whose pulse was 70 and whose basal metabolism was—2, had palpitation and No. 8579 with a pulse rate of 140 had no palpitation.

2. *Dyspnea.* Eleven women complained of shortness of breath. Of these 7 had auricular extrasystoles, but in none of the others could any disturbance of the cardiac or pulmonary mechanisms be elicited, and in none was there any elevation of the basal metabolism.

3. *Headache.* Seven women had chronic or recurring headaches; in 1 sinus infection evidently played a role; in the others no cause for the headache could be found.

4. *Insomnia.* The insomnia was sufficiently marked in 20 patients to demand treatment.

5. *Loss of Weight.* Thirteen patients reported loss of weight.

* We wish to express our appreciation to Miss May Slater, R.N., who, as Superintendent of the Outpatient Department, rendered invaluable assistance in the organization and maintenance of our clinic.

B. Objective Symptoms. 1. *Diarrhea.* Four women, all over thirty years of age, reported attacks of "diarrhea." No dietetic or physiological cause for the intestinal disturbance was present.

2. *Eye Signs.* Von Graefe's sign was present in 19 women and in 12 others there was a definite exophthalmos.

3. *Gastric Disturbances.* Eight women complained of "indigestion." In many of these there was a close simulation of the symptoms of gastroduodenal ulcer or of chronic appendicitis. The relationship of the alterations in the involuntary nervous system to these unclassified gastric disorders will be the subject of a later communication.

4. *Menstrual Disturbances.* Menstrual disturbances of various types were reported by 5 patients.

5. *Sweating.* Abnormal degrees of sweating were present in 17 patients. In 2 instances the profuse night sweats led to the erroneous diagnosis of tuberculosis.

6. *Vasomotor Instability.* Blushing, flushing, or cold extremities pointed to vasomotor instability in 10 patients.

7. *Mental Disturbances.* Emotional instability was common. Psychoneurosis was present in 12; it usually assumed the anxiety or sexual types.

8. *Tachycardia.* Only 2 patients of this group had a pulse rate below 80. In the majority, the most striking objective findings were the tachycardia and the extreme lability of the pulse rate. Thus in patient No. 3598 the range was from 96 to 200. The tachycardia was most marked in the group of the puberty patients, where a rate of from 140 to 160 was not at all uncommon. It is noteworthy that the tachycardia bears no relation to palpitation or to the basal metabolism. Thus patient No. 8539 had a pulse rate of 104, palpitation, and a basal metabolism of −6; No. 8633 had a pulse rate of 120, palpitation, and a basal metabolism of 0; No. 8680 had a pulse rate of 136, palpitation, and a basal metabolism of +10; No. 8547 had a pulse rate of 130, basal metabolism of +8, and no palpitation.

9. *Irregularities of Cardiac Mechanism.* Cardiac irregularities were present in 6 patients. Auricular extrasystoles were the most common (3 patients). One patient (No. 8740) had a paroxysmal tachycardia and another (No. 9235) paroxysmal auricular flutter. All of these patients were referred by Dr. Rothschild from the Cardiac Clinic where they had previously been examined. The absence of any organic cardiac basis for their symptoms was verified clinically, by fluoroscopy and electrocardiogram, before the patients were sent to us. Most of these women had been regarded as "cardiacs" for years. Small doses of atropine gave (Nos. 8498, 8740, 9235) prompt relief. A further study of this group will be made by Dr. Kaufman Wallach and their relationship to the "cardiac war neuroses" studied.

TABLE I.—THE CLINICAL MANIFESTATIONS OF AUTONOMIC IMBALANCE (A. I.)

No.	Age.	Sex.	Goiter noted at age of.	Duration of goiter, years.	Asthenia.	Loss of weight.	Palpitation.	Tachycardia.	Diarrhea.	Bulging eye.	Nervousness.	Dyspnea.	Gastric disturbance.	Menstrual disturbance.	Sweating.	Insomnia.	Irritability.	Headache.	Vasomotor irritability.	Tremor.	von Gräfe.	Exophthalmos.	Pigmentation.	Face oval.	Pulse.	Basal metabolism.	Neck shrink, months.	Consistency of goiter.	Bruit, etc.	Tonsils infected.	Sinus infected.	Apparent etiology of goiter.	Previous removal of thyroid.
															PUBERTY																		
8796	14	♀	?	?	O	O	O	O	O	O	+	O	O	O	O	O	O	O	O	O	O	O	O	..	140	..	1.25 cm 3 mos.	S	O	O	O	Pub.	C
9197	36	♀	34	2	O	O	+	O	O	O	O	O	O	O	O	O	O	O	O	O	+	O	O	..	100	18	Palp.	..	O	O	O	Pub.	Ecto x-ra
8669	15	♀	14	3 mos.	O	O	O	+	O	O	O	O	O	O	O	O	O	O	O	O	O	O	O	..	160	..	Palp.	..	O	+	O	Pub.	
8547	15	♀	14	1	+	O	O	O	O	O	+	O	O	O	+	O	O	+	O	+	O	O	O	..	130	8	Palp.	..	O	+	O	Pub.	
8741	17	♀	?	?	O	O	O	O	O	O	O	O	O	+	O	O	O	O	O	O	O	O	O	..	...	7	Palp.	..	O	O	O	Pub.	
8674	17	♀	15	2	O	+	O	O	O	O	+	O	O	O	+	O	O	O	O	+	O	O	O	..	102	..	Palp.	..	O	O	O	Pub.	
8720	16	♀	?	?	O	+	O	O	O	O	+	O	O	O	O	O	+	O	O	+	O	O	O	..	86	..	Palp.	..	O	O	O	Pub.	
9125	18	♀	15	2½	O	O	O	O	O	O	O	O	O	O	+	O	O	O	O	O	O	O	O	..	...	..	Palp.	..	O	O	O	Pub.	Ops
8031	15	♀	?	?	O	O	O	O	O	O	+	O	O	O	O	+	O	O	O	O	O	+	O	..	96	..	Palp.	..	O	O	O	Pub.	
8569	15	♀	13	2	O	O	O	O	O	O	+	O	O	O	O	O	+	O	O	O	+	O	O	..	...	..	Palp.	..	O	+	O	Pub.	
8565	17	♀	16	1	O	O	O	O	O	O	+	O	O	O	O	O	O	O	O	O	O	O	O	..	88	4	9 cm. 8 mos.	..	O	O	O	Pub.	
9247	15	♀	15	2 mos.	O	O	+	O	O	O	O	+	O	O	O	O	O	O	O	O	O	O	O	..	...	..	....	F	O	+	O	Pub.	
9157	18	♀	16	2	O	+	O	O	O	O	O	O	O	O	O	O	O	O	O	+	O	O	O	..	96	..	....	S	O	+	O	Pub.	
8539	17	♀	?	?	O	O	+	O	O	O	O	O	O	O	O	O	+	O	+	O	O	O	O	..	104	−6	7 cm. 6 mos.	F	O	+	O	Pub.	
8984	16	♀	14	2	O	O	O	O	O	O	+	O	O	O	O	O	O	O	O	O	O	O	O	..	144	..	6 cm. 9 mos.	S	O	+	O	Pub.	
8636	14	♀	Birth	14	O	O	O	O	O	O	O	O	O	O	O	O	O	O	O	+	O	O	O	..	92	10	1.25 cm. 2 mos.	F	O	+	O	Pub.	
9079	14	♀	14	2 wks.	O	O	O	O	O	O	+	O	O	O	O	O	O	O	O	O	O	+	O	..	120	..	Palp.	..	O	+	O	Pub.	
8882	19	♀	19	2 mos.	O	O	O	O	O	O	O	O	O	O	O	O	O	O	O	O	O	O	O	..	...	..	2.5 3 mos.	..	O	+	O	Pub.	
9248	16	♀	14	2	O	O	O	O	O	O	+	O	O	O	O	O	O	O	O	O	O	O	O	..	120	..	Palp.	F	O	+	O	Pub.	
5273	13	♂	13	1 wk.	O	O	O	O	O	O	O	O	O	O	O	O	O	O	O	O	+	+	O	O	...	..	2.5 6 mos.	F	O	O	O	Pub.	
9190	14	♀	14	3 mos.	O	O	+	O	O	O	+	+	O	O	+	O	+	O	+	O	O	O	O	..	120	4	Palp.	S	O	O	O	Pub.	
9159	19	♀	?	?	+	O	O	O	O	O	+	O	O	O	O	O	O	O	O	O	O	O	O	..	96	..	Palp.	..	O	O	O	Pub.	
8716	26	♀	16	10	+	+	+	O	O	O	+	+	O	O	+	O	O	O	O	+	+	O	O	..	112	..	Palp.	..	+	+	O	Pub.	
														POST PARTUM																			
9202	32	♀	32	7 mos.	O	O	O	O	O	O	+	O	O	O	O	O	O	O	O	+	+	O	O	O	114	4	Palp.	..	O	O	O	Preg.	
9195	44	♀	?	?	O	O	O	O	O	O	+	O	O	O	O	O	O	O	O	O	O	O	O	O	104	..	Palp.	..	O	O	O	Preg.	
9124	30	♀	24	?	+	+	+	+	O	O	O	O	O	O	+	+	O	O	O	O	O	O	O	O	96	16	Palp.	..	O	+	O	Preg.	x-ra elect

9077	65	♀	35	30	O	O	O	O	O	O	+	+	O	O	O	O	O	O	O	O	O	O	O	O	...	..	...	..	O	O	O	Preg.	
8559	46	♀	41	5	O	O	+	O	O	O	+	O	O	O	O	O	O	O	O	O	O	O	O	O	104	5	Palp	O	O	+	O	Preg.	
9040	28	♀	20	8	O	O	+	O	O	O	O	+	O	O	O	O	O	+	O	O	O	O	O	O	...	..	Palp.	O	O	+	O	Preg.	
8512	59	♀	45	14	O	O	O	O	O	O	O	O	O	O	+	O	O	O	O	O	O	O	O	O		.	Palp	O	O	O	O	Preg.	
8633	28	♀	21	7	O	O	+	O	O	O	O	O	O	O	O	+	O	O	+	O	O	+	O	O	120	O	Palp.	O	O	+	O	Preg.	X-ray
8582	36	♀	22	14	O	O	O	O	+	O	+	O	O	O	O	O	O	O	O	O	O	O	O	O	.	.	Palp	O	O	+	O	Preg.	X-ray
8592	50	♀	29	21	+	O	+	O	O	O	O	O	O	O	O	O	O	O	O	O	O	O	O	O	88	O	Palp	O	O	+	O	Preg.	
8564	32	♀	27	5	+	O	O	O	O	O	O	O	O	O	O	+	O	O	O	O	+	O	O	O	120	8	Palp	O	O	O	O		
POST INFECTION																																	
8598	48	♀	?	?	+	O	+	O	O	O	+	O	O	O	O	+	O	O	O	+	+	O	O	O	100	..	Palp.	O	O	O	O	Flu	
9235	30	♀	30	1 wk.	+	O	+	O	O	O	+	O	O	O	+	O	O	O	O	O	O	O	O	O	90 210	.	Palp	O	O	+	O	Cold	
POST PSYCHIC TRAUMA																																	
8680	32	♀	27	5	O	O	+	O	O	O	O	O	O	O	O	+	O	O	O	+	O	O	O	O	136	10	3 cm. 9 mos	S	O	O	O	Fright	X-ray
9192	36	♀	32	4	+	O	+	O	O	O	+	O	O	O	O	O	O	O	O	O	O	O	O	O	116	.	Palp	O	O	O	O	Fall	Ops.
9052	22	♀	21	1	+	O	O	O	O	O	+	O	O	O	+	O	O	O	O	O	O	O	O	O	132	.	0.5 cm. 2 mos	O	O	+	O	Tonsillectomy	
ASSOCIATED WITH PSYCHIC TRAUMA																																	
9263	42	♀	?	?	+	+	+	O	O	O	+	+	+	O	O	+	O	O	O	O	O	O	O	O	88	6	Palp	S	O	+	O	b. has goiter	
9233	32	♀	?	?	+	O	+	O	O	O	+	O	O	O	O	+	O	O	O	+	O	O	O	O	..		Palp	F	O	+	O		
8662	26	♀	?	?	+	+	+	O	O	O	+	O	+	O	O	O	O	+	+	O	O	O	O	O	.	17		S	O	+	O		
8705	27	♀	?	?	O	O	O	O	O	O	O	O	O	O	O	+	O	+	O	O	O	O	O	O	.		Palp	O	O	O	O		
8527	25	♀	?	?	O	O	O	O	O	O	+	O	O	O	O	O	O	O	O	O	+	+	O	O	90	4	Palp.	S	O	O	O		
9093	30	♀	30	4 mos	+	O	+	O	O	O	+	O	O	+	+	+	O	O	O	+	O	O	O	O	104	.	0.5 cm. 2 wks.	F	O	+	O		
9249	44	♀	?	?	+	O	+	O	O	O	+	O	O	O	O	O	O	O	O	+	O	O	O	O	104	..	.	S	O	O	O	O	
8860	?	♀	?	?	O	O	O	O	O	O	O	O	+	O	O	O	O	O	O	+	+	O	O	O		8	....	.	O	O	O	O	
ASSOCIATED WITH FOCAL INFECTION OR UNKNOWN																																	
9268	30	♀	30	2 wks.	O	O	+	O	O	O	O	O	O	O	+	O	O	O	O	O	O	O	O	O	120	.	Palp.	O	O	+	+		
8809	33	♀	30	3	+	+	O	O	O	O	+	O	O	O	+	+	O	O	O	O	O	O	O	O		.	....	O	O	+	O	O	
.	43	♀	?	?	O	O	O	O	O	O	O	O	O	O	O	O	O	O	O	O	O	O	O	O		..	....	O	O	O	O	O	
8632	39	♀	31	8	+	+	+	O	O	O	+	O	O	O	O	+	O	O	O	O	O	O	O	O	120	.	....	O	O	+	O	O	2 ect.
9126	26	♀	18	8	O	O	+	O	O	O	+	O	O	O	O	+	O	O	O	+	+	+	O	O	140	12	....	O	O	+	O	O	
8536	46	♀	40	6	O	O	O	O	O	O	+		O	O	O	O	O	O	O	O	+	O	O	O	104	.	....	F	O	+	O	O	
8551	43	♀	31	12	O	O	+	O	O	O	+	+	O	O	O	O	O	O	O	O	O	O	O	O	90	12	3 cm. 4 mos.	O	O	+	O	O	
9024	38	♀	26	12	+	O	+	O	O	O	O	O	O	O	O	+	O	O	O	O	O	O	O	O		.	....	O	O	+	O	O	
8614	30	♀	?	?	+	O	O	O	+	O	O	+	O	O	+	O	O	O	O	O	O	O	O	O	132	.	....	O	O	O	O	O	X-ray
. .	50	♀	26	24	O	O	O	O	O	O	O	O	O	O	O	+	O	O	O	O	O	O	O	O	..	.	....	O	..	O	O	O	
8719	20	♀	?	?	O	O	+	O	O	O	+	O	O	O	O	O	+	O	O	+	O	O	O	O	120	..	3 cm. 3 mos.	O	O	+	O	O	
8765	37	♀	32	5	O	O	+	O	O	O	+	O	O	+	+	O	O	O	O	+	+	O	O	O	72	5	6 cm. 8 mos.	O	O	O	O	O	
8476	33	♀	?	?	O	O	+	O	+	O	+	O	O	O	+	+	O	O	O	+	O	+	O	O	96	10	Palp.	O	O	O	O	O	
5065	27	♂	?	?	O	O	O	+	O	O	O	O	O	O	+	O	O	O	O	+	O	O	O	O	84	10	Palp.	O	O	O	O	O	
8906	23	♀	20	3	O	O	+	O	O	+	+	O	+	O	+	O	O	O	O	O	+	O	O	O	120	18	Palp.	O	O	O	O	O	
8579	23	♀	?	?	+	O	O	O	O	O	+	O	+	O	+	+	O	O	+	O	O	O	O	O	140	14	Palp.	O	O	+	O	O	
8972	41	♀	35	6	O	O	+	O	O	O	+	O	+	O	O	O	O	O	O	O	O	+	O	O	90	..	Palp.	F	O	+	+	O	Ectomy

TABLE I.—THE CLINICAL MANIFESTATIONS OF AUTONOMIC IMBALANCE (A. I.)—*Continued.*

No.	Age.	Sex.	Goiter noted at age of.	Duration of goiter, years.	Asthenia.	Loss of weight	Palpitation.	Tachycardia.	Diarrhea.	Bulging eye.	Nervousness.	Dyspnea.	Gastric disturbance	Menstrual disturbance	Sweating.	Insomnia.	Irritability.	Headache.	Vasomotor irritability	Tremor.	von Gräfe.	Exophthalmos.	Pigmentation.	Face oval.	Pulse.	Basal metabolism.	Neck shrink, months.	Consistency of goiter	Bruit, etc.	Tonsils infected.	Sinus infected.	Apparent etiology of goiter.	Previous removal of thyroid. Result.
3734	47	♀	44	3	O	O	O	O	O	O	+	O	O	O	O	O	O	O	O	O	O	O	O	O	...	..	5 cm. 3 mos.	O	O	+	O	O	
8158	31	♀	25	6	O	O	+	O	O	O	+	O	O	O	O	O	O	O	O	+	O	O	O	O	...	..	Palp.	[illegible]	O	+	O	O	Ectom
8493	28	♀	19	9	O	O	O	O	O	O	O	O	O	O	O	O	O	O	+	O	O	O	O	O	78	O	5 cm. 10 mos.	[illegible]	O	O	O	O	
5567	28	♂	26	2	O	O	O	O	O	O	O	O	+	O	O	O	O	O	O	O	O	+	O	O	...	..	Palp.		O	O	O	O	Ectom
8844	27	♀	20	7	O	O	O	O	O	O	O	O	O	O	O	O	O	O	O	O	O	O	O	O	...	..	Palp.		O	+	O	O	
8591	26	♀	26	3 mos.	O	O	O	O	O	O	O	O	O	O	O	O	O	O	O	O	+	O	O	O	...	..	Palp.		O	+	O	O	
8495	45	♀	?	?	O	O	O	O	O	O	O	O	O	O	+	O	O	O	O	O	O	O	O	O	...	..	Palp.		O	O	O	O	Ectom
9127	44	♀	38	6	+	O	O	O	O	O	+	O	O	O	O	O	O	O	O	O	O	O	O	O	96	..	Palp.		O	+	O	O	
9246	23	♀	?	?	+	+	O	O	O	O	+	O	O	O	+	+	O	O	O	+	O	O	O	O	...	O	Palp.		O	+	+	O	
8643	32	♀	32	3 mos.	+	O	+	O	O	O	O	O	O	O	O	O	O	O	O	O	O	O	O	O	...	..	Palp.		O	O	O	O	
5085	25	♂	?	?	O	O	O	O	O	O	O	O	O	O	O	O	O	O	O	O	O	+	O	O	...	..	Palp.		O	O	+	O	
8057	22	♀	?	?	+	O	+	O	O	O	O	+	O	O	O	O	O	O	O	O	O	O	O	O	112	9	Palp.		O	O	O	O	
8999	36	♀	?	?	+	O	O	O	+	O	+	O	O	O	+	O	O	O	O	O	O	O	O	O	...	..	Palp.		O	O	O	O	
5165	24	♂	?	?		O	O	O		O	+	O	O	O		O	O	O	O	O	+	O	O	O	...	..	Palp.		O	O	O	O	
8663	25	♀	25	6 wks.	+	O	+	O	O	O	O	O	O	O	O	O	O	O	+	O	O	O	O	O	...	..	Palp.	O	O	O	+	O	
8613	34	♀	23	11	+	O	+	O	O	O	+	O	O	O	+	+			+	O	O	O	O	O	70	2	....	O	O	O	O	O	Ectom.
8730	40	♀	?	?	+	O	+	O	O	O	O	+	O	O	O	O	+	O	O	O	+	O	O	O	80	..	n. p.	O	O	O	+	O	
8498	38	♀	?	?	O	+	+	O	O	O	O	O	O	O	+	O	O	+	+	O	+	O	O	O	84	7	n. p.	O	O	O	O	O	
3740	27	♀	?	?	O	+	+	O	O	O	+	O	O	O	+	+	O	O	+	+	+	+	O	O	102	4	n. p.	O	O	O	O	O	
8540	38	♀	?	?	+	O	+	O	O	O	O	O	+	O	O	O	O	O	O	O	+	+	O	O	100	..	n. p.	O	O	O	+	O	
8449	26	♀	?	?	O	O	+	+	O	O	O	O	O	+	O	O	O	O	O	+	O	O	O	O	140	34	Palp.	O	O	O	O	O	Ectomy x-ray.
8644	30	♀	?	?	O	O	O	O	O	O	+	+	O	+	+	O	O	+	O	O	O	O	O	O	132	..	Palp.	O	O	O	O	O	X-ray.
9078	20	♀	17	3	+	+	O	O	O	O	+	O	O	O	+	O	O	+	O	O	O	+	O	O	84	..	Palp.	O	O	+	+	O	

NOTE.—(1) Marked tachycardia in puberty group, (2) absence of relationship between pulse and B. M., (3) absence of relationship between duration or type of thyroid enlargement and sympathomimetic symptoms; (4) preponderance of females; (5) asthenia and diarrhea more frequent in those over thirty-five and eye signs extremely infrequent; (6) eye signs and tremor comparatively frequent in those under thirty-five and asthenia and diarrhea infrequent, (7) no relationship between palpitation and pulse-rate; (8) the frequent occurrence of dyspnea and its independence of tachycardia, elevation of B. M. and cardiopulmonary lesions; (9) two instances of arrested exophthalmic goiter differing in no way except history of crisis from A. I. (10) basal metabolism over plus 18 only once; (11) efficacy of iodides in reducing neck circumference; (12) efficacy of atropin in cardiac group; (13) frequent occurrence of infected tonsils; (14 infrequency of bruit, (15) exciting etiologic role of sex epochs, psychic insult and focal infection, (16) futility of operations on thyroid gland and roentgen-ray in reducing size of gland or symptoms; (17) practically every patient referred as exophthalmic goiter; (18) sympathomimetic symptoms independent of pulse and B. M., and may coexist with myxedema; (18) pressure symptoms from thyroid very rare.

10. *Tremor.* A coarse or fine tremor developed in 23 of these patients when the fingers were extended.

C. MANIFESTATIONS THAT MAY BE INFERRED TO BE SYMPATHOMIMETIC IN THAT THEY ARE FREQUENTLY PRESENT IN AUTONOMIC IMBALANCE AND ARE ACCENTUATED BY ADRENALIN. 1. *Nervousness.* Forty-nine women complained bitterly of "nervousness."

2. *Asthenia.* Asthenia was complained of by 30 patients. This symptom was rarely found in the puberty group but extremely common in the others.

3. *Goiter.* Seventy-two of the 86 patients had a definitely enlarged thyroid gland. The duration of the goiter varied between two weeks to thirty years, and neither the duration nor the size of the goiter bore any relation to the symptoms. There was no uniformity in the consistency of the gland; some were firm, others soft. In 2 patients a bruit was audible over the gland. The relation of the onset of the goiter to the sexual cycle, particularly puberty, was striking in many instances.

Every member of the puberty group (16) had undergone specific but futile treatment referable to the thyroid gland. Ten had been subjected to thyroidectomy; 1 had had two operations. Eight had received roentgen-ray exposures without shrinking the goiter or relieving the symptoms. The effect of small doses of iodine in diminishing the size of the goiter was most striking, even in long standing cases. The earliest change noted was a softening of the gland. The average shrinkage of the neck circumference was about 1 cm. a month.

4. *Basal Metabolism.* Basal metabolism estimations were made on 31 of this group. Because of the fact that these patients were studied in the outpatient department it was necessary for them to come to the hospital before 8.30 A.M. Many had to travel great distances. Consequently a true basal rate was difficult to secure. The conditions under which the basal metabolism estimations were obtained made us regard +18 as within the normal range. Nevertheless, in but one woman (8449) was a striking elevation noted (+34). She was referred to the hospital and carefully studied, but a clinical diagnosis of Graves' syndrome could not consistently be made. Two other readings taken in the hospital were +4 and +8. In all but 5 of the other patients, the metabolism was below +10; the highest was +18.

The elevation of the metabolism bore no relation to the symptoms or to the pulse rate.

Associated Conditions. Many interesting conditions were observed associated with the autonomic imbalance. Concerning their relationship, data are insufficient to warrant definite conclusions. In 2 (8796, 8669) malnutrition appeared simultaneously with the goiter and the symptoms. Two girls presented the picture of Froehlich's syndrome (8674, 8636). One man had the hands of typical acromegalia (5065). The cardiac arrhythmias and the psychoneuroses have already received comment. Four women displayed the clinical picture of myxedema (8592, 8598, 8613, 9127). Thyroidectomy was probably responsible in Case 8613, and this woman had a pulse rate of 70 and a basal metabolism of —2, with a persistence of all of her sympathomimetic symptoms. In all of these, thyroid extract caused a marked improvement. Two women (8632, 9126) gave a history that suggested Graves' syndrome; they were apparently now in the stage of arrest. Except for the crisis their histories differed in no essential respect from those of the other patients.

Correlation of Symptoms. The vast majority (84 per cent) of these patients presented both tachycardia and goiter; *i. e.*, two of the cardinal clinical symptoms of Graves' syndrome. There were 23 with tremor, and of these all but 5 had goiter and tachycardia. Thus 18 patients presented three of the four cardinal symptoms of Graves' syndrome. Twenty-six had either von Graefe's sign or exophthalmos; of these 9 had tremor and 6 had exophthalmos, tremor, tachycardia, and goiter (8716, 9202, 8598, 8860, 9126, 8476). Not one of these patients had a basal metabolism above +10; 1 (8598) had, in addition, some of the characteristics of myxedema. Fifty per cent of the entire group had three or more of the minor symptoms of Graves' syndrome and usually at least two of the four cardinal signs.

100 90 80 70 60 50 40 30 20 10 0

Tachycardia

Tremor

Eye signs

Goiter

Tachycardia plus tremor

Tachycardia plus goiter

Tachycardia plus eye signs

Tachycardia plus tremor plus eye signs

Tachycardia plus tremor plus goiter

Tachycardia plus goiter plus eye signs

Tachycardia plus goiter plus eye signs plus tremor

Sensitiveness to Drugs. In a few of these patients the responses to the subcutaneous injections of atropine and of adrenalin were determined. The incidence of reaction in individuals free from symptoms was first ascertained. Two groups of subjects were chosen—second-year medical students at the College of Physicians and Surgeons, Columbia University, and convalescent medical and surgical patients at Mount Sinai Hospital. Reference to Table II shows that of the medical students 31 per cent responded to adrenalin and 22 per cent to atropine. None of these students had symptoms of imbalance. Table II shows also that of the hospital patients 30 per cent reacted to adrenalin and 22 per cent to atropine. It is evident, therefore, that sensitiveness to these drugs does not imply active autonomic imbalance, and in the article on Graves' syndrome[13] (No. III of the series) it will be shown that autonomic imbalance may exist without drug sensitiveness. We interpret drug sensitiveness in the absence of clinical symptoms of autonomic imbalance as evidence of a latent imbalance and are therefore attempting to keep these individuals under observation. The absence of drug reactions in the presence of clinical manifestations of autonomic imbalance is due to the fact that those particular structures on which the drugs act are in a state of normal irritability. Sensitiveness to adrenalin means nothing more or less than a lowering in the excitability threshold of the myoneural junction of the thoracico-lumbar division; increased reactivity to atropine, which paralyzes the myoneural junction, indicates an increased tonus of the entire bulbo-sacral system. The reactivity to these drugs is therefore no index of the state of the involuntary nervous system as a whole. In the vast majority of patients with autonomic imbalance sensitiveness to adrenalin or atropine is present; this sensitiveness suggests the type of autonomic imbalance. The sensitiveness is not necessarily universal and may be limited to one organ, so that an individual may have either a purely local or a general autonomic imbalance.

Sensitiveness to these drugs cannot therefore be taken as an absolute objective test for the presence of active autonomic imbalance. It is, however, extremely useful as an adjuvant in the diagnosis and together with the clinical impression may serve to corroborate a clinical suspicion. It is probably present as frequently in autonomic imbalance as in Graves' syndrome and is of no aid in this differential diagnosis. To us, these reactions have been of invaluable assistance in our conception of the disturbance and in the management of the patient.

Our technic has been greatly simplified. In order to obtain a basal pulse rate and pressure reading under the prevailing conditions, we first insert the needle into the subcutaneous tissues. The pulse rate and blood-pressure readings are then taken until a constant is obtained on several readings. The barrel of the hypodermic is then attached to the needle and the drug injected. For the adrenalin (0.5 cc) test the pulse rate is taken every minute and the blood-pressure as frequently as possible (two or three a minute) for the first ten minutes. If no reaction occurs after that time the test is usually discontinued and reported negative. For the atropine test 1 mgm. of atropine sulphate is injected and the pulse rate counted every minute for twenty minutes in a negative test. In positive tests, the readings are discontinued at the fastigium.

Many interesting pharmacological data were obtained. The usual adrenalin response occurs within a few seconds and is ordinarily marked by a pressor followed by an accelerator response and

TABLE II.—THE RESPONSES TO THE SUBCUTANEOUS INJECTIONS OF ATROPI ADRENALIN IN TWO GROUPS OF "NORMAL PERSONS" (MEDICAL STUDEN AND CONVALESCENT PATIENTS).

NOTE —No relation between adrenalin and atropin sensitiveness, no relation between subjective sympt objective findings; no relation between original pulse-rate or B. P. and extent of response

Subjects	Before adrenalin		General condition.	After adrenalin.		Subjective symptoms	Atr
	Pulse.	Bl. Pr.		Pulse.	Bl. Pr.		Befor pulse
E. Bessie	....	.	Medical student	....	....	Dry mouth	84*
J. Besel	....	....	" "	....	....	....	82*
H. Bresky	....	....	" "	....	....	....	84
de Merc	....	....	" "	....	....	....	74*
J. Dranit	....	....	" "	....	....	....	72
H. Farnham	....	....	" "	....	....	....	80
Frank	....	....	" "	....	....	....	84
Goldin	....	....	" "	....	....	....	76
Hansen	....	....	" "	....	....	....	70
Lefk	....	....	" "	....	....	....	84
MacDon	....	....	" "	....	....	....	82
Milgrim	....	....	" " (asthma)	....	....	....	66
Mulinos	....	....	Medical student	....	....	....	60
G. Neuman	....	....	" "	....	....	....	60
I. Reich	....	....	" "	....	....	....	78
Rosenblatt	....	....	" "	....	....	....	76
G. S. S.	....	....	Research Ass't.	....	....	....	82*
Talty	....	....	Medical student	....	....	....	88
No. 111	....	....	" "	....	....	....	90
Austrian	76	106	" "	78	106		
Bowen	68	114	" "	80	114	Slight tremor	
Chobat	78	122	" "	110*	156*	Faint; sweat, tremor; irregular respiration, cold	
Foland	80	124	" "	80	124		
Fordyce	80	118	" "	76	118	Pallor; nausea	
Griswold	72	124	" "	88*	156*	None	
H'horn	74	110	" "	108	128	Psychic	
Kohn	80	128	" "	80*	156*	Slight tremor; throb	
MacKie	72	116	" "	96*	160*	Headache; air hunger; tremor; pallor	
Monash	108	140	" "	134	160	Psychic (?)	
Murphy	.	. .	" "	. . .	....	....	68
L. Newman	102	.. .	" "	98	....	Tremor	
O'Brien	78	130	" "	76	138		
Peck	80	134	" "	86	130	Palpitation	
Schroeder	86	116	" "	80	120		
Shafton	80	110	" "	84	124		
Taintor	60	100	" "	110*	114*		
Twiss	64	110	" "	90*	156*		
Wall'st.	80	130	" "	90	134		
Wechsler	90	122	" "	98	130		
Weed	72	110	" "	84	112		
Yaswen	62	114	" "	78	118		
No. 111	90	124	" "	104*	158*	None	
M. Abr.	78	110	Bilateral hernia	88	120	....	72
I. Altman	92	104	Post-pneumonia	120*	144*	Irregular tremor	90
R. Bagno	90	100	Mitral stenosis	96	104	Dyspnea; weakness	96
A. Bass	72	110	???? (Hysteria)	74	120	Weakness	72
A. Below	72	100	Salpingectomy; appendicectomy	100*	130*	Tremor; weakness	78
B. Berlin	60	110	Cancer of colon (?)	60	110	....	60
I. Berman	84	120	Varicose veins	88	112	....	84

lat	....	....	Hernia	....	....		84	90
sky	78	114	Hernia	96*	130*	Tremor	78	72
ne	86	124	Intest. obstruct.	90	130			
hen	88	110	Osteomyelitis	96*	130*		96*	112*
nt.	78	110	Contracture	84	116		72	60
of	60	100	Hyperacidity	72	104		60	54
nan	84	100	Mitral stenosis	108	104	Palpitation	78	84
	84	110	Hemorrhoids	96	116		78	60
nan	60	110	Neuritis	60	110		60	60
	72	110	Post-pneumonia	72	110			
t.	84	112	Catarrhal jaundice	84	116		84	88
erg	96	124	Osteomyelitis	102	114		96	104
at	72	104	Syphilis	76	108		84	88
eb	78	120	Spondylitis	90	120		80	72
s	....	....	Bronchopneumonia	....	....		72	76
n	60	114	Acute appendicitis	96*	144*	Palpitation arythmia	60	64
h	96	116	Cyst of breast	100	120		96	92
	60	110	Ulcer of stomach (?)	60*	130*	None	60	64
an	....	....	Cancer of breast	....	....		90*	132*
fman	96	100	Cholecystectomy	102*	120*		96*	114*
s	104	112	Phlebitis	120*	150*	Dyspnea; palp tremor	100	109
	90	104	Osteomyelitis	120*	130*	Palpitation	98*	110*
sky	92	120	Hernia	96	126		88	92
r	78	114	Fistula	90*	144*	None	78	74
n	60	106	Gastralgia	86*	148*	Palpitation, asthenia	64	66
	84	120	Rheum. fever	120*	140*	Palpitation, asthenia; tremor	78*	90*
f	50	114	Post-pneu.	60	106		50	56
	66	100	Gastric sympt.	84	106		72	66
el	84	100	??	112*	124*	None	66*	86*
s	72	110	Gastric neurosis ?	108*	136*	Epigastric pain; tremor	72	60
r	....	....	Hernia	...	....		88	72
	88	96	Pneumonia	96	100		66*	84*
.	60	90	Arthritis	66	96		68	60
nus	58	120	Lacerations	76	110	Tremor	52	56
an	78	104	Calculus	70	108		72	82
an	60	120	Hernia	64	126		60	64
sk	84	100	Lipoma	96	110		90	80
r	92	98	Hermaphrodite	102	102		84	92
itz	72	112	Acute app.	78	118		66	72
	84	124	Exploratory ops.	120*	166*	Palpitation, pallor, asthenia	72	84
	72	130	Pneumonia	118*	180*	Palpitation	72*	96*
an	66	116	Tonsillitis	98	128	Tremor	72	66
	96	110	Rheum. fever	100	124	Tremor	84*	96*
man	96	110	Pregnancy	116	120	Tremor; asthenia	96	100
	60	108	Gastric (?)	64	110		60	60
	72	110	Breast tumor	76	116		68	76
s	64	94	Acute app.	90*	130*	Nervous tremor; sweat	66	72
man	....	....	Pneumonia	...			84*	126*
	72	124	Breast tumor	80	130		68	60
	92	104	Gastric ulcer	144*	116*	Palpitation; weak.	66*	96*
	....	....	Empyema	...	...		96*	116*
ken	72	100	Pneumonia	78	112		72	60
ck	78	128	Gastric ?	92	140		84	80
	84	130	???	92	130		78*	96*
	84	160	Gastric ulcer	96*	174*	None	84*	108*
nd	78	100	Pneumonia	84	100		80	74
	78	100	Gastric ?	100	110	Tremor	74	74
r	72	104	Nephritis	74	110		72	78
z	80	124	Cholelithiasis	84	128		80	84
ky	90	104	Rheum. fever	96	108		84	90
an	90	140	Hernia	96	144		84	90
l.	106	108	Myositis (?)	118	112		72*	112*

ecapitulation: Of 20 medical students, 4 react to atropin = 20 per cent.
Of 67 patients, 15 react to atropin = 22 per cent.
Of 87 total, 19 react to atropin = 22 – per cent.
Of 22 medical students, 7 react to adrenalin = 31 per cent.
Of 63 patients, 19 react to adrenalin = 30 per cent.
Of 85 total, 26 react to adrenalin = 30 per cent.
Asterisk indicates positive reactions.
Medical students tested by Drs S. Hershfield and Hyman: patients by Dr. K. Wallach.

associated with subjective distress (precordial pain, sense of fulness, fear and an intense and alarming ashen-pallor). Tremor usually occurs later, after the vascular response has ceased. As atypical phenomena we have seen diphasic responses in a few instances (Chart I, A). In these the initial vasodilatation was present followed by the familiar pressor response. We never obtained a pure dilatation. Again, we have seen a pressor response that was intense unassociated with an augmentor response (Chart II) and an acceleration unassociated with elevation of blood-pressure (Chart I, B). A delayed type of curve (Chart I, C) was noted a few times and in these, the reaction did not reach its height for twenty minutes. Corresponding to this "selective" action on the vascular system was variation in the subjective manifestations. There was no relationship between the subjective and objective reactions any more than the pressor and accelerator responses. An intense pressor or accelerator response may occur without subjective distress and subjective distress may be great without

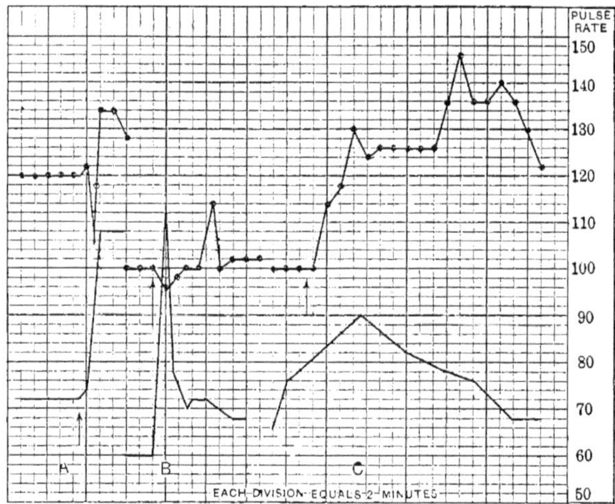

CHART I.—Dotted line is blood-pressure and plain line pulse rate. Arrow indicates time of injection. I—A, B, C and II are adrenalin and III an atropine reaction.

objective phenomena. The delay in the occurrence of tremor was constant. These selective types of reactions suggest an explanation for the variability of the clinical pictures in autonomic imbalance. For it must be evident that alterations may occur within the involuntary nervous system and may not be shared universally.

The atropine response was usually recorded as an initial pulse slowing (Chart III) occurring in the first four to eight minutes (due to vagus center stimulation), followed by a secondary acceleration occurring in from eight to twelve minutes and reaching a fastigium in about thirty minutes (due to peripheral paralysis). Aside from dryness of the mouth and flushing no subjective phenomena were noted and there was never any pressor response. The atropine "reversal" due to the central action was most closely studied and

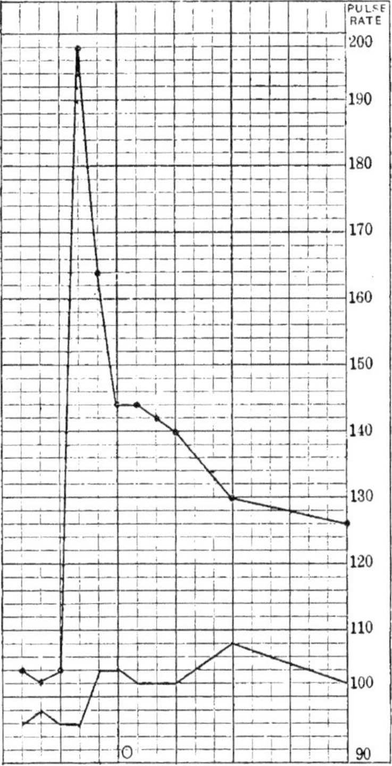

CHART II

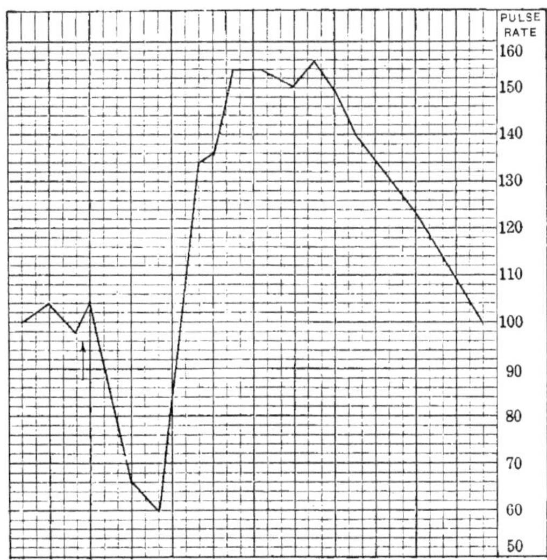

CHART III

an attempt made to utilize this effect therapeutically with some success.

There was no relation between the atropine and the adrenalin responses, between the types of response of one or the other or between any of these and the subjective or objective symptoms of the patients. Neither was there any relation between the presence of reaction and the intensity of the upset clinically.

Diagnosis. The most constant symptoms in these patients are tachycardia and goiter without fever or alteration in the basal metabolism. There is no difficulty in recognizing the syndrome.

The differentiation from Graves' syndrome cannot be made from any one clinical symptom. It has already been pointed out that tachycardia and goiter are present in practically all patients with autonomic imbalance, and that many have in addition tremor, eye-signs, and even all four of the cardinal symptoms of Graves' syndrome. None of our 86 patients had a constantly elevated basal metabolism, and this is the sole objective finding that differentiates autonomic imbalance from Graves' syndrome. However, the diagnosis can be made clinically. After seeing a certain number of these patients one is impressed by the fact that they differ in appearance from those with Graves' syndrome. Our attempts to express this difference in words have failed.

The exciting factor must be carefully sought, for the autonomic imbalance may be the result of some primary condition, such as tuberculosis, or a local pyogenic infection.

Autonomic imbalance is often diagnosed as a form of thyroid or adrenal disturbance; larval hyperthyroidism or formes frustes of exophthalmic goiter or suprarenal insufficiency (asystole). In view of the fact that we have been unable to satisfy ourselves that thyroxin or epinephrin plays any part in maintaining the involuntary nervous system, we consider it misleading to classify these patients as sufferers from thyroidal or adrenal disease.[9] This is important not only from the academic standpoint, but from the standpoint of therapy.

The utilization in diagnosis of the sensitiveness to drugs has been discussed. Drug sensitiveness may be present in about 25 per cent of "normal" individuals. It is present in about 80 to 90 per cent of individuals with autonomic imbalance and Graves' syndrome. It is a helpful but not pathognomonic reaction. The sites of action of the adrenalin and the atropine suggest that they are indicative merely of the tonus of those particular structures in the involuntary nervous system. To read into these reactions an index of thyroid function is misleading and based on erroneous interpretation of laboratory data, as we have shown in our work on the pithed cat.[10] We have also shown that adrenalin sensitiveness may be artificially produced in this preparation, independent of thyroid function. There remains, therefore, no scientific basis for the utilization of the adrenalin test in the diagnosis of thyroid disease. Reliance on this test, as may be seen, would place many of these patients in the category of "exophthalmic goiter" and this in turn might mean subjection to a needless thyroidectomy. Too great emphasis cannot be placed on this point.

Management. Each patient usually comes for the relief of a single symptom. Unless the exciting cause of the imbalance can be removed, the management of these patients is extremely discouraging. When autonomic imbalance is associated with psychic insult much can be done by reassuring the patients and convincing them that their symptoms are not of serious import. When focal infections are present striking results sometimes follow local treatment. In the instances in which the imbalance is associated with the sexual epochs, the administration of gonadal extracts is of no benefit. The symptoms of general autonomic imbalance are most amenable to correction of general hygiene (mental and physical), and to physiological rest. The local symptoms, referable to the bulbo-sacral; are at times alleviated by atropine. If the symptoms are those of increased tonicity, atropine should be administered in large doses to secure the peripheral effects; if the symptoms are those of decreased tonus, atropine is indicated in such small doses that the centers are stimulated while the periphery remains unaffected. Where the manifestations originate in the thoracico-lumbar no specific remedy is available. Adrenalin is so transient in its action that it is useless; furthermore, if sensitiveness to adrenalin exists, the patient may be made extremely uncomfortable.

Course. Autonomic imbalance usually runs a long course. Occasionally it is transitory, as during the establishment of puberty, or when the exciting focus of infection can be removed. Where the exciting cause remains operative, the course is protracted, and even the best hygienic conditions afford no more than a temporary relief, and recurrences and exacerbations are the rule. These patients must be kept under constant observation. Only one patient developed a true Graves' syndrome with elevation of the basal metabolism while under observation. She was a girl of eighteen, and after tonsillectomy under local cocaine anesthesia developed a striking and severe crisis. These patients will be carefully followed during the next few years to learn whether they develop Graves' syndrome.

Conclusions. 1. A study of the clinical manifestations of autonomic imbalance is presented.

2. Such instability of the involuntary nervous system probably constitutes a diathesis.

3. Focal infection, psychic trauma and the sex epochs accentuate the syndrome.

4. The symptoms are strikingly similar to those in Graves' syndrome. Autonomic imbalance may coexist with myxedema.

5. Local manifestations in a single organ, such as the stomach or heart, may attract attention to the organ itself, instead of to the general disturbance of the involuntary nervous system.

6. Hyperplasia of the thyroid gland is a very frequent accompaniment of the syndrome. It is more likely secondary than causative.

7. There is never present in autonomic imbalance a distinct and continuous elevation of the basal metabolism. This serves as a crucial differential point from Graves' syndrome.

8. The recognition of clinical autonomic imbalance is simple. More important, however, is (1) the exclusion of Graves' syndrome, and (2) the determination of the exciting cause of the imbalance.

9. There are no scientific data that substantiate the participation of the ductless glands in the production of this syndrome.

10. While patients with autonomic imbalance usually are sensitive to either atropine or adrenalin, it is possible to have the syndrome without drug sensitiveness; also it is possible without active autonomic imbalance to have drug sensitiveness. The explanation of these facts on a pharmacological basis is recorded.

11. Clear-cut subgrouping of these patients into vagotonic and sympathicotonic cannot be made clinically until some definite information with regard to the tonus of the involuntary nervous system is forthcoming.

12. Autonomic imbalance can rarely be permanently arrested. Usually the symptoms may be alleviated, but the diathesis persists.

13. Hormone therapy is without foundation, and, practically, it is useless.

BIBLIOGRAPHY.

1. Gaskell: The Involuntary Nervous System, Monograph, 1916.
2. Gaskell: The Origin of Vertebrates, 1908.
3. Gaskell: Jour. Gen. Phys., 1920, **2**, 73.
4. Barger and Dale: Jour. Phys., 1910, **41**, 19.
5. Hoskins and McClure: Am. Jour. Phys., 1908, **31**, 59.
6. Cannon: Am. Jour. Phys., 1908, **23**, 356.
7. Stewart and Rogoff: Am. Jour. Phys., 1920, **52**, 305.
8. Idem: Am. Jour. Phys., 1918, **45**, 268.
9. Lieb and Hyman: Jour. Pharm. Exp. Therap., 1922, **63**, 60, 66, 83, 88.
10. Idem:
11. Asher and Flack: Arch. Ges. Phys., 1911, **139**, 562.
12. Cannon and Levy: Am. Jour. Phys., 1919, **49**, 492.
13. Kessel, Hyman and Lieb: Arch. Brit. Med. (to be published).

THE SPONTANEOUS VARIABILITY OF BLOOD-PRESSURE AND THE EFFECTS OF DIET UPON HIGH BLOOD-PRESSURE, WITH SPECIAL REFERENCE TO SODIUM CHLORIDE.

By Herman O. Mosenthal, M.D.

AND

James J. Short, M.D.

NEW YORK.

(From the Postgraduate Medical School and Hospital, New York City.)

The Variability of Blood-pressure. The fact that blood-pressure varies a great deal in the same individual, not only from day to day, but from hour to hour and even from minute to minute, is freely acknowledged in all theoretical considerations of the subject, but is not generally made use of in the practical application of these matters to clinical observation or research. It is very necessary that any one who attempts to gauge the success of therapy applied to cases of hypertension by the sphygmomanometer, should be thoroughly familiar with the rise and fall of blood-pressure readings that apparently occur in a spontaneous fashion, but in reality are brought on by changes in the emotional state of the patient.

A citation of some of the authors who have noted this instability of blood-pressure may serve to indicate how important a factor it is. In 1900, Gumprecht[1] showed that the blood-pressure of laborers dropped with rest in bed during the first week's stay in a hospital; in 1 case the readings dropped from 195 to 125. In the same article this author notes how a student when watching blood-pressure determinations, upon himself, always registered 15 mm. higher than when he did not; after quarreling a rise of 30 to 40 points was common; a patient having a systolic blood-pressure of 170 had one of 202 after a successful hand at cards, and in another the figure rose from 156 to 172 on being amused and laughing. Rolleston[2] finds that nervous influences may constrict the blood-vessels and bring about rapid changes in the blood-pressure. Schrumpf and Zabel[3] in various publications come to the conclusion that blood-pressure is very variable; that psychic causes, thought of good food, fear of pain, etc., are all likely to bring it about; that the nervous, neurasthenic type is more subject to such changes in the arterial tension than the placid individual, and that in normal persons the systolic pressure only varies, while in the arteriosclerotic subject the diastolic fluctuates as much as the systolic. Hecht[4] showed that a low diet associated with physical and mental

[1] Ztschr. f. klin. Med., 1900, **39**, 377.

[2] Clin. Jour., 1905, **26**, 145.

[3] Deutsch. med. Wchnschr., 1910, **26**, 2385. Schrumpf and Zabel: München. med. Wchnschr., 1911, **58**, 1952. Zabel: München. med. Wchnschr., 1910, **57**, 2278.

[4] Ztschr. f. klin. Med., 1912, **76**, 87.

rest reduced hypertension; this view has been endorsed by Janeway.[5] The two last observations indicate the difficulty that any students of this subject encounter. It is impossible to be certain which factor diminished the hypertension, the low diet or the nervous relaxation; it is obviously necessary that in any conclusive clinical observations the psychic elements must first be eliminated before any further data are obtained. Janeway also accentuated the variability of blood-pressure from hour to hour. Oliver[6] claimed rest to be an essential factor in the treatment of hypertension. Maloney and Sorapure,[7] and later Grossman[8] showed how relaxation brought about by breathing exercises and passive motion lowered the blood-pressure; they believe that by these measures the psychic influences resulting in vasomotor stimulation and consequent increase in blood-pressure are done away with. In one of their cases the systolic pressure dropped from 215 to 154. Tixier[9] made the interesting observation that it was rare for blood-pressure readings to remain stationary as long as five minutes. O'Hare[10] found that in most instances, though not in every one, blood-pressure fell during rest; within five to seventy minutes the systolic drop was as high as 46 mm. of mercury and the diastolic 18; excitement in his experience always caused a sharp rise in systolic pressure (as high as 52 mm. of mercury) and a more moderate rise in diastolic pressure (as high as 24 mm.). The most recent effort in this field is that of Boas,[11] who duplicated O'Hare's results and in addition showed how the blood-pressure varied in normal individuals and was particularly prone to fluctuate in those cases described as neurocirculatory asthenia.

The series of observations presented in Table I bears out the contentions of the investigators cited above. These patients were studied at the Vanderbilt Clinic, Outpatient Department; the blood-pressure was read when the subject lay down and subsequently at frequent intervals until it was evident that no further drop in pressure would follow. In all probability these results are less striking than would have been the case if the surroundings had been more conducive to the allayment of physical and mental unrest, since the patients reclined on a rather hard examining table and in most instances must have been more or less annoyed by the coming and going of many persons in the same room. It may be noted that the fall in systolic pressure was usually more marked than in the diastolic, that it occurred in nearly every instance but that at times the change was negligible and occasionally even a rise was present. From the therapeutic point of view it is worth noting that the greatest drop in pressure usually manifested itself well

[5] Am. Jour. Med. Sci., 1913, **145**, 25.
[6] Lancet, 1907, **1**, 1346.
[7] New York Med. Jour., 1914, **99**, 1021.
[8] Ibid., 1905, **102**, 645.
[9] Arch. d. mal. d. cœur, 1919, **12**, 337.
[10] Am. Jour. Med. Sci., 1920, **159**, 373.
[11] Medical Clinics of North America, 1920, **4**, 257.

TABLE I.—CHANGES IN BLOOD-PRESSURE OCCURRING IN THE RECUMBENT POSITION. EACH OBSERVATION WAS CONTINUED UNTIL THE BLOOD-PRESSURE CEASED TO FALL. THE MINIMAL BLOOD-PRESSURE AFTER LYING DOWN IN EACH CASE IS RECORDED IN THE TABLE. IN NEARLY EVERY INSTANCE THE BLOOD-PRESSURE READINGS WERE KEPT UP FOR A CONSIDERABLE PERIOD AFTER THE MINIMAL BLOOD-PRESSURES NOTED ABOVE WERE OBTAINED. THE RESULTS ARE CHARTED IN ORDER, ACCORDING TO THE DROP IN SYSTOLIC BLOOD-PRESSURE.

On lying down.		Lowest noted.		Fall.		Interval minutes.
Systolic.	Diastolic.	Systolic.	Diastolic.	Systolic.	Diastolic.	
244	126	200	96	44	30	10
230	106	188	92	42	14	18
250	120	210	108	40	12	10
215	120	176	115	39	5	90
228	126	190	116	38	10	8
192	104	156	96	36	8	24
280	136	250	122	30	14	30
265	110	235	100	30	10	18
170	104	140	98	30	6	35
184	90	154	88	30	2	15
220	98	190	110	30	12	60
226	102	198	102	28	0	20
226	128	200	118	26	10	12
162	94	136	92	26	2	7
178	100	153	96	25	4	35
220	110	196	120	24	+10	16
202	104	178	94	24	10	6
158	100	135	90	23	10	10
136	84	118	80	18	4	16
212	110	194	114	18	+ 4	17
234	134	218	120	16	14	21
210	104	194	106	16	+ 2	14
220	120	204	118	16	2	18
190	105	175	96	15	9	23
158	94	144	92	14	2	7
200	110	186	108	14	2	15
210	110	196	108	14	2	25
136	66	122	68	14	+ 2	20
140	90	126	85	14	5	38
198	?	184	?	14	?	29
232	132	218	128	14	4	34
160	106	148	108	12	+ 2	24
180	95	168	90	12	5	26
120	75	110	70	10	5	18
200	130	190	126	10	4	3
170	95	160	94	10	1	21
182	115	172	108	10	7	23
166	110	156	110	10	0	19
194	96	185	85	9	11	68
204	110	196	108	8	2	10
216	128	210	126	6	2	12
225	94	230	92	5	2	15
158	98	154	104	4	+ 6	22
156	108	154	106	2	2	33
150	100	150	100	0	0	17
120	84	122	88	+ 2	+ 4	36
126	84	128	88	+ 2	+ 4	11
210	120	214	124	+ 4	+ 4	25
245	140	260	140	+15	0	31

within half an hour, which shows that the customary short nap or rest after meals may have far-reaching results. It is important in this connection to appreciate the fact that subsequent blood-pressure readings, when the sitting or upright position was resumed, often did not return to the initial level of arterial tension, but remained lower for a considerable period.

A very remarkable picture of variations in blood-pressure effected by emotional stimuli is given in Table VII. Every time this patient conversed or was disturbed the blood-pressure rose, only to drop again in a few minutes when the emotional phase had passed away. His heart and arteries were apparently the playthings of his nervous system. Two instances are particularly noteworthy, that on August 11, when the blood-pressure was at a level of 242/116 while he was relating an unpleasant incident, whereas five minutes later the considerably lower reading of 194/114 was obtained, and that on August 20, when the same high systolic tension was again reached (242/120) as a result of the death of the patient in the neighboring bed.

It is perfectly evident from all these data and quotations that very prolonged control observations are necessary before the true blood-pressure (Tixier's "residual blood-pressure") in any case can be determined, and furthermore that the conditions under which the effect of diet, drugs or physical measures are judged, as to their therapeutic value, must be adjusted with scrupulous care.

The mechanism by which these abrupt changes in blood-pressure are brought about is not entirely clear. Cannon[12] states, and this reflects the consensus of opinion, that the main factors determining the degree of arterial pressure are: (1) The energy of the heart as measured by the volume of blood pumped into the arterial system within a given time, and (2) the degree of resistance present in the terminal part of the arterial system. Other considerations appear to be of minor importance. If the individual cardiac contraction becomes quicker and more powerful, though the volume of blood put out with each beat is unchanged, it is obvious that the systolic pressure will rise and that the diastolic will remain stationary; if the peripheral arteries contract and the resistance they present to the blood flow becomes increased, both the systolic and diastolic pressure will be elevated. A corresponding drop in systolic and diastolic pressures will occur if each heart beat becomes prolonged or less forceful and if the arterioles relax. In the blood-pressure changes that occur with rest or emotional stimuli it is probable that both these factors are concerned. It is certain that in most instances the pulse rate does not change and therefore an increased systolic pressure without an augmented diastolic pressure must be due to the increased speed and force of the individual heart beat; if, as

[21] Boston Med. and Surg. Jour., 1911, **165**, 672.

might be assumed, the total volume of blood put out per beat would be raised and the quantity of blood in the arterial system increased, then the diastolic pressure would rise as well. This is, however, improbable and it is much more reasonable to suppose that when the diastolic pressure does rise there is a contraction of the smaller arterioles. It is only natural to suppose that nerve stimuli, brought on by various emotional phases, influence both the heart action and the tone of the smaller bloodvessels so as to bring about the marked variations in blood-pressure which are of such common occurrence and of such great clinical importance.

The Effect of Proteins on Blood-pressure. Recently the results obtained by one of the authors in attempting to modify blood-pressure by protein feeding were published.[13] It is not necessary to reprint these experiments in detail and only a few facts necessary to round out the complete picture as to the relation of diet to blood-pressure will be alluded to.

There is a general impression abroad that proteins in the diet have a tendency to increase arterial tension. It is difficult to find very much carefully gathered evidence to support this contention. Goodall[14] found that in cases of chronic interstitial nephritis the blood-pressure dropped while the patients were taking a low protein diet. Most of the other publications advocating this as a fact are based upon general impressions and not upon properly obtained clinical data.

Recently Squier and Newburgh[15] came to the conclusion that "high protein diet over a short period had no effect on the blood-pressure." Their study included cases of essential hypertension as well as of nephritis. The amounts of protein given these patients were high, well over 150 gm. per day. As the result of the forced protein diet, signs of renal irritation appeared but the blood-pressure remained unchanged. Similar findings in regard to blood-pressure have been reported by Strouse[16] and by Mosenthal.[17]

The purins derived from proteins can not be held responsible for the production of an increased blood-pressure. In this regard possibly it is most conclusive to quote the words of Sir Clifford Allbutt:[18] "Again and again I have placed high-pressure patients on purin-free diets, or on vegetarian diet with cheese, milk and eggs, with no appreciable reduction of blood-pressure within such limit of weeks as to satisfy the conditions of an experiment."

Another phase of the problem of the relation of protein feeding to hypertension has been definitely set aside by the practice of

[13] Mosenthal, H.: Am. Jour. Med. Sci., 1920, **160**, 808.
[14] Boston Med. and Surg. Jour., 1913, **168**, 760.
[15] Arch. Int. Med., 1921, **18**, 1.
[16] Med. Clin. North America, 1921, **5**, 229.
[17] Am. Jour. Med. Sci., 1920, **160**, 808.
[18] Diseases of the Arteries including Angina Pectoris, 1915, **2**, 88.

modern blood chemistry. It was formerly believed that the retention of nitrogenous substances might be responsible for the raised arterial pressure. The experience of everyone practising this branch of medicine is that this idea is incorrect. Recently Williams[19] has again called attention to the fact that, "The height of the blood-pressure bears no relationship to the amount of non-protein nitrogen substances in the blood."

As far as the specific influence of proteins on blood-pressure is concerned there is only one refuge left for those who still believe in this theory and that is the possibility of the production of toxic materials from protein foods within the organism and a consequent pressor action of such substances. The idea that this is a probable explanation of high blood-pressure is widespread. However, there is nothing but circumstantial evidence to favor it; there are no proofs at hand which adequately demonstrate the value of colon irrigations or the control of the intestinal flora in various ways.

The Effect of Carbohydrates on Blood-pressure. It has always been taken for granted that carbohydrates play no role in influencing blood-pressure. It is certainly true that usually neither the amount of starchy food ingested nor the level of the blood sugar apparently change the blood-pressure in any way. On the other hand the liability of cases of diabetes mellitus to develop hypertension is well known. There may be other factors than the disturbed sugar metabolism responsible for this tendency to increased blood-pressure but the coincidence is at least suggestive. Occasionally instances are met with in which an excessive starch intake may either directly or indirectly be the cause of a rise in arterial tension. In certain instances the reduction of the starch intake leads to a definite lowering of the blood-pressure. Thus in a patient fifty-six years old, weighing 215 pounds with a blood sugar of 0.160, who ate a great deal more than his share, the blood-pressure dropped from 146/88 to 112/72 when the carbohydrates in the food were moderately curtailed. The weight at the same time diminished by 25 pounds. It is possible that the loss in weight, remedying of some dyspeptic symptoms or other influence may have been the cause of the fall in arterial tension. Such cases are not common, but they do exist. Dr. W. W. Herrick informs us that he has had two similar ones in whom the change in the level of hypertension was much more marked than in the patient detailed above. One of the present food fads is to avoid meats and to eat starch *ad libitum*. When these precepts are followed without discrimination hypertension, as well as obesity, appear to be among the possible penalties entailed.

The Effect of Sodium Chloride on Blood-pressure. The relation between sodium chloride and hypertension has been urged for

[19] Arch. Int. Med., 1921, **27**, 748.

some time. It is of interest to follow this subject in chronological sequence. In 1904 Ambard and Beaujard[20] claimed that there was a direct relation between retention of sodium chloride and the level of arterial tension. In 8 cases of nephritis studied by them 6 cases conformed to their theory and 2 did not. These 2 exceptions are notable: In the first no rise in blood-pressure occurred in spite of a retention of 60 gm. of salt and an accumulation of 5 kg. of edematous fluid; in the second the blood-pressure rose in spite of the elimination of large amounts of previously retained salt. Subsequently Ambard[21] reiterated his views and defined them a little more closely by expressing the belief that all hypertension is due to retention of sodium chloride and that every case of permanently increased blood-pressure is due to a nephritis. Today when it is a firmly established fact that a permanent rise in arterial pressure is very often not associated with a nephritis, this contention loses much of its force. Combe[22] quotes an interesting observation of Castaigne, that injections of sodium chloride may produce fatal uremia in "chronic atrophic nephritis;" Munk[23] made note of a somewhat similar instance after the administration of a rather large dose of salt. The authors had untoward symptoms occur in a case of nephritis with marked impairment of renal function after a 10 gm. dose of sodium chloride. However, in patients in whom kidney activity was normal, salt in this amount produced no manifestation (with the possible exception of nausea) whatsoever. These observations are set forth in subsequent tables. It is probably to this type of hypertensive disease, associated with marked nephritis, that Allen[24] refers when he remarks that if certain patients with a pressure of 200 received salt there would be fireworks. It must be borne in mind, however, that as shown in the present tables, 10 gm. of salt may be given without fear of harming the patient, provided the hypertension is an essential hypertension, not exhibiting any noteworthy secondary changes or complications.

Loeb,[25] in regard to this problem, makes the obvious but very significant statement that those forms of nephritis—the parenchymatous—that are characterized by a retention of sodium chloride, do not as a rule have a high blood-pressure. Bergouignan and Fiesniger[26] reported one patient who retained salt without a parallel holding back of water, during which period the blood-pressure remained unchanged, while in another instance with salt retention and edema the blood-pressure rose. Bayer[27] reported 6 cases of arteriosclerosis some of which showed a marked increase

[20] Arch. gén. de méd., 1904, **50**, 520.
[21] Thèse pour le Doctorat en Médicine. Semaine méd., 1906, **26**, 361.
[22] Monatschr. f. Kinderh., 1905, **4**, 13, 82.
[23] Pathologie und Klinik der Nephrosen, Nephritiden und Schrumpfnieren, 1918.
[24] Tr. Am. Assn. Phys., 1920, **25**, 76.
[25] Deutsch. Arch. f. klin. Med., 1905, **85**, 348.
[26] Bull. et mém. Soc. méd. d. hôp., 1906, **23**, 425.
[27] Arch. f. exper. Path. u. Pharmakol., 1907, **57**, 162.

in arterial blood-pressure on a high salt diet, whereas others gave evidence of little or none.

Brodzki[28] could produce no increase in blood-pressure with salt in either the experimental uranium nephritis of dogs or the cantharidin nephritis of rabbits. Lowenstein[29] was unable to note any relation of sodium chloride to blood-pressure in 4 carefully observed cases. In one patient the arterial tension diminished in spite of the retention of 50 gm. of salt within a few days. In a general article without definite evidence Oliver expresses the opinion that sodium chloride raises blood-pressure. As the result of the "Karlsbad Cure," in the course of which considerable saline water is taken, Ritter[30] noted his results as follows:

57 cases	Blood-pressure lowered
4 cases	Blood-pressure constant
17 cases	Blood-pressure raised

Allbutt's[31] opinion on one phase of this subject is as follows: "I have found that to cut out salt from the diet of healthy persons for a few days produces no changes of pressure."

Allen,[32] in 1920, made very strong claims for the specific relation between salt and arterial tension. He believes that pure hypertension is essentially a salt nephritis and that the apparent efficiency of salt excretion is purchased at the price of abnormally high blood salt and blood-pressure. The blood-pressure did not vary in direct proportion to the salt concentration of the plasma in all the cases submitted by Allen. This may be due in part to the fact that the sodium chloride was determined in the plasma and not in the whole blood, and in part that the apparently spontaneous fluctuations in blood-pressure brought on by emotional states were not sufficiently controlled. (On standing there is an increase of sodium chloride in the plasma brought about by the passage of carbon dioxide from the plasma to the blood.—Myers, and Myers and Short[33].) These theories concerning the relationship of salt, kidney function and blood-pressure are much like those of Ambard and his associates expressed about fifteen years ago. In one of Allen's cases the blood-pressure rose from 200/100 to 266/110 after the administration of 10 gm. of salt and in another it increased from 215/130 to 254/120 on forcing water. This preliminary report has been the subject of much discussion and there have been several brief comments upon it. McLester[34] failed to reduce the blood-

[28] Berl. klin. Wchnschr., 1906, **43**, 906; Deutsch. Arch. f. klin. Med., 1908, **93**, 310.
[29] Arch. f. exper. Path. u. Pharmakol , 1907, **57**, 137.
[30] Deutsch. Arch. f. klin. Med., 1910, **100**, 11.
[31] Diseases of the Arteries including Angina Pectoris, 1915.
[32] Jour. Am. Med. Assn., 1920, **74**, 652
[33] Practical Chemical Analysis of Blood; Jour. Biol. Chem., 1920, **44**, 47.
[34] Jour. Am. Med. Assn , 1921, **77**, 88.

pressure in nephritis by limitation of the sodium chloride intake. A patient was given 10 gm. of salt every day for ten days by Strouse[35] and the blood-pressure dropped from 260/150 to 200/100.

Christian[36] quotes the work of his colleague O'Hare[37] on 46 patients showing that an increase of blood chlorides occurs in direct proportion as renal insufficiency develops; the blood-pressure apparently was higher in those cases with a low blood chloride than in those with a high. In anemia the blood chlorides rise considerably although the blood-pressure remains constant or diminishes.

In Table II the blood chloride findings are given for 26 patients whose systolic blood-pressure is above 200 mm. of mercury. If we regard 500 mg. sodium chloride per 100 cc of whole blood as the usual upper limit of normal[38] it is seen that in Table II only 2 out of the 26 cases of hypertension are abnormally high. This observation bears out some of the facts quoted to the effect that hypertension and an increased blood chloride do not go hand in hand.

If this problem is approached from another angle it is found that cases in which the blood chlorides are high are not necessarily accompanied by an increased blood-pressure (Table III).

From the above quotations and data it becomes clear that an increase in the blood chlorides does not produce a rise in blood-pressure.

A few experiments were carried out to determine the effect of moderate doses of sodium chloride on patients suffering with hypertension. Those with marked renal insufficiency were avoided, since in them, as previously mentioned, there are untoward and even dangerous manifestations when the body is suddenly flooded with salt in this way. The patients were kept in bed for a period of days and frequent blood-pressure readings were made. It is only by these means that a true control estimate of the arterial tension can be obtained. After the spontaneous variations characteristic of each case of essential hypertension had been recorded, 10 gm. of sodium chloride were given by mouth or through a small stomach tube (to avoid the taste of the bitter solution) and frequent blood-pressure readings were made subsequently. The individual experiments are given in Tables IV, V, VI, VII, VIII and IX.

In Tables IV to IX the individual reactions may be studied in detail. For purposes of discussion only a summary of these observations, as given in Table X, will be alluded to.

[35] Med. Clin. North America, 1921, **5**, 229.
[36] New York State Jour. Med., 1921, **21**, 292.
[37] Proc. Am. Soc. Clin. Investigat., 1921, p. 6.
[38] Practical Chemical Analysis of Blood, 1921, p. 91.

TABLE II.—BLOOD-PRESSURE AND BLOOD SODIUM CHLORIDE IN 26 SUCCESSIVE CASES OF HYPERTENSION (BLOOD-PRESSURE OF 200 OR HIGHER) ARRANGED IN ORDER OF THE LEVEL OF THE BLOOD SODIUM CHLORIDE. IN ONLY A VERY FEW CASES IS THE BLOOD SODIUM CHLORIDE ABOVE NORMAL.

Case.	Blood-pressure.		NaCl mg. per 100 cc whole blood.
	Systolic.	Diastolic.	
I	226	90	627
II	208	94	557
III	214	136	500
IV	200	82	500
V	212	130	500
VI	242	180	495
VII	202	114	495
VIII	224	120	494
IX	224	106	494
X	206	126	488
XI	212	130	488
XII	260	158	488
XIII	235	125	486
XIV	216	132	478
XV	210	114	478
XVI	320	160	474
XVII	210	116	474
XVIII	246	120	462
XIX	240	145	450
XX	250	140	450
XXI	224	140	445
XXII	224	136	429
XXIII	204	128	429
XXIV	224	136	429
XXV	204	126	410
XXVI	265	168	410

TABLE III.—CASES WITH NORMAL BLOOD-PRESSURE AND AN INCREASE OF THE BLOOD CHLORIDES.

Diagnosis.	Blood-pressure.		NaCl mg. per 100. cc whole blood.
	Systolic.	Diastolic.	
Secondary anemia	105	52	660
Parenchymatous nephritis	98	80	625
Carcinoma kidney	120	68	622
Normal	120	71	597
Carcinoma rectum	140	84	588
Cholecystitis	110	80	567
Normal	128	94	561
Obesity	135	85	553
Carcinomatosis	104	78	550
Pernicious anemia	130	70	550
Normal	120	75	540
Normal	112	80	539
Cyclic vomiting	125	80	539
Carcinoma stomach	108	82	538
Diabetes mellitus	108	74	532

The "spontaneous" variations of the blood-pressure occurring during a period of a few days before the test substance is given are shown in Table X (under heading of control blood-pressure).

At the risk of repeating some of the statements made in the introductory section of this paper it is desirable to emphasize the necessity of making these prolonged control observations before plunging into any experiments that are supposed to yield results concerning blood-pressure. The variations in these cases are much more marked than they were in the individuals whose blood-pressure was recorded for short periods of rest only (Table I).

TABLE IV.—E. F., FEMALE, AGED FORTY-EIGHT YEARS. ESSENTIAL HYPERTENSION, RENAL FUNCTION UNIMPAIRED. MARKED "SPONTANEOUS VARIATIONS" IN BLOOD-PRESSURE. GLASS OF COLORED WATER PRODUCES SLIGHT INCREASE IN BLOOD-PRESSURE, COMPARABLE TO THE EFFECT OF 10 GM. OF SALT IN SOME OTHER CASES. A LOW SALT DIET DOES NOT DIMINISH THE BLOOD-PRESSURE.

Date, 1921.	NaCl 24 hrs. urine, gm.	Diet	Blood-pressure			NaCl whole blood, mg. per 100 cc.	Remarks.
			Time.	Systolic.	Diastolic		
Jan. 29		Regular	1.04 P.M.	226	108		
			1.07	210	106		
			1.09	200	106		
			1.10	184	106		
			1.11	182	106		
31	8.10	Regular	1.13 P.M.	224	106	494	
			1.16	228	110		
			1.21	214	106		
			1.23	206	106		
			1.25	192	102		
			1.26	198	106		
			5.53	236	114		
			5.57	230	112		
			5.58	220	110		
			5.59	214	110		
			6.00	214	110		
Feb. 1-4	3.50	Regular	....	230	116		Maximum for period.
	2.24		....	180	102		Minimum for period (12 blood-pressure readings).
4-15	3.20	"Salt-free"	....	238	120		Maximum for period.
	0.78		....	160	90		Minimum for period.
	1.52		....	....			Average for period (42 blood-pressure readings; 7 NaCl determinations).
15	1.60	"Salt-free"	9.08 A.M.	200	96		Felt better than usual.
			9.09	190	100		
			9.12	176	100		
			9.16	184	104		
			10.10				Glass of pink colored water taken by mouth; patient told that it might increase blood-pressure temporarily.
			10.18	208	98		
			10.20	188	96		
			10.52	190	104		Felt distressed, headache.
			10.54	190	100		
			10.57	192	104		
			12.40 P.M.	214	106		Felt worse, headache increased; "hot flashes."
			12.43	190	100		
			7.32	210	110		
			7.35	210	110		
			7.37	204	110		
			7.45	190	110		
16-28	5.00			233	120		Maximum for period.
	0.68			184	102		Minimum for period.
	1.92						Average for period (10 NaCl determinations).

BLE V.—A. K., FEMALE, AGED FORTY YEARS. ESSENTIAL HYPERTENSION, SLIGHT DEGREE OF AORTIC INSUFFICIENCY (NO SIGNS OF LUES, WASSERMANN REACTION NEGATIVE), RENAL FUNCTION UNIMPAIRED. MODERATE "SPONTANEOUS VARIATIONS" IN BLOOD-PRESSURE. MODERATE RISE IN BLOOD-PRESSURE FOLLOWING THE INGESTION OF 7 GM. OF SODIUM CHLORIDE; THE MARKED RISE IMMEDIATELY AFTER THE TAKING OF THE SALT MAY BE ATTRIBUTED TO THE ATTENDANT NAUSEA.

Date, 1920.	NaCl 24 hrs. urine, gm.	Diet.	Blood-pressure.			NaCl whole blood, mg. per 100 cc.	Remarks.
			Time.	Systolic.	Diastolic.		
g. 10	....	Regular	....	200	90	....	On admission to hospital
11–29	7.74	"Salt-free"	....	212	96	485	Maximum for period.
	1.00	....	....	170	84	467	Minimum for period
	3.51	....	....	....	....	....	Average for period (19 blood-pressure readings; 8 urine NaCl and 2 blood NaCl determinations)
30	3.10	"Salt-free"	3.30 P.M.	198	92	....	Sitting up.
			3.35	190	88	....	Reclining and resting
			3.40	188	96	....	Reclining and resting.
			3.42	182	96	....	Reclining and resting.
			3.44	182	96	....	Reclining and resting.
31	2.90	"Salt-free"	10.15 A.M.	192	88	....	After sitting up.
			10.20	180	88	....	Reclining and resting.
			10.25	174	92	....	Reclining and resting
pt. 1	....	"Salt-free"	10.30 A.M.	220	96	....	Sitting up
			10.33	198	96	....	Reclining and resting
			10.40	190	94	....	Reclining and resting
			10.42	186	90	....	Reclining and resting.
			10.44	184	90	....	Reclining and resting
2	2.50	"Salt-free"	1.30 P.M.	212	94	....	Sitting up and conversing.
			1.35	178	92	....	Reclining and resting.
			1.37	180	92	....	Reclining and resting.
3	2.00	"Salt-free"	10.30 A.M.	200	82	500	Sitting up.
			10.32	220	98	....	After conversing.
			10.37	204	96	....	Reclining and resting.
			1.30 P.M.	208	90	....	Sitting up.
			1.35	180	90	....	Reclining and resting
			1.40	178	90	....	Reclining and resting
			3.30	204	88	....	After walking about ward.
			3.35	176	88	....	After resting five minutes.
			3.40	172	74	....	After resting ten minutes.
4	1.47	"Salt-free"	1.00 P.M.	214	90	....	After walking about ward
			1.05	182	86	....	After resting five minutes
			1.10	164	84	....	After resting ten minutes
			4.30	206	86	....	After walking about ward.
			4.40	194	90	....	After resting ten minutes.
			4.42	192	88	....	After resting twelve min.
5	3.70	"Salt-free"	11 30 A M	200	86	....	After resting five minutes.
			11.35	178	90	....	After resting ten minutes.
			11 40	180	84	....	After resting fifteen min
				205	90	....	After walking about ward.
				195	87	....	After resting five minutes
				190	85	....	After resting ten minutes.
6	2.24	"Salt-free"	2.00 P.M.	190	90	....	Reclining and resting
			2.05	179	86	....	
			2.10	178	86		
7	....	....	9.30 A.M.	206	100	....	Reclining and resting.
				190	98	....	
				196	96		
		....	9.45	....	....	....	7 gm. NaCl in 135 cc water taken by mouth; very disagreeable to patient.
			9.58	266	126	....	Patient somewhat nauseated.
	0.97	....	10.00	....	....	....	Output for two hours.
			10.03	247	106		
			10.10	226	110		
			10.14	232	114		
			10.17	232	112		
			10.18	238	114	....	Still nauseated.
			11.32	214	102		

Date, 1921.	NaCl 24 hrs. urine, gm.	Diet.	Blood-pressure.			NaCl whole blood, mg. per 100 cc.	Remarks.
			Time.	Systolic.	Diastolic		
			11.34	214	104		
			11.43	214	98		
			11.54	....	....	497	
	0.75	....	12.00 M.	....	....	....	Output for two hours.
			1.13 P.M.	216	87		
			1.15	190	88		
			1.18	189	92		
			1.20	190	92		
			1.23	190	94		
			1.30	....	....	494	
	2.75	....	1.50	....	....	....	Output for one hour fifty minutes.
			2.25	214	94	....	One visitor (daughter).
			3.00	220	94		
			3.05	220	90		
			3.06	220	94		
			3.09	218	100	....	Visitor left.
			3.15	....	....	490	
			4.00	190	90		
			4.03	200	94		
			4.10	188	88		
			4.17	198	94		
			4.23	190	94		
			5.38	210	94		
			5.41	204	92		
			5.47	210	96		
			5.55	....	....	475	
	3.80	....	6.00	....	....	....	Output for four hours ten minutes
8	1.60						

Furthermore during the interval covering several days of freedom from physical and mental exertion the blood-pressure is not only lowered but it diminishes to such an extent that in some instances it reaches a normal level and in all of them at least approaches it. This fact is of distinct therapeutic importance. In the present series of observations it is very necessary to be informed concerning this marked variability before the effect of the sodium chloride is tested. It is obvious that with such an irregular base-line upon which to build experimental data that all results obtained must to a certain extent at least be interpreted by the observer who is, or ought to be, in the best possible position to render an unbiassed judgment as to what the effect of any given procedure on blood-pressure is and how far results may be influenced by the presence of spontaneous variations in the arterial tension due to the personal equation of the patient or unforeseen disturbances at the bedside. These much-needed control periods have usually been omitted in blood-pressure studies and thus many observations have lost their full value.

The control blood-pressure recorded as taken "just before test" is the final one of a series of readings. A number of observations were made in order that the minimal arterial tension pertaining at the time should be recorded and that the "spontaneous" variations in the blood-pressure occurring at the moment should be set aside. It is of interest to note that in more than half the cases this reading, taken under conditions that were carefully adjusted so as to insure

ABLE VI.—B. Y., MALE, AGED FIFTY-THREE YEARS. ESSENTIAL HYPERTENSION, SLIGHT DEGREE OF CARDIAC DECOMPENSATION ON ADMISSION, NO EDEMA, RENAL FUNCTION UNIMPAIRED. THE ONLY RISE IN BLOOD-PRESSURE NOTED AFTER GIVING 10 GM. OF SALT MAY BE ATTRIBUTED TO "WARD ROUNDS" AND "A VISITOR." ON REPEATING THE EXPERIMENT THERE WAS A SLIGHT RISE FOR A FEW MINUTES, WHICH MAY BE ATTRIBUTED TO THE NAUSEOUS DOSE ADMINISTERED, AND SUBSEQUENTLY THE BLOOD-PRESSURE DROPPED BELOW THE CONTROL LEVEL.

Date, 1921.	NaCl 24 hrs. urine, gm.	Diet.	Blood-pressure.			NaCl whole blood, mg. per 100 cc.	Remarks.
			Time	Systolic.	Diastolic.		
r. 29	....	Mixed	5 00 P. M.	208	114	494	On admission to hospital.
r 30 to	12 30	Low-salt		190	110	....	Maximum for period.
May 5	2 60	....		130	78	....	Minimum for period.
	7 36	....		....	....	....	Average for period (20 blood-pressure readings; 19 NaCl determinations).
ay 5	6 00	Low-salt	11 04 A. M.	168	90		
			11 08	166	90		
			11 10	170	96		
			11 13	....	....		10 gm NaCl in ½ glass of water taken by mouth.
			11.14	174	100		
			11.16	166	90		
			11.18	164	96		
			12.07 P.M.	154	88		
			12.09	162	84		
			12.16	152	82		
			1.14	162	90		
			1.17	150	80		
			1.20	164	88		
			1.30	....	.	544	
			2.08	192	110		Ward rounds.
			2.11	178	98		
			2.16	168	100		
			3.13	188	114		Visitor (wife).
				184	106		
			3.15	184	98		
			3.16	170	96		
				178	98		
			3.22	180	98		
			3.23	184	104		Visitor left.
			4.25	152	80		
			4.28	154	86		
			4.30	152	82	557	
			5.55	1[illegible]5	76		
			5.58	136	72		
			6.00	134	72		
			6.10	....	. .		
			8.15	152	78		
			8.17	150	78		
			8.20	154	80		
ay 11	7.10	Low-salt	10.38 A. M.	150	80		
			10.40	150	80		
			12.12	....	....		10 gm. NaCl in ½ glass of water taken by mouth
			12.14	176	94		
			12.16	158	90		
			12.18	170	90		
			1.20	142	84		
			1.22	140	80		
			1.28	136	80		
			2.14	138	84		
			2.15	134	78		
			2.17	138	82		
			3.20	148	86		
			3.22	142	82		
			3.23	146	82		
			4.24	152	86		
			4.30	148	82		
			5.20	148	80		
			5.24	148	80		
			6.16	132	76		
			6.18	130	70		
			6.19	130	70		
ay 12	7.00	Low-salt		162	90		
13	10.10	Low-salt					
14	8.60	Low-salt		162	96		
15	5.80	Low-salt					
16	3.30	Low-salt		160	88		

BLE VII.—J. H., MALE, AGED SIXTY-TWO YEARS. ESSENTIAL HYPERTENSION RENAL FUNCTION UNIMPAIRED). MARKED "SPONTANEOUS VARIATIONS" IN LOOD-PRESSURE, ESPECIALLY MARKED ON AUGUST 11 AND AUGUST 20 AT 3.35 P.M. SUBSEQUENT TO THE ADMINISTRATION OF 10 GM. OF NaCl THE LOOD-PRESSURE DID NOT VARY IN ANY WAY FROM THE CONTROL PERIOD.

ate, 920.	NaCl 24 hrs. urine, gm.	Diet.	Blood-pressure			NaCl whole blood, mg. per 100 cc.	Remarks.
			Time.	Systolic	Diastolic.		
29	....	"Salt-free"	....	200	100		
30	....	"Soft"	...	172	90		
31	....	"Soft"	1 45 P M	194	104		
1	....	"Salt-free"					
2	7.62	"Salt-free"	10.20 A.M.	180	76	519	Blood NaCl before break-fast.
				176	92		
				188	100		
				160	96		
			8.40 P M.	190	104		
3	8.80	"Regular"	1 40 P M	188	100		
4	5.29	"Regular"	10 20 A M	200	104	....	After exertion
				188	98		
				182	98	....	After resting five minutes.
5	9.84	"Regular"	10.45 A M	194	98	....	After walking about ward.
				180	100	....	After resting.
6	8.56	"Salt-free"	11 30 A M	200	100	....	After conversing
				162	90	....	After resting five minutes
				158	96	....	After resting fifteen min.
				190	100	....	After walking.
[illegible]	....	"Salt-free"	10 15 A M	190	102	....	After conversing
				170	98	....	After resting three minutes
				164	98	....	After resting six minutes.
				168	98	....	After resting nine minutes
9	2.81	"Salt-free"	9 00 A M	172	96	....	After walking about ward.
				160	96	....	After resting five minutes
				178	96	....	After walking about ward.
				160	92	....	After resting.
				218	118	....	After conversing
				204	106	....	After resting five minutes.
10	4.78	"Salt-free"	9.00 A M.	218	110	....	After conversing.
				178	100	....	After resting five minutes
11	3.24	"Salt-free"	11.00 A M	242	116	....	After relating an unpleas-ant incident.
				194	114	....	After resting five minutes
12	4.61	"Salt-free"	2 00 P M.	206	110	....	After conversing five min
				180	100	....	After resting five minutes.
				220	110	....	After conversing three min
13	2.32	"Salt-free"	1 30 P M	176	98	....	After resting
				220	110	....	After conversing.
14	2.50	"Salt-free"	10 30 A M	164	92	....	After resting
				180	96		After conversing
15	2.80	"Salt-free"	9 00 P M	202	110	....	After conversing
16	3.15	"Salt-free"	10 30 A M	200	100	....	After conversing
				196	100	....	After resting three minutes
				178	96	....	After resting six minutes.
17	1.70	"Salt-free"	10.00 A.M	206	110	457	After conversing.
				178	98	....	After resting
18	2.90	"Salt-free"	....	206	114	....	After conversing.
				190	110	....	After resting.
20	11 90	"Salt-free"	8 00 A M	....	....	443	
			8 15	..	..	....	Breakfast.
			9 10	210	104	....	After conversing
				182	98	....	After resting three minutes
			9.15	....	....	....	10 gm NaCl by mouth in 150 cc H_2O
			10 05	210	112	....	After conversing
				190	100	....	After resting three minutes.
				190	100	....	After resting six minutes.
			10.20	....	....	527	
			11.00	170	90	....	Resting
				172	90	....	Resting
			12 00 M.	222	114	....	After conversing.
				202	104	....	After resting five minutes
			12.20 P.M.	...	....	520	
			1.20	200	104	....	After resting.
				184	100	....	After resting.
				210	110	....	After conversing.
			2.45	...	...	494	
			3.35	242	120	....	After death of patient in next bed
				210	110	....	After resting five minutes
				210	112	....	After resting ten minutes.
			4.30	228	114	....	After conversing.
				214	110	....	After resting five minutes.

BLE VIII.—M. D., FEMALE, AGED FIFTY-SIX YEARS. ESSENTIAL HYPERTENSION, SLIGHT DEGREE OF INSUFFICIENCY (WASSERMANN REACTION NEGATIVE, NO SIGNS OF LUES), NO SIGNS OF MYOCARDIAL INSUFFICIENCY, NO IMPAIRMENT OF RENAL FUNCTION (URINARY SPECIFIC GRAVITY VARIED BETWEEN 1.016 AND 1.030). BLOOD ANALYSES AS MG. PER 100 CC: UREA, N 21.4; URIC ACID, 2.8; AND CREATININE, 2.2. VARIOUS EXPERIMENTS AND CONTROL PERIODS. IN NONE OF THE EXPERIMENTS DOES 10 GM. OF SODIUM CHLORIDE PRODUCE A DEFINITE RISE OF BLOOD-PRESSURE.

ate, 921.	NaCl 24 hrs. urine, gm.	Diet.	Blood-pressure.			NaCl whole blood, mg. per 100 cc.	Remarks.
			Time.	Systolic	Diastolic		
il 6	....	Low-salt	8.00 P.M	224	120	494	On admission to hospital
il 7–14	7.83	"Salt-free"	....	232	130	....	Maximum for period.
	1.52		....	180	100	....	Minimum for period
	3.91		....	....	....	....	Average for period.
14	3.20	"Salt-free"	11.30 A.M	....	....	....	30 cc of qitter, pink-colored water taken by mouth *
			12.07 P.M.	190	108		
			12.10	186	106		
			12.12	190	108		
			1.19	176	108		
			1.21	180	110		
			1.22	170	104		
			1.25	184	104		
			4.11	178	109		
			5.17	180	104		
			5.19	178	104		
15	2.24	"Salt-free"	11.50 A.M.	176	108		
			11.56	176	110		
			3.00 P.M.	....	....	....	Small stomach tube introduced; patient somewhat disturbed.
			3.35	190	110		
			3.37	180	110		
			3.40	186	110		
			3.41	180	110		
			3.45	....	....	....	50 cc of colored water introduced through tube *
			47	194	110		
			50	200	114	....	Tube removed.
			39	166	104		
			42	166	104		
16	2.18	"Salt-free"	3.15 P M	192	116	....	Maximum.
			1 39	166	92	....	Minimum (6 readings).
17	3.66	"Salt-free"	12 06 P M.	184	110		
			12 09	180	110		
			12 11	184	110		
			2.15	....	....	....	Tube introduced.
			2.25	197	116		
			2.26	....	....	....	10 gm NaCl in 50 cc colored water given through tube,* nauseated; drank 1 glass of water; no vomiting, tube removed.
			2.27	202	116		
			2.57	197	118	....	Visitors after 3 P M.
			4.13	194	118		
			4.15	185	114		
			4.16	188	114		
			5.42	198	114		
			5.43	192	114		
			5.45	184	114		
			5.47	192	114		
			7.18	200	120		
			7.20	192	116		
			7.23	196	116		
			7.24	188	114		
			8.54	192	106		
			8.57	188	106		
			9.00	180	106		
			9.02	186	108		

ate, 921.	NaCl 24 hrs. urine, gm.	Diet.	Blood-pressure			NaCl whole blood, mg. per 100 cc.	Remarks.
			Time.	Systolic.	Diastolic.		
18	8.00	"Salt-free"	12.23 P.M.	196	118	....	Maximum.
			4.06	182	106	....	Minimum (4 readings).
19	5.30	"Salt-free"	3.00 P.M.	202	134	....	3 visitors (1 reading).
20	3.73	"Salt-free"	10.33 A.M.	166	94		
			10.35	176	104	....	After conversing.
			10.38	164	100		
			1.45 P.M.	....	....	....	Tube introduced.
			1.50	180	106		
			1.53	174	108		
			1.54	174	108	513	
			2.38	....	....	....	10 gm. NaCl in 50 cc colored water given through tube;* tube removed.
			2.41	204	114		
			2.48	190	110		
			3.35	192	104	563	
			3.36	182	110		
			3.38	178	104		
			3.41	178	100		
			6.59	184	106	544	
			7.02	182	110		
			7.03	178	110		
			7,07	180	114		
			9.23	178	114		
			9.25	179	112	525	
21	7.60	"Salt-free"	12.25 P.M.	182	118	....	Maximum.
			4.06	176	114	....	Minimum (5 readings)
22	6.90	"Salt-free"	7.55 P.M.	182	114	....	Maximum.
			7.58	176	106	....	Minimum (4 readings).
23	4.20	"Salt-free"	3.00 P.M.	170	103	....	Maximum.
			10.11 A.M.	158	98	....	Minimum (5 readings).
25	1.50	"Salt-free"	12.15 P.M.	180	112	....	Maximum.
			9.03	166	108	....	Minimum (4 readings).
il 26 to	4.50	"Salt-free"	....	194	120	....	Maximum for period.
lay 5	1.20	....	....	150	100	....	Minimum for period (33 readings).
	3.45	"Salt-free"	....	....	....	....	Average for period.
y 5	....	"Salt-free"	1.01	164	114		
			1.02	164	116		
			1.04	164	112		
			1.50	....	....	....	Tube introduced
			2.45	....	....	....	10 gm. NaCl in 50 cc colored water given through tube; tube removed.
			2.50	167	112		
			2.54	165	112		
			2.58	160	110		
			3.45	162	116		
			3.48	162	116		
			3.49	156	116		
			3.50	156	116		
			3.52	161	120		
			5.04	182	116	....	Patient standing.
			5.08	170	114		
			5.10	178	120		
			5.12	172	124		
			5.13	174	120		
			5.15	173	126		
			8.30	168	126		
			8.31	164	128		
			8.32	168	126		
y 6	....	"Salt-free"	6.55 P.M.	166	106		
			6.57	166	106		
7	....	"Salt-free"	2.40 P.M.	170	110		
9	....	"Salt-free"	8.00 P.M.	176	100		
				182	110		
10	...	"Salt-free"	12.00 P.M.	196	120	....	Patient sitting out on porch.
			12.17	194	120		
11	....	"Salt-free"	11.10 A.M.	196	124		

* Bitter substance used was a few drops of tincture of myrrh; coloring matter was a few drops of nolsulphonephthalein.

TABLE IX.—J. T., MALE, AGED FIFTY-SIX YEARS. ESSENTIAL HYPERTENSION RECOVERING FROM MYOCARDIAL INSUFFICIENCY. NO IMPAIRMENT OF RENAL FUNCTION. THE BLOOD-PRESSURE DOES NOT RISE MORE THAN COULD BE ACCOUNTED FOR BY "SPONTANEOUS VARIATIONS" AFTER TAKING 10 GM. OF SALT IN CAPSULES.

Date, 1920.	Diet.	Blood-pressure.			NaCl whole blood, mg. per 100 cc.	Remarks.
		Time.	Systolic.	Diastolic.		
July 11-29	"Salt-free"	....	238	130	485	Maximum for period
	....	....	190	100	478	Minimum for period (19 blood-pressure readings and 2 blood NaCl determinations).
29	"Salt-free"	9 45 A M	196	110	488	
		10 00	....	....	....	10 gm. NaCl in 5 capsules by mouth with 180 cc of water.
		10.10	194	102		
		10.40	....	....	....	Vomited small amount.
		11.10	208	112		
		11.15	....	....	506	
		11.30	....	....	....	Drank 90 cc of water.
		12.10 P.M.	206	98		
		1.10	192	92		
		2.15	198	102		
		2.20	....	....	513	
		4.05	198	104		
		7.45	208	110		
		8.00	....	....	513	
		9.45	188	104		
30	....	1.30 P.M.	192	100		

TABLE X.—A SUMMARY OF THE DATA CONTAINED IN TABLES IV, V, VI, VII, VIII AND IX. THE VARIABILITY OF THE BLOOD-PRESSURE DURING THE CONTROL PERIOD IS SHOWN. THERE IS NO RISE IN BLOOD-PRESSURE THAT MAY BE ATTRIBUTED TO THE DIRECT EFFECT OF GIVING SODIUM CHLORIDE IN 10 GM. DOSES.

Observation.	Case.	Substance given in test	Control blood-pressure.*			Maximal blood-pressure* after test-substance.			Minimal blood-pressure after test-substance.	
			Several days before test.		Just before test.	Maximal* blood-pressure.	Minutes after test-substance.	Possible cause for maximal blood-pressure.		
			Maximal.	Minimal.					Within 2 hrs.	2 to 4 hrs.
1 . .	E. T.	Colored water	238/120	160/90	184/104	214/106	150	Headache, malaise	188/96	190/100
2 . .	A. K.	NaCl, 7 gm.	220/98	172/74	196/96	266/126	13	Nausea	214/98	189/92
3 . .	B. Y.	NaCl, 10 gm.	190/110	130/78	170/96	192/110	175	Ward rounds	152/82	150/80
4 . .		NaCl, 10 gm	192/110	134/72	150/80	176/94	2	Nausea	136/80	134/78
5 . .	J. H.	NaCl, 10 gm	242/146	158/96	182/98	242/120	380	Patient died in next bed	170/90	202/104
6 . .	M. D.	NaCl, 10 gm	232/130	170/104	197/116	202/116	1	Nausea	185/114	184/114
7 . .		NaCl, 10 gm	202/134	180/106	174/108	204/114	3	Nausea	178/100	
8 . .		NaCl, 10 gm	204/114	150/100	161/1,12	182/116	139	?	156/116	161/120
9 . .	J. T.	NaCl, 10 gm	238/130	190/100	196/110	208/112	70	Vomited	194/102	192/92

* The double figure under each observation indicates the systolic and the diastolic blood-pressure.

the greatest possible degree of mental and physical relaxation, not only at the time but also for a number of preceding days, was considerably higher than the lowest previous observations. This serves to show how uncontrollable a factor the height of arterial tension really is. However, with the control period covering several days and a careful adjustment of conditions immediately before the administration of the sodium chloride, it was felt that as accurate a base-line as possible had been established and the actual experimental periods were instituted.

In none of these patients except one did the salt produce any untoward symptoms; in this instance they were alarming. This point has already been discussed and the conclusion previously arrived at may be repeated here: Sodium chloride may be administered in large doses to cases of essential hypertension provided no sequelæ of the increased blood-pressure are present; if renal, cardiac, cerebral or possibly other complications are present it is not safe to give salt in large quantities. Failure to differentiate between "pure" essential hypertension and the form of the disease in which there is secondary involvement of various important organs has led some authors to conclude erroneously that sodium chloride produced dangerous manifestations in all cases. The patient exhibiting these untoward symptoms is not included in the present series.

If salt effects a rise in blood-pressure this should occur within two hours after the administration of the sodium chloride, because it is within this period that blood chlorides attain their maximum level (Tables VII and VIII); therefore the delayed sudden rise in blood-pressure occurring after 120 minutes in observation 5, Table X, may be discounted. The isolated rise coming on immediately after the dose of salt is in all probability due to the attending nausea observations 2 and 7, Table X. This leaves virtually no distinct rise in blood-pressure that can not be accounted for by other agencies than the postabsorptive effect of the salt. A rise of 30 points in the blood-pressure may be considered as a reasonable increase during the experimental period that may be attributed to spontaneous variations in arterial tension during a period of two to four hours. Observation 1, the control experiment in which colored water was administered instead of salt solution, showed a rise of 30 mm. of mercury, substantiating the above supposition. If the problem is studied from this angle and any rise of arterial tension of 30 or less is regarded as being within the probable unavoidable variation taking place during the period of the experiment, it may be noted that the maximal rise of the systolic blood-pressure was (as given in Table X).

5 mm. of mercury in observation 6
12 " " " " " 9
18 " " " " " 8
22 " " " " " 3
26 " " " " " 4
30 " " " " " 7

This leaves only observations 2 and 5 with a distinct rise in blood-pressure (that is one higher than 30 mm. of mercury) that might be considered as indicating any possible effect of the sodium chloride.

There is another point of view from which the present observations may be analyzed. If salt causes a rise in blood-pressure the arterial tension should not drop while the sodium chloride is exerting its effect. Therefore the study of the minimal blood-pressures obtained would be of as great, if not greater importance, than the maximal. As has already been noted it is within the first two hours after ingestion that the salt is absorbed from the intestine. Neither in the first two or the second two hour period after taking sodium chloride does the minimal blood-pressure rise appreciably above the control reading taken at the time the experiment was started; in most instances the minimal blood-pressure is distinctly lower. Therefore from this point of view, as well as from those previously stated, the ingestion of 10 gm. of sodium chloride does not appear to increase arterial tension.

The observations given in detail in Tables IV to IX have been analyzed from other angles and have not been found to yield any indication that the doses of salt administered were productive of an increased blood-pressure. The difficulties attending the conduction of these experiments, especially in regard to obtaining a proper value for the "spontaneous" variations in blood-pressure, have been studied with some care and it is believed that they have been eliminated as far as this can be done.

Conclusions. Marked "spontaneous" variations occur in the blood-pressure of all individuals. In cases of hypertension a very great diminution of arterial pressure usually occurs during periods of mental and physical relaxation. This variability in blood-pressure has not been accorded sufficient attention when the effect of diet, drugs, etc., upon arterial tension has been studied.

The protein foods do not increase blood-pressure.

The starchy foods may increase blood-pressure indirectly by bringing about obesity.

There is no definite evidence in the literature that sodium chloride raises blood-pressure. The level of the blood chlorides bears no relation to blood-pressure. In a series of experimental observations the ingestion of 10 gm. of salt failed to raise the blood-pressure in cases of hypertension.

DIABETES INSIPIDUS: A CASE REPORT FOLLOWING EPIDEMIC ENCEPHALITIS WITH ENORMOUS POLYURIA.*

By George W. Hall, A.M., M.D.,

Associate Professor of Nervous and Mental Diseases, Rush Medical College, Senior Attending Neurologist, St. Luke's Hospital, Attending Psychiatrist, Chicago Psychopathic Hospital, Chicago.

The patient, J. I., aged sixteen years, a laborer in a packing house, was admitted to the Cook County Hospital, December 16, 1919, complaining of diplopia, marked drowsiness, pain in the back of the neck and night sweats, for one week previous to admission.

Previous Illness. He had chorea at the age of ten years; measles, scarlet fever and whooping-cough in childhood. He gave no history of any venereal infection.

Family History. Negative.

Examination. Examination revealed a slight bilateral ptosis. The pupils reacted to light rather sluggishly. There was a paresis of the left side of the face involving both the upper and lower group of muscles. The spinal fluid was normal. The Wassermann tests upon the blood and spinal fluid were both negative. Urine was normal. Leukocyte count was 15,200.

Diagnosis. Diagnosis was epidemic encephalitis.

The patient made a prompt recovery within three weeks and returned home and to his work. During his stay in the hospital a twenty-four-hour sample of urine measured 3000 cc.

He was admitted a second time to the Cook County Hospital on the service of Dr. J. A. Capps, September 7, 1921, approximately two years later. The complaints on entrance were great thirst, dry mouth, ravenous appetite and frequent micturition.

He said that he had been complaining of this extreme thirst during the past year and that he was compelled to pass urine almost every hour of the twenty-four. This became so annoying that he could not hold a position.

Examination of the eyes, nose and throat was negative. The optic disks were normal. He had one infected tooth. The thyroid gland was negative. Heart, skin and gastrointestinal tract were negative. Muscles, bones, joints and glands were normal. The liver and spleen were not palpable. The blood-pressure was 102 systolic and 80 diastolic.

Examination of the nervous system showed the deep reflexes to be normal and no sensory disturbances or evidences of paralyses were present. Roentgen rays of the sella turcica showed it to be normal in size and contour.

* Read before the Chicago Society of Internal Medicine, April 24, 1922.

This leaves only observations 2 and 5 with a distinct rise in blood-pressure (that is one higher than 30 mm. of mercury) that might be considered as indicating any possible effect of the sodium chloride.

There is another point of view from which the present observations may be analyzed. If salt causes a rise in blood-pressure the arterial tension should not drop while the sodium chloride is exerting its effect. Therefore the study of the minimal blood-pressures obtained would be of as great, if not greater importance, than the maximal. As has already been noted it is within the first two hours after ingestion that the salt is absorbed from the intestine. Neither in the first two or the second two hour period after taking sodium chloride does the minimal blood-pressure rise appreciably above the control reading taken at the time the experiment was started; in most instances the minimal blood-pressure is distinctly lower. Therefore from this point of view, as well as from those previously stated, the ingestion of 10 gm. of sodium chloride does not appear to increase arterial tension.

The observations given in detail in Tables V to IX have been analyzed from other angles and have not been found to yield any indication that the doses of salt administered were productive of an increased blood-pressure. The difficulties attending the conduction of these experiments, especially in regard to obtaining a proper value for the "spontaneous" variation in blood-pressure, have been studied with some care and it is believed that they have been eliminated as far as this can be done.

Conclusions. Marked "spontaneous" variations occur in the blood-pressure of all individuals. In cases of hypertension a very great diminution of arterial pressure usually occurs during periods of mental and physical relaxation. This variability in blood-pressure has not been accorded sufficient attention when the effect of diet, drugs, etc., upon arterial tension has been studied.

The protein foods do not increase blood-pressure.

The starchy foods may increase blood-pressure indirectly by bringing about obesity.

There is no definite evidence in the literature that sodium chloride raises blood-pressure. The level of the blood chlorides bears no relation to blood-pressure. In a series of experimental observations the ingestion of 10 gm. of salt failed to raise the blood-pressure in cases of hypertension.

DIABETES INSIIDUS: A CASE REPORT FOLLOW[illegible] ENCEPHALITIS WITH ENORMOUS POLY[illegible]

By GEORGE W. HALL, A.M., M.D.,

ASSOCIATE PROFESSOR OF NERVOUS AND MENTAL DISEASES, RUSH M[illegible] SENIOR ATTENDING NEUROLOGIST, ST. LUKE'S HOSPITAL, A[illegible] PSYCHIATRIST, CHICAGO PSYCHOPATHIC HOSPITAL, CHICA[illegible]

THE patient, J. I., aged sixteen years, a laborer in [illegible] house, was admitted to the Cook County Hospital, De[illegible] 1919, complaining of diplopia, marked drowsiness, pa[illegible] back of the neck and night sweats, for one week pr[illegible] admission.

Previous Illness. He had chorea at the age of ten years; [illegible] scarlet fever and whooping-[illegible] childhood. He ga[illegible] history of any venereal in[illegible]

Family History. Negative[illegible]

Examination. Examination [illegible] The pupils reacted to light rather slug[illegible] of the left side of the [illegible] involving t[illegible] group of muscles. The spinal fluid was [illegible] mann tests on the blood and spinal flui[illegible] Urine was normal. Leukocyte count was 15[illegible]

Diagnosis. Diagnosis was epidemic encephali[illegible]

The patient made a prompt recovery within [illegible] returned home and to his work. During his stay [illegible] a twenty-four-hour sample of urine measured 3000 [illegible]

He was admitted a second time to the Cook Co[illegible] on the service of Dr. J. A. Capps, September 7, 1921, a[illegible] two years later. The complaints on entrance were [illegible] dry mouth, ravenous appetite and frequent micturitio[illegible]

He said that he had been complaining of this extre[illegible] during the past year and that he was compelled to pa[illegible] almost every hour of the twenty-four. This became so gr[illegible] that he could not hold a position.

Examination of the eyes, nose and throat was negative. [illegible] optic disks were normal. He had one infected tooth. The thy[illegible] gland was negative. Heart, skin and gastrointestinal tract w[illegible] negative. Muscles, bones, joints and glands were normal. T[illegible] liver and spleen were not palpable. The blood-pressure was 10[illegible] systolic and [illegible]

Examination of the nervous system showed the deep reflexes to be norm[illegible] sensory disturbances or evidences of paralyses were present [illegible] of the sella turcica showed it to be normal [illegible]

* Rea[illegible] [illegible] 24, 1922.

TABLE I.

Date, 1921.		Intake in cc.	Output in cc.	Remarks.
Sept.	8	5,730	6,750	
"	9	5,400	no record	Urea N. 13.5 mg.; uric acid, 2; creatinin, 1.51; sugar, 95; chlorides 620 (by Dr. J. Kendall).
"	10	5,710	8,000	
"	11	6,810	6,240	
"	12	5,160	5,000	
"	13	7,080	5,500	Adrenalin chloride gr. $\frac{1}{100}$ t. i. d. in sterile oil.
"	15	2,970	18,800	Mosenthal diet.
"	17	8,200	11,500	Adrenalin as on September 13.
"	18	7,500	9,600	Adrenalin as on September 13.
"	19	8,880	8,160	Adrenalin as on September 13.
"	20	7,500	9,600	Adrenalin as on September 13.
"	21	8,880	8,160	Urea N., 9.34; uric acid, 1.95; creatinin, 1.43; sugar, 83; chlorides, 545.
"	24	7,590	6,500	Pituitrin ½ cc t. i. d., until September 30*. Blood pressure 138–96, twenty minutes after pituitrin.
"	25	8,100	7,500	Relief from extreme thirst.
"	26	8,400	7,000	
"	27	5,940	6,500	
"	28	7,860	6,240	
"	29	7,850	6,240	
"	30	9,900	8,160	
Oct.	2	8,820	7,200	
"	3	6,750	6,720	
"	4	.....	.....	200 gm. glucose given.
"	5	15,660	20,000	
"	6	11,070	8,640	Basal metabolism,—8 5.
"	7	9,960	9,680	
"	14	.....	27,000	
"	20	.....	30,000	
"	23	.....	....	Again given pituitrin as before.
"	27	.....	16,000	
Nov.	2	.....	13,000	

* Following pituitrin, the patient complained of a sensation as though electricity was passing through his body, and of headache and dizziness.

Following the administration of 200 gm. of glucose on October 7, sugar was not detected in the urine after three, six and twenty-four hours. The blood chemistry before the administration of glucose showed 100 mg. of sugar. One hour following the administration of glucose it showed 90.9; after two hours, 66.7 mg.; after three hours, 117.01; after four hours, 55.5 mg.

October 10, 1921, the phenolphthalein test showed 75 per cent elimination during the first two hours. Cystoscopic examination made previously by Dr. Culver revealed a normal mucosa. Phenolphthalein tests were carried out as follows: the right kidney showed the presence of phenolphthalein within three minutes following the injection intravenously. Two ounces of urine were obtained within thirty minutes and showed an excretion of 9 per cent (normal is 25 to 30 per cent). The left kidney showed the appearance of solution in three minutes following injection and 12 per cent excretion within thirty minutes. On this day, 200 gm. of glucose were again given and no sugar appeared in the urine, showing an increased sugar tolerance.

Because of certain peculiar mental manifestations, he was transferred to the Psychopathic Hospital on October 10, 1921. The social service report at that time stated that the patient reached the seventh grade in public school, that he had worked rather steadily as a packer in the stockyards. There was no history of delusions or hallucinations reported. The Binet-Stanford examination, made by Dr. S. H. Tulchin, showed a chronological age of eighteen years, a mental age of eleven years and five months, and an intelligence quotient of 71.3, classifying him as a borderline case mentally. Further mental examination showed orientation as to time, place and person to be good. Memory past and present was good. Retention was good, general information poor,

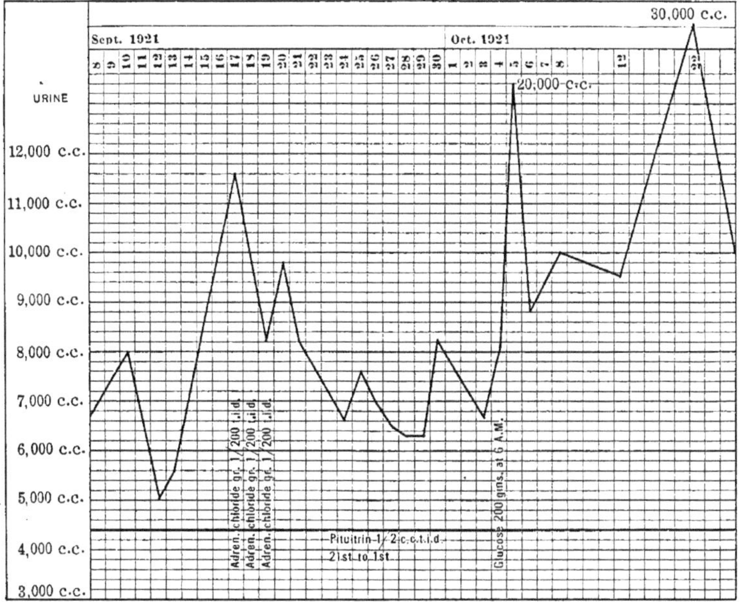

judgment poor and reaction to environment good. Emotional attitude adequate. As to behavior, he was quite coöperative, answered questions promptly, coherently and to the point. No paranoiac trends were elicited. Further investigation showed that the patient had been arrested eight months previous to entering the hospital for making advances to a girl living next door to him, and two weeks later he again exposed himself to the same girl, because he thought she had smiled at him.

Diagnosis. Organic brain disease with a judgment defect, following epidemic encephalitis.

In reference to the extent of the polyuria in diabetes insipidus, Edwards[1] says that it runs from 10 to 40 and even 90 pints per day; Jeanselme and Weil[2] say from 10 to 20 liters per day. In cases reported by Gibson and Martin[3] and Fracassi,[50] the amount of urine reached 15 liters per day; Nasso[5] reported 15 liters; v. Hoesslin,[42] 20 to 24 liters; Herrick,[6] 10 liters; while Trousseau[7] reported an early case in which the urine reached the enormous quantity of 43 liters in twenty-four hours. It will thus be seen that in this case the urinary output in twenty-four hours is one of the largest recorded in the literature.

It is only within the present decade that the morbid entity known as diabetes insipidus or, as it was previously styled, essential polyuria, was definitely removed from the classification of urological diseases, and its pathogenesis referred to some lesion of the nervous mechanism governing the kidney functioning and elimination. However, exact appreciation of the nervous mechanical disturbance is a matter concerning which there is even at the present time no universal agreement, although it is generally conceded that the syndrome of the disease follows a disturbance of the secretion of the pituitary gland, especially the posterior lobe, or some injury to the brain in the region of the pituitary gland. As will be seen later, there are some investigators who believe that the pituitary gland *per se* may be exempted from any direct bearing on the causation of diabetes insipidus and that the brain centers governing the urinary secretion and output are situated outside this gland.

Among the earliest writers who called attention to this morbid condition were Willis,[8] Simmonds[9] and Frank.[10] Willis, in 1682, clearly recognized the distinction between saccharine and non-saccharine diabetes without, however, ascribing any exact cause; Simmonds, more than a hundred years later, described two clinical cases. Frank, in 1792, was the first to give a clear pathological description of the disease. He described it as a long-continued increased secretion of non-saccharine urine, and was convinced that the condition was not due to any diseased state of the kidney. Frank's description is classical and may be accepted at the present day, if we add to it intense polydipsia.

Since that time, the immense literature which has grown up around this subject may be described either as clinical reports, supporting favorite theories regarding the uncertainty of the origin of the condition, or experimental investigations, with a view of discovering the factors concerned with its appearance. It was known that the polyuria was accompanied by polydipsia, but it was not conceded that the former was dependent upon the latter; it was known that the concentration of salts in the urine was disturbed, and different metabolic theories were enunciated to account for it; the blood supply to the kidney and the nervous control of the organ were incriminated and, by degrees, led to a recognition of the higher centers, disturbance of which was responsible for the development of the syndrome.

The disease is uncommon. In the Zurich Medical Clinic, in nearly 36,000 patients observed by Eichhorst during 1876 and following years, he saw only 17 with diabetes insipidus; in the Charité Hospital, Berlin, from 1877 to 1896, Gerhardt observed 55 cases in 113,600 patients. Futcher[20] says that 7 cases of diabetes insipidus were found in over 400,000 patients treated at the Johns Hopkins Hospital, from 1889 to 1904. The disease, therefore, is observed in less than one-tenth of 1 per cent of all cases of disease. It is seen more frequently before the fortieth year of life, and women are affected more than men. Janzen and Brockmann[11] state that it has been observed as a familial disease, and mention 7 instances where the members of families showed a tendency toward or actual development of diabetes insipidus.

In the older views, diabetes insipidus was considered to be of two types: (1) Primary or idiopathic without any evidence of organic lesion, and (2) symptomatic with evidence of organic disease, such lesion being considered as the primary cause. The pathogenic factors concerned are differently estimated as: (1) Primary polydipsia, due to some nervous disturbance; (2) due to pathological condition of the kidneys; (3) due to nervous or vascular disturbance of the kidney function, not, however, dependent upon an organic brain lesion; (4) organic disease of the hypophysis cerebri, especially of its posterior lobe; (5) organic lesion of the centers governing urinary secretion and kidney action—such centers not necessarily being situated in the hypophysis.

The view that diabetes insipidus of idiopathic type exists is scarcely held today; nor is it considered that the polyuria is secondary to a primary polydipsia, which view was supplanted by Ebstein[12] and others. The kidney origin of diabetes insipidus was brought into prominence in 1905 by Meyer,[13] who came to the conclusion that the idiopathic type was primarily a renal polyuria, due to a functional failure of the kidneys which rendered them incapable of secreting concentrated urine, *i. e.*, urine above a certain low specific gravity. Histological examination of the kidneys in cases of diabetes insipidus did not, however, support the view that the condition is due to structural alterations. Further contributions of note concerning diabetes insipidus as being due to a pathological condition of the kidneys were made by Tallqvist,[14] Socin,[15] Forschbach and Weber[16] as well as others.

In 1909, Engel[17] enunciated the view that a prolonged nervous stimulus, possibly in the medulla, excited the glomeruli to greater secretive activity, or the tubules to diminished resorption, or both. Fitz[18] recently discussed the nervous control of the kidney and of its vascular supply. He points out that the researches of Claude Bernard and others have shown that section of the cord at the sixth or seventh cervical vertebra produced an immediate suppression of urine and that section below the twelfth dorsal had practically no effect upon the secretion. In the intermediate sections, the results, as regards the urinary secretion were variable. The studies of Schaefer and Herring[19] have shown that pituitary secretion has a specific dilating effect upon the renal vessels. Fitz thinks that the nerve fibers governing the kidney pass from the medulla to the level of the sixth or seventh cervical vertebra, where they leave the cord, and that an experimentally produced polyuria is an irritative phenomenon or that a brain lesion (even without focal symptoms) may cause hypersensitiveness of the renal vessels either by stimulation of the vasomotor nerves of the kidney or through hypersecretion of the hypophysis. In either case, a polyuria might result from hyperirritability of the renal vessels.

Diabetes insipidus is more usually observed when there is some manifest or implied brain lesion present. The lesion from its symptomatology is usually conceded to be in the hypophysial or closely adjoining region. But, on the other hand, diabetes insipidus may be observed without any clinical showings which would suggest a brain lesion.

The Presence of a Hypophysial Hormone. Bauer and Aschner[21] have very recently expressed the view that diabetes insipidus may find its origin in the kidney or its innervation, dependent upon some disturbance in the nerve centers in the brain. Stimulation of the superior cervical sympathetic ganglion, and a consequential effect upon the brain centers governing the mechanism of metabolism, was enunciated as a hypothesis by Weed and Jacobsen,[22] in 1913. Maranon[23] thinks that the posterior lobe of the pituitary physiologically exercises a controlling action upon the elimination of water through the renal filter and thus produces polyuria through any disturbance. The hypophysial hormone may act partly directly upon the kidney cell or partly by the means of the nervous system. Maranon thinks it probable, as both Cushing and Biedl have suggested, that the hypophysial hormone ascends by the *tuber cinereum* and acts upon the proximal mesencephalic centers.

Bailey and Bremer[24] recently have, as a result of experimentation come to a different conclusion which will be dealt with presently.

Although the brilliant experimental work of Crowe, Cushing and Homans[25] in 1910, had shown that in animals an experimental partial hypophysectomy was followed by polyuria among other effects, yet it cannot be said that a definite connection between the hypophysis cerebri and the syndrome of diabetes insipidus was completely accepted until the findings of Farini,[26] who first, in 1913, showed that injections of hypophysial extract modified polyuria. This finding was confirmed by Rosenbloom,[27] Maranon,[23]

Motzfeldt,[28] Lereboullet[29] and many others since that time. Although the modification is transitory, the effect appears to be absolutely specific for pituitary gland extract, and polyuria recurs as soon as the injections are discontinued or shortly after.

As early as 1901, Magnus and Schaefer[30] had shown that pituitary extract caused an increased urinary secretion and output. Schaefer and Herring[19] showed later that the urinary effects of hypophysial extracts were due alone to derivatives from the pars intermedia and they claimed that the diuretic action was the result of a property of this secretion directly stimulating kidney cell action as well as locally dilating the kidney vessels. They thought that diabetes insipidus might be a manifestation of a superactive hypophysis.

Pars Intermedia. In 1913, Lewis and Matthews,[31] experimenting with dogs, came to the conclusion that the clinical and experimental data showed diabetes insipidus to be due to hypersecretion of the pars intermedia. But Roemer[32] showed that some cases of diabetes insipidus might be due to lack of secretion of the pars intermedia and not to hyperfunction.

Posterior Lobe Secretion. Motzfeldt's important contribution,[29] in 1918, concerning 3 cases of diabetes insipidus, in which all the symptomatology pointed to an insufficiency of posterior lobe secretion of the pituitary, has been generally accepted as showing this to be the part most involved in the syndrome of diabetes insipidus.

The more recent investigations of Leschke, Houssay, Camus and Roussy and Bailey and Bremer have, however, rather tended to focus the cause of diabetes insipidus upon some injury to the brain centers governing urinary secretion other than to the hypophysis.

Tuber Cinereum and the Hypothalamus. Leschke,[33] in 1917, showed that diabetes is not of hypophysial origin because total extirpation of the gland has no influence upon the secretion of urine, when sufficient care is exercised that the *tuber cinereum* and no other part of the brain be touched. When the pituitary gland alone, and without injury to other parts, is removed polyuria is never observed; but, on the other hand, piqûre in the *tuber cinereum* produces polyuria. Leschke thinks it most probable that the brain center for the secretion of urine is situated here near the centers for metabolism and of the sympathetic nerves of the eye, and that very probably diabetes insipidus is produced by a disturbance of this center. The hypophysis has no relation to it and it is only when a hypophysial tumor presses upon the center, or some other such condition, that polyuria arises. Besides, it is known that polyuria may occur in basal meningitis and other pathological conditions, where there is a normal pituitary gland.

Camus and Roussy,[34] in 1913, showed by animal experiments that by puncturing the hypothalamus they were able to produce polyuria. These authors later showed[34] that after removal of the hypophysis of dogs, the administration of pituitary extract did not improve the syndrome of diabetes insipidus, and they, hence, concluded that the essential factor in this disease might be a lesion of some adjacent region in the brain. Camus and Roussy were satisfied from their experimental work upon dogs that it was not the removal of the pituitary gland that determined polyuria but a lesion of the base of the brain corresponding to the optopeduncular space.

Houssay,[35] from experiments reported in 1915–1916, established a cerebral base zone, an injury to which produced polyuria. This zone is bounded in front by the optic chiasm and posteriorly by the peduncle protuberance. The posterior lobe of the pituitary body may constitute a part of this zone, but Houssay does not think it probable.

Bailey and Bremer,[24] quite recently experimenting upon dogs and using the lateral route of approach to the hypophysis devised by Paulesco and Cushing which avoids the probability of injuring it, have found that polydipsia and polyuria are produced with certainty if even a very slight injury to the postinfundibular region of the hypothalamus occurs. The polyuria thus produced may be transitory or permanent. The experimental diabetes insipidus produced does not depend upon a disturbance of a supposed nervous or vascular regulation of the kidney, as it can be induced in animals whose kidneys have been denervated. Lesion of the tuber cinereum has also produced persistent polyuria with adiposogenital dystrophy in dogs. Lesion of the base of the brain outside of the para-infundibular region does not produce polyuria, according to these authors. There is no evidence of any hormone regulating the kidney, especially a pituitary hormone.

It is evident from these findings of Camus and Roussy, Leschke, Houssay and Bailey and Bremer that there is very great divergence of opinion at the present time with regard to the exact location in the brain, injury to which sets up polyuria; general opinion may be taken as in accordance with the editorial view expressed in the *Journal of the American Medical Association*[36] that, in the present conflicting state of evidence, it cannot be accepted that a disorder of the pituitary body is in all cases the cause of polyuria.

Polyuria, seemingly, is a nervous phenomenon, which may be caused by any irritation or lesion of the optopeduncular region; or of the postinfundibular region of the hypothalamus; and in the front rank of such lesions is the pressure produced by enlargement or tumor of the hypophysis. Clinically, although polyuria is modified by hypophysial extract injections, it has never been definitely proved that a lesion of the hypophysis itself is the only cause of diabetes insipidus.

In support of these views are the cases reported by Veil,[37] in which polyuria and increase of chlorides in the urine were caused by piqûre in the floor of the fourth ventricle; when the puncture was made in the midbrain there was polyuria with decreased chlorides. Veil, in fact, called attention to two types of diabetes insipidus, in one of which the chlorine content of the blood is increased and in the other diminished.

Goldzieher,[38] Berblinger[39] and Simmonds[40] have all referred to the relation between diabetes insipidus and lesions in and about the pituitary, especially in its posterior part; the view of Newmark[41] is that polyuria may or may not follow neurohypophysial disease, and that the neurohypophysis is not the only region, disease of which is followed by polyuria and polydipsia. The medulla oblongata figures occasionally in the pathology of diabetes insipidus and v. Hoesslin[42] and Gierke[43] reported cases of diabetes insipidus with tumor or atrophy of the pineal gland. In Gierke's case there was, however, concurrent disease of the third ventricle and of the neurohypophysis as well. Bailey and Bremer, as we have seen, limit diabetes insipidus symptoms to injury of the post-infundibular region.

Despite the experimental demonstrations of Leschke, Houssay, Camus and Roussy and Bailey and Bremer, the fact remains that hypophysial extract injection seems to be specific in the treatment of diabetes insipidus; and, moreover, in many clinical cases of diabetes insipidus, an actual lesion of the pituitary body can be demonstrated. Cushing[44] showed that simple operative manipulation of the posterior lobe led to profuse diuresis and that its ablation caused transitory polyuria. Chiasserini's[45] dog experiments showed that hyperplastic lesions of pars intermedia sometimes induced intense polyuria; bacilli introduced into the sella turcica caused progressive changes in the anterior portion of the gland accompanied by intense polyuria. In Neuberger's case[46] there was destruction of the pars nervosa by a cancerous metastasis; in Maranon and Pinto's case[47] a bullet lodged in the base of the hypophysial stalk; in Luzzato's case,[48] hemorrhage into the stalk; in Catterina's case,[49] a probable compression of the hypophysis relieved by trepanation and disappearance of the symptoms. As previously stated, Crowe, Cushing and Homans[25] reported that a polyuria, either transitory or prolonged, frequently accompanies hypophysectomy. In Franke's case,[51] a bullet was lodged at the base of the pituitary.

The exact etiological factors concerned in diabetes insipidus, if it is to be considered as an independent syndrome, must remain unsettled until more definite knowledge is obtained regarding the precise location of the brain centers governing the action of the kidney, and what conditions affect such centers.

Syphilis as an Etiological Factor. Owing to the frequency with which it invades the brain, syphilis is generally admitted as an important etiological factor, and cases have been reported by Fracassi,[50] Cammidge,[52] Dameno,[53] Chiari[54] among others. In Fracassi's case the patient was passing 15 liters of urine per day, and the polyuria quickly subsided under specific treatment. Chiari's case was very similar. Cammidge thinks that his case was the result of parasyphilitic changes at the base of the brain, which interfered with the passage of the secretion of the hypophysis into the cerebrospinal fluid. The sudden change of pressure under lumbar puncture broke down adhesions and opened a passage again for the secretions. In Dameno's case there was apparently a syphilitic process which had induced diffuse infiltration involving the optic chiasm and pituitary body.

In syphilitic cases the type is either that of a gumma in the floor of the fourth ventricle, in the pituitary or in the brain region outlined by Houssay, which has been previously referred to, or else the syphilitic process may set up a basal meningitis or an endarteritis with connective-tissue proliferation.

Globus and Strauss[58] report a case of teratoid cyst of the hypophysis in a girl, aged six years, who developed polydipsia and polyuria. The tumor was adherent to the optic chiasm and, extending posteriorly, filled up the entire interpeduncular space. The *tuber cinereum* and mammillary bodies could not be identified, the third ventricle was almost obliterated. The hypophysis was small in size and compressed while the infundibular portion of the hypophysis showed no change except compression. They are inclined to think the autopsy findings in this case support the experimental work of Bailey and Bremer.

No Hormone in the Spinal Fluid. It has been considered that the cerebrospinal fluid has some effect upon the inhibitory action of pituitary extract upon the polyuria of diabetes insipidus; or, at least, that the extract was only effective after its discharge into the cerebrospinal fluid. Maranon and Gutierrez's[55] experimental research upon this point is rather convincing. These authors found that by injecting healthy rabbits with cerebrospinal fluid from a normal healthy human subject there was an increase of diuresis. But, if instead of injecting spinal fluid, extract of the posterior or middle lobe of the hypophysis was injected there was considerable diminution in the quantity of urine eliminated in twenty-four hours. If instead of obtaining the injected cerebrospinal fluid from a normal man, it was obtained from a patient with diabetes insipidus the effects on rabbits were the same as in the case of fluid obtained from a normal subject.

The intraspinal injection of pituitrin diluted with patient's own spinal fluid (*i. e.*, 0.5 cc of pituitrin diluted in 2 cc of spinal fluid of the patient injected intraspinally), caused only the same amount of reduction as a subcutaneous injection of the same quantity of pituitrin. This was verified in different experiments.

The general results showed that there was no diffusion of an oliguric hormone in the spinal fluid.

The Effects of Lumbar Puncture. But the spinal fluid can act upon the polyuria by its tension. In the case reported by Herrick,[56] withdrawal of only 5 cc. by lumbar puncture caused an almost immediate gradual reduction of the polyuria from more than 11,000 cc. per day to little over 600 cc. In Graham's traumatic case,[57] lumbar puncture likewise caused an immediate reduction of a polyuria exceeding 5½ liters per day. Graham is unable to explain the increased amount and tension of the cerebrospinal fluid. In his case it increased enough to cause pressure in the hypophysial region and set up polyuria. Three of Maranon and Gutierrez's cases were treated by lumbar puncture with satisfactory results.

Concerning the therapeutics of diabetes insipidus, little need be said. The immediate effects of pituitary posterior lobe extract has already been mentioned. The effects are, however, only transitory and cease when the injections are discontinued or shortly thereafter. Lumbar puncture in some cases has had a salutary effect.

The only treatment outside of surgery that seems to be of permanent value is restriction of the sodium chloride and nitrogen contents of the food. When compression of the brain region in the vicinity of the hypophysis is manifest or suggested by symptoms, surgical operation would, no doubt, give relief, but the difficulty and the dangers of such surgery excludes its application except in very grave cases.

In syphilitic cases antiluetic treatment generally has had little effect upon the diabetic syndrome.

I am indebted to Dr. Jos. A. Capps and his associates for the privilege of using their records in the case reported.

LITERATURE.

1. Edwards: Practice of Medicine, 1916, p. 728.
2. Jeanselme and Weil: Malad. d. reins, Paris, 1909, p. 33.
3. Gibson and Martin: Arch. Int. Med., 1921, **27**, 351.
5. Nasso: Pediatria, Naples, 1920, **28**, 812.
6. Herrick: Arch. Int. Med., 1912, **10**, 1.
7. Trousseau: Lessons on Clinical Medicine (New Sydenham Society Translation), London, 1870, **8**, 528.
8. Willis: De Diuesinimia, Opera Omnia, Amsterdam, 1682, (Sect. IV, Cap. III).
9. Simmonds: Medical Facts and Opinions, London, 1792, p. 73.
10. Frank, Johann: De curandis hominum morbis, Ordo 1, Genus II, (diabetes) Florence, 1832.
11. Janzen and Brockmann: Nederland. Tijdsschr. v. Geneesk., 1921, **1**, 251.
12. Ebstein: Mitth. a. d. Grenzgeb. d. Med. u. Chir., 1912, **25**, 441.
13. Meyer, E.: Deutsch Arch. f. klin. Med., 1905, **83**, 1.
14. Tallqvist: Ztschr. f. klin. Med., 1903, **49**, 181.
15. Socin: Ztschr. f. klin. Med., 1913, **88**, 294.

16. Forschbach und Weber: Ztschr. f. klin. Med., 1913, **67**, 153.
17. Engel: Ztschr. f. klin. Med., 1909, **68**, 112.
18. Fitz: Arch. Int. Med., 1914, **14**, 706.
19. Schaefer and Herring: Phil. Transact. Roy. Soc. of Lond., 1906, **199**, B. 1.
20. Futcher: Bull. Johns Hopkins Hosp , 1912, **10**, 197.
21. Bauer and Aschner: Wien Arch. f. inn. Med., 1920, **1**, 297.
22. Weed and Jacobsen: Bull. Johns Hopkins Hosp., 1913, **24**, 40.
23. Maranon: Endocrinology, 1921, **5**, 159.
24. Bailey and Bremer: Arch. Int. Med., 1921, **28**, 773.
25. Crowe, Cushing and Homans: Bull. Johns Hopkins Hosp., 1910, **21**, 127.
26. Farini: Gazz. d. osped. e d. clin. Milano, 1913, p. 1135.
27. Rosenbloom: Jour. Am. Med. Assn., 1918, **70**, 1292.
28. Motzfeldt: Endocrinology, 1918, **2**, 112.
29. Lereboullet· Bull. soc. méd. d. hôp. de Paris, 1914, **37**, 517, and Paris méd., 1919, **9**. 353.
30. Magnus and Schaefer: Jour. Physiol., 1901–2, **27**, 9.
31. Lewis and Matthews: Arch. Int. Med., 1915, **15**, 451.
32. Roemer: Deutsch. med. Wchnschr., 1914, **40**, 108.
33. Leschke Ztschr. f. klin. Med., 1917, **87**, 201.
34. Camus and Roussy: Endocrinology, 1920, **4**, 507.
35. Houssay: Prensa med., Argent., 1915–16, **2**, 82, 91, 101.
36. Editorial: Jour. Am. Med. Assn., 1920, **74**, .
37. Veil: Deutsch. med. Wchnschr., 1920, **46**, 558; Biochem. Ztschr., 1918, **91**, 317.
38. Goldzieher: Verhandl. deutsch. path. Gesellsch., 1913, **16**, 281.
39. Berblinger: Verhandl. deutsch. path. Gesellsch., 1913, **16**, 272.
40. Simmonds: Munchen. med. Wchnschr., 1913, **60**, 127.
41. Newmark: Arch. Int. Med., 1917, **19**, 550.
42. v. Hoesslin· München. med. Wchnschr., 1896, p. 292.
43. Gierke: Verhandl. deut. path. Gesellsch., 1914, **17**, 200.
44. Cushing: Boston Med. and Surg. Jour , 1913, **148**, 901.
45. Chiasserini: Policlinico, Rome, 1918.
46. Neuberger. Berl. klin. Wchnschr., 1920, **57**, 10.
47. Maranon and Pinto· Nouv. icon. de la Salpêtrière, 1916, **28**, 185.
48. Luzzato: Lo Sperimentale, Florence, 1918, **71**, 405.
49. Catterina: Policlin., Rome, 1921, **28**, sez. chir., 181.
50. Fracassi. Revist. med. d. Rosario, 1918, **8**, 197.
51. Franke: Berl. klin. Wchnschr., 1912, **49**, 393.
52. Cammidge: Practitioner, 1920, **105**, 244.
53. Dameno: Prensa med., Argent , 1919, **5**, 345.
54. Chiari. Wien. klin. Wchnschr., 1920, **23**, 620.
55. Maranon and Gutierrez: Contribucion al studio de la pathogenia hypopisaria de la diabetes insipida, Siglo med., 1919, **66**, 809.
56. Herrick· Arch. Int. Med., 1912, **10**, 1.
57. Graham: Jour. Am. Med. Assn., 1917, **69**, 1498.
58. Globus and Strauss: Arch. Neurol. and Psych., 1922, **8**, 535.

DISFIGURING SCARS—PREVENTION AND TREATMENT.

By George M. Dorrance, M.D.,

and

J. W. Bransfield, M.D.

Surgeons to St. Agnes Hospital, Philadelphia.

In plastic surgery of the head or neck, it is essential to obtain a scar which is not disfiguring. Our observations in the French, English and American Hospitals during the war convinced us of one fact, viz., that simple approximation of the skin edges invariably led to subsequent broadening and dimpling of the scar. Every plastic surgeon in the army has had the disagreeable experience of seeing some of his cases reoperated because of a disfiguring scar. Photographs made a month or so after the first operation showed a scarcely discernible scar. What occurs to cause this late broadening of linear scars and permits the disfiguring umbilications?

To understand this, it is necessary to review our knowledge of wound healing. In a clean aseptic wound where all the bleeding has been carefully controlled and the tissues are properly sewed in layers, we have immediately the production of a small amount of blood ooze which promptly clots. A few migratory corpuscles pass out into the clots and tissues. The fixed connective tissue cells and the endothelial cells of the vessels pass out and promptly multiply, forming embryonic tissue; these cells are known as fibroblasts. At this stage, we have the first splinting of the wound and the cut edges are held in accurate approximation. The fibroblasts destroy any leukocytes present and bridge across the tissues. From each side of the wound, new capillaries are formed; these pass through the clot, joining with their fellows from the other side. The fibroblasts later become spindle cells forming the interlacing fibers. This fibrous tissue formed is very contractile in type and soon obliterates the newly formed bloodvessels. If considerable oozing occurs, we may get the formation of the so-called coagulate lymph clot made up of blood clots, plasma clots, and leukocytes; the same healing process occurs later but the amount of fibrous tissue is materially increased and the extent of the scar is in proportion.

After healing has taken place in a wound approximated by a simple suture under tension, several factors enter into the alteration of the scar. In proportion to their activity, we may classify them in the following order: (1) Muscular pull; (2) contractility of the newly formed fibrous tissue; and (3) low grade infection. We are assuming that proper approximation has been made. If the skin edges are not promptly brought together, this will be a fourth factor in the disfiguring process.

In all wounds about the face or neck, the muscular pull is a potent factor to be constantly reckoned with. The incision as far as possible must be in the line of the muscle fibers. The fact that we have muscles inserting in the superficial fascia and even the skin itself must be considered. In making our closure, a margin of safety is allowed for this fact.

All newly formed scar tissue regardless of its location, contracts and in its early pliable condition is influenced by the muscle pull.

Low grade infection is a fairly rare process, thanks to our modern asepsis and Nature's bountiful blood supply in these areas. When it does occur, we cannot hope for a perfect scar.

Experience has shown us that the best method of preventing noticeable scar formation is to overcorrect as it were, at the primary operation. It is not sufficient to simply evert the skin edges; it is necessary to have accurate approximation of the superficial fascia and to bring fat to fat with the obliteration of all dead spaces. The use of the mattress suture with a skin coaptation button has been most satisfactory in our hands, as it permits us to obtain the conditions essential to proper scar formation.

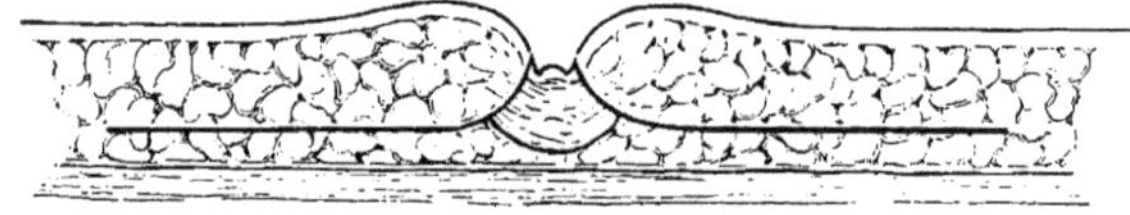

Fig. 1

Repair of Old Scars. When is the opportune time to resect an old scar? As long as the scar tissue is bright red, we know that the fibrous tissue has not finished its contraction, because when full contractility has occurred, the scar will be pale due to the obliteration of the capillaries. No scar should be repaired until

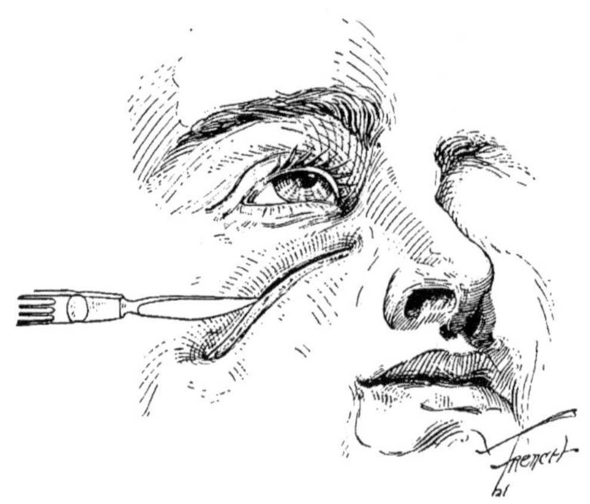

Fig. 2

this pallor exists. The surrounding tissues are then pliable and the scar may be excised. (Figs. 1 and 2.) The edges are undermined as shown in Fig. 3 and the edges are approximated by the mattress sutures with the use of the buttons. (Figs. 4, 5, 6, 7 and 8.)

A failure to use this everted skin-edge method where large flaps are used to repair defects will result in disfiguring scars. In flap cases, it is necessary to evert the skin edges to a greater extent than in normal wounds as we have the shrinking of the flap itself to contend with.

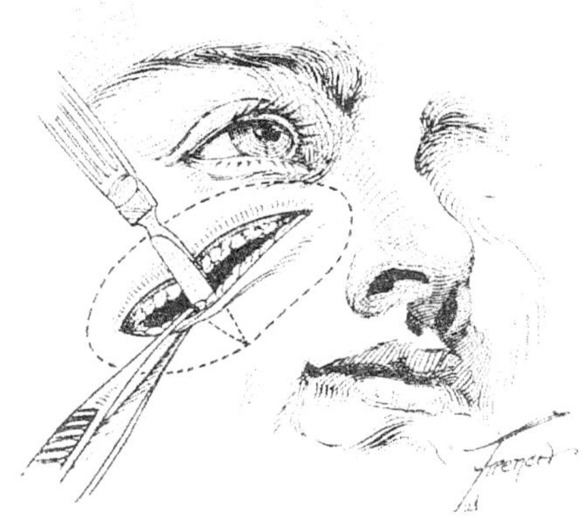

FIG. 3

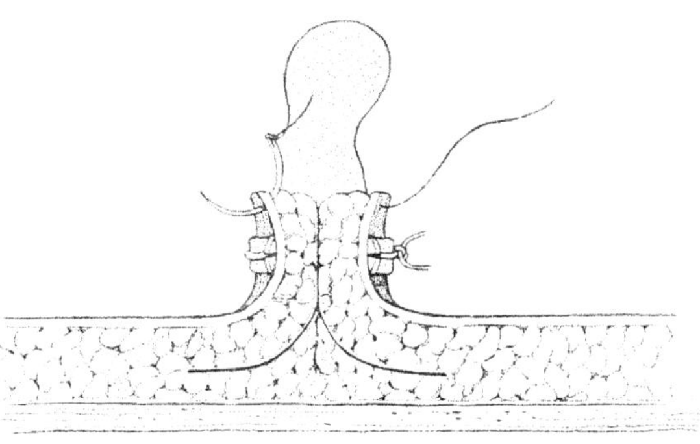

FIG. 4

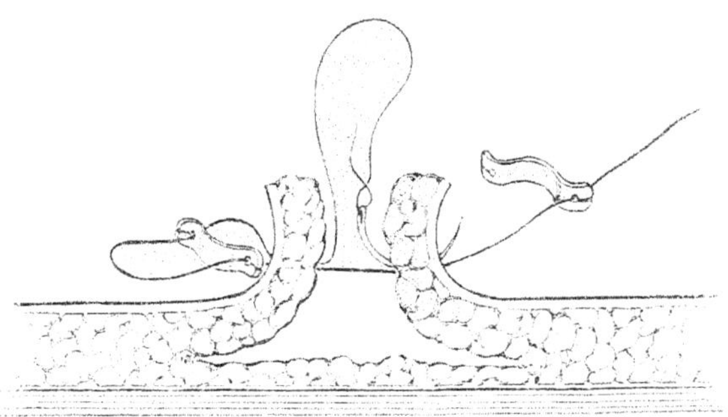

FIG. 5

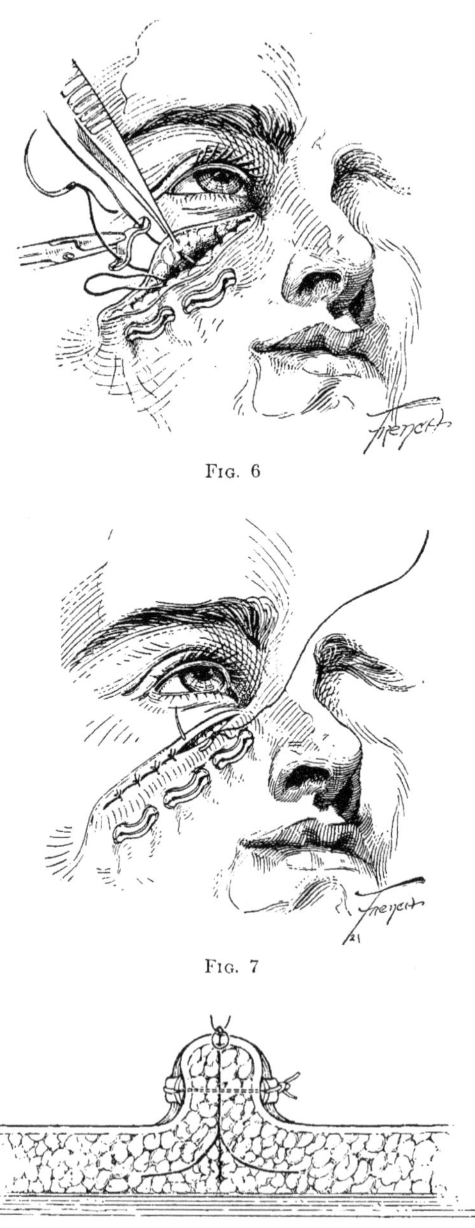

Fig. 6

Fig. 7

Fig. 8

Conclusions. 1. Eversion of the edges places subcutaneou to subcutaneous tissue and as a result, less fibrous tissue is

2. The overcorrected tissue after a comparatively short time will become flat and the scar will be scarcely discernible.
3. Muscular pull and the contractility of fibrous tissue are the most important factors in the production of depressed scars.
4. The use of a coaptation button with a mattress suture is necessary to obtain proper eversion.
5. The use of the button will obliterate all dead space and prevent blood clots' forming.

TRICHINIASIS, ENDEMIC AND SPORADIC, WITH A REVIEW OF THE PRESENT STATUS OF THE TREATMENT OF THE DISEASE.

By M. E. Alexander, M.D.,

ATTENDING PHYSICIAN, WATERBURY HOSPITAL, WATERBURY, CONN.

Although the diagnosis of trichiniasis can be made with absolute accuracy because of the distinctive laboratory findings, the milder cases of this disease frequently still remain undiagnosed. It is only after an eosinophilia is discovered that suspicion of a parasitic disease is oftentimes aroused. Only then are further studies undertaken which lead to an accurate diagnosis. It is the conviction of the writer that trichiniasis is far more common than is generally supposed and that a great many cases escape recognition.

The following case reports are submitted with the aim of drawing attention to the entire absence of clinical symptoms in some cases infected with trichiniasis, indicating the great ease with which instances of the milder types of this disease may remain undiagnosed.

The material is based upon observations made on an outbreak of the disease affecting 35 individuals and on 9 sporadic cases. In the endemic just referred to I had an unusual opportunity to not only make blood examinations on all the individuals known to have partaken of the pork, but to examine sections of muscles from a good number of individuals, including some that presented no clinical symptoms whatever.

Description of the Endemic. On January 15, 1920, a patient was admitted to the Waterbury Hospital with the possible diagnosis of typhoid fever. The patient was a married woman, aged thirty-one years, born in Italy, and six years in this country. The past history was entirely negative.

About two and one-half weeks prior to admission the patient commenced to suffer from indefinite abdominal pain, malaise and slight fever. The symptoms were apparently not very intense, since the patient was able to be up and about for a whole week.

At the end of that time the patient noticed that her eyes were quite swollen, and she also complained of slight soreness in various parts of the body, but particularly in the back. She also complained of considerable abdominal pain. A physician was consulted who prescribed for her and also examined her urine, but found neither albumin nor casts. The patient's temperature at the time of the doctor's first visit was 102° F.; pulse, 112; respirations, 20. The physican saw the patient twice subsequently. The edema of the eyelids had subsided considerably, but the muscular tenderness had increased. The temperature on one visit was 102.6°. On another visit it was 101.8°.

Upon physical examination at the hospital the patient was found to be a well-nourished and well-developed woman of middle age. There was evidence of slight edema of the face, particularly under the eyelids. The tongue was coated. The lungs were negative. The heart showed evidence of a slight degree of dilatation. Apex-beat was in the fifth interspace four inches from the median line. On auscultation a soft, blowing murmur was heard at the apex, but not transmitted to the axilla. The spleen was enlarged and was palpable two fingers' breadth below the costal margin. The uterus was palpable midway between the symphysis pubis and the umbilicus (the patient was about four months pregnant). There was a generalized body tenderness, particularly marked in the extremities. Because of the edema of the face and the muscular tenderness of the enlargement of the spleen a tentative diagnosis of trichiniasis was made. A history of eating pork was obtained, which still further increased the suspicion. A blood count was made immediately, with the following result: Leukocytes, 12,500; polynuclears, 60 per cent; lymphocytes, 3 per cent; mononuclears and transitionals, 5 per cent; eosinophils, 32 per cent. Next day a piece of muscle was excised from the gastrocnemius and trichinæ were found, which finding completed the diagnosis.

Upon further investigation it was found that the pork ingested by the patient was from an animal that was killed on their own premises. Some samples of the remaining pork were procured and trichinæ were demonstrated in abundance in varions parts of the animal, particularly the muscles of the shoulder.

Further investigations of the case revealed the following: The animal was bought in August, 1919, kept for fattening and was killed on December 19, in early preparedness for a Christmas dinner. Two days after the animal was killed a party of 30 partook of the pork. According to the hostess the meat was roasted for about thirty minutes.

All except 3 of the people that partook of the pork that day have eaten of the same many times since, some of them daily. All the 3 that had eaten of the pork but once developed trichiniasis. All together, 40 individuals had partaken of the pork and 5 of these evidently escaped infection; 35 showed evidence of greater or lesser infections as demonstrated by high eosinophil counts; 5 patients were severely ill and 1 of these succumbed to the disease.

TABLE I.—TOTAL AND DIFFERENTIAL WHITE BLOOD COUNTS OF THE PATIENTS THAT HAD PARTAKEN OF THE PORK.

No	Name	Age.	Sex.	Leukocytes.	Polynuclears.	Lymphocytes.	Mononuclears.	Transitionals.	Eosinophils.	Eosinophil myelocytes.	Basophils.
1	B. C.	31	F.	15,200	30	35	4	1	30		
2	L. C.	38	F.	12,800	40	30	5	4	20	..	1
3	Vil.	7	F.	14,600	28	58	2	4	8		
4	Fil.	1	M.	13,400	24	55	13	2	6		
5	D. C.	23	M.	5,800	64	30	5	1			
6	M. C.	36	F.	11,500	64	3	4	1	28		
7	Amb.	36	M.	7,600	62	33	3	2			
8	Mamie	35	F.	11,300	68	20	5	1	6		
9	A. L.	24	M.	6,100	78	20	2				
10	M. M.	34	F.	10,800	65	20	5	1	9		
11	L. M.	42	M.	9,500	47	33	4	3	12	..	1
12	J. M.	34	M.	13,100	39	12	8	4	37		
13	A. V.	8	F.	11,100	46	20	8	2	22	2	
14	M. V.	42	F.	9,400	64	20	2	2	11	..	1
15	Mike	5	M.	13,200	28	23	4	1	42	2	
16	Dan	7	M.	10,800	50	34	2	1	11	2	
17	John	38	M.	12,500	54	30	3	2	10		1
18	T. W.	59	M.	15,100	43	29	5	3	18	..	2
19	L. V.	11	M.	16,200	35	38	4	3	16	3	1
20	H.	22	M.	7,900	62	20	2	3	11	..	2
21	F. M.	17	M.	9,500	54	30	4	2	9	..	1
22	T. M.	25	F.	11,800	43	27	6	6	15	..	3
23	Jim	15	M.	14,100	38	31	5	6	19	1	
24	R. V.	7	F.	12,300	40	36	10	5	7	2	
25	G. M.	16	M.	16,200	50	31	3	5	10	..	1
26	D. V.	6	M.	12,200	42	26	6	3	20	3	
27	E. S.	17	M.	16,200	37	23	4	5	29	..	2
28	C. S.	9	F.	12,300	41	34	6	3	14	2	
29	R. S.	19	M.	12,000	50	21	4	5	18	..	2
30	M. S.	30	F.	7,600	49	24	5	4	17	..	1
31	Eddie	4	M.	10,700	31	26	7	6	27	3	
32	A. M.	6	M.	8,100	46	48	3	2	1		
33	Joe M.	11	M.	6,400	53	30	4	2	10	..	1
34	M. M.	8	M.	11,600	40	32	2	4	19	3	
35	F. M.	35	F.	14,100	52	28	1	6	10	..	3
36	Minn	1½	F.	12,600	16	54	3	2	21	4	
37	Marie	4	F.	9,100	38	44	3	3	9	2	1
38	Lor.	7	M.	12,400	38	48	2	2	8	2	
39	K. M.	24	M.	14,600	48	33	6	11	..	..	2
40	H. M.	40	M.	15,300	25	55	1	3	16		

The blood counts of these cases, along with the data of age, sex and so forth, are to be found in the accompanying tables (Table I). Thirty-five of the cases had an eosinophilia above 5 per cent. The exact figures varied between 6 per cent and 42 per cent. Bits of muscles were excised from 2 of the patients with normal eosinophil counts and no trichinæ were found in either case. In the patients with the higher eosinophil values, the trichinæ were found in the muscles of 7 out of 8 cases examined. The triceps was used in every case.

TABLE II.—WHITE AND DIFFERENTIAL BLOOD COUNT IN THE FOURTEEN CASES OF TRICHINIASIS ANALYZED IN THIS PAPER.

No.	Name.	Leukocytes.	Polymorphonuclears.	Lymphocytes.	Mononuclears and transitionals.	Eosinophils.	Basophils
1	J. M.	13,000	39	12	12	37	0
2	A.	17,600	52	13	5	29	1
3	B. C.	15,200	30	35	5	30	0
4	L. C.	12,800	40	30	9	20	1
5	O. D.	32,400	40	29	5	26	0
6	F. H.	28,200	41	10	7	41	1
7	R. C.	31,100	19	20	6	55	0
8	O. F.	26,400	20	14	4	60	2
9	G. F.	28,200	30	19	7	43	1
10	I. K.	30,600	23	20	6	51	0
11	S. K.	19,800	28	20	11	40	1
12	O. N.	12,400	41	18	5	36	0
13	F. L.	16,100	40	27	12	20	1
14	R. G.	10,600	53	23	9	14	1

All the cases that were not treated in the hospital, with the exception of 5 or 6, could not recall any untoward symptoms and had absolutely no complaints to make during the four weeks prior to this investigation. Of the 5 that had some complaints to make 4 had a recollection of a gastrointestinal disturbance of a very slight degree and for which none sought medical advice because it simulated attacks of indigestion that they had had before. Two of the patients complained of very slight muscular pains, which they attributed to a slight cold. None of them were sick enough to be confined to bed.

Analysis of Symptoms. For this purpose the clinical records and progress notes of 14 cases are used. Four of these belong to the endemic mentioned above. Of the 9 others there were 2 instances each of 2 members of a household being affected, and 5 cases where no other affected individuals could be traced or suspected.

Incubation Period and Onset. In only 2 cases of this series could the incubation period be determined with accuracy. Both these individuals ate of the slaughtered animal on the first day and did not partake of the pork since. In both cases the first symptoms appeared on the seventh day after the ingestion of the meat. Without any dietetic indiscretion to account for it they began to suffer with diarrhea. They also had epigastric distress and nausea, but did not vomit. Edema of the lids and face were noticed by both of these patients on the ninth day after ingestion of the pork.

The disease was ushered in by chilliness in 4 cases; by muscular pains in 6; by nosebleed in 2 and by edema of the face in 4 cases.

Symptoms and Signs. Fever: The patient's temperature varied from 101° F. to 105° F. A marked diurnal variation was quite common in the majority of cases. In 2 cases there was inversion of the usual evening rise, the highest temperature having occurred about 9 or 10 A.M. and the lowest in the evening. This condition persisted throughout the febrile period. In this series of cases the febrile period lasted from ten days to three weeks. A temperature of 106° F. was encountered but once and only lasted three hours.

Gastrointestinal: Dryness of the mouth and thirst were complained of by 11 of the patients. Three of the patients had a protracted diarrhea with traces of blood and mucus in the stools. Eight patients were markedly constipated, while in the remaining 3 the intestinal condition remained apparently normal throughout the disease. They all complained of some abdominal pain, especially during the second week of the disease.

Respiratory: Signs and symptoms of a mild bronchitis were present in 10 of the cases. Three of the patients complained of tightness of the chest, particularly in the presternal region. One case (which terminated fatally) had complete consolidation of the lower right lobe.

Muscular: Twelve of the cases here analyzed had distinct muscular pain and tenderness. In 7 cases it was most marked in the calves of the legs and in the thighs. In 3 cases it was distributed to almost the entire voluntary musculature; mastication was difficult; closing of the eyes was accompanied by a great deal of distress. In 2 cases the muscular pains were slight and inconspicuous.

Cutaneous: Edema of the face was present to a greater or lesser extent in 12 cases of the present series. In 3 of the cases it was very extensive; the face was swollen to unrecognizable proportions and the eyes were so swollen that the lids could hardly be separated. Subconjunctival hemorrhages were encountered in 4 cases, in 1 of which it was very extensive. Erythema was present in 3 cases. The same patients also showed dermographia and evidence of urticaria. Sweating was pronounced in 5 cases. It was most profuse during the second and third weeks of the disease. Pruritus and formication were distressing features in 2 instances.

Pulse: The pulse-rate showed no special changes from other febrile affections except in the striking persistence of arrhythmias in 3 instances. In 1 of these cases a pulsus bigeminus and trigeminus made its appearance on the third day after admission to the hospital and persisted for six days. One patient exhibited three attacks of paroxysmal tachycardia in the course of two days. On one occasion the pulse was 210 per minute.

Heart: In the majority of cases here analyzed the heart showed no particular points of interest. In 1 of the cases the apex-beat was in the fifth interspace, 10 cm. from the median line. A soft murmur was heard at the apex and was not transmitted to the axilla. A systolic murmur, soft in character, was also heard at the pulmonic area. There was no history of rheumatism. This was the same patient that had the attacks of paroxysmal tachycardia described above. At the time of the patient's discharge from the hospital the murmur at the apex could no longer be heard, although the one at the base was still audible. The blood-pressure was not materially affected in any of the cases.

The spleen was definitely palpable in 4 cases. In 2 of the cases it was about 3.5 cm. below the costal margin.

Two of the patients in this series were pregnant women, 1 four months, the other two months. Neither one had miscarried.

Laboratory Findings. Urine: In 5 of the cases the urine was entirely devoid of pathologic elements. In 9 cases albumin was present; in 2 of these it presented a heavy cloud with the heat and acetic acid test. Casts were found in 4 cases, in 2 of which both hyaline and granular casts were present in great numbers. In 2 cases traces of sugar were found. In both cases it was apparently during the third week of the disease. The blood sugar was normal in both of these cases. The diazo reaction was done in 6 of the cases and was found positive in one instance. In this case there was evidence of profound toxemia.

Blood: The hemoglobin and erythrocytes were not appreciably affected in the milder cases but in the severe cases a marked secondary anemia was present. It became especially manifest toward the end of the third or during the fourth week of the disease. No nucleated reds were observed in any of these cases.

TABLE III.—RELATION OF THE EOSINOPHIL COUNT AND THE EASE OF FINDING THE TRICHINÆ IN THE MUSCLES.

No.	Trichinæ in muscles.	Eosinophils, per cent.
1	Abundant	42
2	Abundant	34
3	Very few	27
4	Moderate	14
5	Numerous	11
6	Moderate	19
7	Very few	30
8	Abundant	7
9	Only two parasites seen	28
10	Very few	16
11	Moderate	29
12	Abundant	6

The leukocyte count varied between 10,600 to 32,400. The accompanying tables indicate the details of the blood counts as well as the total and relative eosinophil counts. There was no relationship between the extent of the eosinophilia and the relative number of embryos found in the muscle specimens (Table III).

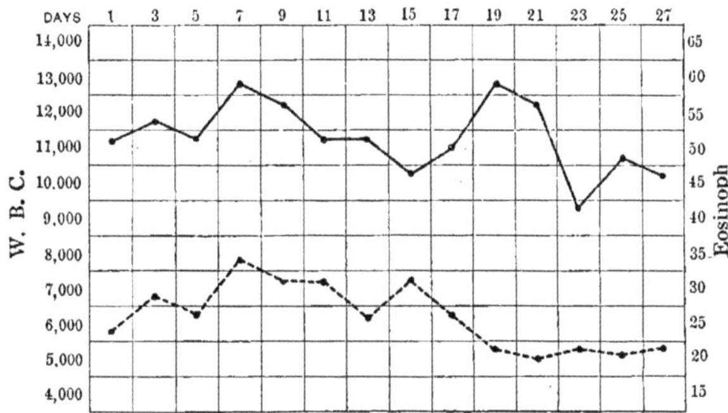

FIG. 1.—Relation of total white cell count to percentage of eosinophiles in one of the cases of trichiniasis.

Observations were made in 9 of the cases as to the persistence of the eosinophilia. (Fig. 1). In all but 1 it was still above 2 per cent at the end of three months. It reached a normal level in all the cases at the end of six months (Table IV).

TABLE IV.—DURATION OF EOSINOPHILIA IN NINE OF THE PATIENTS INVESTIGATED.

Name.	First month, per cent.	Second month, per cent.	Third month, per cent.	Fourth month, per cent.	Fifth month, per cent.	Sixth month, per cent.
J. M.	27	24	18	7	1	1
B. C.	34	29	20	14	7	0
M. C.	20	18	2			
E. S.	29	20	1			
M. M.	32	26	3	2	2	2
D. V.	19	12	5	1	..	1
A. M.	40	22	7	3	1	1
Lor.	18	14	4	2	..	2
W. T.	56	9	7	1	2	1

Finding of the Trichinæ: The parasites were found in the muscles in every one of these 14 cases. In 2 cases, where excision of a piece of the triceps in the second week of the disease showed no parasites, positive results were obtained six weeks later. In several of the cases the embryos were found with no surrounding capsule. In other specimens, removed in the fifth week of the disease, a fibrous capsule was plainly evident. The connective tissue between the muscle fibers was proliferated and the infected muscle fibers showed evidence of granular degeneration.

Trichinæ were found in the blood stream in 2 of 8 patients in which this search was made. In both cases it was in the second week of the affection.

The stools of all the cases were carefully examined for trichinæ but the parasites were not found in any.

Mortality: One of the 14 cases here analyzed terminated fatally (7 per cent). It was apparently due to the complicating lobar pneumonia. It occurred in the third week of the illness. Regretfully, the pneumonia was fully developed before first seen and the influence of the secondary infection upon the eosinophil count could not be observed, since the patient died the next day. The diagnosis of trichiniasis, however, was ascertained by the history of the case and was substantiated by finding free trichinous embryos in muscle specimens.

Summary of the Present Status of the Treatment of Trichiniasis.
Prophylactic. This is still, and ever must be, the most important treatment of this disease. It may be considered under the following headings:

1. Inspection of meat.
2. Prevention of infection in hogs.
3. Proper cooking of pork.

The systematic microscopic examination of pork for trichinæ has been tried extensively in this country and in Germany, but it was given up as unpractical and uncertain. It was pointed out by Stiles and others that not only is the expense enormous and almost prohibitive, but that it did not seem to afford protection. During the years 1881-1898, when Germany had a very rigid method of microscopic examination of pork, there still occurred 2042 cases of trichiniasis with 112 deaths from meat that had been examined and released for trade as free from trichinæ. It illustrates how readily encysted trichinæ may escape detection.

Ransom,[1] of the Bureau of Animal Industry and of the Department of Agriculture, has carried out an extensive investigation on the effect of heat and refrigeration of trichinæ in meat, and has also investigated the efficacy of smoking, salting and other methods of preservation of meat.

The investigations of the various curing processes of meat have apparently not been completed. Inasmuch as smoking and salting would kill the trichinæ in the superficial layers only, it could not be depended upon to penetrate the deeper layers of the ham.

Ransom demonstrated that if a barrel of meat at 0° C. (32° F.) be put in a refrigerator at —15° C. (5° F.), it takes about seven days before the center of the barrel is at the same temperature as that of the refrigerator.

A temperature of —15° C. (5° F.) or below will destroy the trichinæ if exposed to it for about two weeks.

In view of these investigations the federal meat inspection authorities have adopted requirements that all pork that is to be used in the preparation of food products and consumed raw must be kept exposed to a temperature of —15° C. (5°) for at least twenty days or else it must be heated to about 60° C. (140° F.).

In connection with the heating of pork, Ransom has also pointed out the length of time it takes for heat to penetrate large portions of meat. In cooking a 15-pound ham in water at 180° F., it required two and a half hours to raise the temperature of the center of the ham from 78° to 137° F., and it required three and a half hours to raise the temperature of the center of the ham from 46° F. to 137° F.

The extermination of rats and mice near slaughter houses and hog-pens must be insisted upon. Examination of rats from slaughter houses has shown that at least 50 per cent of them are infected with trichinæ. Billings found all the rats from a slaughter house in Boston trichinous. Whether the rat or the hog is the normal host for the trichina has not been established. Staübeli believes that the hog is the normal host for the trichina. There is, however, no doubt but that infected rats help in continuing the infection among hogs. For the same reason hogs should not be fed on slaughter house waste or pork scraps and dead hogs. Rats and mice should be so disposed of that hogs could not come in contact with them.

The proper cooking of pork is the most certain and safest of all precautionary measures. One must remember, however, the length of time it takes for heat to penetrate to the center of a piece of meat. Ransom's observations on this point have been mentioned above. An ordinary sausage requires ten minutes' cooking in water at 71.1° C. (160°F.) to raise the temperature of the center of the sausage from 25.6° C. to 58.3° C. (78° F. to 137° F.) It is very evident, therefore, that pork is frequently insufficiently cooked, and especially when large hams are used one must be very careful that it should be heated sufficiently long for the center of the meat to be likewise affected.

All persons must be educated to the danger of eating raw or insufficiently cooked pork.

It has been pointed out that in the United States most of the local outbreaks of the disease can be traced to a small slaughter house or to a slaughtering of one or more hogs by a family for its own consumption or by a butcher for his own trade. Under such conditions the family or the buyers who partake of the meat get a large dose of trichinous material, while in the large slaughter houses the infected meat is very likely to be mixed with a great deal of meat from other hogs and the person partaking of the pork is not so apt to ingest a large quantity of trichinous material.

Medicinal Treatment. This is still unsatisfactory and is entirely symptomatic. The serum of animals convalescent from trichiniasis has been used with indifferent results. Salzer reported prophylactic and curative effects from such a serum, but Schwartz's investigations did not corroborate these findings. In 2 cases of the series reported in this paper I employed a serum from two individuals in which there was no doubt but what both had recovered from a mild type of the infection. I administered four injections in each case, each of 10 cc intramuscularly, at twenty-four hour intervals. There was no appreciable effect either on the temperature, the eosinophil count or on the duration of the disease.

If the patient is seen soon after eating the suspected meat it may be possible to abort the disease by gastric lavage, by administration of a cathartic and by giving fairly large doses of thymol. Two grains may be given four or five times in the course of the first twenty-four hours and followed by a cathartic.

Thymol has also been employed by intramuscular or subcutaneous injection. Booth reports good results from its employment in 1 case. He dissolved the thymol in sterile olive oil (0.65 gm. (1 gr.) of thymol in 1 cc of oil) and injected 2 to 3 cc subcutaneously or intramuscularly every day for seven days.

Glycerin, on account of its hygroscopic qualities, was recommended by Fielder, a tablespoonful every hour with laxatives. G. Merkel, of Nüremberg, has obtained good results with it.

Arsphenamin and other arsenicals have also been employed, but without any effect. I administered both old and new arsphenamin to 3 cases of trichiniasis, but observed no beneficial effects whatever.

No immunity is conferred by one attack of trichiniasis and no immune substances can be demonstrated in the serum of experimentally infected animals (Schwartz).

Summary. 1. A small outbreak of trichiniasis is reported affecting 35 individuals. Also 9 sporadic cases.

2. A clinical analysis is made of 14 of the more severely ill cases.

3. Blood and other laboratory findings are given with tabulations.

4. High eosinophil blood counts and free, unencysted trichina embryos were found in individuals that have partaken of the trichinous pork and yet have presented no clinical symptoms of the disease.

5. The author wishes to draw attention to the comparative frequency of the disease and to the great necessity of emphasizing the absolute importance of thorough cooking of pork.

BIBLIOGRAPHY.

1. McNerthney, J. B., and McNerthney, W. B.: Trichinosis; Immediate Result Following Intravenous Injection of Neosalvarsan, Jour. Trop. Med., 1916, **19**, 253,

2. Ransom, B H.: Effects of Refrigeration upon the Larvæ of Trichinella Spiralis, Jour. Agric. Research, 1915–16, **5**, 819.

3. Salzer, B. F.: Study of an Epidemic of Fourteen Cases of Trichinosis with Cures by Serum Therapy, Jour. Am. Med. Assn., 1916, **67**, 579.
4. Booth, B. A., et al.: Note on the Treatment of Trichinosis with Thymol, Jour. Am. Med. Assn., 1916, **67**, 2000.
5. Kahn, M.: Thymol Treatment of Trichinosis, New York Med. Jour., 1917, **105**, 1137.
6. Salzer, B. F.: Study of an Epidemic of Trichinosis with Special Reference to Serum Therapy, Med. Record, 1916, **91**, 261.
7. Schwartz, B.: Serum Therapy for Trichinosis, Jour. Am. Med. Assn., 1917, **69**, 884.
8. Hall, M. C., and Wigdor, M.: Experimental Study of Serum Therapy in Trichinosis, Arch. Int. Med., 1918, **24**, 601.

THE BLOOD IN MYXEDEMA*

By Edward S. Emery, Jr., A.B., M.D.
BROOKLINE, MASS.

Although it has been recognized for many years that patients with myxedema may have an altered blood picture, this fact does not seem to be generally known. Doubtless, this may be explained by the lack of constancy in the blood findings, and also the difficulty frequently experienced in making a diagnosis of myxedema from the clinical picture alone. With the introduction of basal metabolism as a clinical test, and the observation that the metabolism is usually lower in myxedema than in any other disease, it is possible to make a much more accurate diagnosis of this condition than formerly. The syndrome of myxedema may be very vague and not infrequently it simulates other diseases, as for instance pernicious anemia. The metabolism likewise may be diminished in the latter disease, as shown by Tompkins, Brittingham and Drinker,[1] though the diminution is not usually as great as observed in myxedema. Inasmuch as the diagnosis of myxedema in each patient at the Peter Bent Brigham Hospital has been confirmed by the determination of the metabolic rate and the diagnosis made thereby as accurately as possible, it seemed worth while to report these cases with their blood findings.

Review of the Literature. In his original paper on myxedema, Gull[2] made no reference to the blood, but Ord,[3] three years later, stated that "the blood examined under the microscope appeared healthy." Four years after this (1881) Charcot[4] while delivering a clinic on myxedema expressed just the opposite view and remarked that those suffering from the disease were "anemic to a high degree," and Horsly,[5] in writing on the function of the thyroid gland, pointed out that marked anemia followed loss of the thyroid gland, and that the anemia included a reduction in the number of red corpuscles.

* From the Medical Clinic of the Peter Bent Brigham Hospital.

In 1888, the London Clinical Society's Report on Myxedema[6] stated that, "Allied with the fall in body temperature are changes in the blood. There is not only anemia due to loss of corpuscles but the relative proportions of these constituents are also altered . . ." However, this statement was based, in part at least, on experiments on cats in which the thyroid had been removed. As these animals later developed tetany the parathyroids were probably extirpated, thus complicating the picture. Nevertheless, 12 cases of myxedema with the blood findings were given at the end of the report, so that there were other grounds for their belief. Enough observations had been made by this time so that those interested in the condition recognized that an anemia was frequently a concomitant finding in myxedema, and in 1892 Putnam[7] wrote, "The point has not attracted as much attention as it deserves that the 'directly' hematopoietic functions of the thyroid, if they are of real importance, ought not to be met by ingestion of the thyroid secretion." From now on numerous cases with data on the blood findings are found recorded in the literature.

There does not appear, however, to be a uniform opinion concerning either the quantitative or the qualitative changes in the blood picture. Some writers[8] have reported normal blood findings; whereas others[9] have reported merely a mild anemia or simply that an anemia exists. Most observers[10]; have reported cases showing red blood counts ranging from 3,000,000 to 4,500,000 cells. Murray[11] in his excellent article on myxedema writes, "Examinations of the blood have shown that the number of red corpuscles may be reduced from between 4,000,000 and 5,000,000 (the average number in health) to between 3,000,000 and 4,000,000." However, lower counts than these occur and McCarrison[12] states that, "The reduction in the red blood corpuscles may amount to 2,000,000 or even to 3,000,000." Pitfield[13] a few years ago reported one case with a red blood count of 2,200,000 cells, and another with a count of 2,030,000 cells. The lowest red blood count found mentioned was in a case reported by LeBreton[14] in which the blood showed 1,750,000 cells per cu. mm.

A reduction of the hemoglobin has been observed which is usually greater in proportion than is the decrease in the number of red cells, so that a color index of less than one frequently obtains.

Falta,[15] Murray,[16] and Ewald[10]; agree that the hemoglobin may be reduced to 60 per cent, or even to 40 per cent of the normal. Howard[17] in discussing the blood in myxedema states that "The hemoglobin is found by most writers to be reduced 10 to 15 per cent below normal," and reports that in 12 cases in his series, "The hemoglobin was normal in 2, between 50 to 75 per cent in 8, and below 50 per cent in 2 cases." In one of Pitfield's[13] cases the hemoglobin was 25 per cent.

Just as the number of red cells appears to vary to a marked degree, their characteristics do not seem to be well defined. In Mendel's[9] case the red blood corpuscles were somewhat smaller than normal; whereas, Kraepelin[8] and LeBreton[14] both found the diameter of the red cells to be increased, the former in spite of a normal count. V. Korczyuski[18] also noticed in one case that the red cells were abnormally large. In most cases, however, there has been reported little or no change in the appearance of the red cells, but this is not surprising in view of the fact that in most reported observations the anemia was of a mild grade. In those cases where the anemia is more severe, evidences of regeneration may be found. Pitfield[13] has found marked stippling of the red cells and other signs of basophilic degeneration. McCarrison[12] remarks that nucleated red blood corpuscles may be found, and Falta[15] goes so far as to say that "In many cases are observed erythroblasts." Minot,[19] who has given the best and the most thorough description of the blood in a case of myxedema states that "The red cells show a definite abnormal variation in size, though they average normal size. Cells slightly larger than normal occur; these are usually round, sometimes a trifle oval in shape, but large macrocytes are not seen. Microcytes are absent. Variation in shape is slight. The red cells stain fairly well, but they appear to be slightly achromic. Polychromatophilia rarely occurs, and the reticulated cells occur in normal numbers. No blasts or other red cell abnormalities are noted. The fragility of the red cells is not definitely abnormal."

All kinds of conditions have been reported as regards the white blood corpuscles. The report of the Committee of the Clinical Society of London[6] was that a "marked leukocytosis occurs." Ewald[10]; remarks, however, that in some cases there is a slight leukocytosis and Murray[16] has stated that "Except for an occasional leukocytosis the white corpuscles are normal in number and appearance." Leichtenstern[8] in a case of myxedema following extirpation of a goiter, found a leukocytosis with increase of lymphocytes. On the contrary, other observers have found a leukopenia of varying degree (Frey,[20]; Bence and Engle,[21] Kocher,[22] Mendel[9]). A third view is that of Howard[17] who believes that the "leukocytes are usually normal in actual numbers as well as relatively." Cabot's[10]; cases also showed the white cells to be normal.

The differential counts show little to go by, although as mentioned above, some observers have found either a relative or absolute lymphocytosis. According to Mendel,[9] Bence and Engle,[21] and Falta[15] the percentage of eosinophiles is said to be increased. On the other hand, Kocher,[22] found the number of eosinophiles to be normal and in Minot's[19] case no polynuclear eosinophiles were seen.

The basophilic cells have been usually reported as normal in number. Mendel[9] found them not to be increased. Kocher[22] found them usually from 0.2 to 0.4 per cent.

The coagulation time is said by Kocher[22] and Kottmans[23] to be decreased, by Bauer[23] to be increased.

As to the cause of the anemia, nothing is known. Horsly,[5] being impressed by the blood picture in cases of myxedema, considered whether the gland might not be a hematopoietic organ. Three years later the Committee of the Clinical Society of London[6] felt that the gland might be "concerned in hematopoiesis and not merely of corpuscles but also of the other elements of the blood." Putnam[24] thought it would be interesting to investigate "whether the cause of the anemia may not persist after the most striking myxedematous conditions have passed away." Nevertheless, little has been done to determine the cause of the anemia; although Esser[25] has found that after the removal of the thyroid in rabbits there was a decrease of myelocytes and an increase of lymphocytic forms in the bone marrow. Minot[19] has pointed out in his case that, "the anemia was apparently dependent upon a decreased formation of blood," and that "this decreased activity of the marrow is entirely consistent with the diminished activity of the other functions of the blood."

Presentation of Data. Fourteen cases of myxedema have been collected from the records of the Peter Bent Brigham Hospital. These represent the cases which through the history and basal metabolic rate* leave no doubt as to the diagnosis. Borderline cases have not been included. Unfortunately, no special studies were done on the blood, the routine examinations only having been made.

Of the 14 cases in the table, 3 had had no red-blood counts done. In the 11 cases in which red-blood counts were done, 3 of them (cases 2, 6, and 7) had essentially a normal number of red cells. Of the 8 cases with an anemia, the red-blood count varied from 4,070,000 to 2,280,000 of which 7 had a count of about 4,000,000 cells.

The hemoglobin was reduced in all the cases, varying from the highest value of 96 per cent to the lowest value of 65 per cent. In 4 cases (3, 5, 12 and 14) the color index was 1 or over. In 6 cases it was less than 1 per cent.

The white count varied from the highest recorded figure of 18,000 cells per cu. mm. to the lowest of 4,850 cells. It averaged about normal although it varied considerably on different days.

Assuming the normal differential count to be as follows:[26]

	Percentage.
Small mononuclears	20 to 25
Large mononuclears	3 to 5
Polymorphonuclear neutrophiles	65 to 75
Polymorphonuclear eosinophiles	2 to 4
Polymorphonuclear basophiles	0 to 0.5

* In obtaining the basal metabolism a 100-liter modified Tissot spirometer was used. After fasting from twelve to fourteen hours, the patient was given a thirty-minute rest period after reaching the laboratory, and the respiratory studies were begun only after the pulse rate had reached a level. Two periods were run in order to obtain a check. Gas analysis was done by Haldane Portable Gas Machines.

TABLE SHOWING CONDITION OF BLOOD IN CASES OF MYXEDEMA.

Case No. and initials.	Med. No.	Date.	Metabolism.	Hemoglobin.	Red-blood count.	Color index.	Remarks.	Smear.								Duration of disease in years.
								W.b.c., per cent.	Neutrophiles, per cent.	Lymphocytes, per cent.	Large mononuclears, per cent.	Eosinophils, per cent.	Mast cells, per cent.	Myelocytes, per cent.	Absolute number of lymphocytes.	
1. H. T.	5849	Jan. 2, 1917	−26	78	4,024,000	0.97	R.b.c. not remarkable	12,000	50	50	0	0	0	0	7400	?
2. G. L. F.	10390	Jan. 28, 1919	−34	94	4,976,000	0.95	Very slight achromia	18,800	67	29	4	0	0	0	5450	2½
		Mar. 2, 1919	−22	80	....	..	R.b.c. not remarkable	7,400	70	30	0	0	0	0	2239	
3. M. J. S.	11260	June 12, 1919	−33	90	....	..	R.b.c. not remarkable	6,600	56	35	4	5	0	0	2310	5
		July 22, 1919	−21	80	3,500,000	1.10	....	4,800								
4. C. T. B.	11541	Aug. 1, 1919	−30	90	....	..	R.b.c. not remarkable	10,000	83	9	6	2	0	0	900	2
5. T. B. F.	12227	Nov. 8, 1919	−34	80	4,070,000	1.00	R.b.c. not remarkable	6,000	60	33	2	3	2	0	1190	7
6. J. F. K.	12805	Jan. 28, 1920	−25	90	5,024,000	0.90	R.b.c. not remarkable	10,200	73	25	1	1	0	0	2521	?
7. K. O.	13295	Apr. 6, 1920	−38	90	4,730,000	0.95	R.b.c not remarkable	7,200	60	15	20	2	3	0	1080	13
8. M. J. B.	4192	Feb. 19, 1916	−49	82	....	..	R.b.c. not remarkable	6,800	61	30	8	1	0	0	2040	2
9. I. C.	11591	Aug. 9, 1919	−34	90	....	..	R.b.c. not remarkable	5,400	65	24	10	1	0	0	1296	5–10
10. D. A. M.	15672	Mar. 19, 1921	−40	70	4,016,000	0.87	R.b.c. not remarkable	6,400	62	35	3	0	0	0	2240	6
		Apr. 4, 1921	+ 1	75	4,280,000	0.88	....	7,100								
		July 6, 1921	−11	115	6,704,000	0.85	R.b c. not remarkable	7,450	58	36	2	2	2	0	2682	
		Sept. 6, 1921	−20	98	5,472,000	0.90	R.b c. not remarkable	9,400	67	21	12	0	0	0	1974	
11. J. F. B.	16697	Aug. 25, 1921	−32	68	4,144,000	0.82	Md. achromia variation in size; slight poikilocytosis	9,900	59	29	9	3	0	0	2871	1
		Sept. 16, 1921	− 4	79	4,480,000	0.88	Slight achromia and slight variation in shape	9,200	64	22	14	0	0	0	2024	
12. S. H. V.	15108	Dec. 31, 1920	−38	65	2,280,000	1.40	R.b.c. not [illegible]able	7,900	65	32	1	1	1	0	2528	.
		Jan. 6, 1921	..	70	2,720,000	1.20	....	4,850	62	36	2	0	0	0	1746	
		Mar. 8, 1921	−16	80	3,004,000	1.20	R.b.c. not remarkable	5,800								
		Oct. 12, 1921	− 5	104	5,644,000	0.93	R.b.c. not remarkable	9,800	71	17	12	0	0	0	1660	
13. T. M.	16907	Oct. 5, 1921	−33	85	4,016,000	1.00	R.b.c. not remarkable	8,650	36	53	5	6	0	0	4594	4
14. H. T. B.	17359	Dec. 12, 1921	−35	80	3,950,000	1.00	Slight anisocytosis and poikilocytosis	5,600	76	20	4	0	0	0	1120	4
		Dec. 19, 1921	−21	83	3,000,000	1.30	Slight anisocytosis	5,600	64	36	0	0	0	0	2016	

1. Hemoglobin was estimated by the Tallquist method in the first 9 cases, by the Sahli method in the last 5 cases.
2. The duration of the disease was judged as well as could be from the history of the symptoms.

it is found that the polymorphonuclear neutrophilic cells fall slightly below the normal values in 9 cases.

The lymphocytes were normal in number in 4 cases (6, 9, 14 and 15) and decreased in 2 cases (4 and 7). Eight cases showed both a relative and absolute increase in the small lymphocytes.

The eosinophiles and basophiles seemed to be about normal.

In 11 of the cases the red blood cells were reported as normal. There was slight achromia in the remaining cases, in 2 of which slight anisocytosis and slight poikilocytosis were also reported.

A study of the table reveals no relationship between the degree of anemia and the metabolic rate. Likewise there appears to be no relationship between the degree of anemia and the duration of the disease. However, it is difficult to place the onset of the disease, as the symptoms begin so mildly.

Following treatment the anemia tended to disappear as is well shown in Case 12 which has been studied more completely than the others.

Conclusions. 1. The blood picture associated with myxedema is not constant and there are no changes which can be cited as typical of the disease. Usually, however, there is a moderate secondary anemia.

2. The hemoglobin is usually reduced.

3. The white blood corpuscles average about normal but tend to vary with the red-blood count.

4. The differential count usually shows the polymorphonuclear neutrophiles to be somewhat decreased in numbers. The lymphocytes may show a relative or absolute increase.

5. There is no relationship between the degree of the anemia and the duration of the disease or the metabolic rate.*

* I wish to express my appreciation to Dr. Cyrus C. Sturgis for his many helpful suggestions and aid in preparing this paper.

BIBLIOGRAPHY.

1. Tompkins, E. H., Brittingham, H. H., and Drinker, C. K.: Arch. Int. Med., 1919, **23**, 441.
2. Gull, W.: Tr. Clin. Soc. London, 1874, **7**, 181.
3. Ord: Med. Chir. Tr, 1877, **61**, 60.
4. Charcot: Gaz. des hôp., 1881, **10**, 74.
5. Horsly, V.: British Med. Jour, 1885, **1**, 111.
6. Tr. Clin. Soc. London, Suppl., 1888, **21**, 70.
7. Putnam, J. J.: Tr. Assn. Am. Phys, 1893, **8**. 333.
8. Kraepelin, E: Deutsch. Arch. f. klin. Med., vol, **49**, 587. Leichtenstern O.: Deutsch. med. Wchnschr., 1893, **49**, 50. Manassa, W: Berl. klin. Wchnschr., 1888, **29**, 595.
9. White, W. H.: Lancet, 1913, **1**, 154. Mendel, E.: Deutsch. med. Wchnschr., 1893, **19**, 25. Bramwell. B.: Edinburgh Med. Jour., 1892–1893, **38**, 895. Gimlette, J. D.: Myxedema and the Thyroid Gland, London, 1st ed., J. C. A. Churchill, 1895, p. 49. Reverdin: Rev. méd. de la Suisse Rom, 1882, **2**, 539.
10. Ewald: Nothnagels Specielle Pathologie und Therapie, 1896, **6**, 247. Hun, H., and Prudden: Am. Jour. Med. Sci., 1888, **96**, 1. Thompson. Tr. Assn. Am. Phys, 1893, **8**, 373. Bramwell, B.: Clinical Studies of Edinburgh, 1907–1908, **6**, 33. Cabot, R.: Clinical Examination of the Blood, New York, 5th ed., Wm. Wood & Co., p. 394.

11. Murray, G. R.: Twentieth Century Practice, 1895, **4**, 691.
12. McCarrison, R.: The Thyroid Gland, New York, 1917, Wm. Wood & Co.
13. Pitfield, R. L.: AM. JOUR. MED. SCI., 1916, **151**, 409.
14. LeBreton. Ref. in Wien. med. Bl., 1895, p. 49.
15. Falta, R.: The Ductless Glandular Disease, Philadelphia, P. Blakiston's Son Company; translated and edited by M. K. Myers, p. 112.
16. Murray, G. R.: Allbutt and Rolleston System of Medicine, vol, **4**, 345.
17. Howard, C. P.: Jour. Am. Med. Assn., 1907, **48**, 1226.
18. v. Korczynski: Wien. med. Presse, vol. **36**, 37.
19. Minot, G. R.: Med. Clin. North America, 1921, **4**, 1733.
20. Frey, H.: Mitt. a. d. Grenzgeb. d. Med. u. Chir., 1915, **28**.
21. Bence and Engle: Wien. klin. Wchnschr., 1908, **21**, 905.
22. Kocher, T.: Arch. f. klin. Chir., 1912, **99**, 280.
23. Ref. from McCarrison: The Thyroid Gland, 1917, New York, Wm. Wood & Company.
24. Tr. Assn. Am. Phys., 1893, **8**, 373 (discussions of Thompson's paper).
25. Esser: Deutsch. Arch. f. klin. Med., 1907, **89**, 576.
26. Webster: Diagnostic Methods, 5th ed., Philadelphia, P. Blakiston's Son Company.

CANCER OF THE COLON.*

BY RAYMOND P. SULLIVAN, M.D.,

NEW YORK.

THE management of cases of cancer of the colon has been a serious problem for generations. In 1716 Pillore of Rouen made use of an artificial anus in the treatment of cancer of the rectosigmoid; Fine of Geneva, in 1797, followed his example. The first successful resection of the pelvic colon for cancer causing obstruction was performed by Reybard, in 1833. Ten years later this operation caused a storm of controversy in the Paris Academy of Medicine, and was rejected by the leading surgeons of the day as too dangerous. Although this operation marks the first step in surgery of the pelvic colon, no less than forty-two years elapsed before the record case was reported by Thiersch who, in 1875, resected the pelvic colon for cancer and the patient died. About the same time, in 1879, Gussenbauer successfully removed the iliac flexure of the colon, in a man of forty-six years, and operated with good results in other cases. Radical treatment for cancer of the colon was soon attempted by a number of surgeons, notably Péan, Guyon, and Nélaton, but the alarming mortality discouraged further attempts along this line of intervention, and colostomy remained the procedure of choice in these cases. It was about 1880 before resection became a recognized procedure in surgery of the large intestine.

The technic of colectomy was modified by Volkmann in 1883 by the application of permanent colostomy. Nine years later, Bloch of Denmark described his procedure of resection for cancer in three stages. His work became better known through the contributions

* Read before the Association of Resident and Ex-Resident Physicians of the Mayo Clinic, Rochester, Minn., May 29, 1922.

of Mikulicz. Results improved at once, but these two methods were not considered the last word in surgery of the colon and, about this time, numerous suggestions were made concerning a better technic of resection and intestinal suture, until enteroanastomosis finally constituted decided progress in the management of cancer of the colon.

The first total extirpation of the rectum for cancer was performed by Lisfranc, in 1826, who utilized the perineal route. Because of grave septic complications, this procedure was soon abandoned in favor of palliative measures such as formation of an artificial anus or rectotomy. However, the value of Lisfranc's procedure was gradually recognized: the operative technic was modified by Denonvilliers, who added to it a posterior longitudinal incision. From 1864 to 1884, several successful resections were reported by French and German surgeons with variable results. However, opinions were widely divided: in England the method of choice was lumbar colostomy. About this time, Kraske recommended the sacral route, a method which extended the surgical indications and under otherwise favorable conditions permitted more or less restoration of function. The results of this method, however, did not entirely meet expectations; some years later, they were investigated by Koenig, and a mortality of 38 per cent, with many recurrences, was shown. In spite of improved technic, Kraske's operation still remains a serious procedure. Excision of the cancerous segment has since become the operation of choice, the surgeon having at his disposal a variety of routes, according to the requirements in a given case, namely the perineal, the perineococcygeal, the sacral, or the abdominoperineal.

From the statistical point of view, it is usually estimated that the relative frequency of gastro-intestinal cancer is equivalent to 50 per cent of cancer in general, while about 16 per cent of the cancers of the digestive tract occur primarily in either the rectum or the sigmoid flexure of the colon. The various segments of the colon are involved as follows: Ascending colon in 11.6 per cent, hepatic flexure in 6.4, transverse colon in 10.2, splenic flexure in 4.9, descending colon in 7.1, and sigmoid flexure, in 27.3. The prognosis is largely governed by the location of the cancer; it is especially unfavorable in cancer of the sigmoid and splenic flexure. A recent report from Hochenegg's Clinic, comprising 779 cases in the last fourteen years, shows that cancer of the rectum represented about 16 per cent of all cases of cancer in the hospital. 44.8 per cent of these cancers were in the ampulla and 25.9 per cent were at a distance of 10 cm. from the sphincter. According to older literature, Boas found, among 500 cases of cancer of the digestive organs, 53 of cancer of the rectum.

Etiology. Local irritation undoubtedly plays an important part in the etiology of cancer in general and of cancer of the colon in particular. The colon is constantly exposed to contamination from stagnating intestinal contents, which may, on good grounds, be suspected of harboring the living cause of cancer. Ochsner has called attention to the alarming frequency of cancer of the stomach in what he picturesquely describes as "manure eating people," meaning the consumers of raw vegetables grown in soil fertilized with barnyard manure and so forth. The question arises if the popular demand for uncooked green vegetables and salads, a by-product of the vitamin controversy, is in part responsible for the increased cancer mortality of the last few years. The increase in occurrence of cancer from the cecum to the rectum, and the predominance of cancer in the anorectal region, is readily accounted for by the common presence of local irritative factors. Heredity as an etiological or rather as a predisposing factor has been considered as an important element, but this view has been discredited. Apparently it played no part in any of the cases of cancer of the colon and rectum in the series of 10 cases herein reported.

Location. Since May, 1919, 10 cases of cancer of the colon have come under my observation. The cancer was in the cecum in 1 case, in the transverse colon in 1, in the splenic flexure in 1, and in the descending colon in 1: in the sigmoid flexure in 2 cases, and in the rectum in 4 (2 growths were in the true anus and 2 were in the lower pelvic colon).

Report of Cases. Case I (St. Vincent's 4489–20). A woman, aged forty-eight years, suffering from cancer of the cecum, complained of indefinite symptoms of biliary and cecal colic.

At the operation, it was found necessary to remove the cecal coil on account of cancerous obstruction of the ileocecal valve. The infected gall-bladder, which contained stones and whose fundus appeared cancerous, was also removed. This was later shown to be cancer. Death resulted four days later from cardiovascular collapse concomitant with acute gastric dilatation.

Case II (St. Vincent's 887–21). A woman, aged sixty-five years, with cancer of the transverse colon had symptoms of incomplete intestinal obstruction, and was kept under observation four days after the acute obstruction had been relieved by enemas.

In this case, the roentgen-ray findings were quite indefinite. The physical signs were variable distension of the right colon, definite borborygmus, and persistent recurrent attacks of intestinal colic. There was no palpable tumor. Under the diagnosis of chronic intestinal obstruction, the patient was operated on, March 16, 1921, and a cancer of the transverse colon found. This was resected and an end-to-end anastomosis made. The patient recovered uneventfully and is now in good health.

Case III (St. Vincent's 3372–20). A man, aged thirty years, with cancer of the splenic flexure, had been operated on twice within two years before I saw him, once for appendicitis and once for adhesions around the cecum. He complained that the symptoms he had had prior to the operation for adhesions persisted, but with predominance of pain in the region of the splenic flexure and left kidney.

The simulation of renal pain necessitated urological examination, in order to exclude renal disease. The findings demonstrated the kidney to be normal, while roentgenograms of the colon were indefinite with regard to obstruction. However, in view of a palpable mass, the persistent colicky pains at the splenic flexure, and the clinical dilatation of the transverse colon and cecum, a diagnosis was made of chronic intestinal obstruction at the splenic flexure.

Operation was performed April 8, 1920, through the left upper abdominal route, and consisted in resection of the splenic flexure, which contained carcinoma. Much difficulty was experienced owing to ankylosis of the splenic flexure by excessive adhesions. A side-to-side anastomosis was made after mobilization of the descending colon with satisfactory results. The patient recovered uneventfully, has gained 30 pounds in weight, is free from all signs of recurrence, and is able to continue his work as my chauffeur.

Case IV (St. Vincent's 4056–21). A woman, aged thirty-five years, with cancer of the descending colon came under my observation complaining of colicky pain in the lower left quadrant of three weeks' duration. She had had intermittent diarrhea, and had lost weight for the last five months. Roentgenograms revealed a defect in the descending colon just above the crest of the ileum suggestive of malignancy.

At operation, November 2, 1921, a carcinoma of the descending colon was found and resected, followed by suture anastomosis. Although an advocate of a two-stage operation, I performed a resection on this patient, because of the short history of obstruction, and because, during mobilization, a small perforation was discovered on the lateral wall close to the mesentery. Usually, however, when there is a history of more or less complete and prolonged obstruction, I prefer the two-stage operation. This patient is alive and well.

Case V (St. Vincent's 2074–19). A man, aged seventy-three years, with an acute perforation through a cancer of the sigmoid was seen in emergency. He had had attacks of intestinal colic and diarrhea for eighteen months. A tumor was palpated in the lower left quadrant.

Operation, May 21, 1919, revealed a large cancer of the sigmoid with perforation on the outer wall. This was mobilized and brought out on the abdomen as a colostomy. Ileostomy was also immediately performed. Death occurred on the fifth day from general peritonitis.

CASE VI (St. Vincent's 426–22). A woman, aged seventy-six years, had an obstructing cancer of the sigmoid flexure. She had had symptoms of intermittent obstruction and progressive starvation for two years, and had been under medical treatment for colitis for eighteen months.

No attempt was made to remove the tumor. Colostomy was performed to relieve the symptoms. Death occurred in six days from starvation, and cardiac collapse.

CASE VII (St. Vincent's 2230–20). A man, aged forty-six years, who had been treated elsewhere for hemorrhoids for one year was referred to me because of a growth in the anus, which proved to be cancerous.

Exploration revealed a metastatic nodule in the right lobe of the liver, and radical removal of the growth in the anus was not attempted. A permanent colostomy was performed.

The patient survived the operation one and a half years with a fair degree of comfort, and died from general carcinomatosis.

CASE VIII (St. Vincent's 3671–20). A woman, aged thirty-nine years, came for consultation on account of diarrhea, anal pain, and tenesmus, of six months' duration. Inspection revealed a small ulcerating growth at the margin of the anus, infiltrating the sphincter muscles and narrowing the lumen of the gut, so as to prevent digital examination. The abdomen was greatly distended, and the patient vomited repeatedly. A slight amount of flatus was finally obtained through the anus by means of a small rectal tube, which considerably relieved the distention.

On the third day, exploratory, laparotomy and permanent colostomy were performed as a first stage. Because of the marginal location, and apparent spreading of the carcinoma into muscles, the patient was subsequently referred to the General Memorial Hospital for intensive radium treatment. She was last seen six weeks ago at which time the colostomy was working well and she was quite comfortable. However, further infiltration of the carcinoma into the perianal region had occurred. Because of the absence of pain, the patient is anticipating ultimate recovery.

CASE IX (St. Vincent's 1224–21). A woman, aged sixty-three years, was referred to me because of chronic intestinal obstruction, rapid loss in weight, and a foul discharge from the anus for one year. A palpable mass could be felt on vaginal examination, and a diagnosis of cancer of the true rectum was made.

Abdominal exploration and a permanent colostomy were performed as a first stage. The growth was mobilized in anticipation of removal later. The patient died on the sixth day from peritonitis.

Case X (St. Vincent's 4981–21). A woman, aged fifty-eight years, was brought to the hospital on account of intestinal obstruction and starvation. A mass in the iliac region extending into the pelvis was palpated. A colostomy was made, and the patient died two weeks later. Extensive metastasis was discovered at necropsy.

Discussion. In reviewing these cases with special reference to diagnosis, it is noteworthy that 1 of the 10 patients had been operated on under the diagnosis of appendicitis. The experience is by no means uncommon, and irritation from obstruction in the colon may actually lead to infection and inflammation of the appendix, as recently pointed out by Beall, whose patient clinically had appendicitis, probably induced by the back pressure of the fluids in a chronically obstructed cancerous colon. The excised appendix was swollen, congested, and contained an excess of fluid in its lumen.

My observations also confirm the well known fact that malignant tumors of the large intestine have a tendency to remain latent for a long time, the function of the bowel apparently remaining undisturbed by the existence of a growth in one of its segments until obstruction actually supervenes. This period of latency may be very protracted; Mikulicz estimated it as lasting from six months to three years and claimed that cancer of the colon first manifests itself clinically by its complications in the form of stenosis, ulceration, and hemorrhage. Occlusion is likely to supervene abruptly, without prodromes, often without progressive aggravation of symptoms. Cancers of the sigmoid flexure and cancers in the rectum sometimes cause sudden obstruction through enterospasm, edema, or invagination, usually preceded by obstinate constipation. In many instances, during the stage of incomplete obstruction, endoscopic examination, may reveal the obstacle to be a slightly protuberant, more or less infiltrating carcinoma. The entire colon can be readily filled with the barium enema, unless the enema is prevented from passing beyond a given obstacle and in this event the seat of obstruction will reveal the focus of the disease.

Roentgenograms are usually the best means for determining the exact location of a cancer of the colon. But in early cases the diagnosis must be made exclusively on the basis of functional disturbances, such as flatulence with colicky pains, diarrhea alternating with constipation, local tenderness, and increased discharge of more or less offensive mucus. The passage of blood is noted earlier in the disease in proportion to the propinquity of the cancer to the anus, on account of injury of the growth during defecation. It is noteworthy that certain cases of cancer of the colon present a more or less distinct picture of renal colic; this was typical of my cases, and indicates the diagnostic advantages to be derived in obscure cases of this description from a carefully conducted urological examination.

Nearly all the segments of the colon are accessible to systemic palpation so that the tumor, its shape, size, and mobility may be often ascertained in favorable cases. Two important sources of error are certain renal tumors, and intermittent segmentary contractions of the bowel, which apparently increase the circumference of the cancer. Bimanual palpation is especially valuable in cancers of the pelvic colon. Percussion and auscultation are serviceable for the detection of local tympanities or incipient dilatation of the cecum, a valuable early sign of stricture lower in the gut. Digital exploration of the rectum, and rectocolonic endoscopy, are among the most useful measures at our command, permitting biopsy and catheterization of the colon in suitable cases. The recognition of cancers of the rectum is based on inspection of the anus, proctoscopy and sigmoidoscopy, vaginal examinations in women, and sometimes cystoscopy.

General Characteristics of Cancer of the Colon. Cancer of the ascending colon and hepatic flexure may be movable or adherent, elongated, or round and nodular, and may develop insidiously or fairly rapidly. Small cancers of the hepatic flexure are usually not palpable; larger growths are likely to extend backward and are more easily discovered. These growths must be distinguished from renal tumors and retroperitoneal neoplasms in general, as well as from tumors of the liver and gall-bladder. Cancers of the transverse colon are more superficially situated, more accessible to palpation, and often more freely movable than the foregoing. Such growths may be found in the vicinity of the stomach or low down toward the pelvis, so that confusion may occur. The splenic flexure and adjacent descending colon are fairly common and well concealed seats of cancer of the colon. The intestinal coil here lies at a greater distance from the anterior surface of the abdomen than any other segment of the colon, and the majority of these cancers remain small, while the other manifestations are not always well marked. The growths become palpable only after they have reached a certain size, or if the splenic flexure occupies an abnormally low position. Under these conditions the findings may suggest tumor of the spleen, kidney, or omentum. According to Madelung, such cancers, because of their anatomical relations, are especially likely to cause intestinal obstruction. With cancers of the sigmoid flexure, the most common in order of frequency, stenosis very often promptly manifests itself by colics, obstipation, and sometimes tenesmus. Large or medium-sized tumors often lie as fairly movable masses in the lower abdomen and may extend as far as the umbilicus, while small hard growths cannot be palpated as a rule. Rectal prolapse is not infrequently noted in the presence of small cancers of the sigmoid flexure, further invagination being prevented by the increasing dimensions of the cancer.

A suspicion of cancer of the colon usually leads to its detection. In the interest of the patient, it is urgently desirable to handle all doubtful conditions as possible malignancies, unless a more harmless cause of the existing disturbances has been positively ascertained. The results of timely operative procedures for cancer of the colon are superior to results of treatment of cancer of any other organ, with the possible exception of cancer of the body of the uterus. Lymphatic involvement is fortunately long delayed, and more or less marked clinical manifestations appear in most cases long before the tumor has become inoperable. The inefficiency of radiation as compared to surgery in the treatment of malignancy of the colon and rectum is illustrated by recent observations in the Vienna Clinic, where roentgen-ray and radium treatment yielded no benefit; in all but 1 of the 28 cases in which it was utilized it seemed to be injurious rather than helpful in its effect on the disease.

According to recent findings of Schoemaker, the operative mortality of cancer of the colon in a large clinic amounted to 6 of 46 cases (13 per cent); 4 of these operations included resection of the colon. Of 30 patients operated on in Utrecht 6 died (20 per cent). In Schoemaker's personal experience, 2 of the 32 patients (6 per cent) died as a result of the operation. The localization of the growth concerned the first segment of the ascending colon, or the terminal segment of the descending colon. Numerous patients were operated on in a stage of acute ileus, others in chronic ileus. The youngest patient was aged forty-four years and the oldest was eighty-four.

Treatment. For a long time, the treatment of cancer of the colon remained palliative, in the form of an artificial anus, for the relief of obstruction, the most common complication of these cases. The remarkable advance of abdominal surgery in general, and the improved technic of intestinal operations in particular, led to resection, in one stage, of the tumor as well as of the affected glands; but the imperfect results soon showed the necessity of two-stage or three-stage operations, which were almost exclusively utilized until a further, and almost phenomenal development of operative technic permitted the resumption of radical treatment in one stage. However, although less brilliant for the surgeon and involving the inconvenience of a temporary artificial anus for the patient, two- or three-stage operations are undoubtedly safer and for this reason preferable in the great majority of cases.

Colectomy in one stage aims at extensive resection of the tumor-bearing segment and its mesentery which, after liberation from adhesions and mobilization of the colonic segment, are removed like a sac with the septic contents. The resection is immediately followed by an end-to-end or side-to-side anastomosis. One-stage colectomy, according to Boyer, is the operation of choice on the right side, whereas two-stage or three-stage operations are indicated on the left segment of the colon. The one-stage colectomy is definitely contraindicated in all cases complicated by intestinal obstruction.

The greatest cause of failure, after primary or secondary one-stage colectomy, is peritonitis. This is due: (1) to the extreme sepsis of the intestinal contents, (2) to the exposure to infection of the raw surfaces created by the detachment of the colonic wall, (3) to some extent, to the technical difficulty of suture application, as well as to the endangerment of the sutures by the passage of hard scybala, and (4) to the peculiarities of the local blood supply.

The adherents of one-stage colectomy consider the cancer to be operable during the entire period of latency, which may extend for from several months to three years, before clinical manifestations occur. The surgical indications for radical interference are therefore governed by a careful anatomical and clinical study of the syndrome. One-stage colectomy often becomes the treatment of choice during the period of tolerance, so that the essential point really is the determination of the most suitable time for the operation. But the clinical findings, as a rule, furnish only more or less indefinite operative indications during the entire period of latency, and an incipient cancer can be revealed only through exploratory laparotomy. This should be performed before the onset of intestinal obstruction, as soon as the patient seeks advice for obstinate constipation, which is accompanied by loss of weight and abdominal pain, alternating with attacks of diarrhea. The greater number of patients come under observation with long standing cancer and stricture, and when first seen are in a state of chronic obstruction or occlusion. In these circumstances two-stage colectomy is distinctly and necessarily indicated. One-stage colectomy, while undoubtedly the ideal procedure, depends for its justification on a timely diagnosis, the essential condition for a safe, rational and radical operation for malignant conditions of the colon.

Technic of Operation. Cancer of the pelvic colon may be treated by several operative procedures; namely, resection of the tumor, reëstablishment of the passage, and suture of the abdominal wall in one stage; resection of the cancerous segment with suture of the afferent and efferent ends into the abdominal wound in another stage, followed later by closure of the resulting artificial anus; or exposure of the affected gut in one stage, resection in the second stage, and closure of the artificial anus in the third stage. According to Schwartz, in Paris, the latter method in three stages is the procedure of choice. The only indication for operation in one stage is an excellent condition of the intestine, which guarantees good anastomosis, but this condition is very uncommon. In all cases in which the gut can be mobilized, it should be exposed; only when this is not practicable, may resection be performed at once, with, or sometimes without, fixation of the two ends in the wound. In order that healthy tissue may be operated on at the second stage, it is of course necessary to mobilize and extensively displace not only the tumor, but also the mesocolon, so as to prevent the tumor from being drawn back into the abdominal cavity by the intestinal mass.

From the operative viewpoint, the sigmoid flexure of the colon presents a segment of bowel extremely well adapted to resection. Being a long organ with a well developed mesentery, which can be drawn out of the abdominal cavity, it offers all the conditions required for surgical interference under favorable prospects. The essential point is the timely recognition of the cancer in this region, before the occurrence of obstruction, adhesions, and glandular involvement. The extirpation of the cancer in one stage is entirely feasible, and under these conditions has a fairly low operative mortality.

The principles which may be considered in the basic technic of the one-stage removal of these cancers are: (1) adequate abdominal incisions, (2) proper mobilization of the diseased segment to insure a serviceable anastomosis without tension, (3) preservation of adequate blood supply to the distal segment, and (4) formation of an efficient end-to-end or lateral anastomosis. However, since experience shows that these cases seldom come to operation early, the two-stage or three-stage operation is the one of choice.

Mortality. Cancers of the terminal sigmoid, as pointed out by W. J. Mayo, cannot be separated surgically from cancers of the upper rectum, on account of the marked tendency for cancer of the sigmoid to invade the rectum, and *vice versa.* In the Mayo Clinic from January 1, 1893 to December 31, 1915, the histories of 753 patients suffering from cancer of the rectum and rectosigmoid were recorded, and 430 of the patients were subjected to radical operation. The operability of the cancers, at the time when the patient was first seen, amounted to 53.1 per cent in the earlier cases, as compared to an operability of less than 25 per cent in the experience of Harrison Cripps (1913) and was subsequently increased in the Mayo Clinic to 71.8 per cent owing to the routine performance of a radical operation in extensive cancers, provided extirpation was not prohibited by the involvement of vital structures. Next to this cause of inoperability, ranked (1) metastasis of the liver, (2) peritoneal retroperitoneal metastasis, and (3) glandular metastasis. According to more recent data, the mortality of the radical operation in the Mayo Clinic averages about 10 per cent. The important causes of operative mortality, as stated by Mayo, who points out that a low mortality is coincident with a low operability, are in order of frequency, sepsis, nephritis, undiscovered metastatic tumors, hemorrhage, postoperative intestinal obstruction and exhaustion.

BIBLIOGRAPHY.

1. Anderson, H. G.: The Three-stage Abdomino-peritoneal Excision of the Rectum for Cancer, Proc. Roy. Soc. Med., (Surg. Sect.) 1921, **14**, 162.

2. Beall, F. C.: Diagnosis of Cancer of the Colon, Texas State Jour. Med., 1921, **17**, 343.

3. Bevan, A. D.: Surgery of Cancer of the Large Intestine, Jour. Am. Med. Assn., 1920, **75**, 283.

4. Bloch, O.: On Extra-abdominal Behandling of Cancer Intestinalis, Nord. med. Ark., 1892, p. 1.

5. Boas, I.: Beiträge zur Kenntniss der Rectumkarzinome nebst Bemerkungen zur Fruhdiagnose, Arch. f. Verdauungskr., 1905, **11**, 574.

6. Boyer, G.: Contribution à l'étude du traitement radical du cancer du colon, Thèse Paris, 1919.

7. Cripps, H.: On Diseases of the Rectum and Anus, Including the Sixth Edition of the Jacksonian Prize Essay on Cancer, London, Churchill, 1913.

8. Denovilliers: Cancer scirrheux du rectum, Bull et mém. Soc. anat. de Paris, 1842, **17**, 15.

9. Fine, P.: Ann. Soc. de méd. de Montpel., 1804, vol. **4**.

10. Gussenbauer, C.: Ein Fall von partieller Resection des Colon descendens zum Zwecke einer Geschwulstexstirpation, Arch. f. klin. Chir., 1878, **23**, 233.

11. Guyon: Epithelioma cylindrique de l'S iliaque—Resection d'une portion de l' S iliaque, De l'intervention chirurgicale dans l'obstruction intestinale, Paris, 1880, p. 184 (quoted by Peyrot, J. J.).

12. Hochenegg, J.: Die sacrale Methode der Exstirpation von Mastdarmkrebsen nach Prof. Kraske, Wien. klin. Wchnschr., 1888, **1**, 254, 272, 290, 309, 324, 348.

13. Koenig: Die Operationen am Darme bei Geschwülsten, mit besonderer Berücksichtigung der Darmresection, Arch. f. klin. Chir., 1890, **40**, 905.

14. Kraske, P.: Zur Exstirpation hochsitzender Mastdarmkrebse, Verhandl. d. deutsch. Gesellsch. f. Chir., 1885, **14**, **464**; also Arch. f. klin. Chir., 1886, **33**, 563.

15. Lisfranc: Tumeur cancéreux du rectum; guérison par l'extirpation, Gaz. d. hôp., 1835, **9**, 621.

16. Madelung: Eine Modification der Colotomie wegen Carcinoma recti, Verhandl. d. deutsch. Gesellsch. f. Chir., 1884, **13**, 118.

17. Mandl, F.: Ueber den Mastdarmkrebs (from Hochenegg's Clinic), Wien. klin. Wchnschr., 1922, **35**, 31.

18. Mayo, C. H.: Resection of the Rectum for Cancer with Preservation of the Sphincter, Surg., Gynec. and Obst., 1914, **18**, 401.

19. Mayo, W. J.: The Radical Operation for Cancer of the Rectum and Rectosigmoid, Ann. Surg., **64**, 304.

20. Mikulicz, J.: Chirurgische Erfahrungen über das Darmkarzinom, Arch. f. klin. Chir., 1903, **69**, 28.

21. Nélaton, A.: Elémens de pathologie chirurgicale, Paris, Germor-Baillière, 1857, vol. **3**.

22. Ochsner, A. J.: Cancer Infection, Tr. South. Surg. Assn., 1920, **33**, 123.

23. Okinczyc, J.: Contribution à l'étude du traitement chirurgical du cancer du colon (Travaux de chirurgie anatomo-clinique), Chirurgie de l'intestin, Hartman, H., Paris, Steinheil, 1907.

24. Pauchet, V.: Signes et traitement du cancer du rectum, Presse méd., 1920, **28**, 705.

25. Pauchet, V.: Diagnostic du cancer du rectum, Jour. de méd. de Paris, 1921, **40**, 29.

26. Pean, J. E.: Diagnostic et traitement des tumeurs de l'abdomen et du bassin, Paris, Masson, 1895.

27. Pillore (Quoted by Amussat, J. Z.): Mémoire sur la possibilité d'établir un anus artificiel dans la région lombaire sans pénétrer dans le péritoine, Paris, Baillière, 1839, p. 84.

28. Reybard: Mémoire sur une tumeur cancéreuse affectant l'S iliaque du colon, Bull. Acad. de méd. de Paris, 1843, **9**, 1031; also Bull. et mém. Soc. chir. de Paris, 1880, **6**, 635.

29. Schoemaker, J.: [Mortality from Operations for Cancer of the Large Intestine.] Nederl. Tijdschr. v. Geneesk., 1920, **1**, 2328.

30. Schwartz, A.: Traitement chirurgical du cancer du colon, Paris méd., 1921, **11**, 272.

31. Thiersch: Ueber einen Fall von Dickdarm Resektion, Verhandl. d. deutsch. Gesellsch. f. Chir., 1878, **7**, 127.

32. Volkmann, R.: Zur Kenntniss des Darmkrebses, Centralbl. f. Chir., 1883, **10**, 153.

REVIEWS.

MANUAL OF GYNECOLOGY. By JOHN OSBORN POLAK, Professor of Obstetrics and Gynecology, Long Island College Hospital, New York. Second edition. Pp. 396; 139 engravings; 10 colored plates. Philadelphia and New York: Lea & Febiger, 1922.

IN revising this manual the author has rewritten entirely some of the chapters and has added many new illustrations from specimens in his collection. It describes the lesions of the female generative organs, omitting irrelevant subjects, and stresses pathology in ample manner, with the result that a remarkably large amount of information is condensed in a small volume, though rhetoric has been sacrificed ruthlessly at times. The book's essential characteristic is the expression of the opinion of a progressive leader in the profession on debatable points, and the presentation of his treatment of gynecologic diseases with a properly detailed description of his technic in the common operations. L.

A MANUAL OF DISEASES OF THE NOSE AND THROAT. By CORNELIUS G. COAKLEY, A.M., M.D., F.A.C.S., Professor of Laryngology and Otology in the College of Physicians and Surgeons, Columbia University, etc. Sixth edition, revised and enlarged. Pp. 635; illustrated with 145 engravings and 7 colored plates. Philadelphia and New York: Lea & Febiger, 1922.

THAT this manual of diseases of the nose and throat by Prof. Coakley has now come to its sixth edition, is evidence of the favorable consideration which it has received at the hands of the medical profession. Prof. Coakley is himself preëminently a clinician and skilful surgeon and it is the clinical and surgical aspect of this book that makes it of distinct value to the laryngologist. The chapters on sinus disease give a very admirable portrayal of the methods of diagnosis and treatment. He is conservative, yet at the same time radical in his suggestions, when radicalism is indicated. In fact, throughout the book where operative procedures are considered, the subject is exceedingly well handled. On the other hand, the anatomical considerations are too brief to be of any especial value, and the treatment of pathology is not as reliable and up to date as we would like. The book, however, would make a valuable addition to the laryngologist's library. W.

Selected Works of Thomas Sydenham, M.D. By John D. Comrie, M.D., F.R.C.P., Edin., Lecturer on History of Medicine and on Clinical Medicine in the University of Edinburgh. Pp. 153; 4 illustrations. New York: William Wood & Co., 1922.

In this small and relatively inexpensive book are combined a brief life of "the prince of English physicians" and extracts from his published works. The selections have been very intelligently chosen and one finds at least a part of each of those which have made the name of Sydenham familiar to all. Among those included are the well-known observations on St. Vitus's dance, gout and on the use of Peruvian bark. No history of medicine nor biography can be a satisfactory substitute for familiarity with a great man's original writings. Unfortunately such works are seldom available in convenient form. Publications such as the present one should be encouraged and should be of interest to both students and practitioners. P.

Ophthalmoscopy, Retinoscopy and Refraction. By W. A. Fisher. Pp. 218; 248 illustrations. Chicago: W. A. Fisher, 1922.

This book is written for the general practitioner, to give him a working knowledge of ophthamoscopy, retinoscopy and refraction. Some exception might be taken to a statement in the introduction that ophthamoscopy and the fitting of glasses belong to the general practitioner The author describes a schematic eye in which lenses can be inserted anteriorly and pictures of the fundus posteriorly, with a shutter diaphragm in front of the lens, to serve as a pupil. It can be made emmetropic, hyperopic, or myopic, and can be used as a human eye for practice in obtaining the fundus reflex, and for learning to recognize fundus details. Retinoscopy and refraction are covered in as full a manner as is possible in a book of this scope, giving the essential fundamentals and methods of making the various examinations for determining the proper glasses to be prescribed for a patient. Attached to the end of the book is a small atlas of 24 colored plates of the fundus, depicting the normal and some of abnormal conditions seen in routine examinations. S.

The Heart as a Power Chamber, (a Contribution to Cardiodynamics). By Harrington Sainsbury, M.D., F.R.C.P., Consulting Physician to the Royal Free Hospital and the City of London Hospital for Diseases of the Chest. Pp. 248; 22 illustrations. London: Henry Frowde, Hodder & Stoughton, 1922.

Relative to the anatomy, physiology, and pathology of the cardiovascular apparatus, the author discusses certain known facts, and speculates upon "the design and foresight which these reveal." The pages present an endeavor to show how these facts "disclose the living principle, the Archæus, working within the organs and tissues." The author's observations upon the relative weights of the muscular walls of the four chambers of the heart comprises his original contribution, and his views regarding the mechanics of the aortic valve, his most interesting presentation. The book as a whole leaves much to be desired; especially are the chapters on heart failure and treatment inadequate. A.

Greek Biology and Greek Medicine. By Charles Singer, University College, London. Pp. 128; 8 illustrations. Oxford: Oxford University Press, American Branch, 1922.

The medical historian will be very much interested in this small volume on the evolution of Greek biology and medicine. It is a series of essays by one who is a student of Greek and the early Grecians, and can be recognized as authoritative. It is very well written, has a tremendous amount of information and is compressed into a comparatively few pages. M.

Reports of St. Andrews Institute for Clinical Research. Vol. I. Pp. 208; 54 illustrations. London: Oxford Medical Publications. Henry Frowde, Hodder & Stoughton, 1922.

In this volume is assembled the first collection of reports from St. Andrews Institute, recently founded by Sir James Mackenzie. The aims and methods of research of the Institute are set forth by Mackenzie and other members of the staff. In addition, there are a number of special articles, including a valuable study of cutaneous sensibility by Waterston. The noval research initiated by Mackenzie, and being carried out with the aid of a staff of specialists and the entire medical personnel of the city of St. Andrews, for the purpose of carefully studying, recording and analyzing all available clinical material in the city, promises valuable results. St. Andrews was chosen for the experiment partly on account of the non-migratory character of the population. It is hoped, therefore, that the records will become increasingly valuable as a source of reliable data bearing on the factors predisposing to disease and the earliest symptoms of disease. The chief merit of this volume lies in the fact that it describes the plan of a splendid research. For the results, we shall have to await future reports. W.

DISEASES OF THE HEART: A HANDBOOK FOR STUDENTS AND PRACTITIONERS. By I. HARRIS, M.D., L.R.C.P., Honorary Physician-in-Charge, Cardiographic Department, Liverpool Northern Hospital. Pp. 196; 50 illustrations. New York: William Wood & Co., 1922.

THE author's practical knowledge of cardiology is apparent to anyone reading this book, but his selective judgment is decidedly open to criticism. He accepts without question, for example, the Diplococcus and Streptococcus rheumaticus as the causes of rheumatic endocarditis, and suggests the use of a diplococcus vaccine. He also recommends vaccine treatment for acute septic endocarditis. In cardiac conditions other than the arrhythmias, too great stress is laid upon the diagnostic value of the electrocardiogram. On page 148 the reference to the hemolytic streptococcus as the cause of subacute endocarditis is evidently a mistake. Discrimination on the part of the reader is therefore required beyond what could be expected of the practitioner or student for whom this book was designed. A.

THE HISTORY OF MEDICINE. By WALTER LIBBY, M.A., Ph.D., University of Pittsburgh. Pp. 427; 9 illustrations. Boston and New York: Houghton Mifflin Company, 1922.

DOCTOR LIBBY has not attempted to make his book an encyclopedia of medicine, but on the contrary has devoted himself entirely to important epochs and periods and to the lives of the greatest of the medical scientists. In this way he has been able to sketch rather superficially the more important features of medicine. He has prepared a volume which makes very much more interesting reading than could be gotten from a book in which the narrative form is not employed. Furthermore, it is a book which should appeal not only to the physician but also to the laity, and can be recommended to anyone who is interested in medicine from the very general point of view, as well as to any individual who is interested in science as a whole. M.

MONTAIGNE AND MEDICINE. By JAMES SPOTTISWOODE TAYLOR, Commander, Medical Corps, U. S. Navy, M.D., F.A.C.S., Membre Société française d'histoire de la médecine. Pp. 244; 32 illustrations. New York: Paul B. Hoeber, 1922.

To a lover of Montaigne this delightful little book will be of great interest. To him who has delved deeply into Montaigne it will recall interesting excerpts from this charming author's works. To one who is not acquainted with Montaigne and his work Taylor's essays will open to him a delightful series of future pleasures. The book is well worth reading and would make a very agreeable remembrance to one's medical friends, as it is nicely bound and attractively gotten up. M.

"BRAIN ABSCESS:" ITS SURGICAL PATHOLOGY AND OPERATIVE TECHNIC. By WELLS P. EAGLETON, M.D., Medical Director, Newark Eye and Ear Infirmary, etc. Pp. 282; 46 illustrations. New York City: The Macmillan Company, 1922.

DR. EAGLETON has written an excellent book on brain abscess and one that fills a real need. In fact, it is not often that a book finds a more ready field of usefulness waiting for it than this book does. The author has taken great care in its preparation and has candidly set forth his own experience in this field, even though not by any means invariably encouraging, as well as a comprehensive review of the literature. No one has known a great deal about brain abscess, so this work will help anyone interested in the subject.

The reviewer is in entire accord with Dr. Eagleton when he states in the beginning that "in no other branch of surgery may the advisability of a major operation depend upon such apparently trivial manifestations; in no other part of the body will neglect of slight hemorrhage play so important a part in the recovery or in the future well being of the patient," etc. As a matter of fact, no one should be allowed, unless in dire emergency, to invade the cranial cavity for brain abscess or any other acute or chronic lesion of the brain who has not taken the trouble to develop a special technic, a large part of which is the proper handling of nerve tissue. It is unusual, therefore, for a specialist in another field, although an allied one, to develop this necessary point of view and technic as unquestionably Dr. Eagleton has done. There are a few little things about the book that the reviewer might have done differently. For instance, he would have changed the order and put Part III, Surgical Diagnosis, and the succeeding chapters up to Chapter XIV, Complications and Results, in the first part, as this seems a more logical sequence. A good deal of stress is laid on technic, perhaps rightly so, since acute brain abscess is an emergency and must be so dealt with wherever it arises. The illustrations for the most part are good and amplify the text. The reviewer extends his congratulations to the author on a book, well done, which he believes is destined to become a classic in its field. R.

Diseases of Women. By Harry Sturgen Crossen, M.D., Clinical Professor of Gynecology, Washington University Medical School. Fifth edition. Pp. 1005; 934 engravings. St. Louis: C. V. Mosby Co., 1922.

Written for the general practitioner, this book describes in ample detail the methods to be used in determining a diagnosis and presents clearly the treatment to be selected and applied by him. The technical description of major operations is not within its scope, but the important features of preparatory and after-treatment are fully covered. The arrangement of the subject-matter has been accomplished with such evident skill that its value for easy reference is readily apparent. Where repetition has been necessary for this purpose it may be not only excused but commended. The liberal use of well selected and appropriately placed illustrations is noteworthy. This edition shows extensive revision and brings up to date the phases of gynecology in which the most recent advances have been made. The emphasis placed on pathology by the addition of new illustrations is in keeping with the character of the text. L.

Chloroform Anesthesia. By A. Goodman Levy, M.D., M.R.C.P., Physician to the City of London Hospital for Diseases of the Chest. Pp. 155; 9 illustrations. New York: William Wood & Co., 1922.

The administration of chloroform is becoming a lost art in many hospitals in this country. The literature of the last few years has aroused a vague fear of its effects, so that, when it is occasionally selected because other anesthetics are strongly contraindicated, it is too often given timidly because the scientific basis of its dangers is not well understood. The author's experience as an anesthetist, his experimental work with animals, and his presentation of the basal sciences as well as the physiology concerned give a stamp of authority to the work that is convincing. The book places chloroform anesthesia on a newer and firmer basis. It commends itself not only to anesthetists but to others interested in the principles of the distribution of a drug in the tissues. L.

THE BASIS OF PSYCHIATRY. By ALBERT C. BUCKLEY, M.D., Medical Superintendent of Friend's Hospital, Frankford; Associate Professor of Psychiatry, Graduate School of Medicine, University of Pennsylvania. Pp. 447; 79 illustrations. Philadelphia and London: J. B. Lippincott Company.

IN this book, relatively small when one considers the subject, Dr. Buckley has placed a world of information regarding mental diseases. The first 115 pages of the book are given over to chapters on biologic phenomena, cerebral development and receptive apparatus, mental development, and psychological processes; in these pages is put forth a real foundation for any student of psychiatry. Dr. Buckley's discussion of the psychoses and psychoneuroses is clear, simple and easy to follow. The work is one of the best on psychiatry and the author should be congratulated on his effort.

W.

PATHOLOGY OF THE NERVOUS SYSTEM. By E. FARQUHAR BUZZARD, M.A., M.D., F.R.C.P., and J. GODWIN GREENFIELD, B.Sc., M.D., M.R.C.P., London. Pp. 334; 103 illustrations. New York: Paul B. Hoeber, 1922.

THIS is one of the few books devoted entirely to the pathology of the nervous system. It is well written, the paper and the illustrations are excellent, and the type clear-cut. From the standpoint of the neurologist it might be said that the book is somewhat elementary; but for students and those practitioners in lines other than neurology, this book will be an excellent guide to the changes brought about in the nervous system by disease. The first 304 pages are devoted to pathology; the remainder of the book takes up the various staining methods and the examination of the cerebrospinal fluid. The authors are apparently little acquainted with the writings of American neurologists, if one is to judge from the references.

W.

DISEASES OF THE THYROID GLAND. By ARTHUR E. HERTZLER, M.D., F.A.C.S., Professor of Medicine in the University of Kansas School of Medicine; Surgeon to the Halstead Hospital, Halstead, Kansas, etc. Pp. 245; 106 illustrations. St. Louis: C. V. Mosby Company, 1922.

IN calling attention to the advantages of the small country hospital for studying such conditions as goiter, which require prolonged observation, the author performs a real service. The present volume is proof that such a study may be of distinct value. It is to be regretted however, that the presentation of statistics has been avoided. If, as the author states, statistics on goiter as now published are misleading in that they present the disease in too optimistic a light, it would seem that a valuable service might be performed by the country hospital in collecting statistics under the more favorable circumstances which may exist in such institutions, and in presenting the disease in its true light.

The first portions of the book are taken up with considerations of goiter which would appeal equally to the physician and the surgeon. The last two chapters are devoted to surgical considerations. The style is interesting, the illustrations good. The book contains points of practical value to the physician or the surgeon, and is decidedly worth reading. A.

Syphilis of the Innocent. By Harry C. Solomon, M.D., Chief of Therapeutic Research, Boston Psychopathic Hospital; Instructor in Psychiatry and Neuropathology, Harvard Medical School, and Maida Herman Solomon, A.B., B.S., Research Social Worker, Boston Psychopathic Hospital, Boston. Pp. 239. Washington: United States Interdepartmental Social Hygiene Board, 1922.

The authors, undoubted authorities upon the social and medical aspects of this disease, here present a study of the social effects of syphilis on the family and the community. To students of social hygiene this work will be of the greatest value, and in it the general practitioner and syphilologist will find a surprising amount of information condensed into a few very readable pages. A.

Regional Anesthesia. By Gaston Labat, M.D., Lecturer in Regional Anesthesia at New York University. Pp. 496; 315 original illustrations. Philadelphia and London: W. B. Saunders Company, 1922.

The author states that "the object of this work is to afford the opportunity of acquiring rapidly a practical knowledge of regional anesthesia and to teach the reader how to use the method successfully," and he has fulfilled that object most abundantly. It is clearly and concisely written in such a way that a person can rapidly gain the desired information about a region of anatomy where he had never used regional anesthesia previously. The last chapter on the "relative value of regional anesthesia" might well have been given a first chapter position for the benefit of those who have had

PROGRESS

OF

MEDICAL SCIENCE

MEDICINE

UNDER THE CHARGE OF

W. S. THAYER, M.D.

PROFESSOR OF MEDICINE, JOHNS HOPKINS UNIVERSITY, BALTIMORE, MARYLAND,

AND

ROGER S. MORRIS, M.D.,

FREDERICK FORCHHEIMER PROFESSOR OF MEDICINE IN THE UNIVERSITY OF CINCINNATI
CINCINNATI, OHIO.

Blood and Bone-marrow Findings During Life in Cryptogenetic Pernicious Anemia, Especially During the Stage of Remission. I. Zadek (*Ztschr. f. klin. Med.*, 1922, **95**, 66) has undertaken a study of the bone marrow during life, together with examinations of the blood, in pernicious anemia. From his comparative studies of the blood and marrow, he arrives at the following conclusions: the characteristic macrocytosis, anisocytosis and hyperchromia, with megaloblasts, observed at the height of an Addisonian anemia, is the expression of a blood regeneration resulting from increased blood destruction; with this, there is a megaloblastic reaction of the bone marrow of the long bones. Close relations exist between the degree of the megaloblastic reaction of the marrow and the number of erythroblasts and macrocytes circulating in the blood. The increased blood destruction may be followed clinically at this stage by the golden-yellow color of the serum with bilirubinemia, by urobilinuria and, at autopsy, by siderosis of the liver. The periods of improvement which occur in most cases of Addisonian anemia are usually *stages of relative remission*, which are related, both clinically and hematologically, to the symptom complex, pernicious anemia, since the hemolysis at this stage of the disease is only slightly decreased, with no, or only few, evidences of regeneration of the blood. During relative remissions, the marrow of the long bones likewise reverts to a more normal state, and in place of red marrow, one finds a yellow marrow, which again becomes red during a recurrence of the disease. The remission is not the result of the megaloblastic marrow reaction, since macrocytes and erythroblasts disappear from both blood and marrow. The megaloblastic marrow doubt about, or no experience with, this form of anesthesia. The diagrammatic illustrations are most instructive as to points in technic and anatomy, and should familiarize one with structures instantly which might be otherwise disregarded.

It seems to the writer that this work would be a most useful addition to anyone claiming to do any type of surgery, for every region of the body is expertly covered, and it is known that regional anesthesia is most desirable in many cases and an absolute necessity in others. Any description of a work summarizing the amount of labor necessary to make it possible, and yet so thorough, so precise and so beneficial to both surgeon and the welfare of his patient, seems totally inadequate. B.

Clinical Medicine: Tuesday Clinics at the Johns Hopkins Hospital. By Lewellys F. Barker, M.D., LL.D., Professor of Medicine, Emeritus, Johns Hopkins University; Visiting Physician to Johns Hopkins Hospital, Baltimore, Md. Pp. 617; 67 illustrations. Philadelphia and London: W. B. Saunders Company, 1922.

It is difficult to estimate the worth of this book, for there is much in it to praise and much to criticize unfavorably. The thirty-one clinics are presented in the form of dialogue between Dr. Barker and one or more hyperstudents; each is a complete exposition of its special topic and displays the author's wide knowledge of clinical and laboratory medicine and of medical bibliography. The clinics, however, are unrelated and in many instances are concerned with rare or at least unusual diseases, for example: "Chronic progressive multiple ossifying myositis." It is difficult in this form of clinical presentation to avoid faulty emphasis, as, for example, occurs in the following sentence on page 186, where in speaking of the roentgen-ray plates it is pointed out that "the stomach is dilated and has not emptied itself at the end of fifteen hours; besides, the duodenal cap is not emptied."

Esoteric words and phrases abound—"the cardiovascular stripe," "smear of the gland punctate," "areflexia," "autoanthropophagus," for the latter of which the author almost apologizes.

As examples of bedside teaching these clinics are inspiring and suggestive to any one who studies the teaching of internal medicine, and this is true even though the careful editing which the clinics must have undergone has somewhat lessened their spontaneity. To Professor Barker's former students the book will certainly achieve its purpose, as stated in its preface, of recalling to them some of the interesting hours spent together. Inherently, however, the book can have but a limited usefulness for the average student or practitioner of medicine. P.

PROGRESS
OF
MEDICAL SCIENCE

MEDICINE

UNDER THE CHARGE OF

W. S. THAYER, M.D.

PROFESSOR OF MEDICINE, JOHNS HOPKINS UNIVERSITY, BALTIMORE, MARYLAND,

AND

ROGER S. MORRIS, M.D.,

FREDERICK FORCHHEIMER PROFESSOR OF MEDICINE IN THE UNIVERSITY OF CINCINNATI, CINCINNATI, OHIO.

Blood and Bone-marrow Findings During Life in Cryptogenetic Pernicious Anemia, Especially During the Stage of Remission.—I. ZADEK (*Ztschr. f. klin. Med.*, 1922, **95**, 66) has undertaken a study of the bone marrow during life, together with examinations of the blood, in pernicious anemia. From his comparative studies of the blood and marrow, he arrives at the following conclusions: the characteristic macrocytosis, anisocytosis and hyperchromia, with megaloblasts, observed at the height of an Addisonian anemia, is the expression of a blood regeneration resulting from increased blood destruction; with this, there is a megaloblastic reaction of the bone marrow of the long bones. Close relations exist between the degree of the megaloblastic reaction of the marrow and the number of erythroblasts and macrocytes circulating in the blood. The increased blood destruction may be followed clinically at this stage by the golden-yellow color of the serum with bilirubinemia, by urobilinuria and, at autopsy, by siderosis of the liver. The periods of improvement which occur in most cases of Addisonian anemia are usually *stages of relative remission*, which are related, both clinically and hematologically, to the symptom complex, pernicious anemia, since the hemolysis at this stage of the disease is only slightly decreased, with no, or only few, evidences of regeneration of the blood. During relative remissions, the marrow of the long bones likewise reverts to a more normal state, and in place of red marrow, one finds a yellow marrow, which again becomes red during a recurrence of the disease. The remission is not the result of the megaloblastic marrow reaction, since macrocytes and erythroblasts disappear from both blood and marrow. The megaloblastic marrow is, therefore, not the primary lesion of the disease, but, rather, the reaction to the toxic, hemolytic poison of pernicious anemia. The examination of the marrow during life serves as an index of the severity of the disease as well as of its stage. In very few cases of Addisonian anemia is the improvement so great that no criteria of the disease are to be found hematologically. In these instances of *complete remission*, the red count and hemoglobin may be normal, though often the hemoglobin is somewhat reduced. Clinically, during such complete remissions, the only sequelæ of the anemia may be the myocardial insufficiency, achylia gastrica and spinal cord changes, which so often form a part of the clinical picture. The marrow of the long bones at this stage of the disease is meeting no unusual demands and is yellow fatty marrow devoid of erythroblasts. The megaloblastic bone marrow of pernicious anemia is one of the processes of the disease which is resolved during remissions. It is to be looked upon as a secondary, labile reaction, conditional—according to the individual resistance of the patient—upon the degree of increased hemolysis; and the degree of the megaloblastic marrow reaction is indicated by the cells in the blood. (Like most of his Teutonic confrères, Zadek is apparently content to remain in blissful ignorance of all work which emanates beyond the Rhine. Without intending to minimize the value of observations upon the marrow during life, it may not be amiss to point out the fact that the most important conclusions of Zadek were arrived at some twenty years ago by Warthin of the University of Michigan, whose results published in this *Journal*, were based upon autopsy findings at various stages of pernicious anemia.)

Reactions of the Cerebrospinal Fluid in Disseminated Sclerosis.—Ch. Achard and J. Thiers (*Compt. rend. Soc. de biol.*, Paris, 1922, **87**, 1006) report findings in the cerebrospinal fluid of disseminated sclerosis which may prove to be of diagnostic importance. In a case reported by Achard recently, a negative Wassermann reaction and a positive colloidal benzoin reaction (réaction du benzoin colloidal) were encountered. The latter test was reported: 122,202,222,000. Targowla and Muttermilch (*Ibid.*, 1922, **87**, 974) have recently reported similar changes in the spinal fluid in a patient ill with this disease. The authors report 2 further cases of disseminated sclerosis, in which the reactions of the cerebrospinal fluid were like those reported above. In a woman who died of the disease, they found a clear spinal fluid, which yielded a negative Wassermann test and a strongly positive colloidal benzoin reaction: 222,222,221,000. In the second patient, a man, whose spinal fluid was also clear and contained no cells, the Wassermann test was negative and the colloidal benzoin reaction was subpositive, in the sense that it gave a precipitate in the first two tubes, *i. e.*, in the syphilitic zone: 111,000,200,000. In this fluid A. Petit demonstrated the presence of spirochetes. If disseminated sclerosis is in reality a spirochetosis, as the researches of Petit seem to show, it would not be surprising, the authors point out, if some of the humoral reactions of another spirochetosis, syphilis, should be met with. One can thus explain a positive Wassermann reaction found at times in the cerebrospinal fluid of patients suffering from disseminated sclerosis, without necessarily concluding that the disease is syphilitic in nature.

THERAPEUTICS

UNDER THE CHARGE OF

SAMUEL W. LAMBERT, M.D.,

NEW YORK,

AND

CHARLES C. LIEB, M.D.,

ASSISTANT PROFESSOR OF PHARMACOLOGY, COLUMBIA UNIVERSITY.

Intestinal Infections and Toxemias and Their Biological Treatment.—N. P. NORMAL and A. E. EGGSTON (*New York Med. Jour. and Med. Rec.*, 1922, **116**, 623) base their treatment on five factors: (1) The removal of foci of infection from the upper digestive and respiratory tracts; (2) the efficient non-surgical mechanical drainage of the colon; (3) sufficient doses of pure cultures of living strains of Bacillus acidophilus; (4) the maintenance of a protective intestinal flora by a proper diet; (5) autogenous vaccines in selected cases.

Phases of Gastrointestinal Infection, Pathology and Treatment.—G. R. SATTERLEE, (*New York Med. Jour. and Med. Rec.*, 1922, **116**, 619) states that chronic intestinal toxemia is a definite entity and is the primary cause of the protean symptoms characteristic of chronic intestinal disease. It may have one or more of the following sources: bacterial by-products of the food in the intestinal lumen; autogenous non-bacterial metabolic products arising from the digestive epithelium; local bacterial foci in the intestinal wall. Of these the last is by far the most important, as inferred from pathological findings and immunity studies. Successful treatment consists in the removal of all accessible foci of infection and the treatment of the bowel focus by antigens prepared from bacteria isolated from the mesenteric lymph glands at the time of operation or from the stools in those patients who have not been operated upon. If this treatment fails the radical operation of colectomy may in special cases be indicated.

The Effect of Magnesium Sulphate on the Secretion of Bile: Experimental Study.—E. B. FRAZIER (*Jour. Am. Med. Assn.*, 1922, **79**, 1594) undertook a series of experiments on dogs to determine whether magnesium sulphate introduced directly into the duodenum or injected intravenously caused any change in the amount or character of the bile secreted. In the control experiments the bile flow was found to be fairly uniform in fasting animals; and since all factors could be controlled, any fluctuation in the secretion could be ascribed to the injection of the salt. After intraduodenal injection, the duodenum, seen through the skin, contracted at first and then during the next thirty to sixty minutes remained in a state of wide relaxation. The initial contraction was probably due to the mechanical stimulation of the muscular wall by the needle. The effects on bile flow were entirely negative. Whether the magnesium sulphate solution was injected directly into the duodenum or into the veins, the bile flow remained practically constant, though in a considerable proportion of experiments the secretion was lessened. When bile was injected into the duodenum there was a definite and prompt increase in the bile output confirming the generally accepted statement that bile itself is the best cholagogue.

The Effects of Thyroxin and Iodides on Metabolism.—F. HILDEBRANDT (*Therap. d. Gegen.*, 1922, **24**, 363) found that the feeding of thyroid extract to rats causes a loss of weight, an increase in O-consumption and a decrease in the respiratory quotient. Since there is no augmentation of urinary nitrogen, the decreased respiratory quotient is intrepreted as an indication of increased oxidation of fat. The intravenous injection of thyroxin causes identical changes in metabolism and the author agrees with Kendall in regarding thyroxin as the active principle of the thyroid gland. Thyroxin contains about 66 per cent of iodine and it occurred to the author that the alterations in metabolism might be due to the splitting off of free iodine; accordingly, the effects of iodine, in the form of potassium iodide and in amounts equivalent to that contained in thyroxin, were determined and were found to be the same as those following thyroid feeding or thyroxin injection. The intravenous injection of potassium iodide into rats fed on thyroid, stopped the loss of weight and flattened the gradient of O-consumption; in some cases there were gain in weight and decrease in oxygen intake. These experiments confirm the clinical findings that minimal doses of iodine lessen the metabolic upset of "hyperthyroidism." If large doses of potassium iodide are injected into thyroid fed rats, the loss of weight and the O-consumption are greatly exaggerated, a reaction that finds its counterpart in the distinctly harmful effects of large doses of iodides in "hyperthyroidism." Further experiments showed that the response to potassium iodide is not altered by thyroidectomy and the conclusion is drawn that the metabolic changes cannot be due to an action of potassium iodide on the cells of the thyroid glands. By a process of exclusion, the author is forced to conclude that the metabolic changes are due to a specific action of iodine on all the cells of the organism.

PEDIATRICS

UNDER THE CHARGE OF

THOMPSON S. WESTCOTT, M.D., AND ALVIN E. SIEGEL, M.D.,

OF PHILADELPHIA.

The Vital Capacity of the Lungs of Children in Health and Disease.—STEWART (*Am. Jour. Dis. Child.*, 1922, **24**, 451) as a result of his exhaustive studies found that at either corresponding age, standing height, sitting height or body weight the vital capacity of the lungs is constantly greater with boys than with girls, the difference increasing with especial rapidity during the latter half of childhood. The curves of vital capacity as plotted against age, standing and sitting height in general pursue a sinuous course showing a fairly uniform increase at first, followed later by a period of more rapid growth in lung capacity, which later diminishes in rate. The curve plotted against body weight for the boys showed a more uniform curve, while that for girls has a definitely convex form. The absolute annual increase in vital capacity in general is fairly uniform during early childhood, but increases in rapidity about the time of puberty and declines later. The relative increase in vital capacity apparently decreases at first, becomes relatively more rapid about the time of puberty and then proceeds at a slower rate again. The period of acceleration in the rate of growth in lung capacity begins and terminates at an earlier age in girls than in boys. Throughout childhood the vital capacity formed a greater proportion of the estimated adult maximum for women with the girls than with the boys. As a whole, as respects lung capacity at corresponding ages, the girls may be considered as relatively more mature than the boys. The vital capacity of the lungs apparently reaches a maximum near the twentieth year with the boys and probably slightly earlier with the girls. On using the proper values for the constant, the vital capacity may be computed accurately from the sitting height, the standing height, the age, or the body weight. The probable error of random sampling increases as the vital capacity increases, but all in all it is relatively small, amounting to less than 25 cc as a rule. Averages obtained from an infinitely large number of comparable series would vary only slightly from those obtained in the present limited series of this observer. The standard deviation or absolute variability increases as a rule as the vital capacity increases and is usually greater with boys than with girls of corresponding age and size. The coefficient of variation or relative variability for each sex decreases during the early years of childhood, increases about the age of puberty and later declines again. The extent of the dispersal of the individual observations from the averages, appears to be smaller when averaged in groups differing 5 cm. in standing height or 2 cm. in stem length, than when averaged according to age in years as estimated from the nearest birthday. Children may have a normal vital capacity even in the presence of a definite insufficiency of the mitral valves, and these individuals show little abnormal tendency to dyspnea on exertion. In more serious cases the vital capacity is greatly reduced, and the tendency to respiratory embarrassment is proportional to the reduction in lung capacity. When the condition of the heart improves the vital capacity gradually increases. Acute bronchitis produces a temporary reduction in vital capacity which in severe cases may be very marked. During the course of lobar pneumonia the vital capacity rapidly undergoes an enormous reduction even in cases free from pleurisy. The reduction is altogether out of proportion to the extent of the pneumonic process in the lungs. Following the crisis, the vital capacity gradually returns to normal in a comparatively short time. Physical signs of the disease may disappear before the normal capacity is reached. In complicated cases the return of vital capacity to normal may be greatly delayed. While bronchial asthma may cause an enormous reduction in the vital capacity immediately following an attack, the reduction promptly disappears as the symptoms subside. Even in children subject to the disease for several years there is apparently

no permanent reduction in the capacity of the lungs. With children showing slight evidence of tuberculosis such as a positive Pirquet reaction, and having a poor health record, and also with those having a definite tuberculosis the vital capacity is as a rule normal. In a few instances there is apparently some subnormal tendency of the lung capacity which leads to the suspicion of tuberculosis. In incipient pulmonary tuberculosis the vital capacity may be practically normal even in the presence of a very active and virulent infection in the lungs. In advanced pulmonary tuberculosis the vital capacity is reduced in proportion to the extent of the disease process. The abnormal tendency to dyspnea on exertion is much more marked where the reduced vital capacity is caused by disease of the heart than when caused by disease of the lung alone.

A Clinical and Chemical Study of Butter-soup Feeding in Infants.—BROWN, COURTNEY and MACLACHLAN (*Am. Jour. Dis. Child.*, 1922, **24**, 368) found that the use of butter-flour mixtures for very young and very small infants was generally attended by rapid gain in weight yet uniform, improvement in vigor, in tissue turgor, in disposition and in resistance to infection. Extraordinarily good results were obtained with many infants suffering from atrophy. It is not indicated, however, for children with diarrhea or other forms of fat or carbohydrate intolerance. The caloric intake with this form of food was usually high, averaging approximately 70 calories per pound. In some cases signs of mild rickets or of a condition simulating rickets, were seen after continuous use of butter-soup. No edema was encountered. If the weight became stationary after long use of butter-soup, the addition of protein to the food or temporary feeding with a cow's milk dilution, was sufficient to bring about a continuation of the rapid weight gain. The stools with this food were acid, strongly resembling those of breast feedings, but were much larger. Like breast milk feces they contained a high percentage of fat. There was generally a poor retention of fat, and sometimes a poor retention of nitrogen and of total salts especially by the older children. There was usually a fair retention of calcium. Sodium chloride was retained in abnormal amounts. The feces contained an excess of inorganic bases over inorganic acids, and the urine showed the reversed condition. The excess of bases in the feces was not to be accounted for by the quantity of fat excreted as soap, but apparently indicated the presence of lower acids.

DERMATOLOGY AND SYPHILIS

UNDER THE CHARGE OF

JOHN H. STOKES, M.D.,

MAYO CLINIC, ROCHESTER, MINN.

Drug Eruptions.—WILE, WRIGHT and SMITH (*Arch. of Dermat. and Syph.*, 1922, **6**, 529) in a preliminary study of iodide and bromide exanthems report that iodide and bromide cannot be found in the purulent material from iodide and bromide acne. They state that cutaneous tests for sensitization to these drugs are invariably negative, so that it is impossible to use such tests to determine a preëxistent sensitiveness. WISE and PARKHURST (*Arch. Dermat. and Syph.*, 1922, **6**, 542) gave a valuable account of the eruptive phenomena associated with the administration of recent medicaments. They cite the observation of Stuhmer that seborrheic eruptions predispose to arsphenamine dermatitis, and that the eruption usually is most persistent at the sites of predilection for seborrhea. The arsphenamine "fixed exanthem," which has attracted much attention in the European literature, is a recurrent plaque of an urticarial or eczmatoid type which appears following each injection of the drug, tending to disappear between injections. The plaques may be solitary or as many as a dozen may appear. Pigmentation becomes marked at the site of the recurrent lesions. The resemblance to the antipyrin and phenolphthalein eruption is obvious. Lichenoid eruptions and actual outbreaks of lichen planus following upon courses of arsphenamine and mercury have been described. MC CAFFERTY (*Arch. Dermat. and Syph.*, 1922, **6**, 591) reports in detail a case of this type in which both the clinical and histological picture conformed to that of lichen planus. The familiar diffuse pigmentation of the skin and hyperkeratoses of the palms and soles which were long thought not to occur with the administration of the arsphenamines, are now known to be among the possible complications, and cases are cited from the literature as reported by Hoffmann, Heller, Philip and others. Herpetic eruptions are recognized as rather frequent after arsphenamine. There are no authentic reports of argyria following silver arsphenamine, according to these authors. The controversy as to whether an arsphenamine dermatitis can favorably influence the course of a syphilitic infection by arousing the defence mechanism of the skin ("esophylaxis" according to Hoffman) is reviewed. While there seems to be a weight of opinion in favor of the belief that an attack of exfoliative dermatitis favorably affects the course of a syphilitic infection, the effect may be only transitory, and too little time has elapsed for the collection of trustworthy figures. Barbital and medinal may give rise to erythematous eruptions suggesting the acute exanthemata and in some cases associated with red blotches, erosins and bullous lesions on the oral mucosæ. The blebs may appear from five minutes to several days after administration and may be confused with pemphigus and erythema multiforme. Itching plaques, generalized pruritus and urticaria have been seen after adalin and bromural. These eruptions may become eczematoid, or tuberose bromodermatous lesions may develop. Old people are especially susceptible. Phenobarbital produces scarlatiniform and rubeolar eruptions, dermatitis and urticaria. Oral lesions are frequent and may in the form of severe stomatitis and bullous lesions, with exfoliation of the mucosa, be the only manifestation of the idiosyncrasy. Cinchophen may produce angioneurotic edema, pyramidon may produce pruritus, swelling of the lip, erythema and purpura. Acetylsalicylic acid eruptions are fairly uniform, and consist of swelling of the face, chiefly the eyelids and lips within an hour, with involvement of the oral and nasal mucosæ. Intense general malaise and urticaria or scarlatiniform erythema may develop. The palms may show a "dyshydrotic eczema." Hexamethylene may produce a burning and itching general eruption. Phenolphthalein eruptions have been previously described by Wise, and present characteristics similar to the antipyrin and fixed arsenical exanthems. The essential lesion is an urticarial plaque or patch which becomes edematous with each dose and subsides in the interim, leaving a residual pigmentation which by accumulation takes on a bluish or livid tinge and persists for months and even years after the ingestion of the drug is discontinued. The tendency to involve the genitalia gives rise to the so-called "blue penis." Erosions are frequent and may be mistaken for venereal lesions.

Effect of Treatment on Viability of Spirochæta Pallida.—RUBIN and SZENTKIRALYI (*Dermat. Wchnschr.*, January 28, 1922, p. 84) undertook to compare the efficiency of four methods of treating syphilis from the standpoint of their effect on the viability of the *Spirochæta pallida* after removal from the body. The purpose of the work was to check the results of Stejskal, who found that the length of life of spirochetes outside the body was shortened in inverse proportion to the time which had elapsed following a neosalvarsan injection, and that this drug caused the rapid disappearance of the organisms. With mercury on the other hand, he found that the essential fact responsible for the disappearance of the organisms was the healing of the lesion, and the drug as such had little effect upon the organisms themselves, but rather on the lesions. The authors further aimed to control the observation of Fantl regarding the resistance of spirochetes in a certain case to the treatment of the patient with inunctions and salvarsan, Fantl having suggested the possibility that the previous mercurialization had rendered the organisms more resistant to the subsequent use of arsphenamine. The series of early cases studied by the authors, 108 in number, were divided into four groups, the first treated only with mercury salicylate intramuscularly, the second with two injections of mercury salicylate followed by neoarsphenamine, the third by neoarsphenamine alone, and the fourth by the Linser mixture of neoarsphenamine and mercury bichloride intravenously. Their findings are of interest. The average life of the spirochete in the moist chamber when taken from untreated cases was twenty to thirty hours. On the other hand they found variations as high as one hundred and twenty-four hours. Living spirochetes were still demonstrable in the lesions of one case as late as twenty-seven days after the first injection of mercury salicylate, and following the sixth injection of the drug. There was a progressive decline in the viability of the organism as the lesion healed and as treatment was continued. They were not convinced that the mercurialization increased the viability or resistance of the organism in any of their cases, although in four they were resistant. In the second series they could elicit no evidence that the previous mercurialization had rendered the organisms resistant. In fact where specimens were taken with frequency, the gradual decline in their viability was apparent. It is of interest to note how small were the doses of neoarsphenamine (0.3 gm.) which caused complete disappearance of all organisms within twelve hours. The spirillicidal superiority of the arsphenamine was obvious. The authors were not impressed with any superiority on this score in the combined injection of neo-salvarsan and mercury bichloride. They were able to confirm the value of the preliminary administration of mercury in preventing the Herxheimer flare-up, but quote Lesser as not regarding this as an unmixed benefit in early cases, which he thinks need the "immunizing shock" of the acute reaction.

Non-specific Therapy of Syphilis with "Mirion." — Non-specific modes of therapeutic attack on syphilis have been engaging the attention of Continental authors. One phase of this discussion has centered around "Mirion," an organic synthetic (Benkö) containing an iodine radical, action of which is supposed to consist in the liberation of nascent iodine in contact with syphilitic lesions for its effect in provoking hyperemia securing a resolving local reaction, and a "mobilization" of the *Spirochæta pallida.* Frölich, Kyrle and Pfanner from Finger's Clinic employed 6000 injections of the drug in 400 cases and credit it with a provocative effect on the Wassermann reaction and the ability to produce a local or Herxheimer flare-up in syphilitic lesions. The iodine content of diseased tissue when this drug is administered is said to be much higher than that of healthy tissue. No spirillicidal qualities are claimed for "Mirion," its use being mainly that of an adjuvant to mercury and arsphenamine to assist in reaching inaccessible foci, much as in the case of iodides. The drug is given intramuscularly in doses of 5 cc but may be used intravenously. The worth of the new preparation is discussed by GAERTNER (*Dermat. Wchnschr.*, January 7, 1922, p. 14). No spirillicidal effects were demonstrable. Some evidence of a provocative effect on the Wassermann reaction was obtained. Urban from Török's Clinic, found in a smaller group of cases that no spirillicidal effect was obtained, that Herxheimer flare-ups were unusual, that early lesions did not respond at all to treatment with the drug and that no convincing provocative effect on the Wassermann could be obtained. Urban noted local flare-ups in trichophytosis under the drug. He feels that none of the effects obtained are markedly different from those obtainable in similar situations with foreign protein, and suggests that the 4 per cent gelatine in "Mirion" may be responsible for much of its action. KYRLE responds warmly (*Dermat. Wchnschr.*, March 18, 1922, p. 256), denying that he has overstated the possibilities of the preparation, and maintaining that the drug subserves its function as a stirrer-up of inaccessible foci and a non-specific therapeutic agent for syphilis.

Sodium Salicylate for Psoriasis.—BRAVO in a brief note (*Brit. Jour. Dermat.*, 1922, **34**, 353), reports favorable results from the use of Sack's method of treating psoriasis with intravenous injections of a 20 per cent sterile solution of sodium salicylate. (SACH's original report is in the *Wien. klin. Wchnschr.*, April 21, 1921.) Sainz de Aja employs a 20 per cent solution giving ½ gm. for the first dose and increasing ½ gm. for each succeeding dose until 3 or 4 gm. are reached. The interval between injections is two or three days. No case reports or details are given.

OBSTETRICS

UNDER THE CHARGE OF

EDWARD P. DAVIS, A.M., M.D.,

PROFESSOR OF OBSTETRICS IN THE JEFFERSON MEDICAL COLLEGE, PHILADELPHIA.

The Prophylactic Rectification of Abnormal Positions.—Ballantyne (*Brit. Med. Jour.*, 1922, **2**, 845) states that, down to the close of 1921, the correction of malpositions and malpresentations in the antenatal department of the Edinburgh Royal Maternity Hospital was not satisfactory. Manipulation was tried and also postural treatment. A modified Trendelenburg was used in some cases with the hope that the presenting part would slip out of the pelvic brim and become movable above it, but this method was but little, if at all, successful. Since the beginning of 1922 a method described by Buist (*Brit. Med. Jour.* 1921, **2**, 782) of using pads for this purpose has been employed, and the results for six months have been satisfactory. Of 509 pregnant women at the clinic, there were 26 cases where the occiput was posterior on the right side, 24 were rectified by pads, and the occiput made to assume anterior positions; the other 2 remained behind. In most of the cases the occiput moved anterior; the back remaining to the right; in some the usual left occipito-anterior position developed. One case was first diagnosed as left occipito-posterior and pads were applied, when it was found that the presentation was a breech, and external version produced a right occipito-anterior. It is thought that the use of pads changed the vertex to a breech presentation. The method as described by Buist is as follows: A binder is laid under the patient and two towel-pads are prepared. The first is rolled to about the thickness of a forearm, the second is folded to a flat pad six or seven inches square. The rolled pad is pinned to the binder in such a position that when the binder is firmly secured the pad will lie close in front of the anterior-superior iliac spine behind and parallel to the trunk. The flat pad is pinned so as to lie on the limbs, pressing them backward. It is sometimes useful to roll the patient to the side opposite the trunk and by hand bring the trunk so far as may be over to that side. The binder is then pulled firmly home. It has rarely been found necessary in the Edinburgh clinic to take the patient to a hospital to apply this method. The patient is asked to bring to the prenatal clinic a binder, two towels and safety pins. The pad and binder are then applied and the patient is allowed after a short rest to go to her home. She returns the next morning when the presenting part is usually found anterior. Occasionally the pads have to be applied again. The two failures are ascribed to the fact that the fetal head was so low in the mother's pelvis that by this method it could not be turned. In the 509 pregnant patients in six months there were 56 pelvic presentations. In 11 of these no attempt at version was made, as the pregnancy was not beyond the seventh month. In 14 cases cephalic version was accomplished by external manipulation, sometimes by one and occasionally by two operators. In 7 chloroform was necessary, and success was obtained in 6 of these. In 3 other cases the attempt failed, because the amount of amniotic liquid was so small that the child could not be turned. In 19 cases spontaneous version occurred. In 2 the patient did not return to the clinic. In the 509, there were 3 cases of transverse presentation; in all of these, external manipulation was successful in securing cephalic presentation. The towel pads are advised in difficult breech and transverse positions.

Eclampsia and its Treatment and the Toxemia of Pregnancy.—Several of the papers upon these subjects recently were read before the British Congress of Obstetrics and Gynecology (*Jour. Obst. and Gynec. of the Brit. Emp.*, 1922, **29**, No. 3). Eden comments upon the reports presented at the meeting of the Congress. Maternal mortality was computed in these reports from 2005 cases at 22.5 per cent. The infant mortality varied from 22 to 44 per cent. The percentage of surviving children varied from 44.4 per cent to 65.6 per cent. As regards the predisposing causes, primiparity was present in 69.3 per cent, multiparity in 30.7 per cent. The mortality is higher among multiparæ than among primiparæ. There is a distinct increase in cases of twin pregnancy, the liability to eclampsia being four or five times greater than a single pregnancy. In the great number of cases (84.7 per cent), there are premonitory symptoms which give warning. In 4 out of 5 cases an opportunity for preventive treatment was present if the significance of the premonitory symptoms was understood. There is an interesting difference in the severity of the disease in various portions of England, in the Midland districts the percentage of severe cases is somewhat higher than in other portions. Indications of danger are coma and pulse above 120; temperature above 103° F.; more than ten convulsions; the urine containing a large quantity of albumin; the absence of edema and the blood-pressure above 200 mm. When any two of these symptoms were present the case was thought to be severe. There was some difference in the results of statistics regarding the presence of edema and its results; this may be disregarded as a positive sign of danger. When methods of delivery are considered, the greater the interference, the higher was the mortality. Medical treatment passed through various periods prior to 1870, venesection, opium, ice pack, cold pack or cold baths, wet cupping in the loins and no obstetric interference was the treatment commonly employed. During the next twenty years narcotics and sweating were most used. Pilocarpin was given very freely and bleeding was abandoned. During this period in Germany maternal mortality was 33 per cent. From 1885 to 1890 the theory of toxemia became common and hepatic toxemia was recognized as a variety. Under early surgical operation in some of the German clinics the mortality fell to 18 per cent. In 1901 Stroganoff described his method which he originally intended should supplant active interference; this gave good results. The writer believes it to be unfortunate that there has been no concerted effort to distinguish between the results of various methods and to bring about an agreement in the use of those which gave the greatest promise of success. From his personal experience he believes that eclampsia and toxemia can usually be prevented, and that prevention is of the most importance. The prophylactic treatment which he advises, consists essentially in confinement to bed and fluid diet only, mostly water, purgatives and diuretics. The case must be closely watched; observe the amount of urine, quantity of albumin and the blood-pressure. If the patient does not do well, or if relapses occur, the pregnancy must be terminated without regard to the interest of the child. The case should be under all circumstances a hospital case promptly, and he would have the patient sent to hospital after the first convulsion. On this, much can be gained by dividing the cases into "mild" and "severe;" so that proper methods of treatment for the two can be adopted and brought into general use. As little obstetric interference as possible should be employed. Simple medical treatment, carefully regulated and closely watched, gives the best results. The methods of the Rotunda Hospital in the treatment of eclampsia and its study are described by Fitz Gibbon. He believes that the toxemia is the primary complication, and that the division of cases under various heads is purely accidental from the development of one dominant symptom. He does not believe that an abnormal condition in pregnancy is the cause of toxemia. Were this so, the conditions found in the placenta would be practically uniform in these cases. So too would be the results in the fetus. In the early stages of the disease the fetus is well, and it is only when the toxemia is severe that the fetus suffers, and even in a large number of the severe cases the fetus is quite unaffected. The pathological findings in toxemia, eclampsia and toxemic hemorrhage are identical. There is a subacute nephritis with a variable degree of focal necrosis in the other organs, especially in the portal symptom of the liver. There is evidently a common irritant substance excreted by the kidneys, injuring their structure, and affecting the other tissues of the body. Two conditions commonly seen in pregnancy favor toxemia. One is the tendency to overeat and the other constipation. Pregnancy greatly increases the activity of the tissues in the body. This naturally throws an increased burden upon the organs of elimination, and where these are damaged before pregnancy occurs, toxemia early follows. In the greater number of toxemic patients they have gained in weight during pregnancy. This is the result of their taking an excessive quantity of food, until the time comes when the eliminative organs rapidly fail and toxemia and eclampsia develop. The writer had never seen personally, toxemia in a primipara who followed a careful hygienic course, has maintained regular action of the bowels with purgatives if needed, and who had avoided excess of eating. Where patients are seen in early toxemia they can be relieved of the symptoms and carried through a pregnancy without recurrence, by attention to diet and the action of the bowels. If the excretory organs are already damaged, the amount of damage is important. He would summarize the causes of toxemia as deficient elimination, excessive ingestion of food and constipation. In treating toxemia the patient is kept in bed, purged, enemata are given and purgatives are continued, 2 or 3 doses daily being administered. The patient must drink at least 6 pints of water in twenty-four hours. When the symptoms have greatly abated, the secretion of urine has increased, and there is a moderate quantity of albumin only, the patient is allowed to take ½ pint of milk and the diet is very gradually increased without meat. If this goes well the patient is allowed to go to her home and to return to the dispensary for treatment. She must follow diet strictly and must secure at least two movements of the bowels daily by the use of purgatives. If the patient does not respond to treatment sufficiently to be tried on a diet, or if she grows worse in trying to follow the diet, or if at any time the child is found to be dead, labor is brought on. This was never done until the eighth day of treatment, and in all the series of cases, was done only 5 times. One toxemic case died, and it was the intention to interrupt the pregnancy three days before she delivered herself. The patient developed a very severe septic pharyngitis and delay was thought to be safer. The majority of cases with live infants were at term or reached term under treatment and came spontaneously into labor. When there is pronounced vomiting nothing is given by the mouth from twenty-four to forty-eight hours. Enemata are frequently administered, lavage of the colon, and a warm solution of bicarbonate of soda was given under the breasts. At the end of forty-eight hours purgatives can always be given by the mouth. In eclampsia, so soon as possible, the stomach is washed out with bicarbonate solution until the fluid returns clear. A saline mixture and about ¾ of a pint of bicarbonate solution are introduced and left in the stomach. A long rectal tube is passed and carried up into the colon. Its introduction may be difficult and may take as long as thirty minutes. The colon is then irrigated with soapy water until the fluid returns well colored with bowel contents. This may require three or four gallons of fluid. The irrigation is continued until the fluid returns clear, when bicarbonate solution is substituted for the soapy water. Saline and bicarbonate solution are then inserted in the colon through the tube. The process of cleansing the colon may require from 8 to 12 gallons in quantity and one and a half hours in time. This is repeated in five hours and again in five hours if the patient does not return to consciousness sufficiently to drink, or the bowels have not begun to act spontaneously. When the patient recovers consciousness the treatment for toxemia is followed. If labor comes on, delivery is completed when the presenting part reaches the perineum, unless the labor ends spontaneously in a short time. No other interference is practised; while the patient is wholly or partially unconscious she is kept lying on her side, so that fluid may run out of her mouth. If the patient is severely ill, 40 ounces of bicarbonate solution are given under the breasts. Large poultices are placed over the loins and maintained until there is a fair secretion of urine. In few cases did the quantity of morphine given exceed in all 0.5 grain. The writer is convinced that morphine does not control the fits, and that it delays elimination and has a tendency to produce respiratory failure. Under the methods described as above, the Rotunda Hospital in twenty years has treated 214 eclamptics with 19 deaths (8.87 per cent). This includes the death of any woman who suffered from eclampsia without regard to the actual cause or time of the death.

GYNECOLOGY

UNDER THE CHARGE OF

JOHN G. CLARK, M.D.,

PROFESSOR OF GYNECOLOGY IN THE UNIVERSITY OF PENNSYLVANIA, PHILADELPHIA,

AND

FRANK B. BLOCK, M.D.,

INSTRUCTOR IN GYNECOLOGY, MEDICAL SCHOOL, UNIVERSITY OF PENNSYLVANIA, PHILADELPHIA.

Conservative Versus Radical Operation for Myoma.—The use of a intelligent follow-up system is becoming more and more apparent to intelligent surgeons throughout the world since it is only by means of some such system that we can have a clear understanding of the results of our treatment. For example, the question of the advisability of removing both appendages when operating for the cure of a fibroid uterus or a chronic metritis is one that has not yet been settled. Indeed it may never be, except by carefully analyzing the end-results in such cases, as has been done by our British colleague Bride (*Jour. Obstet. and Gynec. of the Brit. Emp.*, 1922, **29**, 68). By such methods we shall have some definite facts upon which to base our opinions, rather than by merely stating opinions *per se*. In his series of three hundred cases the most striking feature in comparing the results of the two procedures, *i. e.*, ovarian ablation or conservatism, is the fact that there is so little difference in the percentage of adverse symptoms after either type. One would expect to find the adverse symptoms of the artificial menopause very much more marked after the radical operation, and to find few, if any, after the conservative procedure. With regard to the flushings and the effect on the patient's sexual feelings, there is certainly a larger percentage suffering after the radical operation, and in a lesser degree the physical capabilities of patients seem better after the conservative than after the radical operation. In this investigation the general health was improved in a very large percentage of cases after either operation, but there was a distinct preponderance after the radical operation—91 to 84 per cent. The temperament of the patients after either operation does not seem to have been much affected, but a slightly higher percentage complained of irritability after the conservative than after the radical procedure in the proportion of 28 to 26 per cent. This again is slightly in favor of the radical operation. There is a greater frequency of flushings after the radical than after the conservative operation, although whichever procedure be adopted, a very large percentage of patients will suffer from flushings and sweats for a certain period of time; the less marked as a rule, the more the ovarian tissue that has been preserved. What is surprising is not that 91 per cent had flushes after the radical operation, but that 73 per cent had them after the conservative operation. Pain was noted more frequently after the conservative operation than after the radical in the proportion of 18 to 7 per cent, which seems to the writer to be one of the strongest pleas for the radical operation. Information about the effect of the removal of both ovaries on the sexual relationships of patients is difficult to obtain, but this series shows that these are more disturbed when both ovaries are removed than when some ovarian tissue is left, nearly 40 per cent as compared with 27 per cent: 15 per cent of these radical cases suffered from dyspareunia, chiefly due to narrowing of the vagina from atrophic changes. Briefly summarizing, the author believes that so far as the majority of the manifestations of the artificial menopause are concerned, there is very little to choose between the two types of operation. The advantage lies with the radical operation in every way except the occurrence of flushes and the sexual disability, and the surgeon must decide whether the advantages of the radical operation outweigh these disadvantages, since the radical procedure is easier, quicker and therefore safer for the patient. Furthermore, the final result is better as there remains afterward a smoothly peritonized pelvic floor with a linear scar and there is less risk of the formation of adhesions. Most important of all, the possibility of the ovaries undergoing such pathologic changes as to render necessary a second operation for their removal is done away with.

Milk Therapy of Pelvic Infections.—GELLHORN (*Jour. Missouri State Med. Assn.*, 1922, **19**, 341) calls attention to the fact that from observations made in almost all fields of practical medicine the conclusion has been reached that protein substances, introduced "parenterally," that is, by subcutaneous, intramuscular or intravenous injection, have the faculty of stimulating the cells to greater activity. All cells of the body feel this rejuvenating influence, but none more so than those cells which have been weakened or paralyzed by infection. The protoplasm again develops phagocytic properties, the toxins are neutralized by a fresh production of antibodies and ferments, the local metabolism is intensified, and the pus is absorbed. Under favorable circumstances the infected organ or tissue may thus rid itself of its enemy and normal conditions may be reëstablished. It stands to reason that only those cells can take up the fight for existence with any prospect for success that have not yet hopelessly been damaged, and as a matter of fact, practical experience has shown that foreign protein therapy gives a promise of cure largely in subacute and early chronic cases of salpingitis and pyosalpinx and is apt to fail in cases of very long standing. While this struggle goes on beyond the reach of our eyes, yet there are indications and outward manifestations to the effect that these protein injections have made themselves felt. In most cases there are chills and fever soon after the injections, or there may be nausea or headache. This is the general reaction as distinguished from the local reaction which occurs in the affected part itself and consists of a transitory increase of local pain and occasionally a brief increase in the size of the inflammatory tumors. A number of proteins have been recommended and used to advantage, but the writer has confined his work to the use of milk. The technic is exceedingly simple. Five cubic centimeters of sterilized milk are injected into the gluteal musculature and the injections are repeated at intervals of from three to five days. The amount injected is gradually increased to 10 cc. The average number of injections in the writer's series was eight, although 1 patient received as many as twelve. The injections are not painful and anaphylactic shock has not been observed. Of 10 cases of gonorrhea of the tubes, 6 were cured completely; of these, 2 had large tumors which disappeared entirely; 2 patients were improved and 2 patients were unimproved. Three other patients with rather rare pathologic conditions in the pelvis were cured or materially benefited by the milk injections. It appears that mainly the tubes, the uterus, and possibly the bladder, are favorably influenced by foreign protein therapy. The ovaries seem to remain refractory. Exudates are brought to absorption, but adhesions are left undisturbed. This report of the author is of interest both as a curiosity and as a new method of treatment. However, inasmuch as he states that the treatment is applicable mainly to recent inflammations of the tubes, which very frequently tend toward spontaneous resolution, the editor cannot help but look upon this new trick as perhaps another *post hoc ergo propter hoc.*

Ovarian Organotherapy.—In judging the results of ovarian therapy, most of us have unconsciously succumbed to the familiar "post hoc propter hoc" error, states NOVAK (*Endocrinology*, 1922, **6**, 599) who has made an intensive survey of the literature on the subject in recent times. He believes that if there is any field of medicine in which a healthy skepticism is urgently needed, it is that of endocrinology, and more particulary that of endocrine therapy. Incalculable harm has been done by the trashy superficiality, the ignorance, and, at times, the commercialism which are reflected in much of the enormous literature which has grown up, mushroom-like, within the past decade or so. Especially unfortunate has been the influence of several books published quite recently. We must resign ourselves to the fact that future progress in endocrinology, including, of course, organotherapy, will be a slow developmental process, as it has been in all other branches of medical science. It will mean a tedious search for truth on the part of many men from many lands. Each year will add a few nuggets of knowledge, and now and then a bigger find will spur all the searchers to renewed efforts. It cannot be said that there has been any noteworthy advance in ovarian therapy in the quarter century and more which has elapsed since its introduction. This is especially true as applied to the preparation of the commercial extracts upon which the profession as a whole is dependent. The stellar role in the future development of this branch of organotherapy will unquestionably be played by the biological chemist. The time will almost surely come when we shall be able to place in the patient's circulation the specific secretions of the ovary or corpus luteum, as we now can of the thyroid, and when we shall not be obliged to strain the imagination to see good results from ovarian therapy. The foregoing words of caution from Novak, while admittedly skeptical, are none the less of great value at the present time, happily being in marked contrast to the numerous overenthusiastic reports along this line, many of which are made by careless observers and cannot stand the glare of the scientific searchlight.

OPHTHALMOLOGY

UNDER THE CHARGE OF

EDWARD JACKSON, A.M., M.D.,
DENVER, COLORADO,

AND

T. B. SCHNEIDEMAN, A.M., M.D.,
PHILADELPHIA.

Clinical Significance of Dark Adaptation.—SCHINDLER (*Klin. Monatsbl. f. Augenh.*, June, 1922, p. 710), based upon personal research, substantiates in general Behr's claims as to the behavior of dark adaptation in various diseases of the optic nerve and the basal visual paths. Behr states that inflammatory and chronically degenerative processes markedly lower dark adaptation, whereas processes acting more mechanically upon the optic nerve and the basal visual path, such as tumors, hemorrhages, etc., either do not influence dark adaptation at all or only to a slight extent. Examination of the adaptation may assist in the early differential diagnosis between papillitis and choked disk; such examination may point to early neuritis where the differentiation between neuritis and pseudoneuritis is in question. It may suggest the prognosis in retrobulbar neuritis; it is also of value for the recognition of probable tabetic atrophy in that disturbance of dark adaptation is a constant symptom in this affection. In functional ocular complaints and sympathetic irritation the adaptation test is without value; its normal occurrence in eclampsia bespeaks congestive conditions at the nerve. As regards the value of the examination for clinical purposes, it is not absolutely necessary, not being indispensable either for diagnosis or for therapy; neither is it always reliable, as it demands much time and patience on the part of both physician and patient, and is so largely dependent upon the attention and intelligence of the latter. At the same time the test is of great value clinically in that it supplements the data otherwise determined and enlarges our knowledge of the physiology and pathology of vision.

Syphilis of the Orbit.—RAFFIN (*Klin. Monats. f. Augenhk*, May, 1921, p. 747) refers to the rarity of syphilis of the orbit, amounting in the statistics of Birch-Hirschfeld to but 0.013 per cent of all diseases of the eye. The affection frequently resembles the clinical picture of numerous other diseases of the orbit, especially tumor; for this reason, and from its rarity, its significance frequently remains unrecognized. The periosteum is almost invariably the primary seat of the affection, while the bone is involved only secondarily. The affection presents itself either as an exudative hyperplastic periostitis with thickening of the periosteum, or else as a gummous periostitis with circumscribed nodes of soft, gummous or firmer consistence. The hyperplastic inflammation occurs usually in the late secondary period, the gummous in the tertiary period. Clinically periostitis of the orbital margin can be differentiated from disease of the deeper portion. Every variety of transition occurs between slight, hardly demonstrable thickening of the orbital margin and the formation of circumscribed nodes within the orbit. Three symptoms are of diagnostic importance: Severe cephalalgia with nocturnal aggravation, sensitiveness to pressure at the affected portion of the orbital wall, and, finally, the therapeutic test. The presence of other symptoms of lues is, of course, important; the Wassermann reaction is generally strongly positive.

Diabetic Retinitis.—ONFRAY (*Ann. d'Oculist*, August, 1922, p. 599) summarizes a study of diabetic retinitis with reference to life and vision. He concludes that nine-tenths of diabetics affected with retinitis show vascular hypertension and renal insufficiency, that in half of these patients the renal insufficiency is only just commencing. These patients may be divided into two classes by measuring the vascular tension and by study of the coefficient of urea elimination. Untreated, such cases are liable to a fatal issue in two or three years; subjected to a hypotensile regimen, they may survive five, six and even ten years. Although complete blindness is rare, the prognosis as to sight is grave in all.

PATHOLOGY AND BACTERIOLOGY

UNDER THE CHARGE OF

OSKAR KLOTZ, M.D., C.M.,

DIRECTOR OF THE PATHOLOGICAL LABORATORIES, SAO PAULO, BRAZIL,

AND

DE WAYNE G. RICHEY, B.S., M.D.,

ASSISTANT PROFESSOR OF PATHOLOGY, UNIVERSITY OF PITTSBURGH, PITTSBURGH, PA.

Effect of Hemorrhage on Complement of Blood.—Although it is known that, after hemorrhage, the leukocytes begin to increase within ten minutes, followed by an increase in platelets, that the red cells are made up much more slowly and that the hemoglobin content is the last to return to normal, the relation between these changes and the complementing power of the blood have not been studied. Accordingly, ECKER and REES (*Jour. Infect. Dis.*, 1922, **31**, 361) conducted several experiments to ascertain the changes induced in the complement of the blood of guinea-pigs "by profound and multiple hemorrhages and subsequent blood regeneration and what, if any, were the relations of this change to changes in the cellular elements." By carefully controlling the hematological counts and titrations, before and after bleeding the animals, it was found that complement has a regular curve of decrease and regeneration following a single severe hemorrhage, whereas repeated bleedings, causing extreme degrees of anemia with subsequent recovery, did not alter the level of complement. The complement curve was unaffected by later dilution of the blood by the body fluids. This complement curve did not run parallel to that of any of the cellular elements of the blood nor was there any evidence that any of these cells were a factor in the regeneration of complement. The initial decrease was due to dilution of the blood and was soon overcome and restored to normal by an influx of complement from an unknown source.

Experimental Measles by Inoculation of Monkeys, Guinea-pigs and Rabbits with a Green-producing Diplococcus.—Having described previously a small Gram-positive diplococcus which was isolated from the blood, eye, nose, throat and sputum of patients with measles, during the preëruptive and early eruptive stage of the disease, TUNNICLIFF (*Jour. Infect. Dis.*, 1922, **31**, 382) conducted several experiments on monkeys, guinea-pigs and rabbits, by inoculating these animals intravenously and intratracheally with washings of the nose and throat of patients with measles and with the green-producing diplococci isolated from the blood and respiratory passages of human measles, as well as with control bacteria. It was ascertained that monkeys, guinea-pigs and rabbits were susceptible to measles when the nasopharyngeal washings were introduced and that the same symptoms and lesions might be produced in these animals by the green-producing diplococci. Those rabbits which were inoculated successfully with washings of the diplococci showed no symptoms when reinoculated with fresh virus. The green-producing diplococci from the blood and lung of rabbits which were successfully inoculated with diplococci from measles, produced Koplik spots and exanthems when introduced into other rabbits. Berkefeld N-candle filtrates of the diplococcus cultures, as a rule, showed abundant growth, but old cultures containing large forms sometimes multiplied only after several days incubation or on subculture into a favorable medium. The authoress concludes that "while the experiments indicate that the reaction is due to the coccus itself, and not to a separate virus carried by it, on account of the same symptoms being produced by cultures as late as the seventh generation and the absence of the reaction in rabbits injected with other bacteria isolated from the same plate as the green-producing diplococci, it is possible that the diplococcus possesses the selective power of carrying the specific virus of measles."

Studies upon Experimental Measles. I. The Effects of the Virus of Measles upon the Guinea-pig—Since the demonstration of the virus of measles in the circulating blood by Hektoen and the evidence that the virus is a filter-passer by Goldberg and Anderson, Blake and Trask have added to and confirmed previous knowledge at a time when Sellards shook our confidence in the earlier experimental findings. More recently, DUVAL and D'AUNOY (*Jour. Exp. Med.*, 1922, **37**, 257) conducted various experiments to determine the transmissibility of measles virus from man to the guinea-pig, the possibility of propagation of the virus from guinea-pig to guinea-pig, the effect of such passage on virulence and the relative infectivity of blood obtained from the prodromal, preëruptive, eruptive, and convalescent stages of the human disease. The human blood was collected by syringe, defibrinated and injected into the circulation within fifteen or twenty minutes by cardiopuncture in amounts of 1 or 2 cc. It was found that the guinea-pigs reacted specifically to the intracardiac inoculations of the defibrinated blood from human measles cases, there being a constant rise in temperature and coincident leukopenia after an incubation period of nine to twelve days. This reaction occurred with blood obtained during a period corresponding approximately to the eruptive stage. Those animals which reacted and recovered were not susceptible to reinoculation with measles blood if tested over periods of two weeks to three months after recovery. From the constancy of the reaction, the authors concluded that the virus could be propagated by passage from infected guinea-pig to normal guinea-pig, that such passage apparently increased virulence, death resulting from acute hemorrhagic nephritis, and that intercurrent or secondary infection played no part. Attempts to cultivate the virus were unsuccessful. Later, (*Jour. Exp. Med.*, 1922, **36**, 231) the same authors report observations following inoculation of defibrinated human blood from measles cases into the ear vein of rabbits. A specific reaction analogous in all essential features to that of the human infection was encountered in the experimental animals, which showed after an incubation period of from two to five days definite pyrexia, leukopenia and cutaneous manifestations, consisting of exanthemata and enanthemata, the latter closely resembling the Koplik spots seen in man. Repeated passage of the virus through rabbits seemed to increase its virulence. Here again, those animals, dying presumably as a result of the specific virus, showed grave nephritic changes. The pneumonia so frequently observed in fatal human cases of measles was not seen in the rabbit, a fact which the authors explain "purely on the basis of the destruction of normal defense barriers by the specific excitant of the infectious disease, and the lack of resistance to the ordinary pyogenic microorganism." In a third communication, (*Jour. Exp. Med.*, 1922, **36**, 239), these investigators found that Berkefeld-N filtrates of washings of nasopharyngeal secretions obtained from cases of the human disease at the height of the cutaneous reaction, when injected directly into the trachea or vein of guinea-pigs or rabbits, occasioned a definite and constant reaction. This reaction was characterized "by a complex of objective and subjective signs which very closely resembled the manifestations in man of the acute infectious disease measles." The incubation period for guinea-pigs ranged from nine to fourteen days, while rabbits reacted in from two to seven days, on an average of four days. The reaction consisted, in rabbits, of enanthem, exanthem and fever and, in guinea-pigs, of fever, marked leukopenia and grave nephritis in fatal cases. In other words, the findings following intratracheal and intracirculatory injections of nasopharyngeal secretions secured from human cases of measles were very similar to those obtained when defibrinated blood from human measles cases was introduced into the blood stream of rabbits and guinea pigs.

Pathological Lesions Produced in the Kidney by Small Doses of Mercuric Chloride.—On intravenous injection of mercuric chloride in concentration as low as 0.002 mg. per kilogram of weight, MENTEN (*Jour. Med. Res.*, 1922, **43**, 315) obtained well developed pathological changes in the proximal convoluted tubules and the ascending limb of the loop of Henle of rabbits' kidneys. These changes developed immediately following injection. Attention was called to the possibility of similar degenerative changes resulting from the intravenous use of therapeutic preparations of trivalent mercury.

HYGIENE AND PUBLIC HEALTH

UNDER THE CHARGE OF

MILTON J. ROSENAU, M.D.,

PROFESSOR OF PREVENTIVE MEDICINE AND HYGIENE, HARVARD MEDICAL SCHOOL, BOSTON, MASSACHUSETTS,

AND

GEORGE W. McCOY, M.D.,

DIRECTOR OF HYGIENIC LABORATORY, UNITED STATES PUBLIC HEALTH SERVICE, WASHINGTON, D. C.

School Health Supervision Based Upon Age and Sex Incidence of Physical Defects.—Baker (*Am. Jour. of Public Health*, 1922, **12**, 465) concludes as a result of his study that: (1) The most important physical examination to be made in the school life of the child is the one occurring at the time the child enters school for the first time. (2) In order to make the work of health supervision of school children effective, a complete physical examination of each child should be made before the eight to ten-year period. If this can be done with 100 per cent efficiency, combined with follow-up that is 100 per cent effective and 100 per cent of treatments obtained, it should not be necessary to make regular physical examinations after the eight to ten-year period, reliance being placed after that time upon the routine inspection of the children in the classroom. This routine inspection will permit the nurse, doctor or teacher to pick out the cases of physical defects that have been in any way overlooked during routine physical examinations or which have originated after the eight to ten-year period. (3) An annual test for defective vision is desirable. (4) Unless the amount of money appropriated for school medical inspection is large enough to allow a complete and thorough physical examination each school year, the officials in charge of such work are not justified in spending any money in having physical examinations made after the eight to ten-year period unless the full health needs of the children below that age period have been met. (5) A logical deduction that might be drawn from this study is that great emphasis should be placed hereafter upon the preschool age period as the time when physical defects should be prevented or corrected. (6) To sum up the matter, the study would seem to show that the expenditure of time and money to make annual physical examinations of school children is not warranted and seems to be unnecessary. Analysis of the age and sex incidence of physical defects in this study shows that proper and adequate physical examinations made in the early life of the school child—that is, before the eight to ten-year period—are essential, and if these are properly followed up and suitable treatment obtained, the appropriation for this work will be spent in the most economical way, the child's health will be more thoroughly protected and future disease and the sequelæ of physical defects be more adequately guarded against then by any of the present methods of school health supervision.

Analysis of 123 Cases of Anthrax in the Pennsylvania Leather Industry.—SMYTH and BRICKER (*Jour. Ind. Hyg.*, 1922, **4**, 53) report 123 cases of anthrax connected with the tanning industry in the twelve years from 1910 to 1921, inclusive. They state this number represents almost 12 per cent of the directly exposed employees. The mortality among these 123 cases was over 21 per cent. In the five-year period, for which accurate statistics were obtained (1916–1920, inclusive), there was a yearly morbidity rate of almost 2 per cent of the directly exposed employees. The directly exposed employees include those handling raw stock and those soaking and lining this stock. Anthrax has been contracted from the handling of non-packer cattle hides from Texas, Mexico, China, India and South America, and from goat skins from many regions. Anthrax has been contracted from the handling of both dry and wet, salted hides and skins, and from both certified and uncertified stock, and anthrax bacilli have been isolated from both. The present practice of certification offers little or no protection to the tanner. The mortality of cases treated in hospitals has been considerably less than one-half that of unhospitalized cases. In Pennsylvania apparently the best results of treatment have been obtained by the injection of strong phenol solutions (25 to 50 per cent) locally around the area of the initial lesion, with or without excision of the lesion. The use of antianthrax serum with excision of the local lesion has also given excellent results and its use should not be discontinued. The authors advocate a continued intensive use of a reliable serum, subcutaneously or intravenously, combined with excision of the local lesion and the injection of concentrated phenol solution around the wound. Early diagnosis, prompt hospitalization, if possible, and absolute rest are essential for success in any form of treatment. Anthrax continues to be a decided menace to both the cattle-hide and goat-skin tanner, and will continue to be so until some method is developed whereby tanneries cease to receive anthrax-infested, raw stock. Seymour-Jones advocates for England the prohibition of the importation of any raw stock not previously converted to the wet salt state by means of his formic acid and mercuric chloride method. Whatever method may be finally adopted, the authors state, they feel very strongly that all undisinfected imported stock should be disinfected at one or more centrally located government disinfecting stations before being shipped to the tanners, as the English government is doing at present with wool and hair.

Notice to Contributors.—All communications intended for insertion in the Original Department of this JOURNAL are received only *with the distinct understanding that they are contributed exclusively to this* JOURNAL.

Contributions from abroad written in a foreign language, if on examination they are found desirable for this JOURNAL, will be translated at its expense.

A limited number of reprints in pamphlet form, if desired, will be furnished to authors, *providing the request for them be written on the manuscript.*

All communications should be addressed to—

DR. JOHN H. MUSSER, JR., 262 S. 21st Street, Philadelphia, Pa., U. S. A.

THE

AMERICAN JOURNAL

OF THE MEDICAL SCIENCES

MAY, 1923

ORIGINAL ARTICLES.

TETANY IN THE ADULT, WITH SPECIAL REFERENCE TO ALKALOSIS AND CALCIUM METABOLISM.*

By Wilder Tileston, M.D.,

and

Frank P. Underhill, Ph.D.,

(From the Departments of Internal Medicine and of Pharmacology and Toxicology, Yale University, New Haven, Conn.)

Tetany in the adult occurs in two forms, one endemic in certain parts of Europe and apparently primary in character, the other secondary and occurring in the course of various morbid conditions, especially in connection with disease of the gastro-intestinal tract. We have to report observations on 3 cases of tetany, all of the secondary form.

Case I.—*An Italian woman,† aged thirty-five years, suffering from Weil's disease with acute nephritis and acidosis, is given large amounts of sodium bicarbonate, with a diet poor in calcium. After nine days of alkali treatment, tetany develops, the CO_2 combining power of the blood having risen from 21 to 80 volumes per cent. Recovery.*

This patient, an Italian woman, aged thirty-five years entered the New Haven Hospital, December 17, 1916 (No. 60131), in the

* Presented at the Annual Meeting of the Association of American Physicians, May 2, 1922.

† Reported by one of us (Tileston) at the Annual Meeting of the Am. Soc. for Clinical Investigation, May 1, 1917, and cited by Palmer and Van Slyke, Jour. Biol. Chem., 1917, 32, 499.

service of Dr. H. S. Arnold, to whom we are indebted for the privilege of reporting the case.

Past History. Was negative except for the occurrence of abortion in all of her four pregnancies (Wassermann negative).

Present Illness. The onset was sudden, with fever, ten days previous to admission. She was getting better when on the seventh day jaundice developed. There was diarrhea, with watery stools of a brownish color.

Physical Examination. At entrance showed a well developed and well nourished woman with fever (temperature 103.5°), marked jaundice, and enlargement of the spleen, which was palpable 3 cm. below the costal margin. The liver extended 3 cm. below the ribs.

The blood showed a leukocyte count of 17,200, of which 92 per cent were polymorphonuclears. There was a marked anemia of the secondary type, the red cell count being 2,800,000 and the hemoglobin 55 per cent (Talqvist). The stools were a bright yellowish-brown in color, and gave a very intense reaction for urobilin. The urine at entrance was clear and showed only the slightest possible trace of albumin, and no casts. Bile and urobilin were present in large amounts.

A few days after admission signs of acute nephritis developed, with albumin up to $\frac{1}{3}$ of 1 per cent, granular casts and red cells. The diagnosis of Weil's disease was made on the basis of the presence of the cardinal symptoms, viz.; febrile jaundice, enlargement of the spleen and albuminuria. No search was made for the spirochæta ictero-hemorrhagica.

The temperature fell by lysis, reaching normal on the thirteenth day of the disease, but it rose again two days later, owing to a colon bacillus pyelitis, the result of catheterization. Three days after admission, on December 20, there was nearly complete suppression of the urine, with air-hunger. The non-protein nitrogen of the blood on this day was 178 mg. per 100 cc and the phenolsulphonephthalein output (on the 25th) was only 10 per cent in two hours. The CO_2 combining power of the blood was 21 volumes per cent by the Van Slyke method, indicating a high degree of acidosis, the normal figures ranging from 50 to 60.

The next day the deep breathing continued, and an intravenous injection of 500 cc of a 5 per cent solution of sodium bicarbonate was made. The effect was striking, the dyspnea disappearing completely within twenty-four hours. The CO_2 combining power four hours later was 25.5, and on the 22nd, it had risen to 38. Sodium bicarbonate was given by the mouth, and on the 26th a second intravenous dose of 20 gm. was injected.

The non-protein nitrogen of the blood having risen to 212 mg., on the 26th, the patient was put on a diet poor in nitrogen, and incidentally, also very poor in calcium, with the intention of combating the azotemia. This diet consisted of 6 lemons, 200 gm.

of sugar and 1000 cc of water per twenty-four hours. It caused vomiting, and on the 27th, nothing but water was given. On this day the CO_2 combining power was 80, indicating a considerable increase of the sodium bicarbonate. She had had in all 45 gm. of sodium bicarbonate intravenously and 83 gm. by mouth, in the course of nine days. The temperature was normal.

In the evening of the same day signs of tetany developed. Examination the following morning (the 28th) showed the elbows and wrists flexed and stiff, the fingers flexed at the metacarpophalangeal joints and extended at the others, the thumbs turned in and hyperextended; in short, the classical picture of tetany. The feet showed a similar condition. There was a marked Chvostek sign. Calcium lactate (gr. xx every four hours) and milk were prescribed. During the night of the 28th, two general convulsions occurred, accompanied by screaming. On the 29th, spontaneous spasm had disappeared, but Trousseau's and Chvostek's signs were easily elicited. By the first of January all signs of tetany were gone. The patient made a slow recovery, with gradual disappearance of the jaundice and of the splenic tumor, and was discharged convalescent February 11, 1917.

Discussion. An interesting feature was the remarkably high output of nitrogen in the urine, which began on December 25. During the six-day period from December 27 to January 2, no less than 318 gm. were excreted, or a daily average of 53 gm., on a diet of only moderate protein content. A high non-protein nitrogen of the blood, or "azotemia" has been noted of late in spirochetal jaundice by various French writers.

A somewhat similar instance of tetany occurring after the administration of soda was reported by Harrop[1] in 1919. His case, a colored woman, aged twenty-two years, was suffering from acute mercurial poisoning, with acidosis and suppression of urine. After two intravenous injections of sodium bicarbonate, totalling 60 gm., she developed tetany; the CO_2 combining power of the blood was 80 volumes per cent, and the calcium of the blood serum was "higher than 9 mg. per 100 cc, hence about normal."

Howland and Marriott[2] remark that it is not unusual for tetany to develop in children after the administration of soda for acidosis, and report 3 illustrative cases. In all of them, in contrast to Harrop's case in an adult, the calcium of the serum was much diminished.

Healy[3] saw a series of 6 cases of tetany, 4 of them fatal, developing after gynecological operations in women who had received enemata containing, by mistake, 80 gm. each of sodium bicarbonate. The patients received one enema immediately after operation, and a second four hours later. The 2 cases which recovered were treated with calcium.

Blum[4] recognized the danger of large intravenous injections of soda in diabetic coma, having observed 4 cases in which clonic and tonic spasms developed; though he did not mention tetany, it is probable that the condition was of that nature.

It is evident however that simply increasing the blood alkali is not sufficient to induce tetany; thus to a diabetic man under our observation, who had been operated upon for strangulated hernia, sodium bicarbonate was administered by rectum, to the amount of 49 gm. in two days, and the CO_2 combining power of the blood was raised to 86, yet tetany did not develop, nor could the signs of Trousseau and Chvostek be elicited. P. S. Henderson[5] was unable to produce tetany in children by giving large doses of soda, and the electrical reactions remained unaltered.

It is probable that a second important factor in the production of tetany in such cases is the presence of renal insufficiency, which has been noted in most instances.

CASE II.—*A woman, aged forty-six years, develops tetany following influenza. She is emaciated and suffers from intestinal indigestion with constipation. She has had two previous attacks of tetany. The CO_2 combining power of the blood is 77 volumes per cent, indicating a definite increase in the sodium bicarbonate. The serum calcium, estimated later during a period of latent tetany, is normal.*

Mrs. C., an American woman, aged forty-six years, was first seen by one of us, in the course of private practice, on March 30, 1919, at her home.

Family History. Unimportant.

Past History. She had had two previous attacks of tetany, both unrecognized. The first occurred five years ago while she was convalescing from grippe, the second one year ago after an enema, while suffering from intestinal indigestion. Twelve years ago she had valvular heart disease following acute articular rheumatism, and has been somewhat short of breath on exertion ever since. She has always been poorly nourished, and far from robust. Fifteen years ago she had nervous prostration, and four years ago mucous colitis.

Present Illness. Six weeks ago she had influenza, and has been in bed ever since. During this time she had been on an inadequate diet, very low in calcium, consisting of rice-gruel and Mellen's food, both made up without milk, and of broth. For eight days there was nausea, but no vomiting. The bowels were constipated, and had been moved by enemata. The last catamenia occurred in January (beginning menopause).

Twelve days ago she began to suffer from attacks of numbness and stiffness of the fingers, during which they became flexed. Four days ago, following an enema, she had an attack lasting two hours, in which the legs, arms and back got very rigid. Similar seizures occurred after enemata, three days ago, and again this morning.

Physical Examination. Small, emaciated woman. The thyroid gland was normal. The heart was not enlarged; there was a loud, late systolic murmur at the apex, transmitted to the axilla and to the back. The lungs were negative except for an occasional sonorous rale. The abdomen was negative. The blood-pressure was 94 systolic, 70 diastolic. The superficial and deep reflexes were normal. Trousseau's sign was strongly positive; the Chvostek phenomenon was absent. The urine showed no albumin, sugar or indican; the stools were foul and constipated.

The CO_2 combining power of the blood on March 30, was 77 volumes per cent by the Van Slyke method (Dr. H. W. Haggard). This indicates a distinct increase of the sodium bicarbonate of the blood. The blood sugar was 0.1 per cent, by the Lewis-Benedict method.

The electrical reactions were taken later, and showed the following:

Date.	C. C. C.	A. C. C.	A. O. C.	CC tetanus.
May 16	0.8	1.8	1.2	3.5
May 25	1.0	1.9	2.1	4.0

The cathodal closing tetanus at less than 5 ma. may be taken as indicative of tetany, in the absence of organic disease of the central nervous system; the anodal reversal, while significant in young children, is not infrequently found in healthy adults. The patient was taking 40 grains of calcium chloride a day on the 16th, but the dose was probably too small to affect the reactions; on the 25th, no calcium had been taken for nine days.

The *serum calcium* on May 20, during a period of latent tetany, was 11.3 mg. per 100 cc by the Marriott-Howland method (Dr. L. J. Bogert). This is a normal figure. No calcium had been taken for four days.

The patient was put on a calcium-rich diet consisting of milk, cereals and spinach, and was given calcium chloride, 20 grains, four times a day. Under this regimen the major attacks ceased, but a condition of latent tetany remained, as shown by the occasional occurrence of slight spasms in the right hand, and by a slight Trousseau sign, when the dose of calcium was reduced.

The diet was gradually extended and the patient gained slowly in weight up to 105 pounds. A tendency to stiffness and numbness of the right hand persisted for several months. Up to the present time (1923) she has had no recurrence of tetany.

Comment. Points of interest are the moderate increase in the sodium bicarbonate and the normal figure for the serum calcium, the latter, to be sure, estimated at a time when the tetany was latent, not active.

It will be noted that two of the three attacks of tetany followed acute infections. The exciting cause of attacks was often the taking of enemata, possibly by reflex action from pressure on nerves while on the bedpan.

CASE III.—*An Italian woman, aged thirty-five years, has had for six months fatty diarrhea with marked loss of weight, following influenza. The cause of the diarrhea was not ascertained. Frequent attacks of tetany. Blood analysis shows a high sodium bicarbonate and very low calcium. Study of the calcium metabolism reveals distinct abnormalities. Large quantities of indican in the urine. Progressive emaciation and death four months after onset of tetany.*

A. B., an Italian woman, aged thirty-five years, was first admitted to the New Haven Hospital, April 25, 1919 (No. 71311), discharged May 18, readmitted June 3, (No. 71724) and discharged July 17, 1919. She was on the service of Prof. George Blumer, to whom we are indebted for the privilege of studying the case.

Present Illness. In October, 1918, she had influenza with pleuritic friction rub and persistent cough; she was in bed eight weeks and lost a great deal of weight. Previous to this time she had had diarrhea occasionally, but after the influenza, attacks of diarrhea became very frequent, accompanied by vague generalized abdominal pain, and alternating with short periods of constipation. About four weeks ago she began to have cramps in the feet, hands and neck, lasting for part of a day. Last menstruation four months ago.

Past History. Negative. There were six normal pregnancies.

Family History. Unimportant.

Physical Examination. On April 26 showed a small emaciated woman, weighing only 71 pounds (unimportant details are omitted). Temperature, pulse and respiration normal. The visceral examination was negative. The thyroid gland was small, the isthmus and left lobe were not palpable, the right lobe appeared smaller than usual. There was a constant fine tremor of the upper lip and of the left lower eyelid (later on both sides). Trousseau's sign positive on both sides. Chvostek's sign negative, but was obtained later. The knee jerks and Achilles reflexes absent with reinforcement, the plantar reflexes were also absent. (Later the knee-jerks were obtained, but much diminished.)

The electrical examinations are given below; they showed consistently cathodal closing tetanus with currents much under 5 ma.

Date	C. C. C.	A. C. C.	A O C.	CC tetanus.
May 2	0.4	1.8	0 8	0.7
May 15	0.7	2.3	0 9	1.3
June 4	0.5	1.1	0.8	0.9
June 24	0.8	2.0	1.8	1.5
July 10	0.8	2.0	1.5	1 0

Laboratory Examinations. The blood Wassermann was negative. The urine was negative on routine examination.

Blood. The CO_2 combining power of the blood on April 30, was 90 volumes per cent by the Van Slyke method (Dr. H. W. Haggard), indicating a marked increase in the sodium bicarbonate. (The patient had been taking trifling amounts of soda, up to 2 gm. in twenty-four hours.) The serum calcium by the Marriott-Howland method was 6 mg. per 100 cc on May 10, and 5.4 mg. on May 14 (Dr. L. J. Bogert). Two normal controls showed 10 and 9.5 mg. respectively. The red count was 4,500,000 hemoglobin 68 per cent, leukocytes 10,200, differential count normal.

The stools were liquid throughout the patient's stay in the hospital, about three a day, with a strong rancid odor; they showed many globules of neutral fat and fatty acid crystals, many undigested muscle fibers but no starch. Pus and blood were absent. The trypsin content by the Gross method was 50 units and 250 units on two occasions.

Stomach contents one hour after an Ewald test breakfast: amount 40 cc, total acidity 22, free hydrochloric acid 7, lactic acid and blood absent.

The renal function was good, as indicated by a phthalein excretion of 70 per cent in two hours.

Roentgen-ray examinations of the gastro-intestinal tract and of the lungs were essentially negative.

A number of typical attacks of tetany were observed in the hospital, involving at first only the hands, which assumed the "accoucheur" position, later the feet also. The attacks were controlled at first by dilute HCl (f℥i, three times a day) which was not well tolerated, then by calcium chloride (30 grains, three times a day), for which calcium lactate (40 grains four times a day) was substituted later. A condition of latent tetany persisted, as indicated by the electrical reactions, and by the fact that the attacks recurred when calcium was omitted.

The tremor of the eyelids, so conspicuous a feature in the tetany following parathyroidectomy in dogs, was noted repeatedly, but disappeared under the administration of calcium.

Course of the Disease. The patient continued to lose weight regularly, and became extremely emaciated, the weight falling from 71 pounds on April 28, to 55 pounds on July 16. The diarrhea persisted, except for a period when she was at home for a fortnight between admissions. Large doses of pancreatin and calcium carbonate (45 grains of each three times a day) acted favorably, resulting in a formed stool, with disappearance of the rancid odor and of the acid reaction. But after a while the patient refused to take it, and it was omitted.

She left the hospital July 17, and died at home August 25, 1919. Permission to perform an autopsy was refused.

Diagnosis. The diagnosis of tetany is evident, and requires no discussion. The underlying cause was apparently an obscure disease of the gastro-intestinal tract associated with diarrhea. Disease of the pancreas seemed likely on account of the marked disturbance of fat absorption and the improvement with pancreatin. But the presence of trypsin in the stools in considerable amount is against complete absence of the pancreatic secretion, and in the absence of an autopsy the diagnosis must remain uncertain.

A study of the *calcium metabolism* was made, the details of which are published elsewhere.[6] Three five-day periods were employed, the first and last on a calcium-poor diet, the second on a diet rich in calcium by reason of the addition of milk. Two normal subjects under the same experimental conditions were available for comparison.

The *calcium balance* was slightly negative in the first period, but during the calcium-rich period there was a retention of nearly 3 gm. During the third (calcium-poor) period the stored calcium was partly eliminated, with a negative balance of 1.4 gm. The patient behaved with respect to the calcium balance like a normal person, except that there was a greater tendency to store calcium during the calcium-rich period, and to lose it during the succeeding calcium-poor period. This might indicate an instability in the regulation of calcium in tetany.

A comparison of the figures for the entire fifteen days showed a positive calcium balance of 1.3 gm. in the case of the subject with tetany, as opposed to negative balances of 2.9 gm. in each of the two normal controls.

These results might be taken to indicate a need for calcium on the part of this case of tetany.

The *absorption* of calcium was found to be normal.

The *elimination* of calcium, however, differed from the normal in that in all three periods there was a greatly diminished excretion by way of the kidneys. Thus in the controls 70 per cent of the intake was excreted in the urine during the calcium-poor periods, and 30 per cent during the calcium-rich period, while for the subject with tetany the figures were 10 per cent and 1 per cent respectively, the absolute amounts remaining practically constant at 22 mg. per day during all three periods.

A study of the fat absorption showed the utilization of fat to be very poor, being 78 per cent in the first period, 58 per cent in the second, and 59 per cent in the third. In other words, from 22 to 42 per cent of the fat intake was lost with the feces. These figures are comparable to those met with in total exclusion of the pancreatic secretion from the intestine.

Curiously enough, in spite of the diarrhea and emaciation, the nitrogen balance was positive throughout, and the absorption was unusually good, amounting to 98 per cent of the intake.

The urine analysis showed a high ammonia nitrogen, both relatively and absolutely, the average figures being 22 per cent and 1 gm. per day respectively. The high ammonia is difficult of explanation, for no other evidence of acidosis was to be found, either in the figures for p^H, or for total acidity and organic acids.

The large amounts of indican, indicating increased intestinal putrefaction, are also of interest. A detailed report is to be found in an article by Simpson.[7] It seemed as if the tetany were worse when meat was given and better when it was withheld, but owing to the coincident administration of calcium, these impressions are not conclusive. It has been noted that active tetany is more easily induced in dogs after parathyroidectomy if a meat diet is employed.

Stimulated by the reports of Paton and his coworkers,[8] search was made for guanidine in the urine, using Koch's method. None was found, but a beautifully crystalline salt was isolated in large quantities, which on analysis by P. A. Levene proved to be an ammonium gold salt.

General Discussion. In all of the 3 cases of tetany which we have studied, the sodium bicarbonate of the blood was abnormally high. This is easily explained in the first case by the administration of large amounts of soda. In the second and third cases it is not clear why the bicarbonate was increased. The work of MacCallum[9] is of interest in this connection. He showed that on ligating the pylorus, and removing the HCl by repeated gastric lavage, a condition similar to tetany developed, with marked increase in the blood bicarbonate and diminution of the chlorides; the tetany could be relieved by the administration of sodium chloride. Similar results were obtained by McCann[10] and by Hastings.[11] Loss of HCl by vomiting was not present in our last 2 cases; in the first it may have been a contributory factor.

It is important to note that an increased CO_2 combining power of the blood does not necessarily mean a change in the hydrogen-ion concentration toward the alkaline side, as the increase in bicarbonate can be, and in most cases probably is compensated, so that no change in the reaction of the blood takes place. The term "alkalosis" should be restricted to cases where the p^H of the blood is actually increased.

Interest in the possible relationship of alkalosis to tetany was started by the experimental work of Wilson, Stearns and Thurlow.[12] They found after parathyroidectomy in dogs that the onset of tetany was preceded by a decrease in the hydrogen-ion concentration of the blood, and followed by acidosis. The injection of acids or of calcium relieved the tetany. Their results have been criticized on account of the method employed (Barcroft's dissociation of hemoglobin method). Moreover, their results lack confirmation, for after parathyroidectomy Togawa[13] found acidosis in 10 of

11 dogs, as judged by the CO_2 combining power; Hastings and Murray[14] found a normal alkali reserve and normal p^H of the blood, and MacCallum in two dogs found no alkalosis.

Howland and Marriott[2] found in infantile tetany no increase in the CO_2 combining power of the blood and normal values for p^H.

With the exception of the cases of tetany following the administration of soda, already cited, we have found no published reports of increased CO_2 combining power of the blood in tetany. In future work on tetany of the adult it would seem desirable to determine both the p^H and the bicarbonate of the blood, as well as the calcium, and other elements (Mg, Na. K, P, S).

The relationship of decreased serum calcium to tetany, so well established by MacCallum[15] for tetania parathyreopriva, and by Howland and Marriott[2] for infantile tetany, remains obscure in the case of tetany of the adult, on account of the paucity of observations made by reliable methods. In our third case, and in that of Barach and Murray,[16] there was a notable decrease. In our second case (during a period of latent tetany) and in Harrop's case of tetany after soda, the serum calcium was normal. MacCallum[9] in experimental tetany following ligation of the pylorus found a normal concentration of calcium, and his results should be applicable to the gastric form of tetany in man. Also in the tetany resulting from hyperpnea a normal calcium has been found.

It appears, therefore, that some forms of tetany may occur without any change in the calcium concentration.

From the work of Loeb, Matthews and others* it appears that the excitability of the neuromuscular mechanism varies directly with the ratio $\frac{Na + K}{Ca + Mg}$, so that it is theoretically possible for increased irritability to result either from a decrease of the calcium, or an increase of the sodium. Kramer, Tisdall and Howland[17] have shown that in infantile tetany the increased irritability is due solely to the decrease of calcium, the concentration of magnesium, sodium and potassium in the serum being essentially normal. In the case of tetany following the administration of soda it is probable that the condition is due to the increase in sodium, the calcium remaining normal. Greenwald[18] believes that in these cases it is the increase in the Na ion and not that of the bicarbonate that is responsible.

Greenwald[19] in parathyroidectomized dogs found an increase of the phosphorus of the blood, and Binger[20] was able to produce tetany by the injection of neutral or alkaline phosphates in suitable amount. This was accompanied by a drop in the serum calcium to the extent found in infantile tetany. If, however, he injected *acid* phosphates, although the calcium figure fell to the same degree, tetany did not develop. Howland and Marriott[2] noted a marked

* For a discussion of the literature on this point consult the article by Kramer, Tisdall and Howland.[17]

decrease in the serum calcium, without tetany, in nephritis with acidosis. It is apparent therefore, that decrease of calcium is not enough of itself to cause tetany.

Kramer, Tisdall and Howland[17] found that in infantile tetany the phosphorus of the serum, though variable, was normal or only slightly increased in one-half of their cases. An increase in the phosphorus, therefore, cannot be an important factor in this form of tetany.

Recently Collip and Backus,[21] and Grant and Goldman[22] have noted the occurrence of tetany following overventilation of the lungs in healthy subjects. The urine showed a rapid fall in the titratable acidity, sometimes becoming alkaline, with increase of the basic phosphates and diminution of the ammonia. The blood revealed a decided decrease in the CO_2 combining power, and a definite increase in p^H (decrease in the hydrogen-ion concentration), while the calcium became somewhat increased. They explain the apparent anomaly of an "alkalosis" associated with diminished bicarbonate by the supposition that the CO_2 is washed out of the blood more rapidly than the alkali can be removed, which leads to a decrease of the ratio $\frac{H_2CO_2}{NaHCO_3}$.

Later Goldman,[23] and Barker and Sprunt[24] described tetany as a transitory condition in diseased persons as a result of attacks of hyperpnea. In our cases the tetany could not be attributed to this cause.

The attempts of Paton and his coworkers[8] to connect tetany following parathyroidectomy, and also as it occurs in man under natural conditions, with poisoning by guanidine has not met with confirmation, and owing to possible errors in the method employed, their results are open to question. It must be admitted however, that their production of tetany experimentally by injection of guanidine has been repeated by Watanabe[25] with positive results.

It is quite clear that there is still much to be learned as to the pathogenesis and the ultimate cause of this remarkable condition.

In conclusion it is interesting to note that some of the cases in the literature, and our third case, have been associated with a fatty diarrhea, usually of pancreatic origin; instances in point are the cases of Findlay and Sharpe[8] (almost the precise counterpart of our own), of Barach and Murray,[16] and of Bassett-Smith,[26] the last two occurring in sprue.

Summary. 1. An increase of the bicarbonate of the blood was demonstrated in 3 cases of tetany, 1 of which followed the administration of sodium bicarbonate.

2. A low serum calcium was found in 1 case, another showed a normal figure during a period of latent tetany, the case following soda was not examined as to calcium.

3. A study of the calcium metabolism in 1 case revealed definite abnormalities.

4. Large amounts of indican were found in the urine in 1 case.

REFERENCES.

1. Harrop, G. A., Jr.: Johns Hopkins Hosp. Bull., 1919, **30**, 62.
2. Howland, J. and Marriott, W. M.: Quart. Jour. of Med., 1918, **11**, 289.
3. Healy, W. P.: Am. Jour. Obstet. and Gyn., 1921, **2**, 164.
4. Blum, L.: Ergebnisse d. inn. Med. u. Kinderheilk., 1913, **11**, 480.
5. Henderson, P. S.: Quart. Jour. Med., 1919, **13**, 427.
6. Underhill, F. P., Tileston, W., and Bogert, L. J.: Jour. Metabolic Research, 1922, **1**, 723.
7. Simpson, G. E.: Jour. Am. Med. Assn., 1920, **75**, 1204.
8. Paton, D. Noël and Findlay, L.: Quart. Jour. Exp. Phys., 1916, **10**, 315; Burns D. and Sharpe, J. S., Quart. Jour. Exp. Phys., 1916, **10**, 345; Findlay, L. and Sharpe, J. S., Quart. Jour. of Med., 1919, **13**, 433.
9. MacCallum, W. G. *et al.*: Bull. Johns Hopkins Hosp., 1920, **31**, 1.
10. McCann, W. S.: Jour. Biol. Chem., 1918, **35**, 553.
11. Hastings, A. B., Murray, C. D. and Murray, H. A., Jr.: Jour. Biol. Chem., 1921, **46**, 223.
12. Wilson, D. W., Stearns, T. and Thurlow, M. DeG.: Jour. Biol. Chem., 1915, **23**, 89.
13. Togawa, T.: Jour. Lab. and Clin. Med., 1919, **5**, 299.
14. Hastings, A. B. and Murray, H. A., Jr.: Jour. Biol. Chem., 1921, **46**, 233.
15. MacCallum, W. G. and Voegtlin: Jour. Exp. Med., 1909, **11**, 118.
16. Barach, A. L. and Murray, H. A., Jr.: Jour. Am. Med. Assn., 1920, **74**, 786.
17. Kramer, B., Tisdall, F. F. and Howland, J.: Am. Jour. Dis. Child., 1921, **22**, 431.
18. Greenwald, I.: Jour. Pharmacol. and Exp. Therap., 1918, **11**, 281.
19. Greenwald, I.: Jour. Biol. Chem., 1913, **14**, 369.
20. Binger, C.: Jour. Pharm. and Exp. Therap., 1917, **10**, 105.
21. Collip, J. B. and Backus, P. L.: Am. Jour. Physiol., 1920, **51**, 568.
22. Grant, S. B. and Goldman, A.: Am. Jour. Physiol., 1920, **52**, 209.
23. Goldman, A.: Jour. Am. Med. Assn., 1922, **78**, 1193.
24. Barker, L. F. and Sprunt, T. P.: Endocrinology, 1922, **6**, 1.
25. Watanabe, C. K.: Jour. Biol. Chem., 1918, **33**, 253.
26. Bassett-Smith, P. W.: Lancet, 1919, **1**, 178.

DIFFERENTIAL STUDY OF A CASE OF PULMONARY STENOSIS OF INFLAMMATORY ORIGIN (VENTRICULAR SEPTUM CLOSED) AND TWO CASES OF (a) PULMONARY STENOSIS AND (b) PULMONARY ATRESIA OF DEVELOPMENTAL ORIGIN WITH ASSOCIATED VENTRICULAR SEPTAL DEFECT AND DEATH FROM PARADOXICAL CEREBRAL EMBOLISM.* †

In Three Cases, Aged Respectively, Fourteen, Ten and Eleven Years.

By Maude E. Abbott, M.D., D. S. Lewis, M.D.,

and

W. W. Beattie, M.D.

MONTREAL, CANADA.

(From the Pathological Museum of McGill University, and the Medical Service of the Royal Victoria Hospital, Montreal).

Pulmonary stenosis is one of the commonest of all findings in those forms of congenital cardiac disease characterized clinically

* Presented at the Twenty-third Meeting of the American Association of Pathologists and Bacteriologists, March 31, 1923.
† Published with the aid of a grant from the Cooper Fund for Medical Research.

by the symptom-complex of so-called congenital cyanosis. From the standpoint of etiology and anatomical structure, these cases may be divided into:

1. A small group in which the lesion is purely valvular and has resulted from an endocarditis of the pulmonary segments setting in during relatively late fetal life after the cardiac septa have closed. In these cases, which are considered here first as the less complex anomaly, there is a thickening and usually a fusion of the pulmonary cusps with the production of a small, often funnel-shaped, pulmonary orifice, which opens off the hypertrophied, but otherwise normal, conus of the right ventricle, and the pulmonary artery is usually of normal size, or may even be dilated; the interventricular septum is entire, but the foramen ovale is usually patent and is not infrequently fenestrated. These features prove the origin of the valvular lesion from the action of a fetal endocarditis setting in after the cardiac septa have closed.

2. In the other and much larger group of pulmonary stenoses the lesion is to be traced to an arrest of development in early embryonic life before the division of the heart into its four chambers is completed. In these cases, signs of fetal endocarditis as a complicating or even causative factor in early embryonic life may, or may not, be present but the main lesion is not inflammatory or valvular, but a true hypoplasia of the pulmonary tract, and the interventricular septum presents a defect at the base; while the aorta, which it will be remembered arises in early embryonic life from the *right* side of the common ventricle, usually appears displaced to the right arising from both ventricles above the septal defect, or entirely from the right ventricle; the pulmonary artery is usually small and thin-walled and the pulmonary valve bicuspid or rudimentary, and the conus of the right ventricle is narrowed, or it may (in cases where a septal defect communicates with the conus) be expanded below the cusps into a large chamber connected with the sinus of the ventricle by a constricted orifice (persistent lower bulbar orifice). These associated anomalies definitely prove that the pulmonary stenosis originated in early fetal life before the completion of the cardiac septa, from the operation of some cause which led to an early arrest or deviation of development, whereby an unduly small pulmonary artery has been cut off from a relatively large aorta, or the lumen of the conus of the right ventricle and the pulmonary orifice have become abnormally narrowed or otherwise deformed; and this combination, pulmonary hypoplasia, defect of the interventricular septum at the base, and *Rechtslage* of the aorta, is the commonest of all causes of congenital cyanosis in patients who reach the age of puberty.

The comparison of these two types of pulmonary stenoses and atresia with, and without, associated septal defect, yields considerable information of interest both from the clinical and pathological standpoints. The following communication is based (1) upon the personal observation during life of a case of inflammatory pulmonary stenosis with closed septum (Case I cited below) and (2) the subsequent study of the heart of this patient after death and of the hearts of two other cases in the Pathological Museum of McGill University of (*a*) developmental pulmonary stenosis with associated septal defect and a superimposed inflammatory pulmonary valvular lesion (Case II), presented by Dr. P. P. Smyth of Big Valley, Alberta, and (*b*) developmental pulmonary atresia with associated septal defect and *Rechtslage* of the aorta (Case III) presented from the Pathological Service of the Montreal General Hospital.

The interpretation placed upon the findings in these 3 cases is amplified and corroborated by the results of a statistical study of 82 cases of pulmonary stenosis and 24 cases of pulmonary atresia made by one of us in another connection.[1]

In the 2 cases with associated ventricular septal defect a paradoxical cerebral embolism is suggested. In the light of the literature this surmise becomes a certainty. This interesting subject is discussed further below.

CASE I.—*Pulmonary Stenosis of Inflammatory Origin, Fusion of Cusps and Recent Verrucose Endocarditis. Pinhead Orifice. Ventricular Septum Closed. Patent Foramen Ovale. Death in Dyspneic Attacks.*

Clinical Data: D. S. L., female, aged fourteen years, admitted to hospital with severe dyspnea on exertion and marked cyanosis. Healthy and active until nine years old, when she began having repeated attacks of sore throat each winter. Cyanosis first became noticeable at this time; she became dyspneic on exertion and unable to play. After some three months in bed she improved, and for the next three years was able to attend school. In 1919 her cyanosis and dyspnea increased, and until her death the progress of the disease was steadily downward, and she was confined to bed much of the time. The cyanosis was noted especially about the nose, lips, fingers and toes; cough was troublesome but there was no orthopnea or dropsy. No history of chorea or acute rheumatic fever. Menstruation began at eleven years. Two sisters have dyspnea and palpitation but are of good color.

Physical examination showed a rather undersized girl with marked dyspnea and distinct cyanosis of the cheeks, nose, hands and feet. The mucous membrane of the mouth was a deep purple color. Marked clubbing of the fingers and toes. In the mouth there were many carious roots, and the tonsils showed much scarring and widely gaping crypts. The lungs were relatively normal. There was marked precordial bulging and pulsation; the maximum cardiac impulse being in the fourth left interspace 8.5 cm. from the midline. A rough systolic thrill was felt over the precordium with its maximum intensity in the third left interspace, 5 cm. from the midsternal line. The relative cardiac dulness extended 4 cm. to the right and 10 cm. to the left of the midsternal line. The sounds were loud, regular and very rapid. At the apex, the first sound was very sharp but the second almost inaudible. The second sound was not accentuated at the pulmonic or aortic areas. A long, rough blowing systolic murmur was present at the apex, transmitted to the axilla and through to the angle of the scapula. It was also carried upward to the pulmonic area, its intensity diminishing as the clavicle was approached. The same murmur was audible at the aortic area and to a less degree in the vessels of the neck, and over the tricuspid area. At times there was a presystolic murmur inside the apex beat. Systolic blood-pressure 110, diastolic 60. The liver and spleen were not palpable. A trace of albumin was present in the urine. There was a moderate polycythemia; erythrocytes 7,600,000; leukocytes 22,000; hemoglobin 120 per cent (Sahli). The roentgenograph showed the heart slightly enlarged to right and left, with some fulness about the pulmonary artery. The electrocardiogram marked right-sided preponderance, with auricular hypertrophy.

Progress of Case During the six weeks preceding death the patient had two acute dyspneic attacks, attended with increased cyanosis, but was relatively comfortable during the intervals. She left the hospital and died August 30, 1921, during the third of these paroxysms. The autopsy was performed by Dr. C. T. Crowdy at the home of the patient. Only a small abdominal incision was allowed, through which the heart was removed without the larger vessels.

Description of Heart (W. W. B.) (Fig. 1). The heart of a young adult, greatly enlarged in its right chambers, the apex being formed entirely by the right ventricle. The right auricle is greatly dilated, and its wall is distinctly hypertrophied, and its columnæ carneæ are very prominent. There is a gaping foramen ovale admitting a lead pencil and three small fenestrations exist in the auricular septum along the posterosuperior border of the valvula foraminis ovalis where it joins the limbus Vieussenii. The tricuspid orifice measures 9 cm.; the cusps are slightly thickened and along their line of closure on their auricular aspect is a row of small irregular wart-like vegetations; the chordæ tendineæ are thickened and markedly shortened, the right papillary muscle being directly connected to the valve segment.

The right ventricle is greatly hypertrophied (wall 1.8 cm. thick), and its musculi pectinati and papillary muscles are enlarged and prominent. In its conus the musculature below the pulmonary valve presents a peculiar puckered condition appearing as if the chamber had been at one time of greater diameter, and its wall had been subsequently gathered in at the pulmonary orifice, forming longitudinal pleats. There are six prominent crests and six clefts thus produced. The endocardium over these crests is greatly thickened, appearing as opaque white patches. Viewed from the ventricle, the rim of the pulmonary orifice at the base of the cusps measures 1.2 cm. in diameter.

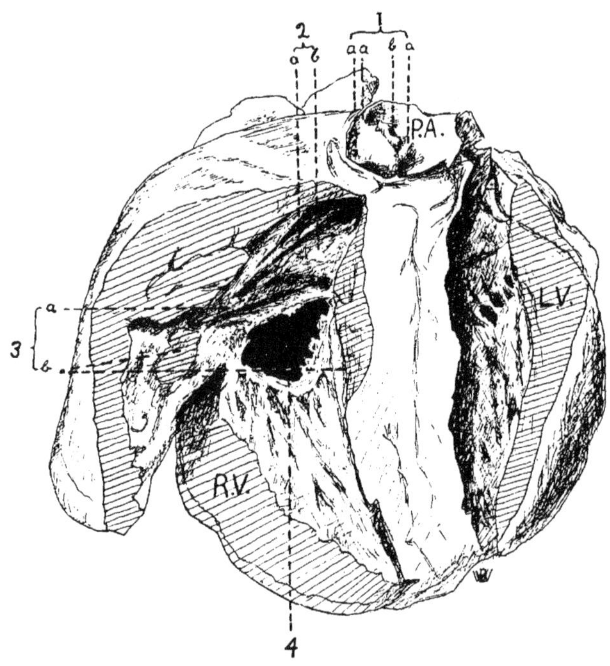

FIG. 1.—*Pulmonary stenosis of inflammatory origin, with fusion of cusps and pinhole orifice surmounted by a ring of warty vegetation.* (Case I). From a specimen in the Pathological Museum of McGill University presented by Drs. Lewis and Crowdy. (1) The fused cusps of the pulmonary valve with raphé *a*, *a*, *a*, showing the line of attachment to each other; *b*, central pinhole orifice with edges surmounted by a row of vegetations; (2) conus of right ventricle showing; *a*, puckering of musculature, and *b*, a white patch of thickened endocardium; (3) lower bulbar orifice formed by; *a*, crista supraventricularis; and *b*, trabecula septomarginalis (moderator band); (4) tricuspid orifice, edges of cusps thickened and surmounted by warty vegetations; *A*, aorta; *P.A.*, pulmonary artery; *R.V.*, right ventricle; *L.V.*, left ventricle.

The pulmonary artery is laid open above the valve; it is of about normal size (2 cm. in diameter), but is very thin-walled. The pulmonary cusps are symmetrically fused along their contiguous borders leaving a central circular orifice 2 mm. in diameter; this is surrounded by a firm brownish-pink colored rim, along the inner edge of which is a growth of small granular, grayish vegetations; the whole forms a structure resembling a partially expanded sea-anemone, the granulations appearing like the partly retracted tentacles. The "sea-anemone" is connected with the wall of the pulmonary artery by three equidistantly placed firm fibrous ridges, 8 mm. in height. These are the remains of the attachments of semilunar cusps to the pulmonary artery. The left auricle is not altered in size or in thickness of wall. The left ventricle appears of normal size and thickness (walls average 1.3 cm.). The mitral orifice is 8.5 cm. in circumference. The aortic orifice measures 1.6 cm. in diameter. The aortic cusps are normal except for two small fenestrations. Both coronary arteries are double.

At the autopsy only a small abdominal incision was allowed. The great vessels, including the ductus arteriosus, were not removed from the body, but were cut away just above the heart, so that their condition cannot be discussed.

Museum Entry No. 7422. Presented by Drs. Lewis and Crowdy.

CASE II.—*Pulmonary Stenosis of Developmental Origin; Narrowing and Deformity of Conus, with Large Defect of Interventricular Septum. Aorta Displaced to the Right Arising from Both Ventricles above it. Fusion of Pulmonary Cusps and Stenosis of Orifice from Valvular Fetal Endocarditis. Patent Foramen Ovale; Phlegmon of Arm; Hemiplegia. Paradoxical Cerebral Embolism.*

Clinical Data (Dr. P. P. Smyth). Male, aged ten years, admitted to hospital with tender brawny swelling of left arm just above the elbow. Has had considerable cyanosis for some years, with dyspnea on exertion. His growth has been stunted and slight injuries have healed slowly. No history of any previous illness or of trauma to the arm.

Physical Examination. Temperature, 102° F. Pulse, 120. Poorly developed child, very marked cyanosis and clubbing of fingers and toes. Lungs and abdomen clear. Heart somewhat enlarged to right and left; sounds regular; soft presystolic murmur over the precordium. The left arm, just above elbow, showed a large fluctuating area, tender to the touch.

Progress of Case. The phlegmon on the arm was incised two days after admission and 100 cc of malodorous, blood-streaked pus was evacuated. Fever subsided under drainage, but the wound healed slowly. On the day of his discharge the boy became stuporous, and shortly afterward had a general convulsion followed by a left-sided hemiplegia. He was taken from hospital the next day but returned ten days later with a persistent left hemiplegia, stupor and incontinence of urine and feces. He passed into coma and died fifteen days after the first convulsion.

Description of Heart (W. W. B.) (Fig. 2). A child's heart of peculiar shape, being very broad transversely in comparison with its longitudinal measurements, and having a broad and flat apex, with a slight indentation (slightly bifid) formed chiefly by the right ventricle. Arising posteriorly at the middle of its base is a large thick-walled aorta, 2.5 cm. in diameter. The pulmonary artery, a

longitudinal pleats. There are six prominent r thus produced. The endocardium over th thickened, appearing as opaque white pat ventricle, the rim of the pulmonary orifi measures 1.2 cm. in diameter.

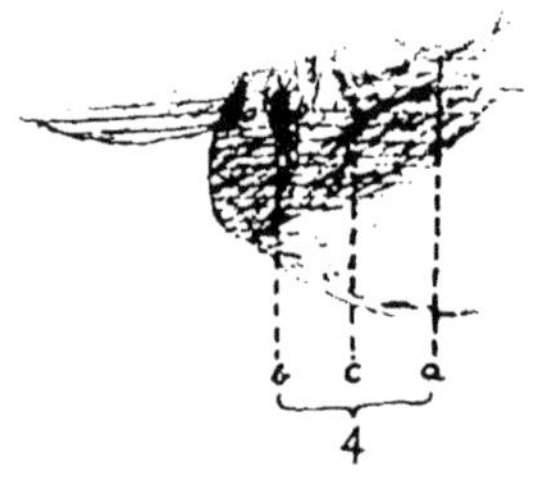

FIG. 2. *Pulmonary hypoplasia of developmental ing and fusion of pulmonary cusps and stenosis of ventricular septum. Rechtslage of aorta and displace left of right posterior aortic cusp.* (Case II). From logical Museum presented by Dr. W. P. Smyth cusps of pulmonary valve with raphé a, a, a, r central circular orifice; (2) hypoplastic ; 1 ste lower bulbar orifice formed by; *a*, crista supraventricularis trabecular septomarginalis here very short: (4) with *a*, chorda tendinea attached to posterior below defect; *b*, chorda tendinea attached to rud from crusta supraventricularis; and *c*, anomal of base of right posterior aortic cusp to free b teriorly; (5) free upper border of ventricular artery in two parts; *A.C.*, anterior aortic cusp cusp; *L.P.*, left posterior aortic cusp; *P.M* right coronary orifice; *L.Cor.*, left coronary or

The left ventricle appears of abo is a peculiar branching aberrant ch interventricular septum to the ba muscle. A second anomalous chord same muscle and passes upward and tricular septum and is inserted poste border of a large defect in the base of

This defect mesures 2 cm. in length; it begins posteriorly just in front of the pars membranacea and 2 mm. below the base of the right posterior (free) aortic cusp, opposite the junction of its middle and left thirds and ends anteriorly 5 mm. behind the anterior (righ ary aortic cusp opposite to the junction of its middle an ds The defect is bounded below by the free superior bo i erventricular septum. which appears as a smooth r crescentic ridge. The chordæ tendineæ of the a mitral valve do not connect with this border n elow it except for the single anomalous chorda m

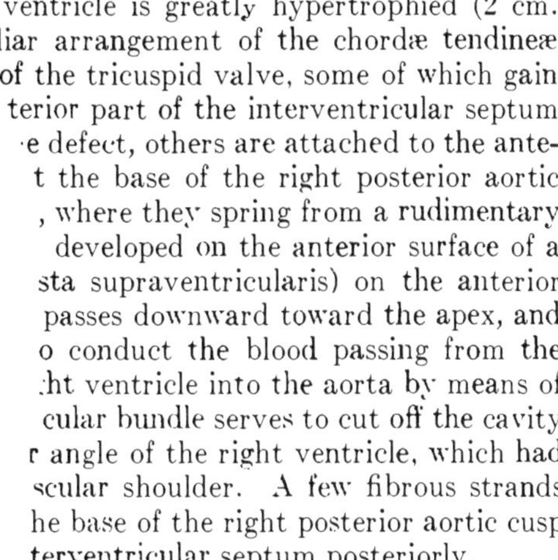

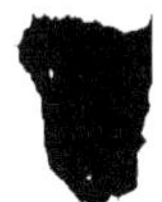

ventricle is greatly hypertrophied (2 cm. th liar arrangement of the chordæ tendineæ f t of the tricuspid valve, some of which gain terior part of the interventricular septum e defect, others are attached to the ante- t the base of the right posterior aortic , where they spring from a rudimentary developed on the anterior surface of a sta supraventricularis) on the anterior passes downward toward the apex, and o conduct the blood passing from the ht ventricle into the aorta by means of cular bundle serves to cut off the cavity r angle of the right ventricle, which had scular shoulder. A few fibrous strands he base of the right posterior aortic cusp terventricular septum posteriorly.

equally from both ventricles, riding over lek-walled and very large for the size of m. in diameter.

tslage or malposition to the right of the ear to the observer by noting the situation ea septi which usually lies at the base of the aortic cusp and between it and the anterior but in this case is seen to lie between the bases or cusp and the left posterior (left coronary) osterior cusp is thus lying in front of, instead of nembranacea septi, as in the normal heart.

he right ventricle leading to the pulmonary orifice ll, appearing when viewed from below, as an elon- anterior upper angle of the right ventricle. It has walls which form projecting pillars on the interior r ntricular wall, and a narrow, straight lumen which b 7 mm. in diameter, and it is lined with opaque lourdium. Its opening into the ventricle is narrowed mforward of the muscular bundles which form its

small inconspicuous vessel with very thin walls, about one-third the size of the aorta and measuring 1 cm. in diameter, arises in front of the aortic trunk, and curves across and around it upward and to the left.

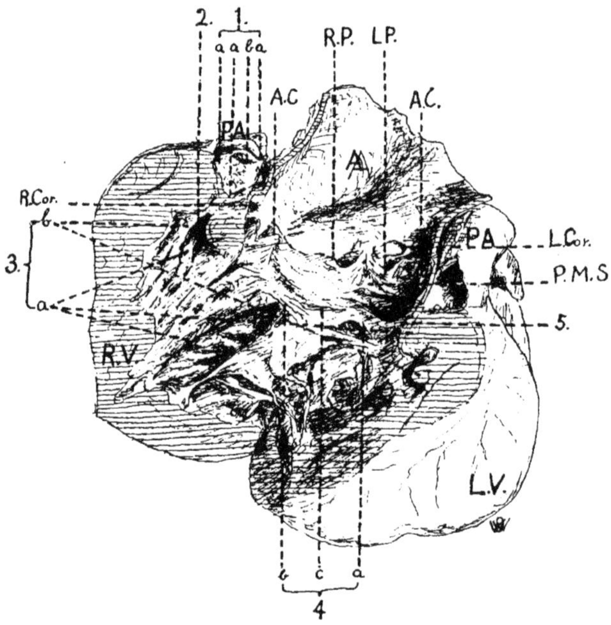

FIG. 2.—*Pulmonary hypoplasia of developmental origin, with inflammatory thickening and fusion of pulmonary cusps and stenosis of orifice. Large defect at base of interventricular septum. Rechtslage of aorta and displacement of pars membranacea septi to left of right posterior aortic cusp.* (Case II). From a specimen in the McGill Pathological Museum presented by Dr. W. P. Smyth, Big Valley, Alberta. (1) Fused cusps of pulmonary valve with raphé *a*, *a*, *a*, representing their attachments; *b*, central circular orifice; (2) hypoplastic and stenosed conus of right ventricle; (3) lower bulbar orifice formed by; *a*, crista supraventricularis here very thick; and *b*, trabecular septomarginalis here very short; (4) infundibular cusp of tricuspid valve with: *a*, chorda tendinea attached to posterior part of interventricular septum just below defect; *b*, chorda tendinea attached to rudimentary papillary muscle springing from crusta supraventricularis; and *c*, anomalous chorda running from right half of base of right posterior aortic cusp to free border of interventricular septum posteriorly; (5) free upper border of ventricular septum at defect. *P.A.*, pulmonary artery in two parts; *A.C.*, anterior aortic cusp, divided; *R.P.*, right posterior aortic cusp; *L.P.*, left posterior aortic cusp; *P.M.S.*, pars membranacea septi; *R.Cor.*, right coronary orifice; *L.Cor.*, left coronary orifice.

The left ventricle appears of about normal size. Near its apex is a peculiar branching aberrant chorda tendinea running from the interventricular septum to the base of the posterior papillary muscle. A second anomalous chorda arises from the apex of the same muscle and passes upward and forward toward the interventricular septum and is inserted posteriorly 1.5 cm. below the free border of a large defect in the base of the interventricular septum.

This defect measures 2 cm. in length; it begins posteriorly just in front of the pars membranacea and 2 mm. below the base of the right posterior (free) aortic cusp, opposite the junction of its middle and left thirds, and ends anteriorly 5 mm. behind the anterior (right coronary) aortic cusp opposite to the junction of its middle and left thirds. The defect is bounded below by the free superior border of the interventricular septum. which appears as a smooth rounded muscular crescentic ridge. The chordæ tendineæ of the aortic segment of the mitral valve do not connect with this border nor with the septum below it except for the single anomalous chorda mentioned above.

The wall of the right ventricle is greatly hypertrophied (2 cm. thick). There is a peculiar arrangement of the chordæ tendineæ of the infundibular cusp of the tricuspid valve, some of which gain an attachment to the posterior part of the interventricular septum just below the margin of the defect, others are attached to the anterior wall of the ventricle at the base of the right posterior aortic cusp opposite its right third, where they spring from a rudimentary papillary muscle, which had developed on the anterior surface of a large muscular column (crista supraventricularis) on the anterior wall of the ventricle, which passes downward toward the apex, and which apparently tended to conduct the blood passing from the right auricle through the right ventricle into the aorta by means of the septal defect. This muscular bundle serves to cut off the cavity in the right upper posterior angle of the right ventricle, which had developed into a large muscular shoulder. A few fibrous strands run from the right half of the base of the right posterior aortic cusp to the free border of the interventricular septum posteriorly.

The aorta arises about equally from both ventricles, riding over the septal defect; it is thick-walled and very large for the size of the heart, measuring 2.5 cm. in diameter.

The condition of *Rechtslage* or malposition to the right of the aorta is further made clear to the observer by noting the situation of the pars membranacea septi which usually lies at the base of the right posterior (free) aortic cusp and between it and the anterior (right coronary) cusp but in this case is seen to lie between the bases of the right posterior cusp and the left posterior (left coronary) cusp. The right posterior cusp is thus lying in front of, instead of behind, the pars membranacea septi, as in the normal heart.

The conus of the right ventricle leading to the pulmonary orifice is extremely small, appearing when viewed from below, as an elongated slit at the anterior upper angle of the right ventricle. It has thick muscular walls which form projecting pillars on the interior of the anterior ventricular wall, and a narrow, straight lumen which admits a probe 7 mm. in diameter, and it is lined with opaque thickened endocardium. Its opening into the ventricle is narrowed by the curving forward of the muscular bundles which form its posterior wall. These represent the moderator band or trabecula septomarginalis medially and the crista supraventricular (Tandler[2]) laterally, the former of which is here much shorter than in the normal heart. The pulmonary orifice is guarded by a peenliar tubular sleeve-like structure which projects into the pulmonary artery for a distance of 1 cm. and which presents at its summit a circular orifice 4 mm. in diameter. This structure is attached to the walls of the pulmonary artery by three raphés, one on the right and the other two on the left side of the orifice; the first reaches the rim of the orifice and the latter two extend to within 4 mm. of this border and are separated at their attachment to the wall of the artery by an interval of 4 mm. This structure is formed of dense white tissue and represents the fused and thickened cusps of an irregularly divided three-cusped pulmonary valve (the left anterior cusp of which is abnormally small), which had evidently been the seat of a chronic fetal endocarditis. The pulmonary artery is very narrow and thin-walled.

The right auricle is dilated but not hypertrophied. The foramen ovale is patent by a valvular opening, admitting a lead pencil, and the posterosuperior border of the valvula foraminis ovalis, shows multiple small fenestrations. The Thebesian valve in the right auricle is represented by a thin thread-like strand which runs across the orifice of the coronary sinus.

Museum Entry No. 7431. Presented by Dr. P. P. Smyth, Alberta.

CASE III.—*Pulmonary Atresia with Associated Ventricular Septal Defect. Aorta from Conus of Right Ventricle. Patent Ductus Arteriosus. Hemiplegia. Appendicitis. Paradoxical Embolism. Cerebral Abscess.*

Clinical Data (Service of Dr. Hutchison, Montreal General Hospital). Male, aged eleven years, admitted to surgical service with severe abdominal pain, vomiting and fever. Had been a bluish color ever since birth; dyspneic on exertion, unable to run, but able to walk slowly. He was thought to have some form of congenital heart disease. Eight days before death the child began having convulsions with twitching of the hands and arms, the head being drawn to the left. Two days before admission he developed a severe pain in the right lower quadrant of the abdomen. Family history negative.

Physical Examination. There was marked cyanosis: definite clubbing of the fingers and toes. Pupils equal and active, tongue dry and coated. Lungs clear. Distinct precordial bulging, a diffuse apex beat and a definite thrill just inside apex beat. Heart extended from right border of sternum to 0.5 cm. beyond the left nipple. Sounds were regular, no accentuation of the first sound, but second was sharply cut and a little accentuated. Rough diastolic murmur at the apex, poorly transmitted toward the axilla. Pulse was full, regular and well sustained. The abdomen showed some tenderness at McBurney's point, and rectal tenderness.

Progress of Case. The appendix was removed on the day of admission. Six days later patient complained of severe pain in head. Temperature 101° F. Pulse 96. Fever continued, but with slow pulse. The following evening he had a definite convulsion followed by a right sided hemiplegia; pupils equal, dilated, inactive double Kernig sign, Babinski on right. Smear of cerebrospinal fluid showed streptococci. Died at 10.30 P.M.

Autopsy (by Dr. Montgomery). This showed abscess of brain, left frontal lobe; acute purulent meningitis; congestion of the organs, recent appendectomy scar.

Description of Heart (W. W. B.) (Figs. 3 and 4). The heart of a child, rather broader than usual in proportion to its length. The apex is rounded and formed equally by both ventricles. There are a few petechial hemorrhages over the right ventricle. A large thick-walled vessel arises from the bulging conus of the right ventricle anteriorly in the position normally occupied by the pulmonary artery, and curves directly upward, giving off the vessels to the neck in their usual situation. This large vessel appears at first sight to be a common arterial trunk, but proves to be the aorta, for dissection in the tissues to its left reveals another very small trunk, the atresic pulmonary artery, arising blindly from the ventricular wall to the left and on a slightly posterior plane.

The aorta measures at its origin 5.5 cm. in circumference. Both coronary arteries are double and the innominate and left common carotid have a common origin. The ductus arteriosus is patent as a thin-walled vessel 1.5 mm. in diameter, arising from a funnel-shaped elliptical orifice 0.4 x 1 cm., guarded in the aorta on the right and left by two low, sharp-edged ridges. It opens into the right branch of the pulmonary artery, which is a vessel 5 mm. in diameter.

The pulmonary artery is a small thin-walled vessel measuring, just above the sinuses of Valsalva, 1 cm. in circumference and broadening out to 1.5 cm. above. Three rudimentary sinuses of Valsalva are recognizable but the cusps are represented only by thin, low, ridge-like folds. The musculature of the conus of the right ventricle is fused 5 mm. below the base of these rudimentary cusps and its lumen at this point is completely obliterated. From here for a distance of 7 mm. above the base of the cusps, the lumen of the pulmonary orifice and artery is occupied and occluded completely below, and partially above, by a cylindrical firm mass of pinkish-white tissue adherent to the posterior aspect of the wall (organized thrombus).

The aorta arises from both ventricles but chiefly from the conus of the right, riding over a defect in the base of the ventricular septum. This condition of "Rechtslage" of the aorta is further made clear by the abnormal relation between the aortic cusps and the pars membranacea, which is the same as that noted and explained under Case II. (See page 643). The septal defect measures 2 cm. in length and is bounded below by the free crescentic upper border of the ventricular septum; this begins posteriorly 1 mm. in front of the pars membranacea septi, being separated from this by a band of musculature, and below the junction of the middle and left thirds of the right posterior aortic cusp, and extends anteriorly to

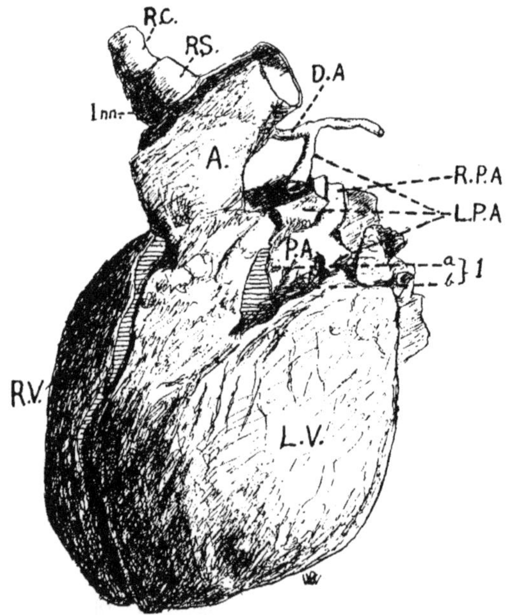

FIG. 3.—*Pulmonary atresia with hypoplasia of pulmonary artery and orifice, and closure of conus below cusps. Persistent lower bulbar orifice (conus a separate chamber). Patent ductus arteriosus; large defect of interventricular septum at base and Rechtslage of dilated aorta.* (Case III). Left anterior surface; heart enclosed: to show relative sizes and position of dilated aorta, atresic pulmonary artery and patent ductus. From a specimen presented to the McGill Museum by Rhea and Montgomery, Montreal General Hospital; (1) Pulmonary orifice obliterated below; *a*, rudimentary sinuses of Valsalva and *b*, partly filled by an organized thrombus; *L.P.A.*, left pulmonary artery divided; *R.P.A.*, right pulmonary artery; *D.A.*, ductus arteriosus patent; *R.S.*, right subclavian artery; *Inn.*, innominate artery; *R.C.*, right common carotid artery.

the cleft between the left posterior and anterior cusps. The left ventricle is dilated and its wall is 8 mm. thick.

The right ventricle is elongated and narrow and greatly hypertrophied. The conus is demarcated from the rest of the cavity by a thick muscular cushion running from the anterior part of the interventricular septum at a point midway between base and apex of the heart, backward and to the right to the middle of the insertion of the right posterior aortic cusp whence it curves forward and downward to the right to the anterior wall producing a semilunar orifice (lower bulbar orifice) 2.2 cm. long leading from the cavity of the right ventricle into the conus. This cushion represents the much accentuated moderator band of the trabecula septomarginalis below, and the crista supraventricularis (Tandler[2]) above, which are present in the normal heart but are less prominently developed. The conus thus forms a separate chamber above the orifice with a

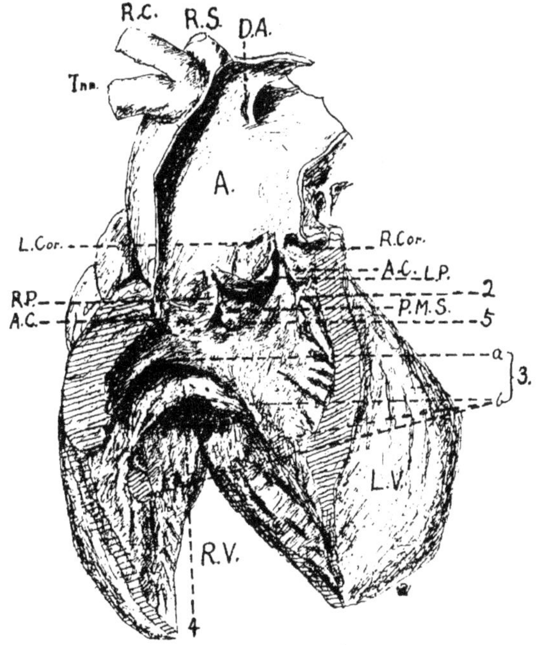

FIG. 4.—*Pulmonary atresia with large defect of interventricular septum at base and Rechtslage.* Right posterior view of the same specimen (Case III) shown in Fig. 3, right ventricle and aorta laid open to expose the interior. (1) (See Fig. 3); (2) obliterated upper part of conus of right ventricle; (3) lower bulbar orifice formed by; *a*, crista supraventricularis; and *b*, trabecular septomarginalis, which form a prominent muscular ridge; (4) infundibular cusp of tricuspid valve; (5) free upper border of ventricular septum at defect; *D.A.*, aortic orifice of patent ductus; *R.C.*; right common carotid, and *Inn.*, innominate artery arising by common trunk; *L.Cor.*, double left coronary; *A.C.*, anterior aortic cusp divided; *R.P.*, right posterior aortic cusp; *L.P.*, left posterior aortic cusp; *P.M.S.*, pars membranacea septi.

thick anterior muscular wall 8 mm. thick. On its superoposterior wall it opens into the aorta by an elliptical orifice 2.2 x 1.5 cm. in diameter.

The conus of the right ventricle ends superiorly and to the right as a blind funnel-shaped cleft in the musculature which represents the obliterated communication with the pulmonary orifice. This cleft is 8 mm. below the anterior aortic cusp and 6 mm. below the anterior limb of the crescentic border of the ventricular septum.

Presented by Dr. Rhea, Museum Entry No. 7286.

Discussion. A. PATHOLOGICAL ANATOMY. Three interesting anatomical points must be emphasized in connection with Cases II and III. (*a*) *The deviation of the aorta to the right, "Rechtslage,"* whereby this vessel rides above the defect rising from the right as well as from the left ventricle, and which is shown in both specimens by the relation of the aortic cusps to the pars membranacea septi. That this is not a deviation of the position of the pars membranacea instead of the aorta as might be thought, is plainly seen in both cases from the fact that on viewing the pars membranacea from the right auricle it is seen to be in its normal situation, *i. e.*, at the base of the medial cusp of the tricuspid valve just posterior to the angle between it and the infundibular cusp, half in the auricle and half in the ventricle. (*b*) The defect in the interventricular septum is not in exactly the same situation in the two hearts, being placed more posteriorly in Case II, than in Case III. This is shown by the fact that in Case II, the defect in the septum leads into the main cavity of the right ventricle being almost entirely behind the crista supraventricularis and only slightly involving this band of muscle. This position of the defect posteriorly is evidenced also by the fact that several of the chordæ tendineæ of the tricuspid valve take their origin from the septum near the edge of the defect. Viewed from the left ventricle the defect impinges directly on the anterior border of the pars membranacea septi. In Case III on the other hand, the defect in the septum leads into the conus of the right ventricle being wholly in front of the crista supraventricularis and, therefore, having no relation to the insertions of the chordæ tendineæ of the tricuspid valve. Viewed from the left ventricle, the defect in the septum is seen to be separated from the anterior edge of the pars membranacea septi by a band of septal musculature about 2 mm. in width and is thus proved to be more anterior than in Case II. (*c*) In Case II, the whole conus is hypoplastic, being much smaller than normal, while in Case III, the conus is as large as, or larger than normal, but is completely aplastic above and is demarcated below from the sinus of the right ventricle by the hypertrophied muscle bands (crista supraventricularis and trabecula septum marginalis) which mark the site of the lower bulbar orifice of the embryonic heart; thus presenting the condition described by Keith[3] as "conus a separate chamber."

The difference in the development of the conus in these 2 cases may be explained by comparing the work that each evidently was called upon to perform. In Case II, the pulmonary orifice was very small and as the defect in the septum did not open into the conus, it is evident that the amount of blood which the conus was called upon to look after was relatively small. Therefore, it did not increase in size and eventually became an unimportant structure as the rest of the heart developed. In Case III, on the other hand, although the pulmonary orifice was not patent, still the defect in the septum opened into the conus and all the blood from the right side of the heart had to traverse the conus before it could enter the aorta. The conus thus was called upon to perform considerable work, and this is reflected in its spacious lumen and thick muscular walls.

B. PATHOLOGICAL PHYSIOLOGY AND CLINICAL ASPECTS OF THE CARDIAC LESIONS. 1. *Cyanosis and Dyspneic Attacks.* As was stated above the clinical picture of pulmonary stenosis or atresia is that of a true *morbus ceruleus*, the patients presenting, in varying degree, but in classic pronouncement, the cyanosis, clubbing, dyspnea and polycythemia that are the expression of deficient aëration of the blood. The prominence and constancy of these manifestations in all cases is explained by the fact that interference with the pulmonary circulation, which is here the pathological condition *per se*, is by far the most serious cause of insufficient oxygenation; a direct admixture of the venous with the arterial stream, such as occurs in a septal defect with raised pressure in the right ventricle, being of quite secondary importance, although of course this is, when present to a sufficient extent, also a factor.

The cyanosis varies in intensity and the date of its appearance, not only with the degree of narrowing of the pulmonary tract, but also with the presence or absence of a defect of the interventricular septum, which introduces a factor of very different clinical significance in the two conditions of (*a*) stenosis and (*b*) atresia of the pulmonary tract.

In *pulmonary stenosis*, where a less acute grade of obstruction exists than in the atresias, cyanosis naturally tends to be less severe and is usually absent at birth, appearing only after the first weeks or months, or in some cases (usually those with closed septum), years of life. Here we find, however, that *an associated defect of the interventricular septum* introduces a mechanical complication that increases the difficulties of the pulmonary circulation and so *intensifies the seriousness of the lesion.* For such a defect in the first place permits the escape of a certain amount of blood from the right to the left ventricle during the heart's systole, and thus reduces the volume of the blood to be transmitted from the right chamber to the lungs through the stenosed pulmonary orifice; and, secondly the venous blood so transmitted enters the arterial stream, thus bringing in another factor to further diminish the lowered oxygenation under which the patient is suffering. In the more favorable condition of pulmonary stenosis with *closed* ventricular septum, the entire force of the right ventricle is expended on pushing the venous blood through the narrowed pulmonary tract; the foramen ovale which is usually patent in these cases appearing to offer less mechanical interference with the development of pressure in the conus of the right ventricle.

A statistical analysis of 83 cases of pulmonary stenosis with autopsy findings in the literature gives the following corroboration of the above statements. Among 19 cases of *pulmonary stenosis with closed septum*, cyanosis was entirely absent in 5; was "slight" or "transient" in 5 others; "moderate" in 3, and in only 2 cases was it "marked." The average duration of life in these 18 cases was *twenty-one and three-tenths years*, the youngest age at death *four*, and the oldest *fifty-seven years*. Case I of this communication is an example of this combination; here cyanosis did not appear until the ninth year, and only became marked with the progress of the inflammatory process, which finally reduced the pulmonary orifice to pinhead size. On the other hand, among 64 cases analyzed of pulmonary stenosis with associated septal defect, the aorta in most cases displaced to the right and, arising from both ventricles above the defect, cyanosis was remarked upon as being "slight" or "absent" in only 4 cases, and was "marked" in 37. The average duration of life in these 64 cases *was eight and seven-tenths years*, the youngest patient dying in infancy at eleven days and the oldest at twenty-eight years. *These figures are conclusive.* Case II of this communication is an example of this more serious and much more frequent type of pulmonary stenosis.

In the group of *pulmonary atresias* an interesting variation from that in pulmonary stenosis is to be observed in that an *associated septal defect* alleviates instead of aggravating the condition, by providing another channel to the lungs for the aërated blood which is here unable to pass through the completely obliterated pulmonary lumen. Especially where the aorta rides over the defect or arises entirely from the right ventricle, we have the greatest amelioration possible, for the current from the right ventricle passes directly into the aorta and thence through a patent ductus to the lungs. Such cases may live to puberty and may be indistinguishable clinically from the graver forms of pulmonary stenosis. A closed or merely slit-like foramen ovale appears further to mitigate the situation, possibly by leaving a greater volume of blood in the right chambers to be transmitted directly into the aorta through the defect. Case III of this communication is an excellent illustration of this relatively most favorable combination in pulmonary atresia, for the aorta arose from the conus of the right ventricle above a large defect in the septum, and the foramen ovale, though patent, was very small. The patient, a well-developed boy, aged eleven years, died of an intercurrent complication (cerebral abscess). Among 18 cases of *pulmonary atresia with defective ventricular septum* analyzed, the average duration of life was three and seven-tenths years, the maximum age at death in the recorded cases analyzed being thirteen years.

On the other hand, *pulmonary atresia* with *closed interventricular septum* is incompatible with life beyond the first weeks or months. The patients are a deep mulberry hue at birth and die in infancy.

Of 6 such cases all died with this intense grade of cyanosis at ages varying from *six days* to *six months*, the average age at death being sixteen weeks. These figures are conclusive.

The following table summarizes the foregoing statements:

Nature of lesions.	Number of cases.	Marked cyanosis	Maximum age.	Average duration.	Precordial thrill.*
Pulmonary stenosis:	83				
(*a*) With closed septum	19	In 2	57 yrs.	21 3 yrs.	In 7
(*b*) With ventricular septal defect	64	In 37 (57.8%)	28 yrs.	8 7 yrs.	In 10
Pulmonary atresia:	24				
(*a*) With closed septum	6	Extreme in all	6 mos.	16 wks.	
(*b*) With ventricular septal defect	18	In 11	13 yrs.	3.7 yrs.	

Dyspneic Attacks. Many of these patients, the subjects of congenital cyanosis, have alarming attacks of dyspnea usually accompanied with temporary increase of the cyanosis, which is often intense. During these attacks there may be loss of consciousness and our first case (pulmonary stenosis with closed septum, the pulmonary orifice of pinhead size) died during one of these paroxysms. There seems to be a curious relationship between the severity of these attacks and the extent of the ischemia in the pulmonary circulation. In another case very similar to our Case I of a pulmonary stenosis with minute orifice (2 mm. wide) and closed ventricular septum reported by Cassel,[4] the patient also presented typical dyspneic attacks of great severity, the cyanosis being absent between the paroxysms during the early part of the illness. Dyspneic attacks with a transient cyanosis are a characteristic symptom also of patent ductus arteriosus, and are probably synchronous here with a temporary reversal of flow, during excitement or exertion from the pulmonary artery to the aorta, through the lumen of the patent vessel. In view of this fact, the special prominence of such attacks in these 2 cases of pulmonary stenosis with pinhead orifice and closed septum appears significant of their explanation as the expression of a temporary acute pulmonary ischemia.

Polycythemia of a moderate grade was present in our Case I, the only one of the three in which a blood count was made. *Hippocratic fingers*, or *clubbing both of fingers and toes*, was present in all three. In Case I the nose was slightly clubbed also.

2. *Atypical Physical Signs.* A *precordial thrill* is of frequent occurrence in pulmonary stenosis and appears to be more frequent in the cases without a defect of the interventricular septum. In a series of 83 cases (M. E. A.) of pulmonary stenosis, a thrill was noted

* This column is from an analysis published elsewhere, and the figures are referred to below.

in 8 out of 19 patients showing an intact septum at necropsy, while a thrill was absent in all but 10 of the 64 patients in whom there was an associated septal defect. (See fifth column in Table above). In our first case as also in that by Lallemand (see below), in both of which the ventricular septum was intact, a marked precordial thrill existed, while in Case II with patent interventricular septum, no thrill was noted. In our third case (pulmonary atresia) the marked thrill that was present was localized near the apex and was undoubtedly produced by the large septal defect and not at the pulmonary orifice.

Murmurs and Accentuations. In this connection the following generalization may be made. In pulmonary stenosis the pulmonary second sound is usually not accentuated and it may be almost inaudible; a rough systolic murmur is practically always present and is usually of maximum intensity over the pulmonary area and transmitted upward along the course of the pulmonary artery; this murmur may be heard loudly over the entire precordium but is usually fainter below, and may be inaudible at the apex and to the right of the sternum; with a patent foramen ovale it may take on a diastolic-systolic phase, or a second murmur, often presystolic in rhythm and variable in its occurrence, may be introduced, with maximum intensity at the third and fourth left interspaces. In an associated septal defect this second murmur has a similar localization, but is more definitely systolic in rhythm, is usually heard also in the left interscapular region and may be propagated, when combined with a pulmonary stenosis, along the aorta into the carotid arteries in the neck (Eisenmenger[5]).

In Case I of this communication (pulmonary stenosis with closed ventricular sepum and patent foramen ovale), the little patient was under the personal observation of one of us (D. S. L.) both in hospital and in private for the last eight months of life and the findings were confirmed by repeated examination. The physical signs are of much interest, not only as illustrating certain characteristic features, namely, the absence of pulmonary accentuation, the presence of a coarse systolic thrill and murmur diffused over the precordium (originating at the pulmonary orifice), and a fugitive presystolic murmur (generated at the patent foramen ovale); but also as emphasizing the fact that it is difficult and frequently impossible to diagnose during life between the various forms of cardiac defects, and especially between these two types of pulmonary stenosis. For here the point of maximum intensity of the thrill (third and fourth left interspace) and the localization and direction of transmission of the murmur (at apex and into the back and vessels of the neck) pointed to an associated ventricular defect, although none was present.

C. Paradoxical Cerebral Embolism. Two of the cases whose histories form the subject of this communication (Cases II and III), both deeply cyanosed subjects, died with unexpected manifestations of a cerebral complication of apparently identical nature, a hemiplegia ushered in by pain in the head, convulsions, stupor and elevation of temperature, death following on the fifteenth and eighth days respectively after the onset of symptoms. In both cases operation upon an inflammatory focus in another part of the body (evacuation of a phlegmon of the arm in Case II and appendectomy in Case III) had taken place shortly before the development of cerebral symptoms. The autopsy in Case III revealed a large abscess of the left frontal lobe and purulent meningitis; in Case II the brain was not examined but a similar condition may fairly be concluded. In both patients the hearts showed a defect of the interventricular septum and a deviation to the right of the aorta, which arose from the right ventricle, thus presenting an easy route for a septic embolus from the thrombosed venules of the periphery to the terminal arteries of the cerebral circulation (paradoxical or crossed embolism).

This combination of events in these two cases, is of interest from several aspects. In the termination by *cerebral abscess* it illustrates in the first place an outcome of congenital cardiac lesions that is far from infrequent, and that was recognized by the older English students of the disease as a part of its classic picture; and they present, in the occurrence of a *paradoxical embolism*, one of the best examples we have of the manner in which the apparently bizarre symptomatology of cardiac defects is reduced, in the light of a complete knowledge of all the facts, to conditions of perfect simplicity. Moreover, the apparent contradiction of an established physiological law by the earliest observations upon the phenomenon of paradoxical embolism, and the subsequent explanation of these by the demonstration of a communication between the two circulations through a defect in the cardiac septum, is a dramatic episode in the history of pathological anatomy in the nineteenth century which claims our instant attention.

Historical. One of the most important of Virchow's early contributions to medical science (1845) was his elucidation of the nature of embolism, as the carrying in the blood stream of fragments broken off from the parent thrombus to the infarction of distant tissues. In a subsequent research, Rindfleisch (1873) pushed these investigations further to the conclusion that an embolus must always go forward in the path of the circulation and that emboli in the right heart or in the lung must, therefore, be derived from the venæ cavæ or their tributaries, and those in the end arteries of the systemic circulation from the radicals of the pumonary veins or the left heart. He explained certain apparent contradictions by supposing that occasionally small emboli could traverse the capillaries of the lung and be stopped in the narrow end arteries of the kidney and other organs. Trousseau (1880) in speaking of ulcerative endocarditis as a cause of cerebral embolism, related a case in which the valves of the right heart only were affected, and suggested that the vegetations had traversed the capillary vessels of the lung by means of ulcerating through the wall of the pulmonary arterioles. The observation made by Hirschberg[6] that cerebral abscess is especially common in gangrenous inflammatory processes in the lungs where there is extensive destruction of tissue may indeed have some such explanation.

The first to trace definitely the path of the embolus through an opening in the cardiac septum was Cohnheim (1877), who demonstrated a recent embolism of the right Sylvian (middle cerebral) artery in a case of widely patent foramen ovale with thrombosis of the veins of the lower extremities, but the valves of the left heart, aortic arch and arterial system proved absolutely free from any thrombus. Litten next, in 1880, autopsied a case of gangrene of the right leg from a large embolus blocking the femoral artery, but was puzzled to account for this and for numerous small infarcts in spleen and kidney, in the absence of any source in the arterial circulation, and finally submitted the organs to Virchow, who demonstrated a patent foramen ovale and thrombi in the right auricle. The conclusions enunciated by Cohnheim and Virchow on the basis of these two cases were substantiated and verified by Zahn[7] (1881), who discovered, in a case of extensive thrombosis of the iliac veins of puerperal origin, a long embolus of pen-handle size sticking through a patent foramen ovale into the left auricle. A similar observation was made by Hauser.[8] In a full analysis of 711 subsequent autopsies in Zahn's service made by his assistant Rostan,[9] the foramen was patent 139 times; in 3 of these cases its orifice was occluded by a thrombus, and in 7 a so-called paradoxical embolism had taken place through it. Of these 7 cases, in 3 the embolism was cerebral. Metastases of tumor masses through a patent foramen were later demonstrated by Zahn;[10] particles from ruptured liver by Schmorl, and the vegetations of malignant endocarditis by Jaeniche, Sänger and others. The above details are cited in a full review of the literature to 1907 as given by Ohm,[11] with the report of a case of his own of patent foramen ovale, thrombosis in the hemorrhoidal veins and two successive attacks of cerebral embolism, the first three weeks before death followed by a left hemiplegia and softening in the left lenticular nucleus and the second a blockage of the right middle cerebral artery, followed by immediate exitus.

Cerebral Abscess. The most interesting publication in connection with the present communication is that by Ballet[12] entitled, "*Des abscès du cerveau consecutifs à certaines malformations cardiaques.*" He collected from the literature 4 cases and published 1 of his own, of cerebral abscess in patients whose hearts showed a communication between the right and left chambers; in 1 (Lallemand) there was a widely patent foramen ovale and pulmonary stenosis of the inflammatory type; in 2 (Ballet, Louis) a ventricular septal defect without other cardiac anomaly; and in 2, those by Farre[13] and Berthody, a condition similar to the authors' Case II of defect at the base of interventricular septum aorta displaced to the right and arising from both ventricles above this and pulmonary hypoplasia. The autopsies in these 5 cases were not detailed and the state of the peripheral veins is not mentioned nor was the possibility of a crossed embolism apparently considered by Ballet, but a causal connection between the cerebral and cardiac lesions was definitely assumed. Stone[14] and Peacock[15] report similar cases. The latter remarked that a cerebral complication is the commonest cause of death in congenital cyanosis, but he also did not try to establish the nature of the etiological sequence which he believed existed.

Several cases of sudden onset of cerebral symptoms followed by death in congenital heart lesions are reported from the clinical standpoint in which a paradoxical embolism may fairly be assumed. Thus Palmer[16] relates the onset of a hemiplegia in a woman, aged twenty-two years, with cyanosis, clubbing, polycythemia and dyspnea in whom physical examination showed a congenital heart lesion. When it is realized how frequent is the occurrence of thrombosis of the right heart and peripheral veins, how direct is the path to the systemic circulation that is presented by a defective septum, especially when associated with deviation to right of aorta, and the fact that small emboli, which would end in the production of relatively harmless infarcts elsewhere in the body, will inevitably lead, on their arrival in the end arteries of the brain, to serious symptoms indicating the disintegration and frequently the septic infection of the delicate nerve tissue, we understand the grave significance of septal defects in this connection.

In further illustration of this interesting subject the 14 cases of cerebral abscess in cardiac septal defect enumerated above, are here summarized:

A. *In defect of interventricular septum.*

(a) *Without other anomaly.*

1. *Louis.* *Arch. gen. de med.* (*quoted by Ballet*), male, aged twenty-five years. Defect V. S. at base, smooth margins. No other anomaly. *Two areas of cerebral softening.* (*a*) In anterior part of corpus striatum, and (*b*) in optic tract behind this.
2. *Ballet.* *Arch. de med.* (1880, **5**, 659), own case, male, aged fifteen years. Defect V. S. at base, malposed septum, aplastic right ventricle, and tricuspid orifice. *Abscess in frontal lobe of brain and purulent infiltration.* Nasal fossæ, bones of cranium and meninges elsewhere free from inflammation. Left hemiplegia twelve days before death.

(*b*) *With deviation to right of aorta and pulmonary stenosis.*

3. *J. R. Farre. Obs.* 3 *in "Malformations of Human Heart," London,* 1814, male, aged nine and a half years. Aorta from both ventricles, pulmonary orifice small. Open between ventricles below aortic cusps. *Abscess in right hemisphere of brain containing ½ ounce of thick pus.* Cyanosis from two and a half years. Left hemiplegia eight days before death.
4. *Berthody. Medical Examiner, May,* 1845, female, aged twenty-one years. V. S. interrupted just below aortic cusps. Pulmonary artery hypoplastic. *Abscess in left posterior lobe of brain* size of pigeon's egg, left lateral ventricle filled also with pus. Slight cyanosis and dyspnea throughout life. Delirium and coma before death.
5. *Stone. St. Thomas' Hosp. Reports,* 1881, **11**, 57. Female, aged nineteen years. Conus stenosis of right ventricle. Acute endocarditis of lower conus orifice. Large defect V. S. at base. Purulent meningitis. *Old cerebral abscess in right occipital lobe containing fetid pus;* burst into horn of right lateral ventricle. Cyanosis and dyspnea from birth. Sudden onset of severe headache. Death.
6. *Peacock. Trans. Path. Soc., London,* 1881, **32**, 65. Male, aged six years and nine months. Aorta to right from both ventricles. Defect V. S. at base. Pulmonary hypoplasia. F. O. closed. Brain not examined. Cyanosis, clubbing from birth. Left hemiplegia with convulsions setting in with pain in head and stupor sixteen days before death. Temperature 101° F.
7. *Authors' Case II (this article).* Male, aged ten years. Pulmonary stenosis, defect V. S. at base deviation to right of aorta. Brain not examined. Cyanosis and dyspnea, clubbing, phlegmon of arm evacuated, left hemiplegia followed and death fifteen days later.
8. *Authors' Case III (this article).* Male, aged eleven years. Pulmonary atresia. Defect V. S. at base. Aorta from conus of right ventricle. *Cerebral abscess of left frontal lobe.* Purulent meningitis. Cyanosis and dyspnea from birth. Appendectomy; six days later headache, temperature 101° F. Right hemiplegia. Death two days later.

B. *In patent foramen ovale. Ventricular septum closed.*

(*a*) *No other anomaly.*

9. *Rostan. Case VII, Thèse de Genève,* 1884. Male, aged sixty-five years. Large patent foramen ovale. Thrombosis of right auricle. *Multiple areas of cerebral softening.* (*a*) In third frontal combination. (*b*) Cicatrized area on anterior surface of left lateral ventricle. No clinical data.

10. *Rostan.* Case X., *Ibid.* Female, aged fifty-four years. Thrombosis in right auricle, *embolism of right Sylvian artery.* Multiple infarcts in lung, spleen and kidneys. Left hemiplegia some days before death. Large patent F. O.
11. *Rostan.* Case XII, *Ibid.* Male, aged twenty-three years. F. O. widely patent. Thrombosis of long saphenous vein. *Multiple infarcts of brain.* (*a*) In left hemisphere. (*b*) In right lenticular nucleus and spleen. No clinical data.
12. *Cohnheim. Allgem. Pathologie,* 1877. *Quoted by Ohm and Rostan.* Adult woman. Thrombosis of veins of legs. Patent F. O. *Recent embolism of Sylvian artery.*
13. *Ohm. Ztschr. f. klin. Med.,* 1907, **61**, 379. Large patent F. O. Thrombosis in hemorrhoidal veins. *Recent embolus in right middle cerebral. Softening in left lenticular nucleus.* Slight cyanosis. Right hemiplegia with facial and hypoglossal paresis and marked dysarthria. Left nasal field of vision defective. Duration one week. Sudden death two weeks later from second cerebral embolus.

(*b*) *Patent F. O. with pulmonary stenosis and closed V. S. (inflammatory type).*

4. *Lallemand. Recherches anat. path. sur l'encephale.* (*Quoted by Ballet*). Patent F. O., tricuspid and pulmonary stenosis; *Cerebral abscess, size of hen's egg in right hemisphere containing* 3 *ounces of yellowish-green pus* enclosed by thick wall. Brain softened around. Cyanosis and dyspnea from infancy, intense last ten years after menopause. Left hemiplegia twelve days before death. Onset with cramped-like feelings in hand and foot. Reason and speech clear. Localized convulsive twitchings on paralyzed side. Coarse precordial thrill.

Summary. 1. Pulmonary stenosis or atresia with closed interventricular septum is of unusual occurrence and is due to a fetal endocarditis setting in after the heart has formed. Narrowing of the pulmonary tract with associated ventricular septal defect is the much more frequent finding and is due to arrested development in early embryonic life and is usually associated with a deviation to the right of the aorta.

2. In pulmonary atresia the degree of cyanosis is naturally more intense and the duration of life shorter than in pulmonary stenosis. In atresia, however, an associated septal defect facilitates aëration of the blood, especially with a deviation to the right of the aorta; such cases have, therefore, a better prognosis and present a more

moderate degree of cyanosis than does pulmonary atresia with closed interventricular septum. In pulmonary stenosis, on the other hand, an associated septal defect is *unfavorable*, for it tends both to reduce the volume of blood passing through the stenosed orifice and to permit the passage of venous blood into the arterial stream. The most favorable prognosis, therefore, in pulmonary stenosis, is in cases where the ventricular septum is closed.

3. Dyspneic attacks are especially frequent and severe in cases where a marked ischemia of the pulmonary circulation is present, as in pulmonary stenosis with pinhead orifice and closed septum and in certain cases of patent ductus arteriosus.

4. Cerebral complications of the nature of abscess or infarction are a frequent complication of congenital cardiac cases presenting defects in the interauricular or ventricular septum, and are in the great majority of cases embolic in origin, from a focus in the venous system (paradoxical or crossed embolism). Two cases of this interesting finding are here added to the literature.

5. Anatomical conclusions on the associated ventricular septal defect and deviation to the right of aorta in Cases II and III.

(*a*) In cases of "Rechtslage" of the aorta the position of the pars membranacea septi is altered in relation to the aortic cusps but is not changed in regard to the right auricle and ventricle.

(*b*) If the defect in the interventricular septum is situated posteriorly just in front of the pars membranacea septi it will open into the sinus of the right ventricle directly under the tricuspid segment, and if "Rechtslage" of the aorta be present, this vessel will appear to arise from the sinus also; while, if the defect be situated more anteriorly, it will open into the conus of the ventricle from which again the aorta will appear to arise.

(*c*) In pulmonary stenosis or atresia with septal defect, the condition of the conus of the right ventricle, whether hypoplastic or not, will depend on whether the defect in the septum opens into the sinus of the ventricle or into the conus; in the former case the conus will be small and aplastic; in the latter it will be large and thick-walled.

REFERENCES.

1. Abbott: Congenital Cardiac Disease, Osler and McCrae's Modern Medicine, 2d edition, 1915, **4**, 323–448 (Pulmonary Stenosis and Atresia, p. 338–398); also, Statistics of Congenital Cardiac Disease, Jour. Med. Res., 1908, **19**, 77–81.
2. Tandler: Anatomie des Herzens, Jena, 1913, p. 60–64.
3. Keith. Malformations of the Bulbus Cordis. From Studies in Pathology, Quatercentenary Publication, University of Aberdeen, 1906.
4. Cassel. Pulmonal Stenose, Berl. med. Gesellsch., November 25, 1891, Berl. klin. Wchnschr., 1891, **52**, 1221.
5. Eisenmenger: Die angeborenen Defecte der Kammerscheidewand des Herzens. Ztschr. f. klin. Med., 1897, **32**, Supp. Heft, I. p. 1.
6. Hirschberg: Beitrag zur Lehre des Hirnabscess (Metastatische) Nach Bronchial drüsenabscess, Deutsch. Arch. f. klin Med., 1913, **109**, 314.
7. Zahn: Rev. méd. de la Suisse, 1881, **4**, 227.

8. Hauser: Ueber einen Fall von embolische Verschleppung von Thrombenmaterial, München. med. Wchnschr., 1888, **35**, 583.
9. Rostan: Contribution a l'étude de l'embolie croissée consecutive à la persistance de trou de botal. Thèse de Génève, 1884.
10. Zahn: Ueber Paradoxe Emboli und deren Bedeutung zur Geschwulstmetastase, Virchows Arch., 1889, **115**, 71.
11. Ohm: Klinische Beobactungen bei offenem Foramen Ovale und deren diagnostischen Bedeutung, Ztschr. f. klin. Med., 1907, **61**, 374.
12. Ballet: Des abscès du cerveau consecutifs à certaines malformations cardiaques, Arch. gén. de méd., 1880, **5**, 659.
13. Farre: On Malformations of the Human Heart, Observation 3, London, Longmans, 1814.
14. Stone: Report of a Case of Tricelian Heart, Cerebral Abscess, St. Thomas Hosp. Reports, 1881, n. s., **11**, 57.
15. Peacock, Thos. B.: Malformation of Heart; Great Obstruction of Orifice of Pulmonary Artery; Aorta Arising from Both Ventricles, Trans. Path. Soc., London, 1881, **32**, 35.
16. Palmer, F. S.: Case of Congenital Heart Disease and Hemiplegia, Proc. Roy. Soc. Med., 1913–1914, **7**, Clin. Sec., 48, 3.

CLINICAL OBSERVATIONS ON HEART BLOCK.* †

BY PAUL D. WHITE,

AND

LOUIS E. VIKO,

BOSTON.

OCCASIONALLY there appears in the clinic a patient with heart block and as such he is examined with a good deal of passing interest. A few striking cases influence greatly our impressions of the incidence, causes, complications and prognosis of the condition. Further study and years of observation may not justify all these first impressions. To obtain more accurate data on heart block we have made a study of all of such cases electrocardiographed in our laboratory at the Massachusetts General Hospital in the past seven and a half years. Without the use of the electrocardiograph the all-important cases of intraventricular block would be missed, as well as certain points of which we shall speak concerning auriculo-ventricular block. From the standpoint of general interest we shall also include the few cases of so-called sino-auricular block that we have seen. Postmortem examinations have not been carried out in a sufficient number of cases to warrant detailed report in this group.

At the outset it is necessary to define briefly the types of heart block:

Complete auriculo-ventricular block consists of complete dissociation between auricular and ventricular contractions not due to excessive irritability of the ventricular pacemaker. Thus it is

* From the Medical Clinic and Cardiographic Laboratory of the Massachusetts General Hospital.

† Read before the Association of American Physicians, Washington, May 3, 1922.

necessary to distinguish between complete heart block and complete auriculo-ventricular dissociation. We have considered an idio-ventricular rate of 60 as the borderline.

Partial auriculo-ventricular block consists of partial dissociation between auricular and ventricular activity in which the conduction time, as expressed electrocardiographically by the *P-R* interval, is abnormally long or in which there are dropped beats, and where ventricular escape is not primarily the cause of the dissociation. For the sake of clearness we have added to this series only those cases with dropped beats or with a *P-R* interval of 0.2 second or over. The borderline group with *P-R* intervals ranging from 0.18 up to 0.20 second we have omitted here, so that there may not be the least question as to the presence of partial block.

Intraventricular block is the expression used for delay or blocking in the arborizations of the auriculo-ventricular conduction system below the bifurcation of the bundle of His. The greater degree is considered to be high-grade block in one of the two main branches of the bundle, which supply left and right ventricles respectively. Such lesions give characteristic electrocardiograms.

Lesser grades of intraventricular block—produced by partial blocking in the main branches of the auriculo-ventricular bundle, or by extensive lesions in the finer arborizations or by both, are also determined electrocardiographically by deformity of the ventricular complexes. In this series only well marked cases have been included. Cases of doubtful aberration have been omitted though without question there is a fairly wide border-line between normal and abnormal electrocardiograms.

Finally "sino-auricular" block is the term generally applied to that condition of the cardiac mechanism in which the sino-auricular node itself fails to function, either at intervals, giving rise to pauses of the whole heart about equal to the interval between two normal beats, or with a distinct halving of the rate of the sino-auricular pacemaker, or with a very slow regular sino-auricular rhythm, or with auricular standstill and idio-ventricular rhythm.

The following table shows the frequency of the various types of heart block found among 3219 cases electrocardiographed at the Massachusetts General Hospital from October 21, 1914, to March 15, 1922. 6719 plates were taken.

TABLE I.

Type of block.	Cases.	Per cent.
Auriculo-ventricular block	156	4.8
Complete	27	0.8
Partial	129	4.0
Intraventricular block	130	4.0
Bundle Branch	41	1.2
Lesser degrees ("aberration")	89	2.8
All cases showing auriculo-ventricular or intraventricular block	252	7.8
"Sino-auricular block"	11	0.3

Complete auriculo-ventricular block we have found 19 times in the male and 8 times in the female. The extremes in age in our series were six years and eighty-three years, but there were only 4 cases under forty years of age. The probable etiological factors were arteriosclerosis in 15 cases, or 56 per cent of the total, syphilis in 4 cases, diphtheria in 3 cases, rheumatic fever in 2 cases and doubtful in 3 cases. Digitalis may have been something of a factor in but 2 cases. Heart failure was found in only 6 cases at the time of the first record of the presence of complete heart block; 3 of these were of the anginal type and 3 of the congestive. Stokes-Adams attacks occurred in only 6 cases, or 22 per cent. The ventricular rates ranged from 25 to the minute up to 60, being in the thirties in 13 cases. Electrocardiograms showed intraventricular block in addi-

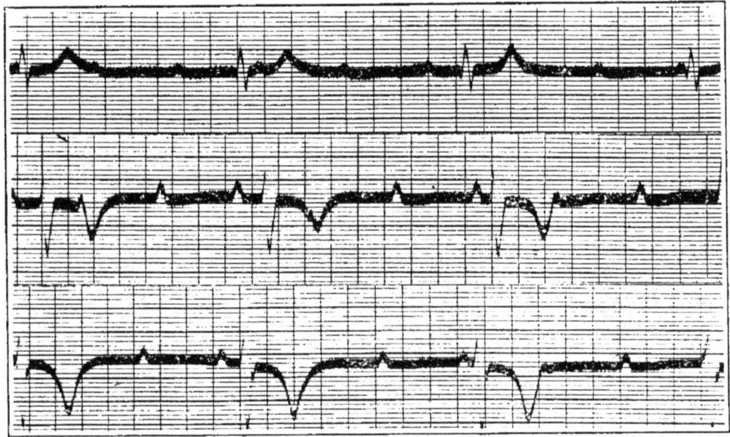

Fig. 1.—Electrocardiogram of S., showing complete auriculo-ventricular block and intraventricular block ("aberration") in addition. Leads I, II and III. In this and in the following figures abscissæ mark the time in 0.2 second intervals and ordinates mark the amplitude in 10^{-4} volts.

tion to complete auriculo-ventricular block in 15 of the patients, or 56 per cent (Fig. 1). Of these 3 showed well-marked bundle branch block. Auricular fibrillation occurred in 2 instances. Of 24 cases followed, 20 of them right up to date, 12 have died from heart failure, 7 of them within one year of the discovery of the complete heart block. Nine cases were "well" or in "fair condition," though still showing heart block when last noted, from one to seven years after the first record of the complete block. Of these 9, 5 had survived over five years, 4 of them being the 4 cases under forty years of age and 3 of these probably diphtheritic in origin. The fifth case was a man about fifty years of age with well treated syphilis.

Of the 129 cases of *partial auriculo-ventricular block*, 91 were male and 38 female. The age limits observed were birth and seventy-nine years. Sixty-two, or 48 per cent, were under forty years. The etiology of the heart disease in the group included rheumatic fever in 57 cases, arteriosclerosis in 34, syphilis in 12, doubtful in 5, miscellaneous (including one congenital block case) in 12, and no heart disease in 9. Digitalis was apparently chiefly responsible for the partial block in 65 cases, or 50.4 per cent, as shown by the characteristic flattening or inversion of the *T* wave of the electrocardiogram (compare Figs. 2 and 3), by the amount of digitalis given and

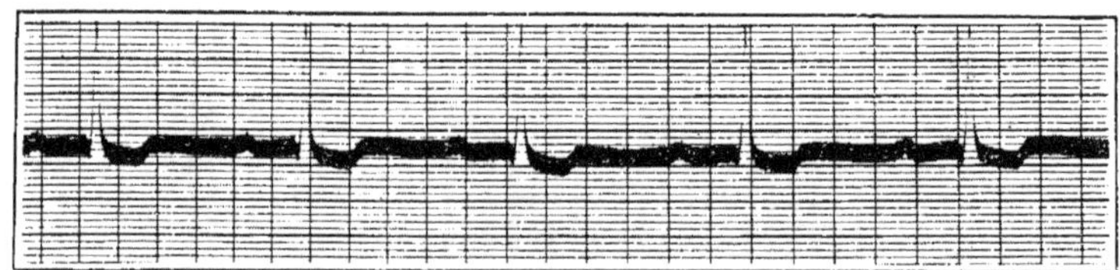

Fig. 2.—Electrocardiogram of C., showing partial auriculo-ventricular block of digitalis origin. Note the long P–R interval and the inverted T wave. Lead II.

by the recovery from the block after digitalis was stopped. Angina pectoris occurred in only 4 cases, and congestive failure in 49. Stokes-Adams attacks were found to have occurred in only 4 cases. The electrocardiogram showed a *P-R* interval varying from 0.20 second to 0.59 second. There was 1 case showing possibly a *P-R* interval of 0.85 second; this is more likely explained, however, by a dropped beat with ventricular escape following. There were a number of interesting variations in conduction time. One patient for example showed a *P-R* interval at times of 0.32 second without dropped beats and at other times with an interval of 0.17 second showed frequent

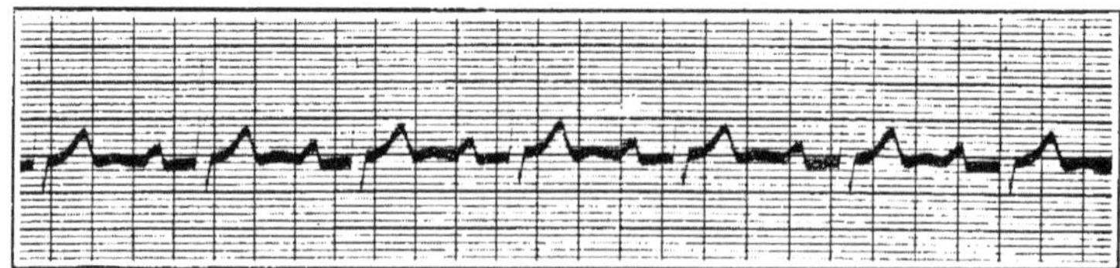

Fig. 3.—Electrocardiogram of M., showing partial auriculo-ventricular block not of digitalis origin. Note the long P–R interval and the upright T wave. Lead II.

dropped beats without any progressive lengthening of the interval. Another patient showed at one time a high grade partial block, with two or three to one rhythm, and on repeated examinations at other times normal rhythm and a *P-R* interval of 0.16 to 0.18 second. The cause of the paroxysm of heart block in this case was not found out, though there was undoubtedly an arteriosclerotic background, for the man had angina pectoris also. Intraventricular block was found in 19 cases of the whole group, or 15 per cent, being of the bundle branch type in 11 cases. Auricular fibrillation was present in 9 cases, in fact all those cases of auricular fibrillation with a ventricular rate of 45 or less being arbitrarily added to the group, but not including 2 cases with the regular idio-ventricular rhythm of complete heart block. Of these 9 cases of auricular fibrillation, 8 showed a well marked digitalization of the *T* wave. Seventy-eight of the 129 patients showing partial auriculo-ventricular block have been followed to date; 47 have had cardiac deaths and 21 are now in fair or good health.

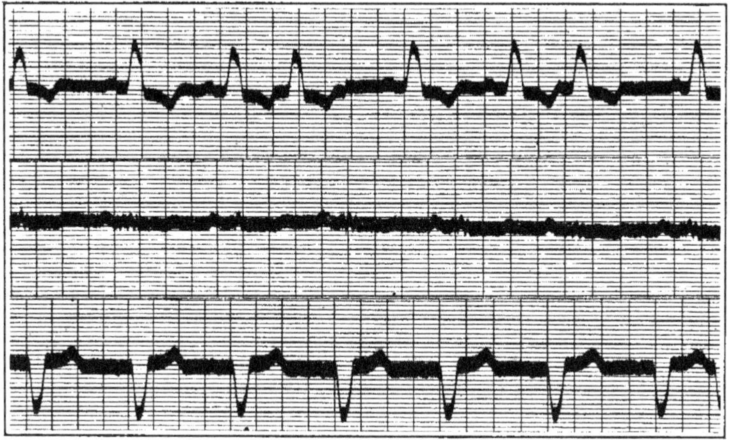

FIG. 4.—Electrocardiogram of Ga., showing intraventricular block of the right bundle branch type. Leads I, II and III.

Intraventricular block of the bundle branch type (Figs. 4 and 5), found in 41 cases of the 3219 electrocardiographed, occurred 34 times in the male and 7 times in the female. All but 2 cases were over forty years of age, the average being sixty years, the highest of all the groups. The youngest case was twenty-nine years of age and resulted temporarily from quinidine. Arteriosclerosis was apparently responsible in 33 of the patients, or 80.1 per cent, rheumatic fever in 4 cases, and syphilis in 3 cases. Although many of the patients received digitalis for congestive failure no relationship could be found which in this group would indicate that digitalis was in any way responsible for the intraventricular block. In 2 cases transient bundle branch block was produced by quinidine sulphate and in 2 other cases there was no change in the block when quinidine was administered. Angina pectoris occurred in 8 cases and congestive failure in 23. Stokes-Adams attacks occurred in 2 cases, one of which had also partial auriculo-ventricular block. Hypertension was found in 24 cases, or well over half. Auriculo-ventricular block occurred in 14 of the 41 patients, complete in 2 and partial in 12. Auricular fibrillation was found in 7 cases, and auricular paroxysmal tachycardia in 2. The block was of the right branch type in 40 cases and of the left branch type in only 1 case.* Of 36 cases followed to date 26 have died, 22 of cardiac failure, 13 of them within one year and 10 within six months of the discovery of the block.

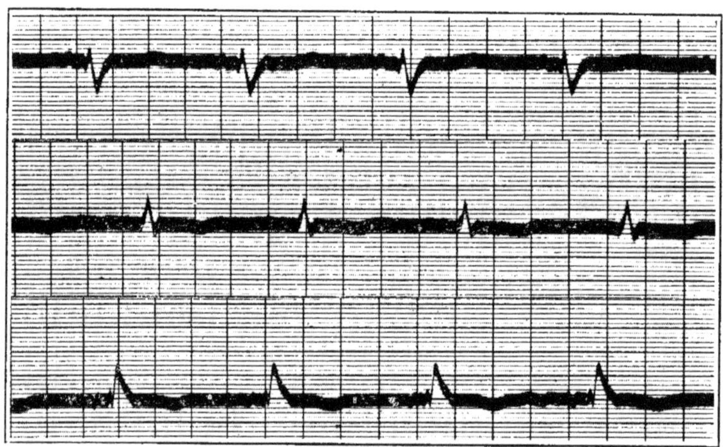

FIG. 5.—Electrocardiogram of Go., showing intraventricular block of the left bundle branch type. Leads I, II and III. (Previously published in the Medical Clinics of North America, January, 1920, **3**, 1035.)

Lesser degrees of intraventricular block (Fig. 6) have been found in 89 cases, 57 male and 32 female. The age limits were twelve and eighty-two years in the group, 17 of the patients being under forty years of age. Arteriosclerosis was apparently responsible in 53 cases, or 59 per cent, rheumatic fever in 22 cases and syphilis in 7. Digitalis did not appear to be a significant factor in any of our cases although it was frequently given because of the presence of heart failure. Quinidine sulphate was the cause of transient aberration in 4 cases, not including the 2 cases of bundle branch block so produced. Congestive failure occurred in 37 patients, at the time of the discovery of the intraventricular block, and angina pectoris in 15 cases. Auriculo-ventricular block coëxisted in 20 of the patients, complete in 12 and partial in 8. Auricular fibrillation coëxisted in 15 cases. Of 69 cases followed to date, 43 have died from heart failure, 25 of them (or 36 per cent of the total number followed) within six months of the discovery of the block.

* During the past year, up to March 23, 1923, 10 more cases have been discovered at the Massachusetts General Hospital in 514 patients electrocardiographed, 8 of the right bundle branch and 2 of the left bundle branch.

"*Sino-auricular block*" was found in 11 cases, 7 male and 4 female. The age limits were seven and seventy-nine years, the majority of the patients being below forty years of age. There was no heart disease in 7 cases, while of the other 4, arteriosclerotic heart disease was present in 2, rheumatic in 1 and hypertensive in 1. Digitalis was primarily responsible in 6 cases, including the 4 with heart disease. There were no Stokes-Adams attacks in this group. In 5 patients the block was complete, giving rise to auricular standstill, in 4 cases there were "dropped beats," in 1 case a very slow regular sino-auricular rhythm of 38, and in 1 case the sino-auricular rate suddenly halved after exercise. The *P-R* intervals when present were within normal limits. The condition was transient in all cases, without effect on life.

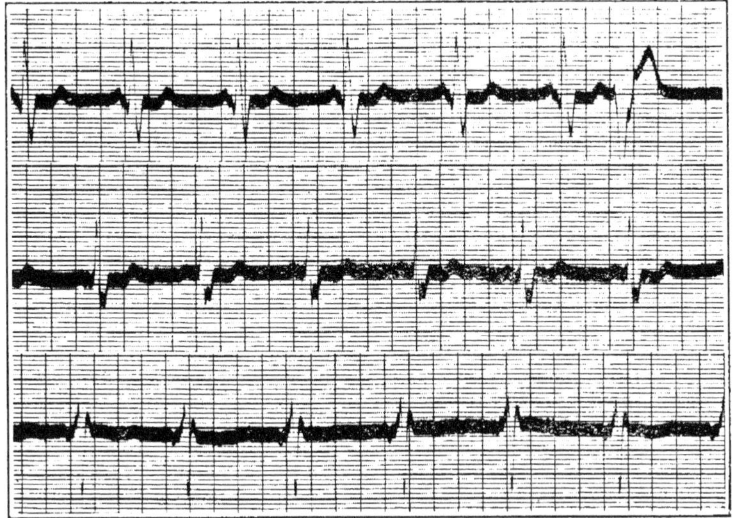

FIG. 6.—Electrocardiogram of W., showing a lesser grade of intraventricular block ("aberration"). Note the wide S_{II}. Leads I, II, and III.

Conclusions. 1. Intraventricular block is almost as frequently seen in a large medical clinic as is auriculo-ventricular block, 4.0 per cent having been found in 3219 cases observed at the Massachusetts General Hospital, as compared with 4.8 per cent of the latter type.

2. Complete auriculo-ventricular block in our series showed one-fifth the frequency of unquestionable partial auriculo-ventricular block.

3. Bundle branch block of high grade made up slightly less than one-third of our total number of cases of intraventricular block.

4. Sino-auricular block was rarely found, less than half as often as complete auriculo-ventricular heart block.

5. Arteriosclerosis was apparently responsible for the majority of our cases of complete auriculo-ventricular block and of intraventricular block of all degrees, but especially of bundle branch type, where it figured as the chief factor in over 80 per cent.

6. In our series syphilis was a probable factor in 16 of 156 cases of auriculo-ventricular block and in 11 of 130 cases of intraventricular block. Antiluetic treatment in a number of these cases which have been followed has not abolished the block, although disappearance of heart block under treatment has been reported and we have seen one such probable case in France during the war.

7. In the series of partial auriculo-ventricular block digitalis seemed to be chiefly responsible in more than half, on a background of rheumatic heart disease more often than arteriosclerotic heart disease. Digitalis was also largely responsible for 6 of the 11 cases of "sino-auricular block." The characteristic flattening or inversion of the *T* wave of the electrocardiogram was here very helpful in the analysis of digitalis effect.

8. Less than one-quarter of the cases of complete auriculo-ventricular block showed heart failure, either anginal or congestive, at the time of discovery, and also less than one quarter gave a history of Stokes-Adams attacks.

9. In every group the male sex was far oftener represented than the female, the ratio being about 5 to 2 in the whole series.

10. In our series the mortality from heart failure in the last seven and a half years has been slightly higher in the group with intraventricular block than in the group with auriculo-ventricular block. Several of the cases with complete heart block were in fairly good condition some years after the discovery of the block, in fact nine being in "good or in fair health" from one to seven years after the first electrocardiographic evidence of complete heart block. Four of the 5 cases surviving in fairly good health over five years after the discovery of the block were the 4 patients under forty years of age.

11. Heart failure was found more often in the patients with intraventricular block than in those with auriculo-ventricular block, especially heart failure of the anginal type. Angina pectoris was found about four times more often in intraventricular block than in auriculo-ventricular block.

12. It appears from this study that intraventricular block is of greater significance than auriculo-ventricular block. For its detection the electrocardiograph is essential.

BLOOD-PRESSURE REACTIONS TO PASSIVE POSTURAL CHANGES AN INDEX TO MYOCARDIAL EFFICIENCY.

By M. A. Mortensen, M.D., F.A.C.P.,
BATTLE CREEK, MICHIGAN.

Experiences during the World War served to emphasize in the minds of the medical profession the importance of the cardiac group of diseases, and the necessity for early recognition of myocardial inefficiency. Previously we exhausted our efforts in trying to make fine diagnoses of the various valvular lesions, and, as a result, often pronounced a heart normal because of absence of murmurs and overlooked a bad myocardium. A proper conception of the efficiency of the myocardium is perhaps the most important function of the cardiologist or the general practitioner. To recognize the heart as a muscle and to be able to evaluate its capacity is a most important art in order to institute proper treatment as well as to make a prognosis. The best of judgment is often put to a test in differentiating between functional and organic disease, whether valvular or myocardial.

Because of these difficulties many tests have been devised to determine myocardial efficiency, the exercise test being the most popular. The interpretation of these tests is based on the response of the pulse rate or blood-pressure to exercise, and the ability of the heart to resume the normal in a given length of time. Most recently the vital capacity of the lungs has been recommended as an index to cardiac efficiency. Our experience in using these tests in a series of cardiac cases resulted in waning enthusiasm because of too much elasticity in their performance. The various exercise tests do not mean the same amount of work for each individual because of variations in dexterity in their performance, and, consequently, the cardiac reaction may easily be misinterpreted. The vital capacity test is also of doubtful value because of the various conditions that have to be eliminated before we are justified in interpreting a deficient vital capacity of the lungs as an evidence of an impaired myocardium.

More than three years ago I became interested in the study of the effect of postural changes in blood-pressure as an index to vasomotor tone. Crampton calls attention to changes in blood-pressure with change of posture and interprets these as evidence of vasomotor status, especially as related to the splanchnic vessels. In his empirical table he refers only to the systolic pressure and pulse rate as the index. I soon became convinced that change in systolic pressure could not be due to vasomotor tone but was, rather, a response of the myocardium to the effect of gravity and to the muscular activity indulged in with changes in posture.

Sewall, in a most excellent article on this subject, states that the relative evaluation of systolic and diastolic blood-pressure leads to the conclusion that the former is an index of cardiac energy expended, a decision in keeping with observations on cardiac strain due to effort. Changes in diastolic pressure with changes of posture are more likely to indicate change in vasomotor tone, and Sewall, in the same article, states that the diastolic blood-pressure is generally admitted to measure the peripheral resistance to the circulation and to be an index of vasomotor tone. In our studies we recognized that even the slight effort of rising from the horizontal to the erect

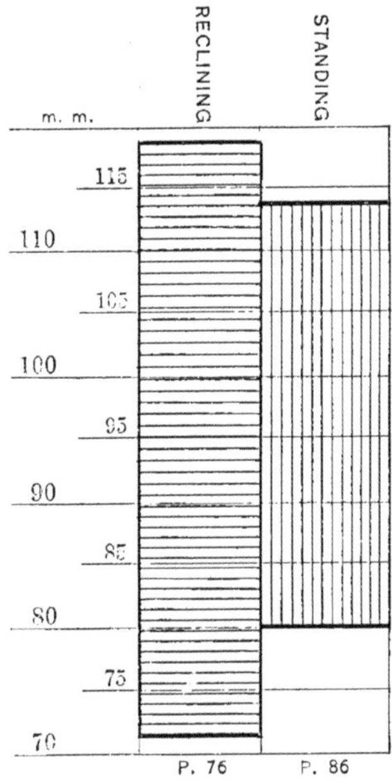

FIG. 1.—The average variation of blood-pressure and pulse rate with passive postural changes in ninety healthy young women.

posture must produce change in systolic pressure, and variation in pulse rate is also to be expected from the same exercise. However, it must be remembered that fundamentally exercise inhibits the vagus and thus tends to slow the pulse rate. In view of these facts, it seemed advisable to continue the study by eliminating the influence of exercise on pressure as well as pulse rate, and for this purpose we devised a tilting table on which a patient could be placed and blood-pressure and pulse rate observations made in both the reclining and the erect posture without effort or anxiety on the part of the patient, and with ease to the observer. An effort was also made to eliminate all possible variation in technic and, consequently, the mercurial sphygmomanometer was used in our observations as well as Bowles' stethoscope with an armband to hold it in position to maintain a uniform pressure on the brachial artery. The readings were made within thirty seconds after placing the patient in the upright position, and the pulse rate was based on quarter minute observations. In this way we limited our study to the influence of gravity on the blood volume, and the effort of the circulatory system to overcome this factor and to maintain a proper circulatory equilibrium.

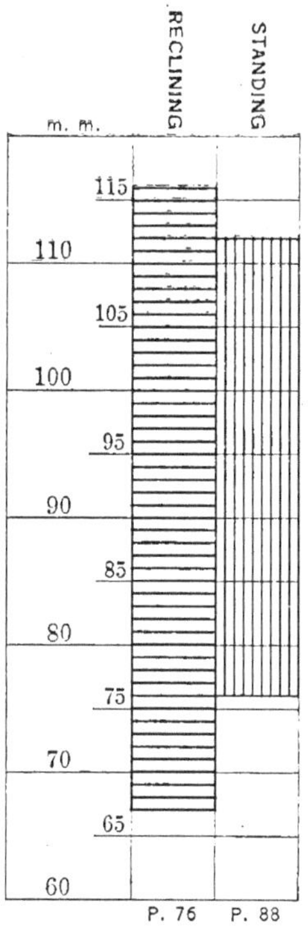

FIG. 2.—Miss M. B., No. 135746. Mitral lesion (tonsillar infections). No symptoms of cardiac inefficiency. Normal responses.

First, an effort was made to find the normal reaction of blood-pressure and pulse rate to this passive postural change in the healthy individual. For this purpose we took 90 young women from our Normal School of Physical Education, who had been in training for some months, and who, on entrance to the school had been carefully examined in order to eliminate all possible cardiac cases. To our surprise we found a marked uniformity in the reactions to passive postural change, fully 80 per cent showing a *slight decrease in systolic pressure and a slightly greater rise in diastolic pressure, thus cutting the pulse pressure at both extremes.* The pulse rate also increased uniformly, as much or more than in the change of position when assumed actively. In very few cases was the systolic higher in the erect posture and in no case was the diastolic found to

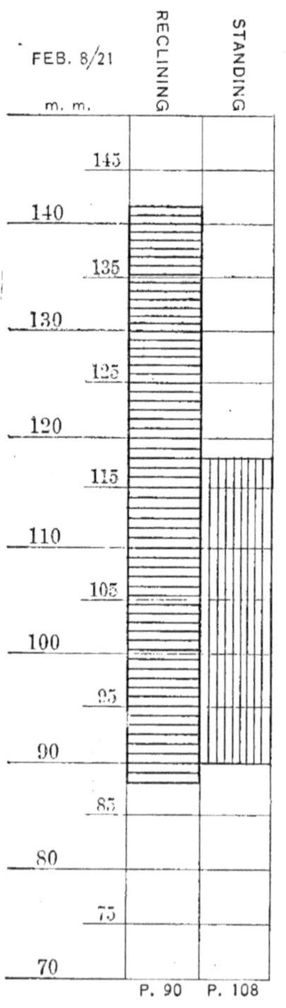

Fig. 3.—J. D. O., No. 136383. Chronic myocarditis. Attacks of acute dilatation associated with alcoholism. Note marked change in pulse pressure.

be lower. The *average maximum pressure in the 90 girls was* 118, *minimum* 72, *pulse rate* 76, as observed in the reclining position. After putting them in the erect posture the *average maximum pressure was found to be* 114, *minimum* 80, *pulse rate* 86. Since this definite series of normals was studied many normal individuals have been observed, both men and women, and with parallel results,

My findings in hundreds of cases have been so uniform that I feel confident that a marked deviation from these figures is an indication of some pathological condition. I have never found anything but very slight increase in systolic pressure when placing the individual in the erect position, and only once a decided drop in diastolic pressure with change of posture, and that individual complained

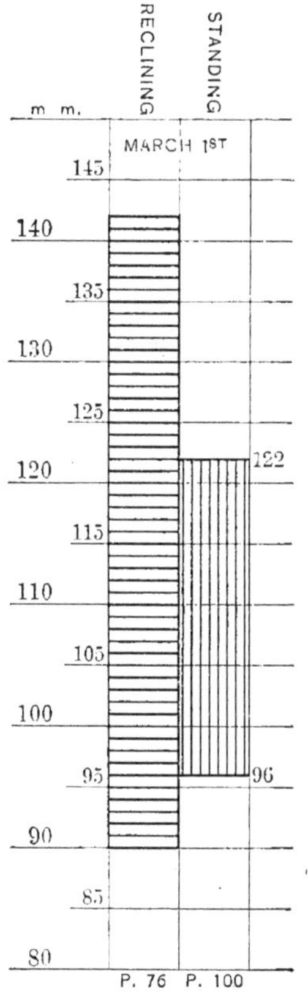

FIG. 4.—Mrs. N., No. 135192. Arteriosclerosis, hypertension, myocarditis with alternating pulse. Symptoms of angina. Note marked drop in systolic pressure with alteration.

of feeling faint and her appearance indicated this, which would tend to prove a sudden loss of vasomotor tone.

After obtaining these findings for the normal a systematic study was made of cases with definite cardio-vascular disease, especially those borderline cases where exercise tests were contraindicated, such as in angina pectoris. We were impressed with the fact that the drop in systolic pressure was definitely greater than in the normal cases, but the diastolic pressure behaved very much the same as in the normal case or in a few cases remained stationary. The drop in systolic pressure in the various types of cardiac cases studied ranged from 10 to 40 or 50 mm., depending, of course, on the degree of arterial tension, and impairment of the myocardium. I might interpolate that in cases of marked arterial hypertension with symptomatic evidence of myocardial inefficiency the change

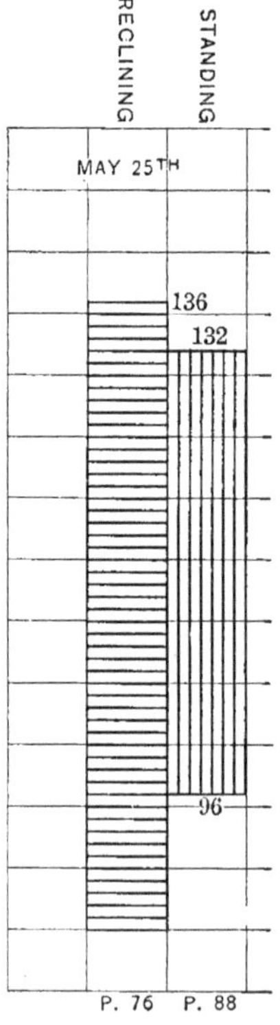

Fig. 5.—Dr. M. T., No. 136988, aged fifty-two years, chronic myocarditis. In college a sprinter and athlete. Symptoms of tachycardia, precordial discomfort with exertion. Note small pulse pressure with pronounced increase in pulse rate. Observation March 1, 1921.

in systolic blood-pressure with change of position was only a few millimeters, so that I feel justified in stating that an efficient myocardium, even in arterial hypertension, maintains the systolic pressure within 8 or 10 mm. of that found in the reclining position. As a result of three years' observation of almost daily use of this test I feel warranted in offering it as a test for estimating the efficiency of the myocardium. Graphic figures are presented showing the changes noted in different types of cases of cardiac disease with or without symptomatic evidence of cardiac inefficiency. In these studies changes also in pulse rate should always be noted and can be taken as additional evidence of myocardial embarrassment, as in all cases there is a greater increase in rate than would

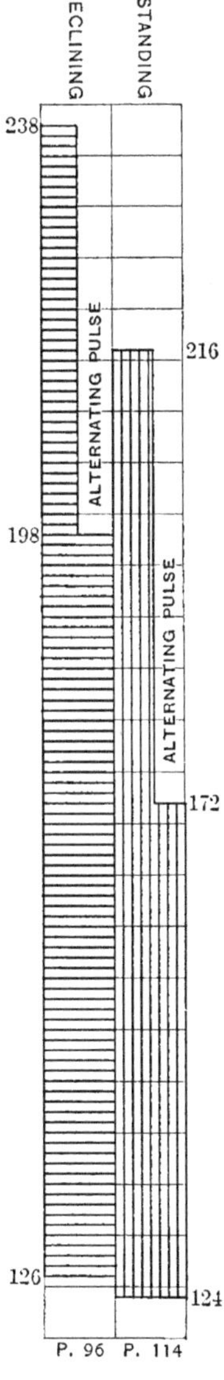

Fig. 6.—Dr. M. T. (same). Observation May 25, 1921, after carrying out program of graduated exercise and digitalis therapy.

be expected in the normal even without effort on the part of the patient in changing positions. Moreover, I have found the test of value when used at intervals to note a definite evidence of improvement while the patient is under treatment, whether this be in the form of digitalis therapy or graduated exercise. In a number of cases we have been impressed with the gradual improvement in the systolic pressure with digitalization indicating a better efficiency of the heart muscle, and in our opinion, corroborating the value of the test.

In a graphic representation of these studies the most striking feature is the decided change in pulse pressure, since with the passive postural change it is curtailed at both extremes, and a small pulse pressure, I believe, is accepted as definite evidence of circulatory inefficiency and might be compared with the so-called secondary low pressure.

Since beginning these studies Max Ellis reports a series of observations in normal individuals and his findings of changes from reclining to erect postures correspond in the main with our results. In our opinion the uniform range in systolic pressure is an indication of the ability of the heart to respond to a sudden demand to maintain the proper distribution of blood, especially to the brain, and the rise in diastolic pressure is the response of the vasomotor system to further help resist the influence of gravity on the distribution of blood. In the great majority of my cases the diastolic pressure was maintained or rose several millimeters, indicating a uniform response of the vasomotor mechanism. Consequently, in all types of heart disease, with or without arterial hypertension, three striking features are manifested with the passive postural changes. First, a decided fall in systolic pressure and a uniform maintenance or rise in diastolic pressure. Second, marked decrease in pulse pressure, which is the most striking evidence of inefficiency of the circulation. Third, the decided increase in pulse rate which, in spite of the absence of muscular effort, is further evidence of a decided effort on the part of the heart to maintain a circulatory equilibrium.

In performing the test it is necessary to have a tilting table so constructed that the patient can be changed from the horizontal to the erect posture without great effort on the part of the observer and without anxiety to the patient, and the mechanism for manipulating the table should be such that the change of posture can be made within a few seconds. Our table operates with a crank and is steadied by springs in the pulley chain so as to avoid jarring or sudden jerking of the patient.

Summary. 1. Very little has been recorded in literature relative to passive postural change of the blood-pressure in the normal individual, and none, as far as I have been able to determine, relative to these changes in heart disease.

2. A drop of more than 6 to 8 per cent in the systolic pressure, in changing from the reclining to the erect posture, may be viewed as an evidence of myocardial inefficiency. Careful history and physical examination will usually add support to this conclusion.

3. The rise in diastolic pressure is an index to the response of vasomotor mechanism to assist the heart to maintain circulatory equilibrium against the influence of gravity.

4. Pulse rate increase with change of position is greater than that noted with active postural change, indicating increased effort on the part of the heart to work against the influence of gravity.

5. This test is applicable in cases of angina pectoris or advanced arteriosclerosis where exercise tests are contraindicated. Cases of angina pectoris uniformly show a decided drop in systolic pressure.

6. The test is uniform for all individuals as it practically climinates all but the factor of gravity in the circulation. It is easily applied without discomfort to the patient and can be used at intervals for the purpose of noting progress in the management of cases and as an index to the influence of digitalis or exercise on myocardial efficiency.

BIBLIOGRAPHY.

Sewall, H.: Clinical Significance of Postural Changes in Blood-pressures and Secondary Waves of Arterial Blood-pressure, Am. Jour. Med. Sci., 1919, **158**, 786.

Barringer, T. B., Jr.: Heart's Functional Capacity, Arch. Int. Med., 1917, **20**, 829; Cardiac Insufficiency, Am. Jour. Med. Sci., 1918, **155**, 864.

Ellis, Max: Pulse Rate and Blood-pressure Response of Men to Passive Postural Changes, Am. Jour. Med. Sci., 1921, **161**, 568.

Crampton, C. W.: Blood Ptosis; a Test of Vasomotor Efficiency, New York Med. Jour., 1913, **98**, 916.

A CONSIDERATION OF THE VARIOUS LAWS OF HEREDITY AND THEIR APPLICATION TO CONDITIONS IN MAN.*

By J. Arthur Buchanan,

FELLOW IN MEDICINE, THE MAYO FOUNDATION, ROCHESTER, MINNESOTA.

Heredity is a science devoted to the study of the phenomena of breeding.

The mechanism of heredity came into play with the appearance of bisexual life on the surface of the earth. Its laws will continue to function until such life becomes extinct. The efforts of ancient, of medieval, and of modern investigators, to unravel the workings of the mechanism of heredity, form an interesting chapter in the development of biological knowledge.[12]

* Submitted to the Faculty of the Graduate School of the University of Minnesota in partial fulfilment of the requirements for the degree of Master of Science in Medicine, March, 1922.

The physico-biological characters, which are transmitted to subsequent generations by means of the germ plasm, furnish the concrete evidences for studies in heredity. A biological character signifies a type of physical and chemical composition possessed by individuals, by which they may be differentiated. Characters are rendered physically immortal by heredity, and the study of heredity becomes, in consequence, an investigation of the mechanism of physical immortality. The vehicles on which the transmission of the characters depends are the nuclear structures, chromosomes in all germ cells, and in certain instances the cytoplasm of the germ cells. The hereditary substances in the chromosomes and cytoplastic substances together comprise the germ plasm. The germ cells or gametes in man are the ova and the spermatozoa.

Heredity never deals with the etiological factors of disease. Any characters appearing in man that can be proved hereditary are normal, biologically speaking, regardless of how the characters may unfit their bearer for harmonious coöperation in the economical and social programs of civilization. This conception becomes clear when it is remembered that characters are brought to their bearer as an integral part of the stuff from which he developed, and that there is no alteration from the normal course of life. The factor on which the character depends is in the germ plasm. The character undergoes development along a fairly fixed line, as a component part of the body in which it appears. Hereditary characters in all plants and animals, and even in man in certain instances, are considered as expressions of normal features. The characters in man which embarrass his participation in all or certain parts of his duties and pleasures are looked on as expressions of disease. A man with an untoward hereditary character cannot be otherwise from a biological and physiological standpoint. The embarrassing characters are the physical expression of the type of stuff of which he is composed genetically, and not the expression of pathological processes.

By heredity the quantitative and qualitative characters in all bisexual species are kept extant and limited. Under similar conditions of reproduction, the numerical expression of the transmission of these characters follows very closely, or is reducible to, a fairly definite ratio. A character once proved hereditary is always hereditary, and not hereditary on a percentage basis.

The science of heredity includes the study of the intermediate as well as of the immediate stage of certain features of the life cycle. The ova and spermatozoa form the intermediate stage of the life cycle in man. The rearrangement of chromosomes which occurs following their union furnishes the fundamental basis for the study of the method of production of the tangible evidences of heredity in the immediate stage, the corporal stage, of the life cycle.

It is remarkable that heredity, a science so familiar not only to physicians, but to all reading men, whose principles are so easily gathered from the works of biologists, should be characterized by a lack of accuracy in medical literature.

Heredity as ordinarily used by medical writers means the presence of a like condition in parent and child. This occurrence is usually described as one of the etiological factors for the disease under consideration. The laws of heredity which have been established are at variance with this usage.

Kölreuter[23] made the first systematic investigation of hybridization, which is the first stage resulting from the crossing of parents with different inheritable characters. By his experiments he estabblished the fact that the hybrid offspring generally looks as like the male as the female parent.

Mendel[29] carried the work of Kölreuter one step farther by mating hybrid with hybrid. When the products of this mating were examined, he found that the parental characters which entered into the formation of the hybrid were separated in a peculiarly striking manner, and that the hybrid reappeared in its identical form. To this phenomenon Mendel applied the phrase. "segregation of characters." This is now known as the first law of heredity. Mendel believed that in the offspring of a mating all characters are segregated independently, and that there is no interrelationship in the transmission of characters. This belief is usually spoken of as the "independent assortment of characters," and is the second law of Mendel and of the science of heredity. This law has been found to be only partially true.

Since the time of Mendel four other laws have been derived from experiments carried out on plants and animals. They are known as: (1) Linkage, and its corollary, crossing over; (2) linear order of genes; (3) interference, and (4) limitation of the linkage groups. They have been carefully studied by Morgan.[30] Linkage of characters has been found to occur in man. The corollary and the other three laws have not yet been worked out in man.

The discovery of the spermatozoön in man by Leeuwenhoek,[24] the ovum in mammals by von Baer,[5] the cell by Schleiden and Schwann,[41, 42] the chromosomes by van Beneden,[4] the theory of cellular continuity by Virchow,[44] the theory of germinal continuity by Nussbaum,[34] furnished the material on which Weismann[46] evolved the theory of the germ plasm. This theory clearly isolated the ultimate units on which physico-biological characters must depend. The theoretic units are located in the germ plasm, and in their finest division are known as "biophors;" aggregations of biophors are known as "determiners," and the latter when grouped together are known as "ids." Groups of ids are called "idants," which are identical with chromosomes. Determiners are the fundamental aggregations of hereditary units in the germ plasm. Weismann vivified the significance of the spermatozoön and ovum with their nuclear and cytoplastic structures as the medium for the transmission of the ultimate units of hereditary characters.

The terminology used in studies in heredity is very simple. The parental generation, or the stock from which a series of studies has been made, is expressed by the symbol, *P*. The first product resulting from a mating of the parental generation in which unlike characters are crossed is known as the hybrid, and this stage is spoken of as the first filial generation. By mating members of the first filial generation, the second filial generation is obtained. This generation was the important one in the studies of Mendel. All generations, except the parental, are designated by the letter *F*, and a subnumeral which indicates the generation under consideration. The term homozygote is used to designate individuals who are pure bred for a particular character. The homozygote. when crossed with a homozygote with like characters, always breeds true to the characters present. The term heterozygote refers to an individual who, while possessing a certain character in his somatic cells, because of certain properties in the germinal cells, has the ability of transmitting not only a character present in the somatic cells but a character which is concealed or dormant in the germinal cells. The determiners for the dormant and evident characters are located in the germ plasm.

The discovery of the heterozygous property of plants was one of the most fundamental discoveries made by Mendel. In man the heterozygous person can be determined only by breeding, whereas in plants the knowledge of the nature of the parental generation furnishes information which enables an observer of plant breeding to determine, in certain instances, by physical inspection the homozygous and heterozygous types.

The property of the hybrid in plants to conceal one character while another was evident led Mendel to introduce the words "dominant" and "recessive." The character which is visibly represented in the hybrid is spoken of as dominant, while the other is spoken of as recessive. These words have been used in connection with the study of heredity in man, but erroneously so, as there is no direct way of determining which of the two characters will be dominant, because when two persons are mated to produce a cross of different characters, instead of a hybrid generation, there is an immediate progression to the segregation of the characters introduced in the cross with the production of both homozygous and heterozygous individuals, just as occurs in plants and fowls in the second filial generation. The first filial generation, or hybrid stage, in man is absent. The terms "dormant" and "evident" are more expressive when speaking of hereditary characters in man.

Mendel left no graphic illustration of his work which was carried out on species and subspecies of the edible pea (Pisum sativium) and species of the hawkweed (Hieracium) but Correns,[14] who discovered Mendel's work, confirmed and extended it, and visualized the parental generation, the first filial generation, and the second filial generation during which the segregation of characters took place (Fig. 1). In this experiment the four o'clock was used. A red flower (character red) was crossed with a white flower (character white). The result was a pink hybrid. When two of the hybrids were mated together, their offspring consisted of one red flower, one white, and two pink flowers, commonly spoken of as heterozygotes. The separating was the clearest possible example of what Mendel meant by the expression, "segregation of characters." The red and white if crossed with red and white respectively breed only red and

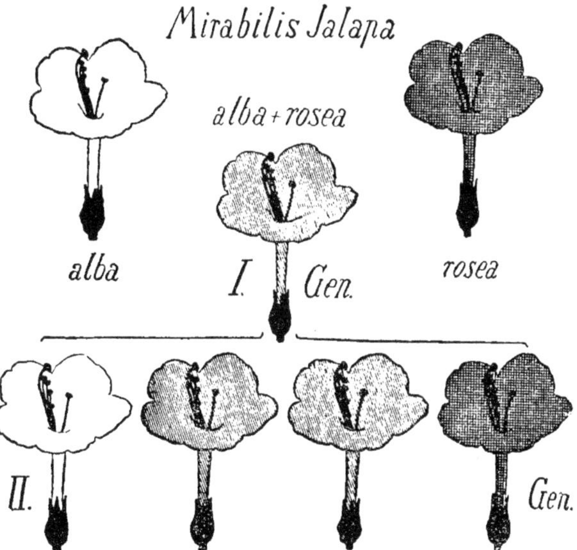

FIG. 1.—A diagram to show inheritance of flower color in crosses of Mirabilis, the "four-o'clock." *Alba*, white parent; *rosea*, red parent; *alba-rosea*, the unfixable F_1 heterozygote of intermediate color, pink. First generation = F_1. Second generation = F_2. (After Correns).

white respectively, whereas if the pink flowers of the second filial generation are crossed with pink flowers the segregation of characters repeats itself.

By a statistical investigation of many crosses Mendel established the now famous 3 to 1 ratio which is approximate and not absolute, as shown by his investigations. He found in Experiment 1, a ratio of 2.96 to 1; in Experiment 2, 3.01 to 1; in Experiment 3, 3.15 to 1; in Experiment 4, 2.95 to 1; in Experiment 5, 2.82 to 1; in Experiment 6, 3.14 to 1; and in Experiment 7, 2.84 to 1. These figures show a rather narrow range of possibilities.

In the study of heredity in man, the absence of the hybrid stage presents distinct obstacles to the direct application of the scheme used by Mendel in his investigations. The heterozygote in man is identical genetically with the hybrid of plants. Mendel demonstrated the segregation of characters by mating hybrids, which were the offspring of the same parents. The only similar biological and genetic situation in man would be the crossing of sister and brother heterozygotes, provided their heterozygous nature could be proved beforehand. Such a cross in man is clearly impossible. Furthermore, it is quite impossible to say in advance of a mating, whether or not a cross is of heterozygotes, or of homozygotes and heterozygotes. The evident character is always discernible, but the dormant character in man exists without any evidence. It is also often impossible to determine after studying the offspring resulting from a cross between two persons whether the parental generation was heterozygous or homozygous. The homozygous nature of both parents is demonstrated when all the children possess the same characters as the parents.

These difficulties make it impossible to derive Mendelian ratios directly by tabulating the products of crosses in man. Through a long period of time, it may be possible to demonstrate which characters may appear in certain combinations only as evident or dormant characters. Hitherto, no attempt has been made to prove this essential possibility in man, but by such an indirect procedure dominant and recessive characters can be determined. After the relationship of the dormant and evident characters in the heterozygote has been worked out, it will still be impossible to determine in advance of mating the homozygous or heterozygous nature of any particular person, unless his ancestors have been previously proved to be homozygous for the character under consideration. The accuracy of Mendelian ratios in man will be lessened for a long time to come on account of these obstacles.

Certain requirements are necessary in order to determine if a character or condition in man is hereditary and to establish its relationship to another character. The character must be arbitrarily defined, and a contrasted character must be selected. When two characters are crossed, at least three, and preferably four or more, children must result in order to observe the segregation of the characters and to establish their numerical relationships. A cross in man where only two characters are concerned needs investigation through but two generations. The evident characters will be discernible, but the recipients of the dormant characters cannot be distinguished. This fact must be borne in mind constantly, for heterozygous mates will reproduce their ancestors; unless this faculty is recalled, many conditions will be considered hereditary on a percentage basis or else not considered hereditary at all. The heterozygous principle has been responsible for immeasurable misunderstandings in the study of heredity in man. In cases in which three or four characters are under investigation the four grandparents, the parents, and a final generation of preferably four or more children must be studied; a final generation of less than three children furnishes data of no conclusive value. The *sine qua non* of a hereditary investigation is the knowledge of the characters represented in the germ plasm of the ancestors of the individuals under consideration.

THE INHERITANCE OF THE BLOOD GROUP: STUDY I. In 1900, Shattock[43] observed that the serum of patients suffering from certain diseases agglutinated the red blood cells of healthy men. He also noted the persistence of the agglutinative phenomena during the convalescence from the diseases. In 1901, Landsteiner[24] discovered that the red blood cells of healthy men, because of certain agglutinative properties of the serum, could be classified into three groups. A fourth blood group, Group 1 of the Moss classification, was dis-

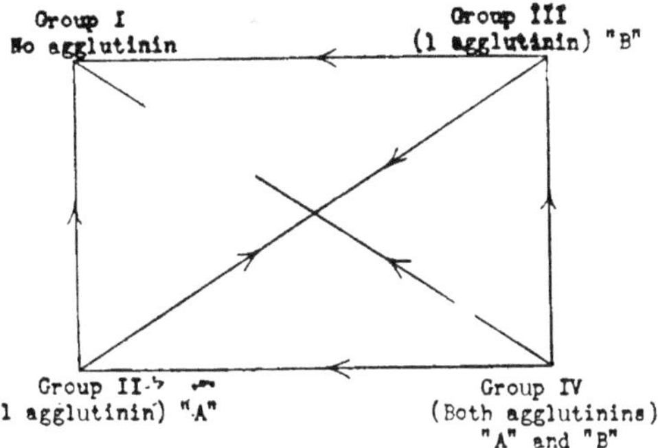

FIG. 2.—The corpuscles of the various groups are agglutinated by the serums of the groups from which the arrows lead. (After Sanford.)

covered by Decastello and Sturli in 1902.[16] In 1907, Jansky[22] made independent observations and reported the existence of four blood groups. The observations were reported independently by Moss[31] in the United States in 1909. The four blood groups known today are arbitrarily designated as Group I, Group II, Group III, and Group IV. They have been classified by Jansky and by Moss. Their classifications differ in that Jansky's Group I is the Group IV of Moss and *vice versa*. The scheme of Moss has been concisely presented by Sanford[40] (Fig. 2). I have followed the Moss classification, although the priority of Jansky is recognized as adopted by the American Association of Immunologists, the Society of American Bacteriologists, and the Association of Pathologists and Bacteriologists.*

The Mendelian transmission of blood group to subsequent generations by the germ cells has been suspected;[37] some definite evidence

* Article on Isohemagglutination: Jour. Am. Med. Assn., 1921, **76**, 130.

has been presented, but certain difficulties remain. This study was made in an attempt to obviate these difficulties.

The material studied was obtained in a unique manner. In discussing my desire to add further data concerning the inheritance of blood group with Dr. W. A. Evans, he suggested that a notice (Fig. 3) be inserted in his health column in the *Chicago Tribune*. It appeared on April 26, 1921. The same request subsequently appeared in all the publications of the Tribune Syndicate. Through the kindness of the Eugenics Record Office, the interests of Mr. A. E. Wiggam was aroused, and a similar request appeared in the *Physical Culture Magazine*, August, 1921. The replies to these requests were mailed to me. Each member of the family was mailed a 3 cc glass tube which contained 1 to 2 cc of 2 per cent sodium citrate solution. The tubes were well corked, packed in cotton in an ordinary mailing tube, and sent by first-class mail. At the same time, instructions were followed for collecting blood from a needle stab in the finger,

It's a Bona Fide Inquiry.

J. B. writes: "I would like to get the names and addresses of a few families in which four grandparents, both parents, and four or more children of the present generation are living and within reach. Will any one knowing of one or more such families write me the facts? The promise is that no improper use of the information will be made. The object is to get light on a question of family resemblance."

Difficult to Diagnose Comment.

I know the person inquiring and the object of the inquiry. If letters are sent to me I will see that they reach J. B. In violation of our rule we are keeping his name and address on file.

Fig. 3.—Insert from *Chicago Tribune*, April 26, 1921. Kindness of Dr. W. A. Evans.

and for labelling and remailing the tubes. The instructions were accompanied by a letter requesting the coöperation of the family in the work. If the first letter failed, a follow-up letter was sent. One tube was broken; twice hemolysis of the red cells occurred, so that second specimens had to be obtained. The cells were grouped with known Groups II and III serums and checked with homologous serums. Families suitable for this study are very scarce. There is not such a family on record at the Eugenics Record Office, Cold Springs Harbor, New York.*[11]

In 1908, Ottenberg[37] first suspected that the blood group was hereditary and transmitted to subsequent generations according to the laws of Mendel. In 1910, von Dungern and Hirschfeld[18] reported 72 families (348 persons) in which the grouping of the blood had been carried through two generations. They concluded

* I owe my thanks to Mr. E. C. Myers and Dr. J. I. Mershon, Mt. Carroll, Illinois, Dr. H. B. Cole and Dr. B. P. Flinn, Redwood Falls, Minnesota, Dr. R. A. Jacobson and Dr. C. F. Crow, Exira, Iowa, Dr. Greenleaf, Atlantic, Iowa, and Dr. C. C. Bassett, Goodland, Indiana, for their assistance in the work.

that blood group was hereditary and transmitted according to the Mendelian rules. Ottenberg,[38] in 1921, established certain formulas which he considered to be representative of the blood groups. In this study, in contradistinction to Ottenberg's formulas, I have used the terms Group I, Group II, Group III, and Group IV as expressive of a specific biological property of the blood of man. The factor for blood group is considered as comparable to those unexplained factors on which the unit characters height, shape, size, color, etc., in plants and animals depend. The exact formulas of the ultimate units on which hereditary characters depend are unknown.

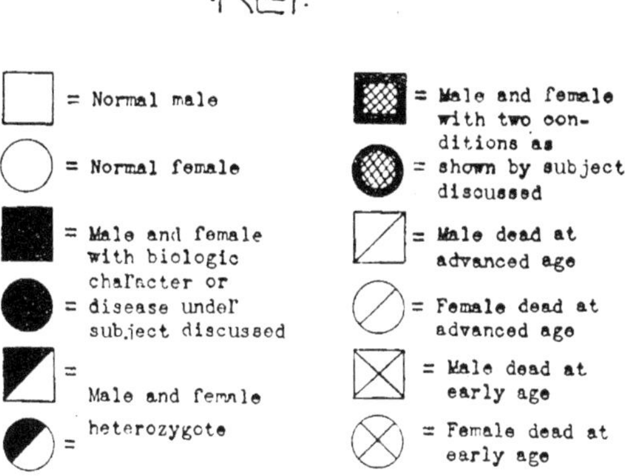

KEY TO FIGS. 4 TO 41.

If it is assumed as a premise that blood group is expressive of a hereditary character dependent on a unit factor comparable to that for color of flowers, height of plants, etc., it becomes necessary to present data to ascertain if blood group is transmitted

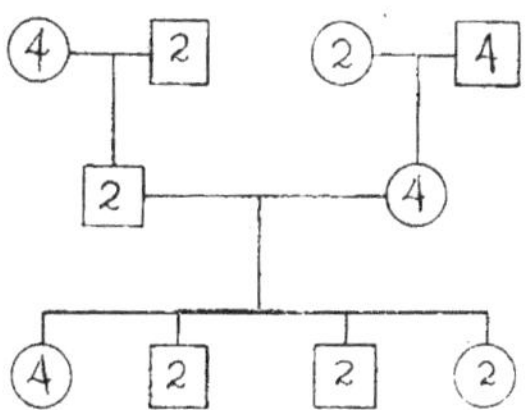

FIG. 4.—Transmission of blood Groups IV and II through three generations.

between generations in a manner similar to that occurring in plants and flowers. The data presented in Fig. 4 consist of the crossing of Group II with Group IV through three generations. If Fig. 4 is compared with Fig. 1 the absence of the hybrid stage or stage of the first filial generation in Fig. 4 will be noted; otherwise a new blood group having, to a certain extent, the characteristics of both parents would result. In the third generation of the family studied 1 child in Group IV and 3 children in Group II appeared. The blood groups present in the previous generations appeared in the final generation. No other blood groups appeared. If the phenomena observed in the third generation of this family were considered as illustrative of the first law of Mendel, it might be assumed that 2 of the children were homozygous and 2 were heterozygous, as occurs in the Mendelian segregation of characters. It was impossible to demonstrate a basis for the assumption in this family, as it would have been necessary to group the progeny of all 4 children in the family. The result would have been influenced by groups introduced by marriage, and the data obtained might or might not have been of any conclusive value.

The evidence that there are heterozygous individuals for blood group produced by the crossing of Group II and Group IV is shown in Fig. 5. The parental generation on both sides of the family consisted of the union of Group II with Group IV. Both families

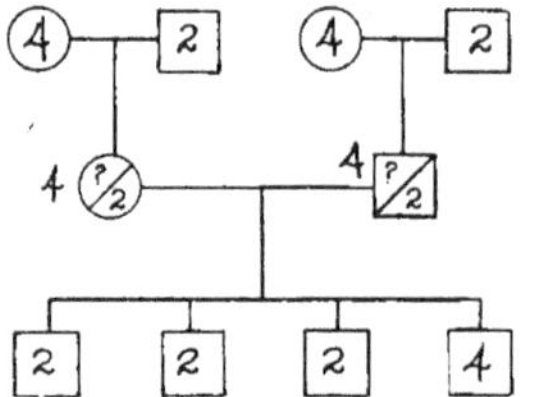

Fig. 5.—Transmission of blood Groups IV and II to the third generation because of the heterozygous nature of one of the parents in the second generation.

had a child in Group II. The mating of these children resulted in 3 children in Group II and 1 child in Group IV. If the blood group is hereditary, the factor for the Group IV must have been present in the germ plasm of either the male or the female parent, for there is no other mechanism in heredity by which it could have appeared in the final generation. A like situation is shown in Fig. 6. The blood of a heterozygote is not different from the blood of a homozygote. The difference is in the germ plasm alone.

The heterozygous property is illustrated in Fig. 6. In the parental generation on the left, the cross consisted of presumably homozygous Group II parents, and on the right a Group IV was crossed with a Group I. The result was a Group II on the left and a Group IV on the right. The final generation showed 2 children in Group II, 1 in Group I, and 1 in Group IV. This happened because of the heterozygous nature of the parental Group IV on the right. Figs. 7 and 8 are also a very clear demonstration that blood group is a distinct hereditary character, as all the characters concerned in the primary generation reappeared in the final generation. The same phenomenon is observed in Fig. 9, where Groups III and IV appear as the expression of the heterozygous principle.

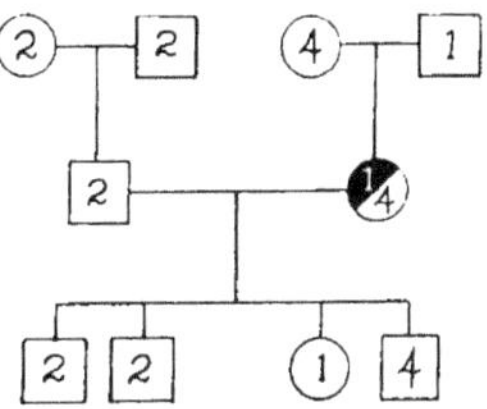

Fig. 6.—The segregation in the third generation of all the characters introduced by the ancestors. The female in the second generation was a heterozygote.

The homozygous nature of blood group is illustrated in Fig. 10. In this family the parental crossings on both sides resulted in children in Group II, which on being crossed produced 4 children in Group II. The same situation is shown in Fig. 5 where Group IV is the

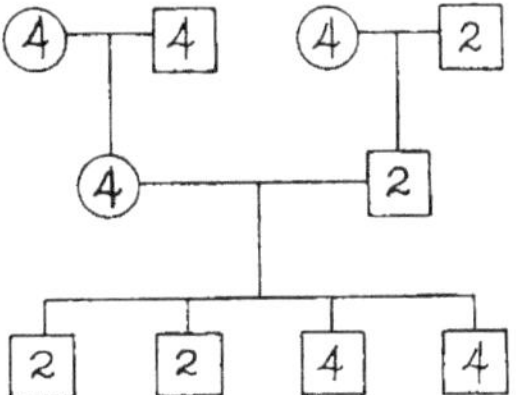

Fig. 7.—Transmission of blood Groups II and IV through three generations. There is no method of demonstrating the homozygous or heterozygous status of the male in the second generation.

homozygous character. Ottenberg,[37] in 1908, demonstrated the homozygous nature of Group III. He reported a father, mother, and 4 children all in Group III. The effect of crossing Groups III and IV is shown in Fig. 11. The homozygous nature of Group I

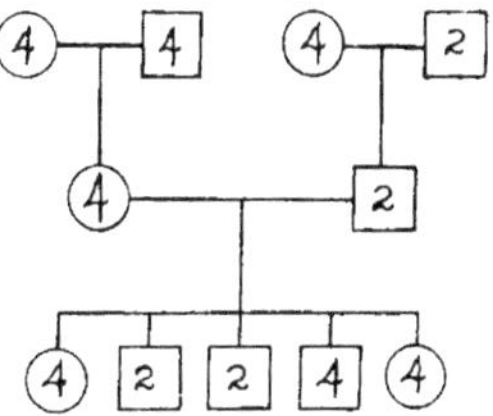

Fig. 8.—Transmission of Groups IV and II through three generations.

has not yet been demonstrated, but it seems reasonable to suppose, from its behavior when crossed with other blood groups, that it could appear in the homozygous state as well as in the heterozygous state (Figs. 6, 12 and 13).

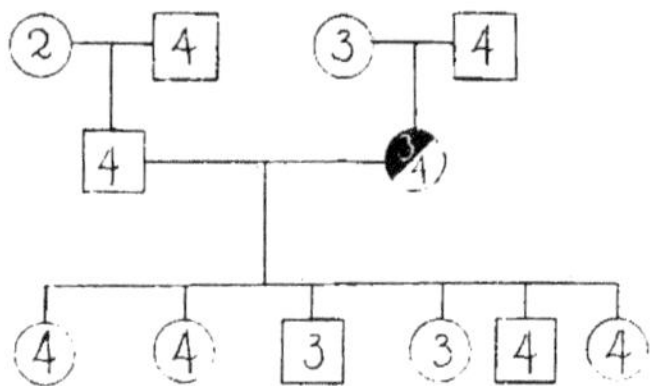

Fig. 9.—Transmission of blood Groups IV and III through three generations by means of a heterozygous female in the second generation.

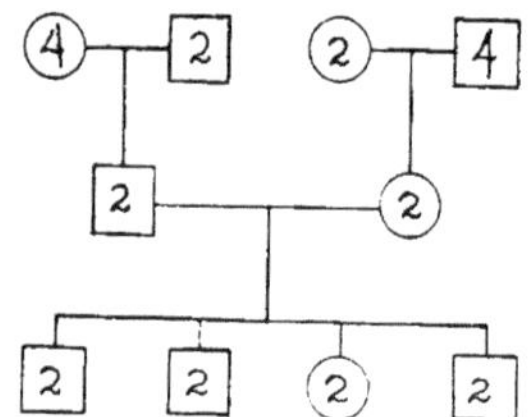

Fig. 10.—Segregation of pure Group II in the second generation as indicated by all the children of the third generation being in Group II.

The expressions, dominant and recessive, are frequently heard in discussing the inheritance of any character. Mendel described

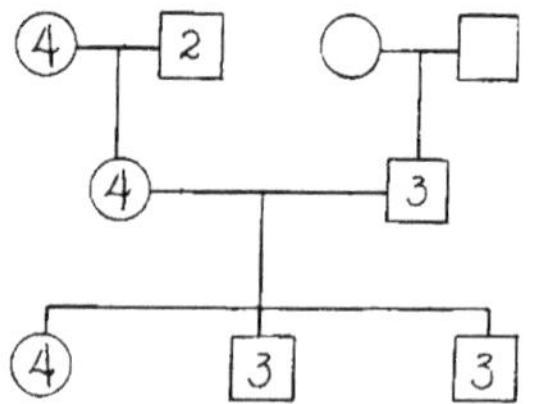

Fig. 11.—Result of crossing pure Groups IV and III through two generations.

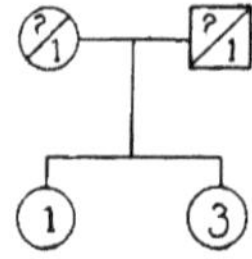

Fig. 12.—The value of the three-generation study for determining the origin of blood group. The Group III is explainable only by information obtained through families as in Fig. 6.

this usage thus: "Those characters which are transmitted entire or almost unchanged in the hybridization and, therefore, in themselves constitute the characters of the hybrid, are termed the dominant, and those which become latent in the process, recessive. The expression recessive has been chosen because the characters thereby designated withdraw or entirely disappear in the hybrid, but nevertheless reappear unchanged in their progeny." The hybrid state is absent in all families I have studied, as well as in all the families grouped by von Dungern and Hirschfeld,[18] and by Ottenberg.[39] The absence of the hybrid stage in man is shown in the study of all families reported as illustrative of the transmission of hereditary characters of all kinds, unless the sex linkage phenomenon as seen in hemophilia and in color blindness, may be interpreted as expressive of the hybrid stage. It is, then, improper to use the term dominant and recessive in connection with heredity in man until further studies are made. As the heterozygotes in plants are identical physically and genetically with the plant hybrid, and as the heterozygote in man behaves in the same manner as the heterozygote in plants, it may be possible to work in a reverse manner in order to determine which blood groups in various combinations can appear only as the dormant and evident combinations. If there is no reversal in the relationship of the dormant and evident characters, dominance of one character to another may be spoken of in its true sense. If there is reversal, the use of the expressions, dominant and recessive will remain meaningless. The settlement of this point is, however, not of vital importance in the study of heredity in man; it is more a matter of accuracy and correct usage. It could be of importance, however, in the use of the blood group in the adjudication of medico-legal disputes. Until it is proved which character may appear as dormant in certain unions, the use of blood group in medico-legal affairs will be fraught with great danger, unless the blood grouping is carried in a definite scheme into the preceding generations, and even then the result may be inconclusive (Fig. 18). The possibilities of the medico-legal value of the blood group were mentioned by von Dungern and Hirschfeld in 1910,[18] and by Giraud in 1919.[21]

Ottenberg[38] has presented data in an endeavor to demonstrate the possible blood groups that may result from crossing two persons in the same or different groups. His conclusions were made in conformity with formulas which he had outlined as representative of the various blood groups.

The acceptance by Ottenberg of the hypothesis that in the inheritance of the blood group agglutinogens *A* and *B* of the red cells behaved as dominant characters while the agglutinins, *a* and *b* of the serum behaved as recessive characters is stimulated by the belief that Group IV (Group I of Jansky) can exist only in a pure state (recessive). Ottenberg also believes in the existence in man of a hybrid for blood group, in a variable relationship in the groups of the supposed dominant and recessive characters, and in the union of *A* and *B* to produce Group IV (*A. B.*) These beliefs are entirely groundless in the light of Mendel's experiments. The dominant and recessive characters are determined by means of the hybrid. A hybrid stage for the blood group is absent in man. Even if Group IV (Group I of Jansky) were a recessive character to one blood group, evidence would have to be presented to establish its relationship to the remaining two groups. My study clearly shows that unions of Group IV (Group I of Jansky) may result in offspring in the other three groups, depending solely on the groups present in previous generations. By crossing a Group II with a Group III it is shown that Group IV (*A, B*) is not the result of the union of *A* and *B*. If a hybrid stage in man existed this result would be possible, and all the children would be in Group IV (*A. B.*). The serum of this hybrid would agglutinate the cells of Groups II and III, and the cells would be agglutinated by the serum of Groups II and III. Such a combination does not exist. Furthermore, if Group IV were to be considered as a hybrid resulting from unions of Groups II and III, crosses of Group IV would always result in children in Groups II, Group IV and Group III. In sufficiently large families the groups would be distributed numerically so as to maintain the relationship of one Group II, two Group IV, and one Group III. Crosses of Group IV may result in only Group IV children. There is no way by which a union of *A* and *B* can explain the origin of Group IV. The conclusions of Moss in reference to the existence of three specific iso-agglutinin combinations, *A, B, C*, in the serum, and three distinct receptor substances *a, b, c*, in the red blood cells, as arranged by that author into four groups comply exactly with data obtained in my study of the germinal transmission of the blood group to subsequent generations. The constitution of each blood group is specific whether present in the blood or represented by a determiner in the germ plasm. Any variability in the hypothetic structural formula for a blood group is untenable. There are four blood groups known today and, as the theory of heredity is based on the belief of a specific determiner for each hereditary character, transmissible through the germ plasm, I believe in the existence of four separate and distinct biological determiners for the blood groups. The whole story of the origin of the blood group is not told in the blood of the parents of a family, and the fact must ever be kept in mind that ovaries and testes are the vehicles through which past and present biological characters of man are linked together. If the function of germinal tissues to segregate and transmit characters to subsequent generations is ignored, worthless hypotheses and formulas will be established in order to explain an evident character occurring in man. A curious situation would exist in the family represented in Fig. 5, if the criteria of Ottenberg were accepted. The twins were in different groups, and one was in a group different from that of either parent. The danger of drawing conclusions from

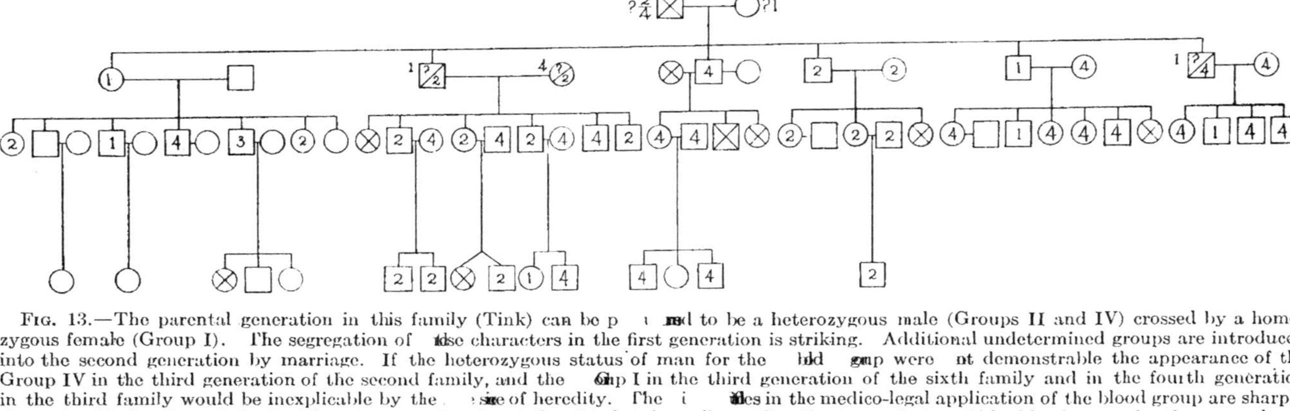

Fig. 13.—The parental generation in this family (Tink) can be presumed to be a heterozygous male (Groups II and IV) crossed by a homozygous female (Group I). The segregation of these characters in the first generation is striking. Additional undetermined groups are introduced into the second generation by marriage. If the heterozygous status of man for the blood group were not demonstrable the appearance of the Group IV in the third generation of the second family, and the Group I in the third generation of the sixth family and in the fourth generation in the third family would be inexplicable by the laws of heredity. The difficulties in the medico-legal application of the blood group are sharply shown in this family and the inability to prove by the study of isolated small families the transmission of the blood group by the germ plasm. (Information obtained through the courtesy of Mr. F. T. Jung, Sheboygan, Wisconsin.)

two-generation studies is shown in Figs. 13, 14, 15, 16, and 17. Such families are without conclusive value in the study of the inheritance of the blood group, (Figs. 19 and 20) and dangerous when

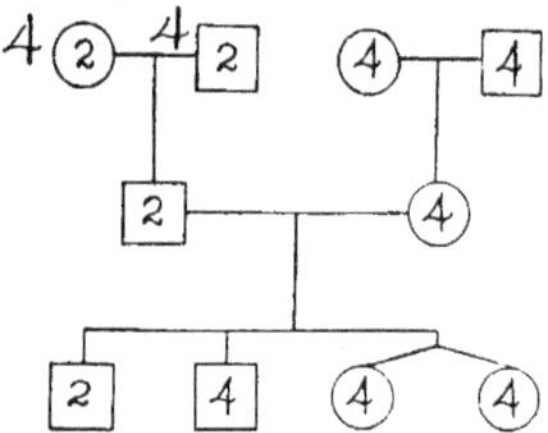

Fig. 14.—Transmission of blood Groups II and IV through three generations and the occurrence of twins of the same blood group.

utilized as criteria to establish the usage of the blood group in medico-legal affairs. There are more than 200 small families or parts of families on record at the Mayo Clinic.

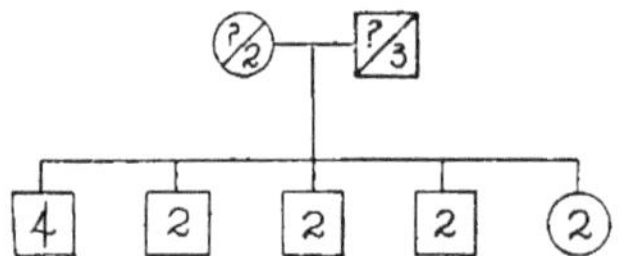

Fig. 15.—Crossing of blood Groups II and III. The result demonstrates the inability to determine parentage from a two generation study of the blood group.

Alexander,[2] in 1921, made an investigation in order to determine if Mendel's second law was fulfilled in the transmission of blood group. He came to the conclusion, in malignancy in particular, "While persons belonging to all four groups are liable to malignant disease, those in Groups I and III appear to be peculiarly susceptible,

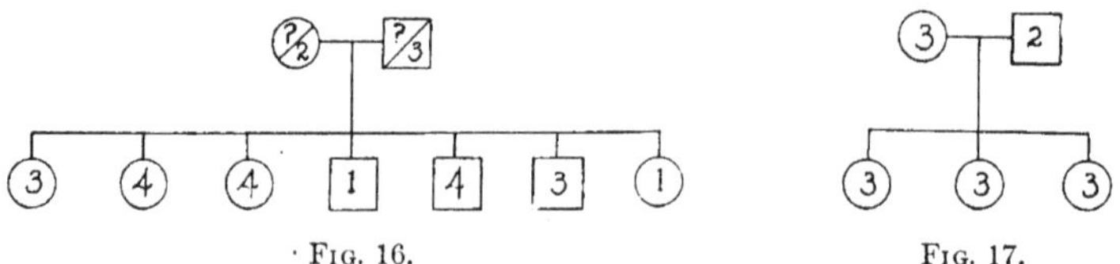

Fig. 16. Fig. 17.

Fig. 16.—The frequency of additional groups besides those represented in parents is due to scarcity of pure Group III and the frequency of heterozygous Group II.

Fig. 17.—Demonstrates the necessity for at least four children for the study of the segregation of characters.

and the clinical type of disease is, generally speaking, more malignant." He believed this situation arose by linkage of the factors for cancer and for blood group. The investigations of Higley and myself[8] on material collected by Sanford in the Mayo Clinic showed this conclusion to be incorrect. In a study of 2446 persons with various diseases we found that there were no evidences of linkage. There was no evidence that a person in a particular blood group

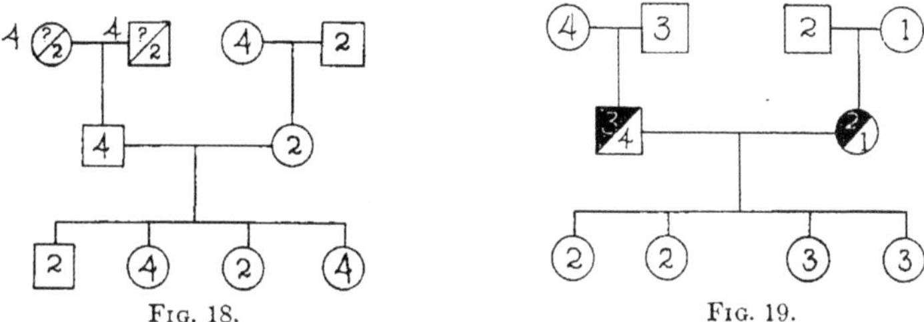

FIG. 18. FIG. 19.

FIG. 18.—Transmission of blood Groups II and IV through three generations demonstrating the heterozygous nature of one of the parents on the left in the parental generation.

FIG. 19.—If this family had been grouped through two generations only, it could be believed that the resulting groups were simply the product of a rearrangement of specific substances *A* and *B*, and *a* and *b*. A review of an earlier generation gives the clue to the groups to be expected in subsequent generations. The blood of parents in the second generation was in Groups IV and I, but all four groups were present in the germ plasm. The dormant characters reappeared and, it must be admitted that the evident characters would have appeared had the family been sufficiently large to permit of segregation of all the determiners for blood group in the germ plasm. If not, blood group is not hereditary. An attempt to state that unions of Groups I and II, and Groups I and III can only give rise to similar groups is to ignore the possible heterozygous state of a parent. Unions with Group IV or of Groups II and III give rise to all groups because persons who are pure for the common groups, Groups II and IV, are very difficult to find; it is still more difficult to find persons who are pure for the rare groups, Groups I and III.

was more susceptible to a certain disease and the reactions to disease were practically the same in all blood groups.

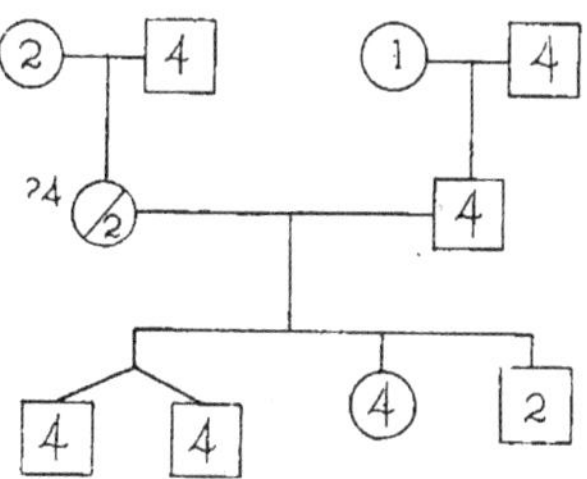

FIG. 20.—In this family three groups were crossed in the first generation. The members of the second generation showed only one group in their blood unless the blood group of the third generation is studied, there is no way of determining the heterozygous or homozygous nature of the parents in the second generation. If the numerical superiority of one character to another is a fixed thing in man, either Group II or Group IV should constantly recur in greater numbers when they are crossed. Other families studied indicate that Group II appears with greater frequency when crossed with Group IV. The female of the second generation may have Groups II and IV in her germ plasm but at present this cannot be proved.

The percentage relationships of the blood groups in the two sexes did not vary in 2176 groupings of 1245 males and 931 females.

The percentage distribution in the males was Group I, 3.69 per cent; Group II, 40.97 per cent; Group III, 9.39 per cent; and Group IV, 45.77 per cent. In the females the distribution was Group I, 3.97 per cent; Group II, 41.46 per cent; Group III, 8.69 per cent; and Group IV, 45.85 per cent. The families represented in Figs. 1 to 21 demonstrate the transmission of the blood group between males and females without regard to sex. There are no evidences of sex linkage in the transmission of the blood group.

The second law of Mendel, namely, the independent assortment of characters, so far as data at present are concerned, is fulfilled by the blood group.

Comment. The blood group is an expression of a hereditary character of man. There are four characters known at present which are arbitrarily designated Group I, Group II, Group III, and Group IV. The blood is transmitted by the germ plasm according to the first and second laws of Mendel. The hybrid stage is absent.

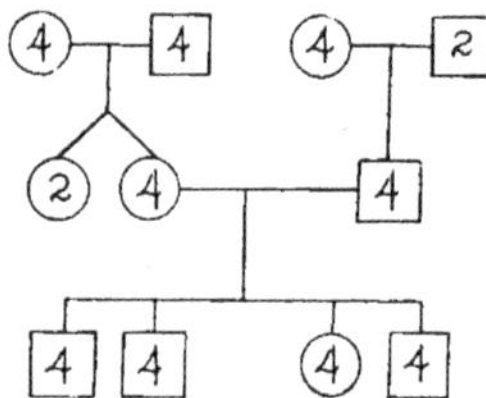

Fig. 21.—Segregation of pure blood Group IV from the parental generation as shown by all the children being in the same group. The twins are in different groups which demonstrates the heterozygous nature of one of the parents, and the peculiar segregative power of the germ plasm.

Whether the Jansky or Moss classification is used in this study of the inheritance of the blood group is not of importance. The groups may be classified by either method and are transmitted between generations in accordance with the same rules. There is no method available at this time by which a strict or presumptive delimitation of the blood group possible in children resulting from the union of two persons can be made. Careful investigation conducted into the ancestry of every generation must be carried out in order to ascertain the blood group possibilities in any family, and even then the medico-legal application of blood groups will be surrounded with many difficulties.

The blood group offers a concrete means for the study of heredity in man.

Inheritance of Migraine: Study II. The demonstration of the transmission of migraine through generations by means of the germ plasm transfers the condition from the category of disease to that of biological character of man. The term "migraine" designates an unknown physiological process which is recognized by periodic attacks of pain, usually in the head, either unilateral or bilateral, but occurring also in the abdomen, and in either location frequently associated with nausea, vomiting, mental depression, visual phenomena, and many vague somatic disturbances. One or all of the symptoms may occur in an attack, which lasts from a few to several hours or days. The first expression of the character appears early in life, and as a rule, the manifestations disappear during the fourth decade.

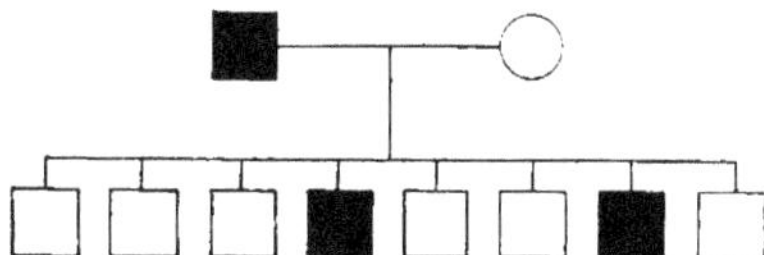

Fig. 22.—The segregation of the migraine character in families in which a person with migraine and a person without migraine have been crossed.

Studies instituted to prove migraine expressive of a hereditary character must of necessity include the investigation of parents and at least four children in families in which there were unions of a person with migraine to a person without migraine, of known heterozygous persons, or of two persons with migraine. "Without migraine" is the contrasted character. Under like conditions, the segregation of the character will occur among the children in a fairly definite manner.

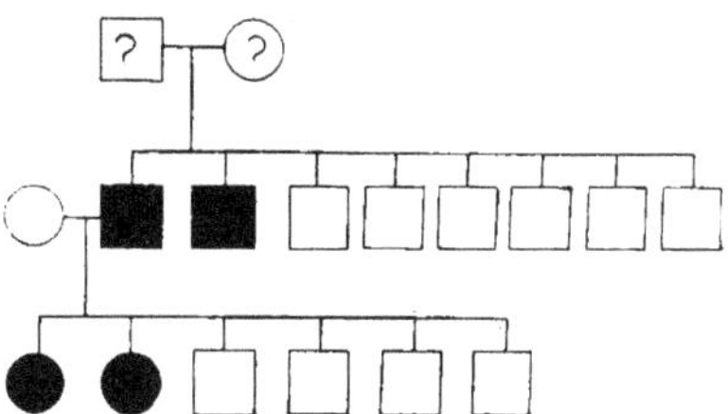

Fig. 23.—The value of searching for all the evidence available in a family in which one member has migraine. It can be presumed that a parent in the first generation had migraine because of the distribution in the second generation. The segregation is carried into the third generation.

The Distribution of Migraine in Families.[9, 10] A study was made of 127 families, one or more representatives of which were examined in the Mayo Clinic in 1919. Migraine followed the two laws of Mendel (Figs. 22, 23 and 24). Of the total number of children in the 127 families, 198 had migraine and 610 had the character, without migraine. At the time the study was reported a combined Mendelian ratio was calculated for all the families studied. This ratio was incorrect, as amalgamation of the crosses was contrary to the scheme of Mendel. The ratios were correct for the individual groups. The same difficulties exist in working out a Mendelian ratio for migraine as exist for the blood group.

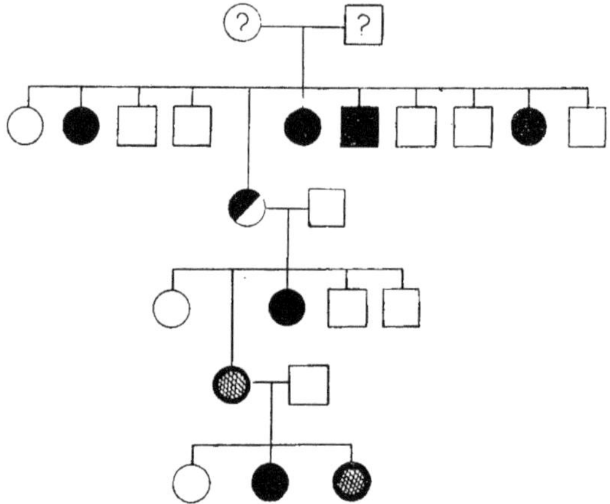

FIG. 24.—Transmission of migraine with abdominal crises.

Like all hereditary characters migraine exists in either the homozygous or the heterozygous state. The heterozygous state (Fig. 25) has led many writers to say that migraine is hereditary in 90 per cent of instances and in various other percentages, because it occurs in a number of families in which it is not demonstrable in the parents. During the last two years many cases in the Mayo Clinic have been

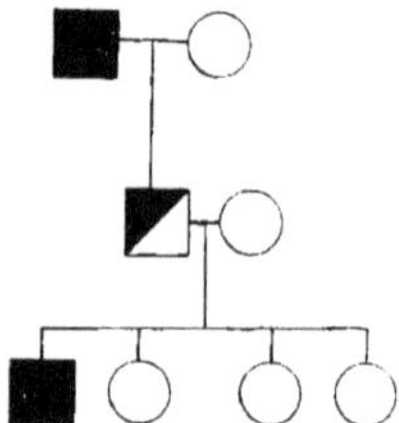

FIG. 25.—The heterozygous status of the male of the second generation as shown in the appearance of the character in the final generation.

observed, in which migraine was not present in the parents, but present in the brothers or sisters, if the family was sufficiently large or present in one or the other of the grandparents. Data derived from patients having no knowledge of their parents and grandparents are not usable as evidence for or against the Mendelian transmission of migraine. Such information is valueless on either side of the question. It is to be remembered that by means of the heterozygous status of certain persons a character may be transmitted through many generations of small families without any signs of its presence. The character may appear in the first large family.

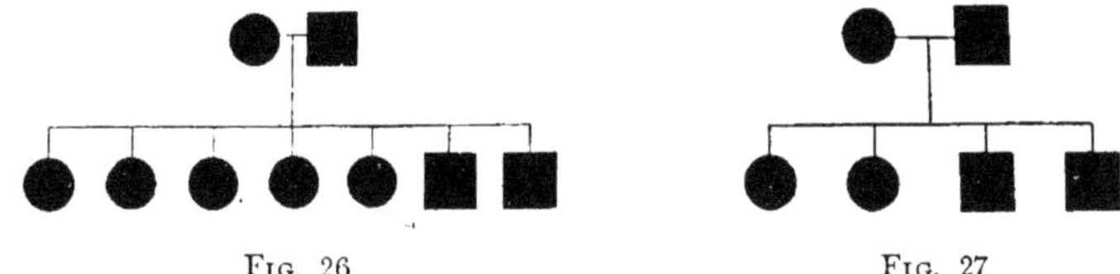

Fig. 26 Fig. 27

Fig. 26.—Cross of persons with the pure migraine character.
Fig. 27.—The union of homozygotes results in all offspring having the same character.

The homozygous state of migraine has been studied in three families in which both parents had migraine. If migraine exists in a homozygous states, all children resulting from such unions should have migraine. This occurred in the three families studied (Figs. 26, 27 and 28). Although this is an interesting observation,

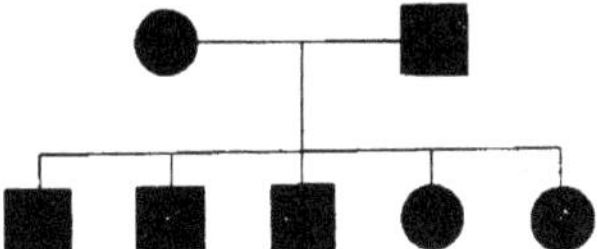

Fig. 28.—If migraine is heterozygous for families without migraine, individuals without the character should be segregated in families of four or more children. The absence of such segregation is illustrated in this family.

the data are too meager to be of value in determining if the relationships of the dormant and evident phases of migraine are reversible. It may be that a person with migraine may become the parent of children without migraine, just as it has been shown that the relationships of the blood group in the heterozygote are reversible. This subject requires careful study.

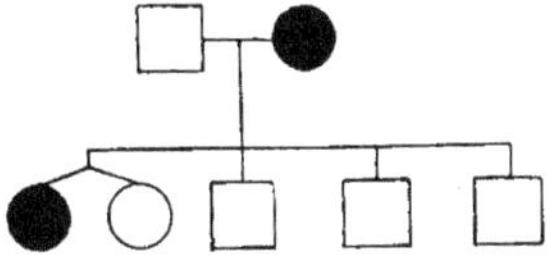

Fig. 29.—The segregative power of the germ plasm. One twin had migraine the other was without migraine.

One family has been studied (Fig. 29) in which there were twins; one had migraine and the other did not have migraine. This is interesting when compared with the appearance of different blood groups in twins (Fig. 5).

In the description of the causal factors for a number of diseases, various writers have given migraine as one of the etiological factors. So far as is known, the determiner in the germ plasm for migraine has nothing to do with the production or evolution of any character other than itself. The migraine determiner is as specific for itself as the determiner for a particular blood group is for itself. Any disease may occur in the person with migraine. It is an association and not an etiological relationship.

Comment. Migraine is the expression of a hereditary character, but the physiological processes which occur at the time of the manifestation of its phenomena are unknown. It is not possible to change the blood group by either surgery or drugs, so it does not seem reasonable to expect that migraine which is a similarly derived character could be influenced by any of the procedures recommended. Patients with migraine who have been examined in the Mayo Clinic demonstrate the futility of all sorts of treatment. Evidence has not been accumulated to substantiate the belief that a "tendeney to migraine" is inherited; "migraine" and "without migraine" are the inheritable characters. A person either has or does not have migraine, just as a person always belongs to a blood group.

INHERITANCE OF ESSENTIAL EPILEPSY: STUDY III. There is no gross pathological basis for the explanation of the seizures of essential epilepsy. It is characterized in man by periodic seizures in which there is loss of consciousness, preceded by more or less marked prodromal sensations, and followed by and associated with tonic or clonic spasms of the general musculature. The seizures last from a few minutes to one hour or more, and their frequency is variable. A seizure in which there are severe convulsions and loss of consciousness is termed "grand mal." A milder form in which vertiginous or momentary blank sensations replace the convulsions is termed "petit mal." Hippocrates believed that essential epilepsy began in utero, and as a consequence of this belief and the absence of a pathological basis, many diseases such as neurasthenia, hysteria, insanity, and the undefined group of diseases known as nervous disorders or neuropathies have been incriminated as causal agents. St. Hildegard seems to have been one of the earliest writers to suspeet that migraine and essential epilepsy were expressive of the same entity.

The Relationship of Migraine to Essential Epilepsy. In order to obtain data on the relation of the various neuropathic influences to essential epilepsy, two series of cases observed in the Mayo Clinic were analyzed. The results warranted the dismissal of all of the so-called nervous disorders as related factors, since they occurred not more often in the ancestral history of persons with essential epilepsy than in the ancestral history of persons with diseases of known etiology. Migraine is the only character which appeared with enough frequency to attract attention. In the first

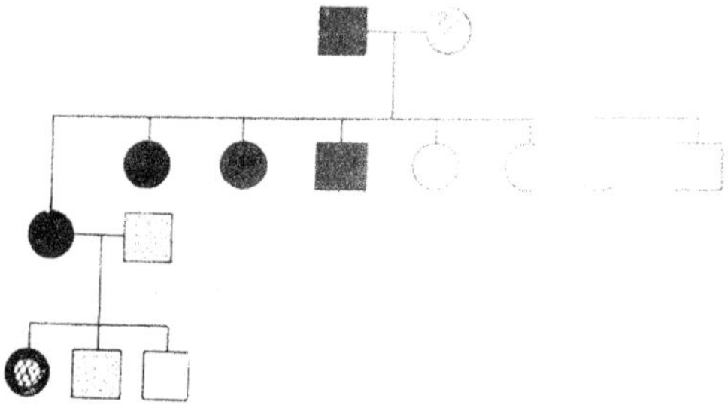

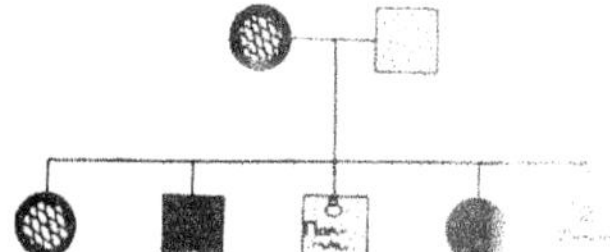

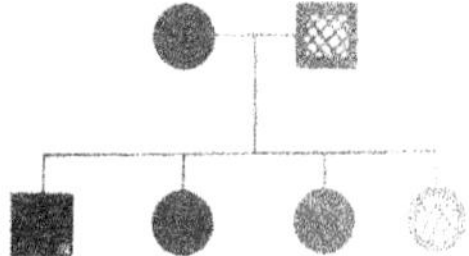

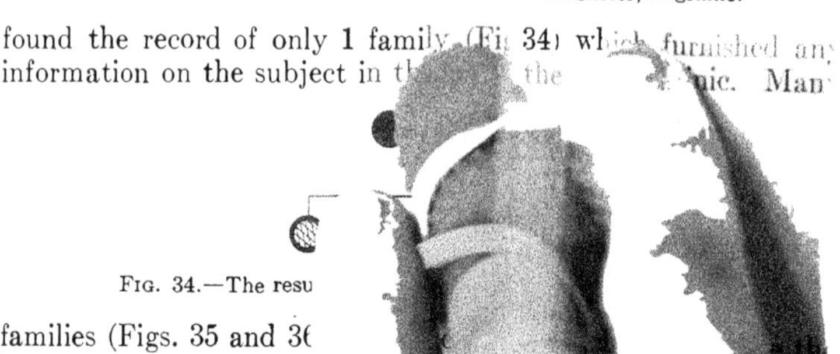

In the description of the causal factors for a number of diseases, various writers have given migraine as one of the etiological factors. So far as is known, the determiner in the germ plasm for migraine has nothing to do with the production or evolution of any character other than itself. The migraine determiner is as specific for itself as the determiner for a particular blood group is for itself. Any disease may occur in the person with migraine. It is an association and not an etiological relationship.

Comment. Migraine is the expression of a hereditary character, but the physiological processes which occur at the time of the manifestation of its phenomena are unknown. It is not possible to change the blood group by either surgery or drugs, so it does not seem reasonable to expect that migraine which is a similarly derived character could be influenced by any of the procedures recommended. Patients with migraine who have been examined in the Mayo Clinic demonstrate the futility of all sorts of treatment. Evidence has not been accumulated to substantiate the belief that a "tendency to migraine" is inherited; "migraine" and "without migraine" are the inheritable characters. A person either has or does not have migraine, just as a person always belongs to a blood group.

Inheritance of Essential Epilepsy: Study III. There is no gross pathological basis for the explanation of the seizures of essential epilepsy. It is characterized in man by periodic seizures in which there is loss of consciousness, preceded by more or less marked prodromal sensations, and followed by and associated with tonic or clonic spasms of the general musculature. The seizures last from a few minutes to one hour or more, and their frequency is variable. A seizure in which there are severe convulsions and loss of consciousness is termed "grand mal." A milder form in which vertiginous or momentary blank sensations replace the convulsions is termed "petit mal." Hippocrates believed that essential epilepsy began in utero, and as a consequence of this belief and the absence of a pathological basis, many diseases such as neurasthenia, hysteria, insanity, and the undefined group of diseases known as nervous disorders or neuropathies have been incriminated as causal agents. St. Hildegard seems to have been one of the earliest writers to suspect that migraine and essential epilepsy were expressive of the same entity.

The Relationship of Migraine to Essential Epilepsy. In order to obtain data on the relation of the various neuropathic influences to essential epilepsy, two series of cases observed in the Mayo Clinic were analyzed. The results warranted the dismissal of all of the so-called nervous disorders as related factors, since they occurred not more often in the ancestral history of persons with essential epilepsy than in the ancestral history of persons with diseases of known etiology. Migraine is the only character which appeared with enough frequency to attract attention. In the first series of 128 cases,[7] migraine occurred in the ancestral or personal history or in that of the brothers and sisters in 53.9 per cent of the cases. The 128 cases comprising the second series had been carefully studied in the Section on Neurology of the Clinic and of these cases 66.4 per cent gave a history of migraine in ancestors, brothers or sisters or in the personal history. In the former series migraine was present before the onset of essential epilepsy and alternated with or continued with epilepsy in 14 per cent of the cases studied. In the latter series, this occurred in 10.5 per cent of the cases. The genetic relationship of migraine to essential epilepsy seemed to be quite striking.

The Familial Distribution of the Migraine-epilepsy Character. If essential epilepsy is expressive of the same underlying biological factor on which migraine depends, its appearance in families would not disturb the relationship of persons with migraine to persons without migraine; it would simply replace or alternate with the migraine character in certain persons. The same laws and requirements that govern the transmission of the blood group or migraine alone would be followed and fulfilled.

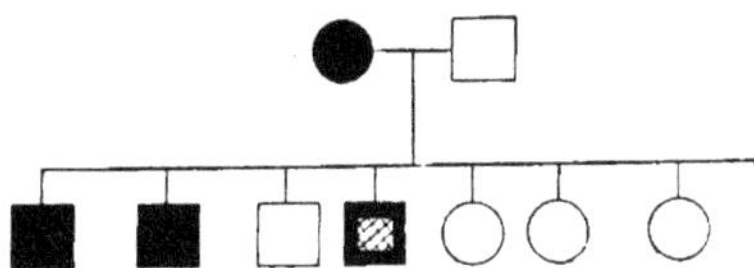

FIG. 30.—The failure of essential epilepsy to disturb the numerical relationship of normal persons to those with the inherited character. Essential epilepsy is superimposed on an individual with the migraine character.

Essential epilepsy on empirical grounds was considered as simply another phase of the phenomena of the migraine character in a study of 47 families whose histories were complete for ancestral data. The contrasted character was "without migraine-epilepsy," or what is commonly called the normal. The same segregation of characters was seen as when considering migraine alone (Figs. 30, 31 and 32). At a subsequent date, 35 similar families were studied, and the data obtained in the first families were altered in no way. In a certain number of the patients studied, varying in all series from 10 to 14 per cent, migraine and epilepsy alternated irregularly.

If essential epilepsy is expressive of the same phenomena as migraine, the marriage of an epileptic person to a migrainous person would result in all of their children having migraine or all or part having essential epilepsy. One family has been found to fulfil this condition; all the children had migraine, and in 1 the migraine alternated irregularly with epileptic attacks (Fig. 33).

If essential epilepsy depends on the factor of migraine for its evolution, the marriage of homozygotes or heterozygotes for migraine should result in the production of a certain number of children

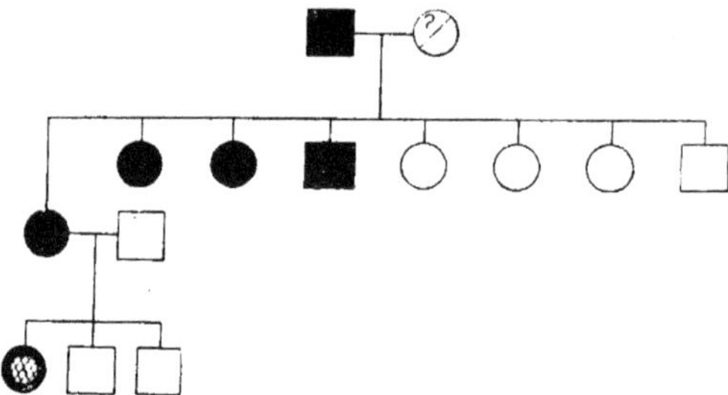

FIG. 31.—The number of persons in the second generation with migraine is greater than is to be expected from a cross of a pure migraine with a pure normal. This has been observed in several families and is considered due to the heterozygous, although unproved, status of the apparently normal parent. The character appears as essential epilepsy in the final generation.

subject to seizures of essential epilepsy. The marriage of two persons with migraine is quite rare and as a consequence the opportunity

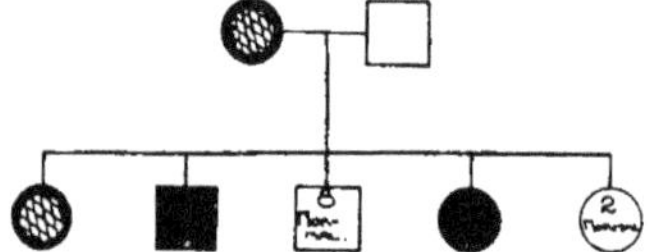

FIG. 32.—The mother had epilepsy in early life, replaced by migraine. The same segregation of the characters occurred as if the mother had always presented migraine.

to observe the frequency with which a child with essential epilepsy should result from such unions would be very infrequent. I have

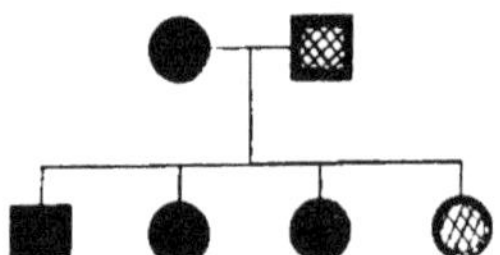

FIG. 33.—The crossing of a migrainous person with an essential epileptic person. The character, epilepsy, behaves as does the character, migraine.

found the record of only 1 family (Fig. 34) which furnished any information on the subject in the files of the Mayo Clinic. Many

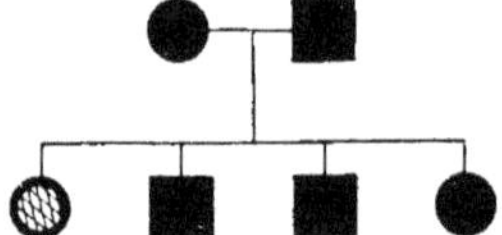

FIG. 34.—The results of crossing two persons with migraine.

families (Figs. 35 and 36) have been found which demonstrate the heterozygous property of the normal to transmit migraine, essential epilepsy, or both to their children, because of the strain which had been introduced into their germ plasm by the grandparents.

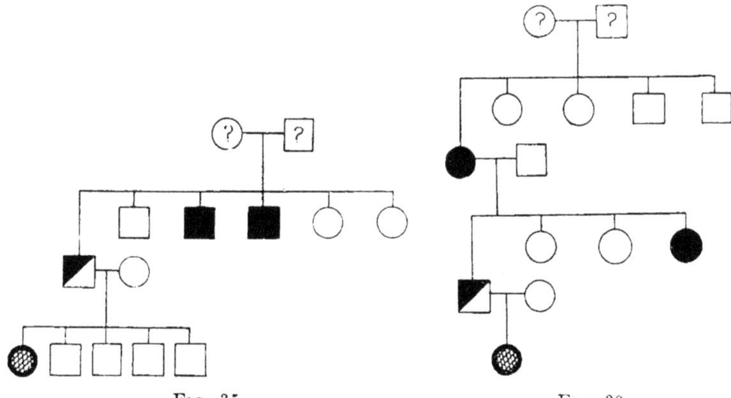

FIG. 35 FIG. 36

FIG. 35.—The transmission of the migraine-epilepsy character because of the heterozygous status of the male parent.

FIG. 36.—The heterozygous status of the germ plasm and its segregative power. The final generation studied would have no value if considered by itself without information obtained from other families.

Comment. Essential epilepsy and migraine are transmitted from generation to generation as the expression of the same underlying factor in the germ plasm. The mechanism for the production of the seizures is unknown. The organic factors capable of producing phenomena similar to those of essential epilepsy are so numerous that the classification of an individual in the class with essential epilepsy demands extreme caution.

A diminution in the number of essential epileptics by segregation in colonies is not to be hoped for, as the person with migraine is more likely to produce epileptic offspring than the epileptic person himself.

The theory that essential epilepsy and migraine are the expression of a biological character, and their manifestations are, therefore, physiological needs offer no insurmountable obstacles in its acceptation. If it is possible for such striking characters as waltzing in a mouse and tumbling in a pigeon to be hereditary there is no reason why characters equally striking might not appear in man. The management of migraine and essential epilepsy as expressions of biological characters undoubtedly will result in a greater degree of happiness and health than has hitherto been possible for those individuals because of the unlimited and ever-varying type of operation and drug therapy which has been carried out without benefit.

DIABETES MELLITUS: STUDY IV. From the earliest history of diabetes mellitus references have been made to heredity as an explanation for the occurrence of a varying percentage of cases of the disease. The reported families were compiled, in 1912, by Foster[19] who at the same time reported a family observed by himself. In practically all of the articles on the subject, mention is made of the number of persons in the family who were afflicted, but no mention is made of those who were in good health. The 3 families reported by Long[26] are noteworthy exceptions. Von Noorden,[33] Naunyn,[32] May[28] and more recently, Allen[3] have called attention to the importance of heredity in diabetes. Allen suggests that the subject should be studied by the methods used by biologists in determining hereditary characters, as no attempt has been made to study the condition in the light of the laws of heredity.

If diabetes mellitus is to be considered as representative of a unit character, it would be interpreted as a physiological expression of a cycle in the life of certain persons, whereby they would lose the power to metabolize carbohydrates and as a consequence a portion or all of the sugar ingested, the stored carbohydrates, and a portion of the body protein and ingested protein are converted into sugar and excreted as such in the urine. At the same time the chemical changes which result in coma and death would be the final expression of this lethal cycle. The contrasted character would be what is called "normal," or that possessed by a person whose carbohydrate metabolism is constituted so that the phenomena of diabetes mellitus do not appear. The families should be studied through two generations, and at least three and preferably four children should be present in the families used for study.

Diabetes Mellitus not a Mendelian Character. Diabetes mellitus, if hereditary, must conform to the known laws of heredity. To determine if such be the case, the progeny of persons with diabetes mellitus married to persons without diabetes mellitus have been studied. The material consisted of 34 families, 17 of which were studied through two generations and 17 throught three generations. The total number of diabetic offspring was 65; 274 were without any evidence of diabetes mellitus at the time the data were collected. Sixty-five children (16.08 per cent) died in early life.

The results of unions (Figs. 37, 38 and 39) of diabetics (homozygotes) and non-diabetics in the cases studied revealed no information to show that the condition was transmitted through the germ plasm. The occurrence in the children did not conform to the Mendelian laws. Further investigation in these same families may reveal information of great value.

Occasional families have been observed (Fig. 38) which suggested the possibility that diabetes mellitus might be transmitted to a subsequent generation because of the heterozygous state of a parent. A study to throw definite light on this subject was made in 18 families, of which 11 were studied through two generations, and 7 through three generations. There were 18 children with diabetes, and 126 without. Thirty-five of the children (19.05 per cent) died in early life. The impression that diabetes might be transmitted through the germ plasm on account of the heterozygous

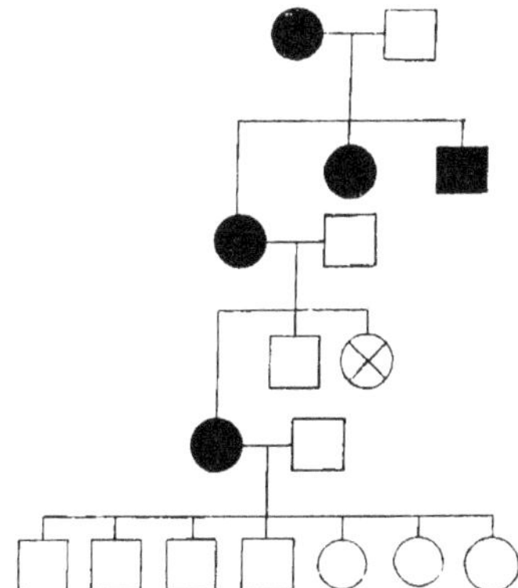

FIG. 37.—A family in which diabetes mellitus has occurred for three generations. It appeared in the mother of the last generation at the thirty-third year. None of the children were affected at the time the patient was investigated.

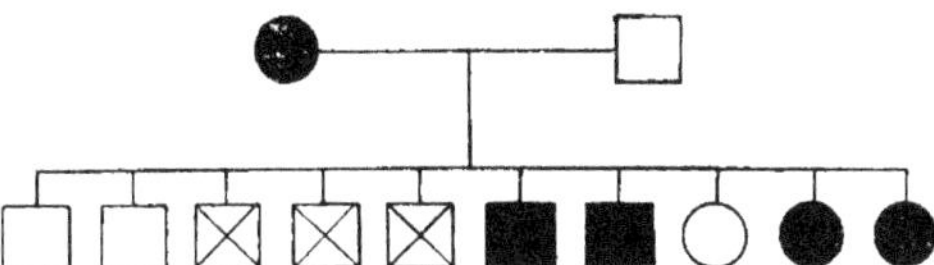

FIG. 38.—The results of crossing the diabetic and non-diabetic persons. The number of diabetic offspring is too large, as the father's family was free from diabetes. Three children died in early life, presumably free from diabetes mellitus.

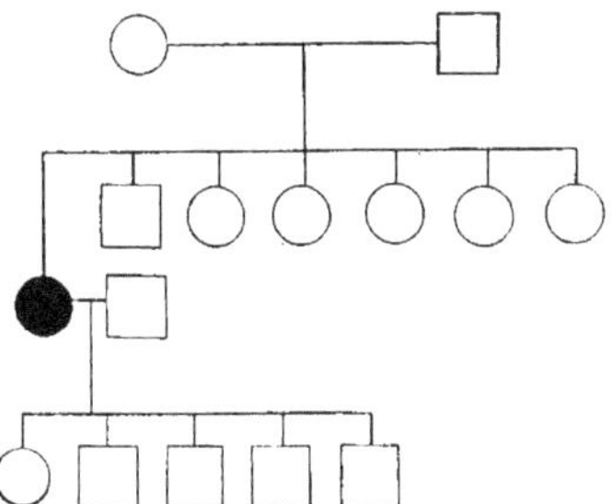

FIG. 39.—The failure to conform to known laws of heredity is shown in this family Diabetes if hereditary would have appeared at the age of sixty-two or thereabouts in at least two children in the second generation.

nature of a parent was not supported by the data obtained from the 18 families studied. These families are typified in Fig. 41.

If diabetes mellitus were hereditary, homozygous and heterozygous individuals would result from the crossing of a diabetic person with a non-diabetic. The failure of the homozygous principle to be supported has been shown in the cases of diabetes reported by Crofton and others in which it has been found that both parents may have diabetes mellitus and none of the children be afflicted.

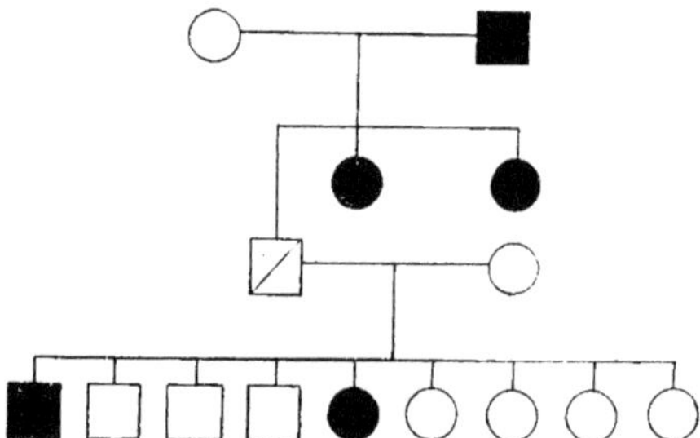

FIG. 40.—This group suggests that diabetes mellitus might be transmitted through the germ plasm because of the heterozygous nature of the male parent of the second generation.

The lack of conformity to the laws of dominance and recessiveness in man because of the absence of the hybrid stage may explain certain discrepancies in the familial occurrence of diabetes, but neither the homozygous nor the heterozygous principles in heredity have been fulfilled by diabetes mellitus.

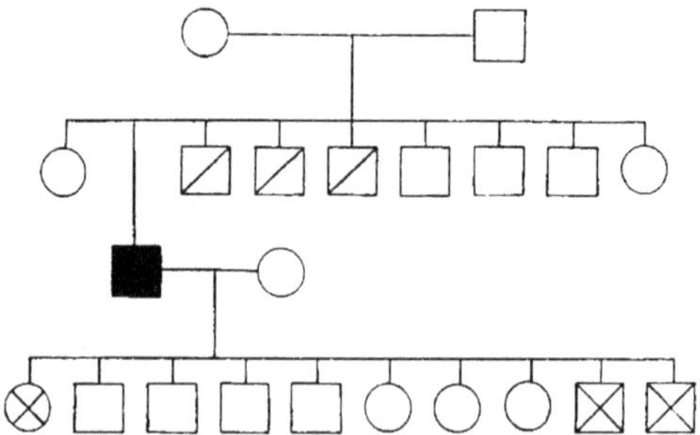

FIG. 41.—A family illustrating the families studied to determine if diabetes mellitus is transmitted by a heterozygote.

Method for Collection of Data. The methods used today for the collection of data in families where diabetes mellitus occurs are not such as will ever result in obtaining data of conclusive value. To prove diabetes mellitus hereditary, a cyclic nature of the disease would have to be postulated, that is, the condition would make its appearance at approximately the same age and have a definite progress in a certain number of the members of the family. Therefore, data should be obtained in each family concerning: (1) The time of onset in the parents; (2) the number of brothers and sisters of the parents and the age of each; (3) the age of each at onset of diabetes; (4) the number of children in the last generation; (5) the age of each child when the condition appeared; and (6) the ages of those at or beyond the age at which it appeared in the parents. The collection of the data would necessitate a follow-up system of investigation and a study of the children as they arrived at the proper age. In no other way will it be possible to prove that conditions like diabetes mellitus should be transferred from the status of a disease to the list of conditions in man which are expressive of a biological character transmissible through the germ plasm. The data presented in my study did not fulfil these requirements. So far as the data collected are reliable, there is not the slightest evidence to justify the statement that diabetes mellitus is at times hereditary. There is also insufficient evidence to show that the condition is not hereditary, but the evidence does point more toward the quantitative action of some causal factor rather than the expression of the segregative properties of the germ plasm.

The high mortality in early life of children born of diabetic parents is striking.

Essential Asthma: Study V. In essential asthma, as in all conditions in man the etiology of which is obscure, the mechanism of heredity has been believed to play an etiological role. Geddings[20] reviewed the statistics of the earlier writers, and came to the conclusion that the tendency to essential asthma is hereditary. All of the earlier writers, with the exception of Drinkwater,[17] reported a percentage of inheritance of essential asthma varying from 10 to 50 per cent. Drinkwater reported his families as expressive of the segregative power of the germ plasm. The more recent literature has been reviewed by Adkinson,[1] who at the same time presented data obtained from a large number of cases. She found a family history of essential asthma in 48 per cent of the 400 cases studied, and came to the conclusion that asthma is hereditary in a varying percentage of cases. She also concluded that asthma appeared at an earlier date in the children than in the parents. If asthma is a hereditary character it must have been present in man since his appearance on earth, as there is no way for hereditary characters to be kept extant except by breeding of those in whom the character is present. The known period of man on earth has been computed to be millions of years. Essential asthma was distinguished as a distinct clinical entity by Willis[47] about 1600. If a character were present in primeval man, or even since 1600, and appeared at a perceptibly earlier age in the children of each generation, the cycle required for its appearance would eventually be brought down to a period earlier than the performation of the embryo, or in the germ plasm, and after it had arrived at that state would of necessity either have to disappear, or by some miraculous process again revert to appearance in old age. This claim is made for other conditions in man, but there is no evidence in heredity to support such a hypothesis.

An investigation to demonstrate the transmission of essential asthma to subsequent generations by the germ plasm must be conducted in the same manner as that for migraine. It would be transmitted in exactly the same manner, and follow the same rules of heredity. For this reason a small number of families would be sufficient to establish the hereditary character of the condition. The contrasted character would be "without asthma."

The families presented in Tables I and II are sufficient to justify a conclusion in regard to the hereditary nature of essential asthma. In families used for the study the children had reached the age at which the condition appeared in the parent. In the 17 families in Table I there was evidence of asthma in parent and offspring. This does not warrant the conclusion that asthma is hereditary. The law for the segregation of characters is not followed to a degree in any way approximating the numerical ratio for hereditary characters. In Table II the data presented does not lead to the conclusion that asthma was transmitted in these families as a result of a heterozygous state of one or the other parent. If a character or condition under consideration does not follow the course of either the homozygous or heterozygous type for hereditary characters, it is safe to conclude that the condition is not hereditary. The study of a larger group of similar families would show the same figures.

TABLE I.—TRANSMISSION IN SEVENTEEN FAMILIES IN WHICH FATHER OR MOTHER HAD ASTHMA.

	CHILDREN.	
Asthma in.	With asthma.	Without asthma.
Mother	1	14
Father	..	5
Mother	2	7
Mother	1	4
Mother	1	3
Mother	1	8
Mother	..	6
Father	..	4
Father	..	4
Mother	..	3
Father	..	5
Mother	..	8
Mother	..	9
Father	..	5
Mother	2	6
Father	..	7
Father	..	4
	8	102

TABLE II.—TRANSMISSION IN THIRTY-NINE FAMILIES IN WHICH NEITHER FATHER NOR MOTHER HAD ASTHMA.

CHILDREN.

With asthma.	Without asthma.	With asthma.	Without asthma.	With asthma.	Without asthma.
1	7	1	5	1	12
1	7	1	7	2	3
1	3	1	6	1	4
1	3	1	5	1	5
1	7	1	9	2	3
1	4	1	4	1	5
2	3	1	6	1	5
1	3	3	4	1	6
1	3	2	12	1	5
1	12	1	6	1	5
1	6	1	7	1	7
1	3	1	8		
1	9	2	4	—	—
1	9	1	4	46	226

Comment. Essential asthma in its familial appearance follows none of the known laws of heredity. It is not the expression of a specific hereditary biological character of man.

Protein Sensitivity: Study VI. Protein sensitivity has been attributed by Osler,[36] Oppenheimer and Gottlieb,[35] Walker,[45] Longcope,[27] Barber,[6] Cooke[13] and others to the inheritance of a particular type of sensitive cells which react in a particular way when subjected to the influence of various protein substances. This belief permits of a very important investigation in man.

For many years "the inheritance of suceptibility to certain states" has been believed. If such be the case, the suceptibility must be transmitted in accordance with the laws which govern the inheritance of all characters. The mating of a person with protein sensitivity to a person without protein sensitivity, if the condition were dependent on the transmission by the germ plasm of a particular type of cellular protoplasm, would result in the production of a certain number of children of this susceptible type, some of whom would be heterozygous, others homozygous. If the children of such crosses were exposed to the same conditions of protein influence, and they would be so long as they lived under the same climatic and seasonal environments, those who inherited the peculiar type of somatic cells would react to the foreign substance in such numbers as to fulfil the Mendelian law for the segregation of characters. The possibility of the inheritance of a type of cellular structure that is susceptible to certain influences could be demonstrated under no more propitious circumstances.

The Familial Occurrence of Protein Sensitivity. In order to investigate the possibility of inheritance of the susceptibility to foreign protein, I have studied a small number of families in which there was parental protein sensitivity, and a larger group in which there was no parental sensitivity to proteins.

The number of families studied in Table III is very small, but the segregative property of the germ plasm does not wait until the hundredth family. The segregation will appear in the first family studied as well as in the last. There is no evidence in these families that the germ plasm carried any factor on which the protein sensitivity depended.

The 24 families of Table IV consisted of 28 children with protein sensitivity and 126 without. The families might be considered as expressive of the transmission of the condition by a heterozygous parent. This assumption is disproved by the failure of protein sensitivity to reappear in the third generation of certain families of Tabes III and IV. Hereditary characters are carried on forever, otherwise, the theory of germinal continuity would be false, and there is no obvious reason why an exception should be made in the case of protein sensitivity.

Comment. A consideration of the families represented in Tables III and IV leads me to the conclusion that protein sensitivity is not dependent on the transmission through the germ plasm of a factor which is responsible for the appearance of the condition in man. Furthermore, the data presented are criteria against the continuation of the use of the expression, "inheritance of susceptibility to disease." No evidence has been presented in the study of heredity to show that characters are susceptible of appearing or that there is a tendency for them to appear. They are either present or absent. There is no uncertainty.

TABLE III.—THE FREQUENCY OF PROTEIN SENSITIVITY IN CHILDREN OF SEVEN FAMILIES WHEN PRESENT IN ONE PARENT

Protein sensitivity in.	CHILDREN. With protein sensitivity.	Without protein sensitivity.
Mother	1	3
Mother	..	6
Mother	1	11
Mother	..	4
Mother	..	4
Father	..	4
Mother	..	4
	2	36

TABLE IV.—THE FREQUENCY OF PROTEIN SENSITIVITY IN CHILDREN OF TWENTY-FOUR FAMILIES WHEN ABSENT IN PARENTS.

CHILDREN.

With protein sensitivity.	Without protein sensitivity.	With protein sensitivity.	Without protein sensitivity.	With protein sensitivity.	Without protein sensitivity.
1	5	1	6	1	7
1	4	1	6	1	5
1	9	1	3	1	5
2	2	2	5	1	4
1	4	2	2	1	3
1	3	1	3	1	6
1	5	1	6	1	5
1	9	1	7	1	6
				28	126

BIBLIOGRAPHY.

1. Adkinson, J.: The Behavior of Bronchial Asthma as an Inherited Character, Genetics, 1920, **5**, 363.

2. Alexander, W.: An Inquiry into the Distribution of the Blood Groups in Patients Suffering from "Malignant Disease," Brit. Jour. Exp. Path., 1921, **2**, 66.

3. Allen, F. M.: Diabetes Mellitus. Nelson's Loose Leaf Medicine, New York, 1920.

4. Beneden, van E.: Récherches sur la maturation de l'œuf la fécondation et la division cellulaire, Gand, Leipzig et Paris, 1883.

5. von Baer, K. E.: Commentar zu der Schrift: De ovi mammalium et hominis genesi, Leipzig, Heusinger, Ztschr., 1828, **2**, 125.

6. Barber, H. W.: Protein-sensitization and Focal Sepsis in the Etiology of Certain Skin Affections, Guy's Hosp. Rep., 1921, **71**, 385.

7. Buchanan, J. A.: A Study of the Hereditary Factors of Epilepsy, Minn. Med., 1920, **3**, 536.

8. Buchanan, J. A., and Higley, Edith T.; The Relationship of Blood-groups to Disease, Brit. Jour. Exp. Path., 1921, **2**, 247.

9. Buchanan, J. A.: (1) Mendelism of Migraine, Med. Rec., 1920, **98**, 807. (2) The Abdominal Crises of Migraine, Jour. Nerv. and Ment. Dis., 1921, **54**, 406.

10. Buchanan, J. A.: The Familial Distribution of the Migraine-epilepsy Syndrome, New York Med. Jour., 1921, **113**, 45.

11. Buchanan, J. A.: Medico-legal Application of the Blood Group, Jour. Am. Med. Assn., 1922, **78**, 89.

12. Buchanan, J. A.: Theories and Theorizers Connected with the Development of the Laws of Heredity. (In press.)

13. Cooke, R. A. and Vander Veer, A.: Human Sensitization, Jour. Immunol., 1916, **1**, 201.

14. Correns, C. G.: Mendel's Regel über das Verhalten der Nachkommenschaft der Rassenbastarde, Ber. d. deutsch. botm. Gesellsch., 1900, **18**, 158.

15. Crofton, A. C.: A Note on Conjugal Diabetes, New York Med. Jour., 1908, **88**, 162.

16. Decastello, A. and Sturli, A.: Ueber die Isoagglutinine im Serum gesunder und kranker Menschen, München. med. Wchnschr., 1902, **49**, 1090.

17. Drinkwater, H.: Mendelian Heredity of Asthma, Brit. Med. Jour., 1909, **1**, 88.

18. von Dungern, E. and Hirschfeld, D. L.: Ueber Vererbung gruppenspezifischer Strukturen des Blutes, Ztschr. f. Immunitätsforsch. u. exper. Therap. Orig., 1910, **6**, 284.

19. Foster, N. B.: Consanguineal Diabetes Mellitus, Bull. Johns Hopkins Hosp., 1912, **23**, 54.

20. Geddings, W. H.: Bronchial Asthma. Pepper's System of Medicine, Philadelphia, Lea Brothers, 1885, **3**, 190.

21. Giraud, G.: Les Groupes Sanguins, Presse méd., 1919, **1**, 21–22.

22. Jansky, J.: Hämotologische Studien bei Psychotiken, Jahrsch. f. Neurol. u. Psychiat., 1907, **11**, 1092.

23. Kölreuter, J. G.: Quoted from Lock, R. H., New York, Macmillan, 1907, 150.

24. Landsteiner, K.: Ueber Agglutinationerscheinungen normalen menschlichen Blutes, Wien. klin. Wchnschr., 1901, **14**, 1132.

25. van Leeuwenhoek, A.: The Selected Works of. Translated by Samuel Hoole, London, Nicol, 1798-1807, p. 40.

26. Long, F. A.: A Contribution on the Study of the Familial Aspect of Diabetes Mellitus, Western Med. Rev., 1914, **19**, 30.

27. Longcope, W. T.: The Susceptibility of Man to Foreign Proteins, Harvey Lectures, Philadelphia, Lippincott, 1915–1916, **2**, 371.

28. May, O.: The Significance of Diabetic Family History in Life Insurance, Lancet, 1914, **1**, 679.

29. Mendel, G.: Versuche über Pflanzen-hybriden, Verhandl. Naturf. Ver. im Brünn, 1865, **4**, 1. Ueber einige aus künstlichen Befruchtung gewonnene Hierecum Bastarde, Verhandl. Naturf. Ver. im. Brunn, 1869, **8**, 26.

30. Morgan, T. H.: The Physical Basis of Heredity, Philadelphia, Lippincott, 1919, 15.

31. Moss, W. L.: Studies on Isoagglutinins and Isohemolysins, Tr. Assn. Am. Phys., 1909, **24**, 419.

32. Naunyn, B.: Der Diabetes Mellitus, Wien, Holder, 1906, p. 108.
33. von Noorden, C.: Die Zuckerkrankheit und ihre Behandlung, Berlin, Hirschwald, 1917, 75.
34. Nussbaum, M.: Zur Differenzirung des Geschlechts im Thierreich, Arch. f. mikr. Anat., 1880, **18**, 1.
35. Oppenheimer, S. and Gottlieb, M. J.: Pollen Therapy in Pollinosis; with, Results of Treatment by Immunization Methods during 1915, Med. Rec., 1916, **89**, 505.
36. Osler, W., and McCrae, T.: The Principles and Practice of Medicine, 9 ed., New York, Appleton, 1920, p. 620.
37. Ottenberg, R. and Epstein, L.: Discussion, Tr. New York Path. Soc., 1908, **8**, 117.
38. Ottenberg, R.: Medico-legal Application of Human Blood Grouping. Jour. Am. Med. Assn., 1921, **77**, 682.
39. Ottenberg, R.: Medico-legal Application of Human Blood Grouping, Second Communication, Jour. Am. Med. Assn., 1922, **78**, 873.
40. Sanford, A. H.: A Modification of the Moss Method of Determining Isohemagglutination Groups, Jour. Am. Med. Assn., 1918, **70**, 1221.
41. Schleiden, M. J.: Beiträge sur Phylogenesis, Arch. f. Anat. u. Physiol., 1838, 137.
42. Schwann, T.: Mikroscopische Untersuchungen über die Uebereinstimmung in der Structur und den Wachstum der Thiere und Pflanzen, 1839, Trans. London, Sydenham Soc., 1837.
43. Shattock, S. G.: Chromocyte Clumping in Acute Pneumonia and Certain Other Diseases, and the Significance of the Buffy Coat in the Shed Blood, Jour. Path. and Bacteriol., 1900, **6**, 303.
44. Virchow, R. L. K.: Cellular Pathology as Based upon Physiological and Pathological Histology, Theory of Cellular Pathology, Translated by Frank Chance, New York De Witt, 1860, p. 23.
45. Walker, I. C.: Studies on the Cause and the Treatment of Bronchial Asthma, Jour. Am. Med. Assn., 1917, **69**, 363.
46. Weismann, A.: The Germ Plasma. A Theory of Heredity, New York, Scribner's Sons, 1921, 37.
47. Willis, T.: Quoted from Auld, A. G., Asthma, Brit. Med. Jour., 1908, **2**, 1850.

TOLYSIN IN ACUTE RHEUMATIC FEVER AND OTHER CONDITIONS.

By H. G. Barbour, M.D., E. Lozinsky, M.D.

AND

C. Clements, M.D.

MONTREAL, CANADA.

(From the Department of Pharmacology, McGill University, and the Montreal General and Royal Victoria Hospitals.)

Ethyl ester of paramethylphenylcinchoninic acid (tolysin) has received recent recognition as an improvement over salicylates in acute rheumatic fever and other conditions. In particular, Hanzlik, Scott, Weidenthal and Fetterman[1] employed it in 3 cases of acute rheumatic fever and observed complete relief after 11 to 16 gm. had been given. These authors point out that the drug appears to be quite innocuous in large doses and is less irritating than cinchophen or the salicylates that are usually given. According to their evidence and that of Chace, Myers, and Killian[2] the function of the kidneys appears to be stimulated in some cases by tolysin.

Two of the present authors[3] have recently demonstrated that tolysin exhibits an unusual lack of toxicity. It is impossible to injure dogs in any way with doses amounting to 5 per cent of their body weight; it is nevertheless an efficient antipyretic in these animals in small doses. It was found that this is due to an unusual coincidence between the maximum therapeutic dose of tolysin and the maximum amount which can be absorbed from the intestine.

Such a drug seems to offer possibilities as a partial, if not a complete, substitute for the salicylates which are now in use, all of which require constant attention to the avoidance of toxic symptoms. In the following report, therefore, we shall present evidence as to the clinical value of tolysin.

The cases herein described are from the wards of the Montreal General Hospital, service of Dr. F. G. Finley, and the Royal Victoria Hospital, service of Dr. C. F. Martin, and include also a number of private observations.* They will be presented under the headings:

1. Acute and subacute rheumatic fever.
2. Other cases of arthritis.
3. Observations on tolysin as an antipyretic and analgesic.

1. Acute and Subacute Rheumatic Fever. 12 individuals suffering from rheumatic fever were treated with full doses of tolysin; one of these received two courses of the drug, having suffered a relapse in the interval, for which he was unsuccessfully treated with salicylates. The routine dosage finally determined upon was 2 gm. every two hours for three doses, followed by 1 gm. every four hours (four or five times a day). In a few of the earlier cases were made some unimportant differences in the dosage and interval. The details of this series are presented in Table I.

It will be noted from the above that, with two exceptions, the amount necessary for complete relief (by which is meant cessation of fever, pain and swelling) varied from 10 to 16 gm. To this may be added the fact that partial relief was usually noted after 7 to 8 gm. had been given.

In several cases the drug was continued over a longer period of time than absolutely necessary in order to demonstrate its non-toxicity. 2 different patients received 50 gm. of tolysin within eight days. Similarly, a patient not included in the present series received 24 gm. within forty-eight hours. As reported in our laboratory paper, this 24 gm. of tolysin was completely absorbed, none being recoverable from the feces. In none of these 3

* The authors desire to express their appreciation of the coöperation of Professors Finley and Martin and their respective staffs, including especially Miss Jackson of the Montreal General Hospital.

Case No.	Name.	Age.	Sex.	Clinical diagnosis	Tolysin giving complete relief.	Total number of grams administered in number of days.		Gastric symptoms.	Albuminuria.	
					Gm.	Gm.	Days.		Before treatment.	After treatment.
1	A. C.	40	M.	Acute rheumatic fever	16	26	7	None	0	0
2	J. F.	14	M.	Relapse, acute rheumatic fever	6 5□	6 5□	3	None	0	0
3	S. M.	49	M.	Acute rheumatic fever	16	38	5	None	0	0
4	N. D.	28	M.	Acute rheumatic fever	12	54	7	None	++	Trace
5	H. B.	35	M.	Acute rheumatic fever	14	50	8	None	Faint trace	0
6	E. B.	24	M.	Subacute rheumatic fever	10	13	4	None	0	0
7	A. S.	17	F.	Acute rheumatic fever	10	21	7	None	0	0
8	R. S.	23	M.	Acute rheumatic fever	16	24	6	None	Faint trace	0
9	J. M.	24	M.	Acute rheumatic fever	40[1]	40	10	None	Faint trace	0
10	H. C.	38	M.	Acute rheumatic fever	16	24	6	None	0	Faint trace
11	L. F.	18	F.	Acute rheumatic fever	14[2]	18	6	None	Faint trace	0
12	W. W.	37	M.	Acute rheumatic fever	16[3]	60	14	None	Faint trace	0
"	"	"	"	Relapse[5]	16[4]	24	8	None	0	0

[1] Sodium salicylate, 3 grams per diem for six weeks, had given partial relief.
[2] Sodium salicylate, 4 grams per diem for eight days, had given partial relief.
[3] Every symptom relieved except one slightly painful shoulder.
[4] Preceded by eleven-day interval of sodium salicylate treatment (48 grams in all).
[5] Occurred during salicylate treatment.

instances of high dosage were noted any untoward symptoms whatever.

In fact, in all cases in which we have followed the results of tolysin treatment, nausea, vomiting, excessive sweating and cardiac depression have been absent. So-called "salicylism" is not induced even by relatively large doses. Complaints of gastric disturbance were not elicited, although carefully sought.

Albuminuria, which was present in 6 of the 12 patients on admission, disappeared in 5 of these during treatment; in the sixth the albumin became diminished to a trace. Improvement in this respect may presumably be attributed to rest in bed and restricted diet. In only 1 of the 12 cases did albumin first appear or increase in amount during treatment with tolysin.

Below are given the chief points in the clinical histories of patients with acute rheumatic fever. Temperature Charts I to III are also illustrative.

Case Reports. Case I.—A. C., male, aged forty years. March 3, 1922. Admitted to hospital complaining of pain and swelling in joints.

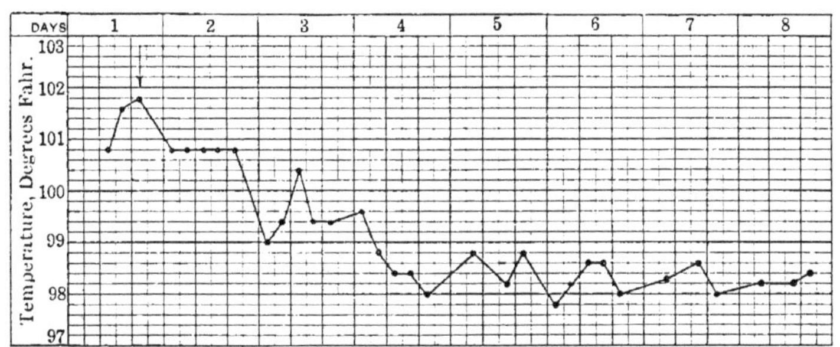

Fig. 1.—Case 1. Acute rheumatic fever. Readings every four hours. Tolysin 1 gm. every two hours for 3 doses, then 1 gm. every four hours started at arrow. Relief from symptoms coincident with fall in temperature.

Present Illness. On February 11, 1922, patient got his feet wet and three days later pain and swelling of right ankle and foot caused him to take to bed where he remained for three days when he apparently recovered and returned to work. Two days later left knee painful for three days but not severe, morning of fourth day left knee very painful, tender and swollen and patient was again forced to his bed. March 22, 1922 pain and swelling of left shoulder, elbow and wrist. March 3, 1922, admitted to hospital.

Treatment. Patient had no treatment at home except iodine painted over painful joints. March 3, Tolysin 1 gm. every two hours for 3 doses then every four hours. March 4, slight fall in temperature with some relief from pain. March 6, patient free from all pain. March 11, patient discharged, cured. He received in six days a total of 26 gm. of tolysin. Temperature Chart I, is the temperature record of this patient.

CASE II.—J. F. male, aged fourteen years, was admitted to hospital February 17, 1922 with diagnosis of acute rheumatic fever. Treated with salicylates for three days with good results. March 1, patient suffered a relapse, pain and swelling returning in several joints. For this relapse he was given tolysin 0.7 gm. every four hours for 10 doses which gave him complete relief.

CASE III.—S. M., male, aged forty-nine years, was admitted to hospital March 12, 1922, complaining of pain and swelling in joints.

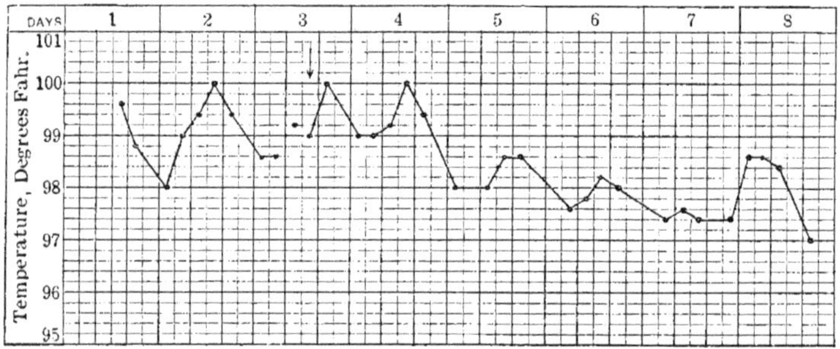

FIG. 2.—Case 3. Acute rheumatic fever. Readings every four hours. Tolysin 2 gm. every two hours for 3 doses, then 2 gm. every four hours started at arrow. Relief from symptoms coincident with fall in temperature.

Present Illness. Patient gives history of recurring attacks of acute rheumatic fever. Present attack started nine weeks ago. Pain first felt in right foot which became swollen, red and tender and remained so for four or five weeks. The joints next involved were the right knee, right hip, left wrist, left knee and right wrist.

Treatment. For first two days in hospital patient was on a sugar tolerance test and he received no medication. On third day 2 gm. of tolysin every two hours, 3 doses, then every four hours; complete relief with subsidence of temperature after receiving 16 gm.; total administered, 38 gm. in five days—no signs of toxicity. Discharged March 30, 1922. Temperature Chart II, temperature record of the patient.

CASE IV.—N. P., male aged twenty-eight years, was admitted to the hospital, March 15, 1922.

Present Illness. Patient's history difficult to get. Diagnosis of acute rheumatic fever made.

Treatment. Tolysin 2 gm. every two hours for 3 doses, then every four hours. Complete relief from 12 gm.; the drug was pushed for seven day during which time he received 54 gm. No toxic effects. Discharged March 31, 1922.

Case V.—H. B., male, aged thirty-five years, was admitted, March 19, 1922, complaining of pain and swelling of joints.

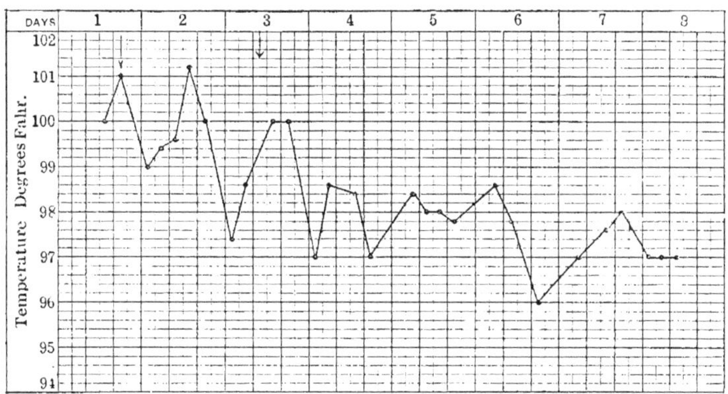

Fig. 3.—Case 5. Acute rheumatic fever. Readings every four hours. Tolysin 2 gm. every two hours for 3 doses, started at first arrow, then 1 gm. every four hours started at second arrow. Relief from symptoms coincident with fall in temperature.

Present Illness. Two weeks ago left foot became painful and swollen, that night he had chills and some fever. Next morning pain less severe in foot but left knee very painful and swollen. In course of next four or five days left shoulder, left wrist and hand involved. Several days later left elbow and right knee involved.

Treatment. Tolysin 2 gm. every two hours for 3 doses, then 2 gm. every four hours. Patient relieved of all symptoms after 14 gm. Drug pushed until 50 gm. had been given; no toxic effects were manifest. Patient discharged March 29, 1922. Temperature Chart III, temperature record of this patient.

Case VI.—E. B., male, aged twenty-four years, was admitted March 16, 1922, complaining of pain and swelling in joints.

Present Illness. Three weeks ago pain in left big toe, next left ankle then right hip painful. Some fever at onset, pain has persisted until present.

Treatment. Tolysin 0.7 gm. every three hours for 4 doses, then every four hours for four days. Complete relief in four days.

Case VII.—A. S., female, aged seventeen years, was admitted to hospital, May 10, 1922, complaining of stiffness and pain in joints.

Present Illness. Illness began about six weeks ago with pain in both shoulders and both elbows. Pain more severe at night than during day. Four weeks ago knee-joints involved, followed by left foot and ankle. Since onset of pain, shortness of breath on exertion.

Treatment. Tolysin 1 gm. three times a day, complete relief after 10 gm.; total administered 21 gm.

Case VIII.—Male, aged twenty-three years, was admitted to hospital, May 20, 1922, complaining of pain and swelling of left wrist-joint, both shoulder-joints, knee-joints and ankle-joints.

Present Illness. Well until two weeks ago. On May 6, 1922, developed pain and swelling in right ankle-joint. Since then pain and swelling with slight redness in joints enumerated above. Some fever and profuse perspiration.

Treatment. Tolysin, 1 gm. every four hours, partial relief after 8 gm.; complete relief after 16 gm. Total administered twenty-four gm.

Case IX.—J. M., male, aged twenty-four years, was admitted to hospital, February 25, 1922, complaining of swelling, redness, pain and tenderness in ankles, shoulders, wrist and hip-joints. Onset was acute with progressive involvement of the various joints.

Treatment. Sodium salicylate, 1 gm. three times a day was given continuously over a period of six weeks with considerable relief from symptoms. A relapse occurred and sodium salicylate produced some relief from symptoms, but never complete. May 13, 1922, tolysin 1 gm. every four hours, marked improvement after 6 gm. had been given. Administration continued for ten days, with total relief from pain, but some stiffness still present.

Case X.—H. C., male, aged thirty-eight years, was admitted to hospital, May 18, 1922, complaining of pain in ankle and knee-joints.

Treatment. Tolysin 1 gm. every two hours for 3 doses, then 1 gm. every four hours. Partial relief after 8 gm.; complete relief from pain after 16 gm. although some stiffness still present. Total tolysin administered 24 gm. with continued improvement.

Case XI.—L. F., female, aged eighteen years, was admitted to hospital, May 9, 1922, complaining of: (1) Pain in soles of feet, ankles, left thumb, left shoulder and small of back; (2) shortness of breath on exertion.

Present Illness. About three weeks ago developed dull aching pain in toes, heels and ankle-joints. The pain was not severe enough to confine patient to bed but was persistent. Later, shoulder and wrist-joints involved, also small of back.

Treatment. On admission, sodium salicylate 1 gm. every four hours for eight days with some relief. May 18, 1922, tolysin 1 gm. three times a day. Patient entirely free from pain after 14 gm.; total administered 18 gm.

Case XII.—W. W., aged thirty-seven years, was admitted to hospital, April 12, 1922, complaining of pain, swelling and tenderness in joints.

Present Illness. Illness began two weeks ago with a chill, following day pain and swelling of right elbow, and stiffness of finger joints. Two days later both feet and ankles were swollen and painful, then knees and left wrist. On admission, right shoulder shows moderate swelling, tender and very painful on movement. Left wrist, left ankle and right knee also tender but not swollen.

Treatment. April 12, 1922. Tolysin 2 gm. every two hours for 3 doses, then 1 gm. every four hours. Partial relief after 10 gm., patient relieved from all pain after 16 gm. except shoulder, which persisted slightly painful. Tolysin discontinued April 26, 1922, and sodium salicylate 1 gm. three times a day commenced. May 6, 1922, relapse, temperature 101° F., pain and swelling of joints. May 8, 1922, tolysin 1 gm. every four hours, relief after 8 gm.; free from pain after 16 gm. May 15, discharged, free from pain.

2. Other Cases of Arthritis. In 7 further cases of arthritis tolysin was given. The series includes a somewhat ill-assorted list of conditions, especially cases of infective arthritis and chronic joint pains. As will be seen from the following case reports, tolysin gave satisfactory results in all of these except Case XIX, in which severe chronic pains in back and legs were not relieved.

Case XIII.—L. O'B., female, aged thirty-two years, was admitted to hospital January 19, 1922, complaining of pain in joints and feverishness.

Clinical Diagnosis. Multiple arthritis, infection (tonsil).

Present Illness. On January 15, 1922, headache, sore throat, pain in back, following day severe and steady pain in right shoulder and both elbows with tenderness and slight swelling. January 17, 1922, elbows improved, right knee painful. January 18, 1922, left knee involved also right hand painful and swollen.

Physical Examination. On day of admission, January 19, 1922, Temperature 103.3° F., pulse 128. Both knees and both elbows painful and tender, no redness or swelling; right hand is painful and stiff, right shoulder painful.

Treatment. Sodium salicylate 2 gm. every four hours for 6 doses, then 1 gm. three times daily. During the first few days patient was greatly relieved but pain soon returned varying in severity from day to day, there was a slight degree of pyrexia.

This continued for three weeks. Tolysin February 13, 1922, 2 gm. every six hours was started. At time of administration temperature 100° F., the following day temperature down to 98° and joints less painful. The patient was kept comfortable as long as tolysin was given but pain returned after drug was stopped for two or three days. Relief was again obtained when tolysin was given. Patient discharged March 5, 1922.

Case XIV.—M. S., female, aged twenty-eight years, was admitted to hospital March 7, 1922, complaining of pain in joints.

Present Illness. Well until five weeks ago, first symptom was pain in the right ankle which became swollen and painful during the past five weeks, one joint after the other became involved, including both sternoclavicular articulations. She was treated with salicylate from the start without improvement. Admitted to hospital March, 7, 1922, temperature 99.4° F., pulse 104, respiration 22.

Treatment. Tolysin, 1 gm. every four hours. Temperature did not become normal until after one week's treatment; pain in joints slowly but certainly relieved, patient ready for discharge April 4, 1922.

Case XV.—M. J., a female with chronic multiple arthritis of long standing. Patient has taken aspirin for relief of pain but without much alleviation, lately she has been taking tolysin 0.7 gm. four times a day and she feels a great deal of improvement.

Case XVI.—A female aged sixty-eight years, reported by courtesy of Dr. D. S. Lewis.

Clinical Diagnosis. Diabetes and rheumatoid arthritis, neuritis. Has had severe lancinating pain in right leg for six weeks.

Treatment. Phenacetin 5 gr. three times a day without result; aspirin 5 gr. four times a day, without result; a combination of aspirin, phenacetin and codein with very slight relief. Tolysin, 1 gm. every four hours, began to sleep well again. Pain controlled by 1 gm. twice a day after first forty-eight hours. After two weeks 1 gm. three times a day. After ten weeks 1 gm. four times a day, gave fair control of pain.

Case XVII.—E. E., female aged forty-seven years, was admitted to hospital, March 31, 1922, complaining of pain and swelling of joints.

Present Illness. Illness began one month ago with a chill following which pain and swelling in left ankle-joint and left knee-joint developed. Patient felt very ill and had some fever, soon right knee, left wrist and right shoulder-joint became swollen and painful. Temperature on admission 99.4° F.

Treatment. Tolysin 2 gm. every two hours for 3 doses, then 1 gm. every four hours. Temperature started to fall after 10 gm. Normal in seven days. Acute pain and swelling rapidly subsided, but patient still complained of stiffness and some pain. Treatment continued over a period of four weeks, with only intermittent relief from symptoms. Urine albumin free and no gastric disturbances.

CASE XVIII.—A. O., male, aged forty-five years, was admitted to hospital, May 8, 1922, complaining of pain in knees, feet, back, elbow and hands.

Present Illness. Well until May 1, 1922, when he developed pain and swelling in left wrist. Four days later pain and swelling in left knee, and both ankle-joints, also pain in back.

Treatment. Tolysin 2 gm. every two hours for 2 doses, then 1 gm. every four hours. Temperature normal after 7 gm. Complete relief from pain after 24 gm. Total drug administered 56 gm. in fifteen days.

Clinical Diagnosis. (1) Multiple arthritis; (2). prostatitis and seminal vesiculitis; (3) chronic urethritis.

CASE XIX.—H. M., male, aged fifty-two years, was admitted to hospital May 9, 1922, complaining of pain in back and legs.

Present Illness. Well until one year ago, when he began to have pain in back and legs, this condition while persistent at all times since then became very severe on several occasions, forcing patient to remain in bed. On admission temperature 98° F., pulse 80.

Treatment. Tolysin 1 gm. three times a day for six days without appreciable relief.

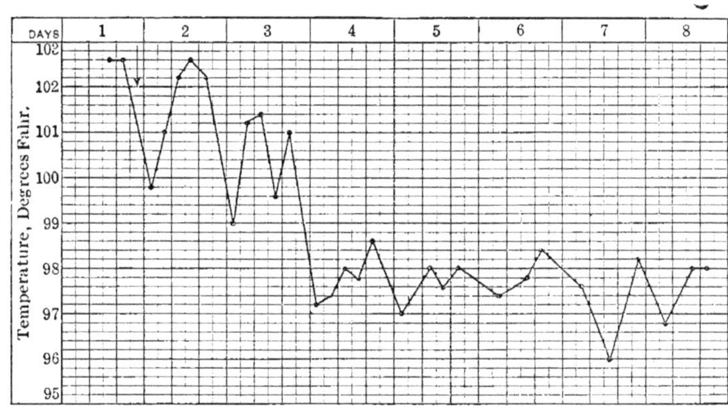

FIG. 4.—Acute tonsillitis. Readings every four hours. Tolysin 1.3 gm. every two hours, then 1.3 gm. every four hours, started at arrow.

3. FURTHER OBSERVATIONS ON TOLYSIN AS AN ANTIPYRETIC AND ANALGESIC. Tolysin has been further studied in 3 cases of

acute tonsillitis, 4 of ordinary "cold," and upward of 15 headaches, types of cases in which antipyretics, especially aspirin are generally used. As an analgesic for the relief of headache tolysin requires somewhat longer to act than do the salicylates. Doses of 0.7 to 1.0 gm. were usually found effective. The malaise and fever associated with the onset of a "cold" were relieved by tolysin in doses of 0.7 to 1.0 gm. every three hours for 2 or 3 doses. In the 3 cases of acute tonsillitis tolysin proved an efficient antipyretic in doses of 1 to 2 gm. repeated every three or four hours.

Temperature Chart IV is the fever record of a case of acute tonsillitis, showing the action of tolysin.

Summary. 1. Tolysin (ethyl ester of paramethylphenylcinchoninic acid) appears to be a very safe drug.

Two different patients received each 50 gm. of tolysin within eight days without any untoward symptoms whatever. Our recent laboratory investigation has shown that the body is unable to absorb much more than the therapeutic dose.

2. In a series of 12 cases of acute rheumatic fever tolysin was found a fully efficient therapeutic agent. The usual dose required for complete relief of symptoms is 10 to 16 gm. Partial relief was obtained with 7 to 8 gm. A satisfactory routine is to give 2 gm. every two hours for 3 doses, followed by 2 gm. every four hours. No gastric symptoms were elicited, and albuminuria was increased in only one case.

3. Satisfactory results were further obtained in 6 out of 7 cases of arthritis of other types, including acute infections and chronic joint pains.

4. Tolysin has been employed in cases of ordinary "colds" and headaches with effects apparently equivalent to those of aspirin, but the action appears slower and somewhat larger doses are indicated.

5. In acute tonsillitis 1 to 2 gm. tolysin (which can be repeated) exert a good antipyretic action.

6. The employment of tolysin may be substituted for any internal salicylate medication. It is particularly efficient in acute rheumatic fever and, on the basis of the evidence at present available, apparently can be administered constantly in this and other forms of arthritis without harmful effects.

REFERENCES.

1. Hanzlik, P. J., Scott, R. W., Weidenthal, C. M., and Fettermann, J.: Jour. Am. Med. Assn., 1921, **76**, 1728.

2. Chace, A. F., Myers, V. C., and Killian, J. A.: Jour. Am. Med. Assn., 1921, **77**, 1230.

3. Barbour, H. G., and Lozinsky, E.: Jour. Lab. and Clin. Med., 1923, **8**, 217.

THE EARLY SYMPTOMS AND THE DIAGNOSIS OF TUMORS OF THE SPINAL CORD, WITH REMARKS ON THE SURGICAL TREATMENT.*

By Charles A. Elsberg, M.D.,
NEW YORK.

In the progress of our understanding of disease, as in the story of the forward march of other branches of human knowledge, history repeats itself. Symptoms were again and again described as a disease but were found to be only a result or a symptom. The diagnosis "primary peritonitis" became more and more rare with the advances in our knowledge of the pathology of the intra-abdominal organs. We are beginning to realize that primary inflammations of the pleural membranes are unusual and that the pleural lesion is most often secondary to a pathological process in the cortical portions of the lungs. Who knows but that meningitis will one day be shown to hold the same relation to affections of the brain and spinal cord that peritonitis does to the abdominal viscera and inflammation of the pleura to the lungs.

Not so many years ago "chronic transverse myelitis" was considered a disease of frequent occurrence; we now know that it is rare. That this supposed affection has been relegated to the background of the past is mainly due to the advances in our knowledge of local spinal compression, and more especially to our understanding of the pathological effects and the symptoms of tumors of the spinal cord.

The history of the marvellous progress made in this field is one that must deeply impress the student of the subject. In 1882, a great clinician made the statement that "the existence of an intraspinal tumor can hardly be determined with certainty, and, assuming that a tumor exists, to determine its character from the symptoms is impracticable."[1] And a surgeon, famous in his day, had declared that "the operation of trephining the spine is an operation not within the range of practical surgery."[2] At the same period, however, Gowers, Leyden, Erb and Osler voiced the belief that tumors of the cord could be recognized and were, perhaps, amenable to surgical treatment. How quickly was the darkness and doubt dispelled when, in 1887, Horsley successfully removed a spinal cord tumor that has been correctly diagnosticated and localized by Gowers.

In the thirty-five years that have passed since Horsley and

* Read before the Section of Neurology at the Stated Meeting of the New York Academy of Medicine, March 16, 1922.

[1] Flint, Austin: Practice of Medicine, 1882.

[2] Heath: History of Surgery, 1881.

Gowers' epoch-making operation[3] our knowledge of the symptomatology of spinal tumors and of their surgical treatment has made rapid strides. Then, the neurologist was victorious if he successfully determined the level of a spinal new growth. Now, we are able to diagnose from the progress of the symptoms and the signs of interference with function—not only the level of the cord lesion, but also the location of the growth in relation to the cord, the ventral and dorsal roots, and the dentate ligament. Then, spinal tumors were considered very rare; now, they are met with frequeney. Then, the symptomatology was considered invariable—a beginning with root pains and a progress with increasing sensory and motor paralysis. Now, we know that many cases begin without pain and progress with irregular motor and sensory disturbances. Then, a diagnosis could be made only when the signs of motor and sensory loss were far advanced. Now, we can often make the diagnosis before much paralysis or sensory disturbance has occurred if the patient comes under observation early enough. Then, the operation of laminectomy was a hazardous procedure; now, the exposure and removal of a spinal neoplasm is an operation devoid of great danger.

The story of the stages in the progress is of absorbing interest. As the time is short, I can only speak of some aspects of the subject, and have selected the subject of the early symptoms of spinal cord tumors.

Pain and Other Subjective Sensory Disturbances as Early Symptoms. As our understanding of pain due to irritation of sensory spinal roots became greater, we began to have a fuller realization of the significance of this symptom. At the present time the very word neuralgia, if the cranial nerves are excepted, should bring to the mind of the physician the possibility of a root pain. This subject is not only of importance to the neurologist and the neurological surgeon, but also to the general practitioner and the general surgeon. Many patients with spinal cord tumors have a long period lasting from many months to five or even eight years, during which they complain of pain in one or other part of the body, due to irritation of one or more sensitive posterior roots. These patients are treated for long periods for neuralgia. If the pain affects an upper extremity, it is considered a brachial neuritis, if in the thorax it is called intercostal neuralgia or perhaps pleurisy; if the lower extremities are affected, the cases are called sciatica. When these painful symptoms occur in the abdomen, an intra-abdominal lesion is thought of and only too often an abdominal operation of one kind or another performed. I am repeatedly seeing patients with disease of the thoracic cord who have had

[3] No one who is interested in spinal-cord tumors should fail to read the original report of the case. It was published in the Medico-Chirurgical Transactions, London, 1888.

one or more laparotomies or other operations for supposed abdominal or pelvic disease.

The following are a few cases of this nature:

Case I.—Mrs. W. (Neurological Institute, 1916). In 1910, the patient complained of sciatica and was treated for it. As she had large hemorrhoids, these were supposed to be the cause and the hemorrhoids were removed by a surgeon. The symptoms continued and there were added pains in the lower portion of her back and extending into the rectum. As she had a movable coccyx, this was removed in 1911. In 1912, the sphincter ani was stretched and partly cut. In 1913, a sigmoidopexy was done. In 1914, a ventral suspension was done. But none of these operations relieved the symptoms. The patient became more and more miserable, complaining constantly of a sensation of pressure in the rectum with continual desire to move her bowels, pain high up in the rectum and in the bladder and pain in the lower portion of her back. She noticed that when she took a cathartic, she sometimes did not have perfect control of her bowels and occasionally of her bladder. There were no disturbances in the lower extremities. Finally, a lumbar puncture was done and yellow fluid was withdrawn under pressure, and then neurological examination revealed that there were very slight sensory disturbances over the lower sacral areas. At the operation a small tumor, about the size of an almond, was removed from between the roots of the cauda equina.

Case II.—Samuel T. (Neurological Institute No. 12,955). Four years previously the patient suffered from rheumatism in both legs. For one year he noticed that sneezing caused him severe pain in the rectum. At the same time be began to have difficulty in passing his water. He was told that he had a slight amount of cystitis, a small amount of residual urine and a markedly large prostate and he was advised to have his prostate removed. Before subjecting himself to this operation, examination showed that the lower abdominal reflexes were weak, that the ankle jerks were slightly exaggerated and that there were very slight sensory disturbances. A lumbar puncture was then done and the typical fluid of spinal cord tumor found. At the operation, a tumor about the size of a small olive was removed, lying in front of the cord at the level of the tenth thoracic segment.

Case III.—Mrs. B. (Mount Sinai Hospital No. 173,333). Two years' history of pain in the right hypochrondrium and right side of the abdomen. Cholecystectomy, later appendectomy; no relief. Finally, spinal symptoms discovered. Laminectomy and removal of lobulated tumor from underneath the sixth, seventh, and eight thoracic spinal roots on the right side.

Case IV.—Alexander B. (Mount Sinai Hospital No. 214,385). Twenty-one months' history of attacks of pain in the left hypochondrium and left lumbar region, usually worse after meals. After thirteen months, tingling in the soles of both feet and slight weakness. Five months before admission, laparotomy for suspected gastric ulcer. November 22, 1921: laminectomy and removal of spinal cord tumor from the anterior and left side of the cord at the seventh thoracic segment.

Instead of beginning with neuralgic pain, some patients first complain of a persistent pain in the back of the neck or in the thoracic spine. The pain is usually strictly localized and does not radiate for a long time. Later it may radiate around the body or down one or both limbs. The pain is very similar to that of malignant disease of the vertebræ, but the pain of malignant disease is more apt to be felt in front of the chest as well as in the back and is more often made worse by movement. On the other hand, patients with extramedullary spinal tumors often state that the pain in the back is made worse by coughing or by sneezing. In not a few of these patients, the roentgen-ray picture shows more or less marked arthritis of the vertebræ and the roentgen-ray changes may be so marked that the patient is actually treated for Pott's disease. In the early stages, it is often difficult to differentiate the pain in the back from that which occurs in primary or secondary vertebral disease or from aneurysm of the aorta. For a long time the symptoms may be perplexing. In every patient who complains of persistent pain in the back, repeated neurological examinations should be made.

Pain in the lower part of the back is one of the earliest and most continuous symptoms of the large intradural tumors of the lumbosacral parts of the cord and of the roots of the cauda equina. This "pain in the small of the back" is usually made worse by movement and by coughing and sneezing, and may for years be the only symptom. The pain is either continuous or occurs in attacks and the patients are supposed to be suffering from lumbago. After a period of, perhaps, years, the knee jerks are found to have been lost, and then the diagnosis of locomotor ataxia may be made. Finally, the characteristic symptoms and signs of conus or cauda become evident.

The late Dr. Pearce Bailey was one of the first to call attention to the fact that in a certain number of instances, spinal cord tumors develop without any painful symptoms. These cases are of sufficient frequency to demand consideration. It has been my experience that tumors with a painless onset occur either with a growth of small size which has developed from the pia or arachnoid on the anterior or antero-lateral aspect or on the posterolateral surface of the cord between two nerve roots. In these patients, root symptoms may appear late instead of early in the disease.

Bailey was correct in his statement that there is a group of spinal cord tumors which begin without pain. Dr. Stookey and I, studying my spinal tumor records, have found that the large majority of cases of spinal tumor have some kind of subjective sensory disturbance as an early symptom. The accompanying table (see Table I) gives the early sensory complaints in the patients.

TABLE I.—SENSORY SYMPTOMS AT ONSET.

	Extra-medullary.	Extra-dural.	Conus and cauda.	Intra-medullary.
Root pains	19	3	0	2
Pain in back or in neck	6	4	1	4
Pain in back extending down limbs	1	2	7	0
Pain in homolateral limb below level	1	1	0	0
Pain in contralateral limb below level	2	1	0	0
Pain in both legs below level	2	0	2	0
Pain in rectum	1	0	1	0
Pain in chest or abdomen	2	2	0	1
Tingling, burning, heaviness, pin-and needle sensation or numbness of homolateral limb below level	1	0	0	4
Tingling, burning, heaviness, pin-and-needle sensation or numbness of contralateral limb below level	5	0	0	0
Tingling or numbness of both lower limbs	3	0	0	2
Tingling without pain, on same side	1	0	0	0
Tingling without pain, on opposite side	2	0	0	0
Numbness or heaviness, but no pain	1	1	0	0
Feeling of stiffness, but no pain	1	0	0	0
No sensory symptoms	1	0	2	2

A number of different sensations are recorded as early symptoms. Many complained of a pain that was evidently radicular in character; others of a localized or radiating pain in the back, others of a visceral pain. Tingling, burning, heaviness, numbness, stiffness or a "pin- and needle" sensation, were very often complained of. Total absence of complaints regarding some kind of abnormal sensation was very rare in extramedullary and extradural growths, and was somewhat more frequent in intramedullary growths. It is especially noteworthy that a considerable number of patients with extramedullary tumors complained of paresthesiæ of some kind—a symptom which was once considered characteristic of intramedullary growths.

Diminution or loss of articular sense, which is seen whenever one or both posterior columns are involved, was never recognized as such by the patients; they are apt to interpret the disturbance as a motor weakness. In not a few instances the patients stated positively that one limb was much weaker than the other, although the examination showed that there was no loss of motor power but only loss of the sense of position of the affected limb.

Early Subjective Motor Disturbances. In the majority of the patients, the motor disturbance that is first noticed by the patient occurs in the upper or lower extremity on the side of the tumor. If the growth is situated in the lower cervical (C VI—C VIII) and upper thoracic segments, the sequence of the limbs is usually (1) homolateral upper extremity, (2) homolateral lower extremity, (3) contralateral lower, and (4) contralateral upper extremity. Sometimes, however, the contralateral upper limb is affected before the lower limbs, and sometimes weakness of the contralateral lower limb is noted before the homolateral one.

In order to understand the apparently paradoxical weakness of the limb on the side opposite to that of the tumor, the mobility of the cord and the mechanical effects produced by spinal new-growths should be thoroughly understood.

In extradural and intradural growths which are adherent to the dura, the cord is often pushed to the opposite side of the dural sac by the fluid between the cord and the growth. When this occurs there is a period during which the side of the cord opposite to that of the tumor is pressed against the dural sac and the bony wall of the spinal canal. As a result, contralateral motor symptoms may be observed, and on examination the contralateral limb may be weak and spastic and the reflexes on that side exaggerated as the result of the compression of that side of the cord against the dura and bone wall of the vertebral canal.

Early Objective Sensory Disturbances. The mobility of many segments of the spinal cord is such that sensory disturbances may also occur as the result of the mechanism above described. Unless correctly evaluated, these sensory disturbances may lead to an incorrect localization of the tumor in relation to the cord. In tumors adherent to the dura (both extradural and intradural) there is often a stage during which the sensory disturbances (especially as regards pain and temperature) are more marked on the side of the tumor while the motor signs are most distinct on the opposite side. We have become accustomed to call this clinical picture a "reverse Brown-Séquard." Similarly we have seen early posterior column disturbances with tumors on the ventral aspect of the cord, from the backward dislocation of the affected part of the cord and the impact of the posterior column against the bony walls of the spinal canal. The reasons why these disturbances have not been more often observed, is that the patients are not more often seen by a neurologist in the earliest stages of spinal compression.

In extramedullary tumors of the spinal cord, the earliest evidence of diminution of superficial sensibility is to be found either over root areas at the level of the growth or in the peripheral parts of the limbs. Sensory disturbance in the toes or fingers should be carefully looked for in early suspected spinal disease. It is especially apt to occur in tumors on the posterior or postero-lateral aspect of the cord, and is more rare in anterior growths. In the latter, as well as in intramedullary tumors, the earliest and most marked sensory disturbance involves the dermatomes just below the segmentary cord level.

The Diagnosis of the Location of Tumors in Relation to the Cord. It is no longer sufficient to make a diagnosis of an extramedullary tumor at one or another level of the cord; we must now diagnose the exact relation of the tumor to the cord. In order to make this more precise localization, a general plan of classification of the relations of such growths is necessary.

We are accustomed to classify tumors, in their relation to the cord, in the following manner: Tumors behind the posterior roots we call posterior; those between the posterior roots and the dentate ligament are postero-lateral; those between the dentate and the anterior roots are antero-lateral; finally, those in front of the anterior roots are anterior growths.

The following two tables (Tables II and III) give the segmentary level and the local relations of the growths in our patients. In the second table (Table III) the tumors of the conus and cauda equina are not included because these tumors usually surround and lie between the caudal roots and exact classification as to their relation to the structures is not possible. This second table shows that in our experience 62 per cent of the extramedullary growths lie, according to our method of classification, on the posterior or postero-lateral aspect of the cord, while 36 per cent lie anterior or antero-lateral. This high relative proportion of ventral or ventro-lateral growths is of considerable importance because it is the growths in these locations that often give indefinite symptoms and signs for a considerable period of time.

TABLE II.—SEGMENT LEVEL OF TUMORS.

	Extramedullary.	Extradural	Intramedullary
Cervical—1-4	3	0	0
4-8	11	4	8
Thoracic—1-4	7	2	2
4-8	10	5	2
8-12	9	2	3
Lumbosacral and cauda	15	0	0
Totals	55	13	15

TABLE III.—RELATION OF TUMORS TO SURFACES OF CORD.

	Extramedullary. (Not including conus and cauda)	Extradural.
Anterior and median	1	1
Anterior and lateral	6	4
Antero-lateral	6	2
Posterior and median	2	0
Posterior and lateral	12	2
Postero-lateral	14	3
Lateral and posterior	1	0
Anterior and posterior	0	1
	42	13

Posterior tumors are characterized, above all, by root pains and by very marked posterior column disturbances. In growths on the dorso-lateral side of the cord, the root pains are apt to be very severe, and the Brown-Séquard type is apt to be very distinct. If a suspected spinal tumor causes root signs on one side of the body, sensory disturbances on the same side, and motor disturbances on the opposite side of the body (excluding, of course, tumors between the roots of the cauda equina) there is considerable probability that the tumor is either extradural or intradural and primarily from the dura itself.

Growths on the ventro-lateral aspect are apt to have a beginning without root pains with a Brown-Séquard picture and early local muscle atrophies. Growths in this location may also give signs of a reversed Brown-Séquard picture, and in such instances, also, the diagnosis of a dural origin is probable.[4]

Tumors on the anterior aspect of the cord very frequently have a painless beginning, with tingling in one or both lower limbs and relatively late sensory disturbances.

If we exclude root signs, hyperesthesia and diminution of sensation, there is no doubt that in a large number of the patients, if seen early enough, the first objective sensory disturbances will be found in the most peripheral part of the lower extremities in posterior or postero-lateral growths, and over the trunk in anterior or antero-lateral tumors. A sensory disturbance, most marked near the level of the spinal lesion, is characteristic also of intramedullary growths, but in these patients a Brown-Séquard syndrome or even an indication of this clinical picture is rare. We have not, I believe, paid sufficient attention to this subject and have not, in suspected spinal tumors, made a thorough search for the slightest evidence of diminution of sensation in the peripheral parts of the lower extremities.

In direct contradiction to the belief which is general and which is to the effect that there is no arrangement of fibers in the tracts of the cord corresponding to extremities and to different parts of the extremities—a belief which for many years has been grounded on clinical and pathological evidence—I have become convinced that there is a grouping of fibers for the different parts of the body in most if not all of the pathways of the cord. It is only on such a basis that it is possible to explain the not infrequent occurrence of motor and sensory disturbances in the lower limbs as the earliest signs and symptoms of extremedullary cord tumors in the cervical region.

If all the facts to which attention has been called in the foregoing remarks are taken into account, they will be found to aid

[4] This subject is of considerable diagnostic importance, and we shall, in another paper, discuss the mechanical effects of spinal-cord tumors and the resulting variations in the symptomatology.

in the differentiation between extramedullary and intramedullary, and also between extradural and intradural growths.

From the surgical standpoint, the finer localization of a tumor with reference to the cord is of importance, for it will allow the surgeon to plan and execute his operation in accordance with the conditions that exist. Thus, if a tumor is supposed to lie on the anterior aspect of the cord and more to one side, more of the laminæ on that side will have to be removed in order to gain the best access to the front of the spinal cord, and the number of vertebral arches to be at first removed will have to be larger, as it is probable that the cord will have to be dislocated in order to expose and remove the tumor.

If, on the other hand, the growth lies on the posterior aspect of the cord, the number of vertebral arches and the amount of each arch that is removed in the laminectomy may be reduced to the minimum.

LARYNGEAL PARALYSIS ASSOCIATED WITH THE JUGULAR FORAMEN SYNDROME AND OTHER SYNDROMES.*

By Gordon B. New, M.D.,

SECTION ON LARYNGOLOGY, ORAL AND PLASTIC SURGERY, MAYO CLINIC, ROCHESTER, MINNESOTA.

Complete unilateral paralysis of the recurrent laryngeal nerve is not uncommon and is usually due to aortic aneurysm, carcinoma of the esophagus, or pressure on the nerve from some type of neoplasm.

Jackson, in 1864, first described complete unilateral laryngeal paralysis associated with paralysis of the soft palate, tongue, trapezius and the sternocleidomastoid muscles. Since the lesion occurs in the region of the jugular foramen where the ninth, tenth, and eleventh cranial nerves leave the skull and the hypoglossal foramen, through which the hypoglossal nerve passes, the syndrome has been called the jugular foramen syndrome of Jackson. Jackson's original description does not contain details with regard to the involvement of the ninth cranial nerve, as shown by the change in the sensation of taste on the posterior part of the tongue and by involvement of the pharynx.

Mackenzie, in 1883, reported a patient with a syphilitic lesion of, or near the medulla causing paralysis of the soft palate, tongue, vocal cord, and the sternocleidomastoid and trapezius muscles. The patient did not respond to treatment for syphilis. He had constant headache and vomited occasionally. A swelling of nine

* Thesis submitted to American Laryngological Association, May, 1922.

months' duration involved the left side of the soft palate and the tonsil, and displaced the uvula to the right. It is possible that this patient had a nasopharyngeal tumor with secondary affection of the jugular foramen and intracranial involvement. Mackenzie, in discussing Jackson's case, at the Harvaine Society, in 1886, said that he had seen 8 patients with unilateral paralysis of the tongue, soft palate, and vocal cords.

Collet, in 1915, reported a case of what he called, "The total syndrome," in which the ninth, eleventh, and twelfth cranial nerves were affected. The patient was a soldier who had received a bullet wound in the right mastoid region. He complained of difficulty in swallowing, deafness, and noises in the ear. The roentgen-ray showed a shrapnel ball situated at the base of the skull. There was hemiplegia of the tongue, larynx, palate, and pharynx and of the sternocleidomastoid and trapezius muscles, and lack of perception of taste at the base of the tongue on the side involved.

Avellis, Schmidt, and Tapia have reported syndromes associated with laryngeal paralysis in which certain variations have occurred. Avellis reported paralysis of the tenth cranial nerve, Schmidt of the tenth and eleventh nerves, and Tapia of the eleventh and twelfth.

Lannois and Vernet reported 2 cases of war wounds; in 1 the bullet entered the malar region and in the other it entered the preauricular region. In both cases the ninth, tenth, eleventh, and twelfth nerves were affected, and in the second case the cervical sympathetic as well.

Lannois and Jouty reported a case of a soldier injured back of the angle of the jaw; the last four cranial nerves were affected. These authors found that 17 instances of the jugular foramen syndrome had been reported.

Vernet reported a case in which a soldier was injured by a shell fragment passing through the external auditory canal. Roentgenograms revealed the fragment in the prevertebral region. Besides the total syndrome the seventh nerve on the injured side was paralyzed by the wound.

Hall, in a consideration of the etiology of unilateral paralysis of the recurrent laryngeal nerve, collected 116 cases and found that in 10, besides the laryngeal paralysis, there was hemiplegia, paralysis of the face, palate, pharynx, and trapezius and sternocleidomastoid muscles.

Thomson, in an analysis of the 360 cases of unilateral paralysis of the larynx, found 1 in which symptoms were due to an extracranial growth close to the exit of the vagus.

Guder and Dufour reported 63 cases of unilateral paralysis of the recurrent laryngeal nerve, but none were associated with the jugular foramen syndrome.

Aloin reported a case of acute phlegmon of the pharynx and neck;

the patient developed paralysis of the soft palate, vocal cord and tongue with weakening of the shoulder muscles due to neuritis of the tenth, eleventh, and twelfth cranial nerves. He noted that involvement of the tenth nerve was shown by intense salivation, pulse 140, and difficulty in breathing not accounted for by any mechanical cause. Several months passed before the paralyzed muscles returned to normal.

Cauzard and Laignel-Levastine reported a syphilitic lesion of the right bulb with involvement of the fifth, seventh, ninth, tenth, eleventh and twelfth cranial nerves.

Beck and Hassin reported a case of tuberculosis of the cervical glands and secondary invasion of the ninth, tenth, eleventh, and twelfth nerves. The symptoms improved markedly following removal of the glands. The symptoms recurred, and a second operation was performed to free the nerve from the scar tissue.

Pollock reported a similar case in a man in whom the last four cranial nerves and cervical sympathetic nerves were affected owing to tuberculous adenitis. There was no change in pulse, respiration, secretion or sensation.

It is seen that many varieties of symptoms may result from involvement of the last four cranial nerves in the region of the jugular foramen.

Lannois and Bourcart reported the involvement of the cervical sympathetic nerve associated with laryngeal paralysis.

TABLE I.—SUMMARY OF CASES.

Case.	Age, sex	Duration.	Cause.	Primary nasopharyngeal tumor.	Secondary nasopharyngeal tumor.	Cranial nerves										Cervical sympathetic nerve.
						Second.	Third.	Fourth.			Seven h.		T	E ent.	T	
A81249	62 F.	3 years	Indeterminate, neoplasm (?)										+		+	
A165869	52 M.	8 years	Epithelioma	....	+			+	+	+	+	+ (?)		+		
A271166	47 M.	6 weeks	Neoplasm (lymphosarcoma?)	+ and pharynx					..			+ (?)	+		+	+
A285410	35 M.	2 years	Carcinoma (mixed tumor type)									+	+			+
A348444	43 F.	12 years	Neoplasm (mixed tumor type?)									+	+			+
A350568	54 F.	3 months	Neoplasm (lymphosarcoma?)	+			+	+	+	+				+	+	+ (larynx not involved).
A361632	40 F.	4 years	Neoplasm (mixed tumor type?)									+	+		+	

Vernet gives a complete table showing the effect of paralysis of the ninth, tenth, eleventh, and the twelfth cranial nerves. What he considers the internal branch of the eleventh nerve is usually classified in this country as part of the tenth. This, however, is a matter of nomenclature. The distribution of the ninth and tenth nerves, as seen in Table II, is not absolute. The affection of the cervical sympathetic nerve is shown by myosis, narrowing of the palpebral fissure, and enophthalmos.

TABLE II.—PARALYSIS OF THE LAST FOUR CRANIAL NERVES.

	Vernet.	Oppenheim..
Paralysis of the ninth	Paralysis of the superior constrictor of the pharynx (curtain movement of the posterior wall, disturbances in deglutition of solids). Disorders in taste, posterior one-third of tongue.	Loss of taste over the posterior part of the tongue. Difficulty in swallowing owing to paralysis of some of the pharyngeal muscles. Abolition of reflex excitability of the pharyngeal mucosa.
Paralysis of the tenth.	Disorders in sensibility of half of the soft palate, of the pharynx, of the larynx and of the auricular branch. Disorders of salivation. Coughing crises. Disorders of respiration (intermittent dyspnea and pseudo-asthma).	Unilateral paralysis of the palate, pharynx and larynx. Anesthesia of the pharynx, larynx and external auditory meatus, rarely found. Sometimes slowing, sometunes acceleration (irregularity) of breathing. Heart symptoms not constant, sometimes slowing but most often accelerated.
Paralysis of the eleventh internal branch.	Paralysis of half of the soft palate and larynx. Acceleration of the pulse.	Paralysis of the sternocleidomastoid and trapezius muscles.
Paralysis of the eleventh external branch.	Paralysis of the sternocleidomastoid and trapezius muscles.	
Paralysis of the twelfth.	Hemiparesis of the tongue.	Hemiparesis of the tongue.

Report of Seven Cases Observed in the Mayo Clinic. CASE I (A81249).—Mrs. T. J. D., aged sixty-two years, came to the Clinic, June 29, 1921. She had had two operations for exophthalmic goiter, February 3, 1914, and January 6, 1915, respectively. For the last two or three years she had noticed shrinking and weakness of the right side of the tongue. The last nine months she had had hoarseness, and breaking of the voice, difficulty in swallowing, regurgitation of food, breathlessness on exertion, and pronounced tachycardia and palpitation. She had had pain in the left arm for three or four months.

Examination revealed the middle line of the palate displaced to the left, and partial paralysis of the right side of the palate. The right side of the tongue was atrophied and protruded to the right. The right vocal cord was fixed in the intermediate or cadaveric position. No pathological changes were demonstrable in the nasopharynx, nor was change in sensation demonstrable in the pharynx or larynx. The right sternocleidomastoid and trapezius muscles were partially paralyzed and atrophied.

Summary. In this case the tenth, eleventh, and twelfth nerves on the right side were affected partially. The etiological factor was questionable but the condition was probably due to a neoplasm in the region of the jugular foramen.

Case II (A165869).—Mr. H. N., aged fifty-two years, came to the Clinic, July 13, 1921, because of recurring epithelioma of the right cheek. He had had syphilis thirty years before. When a child he had been injured on the right cheek at the site of the present lesion. The area had remained discolored until twelve years before when a sore had developed. In 1918, this area was plastered by a cancer quack and, in 1920, it was excised. Roentgen-ray treatments had been carried out four months before; the cheek had been cauterized and medicinal treatment given by the local physician one week before.

Examination showed a recently cauterized opening in the right cheek just below the malar bone, 3.75 cm. in diameter and 2.5 cm. deep. A specimen removed from the margin revealed basal-cell epithelioma. The Wassermann reaction was strongly positive, amounting to total inhibition.

July 20, 1916, the area on the right cheek was thoroughly cauterized with soldering irons and treatment for syphilis instituted.

The patient returned June 6, 1919, complaining of diplopia and pain over the right side of the head. Examination showed paralysis of the right external rectus muscle and involvement of the fifth nerve. August 8, 1919, almost complete paralysis of the right fourth, fifth, and sixth nerves had developed.

February 24, 1921, the patient returned and requested a plastic closure of the opening in the right cheek, about 5 cm. in diameter, which connected the nose, the antrum, and the mouth. Since our last examination, August 1919, two operations had been done elsewhere, one, fifteen months before, and one, twelve months before. The right eye had been removed with the orbital growth and a plastic operation attempted. Examination then showed a recurring basal-cell epithelioma at the right margin of the orbit. The left eye was normal, the fundus negative, and vision 6/6. There was a definite fulness in the right nasopharynx. The small recurrent growth was removed and treatment for syphilis was given.

December 27, 1921, the patient returned complaining of pain on the right side of the head, hoarseness, and difficulty in swallowing. The right side of the soft palate and pharynx was paralyzed and the right cord was fixed in a cadaveric position. There was diminished sensation over the right side of the pharynx and a collection of mucus in the hypopharynx. There was paralysis of the right sternocleidomastoid and trapezius muscles. The right nasopharynx was filled with a sloughing area, malignant in appearance. The patient was deaf in the right ear owing to involvement of the nasopharynx. There was complete facial paralysis on the right with areas of anesthesia on the affected side.

Roentgenograms of the skull were negative; examination of the left fundus was negative. The pulse was 88, and there was no respiratory trouble. Examination showed involvement of the fifth, seventh, ninth, tenth, eleventh, and twelfth cranial nerves.

Summary. The right third, fourth, fifth, sixth, seventh, ninth (?), tenth, eleventh, and twelfth cranial nerves were affected owing to direct extension from an epithelioma of the cheek to the region of the jugular foramen and possible extension intracranially.

Case III (A281166). Mr. M. F. M., aged forty-seven years, came to the Clinic, February 2, 1921. Six weeks before, the patient had had pain over the right mastoid region and had noticed something wrong with his throat which seemed sore. His home physician had lanced it, expecting to find an abscess, but no pus was found. Pain in the right ear had been accompanied by slight deafness. The patient had been unable to swallow for a week, as fluids strangled him and regurgitated into his nose. He had lost 17 pounds in the last six weeks.

Examination showed drooping of the right upper eyelid and a small right pupil. A non-ulcerating mass in the right side of the nasopharynx extended into the pharynx and partially into the hypopharynx. Metastatic glands were present at the right angle of the jaw. The muscles on the right side of the palate were paralyzed. There was a great deal of mucus in the right pyriform fossa and the right cord was fixed in the intermediate or cadaveric position. The right side of the larynx was somewhat insensitive and paralysis of the muscles of the right side of the pharynx and of the sternocleidomastoid and trapezius muscles was noted. The tongue protruded to the right. There were no respiratory or cardiac disorders. The ninth, tenth, eleventh, and twelfth nerves were affected by the nasopharyngeal and the pharyngeal tumor.

Summary. This patient presented a rapidly growing tumor, probably lymphosarcoma, of the right nasopharynx and pharynx, and affecting the ninth (?), tenth, eleventh, and twelfth nerves and the cervical sympathetic nerve.

Case IV (A285410).—Mr. A. W., aged thirty-five years, came to the Clinic, August 29, 1919, on account of roaring and pain in the right ear of two years' duration. A year before he had become deaf. Since then he had had attacks of sharp pains in the right ear which had lasted only a few minutes. There was no discharge from the ear, but about one year ago a small tumor had appeared below it. The patient's general health was good.

Examination revealed a small, rounded, pedunculated tumor on the floor of the right auditory canal, 1.5 mm. in diameter, and a tumor in the right parotid region just posterior to the ascending ramus of the jaw, which was about 3.75 cm. in diameter and "felt" malignant. The tumor in the auditory canal was removed, but malignancy was not demonstrable microscopically. The ear drum was normal. A roentgenogram of the skull was negative and the neurological examination afforded nothing of note. September 3, 1919, the mass in the parotid region was explored by Dr. Sistrunk, but the tissue removed did not show malignancy.

The patient returned October 21, 1920, complaining of loss in weight, hoarseness, and difficulty in swallowing of eight weeks' duration. He had pain lasting for a few minutes at a time in the right shoulder and right side of the neck. The right cord was fixed in the cadaveric position with a collection of mucus in the pyriform fossa. Paralysis of the soft palate, pharynx, and vocal cord was complete on the right side. Neither edema nor neoplasm was visible. The tumor below the right ear in the parotid region was still present. The sternocleidomastoid and trapezius muscles were partially paralyzed.

The ninth, tenth, eleventh, and twelfth cranial nerves were affected, due to a tumor arising in the right parotid region and extending to the jugular foramen.

November 13, 1920, Dr. Adson explored the area and found a carcinoma of the mixed-tumor type, 3 cm. in diameter and 17.5 cm. in length, situated in the region of the jugular foramen outside of the skull with some extension into the cranial cavity through the foramen. The tumor was removed. The patient recovered uneventfully, but with no change in the nerve, as had been expected.

Summary. In this case the tumor was a carcinoma of the mixed-tumor type in the right parotid region. The carcinoma involved the jugular foramen extracranially, and the ninth, tenth, eleventh, and twelfth cranial nerves.

Case V (A348444).—Mrs. W. B., aged forty-two years, came to the Clinic, February 3, 1921. She complained of weakness, hoarseness, choking sensation, and drooping of the right eyelid of about two years' duration. When swallowing, she had noticed a choking sensation in the throat, and coughing had brought food back into her mouth. Sixteen months before, she had noticed that the right side of her tongue was thick and stiff. When eating she had perspired freely over the right side of the face and scalp so that drops of water fell to her shoulder. Her heart had palpitated at times and she had become dyspneic when climbing stairs. She had lost 32 pounds in weight, 10 during the last month.

Examination revealed a very slight ptosis of the right upper eyelid; the right pupil was myotic. Vision was normal. Examination of the nasopharynx was negative. The right half of the tongue, the right side of the soft palate, and all of the pharyngeal muscles were paralyzed and atrophied. The right vocal cord was fixed in an intermediate position. There was marked anesthesia over the soft palate, the right pharynx, and the larynx. The sternocleidomastoid and trapezius muscles were not paralyzed. A firm mass 3.5 cm. in diameter was found between the right angle of the jaw and the mastoid process. Examination of the heart revealed a loud systolic murmur, heard best at the apex and transmitted to the axilla. Anemia was marked. The hemoglobin was 30 per cent, the erythrocytes numbered 3,170,000 and the lenkocytes 5800. The color index was 0.4; polynuclear neutrophils, 67.5; small lymphocytes, 27.5; large lymphocytes, 4.5; basophils, 0.5; anisocytosis and poikilocytosis were slight.

Summary. This case illustrates involvement of the ninth, tenth, and twelfth cranial nerves and possibly partial involvement of the cervical sympathetic nerve by a mixed tumor in the region of of the jugular foramen.

Case VI (A350568).—Mrs. F. O. B., aged fifty-four years, came to the Clinic, February 25, 1921. Three months before, she had noticed pain above and behind the right eye and deafness in the right ear. Two months before, she had had difficulty in opening the mouth wide, a swelling had appeared on the right side of the face, and the right nostril had become obstructed. Three weeks before, the corner of the mouth and the upper eyelid on the right side had begun to droop. Two weeks before, she had noticed that she could not move the right eye; it became more prominent, and blindness developed gradually.

The general examination showed nothing of note. Examination of the eyes revealed a proptosis of the right with drooping of the upper eyelid, complete ophthalmoplegia, and blurring of the disc. Pupillary reflexes were absent; the right pupil was dilated. Vision of the right eye was 0, of the left 6/4. There was bulging of the right temporal region. A tumor, ulcerated and bulging to the middle line, filled the right side of the nasopharynx. The Eustachian tube could not be seen. The right side of the palate and pharynx was paralyzed. The tongue deviated to the right. There was no laryngeal paralysis. Sensation was decreased over the right cheek, the forehead and chin, and the action of the muscles of mastication was impaired. The trapezius and the sternocleidomastoid muscles were not paralyzed. Deafness was complete in the right ear.

Summary. This case illustrates involvement of the third, fourth, fifth, sixth, ninth, tenth, and twelfth cranial nerves and probably the cervical sympathetic nerve by a rapidly growing nasopharyngeal tumor, probably lymphosarcoma. The deafness was owing to encroachment of the tumor on the Eustachian tube.

Case VII (A361362).—Mrs. G. L., aged forty years, came to the Clinic, June 15, 1921. Seven years before, following childbirth, the patient had noticed difficulty in swallowing. Three years later, she had become suddenly hoarse; this persisted. She had not coughed, but in swallowing she had difficulty in keeping food from falling into the windpipe or passing into the nose. Six years before, she had noticed gradual wasting and weakening of the right shoulder and arm which had continued to ache since the onset of the trouble. The tonsils and many teeth had been removed without relief. She had had headache over the right occipital region often. The right side of her tongue had felt thick and at times she had difficulty in speaking.

Examination of the right side of the tongue revealed paralysis and atrophy. The right side of the palate, pharynx, and larynx was paralyzed, and the right trapezius and sternocleidomastoid muscles were atrophied. The right vocal cord was in the intermediate position. There was a collection of food in the right hypopharynx. Roentgen-ray examinations of the head and of the cervical spine were negative; examination of the eyes and the Wassermann reaction on the blood were negative.

Summary. This case illustrates involvement of the ninth, tenth, eleventh, and twelfth cranial nerves on the right side, probably owing to a mixed tumor in the region of the jugular foramen.

Discussion. In 6 of the 7 cases in the series there was unilateral complete laryngeal paralysis associated with the jugular foramen syndrome or other syndromes, and in 1 case (Case VI), there was paralysis of the right side of the palate and pharynx, and involvement of the second, third, fourth, fifth, sixth, eleventh, and twelfth cranial nerves and of the cervical sympathetic nerve, without laryngeal paralysis. In all the cases in which the larynx was paralyzed the vocal cord was in the intermediate or cadaveric position and not in the middle position usually taken by it after an injury to the recurrent laryngeal nerve.

Cases II and VI are unusual on account of the extent of the involvement of the nerves. In Case II the third, fourth, and sixth nerves were probably affected in the orbit owing to extension of the epithelioma. The fifth and seventh nerves were probably affected intracranially, and the ninth, tenth, eleventh, and twelfth nerves by direct extension of the tumor to the region of the jugular foramen. The patient was deaf on the side involved because of encroachment on the Eustachian tube in the nasopharynx. In

Case VI a nasopharyngeal tumor affected the second, third, fourth, fifth and sixth nerves, probably intracranially, and the ninth, tenth, eleventh and twelfth, and the cervical sympathetic nerves in the region of the jugular foramen.

The cervical sympathetic nerve was affected in 4 cases as shown by myosis and narrowing of the palpebral fissure.

In a review of the entire group several points of interest may be noted. In all of the cases, except possibly Case I, involvement of the nerves was due to neoplasm in the region of the jugular foramen, and even in this case such involvement is the most probable cause, although it is possible the medulla was affected.

In 6 cases the nerve involvement was caused by a tumor. In 4 of these cases the tumor was slow-growing and of a low grade of malignancy; the duration of symptoms ranged from two to twelve years. One lesion of the series was microscopically proved to be carcinoma of the mixed-tumor type. Two growths were clinically mixed tumors and 1 a recurring basal-cell epithelioma. In 2 of the 6 cases the pathological lesion was a rapidly growing tumor, probably a lymphosarcoma, the symptoms of which were present from three to six months only. In these cases the tumor originated in the nasopharynx and pharynx.

The age of the patients was from thirty-five to sixty-two years and the duration of the symptoms from six to twelve years. The males and females were about equally affected.

Definite cardiac or respiratory disorders did not occur, except in Cases I and V. The patient in Case I complained of palpitation and dyspnea on exertion; but she had been operated on for toxic goiter. In Case V the patient complained of pounding of the heart and dyspnea when climbing stairs. Examination of the heart showed loud systolic murmurs at the apex, transmitted to the axilla.

In examining the patients it was noted that those with paralysis of half of the tongue had trouble in swallowing liquids, an act effected by means of pressing the tongue against the hard palate. Paralysis of the palate caused food to become lodged back of the nose. Paralysis of the muscles of the pharynx interfered with the swallowing of solids.

In some of the 7 cases in the series it was difficult to determine definitely the degree of involvement of the ninth and tenth nerves, but this is because of our vague understanding of the anatomy and physiology of this region.

Summary. It may be seen from a review of the cases in the literature and of my group of cases that laryngeal paralysis associated with a syndrome due to involvement of the last four cranial nerves and the cervical sympathetic nerve in the region of the jugular foramen is quite unusual. When this occurs it is usually owing to a neoplasm, although a tuberculous process in the glands of the neck or an acute phlegmon may be the cause. During the World War cases were reported due to bullet or shrapnel wounds. The vocal cord is in the intermediate or cadaveric position in vagus involvement.

BIBLIOGRAPHY.

1. Aloin, H.: Phlegmon latéropharyngien avec névrite des trois derniers nerfs crâniens (syndrome de Jackson), Paris méd., 1918, **29**, 209.

2. Avellis, G.: Klinische Beiträge zur halbseitigen Kehlkopflähmung, Berl. klinik., 1891, **40**, 1.

3. Avellis, G.: Die Frage der motorischen Kehlkopfinnervation, analysirt nach einem neuen Falle von traumatischer Zungen-, Gaumen-, Kehlkopf- und Nackenlahmung und den neuesten Arbeiten der Gehirnanatomie, Arch. f. Laryngol. u. Rhinol. 1900, **10**, 1.

4. Beck, J. C. and Hassin, G. B.: A Case of Combined Extracranial Paralysis of Cerebral Nerves, Med. Rec., 1915, **88**, 308.

5. Cauzard, P. and Laignel-Levastine: Paralysie du récurrent d'origine bulbaire. Bull. de laryngol., otol. et rhinol., 1904, **7**, 274.

6. Collet, M : Sur un nouveau syndrome paralytique pharyngolaryngé par blessure de guerre (hémiplégie glosso-laryngo-scapulopharyngée), Lyon méd., 1915, **125**, 121.

7. Guder and Dufour: Discussion on Unilateral Paralysis, Proc. Roy. Soc. Med., Laryngol. Sect., 1913, **6**, 152.

8. Hall, F.de H., Ferrier, D. and Permewan, W.: Discussion on the Etiology of Unilateral Paralysis of the Recurrent Laryngeal Nerve, Proc. Roy. Soc. Med., Laryngol. Sect., 1913, **6**, 139.

9. Jackson, J. H.: Quoted by Mackenzie.

10. Jackson, J. H.: Paralysis of Tongue, Palate, and Vocal Cord, Lancet, 1886, **1**, 689.

11. Jackson, J. H.: A Case of Hemianopsia, and of Wasting and Paralysis on One Side of the Tongue in a Syphilitic Patient, Brit. Med. Jour., 1887, **1**, 729.

12. Lannois and Jouty: Un cas d'hémiplégie des quatre derniers nerfs crâniens, Lyon méd., 1917, **126**, 424.

13. Lannois, Sargnon and Vernet: Sur le "Syndrome total" des quatre derniers nerfs crâniens (deux observations nouvelles de blessés de guerre), Rev. neurol., 1916, **23**, 943.

14. Lannois and Boucart: Un nouveau cas de paralysies multiples des nerfs crâniens, Lyon méd., 1917, **126**, 41.

15. Mackenzie, S.: Case of Intracranial Disease Involving the Medulla Oblongata, Brit. Med. Jour., 1883, **1**, 408.

16. Oppenheim, H.: Diseases of the Nervous System, Philadelphia, Lippincott, 1900, pp. 899.

17. Pollock, L.: A Case of Multiple Cranial Nerve Palsy Due to Extracranial Disease, Jour. Am. Med. Assn., 1922, **78**, 502.

18. Schmidt, M.: Die Krankheiten der oberen Luftwege, Berlin, Springer, 1897, pp. 883.

19. Tapia: Un nouveau syndrome; quelques cas d'hémiplégie du larynx et de la langue avec ou sans paralysie du sterno-cléidomastoidien et du trapèze, Arch. internat. de laryngol., 1906, **22**, 780.

20. Thomson, St. C.: Discussion on Unilateral Paralysis, Proc. Roy. Soc. Med., Laryngol. Sect., 1913, **6**, 150.

21. Vernet, M.: Sur le syndrome des quatre dernières paires crâniennes, d'après une observation personnelle chez un blessé de guerre, Bull. et mém. Soc. méd. d. hôp. de Par., 1916, **40**, 3.s., 210.

22. Vernet, M.: The Classification of the Syndromes of Associated Laryngeal Paralysis, Jour. Laryngol., Rhinol., and Otol., 1918, **33**, 354.

THE PATHOLOGY OF NODULAR (ADENOMATOUS?) GOITERS IN PATIENTS WITH AND IN THOSE WITHOUT SYMPTOMS OF HYPERTHYROIDISM.*

By Louis B. Wilson, M.D.,
ROCHESTER, MINN.

The pathologic changes met with in the thyroid in true exophthalmic goiter are now well agreed on. Briefly, the disease as indicated in the changes in the thyroid may be divided into three general stages:

1. Early exophthalmic goiter, with moderate increase in basal metabolism and usually moderate exophthalmos. In this condition there is moderate thyroid enlargement. The parenchymal cells show marked hypertrophy and moderate hyperplasia. There is diffuse hyperemia throughout the gland.

2. Advanced exophthalmic goiter with high metabolic rate, usually marked exophthalmos and a well-marked nervous syndrome. There is usually marked thyroid enlargement. There is advanced parenchymal cell hypertrophy and hyperplasia. There is little if any stored colloid. There is diffuse hyperemia throughout the gland.

3. Late exophthalmic goiter with high but sometimes declining metabolic rate, exophthalmos and a well-marked nervous syndrome. Pathologically the changes in the gland are similar to those in the earlier stages of exophthalmic goiter but with beginning or well-marked storage of colloid. Many follicles containing colloid are lined with flattened parenchymal cells. In some instances newly developed follicles are numerous. Hyperemia is usually materially less than in glands in the previous groups.

The parenchymal changes in the thyroid in true exophthalmic goiter are almost always diffuse and, therefore, the gland is rarely nodular in its gross appearance.

As pointed out by H. S. Plummer, related to, but clinically distinct from, exophthalmic goiter is a large group of patients with symptoms usually of slow development or, if rapidly developing, only after a long period of non-symptomatic thyroid enlargement, with basal metabolism increased as much as in exophthalmic goiter but usually with no ocular symptoms, and without the nervous syndrome peculiar to exophthalmic goiter. This type of hyperthyroidism is so often associated with nodular thyroids that Plummer tentatively designated the disease first "toxic non-hyperplastic goiter," then "toxic adenoma" and now "hyperfunctioning adenoma."

* Presented before the Association of American Physicians, Washington, D. C., May 2, 1922.

Before the routine determination of basal metabolic rates was established in the Mayo Clinic it was difficult to select groups of patients representing on the one hand well-marked stages of this syndrome and on the other, patients entirely free from the symptoms. Since 1908, I have made several attempts at a comparison of specimens from groups of such cases selected on a clinical basis only, but previously I have never been able to determine any marked general difference between groups of thyroids from the two types of cases. This was due in part to the necessary shifting of the group as it was being clinically differentiated, and in part to the failure first to compare thyroids from patients with extreme symptoms with those from patients without symptoms. During the last year, however, I have been able to study two groups at the extremes of the metabolic series selected in chronologic order of occurrence by Dr. Boothby.

Group A. Patients with enlarged nodular thyroids, with symptoms of hyperthyroidism but without exophthalmos, without the nervous syndrome peculiar to exophthalmic goiter, and with basal metabolic rates of 20 or more points above normal.

Group B. Patients of approximately the same age with enlarged nodular thyroids, without symptoms of hyperthyroidism and with basal metabolic rates within 10 points of normal.

I have studied the thyroids from about 250 patients in each series, or a total of over 500 thyroids.

The specimens were all placed in 10 per cent formalin within a few minutes after their removal and, after complete fixation, sectioned by freezing and stained with hematoxylin and eosin. Some of them were also imbedded in paraffin and the sections stained by other methods. Every effort was made to adhere to parallel processes throughout the technic of preparing the sections. The cases were numbered chronologically and the two series placed in separate trays beside each other for convenience in comparison. This work was done for me by Dr. C. W. Barrier, of the Mayo Foundation, in the course of a piece of research on the thyroid he was carrying on for himself.

The examination of the first twenty specimens, that is, ten from each series, showed such a marked difference between the two series that I immediately took the specimens numbered 51 to 60, 101 to 110, 151 to 160, 201 to 210, and so forth from each series and carefully compared them. The results in these widely separated decimal groups were so parallel with those in the first ten that I was satisfied no error of technic could explain the findings. I therefore went back and studied more leisurely all the specimens in each series, comparing each number not only with the corresponding number in the other series but also with many others. The results of this examination are as follows:

1. About 90 per cent of all thyroids in Group A show in one or

more of the areas from which sections were examined distinct evidence of increased activity of the parenchymal cells. This is indicated by moderate degrees of cell hypertrophy and hyperplasia associated usually with some colloid storage. In many there are areas in which the follicles are closely packed with dense colloid, but there are also many areas showing follicles containing little or no colloid, and lined with hypertrophic parenchymal cells. Where colloid is present it has a distinctly lighter staining reaction than that in thyroids in Group B. In many instances there is considerable parenchymal cell hyperplasia.

Grossly many of the glands are (*a*) diffuse colloid goiters without any evidence of new follicle formation, but whose nodular character is the result of increased and contracting interlobular connective tissue usually associated with round-cell infiltration indicating chronic inflammation; or (*b*) colloid goiters with definite new follicle formation but without definite capsule formation, (adenomatosis) with many of the new follicles lined with parenchymal cells of functioning type which are hypertrophic, or (*c*) definitely encapsulated areas of new follicle formation (adenomas) with hypertrophic and often hyperplastic parenchymal cells lining follicles which contain little or no stored colloid. All of these hypertrophic and hyperplastic changes are so moderate in degree and in amount as readily to escape notice except by careful comparison of a large number of thyroids from patients with high metabolic rates side by side with a like number of thryoids from patients exhibiting no increase in basal metabolic rate.

In comparing the changes in the thyroids in Group A with the changes in the thyroids in a series of typical exophthalmic goiter cases it is found that in general the difference is not only one of degree but in most instances also of kind. The most advanced parenchymal cell hypertrophy and hyperplasia found in any case in Group A, is about the equal of the more moderate degrees of parenchymal cell hypertrophy and hyperplasia in thyroids from the true exophthalmic goiter series; but in most of the thyroids in Group A the histologic picture shows that there has been marked colloid storage in most of the follicles and that now the stored colloid is apparently being taken up by the parenchymal cells and passed into the circulation. The parenchymal cells are apparently not, under high functional pressure, discharging their secretion directly into the vessels as is the case in exophthalmic goiter, but are first storing it in the follicles. A very common picture in these specimens is the presence in one portion of a large follicle, most of which is filled with dense stored colloid, of small areas of very lightly staining colloid in immediate opposition to hypertrophic or hyperplastic parenchymal cells, while the parenchymal cells lining other portions of the follicle are flattened and atrophic. The chief departure from this picture in thyroids in Group A is in those instances in which there is very marked formation of new follicles. These, in definitely encapsulated "adenomas," may contain dense stored colloid. Where there is diffuse new follicle formation without definite encapsulation the follicles are not likely to contain colloid, or if any, it is feebly staining. The number of the former type of glands is, however, much greater than of the latter. From the pathologic evidence alone we are not warranted in concluding that the formation of new follicles is the essential factor in the production of hyperthyroid symptoms, since in almost all glands, even in which this is the predominating picture, there are to be found as well many areas which indicate absorption of colloid by reactivated parenchymal cells.

About 95 per cent of the thyroids in Group B, that is from patients with nodular goiters with the clinical diagnosis of adenoma without increased basal metabolic rates or other symptoms of hyperthyroidism, showed in none of the sections from any of the areas examined evidence of even moderate degrees of cell hypertrophy and hyperplasia. The parenchymal cells in follicles of adult type were uniformly flattened or atrophic. In most follicles in adenomas they were of very undeveloped embryonic type. The intra-follicular colloid stained much more densely than that in thyroids in Group A. Grossly the thyroids from these patients could readily be divided for the most part into three groups closely paralleling those of glands from the hyperthyroid series. A few of the specimens consisted of proliferating adenomas, Langhans wuchernde Struma. It should be noted that the patients from whom these thyroids were removed had been grouped clinically on the basis of nodular goiters. Had the marked nodular character of the thyroids not been recognized clinically no doubt some thyroids would have been found in which the colloid was evenly distributed throughout all the follicles which were lined with flattened or atrophic parenchymal cells, and their interlobular bands of connective tissue would not have been found to be abnormally increased or contracted.

Owing to the work of Boothby and others we may now safely assume that in thyroid disturbances the basal metabolic rate is a true index of the degree of hypothyroidism and hyperthyroidism. It follows then that the high incidence of moderate parenchymatous cell hypertrophy and hyperplasia in thyroids from the patients in Group A and its absence from almost all thyroids of patients in Group B can be rationally explained on the basis of a causative relationship. That is, the hypertrophic and hyperplastic parenchymal cells in Group A are apparently secreting a substance which is probably responsible for the symptoms and the increased metabolie rate, and on the other hand no substance in sufficiently large amounts to excite symptoms or increase the metabolic rate apparently is being secreted by the parenchymal cells in the follicles of the thyroids of Group B. No doubt some of the instances of non-conformity in Group A and also those in Group B may be explained by technical errors, for example: Failure thoroughly to search sufficiently numerous areas in the glands for evidence of increased cell activity. It would seem reasonable to assume, however, that the finding of moderate degrees of cell hypertrophy and hyperplasia in about 5 per cent of the thyroids in Group B may be explained by the supposition that not enough increase in cell activity had occurred to induce symptoms of hyperthyroidism or to increase the metabolic rate.

It is a very inviting hypothesis that the symptoms of non-exophthalmic hyperthyroidism are caused by the adsorption of complete thyroxin in previously stored colloid which is being manufactured more rapidly than in the normal gland but much more slowly than in the thyroid of exophthalmic goiter. This hypothesis receives support from the facts that the symptoms produced by the administration of thyroxin in large doses to human beings are essentially those of non-exophthalmic hyperthyroidism, that stored colloid does contain thyroxin and that the histologic picture indicates that colloid is being transferred from the follicles to the circulation.

On the other hand we might go a step further and speculate on the probability that true exophthalmic goiter is caused by an incompletely elaborated thyroid secretion, an antecedent of thyroxin but not with its normal quota of its atoms of iodine in the molecule, for example. Such a hypothesis would harmonize many of the clinical and pathologic findings. However, an equally alluring hypothesis is that in true exophthalmic goiter the primary onset of the disease is in the nervous system and that the more significant thyroid hyperfunction is nevertheless a secondary development.

THE CLINICAL CRITERIA OF ACTIVITY IN PULMONARY TUBERCULOSIS.*

By Paul H. Ringer, A.B., M.D.,
Asheville, N. C.

Every physician having to do with the diagnosis and treatment of pulmonary tuberculosis is asked by his patients whether they have *any* activity, *more* activity, or *less* activity. To these questions an answer must be given, as in that answer is contained that which is most important to the patient, his improvement or the

* Read (by invitation) before the Medical Association of the State of Alabama at its Meeting in Birmingham, April 18–21, 1922.

reverse. Conflicting statements are not infrequently made to patients by competent examiners at periods so close one to another that a change in pulmonary conditions is out of the question. There is evidently a difference in the conception of activity on the part of many well qualified men, and there is also evidently a lack of standardization with regard to what actually constitutes the existence of activity.

First of all activity must be defined. This is not so easy. "Infection greater than resistance." "Evidence of poisoning, local and general, by the toxins of the tubercle bacillus." "Onward progress of the tuberculous process." "The picture presented and the physical signs elicited as a result of intoxication with the poisons of the bacillus of tuberculosis." "Tuberculous disease as opposed to tuberculous infection." These are a few of the definitions that present themselves.

There are, broadly speaking, five bases for the estimation of the presence of activity. These are:

1. Palpatory.
2. Radiological.
3. Auscultatory.
    - Rales.
        - Dry.
        - Moist.
4. Laboratory methods.
    - Bacilli in sputum.
    - Arneth's differential leukocyte count.
    - Complement-fixation.
5. Symptomatic.

1. *Palpatory.* The palpatory estimation of activity has found but little favor at the hands of the profession as a whole, though its few adherents are enthusiastic as to its value. Pottenger who has lauded it most highly, claims that by the rigidity of the muscles overlying the lungs which can be appreciated by the palpating fingers, the site of the lesion can be accurately determined, and moreover, that by the intensity of this rigidity the grade of activity can be estimated. Such a highly developed palpatory sense is vouchsafed to few, and just as to the man doing but little lung work, percussion is not as a rule of much aid, so to the majority of workers in tuberculosis the palpatory determination of activity has remained a sealed book.

2. *Radiological.* In the past decade the routine use of stereoscopic roentgen-ray plates in chest diagnosis and study has opened a tremendous field for good and also for confusion. There is at present between the radiologist and the clinician much dispute as to the true significance of the picture. The radiologist with his greater mechanical and technical knowledge, often avers that he has discovered evidences of pulmonary activity where the clinician,

fortified by his general knowledge of the patient and by his physical examination, feels that such activity does not exist. Many patients have been declared actively tuberculous by the radiologist in whom the subsequent evolution of their condition showed them to be at most subjects of tuberculous infection and not victims of tuberculous disease. The roentgen-ray as the sole evidence of tuberculous activity should not be relied upon. As an adjuvant, and as a corroborator of other pathological evidences or of merely suggestive symptoms, it is in the very forefront of diagnostic aids. The roentgen-rays will almost invariably shame the examiners' fingers and ears, but comfort can be derived from the fact that the plate may be said to present a pathological picture, while the other methods of physical examination may be said to present a clinical picture. How often in the absence of any detectable change in the breath sounds and in the absence of any adventitious sounds will the plate show not alone peribronchial thickening but also cotton-ball shadows of various sizes! These latter we know usually betoken the coalescence of tubercles with consequent softening, and indicate active disease. If other evidences of activity are at hand, we must unquestionably accept these radiological signs as evidences of active trouble; if, on the other hand, all other evidences are wanting, we must be cautious in discarding these shadows as unimportant, and while perhaps not coming out openly and saying that no activity exists, we must keep the patient under careful supervision for many weeks until certainty of judgment can be reached.

3. *Auscultatory.* The appreciation of the presence of activity by auscultation is the method of examination at present most relied upon, and that which, in the long run, will be of the greatest service to the greatest number of physicians. Valuable it is indeed, and yet the interpretation of the auscultatory signs is so varied that differences of opinion are often forthcoming even between men widely recognized as experts. Estimation of activity by auscultation should be restricted to the presence, location and character of rales, and should not be concerned with the breath sounds. Rales are in themselves a great stumbling block. Much depends upon their location and their character, it being really superfluous to repeat that basal rales are of infinitely less importance than apical rales. This observation would indeed not have been made had it not been for an experience of the writer while in the service, when requested by the head of the tuberculosis board at one of the camps to go over six men that had been slated for an S. C. D. (Surgeon's Certificate of Disability), to find the only abnormality to be a few fine marginal rales at both pulmonary bases. These signs and these alone were the evidence upon which discharge from the service had been deemed wise. The moist rale has ever been the one that is held to betoken activity. It matters not whether it be a fine or a coarse moist rale. Well and good as far as it goes, but it is by no means always easy even for men of large experience to distinguish

between a moist and a dry rale. To be sure, extremes of either variety can easily be recognized, but in the appreciation of the borderline sounds the personal equation plays such a part that an absolute standard is not obtainable. None the less, it is an indisputable fact that moist rales, not sibilations or large ronchi, but true moist rales, denote an active process. The pleuritic friction, when accompanied by other evidences of illness, is also a physical sign of paramount importance.

4. *Laboratory Methods*. Tubercle bacilli in the sputum, while diagnostically the one positive proof of pulmonary tuberculosis, have been held by some to be an evidence of activity. This has never impressed the writer as being a tenable position. Tubercle bacilli in the sputum merely indicate the presence of an ulcerated tuberculous process in the lung, through which the bacilli are enabled to reach the bronchial tree. To be sure, if 100 patients with positive sputum be compared with 100 patients with negative sputum, the majority of actively ill individuals will be found in the positive group; but all men doing lung work see not infrequently patients with a quiescent lesion doing a full day's work right along, and having a teaspoonful of sputum per day, even per week, in which tubercle bacilli are constantly to be found. If such individuals are to be classed as "active" cases, they have at any rate achieved an "economic recovery" which is the great goal of all the tuberculous, and the question of "activity" becomes one of merely academic interest.

The Arneth differential leukocytic count, simple to make, has had numerous followers. The count is a differential one of the polymorphonuclear neutrophiles based upon the number of nuclear lobes that they possess, namely whether 1, 2, 3, 4, or 5. Arneth claims that in active cases the preponderance of the cells are found to have one or two lobes, whereas in inactive or negative cases the majority have three, four or five lobes. Thus in active cases there results a "shift to the left" (Verschiebung nach links) of the dominating percentages, classes 1 and 2 being naturally to the left of the percentage table as it is recorded on the paper. Several years ago my associate, Dr. C. L. Minor,[1] and myself[2] did fairly extensive work with this method, studying some 475 cases with a total of almost 800 counts. An initial enthusiasm for the method gradually waned with increasing experience, and a final conclusion was reached that, while generally corroborative, the method was too unreliable to secure for itself a place among the true criteria of activity.

The complement-fixation test, while it has had some supporters, is not to be compared in reliability to its kinsman the Wassermann

[1] Arneth's Method of Blood Counting—Its Prognostic Value in Pulmonary Tuberculosis, AM. JOUR. MED. SCI., 1911, **141**, 638.

[2] Ringer, P. H.: A Further Study of the Prognostic Value of Arneth's Leukocytic Blood Picture in Pulmonary Tuberculosis Based upon 729 Counts in 475 Patients, AM. JOUR. MED. SCI., 1912, **144**, 561.

reaction, and has hardly stood the acid test as a criterion of activity in tuberculosis.

5. *Symptomatic.* The realm of symptomatology, in the writer's opinion, is that furnishing the most valuable evidences of tuberculous activity. In our routine and periodic examination of patients, while all possible care is taken to keep track of both extent and character of adventitious sounds and of variations in the stereoscopic picture, the opinion given to the patient as to improvement or the reverse (in other words as to lessened or increased activity), is based mainly upon the contents of the column labelled "Symptoms" on the examination chart. A patient whose temperature is lessening, whose pulse is slowing, whose appetite and sleep are growing better, whose weight is going up, must be and is improving even though cough and sputum may be practically unaffected and physical signs stationary. It is rare to find marked lessening of cough and especially of sputum in the absence of some change for the better in the physical signs, but even if this change is not demonstrable, a betterment in symptoms justifies a frank expression of opinion to the effect that activity is on the wane. Changes in physical signs are not of such prime importance as they were once conceived to be. As an example of this may be quoted the interesting statistical study made by Dr. Francis B. Trudeau[3] of a total of 979 cases discharged from the Trudeau Sanatorium with special reference to the physical signs.

RESULTS OF 979 CASES AT TRUDEAU SANATORIUM.

	No.	Per cent.	Per cent well.	Per cent living.	Per cent dead	Per cent unknown.
Increase in physical signs . .	422	43.1	52 9	14.7	31.0	1.4
Decrease in physical signs .	398	40.6	69 8	12.8	15 8	1.5
No change in physical signs .	159	16.3	78 0	10.7	10 1	1.2

This study shows of course that in general an increase in signs is of bad import and signifies progressive activity, which is really self-evident, but it also shows that it matters much less whether the physical signs decrease or remain stationary. As a matter of fact, Dr. Trudeau's figures for the "well" class in those showing "No Change" are better than in those showing "Decrease" in signs (78 per cent as against 69 per cent), though this is probably accounted for by the far greater number (398 as against 159) that were included in the "Signs Decreased' table. I would not be thought to wish to give little or no importance to extent of, character of, and changes in physical signs, but I do wish to stress the point that in the estimation of pulmonary activity symptoms have vastly greater weight. Moreover, symptoms are tangible, palpable facts in which the personal equation of the physician, the acuity of his hearing, the technic of his roentgen ray or of his laboratory play

[3] The Importance of Physical Signs in the Prognosis of Pulmonary Tuberculosis, Trans. Nat. Tuberc. Assn., 1920, p. 283.

no part. Variations in weight, range of temperature, fluctuations of pulse, measurement of daily sputum, amount of food consumed, hours of sleep, improvement in hemoglobin and red cells, general increase in vitality and good feelings on the part of the patient, all these save the last can be determined by instruments of precision requiring no special training for their use, and nothing beyond ordinary common sense for their correct interpretation. It is on these data that a correct basis for the estimation of activity of tuberculous disease can best be established.

I will not bore you by citing examples illustrative of all the points I have made, but will limit myself to reporting three widely differing cases, each of which stresses a certain phase of the subject.

The first of these shows the danger in relying solely upon a radiological diagnosis of tuberculous activity when symptomatic corroboration is lacking. This patient consulted her family physician, who made no examination but referred her to a very prominent radiologist, who took and interpreted the plates and sent in a report of peribronchial thickening suggestive of active tuberculosis. On the basis of this report alone she was adjudged actively tuberculous and sent to us.

Case I.—Mrs. X., aged thirty-six years. Paternal grandfather and grandmother and one uncle died of tuberculosis. One brother now in the West because of tuberculosis. Childhood history negative. Was never exposed to any of the tuberculous members of her family. Married at twenty-one, has one child, aged eight years. Never well since the birth of this child when she had a very difficult labor. Suffered a third degree perineal tear which was repaired at the time, but not satisfactorily. Four years later a trachelorrhaphy and perineorrhaphy were done. For a while she felt better, but then began to flow profusely for eight days every three weeks. Finally a hysterectomy was done in June, 1919, the ovaries and tubes being left. (I am not sure whether both ovaries were left or only one). There was no particular improvement in her feelings after this operation. For the past year has lost all energy and enthusiasm. Has taken every kind of tonic but to no avail. Is exceedingly nervous, crying frequently. For the past few months has run some temperature, between 99 and 100 °F., the latter rarely. Teeth have been pronounced sound after being radiographed twice. *At no time has there ever been any cough* or *sputum*. Spirits very poor. Nutrition bad; sleeps poorly; perspires very freely; appetite poor; bowels constipated. Physical examination of the lungs was absolutely negative. Stereograms showed some peribronchial thickening but not enough in our opinion to warrant a diagnosis of active tuberculons disease in view of the history and symptoms. The patient was told she did not have any active tuberculosis, and a diagnosis of psychasthenia with possibly some endocrine disturbance was made. She was placed in a neurological sanatorium on a rest cure for a period of three weeks and received as medication ovarian extract and thyroid extract. In addition she was given psychotherapy, in the course of which a domestic infelicity was brought to the surface and largely cleared up. In four months she had completely recovered. All symptoms had disappeared and she returned home happier and better than she had been in years. This condition of health had persisted for over two years when she was last heard from at Christmas, 1921. The history in this case, mainly nervous and gynecological, the long duration of asthenia, the absence of any focal symptoms or signs of tuberculosis, did not warrant a diagnosis of activity on the peribronchial thickening demonstrable in the stereograms. In addition to her endocrine disturbance and functional nervous disorder, this woman had a tuberculous infection, to which she was entitled, being thirty-six years of age, but she did not have tuberculous disease.

The second case illustrates the diagnosis of tuberculous activity on symptoms in the complete absence of physical signs, but with definitely positive stereograms.

Case II.—Mr. Y., aged twenty-six years. Family and childhood history negative. In U. S. Army, 1917–1919; overseas eighteen months, slightly gassed. Average weight, 150. Has dropped to 132. Discharged from the service in 1919 as physically fit. Has not felt perfectly well since his discharge. Tires very easily and has frequent and repeated colds with cough and sputum. There has been some blood in the sputum at times, but never any frank hemoptysis. In September, 1921, had bronchopneumonia and was ill three weeks. Has not been able to work since with any regularity, owing to rapidly appearing fatigue. Now there is slight cough, slight sputum, which is constantly negative for tubercle bacilli, temperature ranging at its maximum from 99.2 to 99.6, daily, very little endurance and dyspnea on slight exertion. Physical examination of the lungs, both at my hands and at those of Dr. Minor was absolutely negative, but the stereograms showed very distinctly a lesion at the right apex, appearing as a group of ten or twelve cotton-ball-like masses. A diagnosis of active tuberculosis would, in my opinion, have been justifiable on the symptoms alone, though I confess it was a comfort to find that our surmise was borne out radiologically.

It is interesting to note that during the three months that have elapsed since this diagnosis was made, a few fine rales have made their appearance first opposite the spine of the right scapula, and later in the first intercostal space on the same side, so that now this patient presents both symptoms, radiological evidences, and physical signs.

The third case illustrates marked improvement in general condition with consequent lessening of activity, according to the premise of this paper, and yet with no change to speak of in the physical signs at the end of seven months.

Case III.—Mrs. Z., aged forty-one years, came to us September 9, 1921. It is unnecessary to go into the details of her history. She had a definite advanced right-sided pulmonary tuberculosis without complications. On arrival her weight was 96 (average weight in health, 125; best weight, 130; standard insurance weight, 135). She had considerable cough and a little over one ounce of sputum. Temperature ranged from 99 to 100°F. She was weak and dyspneic. Her pulse was not unduly accelerated. On physical examination, she showed dulness on the right side to the third rib in front and to the fifth vertebral spine behind. Auscultation revealed broncho-vesicular breathing over a similar area with feeble breathing over the rest of the lung. Fine moist and dry rales were to be heard over the entire front of the right lung, and over the back to about an inch above the angle of the scapula. There were tubercle bacilli in the sputum. Her present condition is: Weight, 128¼, a gain of 32¼ pounds; temperature absolutely normal; cough very slight; sputum about half an ounce in twenty-four hours; no dyspnea; strength so much improved that she can walk from forty-five minutes to one hour at a stretch without becoming fatigued. Physical and radiological examination, however, reveal conditions to all intents and purposes identical with those found in September as regards dulness, broncho-vesicular breathing, extent and quality of rales, and roentgen-ray shadows. This patient is, nevertheless, a totally different woman from what she was seven months ago; her friends would not recognize her—she has improved wonderfully. Her symptoms are all better, and many of them have disappeared entirely. Unquestionably we must assume that activity has greatly lessened and this assumption is based not on changes in physical signs or radiological findings, but on changes in symptoms the intensity of which are the main criteria for estimating the potency of the general infection.

Summary. Thus we see that the more we study the various forms of pulmonary tuberculosis, the more we are driven to symptoms in our estimation of the presence or absence of activity. Refinements of physical diagnosis lie in the province of the pulmonary expert; refinement in plate reading in that of the radiologist; refinements in laboratory methods in that of the clinical pathologist; they are all useful, and each one of us should master all of them that he can; but for the man doing general work, the estimation of the presence or absence of activity in tuberculosis will be based in the main upon the careful consideration of symptoms which alone point out the relative strength of the two great fundamental biological factors in any infectious disease; virulence of the invading parasite, and resisting powers of the invaded host.

REVIEWS.

MINOR SURGERY AND BANDAGING. By HENRY R. WHARTON, M.D., Consulting Surgeon to the Presbyterian Hospital. Ninth edition. Pp. 647; 450 illustrations. Philadelphia: Lea & Febiger, 1922.

THIS edition is a distinct improvement over the last. The book is well arranged, the reading matter easy and the style clear and concise. Illustrations are excellent and profuse. The table of contents and index are so arranged as to make the subject-matter easily accessible with a minimum of effort. The parts dealing with bandaging, asepsis and antisepsis, fractures and dislocations are full and well handled, giving the optimum of instruction with the minimum of verbal effort. Ligation of arteries and minor operations are treated under separate chapters. The subjects of anesthesia and transfusion are covered in great detail, but certain parts dealing with a number of minor surgical affections are a trifle brief.

This work has made and should continue to make an excellent and handy text-book for the general practitioner.

H.

DISEASES OF THE NERVOUS SYSTEM. By SMITH ELY JELLIFFE, M.D., PH.D., formerly Professor of Psychiatry, Fordham University, and WILLIAM A. WHITE, M.D., Professor of Nervous and Mental Diseases, Georgetown University. Fourth edition, revised, rewritten and enlarged. Pp. 1119; 475 engravings and 13 plates. Philadelphia: Lea & Febiger, 1923.

THIS new edition of such a well-known book does not require a great deal of comment. The authors have kept in view the idea of producing a work which is not merely a collection and arrangement of a mass of facts, but one which will stimulate the thought of the student using it conscientiously. And in this they have succeeded most admirably. Doubtless, neurologists may differ in regard to some of the opinions expressed by the authors, but no one of them can deny the thought-stimulating power of the book.

The high standard reached in the earlier editions has been made still higher in this one, not only by the new matter which has been added and the parts which have been rewritten, but more especially by the character of the work in general and the method of treatment of the subject as a whole.

A prominent feature of the book is the number of excellent figures and charts which help to a much clearer understanding and more exact diagnosis of the various conditions considered. M.

AN INTRODUCTION TO THE PRACTICE OF PREVENTIVE MEDICINE. By J. G. FITZGERALD, M.D., F.R.C.S., Professor of Hygiene and Preventive Medicine and Director of Connaught Laboratories, University of Toronto; assisted by P. GILLESPIE, M. Sc., and H. M. LANCASTER, B.A.Sc. Pp. 826; 129 illustrations. St. Louis: C. V. Mosby Company, 1922.

As the title of this book indicates, it does not pretend to be a complete exposition of the whole field of preventive medicine in all its details, but is merely an introduction to the practice of that branch of medicine. The idea in the mind of the writer would seem to have been to produce a book which would not frighten the general practitioner by its bulk, but which would rather stimulate his interest in the subject and help him to realize the importance of the part he should play in the campaign for the prevention of disease.

If viewed in this light, the book takes on a different character from that which otherwise might be given to it, and the value of having the various questions presented in a fairly brief, but very clear manner, is at once perceived. The author has received the assistance of certain authorities in writing special sections, such as those relating to water, milk, diet, sanitation, etc., so that one appreciates that the book presents the most recent ideas in preventive medicine. M.

TWELVE ESSAYS ON SEX AND PSYCHOANALYSIS. By WILHELM STEKEL, M.D., Vienna: translated and edited by S. A. TANNENBAUM, M.D., New York. Pp. 320. New York: The Critic & Guide Company, 1922.

THESE essays cover a period of ten years, most of them having appeared in print between 1909 and the beginning of the War. In the theses presented by the author, there is plenty to offend some, who, through ignorance or conviction, are opposed to the doctrines of psychoanalysis. Among those more sympathetic, some do not agree in detail with all the conclusions of the author, for highly controversial matter is involved. The style is vivid, but perhaps not so conspicuously epigrammatic as some later works of the same author. These studies contain much sound truth and much that challenges the psychiatrist's attention; they should not be overlooked by any physician who deals with neurotics, exhibitionists, thieves or suicides, especially if he is concerned to protect the young from joining any such group. What is said of onanism is to be heeded in quarters whence comes much sincere but badly devised propaganda on sexual themes.

The essay on "Sexual Abstinence and Health" has been widely quoted since its publication in 1909. The author sets forth characteristics of the "supposedly innocent child," the power of instinct and the demand for sexual activity. He presents a situation involving practical difficulties for the conscientious physician of this land, though perhaps the difficulties are less under Continental culture. He would punish one who knowingly infects another, and legalize abortion before the fourth month. He would enlighten children gradually and postpone gross sexual stimuli as long as possible. Onanism is discussed, its implications, frequency and comparative harmlessness. His views on sleep and insomnia differ in some points from those traditional; for instance he asserts that sleep does not strengthen the nerves. Happy persons, he says, never complain of insomnia. Homosexuality is presented as frequent but tremendously repressed. Suicide is not considered a logical or philosophical act, but one determined fundamentally by a sense of guilt. It was growing more frequent among children when this essay was written, and particularly among the children reared in small families. Obsessions are presented as results of the repression of an unacceptable idea. The obsessed neurotic's character is discussed. Exhibitionism is next considered and its relation to the neurotic character and to onanism. The dramatic instinct of the neurotic and his piety and belief in his mission are described, together with notes on treatment. The neurotic's obscuration of the border between fantasy and reality, the annulment of reality and his attitude toward time are ingeniously presented. The book ends with a discussion of the psychology of kleptomania, relating it to early sexual stimulation and the temptation to do something forbidden. The translator has interlarded many comments of his own, bracketing them from the rest of the text. These comments amplify the subject and rarely suggest a different view or a feeling that the original statement needs defense. If one must add to a text this is perhaps the best way, through brackets sometimes offend the eye of the reader.

Fortunately we are now in a period when psychoanalysis is discussed with less bitterness than used to be aroused. The author has done important work in this field and his formulations are still important. H.

CHARLES WHITE OF MANCHESTER (1728–1813), AND THE ARREST OF PUERPERAL FEVER (the Lloyd Roberts Lecture, Manchester Royal Infirmary, 1921). By J. GEORGE ADAMI, C.B.E., M.D., F.R.S., Vice-Chancellor of the University of Liverpool. With which are reprinted Charles White's published writings upon puerperal fever. Pp. 142; 4 illustrations. Liverpool: The University Press, Ltd.; London: Hodder & Stoughton, Ltd., 1922.

THIS scholarly lecture is a most delightful historical sketch of that famous British surgeon, obstetrician and hygienist, Charles White, whose far-sighted teaching and keen analysis of the cause of puerperal fever clearly establishes a prior claim for him in the matter of prophylaxis and prevention of that malady.

To the lecture are appended chapters from the writings of Charles White. Would that every parturient today might be delivered under the safe, sane and sensible directions he laid down in the year 1773. Then one of the scourges of child-bearing would be minimized. This book will be of interest to all medical historians and obstetricians. W.

SOME MEDICAL ASPECTS OF OLD AGE. By SIR HUMPHRY ROLLESTON, K.C.B., M.D., D.C.L., LL.D. Being the Linacre Lecture 1922, St. John's College, Cambridge. London: The Macmillan Company, 1922.

IN this "*De Senectute*," Sir Humphry Rolleston has skilfully combined a discussion of some of the general features of old age with considerations more strictly medical. It is a subject in which we all will be interested if we live long enough. The basis of the book is the material collected for the Linacre Lecture at St. John's College, Cambridge, of which Sir Humphry was at one time a Fellow.

The duration of life in higher and lower forms is discussed in a general way and there are portraits of several traditional "oldsters" who are reputed to have lived beyond the usual time, including Henry Jenkins with one hundred and sixty-nine years and a Hungarian with one hundred and eighty-seven years. The author is sceptical as to the correctness of certain of these records. He gives explanations but does not decide the question as to the duration of the life of Methuselah.

When does old age begin? The author points out that it is often unrecognized by the victim himself until perhaps some chance remark or occurrence brings it home to him. The influence of heredity, environment and past diseases on longevity are considered and the evil effect of syphilis is emphasized. Much stress is placed on functional activity and the evil of autosuggestion is mentioned;

"I am getting older and older every day" has its harmful influence. The often injurious effect on a healthy old man of giving up work is pointed out. This is a subject on which our advice is not infrequently asked and the decision is often difficult. Perhaps of chief importance is whether or not there is an *avocation* to which he can turn when the *vocation* is given up. The wise man cultivates a hobby in his maturity. Some have held that the attainment of old age is in great part a matter of the will. As Strachey says of one circle, "They refused to grow old; they almost refused to die." As to personal habits, the observation that the majority of those who have reached old age are small eaters of meat is noticed and the use of alcohol even in moderation is regarded as unfavorable. Among the causes of senescence the influence of the endocrine glands is discussed. The conclusion is reached that changes in the interstitial cells are not the cause but an accompaniment of old age. As to the use of thyroid and other gland extracts a word of caution is given, for harm may be done by stimulating metabolism overmuch. The discussion of the normal structural changes and physiology of old age dwells more on the purely medical aspects. The attitude toward death is described as rarely showing a desire for rest, as one might long for sleep, but rather there is "a passionate, absorbing, almost bloodthirsty clinging to life."

This is a delightful little book, not strictly medical but taking us along a bypath which is sometimes a pleasant change from the straight road of professional writing. Whether old age in itself should be regarded as a disease is a question about which there has been much debate. Its definition as "the period at which a man ceases to adjust himself to his environment" the author regards as true only of senility or morbid old age. Certainly a study of those who have reached a sunny old age to discover their method and philosophy of life is worth while, so that those who come after may profit thereby. What more delightful character is there than the genial old man who has seen many years but has not lost the savor of life?

McC.

Surgical Clinics of North America. St. Louis Number, Vol. II, No. 6. Pp. 289; 105 illustrations. Philadelphia: W. B. Saunders Company, 1922.

This, the St. Louis number, is presented to the readers as the work of twelve of the big men of that city. They have well maintained the high standard of the contributions for which the *Clinics* are famed. Each article adds something that is new, useful and instructive. The great feature in these *Clinics* is not the reported cases so much as it is the description of the way they are handled. Here, we readers can obtain the many little tricks in technic that can be obtained only by such articles so presented.

E.

Blood Transfusion. By Geoffery Keynes, M.A., M.D. (Cantab.), F.R.C.S. (Eng.), Second Assistant, Surgical Professorial Unit, St. Bartholomew's Hospital. Pp. 166; 13 illustrations. London: Henry Frowde, Hodder & Stoughton, 1922.

The first chapter is devoted to a very complete and interesting review of the history of transfusion. The following chapters include the indications for transfusion, and the dangers incident to its employment are thoroughly discussed. The methods of direct and indirect transfusion are described, and the principles underlying the various technic are described in detail.

The volume is compact and gives all the information necessary to a complete understanding of the subject. A very complete bibliography is appended. S.

A Text-book of the Practice of Medicine. By Various Authors; edited by Frederick W. Price, M.D., F.R.S. (Edin.), Senior Physician to the Royal Northern Hospital; Physician to the National Hospital for Diseases of the Heart, London; formerly Physician and Honorary Pathologist to the Mount Vernon Hospital for Consumption and Diseases of the Chest; Examiner in Medicine at the University of St. Andrews. Pp. 1753; 96 illustrations. London: Oxford Medical Publications, 1922.

The editor of this volume states in his preface that, on account of the great advance in knowledge throughout the domain of medicine, it is impossible for any one authority to do full justice to the ever-widening field of medicine and that, therefore, a useful purpose might be served by the publication of a work of moderate compass and in one volume, compiled by specialists in the different branches of medicine. To the reviewer this seems eminently fit. It is certainly impossible for any one man to speak authoritatively on all the phases of internal medicine, and while such a man may be able to write on the various phases of medicine from his knowledge of the literature, he certainly cannot do it from first-hand practice in all the special branches of medicine. For this reason, it seems quite possible that the old style text-books of medicine may in time disappear, and be replaced by volumes such as the present one, which deal with the various diseases from the viewpoint of those who have made special study of this or that disease. This plan has been followed out in the large systems of medicine and the same scheme is followed in this one volume presentation of the subject of medicine. It is, in reality, a small system, although one hardly could call it small, as there are packed between the covers nearly two thousand pages of small print.

As with all systems, some of the sections are superior to others and some of the authors are better known than others but it does not follow that the best sections are always by the best known authors. In going over some of the diseases in most cases there seems to be a very complete exposition of the disorder. There is really a greater uniformity in the sections than one would think possible, when you consider that twenty-six different authors contributed to the volume. Taken as a whole the book can be recommended as an authoritative, complete and thorough handbook of medicine. M.

MEDICAL RESEARCH COUNCIL OF GREAT BRITAIN (REPORT FOR THE YEAR 1921–1922). Edited by SIR WALTER M. FLETCHER, K.B.E., M.D., Sc.D., F.R.S., Secretary. London: H. M. Stationery Office, 1922.

THE great value of the research work fostered by the Medical Research Council has been more and more appreciated throughout the scientific world since its first publications in 1915. Not, however, until one carefully studies its latest annual report of 125 pages, does one realize the truly astounding amount of work that the Medical Research Committee (later Council) has been able to achieve or stimulate. From the first publication of their special report series in 1915 on "The Boot and Shoe Industry," this phase of their work alone has produced 72 careful studies, averaging from 30 to 300 pages in length, and scattered over such topics as tuberculosis, cerebrospinal fever, dysentery, alcohol, rickets, shock, venereal disease, industrial hygiene, pathological methods, biological standards, radium, etc., etc. In addition, they have aided many institutions and individual investigators with part-time grants, so that the present report alone names over 500 persons and 150 institutions with which they have had associations in the past year.

The National Research Institute, with which the Council is most directly concerned, received about one-quarter of the total budget for work in its six departments of Biochemistry and Pharmacology, Experimental Pathology, Bacteriology and Protistology, Applied Physiology, Applied Optics, Statistics and Library Publications, under the direction of eminent scientists, such as H. H. Dale, Capt. S. R. Douglas, Leondar Hill and J. E. Barnard.

The national collection of type cultures at the Lister Institute, the Standard Laboratory at Oxford, the Department of Clinical Research and the Cardiographic Department of the University College Hospital Medical School, the clinical research units at the London and St. Bartholomew's Hospitals, the work of Mellanby, Sir Almroth Wright, MacLean, Meakins, Starling; Laslett and Ivy Mackenzie are only a few of the important projects subsidized by the Medical Research Council.

Truly can one say that the annual grant of £130,000 has been wisely administered and that Parliament's Committee on National Expenditure showed wisdom in not cutting down their grant-in-aid even in these days of general retrenchment. K.

A CLINICAL TREATISE ON DIABETES MELLITUS. By MARCEL LABBÉ, M.D., Professor of General Pathology at the Faculty of Medicine of Paris and Physician to the Charité Hôpital: translated, revised and edited by CHARLES GREENE CUMSTON, M.D., Lecturer at the Faculty of Medicine of the University of Geneva and Fellow of the Royal Society of Medicine of London. Pp. 382. New York: William Wood & Company, 1922.

It is like carrying coals to Newcastle to translate such a book as this from the original French into English at the present time. The rapid advance of our knowledge concerning many aspects of the diabetic problem results in a book becoming out-of-date very quickly. It is true that the author has had a very large experience with diabetes, and his observations on the symptomatology of diabetes are valuable. For example, the chapters on "Diabetes and Tuberculosis," on "Edemas in Diabetes" and on the "Painful Syndromes in Diabetes" are all interesting but there is little mention of many of the chemical methods which we have learned to depend upon in this country. The translator also has unfortunately used many unusual words and phrases, as for example, "Social midst," "acromegalia," "larvate," "undosable," "ammonuria," and "hyperglycistia." In fact, there is little to recommend in this book. P.

MALADIES DE LA PLÈVRE ET DU MÉDIASTIN. By MARCEL LABBÉ, M.D., Professor, Faculty of Medicine of Paris; P. MENETRIER, Professor, Faculty of Medicine of Paris; L. GALLIARD, Honorary Physician to the Hospital of Paris; F. BALZER, Physician to the Hospital St. Louis; and E. BOINET, Professor of the School of Medicine of Marseilles. Pp. 596; 114 illustrations. Paris: J. B. Baillière, 1922.

THIS extensive study offers much that is of value from a clinical point of view, while at the same time suffering from a failure to include references to the recent literature. There are many references given, few of which are to other than French literature. Most of the references date back ten or twenty years and the only recent ones are from the French literature. French clinicians have always been peculiarly interested in diseases of the pleura and this present work is essentially a review of their studies. The article on pulmonary syphilis is especially interesting, for the French place much more emphasis on this subject than do our own writers. Another interesting chapter concerns adenopathies of the mediastinum. On the whole, however, the work offers little which cannot be obtained equally well from any one of the recent systems published in the English language. P.

RICKETS. By J. LAWSON DICK, M.D. (EDIN.), F.R.C.S. (ENG.), Deputy Commissioner of Medical Services, London Region, Ministry of Pensions. Pp. 488; 7 full-page illustrations and numerous figures in text. New York: E. B. Treat & Co., 1922.

IN this book the author has endeavored to build a background for the present-day scientific understanding of rickets. He has collected a wealth of information, geographical, ethnological, sociological and economic, to show that rickets is a disease pursuant to modern industrialism. While the latest studies on the effects of light deprivation are not included in the book, the author is convinced that housing conditions, which compel deficient light and fresh air, constitute the important factor in the etiology of the disease. The history of rickets is well considered; it is especially interesting how the disease, at first most common among the cultivated classes, came to be a disease of the laboring man's child. The book is very readable, being free of tedious tables of experimental data. The author presents his work as evidence to justify the sweeping reforms necessary for the elimination of rickets, if this theory of its causation be proved correct. S.

PHYSICAL EXERCISES FOR INVALIDS AND CONVALESCENTS. By EDWARD H. OCHSNER, B.S., M.D., F.A.C.S., President, Illinois State Charities Commission; Attending Surgeon, Augustana Hospital, Chicago. Second edition. Pp. 56; 42 illustrations. St. Louis: C. V. Mosby Company, 1922.

THERE are described forty-two exercises especially designed for the use of convalescents and invalids and persons engaged in sedentary occupations. They are so arranged as to give well-balanced exercise to the whole body, and no apparatus is required. The descriptions are clear and the illustrations adequate. K.

PROGRESS

OF

MEDICAL SCIENCE

MEDICINE

UNDER THE CHARGE OF

W. S. THAYER, M.D.

PROFESSOR OF MEDICINE, JOHNS HOPKINS UNIVERSITY, BALTIMORE, MARYLAND,

AND

ROGER S. MORRIS, M.D.,

FREDERICK FORCHHEIMER PROFESSOR OF MEDICINE IN THE UNIVERSITY OF CINCINNATI, CINCINNATI, OHIO.

Phenoltetrachlorphthalein Liver Function Test.—ROSENTHAL (*Jour. Am. Med. Assn.*, 1922, **79**, 2151) has introduced an important modification of the technic of the use of phenoltetrachlorphthalein in the estimation of liver function, depending on the study of the rapidity of the removal of the dyes from the circulation. After detailing the technic of the phenoltetrachlorphthalein test, he gives the results in 37 instances, comprising cases of known degree of liver damage. Ten cases are used as controls which were normal from a point of view of liver function, but which comprised diseases of practically all the other organs of the body. Five cases of carcinoma of the liver were tested; 3 cases of cirrhosis of the liver; 2 cases of acute hepatitis; 1 case of cholangitis and 1 of chronic passive congestion. Several cases of toxemia of pregnancy and 1 of acquired hemolytic jaundice were also tested. Rosenthal makes the following comment: "The normal liver removes phenoltetrachlorphthalein from the blood stream with rapidity and uniformity. The damaged liver takes up the dye much more slowly; large amounts may remain for a prolonged period in the plasma, where the dye can be accurately and quantitatively estimated. Experiments have shown that practically none of the dye is taken up by the red cells. In this series of cases of liver disease the abnormal results have not paralleled the degree of jaundice or hepatic enlargement. The highest degrees of retention have been present in acute hepatitis, in a case of cirrhosis in which there was a small liver, and in advanced cases of hepatic carcinoma. A fixed dosage of tetrachlorphthalein according to the body weight is used, so that a unit of work is imposed on each unit, by weight, of liver tissue. The normal curves show the time required for the entire liver to perform this task. For these reasons, borne out by clinical and experimental observation, it seems probable that the test gives an index of the total amount of functioning liver tissue." This communication would appear to be of real importance, describing apparently a method of study of hepatic function decidedly more satisfactory than any which has yet been devised.

Relapsing Pyrexia in Hodgkin's Disease.—HALL and DOUGLAS (*Quar. Jour. Med.*, October, 1922, p. 22) report a case of anatomically proved Hodgkin's disease which showed regularly recurring attacks of pyrexia. They have examined the temperature records of other cases extending over long periods of time. They show that the time from the middle of one period of fever to the middle of the next (the pyrexial span) was found to vary between fifteen and twenty-five days in 80 per cent of the cases. In individual cases, however, the periodicity did not vary by more than five days and in many cases was of remarkable regularity. The *form* of the pyrexial wave in each individual case was fairly constant. Very low temperatures were often recorded in the apyrexial periods, at which time there was often an apparently complete symptomatic recovery. The charts show a gradual stepping upward and downward of the pyrexial waves. The authors observed in these characters of periodicity gradual ascent of fever, and low temperatures with apparent complete recovery between pyrexial periods. The disease shows a similarity to certain recurring fevers such as malaria, relapsing fever, rat-bite fever and trench fever. It differs from these in greater length of span. The similarities suggest the possibility of an organismal infection as the cause of this type of relaxing pyrexia.

Family Association of Cardiac Disease.—ST. LAWRENCE (*Jour. Am. Med. Assn.*, 1922, **79**, 2051) studied 100 families, each of which contained at least 1 child enrolled in the cardiac clinic of St. Lukes Hospital. Exclusive of the 100 children who formed the basis of study, there were 480 persons known to have had close and long-lasting contact with patients suffering from rheumatic heart disease. Seventy-one (14.8 per cent) of these "exposed" persons had a definite infection of the rheumatic group. 38 (8 per cent) had definite cardiac disease. These figures are much greater than those given for the incidence in the general population. A similar study of 100 families, each of which had at least 1 member the subject of tuberculous infection, showed very similar figures. The results of the investigation suggest that the intimate association of family groups may have an important relation to the spread of rheumatic heart disease, and that the family offers a place for the application of the available preventive measures.

Psychologic Tests Applied to Diabetic Patients.—MILES and ROOT (*Arch. Int. Med.*, 1922, **30**, 767) report the results of psychologic tests made on 39 diabetic patients, and give the figures for a corresponding number of controls. Diabetic patients frequently complain of poorer memory and power of attention, but objective proof of this has been lacking up to the present time. By certain psychologic tests applied in such cases as well as to suitable controls it was found that diabetic patients with hyperglycemia and glycosuria at the beginning of treatment show a decrement of about 15 per cent or more in memory and attention tests. The loss is in amount rather than in quality. With treatment the diabetic improves rapidly in his psychologic status, approaching, but not quite reaching normal. In accuracy and quickness of movement 5 treated diabetics, each case of long duration, were 20 per cent below normal.

Chronic Nephritis Anemia.—BROWN and ROTH (*Arch. Int. Med.*, 1922, **30**, 817) from their study of 187 cases diagnosed chronic glomerular nephritis at the Mayo Clinic, report their observations on 105 of these cases which showed anemia. They present evidence to show that the anemia of uncomplicated chronic nephritis develops in the absence of blood loss (microscopic blood in the urine having no relation to the degree of anemia) and this anemia is not due to excessive hemolysis. They point out that this type of anemia cannot be attributed to increased concentration in the blood of any known nitrogenous substance. They believe that the bone marrow suffers damage concomitantly with renal, retinal and cardiac tissues. In a group of cases studied during the development of renal insufficiency, anemia developed four to six weeks after the onset of the renal injury. The tardiness of the anemia is explained on the basis of decreased formation of erythrocytes. The injury to the bone marrow concerns only its erythrogenetic function. Leukocytogenesis is not involved. They believe that the unknown agent causing renal insufficiency is probably the etiological factor in the disturbance of hematopoiesis, in other words, a common cause is present. Twenty cases of chronic glomerular nephritis in whom the red blood cell count was found to be below 3,500,000 per cm. showed a remarkably high death rate, 18 of the 20 dying within ten months and many of them within one month. The authors point out that an anemia of this degree has a prognostic value similar to that of creatinin retention.

SURGERY

UNDER THE CHARGE OF

T. TURNER THOMAS, M.D.

ASSOCIATE PROFESSOR OF APPLIED ANATOMY IN THE MEDICAL SCHOOL AND ASSOCIATE PROFESSOR OF SURGERY IN THE SCHOOL FOR GRADUATES IN MEDICINE IN THE UNIVERSITY OF PENNSYLVANIA; SURGEON TO THE PHILADELPHIA GENERAL AND NORTHEASTERN HOSPITALS.

A Case of Congenital Osteosclerosis.—GHORMLEY, (*Johns Hopkins Hosp. Bull.*, December 1922, p. 444) says that the patient limped and complained of pain in the left hip. Repeated roentgenographs of all the bones were then made and showed much the same condition throughout the skeleton. Besides the curious density of the flat bones and the rather hazy outline along all the bones, the vertebral bodies showed a marked density at either pole. Definite thickening of the cortex of all the long bones was noted as more marked in the femora and humeri. The skull was thicker than normal. In the femoral necks and especially in the left, there seemed to be a breaking down of the bone just below the epiphysis, so that the epiphysis had slipped inward and downward. Roentgenographs of the mother and father were then made, which showed the mother's bones to be normal; but practically the same condition existed in the father.

Salivary Glands in Carcinoma.—Dudgeon and Mitchiner (*Lancet*, September 2, 1022, p. 558) say that in the vast majority of cases of carcinoma of tongue and floor of mouth these glands are not the seat of carcinoma. In nearly all cases, the changes present in these glands are of a chronic inflammatory nature somewhat analogous to the changes met with in the pancreas in chronic pancreatitis and are apparently due to infection from the mouth along the ducts. In other cases, no microscopical change can be seen. The lymph nodes in this area show malignant change in only 27.3 per cent of early and 50 per cent of late cases, though inflammation is always present. It would appear, therefore, in certain cases with early carcinoma of the tongue, to be justifiable to leave the submaxillary area untouched at operation, though clinical experience teaches that the risk of the subsequent appearances of metastases is very great.

The Healing of Gastric Ulcer.—Stewart (*Brit. Med. Jour.*, 1922, **2**, 1164) says that healing of gastric and duodenal ulcer is a common event. Statistics are given to show that in the postmortem room scarring is met with almost as frequently as ulceration, while duodenal scars occur with about one-half the frequency of duodenal ulcers. This difference may be partly accounted for by the greater liability of duodenal ulcers to perforate. Single and multiple gastric scars are met with in the ratio of 4 to 1, which is exactly the same as the ratio of chronic to acute ulcers. It is suggested from this, that acute and chronic ulcers have an equally good chance of healing. Hour-glass contraction of the stomach is met with in about 6.5 per cent of all cases of completely healed gastric ulcer. There is no evidence from present observations that carcinoma arises in connection with gastric scars, whereas in a series of 98 stomach specimens received for microscopical examinations, the incidence of carcinoma in cases of simple chronic ulcer was 11.5 per cent.

The Diagnosis and Treatment of Bone Lesions.—Bloodgood (*Am. Jour. Roentgenol.*, 1923, **10**, 42) says that roentgenograms immediately after trauma to bones and joints are highly essential for a record of comparison if the trauma excites some benign or malignant pathological process. Moreover, roentgen-ray examination of multiple bone lesions would aid in differential diagnosis. When the roentgen-ray show multiple distinctly central lesions, one can practically exclude primary sarcoma. When distinct periosteal multiple lesion is found, malignancy can be excluded. Roentgenograms of the chest should be made routinely, for the author can cite evident metastases to lungs within three months of first symptoms of sarcoma. Moreover, he has not found tuberculosis of the lung in cases of sarcoma of bones.

Renal Torsion.—Brasch (*Jour. Urolog.*, 1923, **9**, 12) says that incomplete congenital rotation and acquired torsion of the kidney, while of anatomical interest, are of no clinical importance *per se*. The anomalous position of the renal pelvis and its relation to the ureter may, in certain cases, permit urinary obstruction by some extrarenal factor. Traumatic hydronephrosis without direct injury to the kidney, may occur following a fall or blow which is accompanied by renal torsion and fixation of the upper ureter by adhesions. Renal torsions without evident ptosis or other known etiological factors, may occasionally occur with a moderate degree of hydronephrosis.

Surgery in Patients with Obstructive Jaundice.—Walters (*Am. Jour. Surg.*, 1923, **37**, 2) says that postoperative intra-abdominal hemorrhage is often the cause of death in patients with obstructive jaundice. Moreover, the coagulation time of the blood should be determined before operation and if the time is lengthened beyond six minutes, an attempt should be made to reduce it by intravenous injections of calcium chloride. Calcium chloride given intravenously, reduces the coagulation time of the blood and combines with the bile pigments circulating in the blood stream, rendering them less toxic. The diminution in the supply of glucose to the tissues in the body as a result of the toxemia of the liver cell, is overcome by supplying glucose directly to the tissues by means of proctoclysis and subcutaneous injection.

Diverticula of Bladder in Children.—Hyman (*Surg., Gyn. and Obst.*, 1923, **36**, 27) says that vesical diverticula are rare findings in childhood, not more than 30 being found in a review of over 600 cases. However, diagnosis of this condition in children should present no difficulties. Little value can be placed on history. Physical examination of the abdomen is important. A chronically distended bladder, especially asymmetrical in outline, should make one suspicious of a diverticulum. The cystoscope and cystogram are absolutely essential in making a correct diagnosis. In the 3 reported cases there were no evidences of obstruction, either vesical or urethral. All 3 diverticula were in immediate proximity to the ureter; in 1, the ureter opened into the sac and as a result, the ureters were compromised to such a degree, as to cause obliteration of the lumen with resultant dilatation. Division of ureter with reimplantation was performed in all 3 cases, with recovery of the patients. The author feels that there will be an increase in the number of cases reported, as soon as cystoscopy in children is done more routinely. He feels that the presence of diverticula in patients so young without evidences of any obstruction, leads one to conclude that they were congenital and that in all probability, many of the diverticula in adults have also a similar origin.

Cancer of the Pharynx.—Jackson (*Ann. Surg.*, 1922, **77**, 1) says that certain curable laryngeal conditions are in some cases the sequential predecessors of frequently incurable cancers. The author feels that it is justifiable to use the word precancerous for such conditions as continual laryngeal irritation from chronic laryngitis, keratosis, syphilis, pachydermia, so-called prolapse of the ventricle and benign growths (occurring in a person of cancerous age). All these should be cured surgically or otherwise. It is no argument against this life-saving rule to contend that these conditions are too rarely predecessors of cancer to justify regarding them as etiological factors in cancer. There is no known agent causative of any disease that will always, in all individuals under average conditions of exposure, produce that disease. There will be few deaths from laryngeal cancer when every member of the medical profession fully realizes the frequently malign nature of chronic hoarseness.

Pyelonephritis.—STERLING (*Jour. Urolog.*, 1923, **9**, 29) says that a large number of so-called surgical kidneys can be saved an operation by drainage and lavage of the kidney pelvis. At least 50 per cent of the cases of pyelonephritis are being treated for other conditions such as appendicitis, cholecystitis, duodenal ulcers, without the formality of a urinalysis. Careful elimination of the foci as well as other accessory factors, will clear up the majority of the kidney infections. Repeated search should be made of the urine for pus, as one negative urinary examination does not always eliminate the urinary tract. The colon bacillus usually crowds the streptococcus out, which has been demonstrated culturally, making it difficult to demonstrate it in the urine in these infections.

The Relation of Calcified Abdominal Glands to Urinary Surgery.—WALKER (*Lancet*, 1922, **2**, 1213) says that operation in 11 of 42 cases of painful calcified abdominal glands, resulted in the disappearance of the pain whether it had the form of constant aching or recurrent attacks of colic. Moreover, all these cases have remained free from pain since operation. The author believes that there is no longer any danger of general dissemination of the tubercle bacillus which is usually responsible for the condition, or probability of infection in the urinary tract. Tuberculous peritonitis is not a concomitant or a sequel of this condition and adhesions which might interfere with the action of the bowel, or form obstructing bands, do not form. Against any general rule of operation of these cases in children, is, however, the knowledge that recovery without operation must take place in the great majority of these cases without further trouble. Therefore, operation is only justifiable in those cases in which symptoms are severe and are proved to be directly due to the calcified glands. These cases can be selected only after investigation by thoroughly modern methods of examination.

The Question of Recurrent Calculi.—BARNEY (*Surg., Gynec. and Obst.*, 1922, **35**, 743) says that there is an unfortunate paucity of investigation on the matter of recurrent or overlooked renal calculi and it would be desirable to have various observers in different clinics undertake such investigations. Roentgenographic examination during or shortly after convalescence, is essential for the accuracy of the results in such work. The data at hand show that stones are subsequently found in the kidney after operation in a surprising number of instances. It is however impossible to say which are "recurrences" and which are "left overs." Actual recurrence is unquestionably very frequent. The complex character of the interior of the kidney, hemorrhage from its mucosa and the comparative inaccessibility of this organ in many cases, contribute to the difficulties in removing all stones. The fluoroscope offers the most promising prospects for success in this work. Moreover, preoperative study cannot be too painstaking, nor must the possibility of superimposed shadows of calculi be overlooked. A second operation for the removal of remaining stones is advisable in most cases and should be done soon after first operation. Pyelotomy is unquestionably the operation of choice and is often advantageously combined with partial nephrectomy.

THERAPEUTICS

UNDER THE CHARGE OF

SAMUEL W. LAMBERT, M.D.,
NEW YORK,

AND

CHARLES C. LIEB, M.D.,
ASSISTANT PROFESSOR OF PHARMACOLOGY, COLUMBIA UNIVERSITY.

Balancing the Diabetic Diet.—Strouse (*Jour. Am. Med. Assn.*, 1922, **79**, 1899) summarizes the recent metabolic work in diabetes and presents a simple procedure for applying these principles clinically. It is necessary that certain data be first obtained. The basal metabolism, the basal caloric requirement calculated therefrom, the daily urinary sugar and nitrogen and the glucose tolerance must be determined. The protein ratio is then 0.66 gm. per kilogram of body weight. Inasmuch as 56 per cent of the protein is burned as carbohydrate, the carbohydrate ratio may be calculated by subtracting from the glucose tolerance 58 per cent of the protein. The basal caloric requirement being known from the determination of the basal metabolism plus 20 per cent for the specific dynamic action of protein and the energy requirements for a bed existence, the calories supplied by the protein and carbohydrate to be fed are calculated by multiplying the total grams of these two substances by 4.1. The remaining calories must then be supplied in fat and the fat in grams is calculated by dividing the caloric requirement by 9. This ratio of fat is comparatively high in proportion to the amounts used by Allen. The danger of acidosis must be guarded against and this is accomplished by the antiketogenic substances resulting from the combustion of protein and especially carbohydrate. The acidosis producing substances are ketogenic and there exists a definite relationship between the ketogenic substances of fat metabolism and the antiketogenic substances of protein and carbohydrate metabolism. This ratio may roughly be approximated when the ratio of fat in grams is to the available carbohydrate in grams (equal to carbohydrate tolerance as calculated above) as 2.5 to 4 is to 1. A diet so calculated will provide a comparatively low protein and high fat allowance. The patients maintained on such a diet were without significant clinical acidosis.

Cardiac Functional Tests.—Brittingham and White (*Jour. Am. Med. Assn.*, 1922, **79**, 1901) have eliminated as of small value all but two of the many cardiac functional tests. These two were submitted to further study. Vital capacity determinations were made on 144 patients, 48 of whom had some cardiac complication; 16, some pulmonary complication and 80 had neither cardiac nor pulmonary disease. Of the 80 with no intrathoracic disease, 50 per cent had vital capacities at least 20 per cent below the calculated normal; in the cardiac group "most of those who had no congestive heart failure had normal vital capacities" while every one of the patients with congestive failure had a low vital capacity. The conclusion is reached that vital capacity determinations furnish measures of dyspnea more definite than "marked," "slight," etc., but rarely aid in the management or "sizing up" of the patient. The exercise tolerance test consisted in swinging from floor to overhead, two 20-pound dumbbells, a given number of times (15 and 20) in a given number of seconds (40 and 50), and determining the effects on blood-pressure. The test proved of no value for diagnostic or prognostic purposes generally, so far as the heart is concerned and is useful only in following the progress of the individual case. The test is therefore unsatisfactory as a cardiac efficiency test. Vital capacity and exercise tolerance determinations were markedly at variance in 14 per cent of the cases in which both tests were performed. The final conclusion reached by the authors is that there is no satisfactory test of cardiac functional efficiency at the present time.

PEDIATRICS

UNDER THE CHARGE OF

THOMPSON S. WESTCOTT, M.D., AND ALVIN E. SIEGEL, M.D., OF PHILADELPHIA.

Intraperitoneal Transfusion with Citrated Blood. An Experimental Study.—Siperstein and Sansby (*Am. Jour. Dis. Children*, 1923, **25**, 107) have shown that freshly citrated blood injected into the peritoneal cavity of rabbits is absorbed. Necropsies at various intervals following the operation reveal that the quantity present in the abdominal cavity rapidly decreases in amount and that absorption of comparatively large amounts of blood is completed in three or four hours. Estimation of blood values demonstrates definite increases from the time the blood is transfused until the animal is killed. They have shown that the erythrocytes enter the blood stream without undergoing any morphological changes. Smears of the fluid in the abdominal cavity taken at necropsy show no change in the size, shape, and structure of the corpuscles, and no evidence of hemolysis. A rise in hemoglobin and cellular elements was seen following transfusion in normal and anemic animals, which cannot be accounted for by a mere concentration of the blood. Nucleated red blood cells of pigeons when injected intraperitoneally into rabbits can be recovered from the general circulation in fifteen minutes, and can persist for at least twenty-four hours. They found that the erythrocytes enter the blood stream very rapidly. The increase in the blood values of the animals persisted for days. After severe hemorrhage the animals improved after the transfusion. No hemoglobinuria could be demonstrated. Autotransfusion and retransfusion have been successfully used in man. Clinical experience with cases of internal hemorrhage as compared to external hemorrhage tends to show that the blood is absorbed in a functioning condition. The intraperitoneal transfusion of citrated blood in rabbits is a safe procedure, simple to apply and efficient. Absorption of the blood takes place very rapidly, and a rabbit can apparently absorb approximately one-fifth of its own blood value in four hours. The intraperitoneal transfusion of citrated blood acts as a true transfusion, and not as the absorption of nutrient material.

The Effect of Olive Oil on Gastric Function as Measured by Fractional Analysis.—LOCKWOOD and CHAMBERLIN (*Arch. Int. Med.*, 1923, **31**, 96) in their experiments demonstrated that olive oil given before meals, as is usually done clinically, reduces the average total acidity about 12 per cent, and lowers the high point of the curve about the same degree. It causes a marked delay of the test meal in the stomach, and the oil is the last portion of the meal to be evacuated. When oil is given regurgitation of bile is five times as frequent as without it. They feel that the oil coats the food and mucous membrane whereby the usual local reflex action of the food is lessened. The presence of bile in the stomach usually means reversed peristalsis. This alone might account for the delay in emptying time. Alkaline duodenal regurgitation might also lower the acidity to the extent found.

Intracutaneous Reaction in Pertussis.—REISENFELD (*Jour. Am. Med. Assn.*, 1923, **80**, 158) studied 400 children in a large institution over a period of four years through several epidemics of pertussis. He had the opportunity of observing the disease with special reference to natural immunity, acquired immunity, and the diagnosis of the disease in its earliest stages and before the development of the characteristic spasmodic cough, whoop and vomiting. Children exposed in previous epidemics and not acquiring the disease were considered as possessing a natural immunity. Those giving the history of having had the disease before admission, or having had an attack of pertussis while in the institution, were grouped as those possessing an acquired immunity. The value of a method whereby it would be possible to designate children who had natural or acquired immunity, and to be able to diagnose pertussis in its earliest stages, can be readily appreciated. This was the motive of the author's study. Various preparations of Bordet-Gengou bacillus were employed. The reactions occurring in the Schick test for diphtheria were the standard of comparison. He injected 2 minims intracutaneously into the upper part of the flexor surface of the forearm. Sixty cases tested with pertussis vaccine gave 53 positive and 7 negative reactions. Thirty-nine cases tested with staphylococcus vaccine gave 35 positive and 4 negative reactions. Of 26 cases of active pertussis tested with pertussis vaccine, 14 reacted positively within three hours, 19 in twenty-four hours and 7 in forty-eight hours. Twenty-five cases of active pertussis tested with staphylococcus vaccine gave 13 positive reactions in three hours, 20 in twenty-four hours, and 15 in forty-eight hours. No reaction was considered positive unless at least 5 mm. in diameter. As a result of his observations Reisenfeld found that no specific reactions were obtained by the use of various preparations of Bordet-Gengou bacilli injected intracutaneously to prove presence of the disease, or of a natural or of an acquired immunity. Positive and negative results alike were obtained in children having the disease, in children with an immunity, and in children developing the disease after the injection.

Malignant Tumors of the Suprarenal Gland.—STEVENS (*Jour. Am. Med. Assn.*, 1923, **80**, 171) reports a case in which there seemed to have been a definite connection between the trauma and the development of the hypernephroma. An early diagnosis was rendered difficult by the appearance of symptoms so soon after the injury, by the bleeding and hematoma found at the first operation, and because of the negative findings in the second operation. The patient's later symptoms, pigmentation of the skin, tumor mass, weakness and gastro-intestinal symptoms were suggestive of a tumor of the suprarenal gland. An interesting feature of this case was the brownish discoloration of the skin although only one of the suprarenal glands was affected. Another unusual feature was the comparatively slow progress of the disease. The majority of adrenal tumors progress rapidly after the first symptoms appear. Adenocarcinoma is infrequent in a patient so young. Until comparatively recent times the majority of both cortical and medullary growths were classed as sarcoma or lymphosarcoma. The latter are now considered to be of neuroblastic origin, and are termed neuroblastoma or neurocytoma. They are derived from the medullary portion of the gland and are seen during infancy or early childhood. In a study of 74 cases in which this case is included the following facts were elicited: Of 70 cases in which sex was mentioned, 42 males and 28 females were affected. Thirty-four per cent occurred in infants or young children, 18 per cent between six and forty years, and 48 per cent after forty years. The right suprarenal was involved in 41 per cent of the cases, the left in 45 per cent and both in 14 per cent. Tumor mass was palpated in 38 per cent; pigmentation occurred in 20 per cent; loss of weight was noted in 12 per cent; hematuria was observed in 9.5 per cent; elevation of temperature was seen in only 8 per cent. Premature sex development, principally overgrowth of hair, occurred in 8 per cent. Pus, albumin or casts were found in 7 per cent. Cases of successful extirpation have been reported.

After-care of Infantile Paralysis Cases of the 1916 Epidemic in Brooklyn.—DUNHAM and RILEY (*Jour. Am. Med. Assn.*, 1923, **80**, 224) report the results of their work in 300 cases. These patients did not come under care from the acute onset. The care of these individuals began from one to two years after the initial period of their illness, and as a result there was a great variety of physical defect, depending on the severity of the attack, the type of early treatment and the manner in which the parents coöperated with the physician. In this group only 14 families had more than 1 child ill with this disease at the same time, which would strongly suggest that its contagion is not transmitted by methods obtaining in the common infectious diseases, since the vast majority of all other cases were in families with 2 or more children in the same household. The experience of that large epidemic should have taught that during an epidemic of infantile paralysis of any size of children with obscure indispositions should be kept at rest in bed for days until the exact nature of the condition can be determined. When paralysis occurs it usually appears a short time after the initial upset, the average in this series being three days. Often the paralysis comes on in from twenty-four to forty-eight hours. Early neglected cases should never be ignored in treatment later regardless of the degree of involvement. This is essentially a disease of childhood and every acute illness warrants a reserved diagnosis of acute poliomyelitis until later developments overrule this. Sporadic cases occur every year. In this series the back and abdomen, with both lower extremities, was the combination of involvement most frequently found. In the lower extremities the tibialis anticus was most often affected, next in frequency being the muscles of the calf and the tibialis posticus. In the upper extremities the biceps and the triceps were involved most frequently. The more severely involved upper extremities did not respond to treatment as readily as the equally involved lower extremities. Those patients made the best recoveries in return of function who had the least interference during the initial stage of the disease, and when treatment in the subacute and chronic stages was intelligently advised and faithfully carried out.

DERMATOLOGY AND SYPHILIS

UNDER THE CHARGE OF

JOHN H. STOKES, M.D.,

MAYO CLINIC, ROCHESTER, MINN.

Clinical Test of a New Mercurial.—An excellent example of clinical approach to the problem of the efficiency of an antisyphilitic medicament is afforded by the report of COLE, DRIVER and HUTTON (*Jour. Am. Med. Assn.*, 1922, **79**, 1821) on Mercurosal, a proprietary mercurial for intramuscular and intravenous use, recently advertised to the profession as possessing special efficiency. The drug was employed on 38 patients in general accordance with the manufacturers' recommendations, but it was found it could be given somewhat more frequently. It was found to cause pain on intramuscular injection, to have some sclerosing effect on the vein, no general ill effect on the patient, less effect on syphilitic lesions than other familiar mercurials such as the biniodide and inunctions, no marked spirillicidal powers, in contradiction of the claims of the manufacturers, and no striking effect on the Wassermann reaction. In certain cases it failed to produce improvement and was then replaced by the more familiar medicaments with benefit. In general it was apparent that the drug had no superiority and was in fact in some respects inferior to familiar non-proprietary preparations.

The Mechanism of Mercurial Stomatitis.—Two recent communications recall the important contributions of ALMKVIST to mechanism and treatment of mercurial stomatitis. *Acta Dermato-venereologica*, 1923, **1**, 312, contains an exceptionally complete review by this author of recent knowledge including the author's contributions (*Dermat. Wchnsch.*, 1922, **7**, 152) and an extensive bibliography. In a recent reply to a misquotation by Schreus, the author points out that a mercurial stomatitis is not produced by the irritant action of mercury in the saliva, as is so often supposed, but that bacterial action on the mucous membrane with the production of erosions and pockets is essential. The proteolytic bacteria, acting on food remains and accumulations about these pockets produce hydrogen sulphide, which penetrates or is absorbed by the mucous membrane. It then acts upon mercury in the tissue lymph, resulting in accumulations of mercury sulphide in the tissues, with subsequent necrosis and heightening of the bacterial action upon the necrosed tissue. The mercury sulphide formed in the blood is carried to the kidneys and excreted. A vicious circle is developed, with ulceration and extension. The proper point at which to attack the process is not by way of the mercury, but by way of the bacterial infection, through the cleaning and disinfection of the gum pockets and other accessible foci of bacterial infection in the mouth cavity, including the tonsillar crypts. Schreus advocates for treatment the Pfannenstiel method of administering sodium iodide and liberating nascent iodine in contact with the affected tissues by the local use of hydrogen peroxide, but the author states that this method has had extensive trial without any demonstrated superiority over peroxide alone. In the same issue of the *Dermatologische Wochenschrift* appears a communication from HAMMER (p. 158), describing a technic of treating the pockets, and suggesting that inhalation of mercury vapor such as occurs in the use of inunctions probably explains a greater frequency of stomatitis in this mode of administration. He has seen a case in which a laboratory worker developed the clinical picture of mercurial stomatitis from the inhalation of hydrogen sulphide. He has noted variations in the virulence of the mouth flora which he believes explain the occasional epidemic character of mercurial stomatitis.

Syphilis in French Africa.—In an elaborate study of syphilis in a subtropical country (French Africa) LACAPERE, (*Ann. des malad., vener.*, 1922, **17**, 561), discusses the incidence of neurosyphilis among the Mohammedans of Morocco, as compared with the incidence of neurosyphilis in France. He confirms earlier observations on the comparative rarity of late neurosyphilis among the Arabs, giving the incidence as approximately 5 per cent as compared with 30 per cent in Fournier's estimates for France. He points out that in early syphilis there is a much less striking difference in the incidence of involvement of the nervous system in the two races; but that in later years of the infection, the two types seem to diverge, syphilis of the bones and skin becoming more common among the Arabs and syphilis of the nervous system among the Europeans. Among the early clinical manifestations, meningeal and cerebral lesions are approximately as common as in Europe. Hemiplegias, ocular paralysis, lesions of the cranial nerves and spastic paraplegia are the common late forms of neurosyphilis. Tabes and paresis are rare among the rural Mohammedan population and confined almost entirely to the mixed types of the large cities along the coast. Among the possible causes for this rarity of late neurosyphilis among the Arabs, the author rates the extremely early age at which the infection occurs. He considers that the embryonic and inactive condition of the nervous system at this earlier age diminishes the tendency to involvement. He emphasizes moreover, the absolute serenity and calm of the Arab life. He feels that the complete absence of nervous strain is influential in protecting the nerve structures. The extreme rarity of chronic alcoholism among native Mohammedans is also credited with some influence in protecting them from neurosyphilis. While none of these theories appear quite convincing, the statistical difference between the two races is apparent enough to need explanation.

Occupational Dermatitis.—GARDINER (*Brit. Jour. Dermat. and Syph.*, 1923, **34**, 297) discusses at considerable length the characteristics of occupational dermatitis. Among the interesting individual cases is one in which a lupus erythematosus-like eruption developed in a T. N. T. worker. Housewives, general laborers, iron and steel workers and colliery workers were most numerous among his patients in the order named. 63.6 per cent were found to have had preceding eruptive conditions on the skin. Seborrhea was the most important (28 per cent), and hyperhidrosis next (27 per cent). 77.4 per cent of the patients were shown to have some predisposing background in previous cutaneous conditions or general ill health. Alterations in materials in use in a given occupation may cause the development of the dermatitis in the case of a worker employed for many years at the same occupation. An attack of dermatitis may render a worker susceptible to something which he could previously resist. Spreading of the dermatitis may be from the irritant itself, or secondary infection. While attacks may commence in youth, they are more common over forty. In the less pronounced irritants, the gradual onset of the dermatitis may occupy a period of years and is usually most delayed in those types associated with seborrhea. Local traumatism is an important factor, and illness, the climacteric and old age are influential causative influences.

OBSTETRICS

UNDER THE CHARGE OF

EDWARD P. DAVIS, A.M., M.D.,

PROFESSOR OF OBSTETRICS IN THE JEFFERSON MEDICAL COLLEGE, PHILADELPHIA.

Fetal Death Before, During and After Birth.—This subject was discussed in the section on Obstetrics and Gynecology of the British Medical Association at its last meeting (*Brit. Med. Jour.*, 1922, **2**, 583). Ballantyne considered the difference in the method of respiration in the child before and after birth to be so great as to influence very markedly its pathology. The same difference in varying degree may be found between the functions of nutrition before birth and those established after birth. There is a period while the child is passing from its connection with the mother to its life in the external world, which is neither typically intra-uterine nor postnatal life, and during this period conditions originating in the uterus may develop. Such would be an infection or a process of degeneration. A fetus may also be so constituted as to be able to live within the mother's uterus, but unable to establish an independent external life. Stillbirth is commonly defined as the death of the fetus when viable, and in these cases maceration is often present. The causes of death in the fetus are those affecting the mother and transmitted to the child, such as the acute infections; those conditions developing in the mother which affect her ability to nourish the child, such as maternal toxemia and active and external poisons, like lead and alcohol. One recognizes that conditions developing in the appendages of the child, for example, the placenta and membranes, may cause its death; so may malformation. With a healthy placenta the child in the uterus is much safer from disease than after birth. The most important cause of fetal death during labor is prolonged and early rupture of the membranes. This not only tends to death from mechanical causes, as hemorrhage following pressure, but is especially apt to be followed by infection. The so-called complications of labor, placenta previa, separation of the placenta, prolapsed cord, disproportion, and unusual presentations and mechanisms, naturally influence fetal mortality during labor to a very great extent. As modern obstetric surgery has developed, direct injury to the fetus through unskilful interference and improper operations has very much lessened. So the destructive operations upon the child have been greatly reduced in frequency by the perfection of Cæsarean section. From all causes, the actual mortality of the fetus during labor has grown less. Fetal death any time during the stage of transition from intra-uterine to extra-uterine life has a pathology at present but little understood. The intra-uterine death of the fetus seems to depend in a considerable degree upon the pathology of the placenta; in proportion as this is sound the fetus is secure within the womb. It is not yet explained why the dead and retained fetus does not undergo putrefaction, and one does not know how a child can apparently be on the verge of death after delivery, and yet, ultimately develop to adult life. If maceration were understood, we should know much more about the pathology of fetal death. In preventing the loss of the fetus, unusual and diseased conditions in the mother must be studied, and so far as possible remedied during pregnancy. Whatever points to an unnatural development of mother or child, whether from mechanical or other causes, must be rectified if possible. Too little importance has been placed in the past on the value of fetal life and with advances in obstetric science, it should be possible to greatly lessen fetal mortality. Syphilis threatens the fetus by rendering its bloodvessels so fragile that pressure or traumatism during labor is quickly fatal. While treatment during pregnancy may benefit the mother, if the child is subjected to mechanical interference during labor, the result may be fatal. In caring for the newborn child, especial attention must be given to the circumstances and character of its birth. After difficult labor not only does the mother but also the child demand unusual attention. In the city of Edinburgh under Ballantyne's supervision 138 women having venereal diseases were treated during pregnancy, and these women gave birth to 7 stillborn children. In contrast to these is a group of 33 who had no treatment during pregnancy, and who gave birth to 20 stillborn children. The lowest mortality rate was in patients cared for at prenatal clinics, free from venereal disease and delivered by the staff of the hospital. Among these patients the rate of fetal death was 5.9 per 1000; including patients with venereal disease under treatment during pregnancy the rate of fetal loss was 13.5 per 1000. One can form some idea of the results of treatment, by contrasting those cases where the mother had venereal disease during pregnancy, without treatment, with a fetal stillbirth rate of 606 per 1000, compared with those women who had no venereal disease and who received proper attention before the birth of the child, 5.9 per 1000. The success of treatment addressed to syphilis complicating pregnancy may be inferred from the rate of stillbirth in the children of such patients, which was 50.7 per 1000. In comparison with these may be taken the average percentage of stillbirth for the entire city, which was 47.7 per 1000. Although it is very difficult to obtain accurate statistics from the average hospital record, it is evident from every source that venereal disease and especially syphilis greatly increases fetal death, and that this condition can be greatly improved by prenatal care and by treatment addressed directly to the venereal disease.

Fetal Deaths During Labor.—HOLLAND (*Brit. Med. Jour.*, 1922, 2, 588) asserts that more children are lost from complications in labor than from disease in either mother or child. In these cases there is no inherent pathological condition in the fetus, so that they might live and develop, if they could be carried through the dangers of birth. If these cases were classified so that the cause of death was given as maternal, placental or fetal, it might be of service. More than half (51 per cent) of deaths of the fetus are caused by some abnormal condition in the delivery, and hemorrhage is the most frequent of these, whether cerebral or visceral. That portion of the brain most injured is the tentorium cerebelli, and pertains especially to labor in breech presentation where, although delivery may be spontaneous, the child dies during or soon after birth. So frequent is this that 88 per cent is stated as not an undue calculation. This suggests that in the birth of the aftercoming head, abundant time should be taken to guard the interest of the child. At least ten minutes should be allotted to this portion of labor.

The Influence of Toxemia in Causing the Death of the Child.—McIlroy (*Brit. Med. Jour.*, September 30, 1922) in treating of toxemia as a cause of death of the child reverts to the modern explanation of the toxemia of pregnancy, as the absorption of trophoblastic elements into the mother's blood, producing toxins, whose effects are better known than their composition. It is a familiar observation that the process of toxemia in the mother is shared by the embryo and fetus. Where the child is macerated this condition applies properly to changes in the tissues of the fetus only, and to understand the process present in the mother and child the placenta and membranes must be examined, when evideuces of processes of degeneration will be found. The writer joins in the previous writer's plea for greater importance upon the life of the fetus as compared with the life of the mother. Without in any way desiring to neglect the mother, the interest of the fetus should receive more consideration. Of all the abnormal states which predispose to maternal toxemia, the retention of waste material in the bowels is held to be the most important. The modern theory of foci of infection is acknowledged as important; and not only constipation but deficiency in the action of the kidneys is recognized as having a powerful effect in the production of toxemia. That the ductless glands are important in determining the metabolism of mother and child is a familiar observation. The writer in making diagnoses in these cases would have the usual analyses of the urine and the blood supplemented by examination of the feces to determine the presence or absence of bacteria. The examination of the urine by chemical methods is far less important and satisfactory than has been believed. In the present stage of our knowledge a large percentage of urea in the blood is an indication of danger.

Disturbances of Vision Complicating Eclampsia.—Hirsch (*Monatsschr. für Geburts. u. Gyn.*, 1922, **59**, 141) describes the case of a woman suffering from eclampsia who was suddenly taken with loss of vision. This was temporary, lasting during the shortest interval for one hour and at the longest time for three days. No cause except the eclampsia could be found for this condition, and the examination of the eyes was negative. The question arose as to whether intrà-cerebral condition might be present. Of this there is no positive proof. Prognosis in these cases so far as the vision is concerned is excellent, as patients regain fully normal vision. In none of these cases has there been a permanent injury to the sight. In 28 of these patients, 2 died from the eclampsia, 1 with rupture of the uterus as a complication. The disturbance of vision varies in degree with the severity of the eclamptic process, and from this ocular complication no idea can be gained of the severity of the eclampsia. It may be mild or excessively severe.

PATHOLOGY AND BACTERIOLOGY

UNDER THE CHARGE OF

OSKAR KLOTZ, M.D., C.M.,

DIRECTOR OF THE PATHOLOGICAL LABORATORIES, SAO PAULO, BRAZIL,

AND

DE WAYNE G. RICHEY, B.S., M.D.,

ASSISTANT PROFESSOR OF PATHOLOGY, UNIVERSITY OF PITTSBURGH, PITTSBURGH, PA.

Effect of Injection of Active Deposit of Radium Emanation on Rabbits, With Special References to the Leukocytes and Antibody Formation.—Following previous studies on the effects of benzene, roentgen ray and thorium X on antibody formation, HEKTOEN and CORPER (*Jour. Infect. Dis.*, 1922, **31**, 306) inoculated rabbits intravenously with various-sized doses of the "active deposit" of radium emanation as used by Bagg. Total and differential counts were made of leukocytes before and at regular intervals after injection of the active deposit and if the animal died the tissues were carefully studied. The effect of the radium on antibody formation was determined by injecting 30 rabbits, intravenously, with 1.5 and 10 mc. four days before, coincident with, or five days after the intraperitoneal injection of about 10 cc of citrated sheep blood per kilo of body weight, and ascertaining the specific precipitin and lysin for sheep blood at regular periods afterward. The active deposit of radium emanation, given into the vein in salt solution, was lethal to rabbits in about six days in quantities exceeding approximately 8 to 10 mc. per kilogram weight. In lethal doses, the active deposit produced an initial leukocytosis, (as high as 34,600) which was followed by a marked diminution in the circulating leukocytes especially of the polymorphonuclears. This was associated with congestion in the liver, lungs, lymph glands, spleen, suprarenals and kidneys, frequently accompanied by capillary hemorrhages. The cells of the spleen, lymph nodes and bone-marrow often were decreased in number. It was noted, also that "the active deposit in non-lethal amounts may have a depressing effect on the formation of lysin and to a less extent on precipitin for sheep blood."

Study of the Action of Four Aromatic Cinchona Derivatives on Pneumococcus. A Comparison with Optochin.—FELTON and DOUGHERTY (*Jour. Exp. Med.*, 1922, **35**, 761) report the results of *in vitro* and *in vivo* experiments to ascertain the bactericidal activity and organotropism of chloroacetylanilide, p-chloroacetylaminophenol, m-chloroacteylaminophenol, 4-chloroacetylaminopyrocatechal and optochin, when pneumococci, Type I (Neufeld) was employed. The experimental animals were young white mice and rabbits. To avoid repetition of the long names of the first four drugs, which represent a uniform series of hydroquinine derivatives, the laboratory numbers, C 29, C 36, C 40 and C 110, respectively, will be used to refer to them. After extensive observations and comprehensive protocols, the authors conclude in part, that all four of the aromatic cinchona derivatives have a rapid pneumococcidal activity both *in vitro* and in the peritoneal cavity of mice, and to a lesser degree in rabbits. In comparison, optochin (ethylhydrocuprein) is slower in action but its power is not so easily destroyed either *in vitro* or *in vivo*. In comparing the rapidity of *in vitro* bactericidal action and the intraperitoneal toxicity, C 29 exhibited the most rapid pneumococcidal action and was the most toxic for mice. C 36 was one-fifth as toxic as C 29 and only one-tenth less active bactericidally. C 40 was one-half as toxic and had about the same bactericidal power, while C 110 was one-eighth as toxic and one-fifth as pneumococcidal. Optochin was one-sixth as toxic and had one-fifth the bactericidal action. Arranged in the order of their ability to kill pneumococci when injected simultaneously with them into the peritoneal cavity, the drugs were C 40, C 110, C 36, optochin and C 29. While the chemotherapeutic action of the aromatic compounds was essentially local in character, a certain degree of diffusion was shown by administration per os, C 40 and C 110 having approximately the same value as optochin. When injected intravenously in small doses the drugs destroyed to a greater or less extent the natural defenses of the animal, optochin being perhaps less injurious than the others. The maximum tolerant dose, given intraperitoneally in a single dose, was not so efficacious as the same dose divided in fifths and inoculated at hour intervals. Under these conditions, optochin was not so active as the aromatic compounds. There was found to be a zone between the therapeutic and toxic doses, both single and repeated, for all the chemicals alike, where the natural resistance of the animal to an infection was reduced. This effect was noted particularly with C 29, C 36 and C 40. With optochin, the therapeutic dose was nearer the toxic than with C 110, C 36 and C 40.

Distribution of Potassium in Normal and Pathological Kidney.— By means of the Macallum potassium reagent, MENTEN (*Jour. Med. Res.*, 1922, **43**, 323) compared the microchemical distribution of potassium in kidneys from normal rabbits with those from animals receiving mercuric chloride. In the former a preponderance of potassium was observed in the convoluted tubules and ascending limb of the loop of Henle, while a relatively small amount was noted in the glomeruli and collecting tubules. The rods of Heidenhain were enveloped in a thin film of potassium. The normal nuclei were invariably free from any trace of this element. Furthermore, the minimum reaction occurred in the resting condition of the cell. After degenerative changes had been produced in the kidney by intravenous injections of mercuric chloride (and many other heavy metals), the amount of potassium was much augmented and the increment of increase was found always to be greatest in the convoluted tubules. No appreciable increase was noted in the glomeruli, which fact would seem to favor the theory of secretion of the urinary potassium salts by the tubules rather than of their filtration in dilute aqueous solution through the glomerulus with subsequent reabsorption of the excess water by the tubules. The cytoplasm of the necrobiotic cell contained a maximum amount of potassium, which substance could also be demonstrated in variable amounts in the nuclei of such cells. Experiments showed that the increased amount of demonstrable potassium salts found in the injured cells was due to a liberation of the so-called "masked" salts, that is, those absorbed in the normal state, and that the transformation of these absorbed inorganic salts from the un-ionized to the ionized condition was intimately related to changes in surface tension of certain structural elements within the cells.

Device for Tubing Cooked Meat Medium.—To introduce meat medium into test tubes in a clean and rapid manner, HOLMAN (*Jour. Bacteriol.*, 1923, **8**, 47) uses the ordinary automobile grease gun. The front cap and nozzle are unscrewed and the barrel filled with the meat. The nozzle must not have too small a diameter, and must reach past the middle of the tube. The fluid portion is added to the meat particles through the ordinary tubing funnel. The medium is made from ground meat, preferably skeletal muscle, to which is added an equal quantity of water. This is mixed, sterilized, neutralized, and allowed to stand over night. The fat is then skimmed off, the medium tubed as described above, the fluid being added last, and it is then autoclaved at 120° C. for thirty minutes. The author points out that this medium keeps sterile for days, and that it is not necessary to boil and cool immediately before use as was formerly believed. "(Unless for very special purposes) Nor need the surface be covered with oil or paraffin. Complete mixing of the seeded material with the meat particles is the most important point." The author believes that "the simplicity of preparation, tubing and sterilizing, its wide range of use in the growth of bacteria, and its keeping qualities should make cooked meat the medium of choice for routine bacteriological studies."

The Use of Phenol-red and Brom-cresol-blue as Indicators in the Bacteriological Examinations of Stools.—After a series of investigations to determine the efficacy of phenol-red and brom-cresol-purple as indicators in differentiating between B. coli and members of the typhoid-dysentery group, CHESNEY (*Jour. Exper. Med.*, 1922, **35**, 181) found that a 3 per cent beef-extract agar cleared with egg to which 1 per cent lactose had been added from sterile 20 per cent solution, gave the best results. In the instance of phenol-red, the optimum reaction was a hydrogen-ion concentration of pH 7.6 to 7.8 and the optimum amount was 10 cc of a 0.04 per cent aqueous solution for every 100 cc of agar. With this indicator, the typhoid, paratyphoid and dysentery (Shiga, Flexner and His-Y) bacilli produce pink colonies, while the colon bacilli assume a bright green or yellow-green colonies, and the colonies are more opaque. The optimum reaction for brom-cresol-purple was pH 7.2 to 7.4, and the optimum amount was 5 to 8 cc of a 0.04 per cent aqueous solution for every 100 cc of agar, the colon bacilli producing greenish-yellow colonies, with a yellow zone, while the typhoid-dysentery group produced bluish colonies. It was found that either indicator could be used in conjunction with brilliant green in the amounts advocated by Krumwiede, without exercising any inhibitory effect upon the restraining powers of the brilliant green. Of the two indicators, brom-cresol-purple gave the sharper differentiation, and, the author states, is to be preferred.

HYGIENE AND PUBLIC HEALTH

UNDER THE CHARGE OF

MILTON J. ROSENAU, M.D.,

PROFESSOR OF PREVENTIVE MEDICINE AND HYGIENE, HARVARD MEDICAL SCHOOL, BOSTON, MASSACHUSETTS,

AND

GEORGE W. McCOY, M.D.,

DIRECTOR OF HYGIENIC LABORATORY, UNITED STATES PUBLIC HEALTH SERVICE, WASHINGTON, D. C.

The Effect of Gasoline Fumes on Dispensary Attendance and Output in a Group of Workers—SPENCER (*Public Health Reports*, 1922, **39**, 2291) states that the gasoline fumes liberated in the workroom studied had produced cases of mild chronic gasoline poisoning. In workrooms where the ventilation is not adequate the liberation of gasoline fumes from open containers or from processes will, sooner or later, depending upon the amount and the concentration of the fumes, produce cases of acute, mild chronic or chronic gasoline poisoning. The liberation of gasoline fumes above an undetermined concentration, in an improperly ventilated workroom, will result in increased dispensary attendance and absenteeism among the workers exposed. Increased production and a lower rate of dispensary attendance were obtained by the removal of the gasoline fumes.

Malaria Control Operations in Relation to the Ultimate Suppression of the Disease.—BASS (*Jour. Am. Med. Assn.*, 1922, **79**, 277) states that malaria has disappeared from large areas in this country and in other parts of the world, chiefly as a result of development of the country, including drainage and clearing of the forest, incidental to agricultural and other industrial pursuits. Malaria prevalence is slowly but surely decreasing over practically all of this country, as a result of the steady march of civilization and settlement of the country. This process may be aided and hastened by anti-mosquito measures or the proper use of quinine. Health agencies are interested in encouraging these measures. The only part of the present malaria control activities that actually lead to ultimate suppression of the disease is permanent drainage and filling operations. All others are temporary and must be continued indefinitely, or the tendency will be toward a return to former conditions. The cost of intensive anti-mosquito operations for malaria control is so great that they have not been applied to a sufficiently large part of the total malarious area of the country to affect seriously the total prevalence of the disease. The cost of such malaria control as results from infected persons taking proper quinine treatment does not involve any cost over the amount that would be spent for other remedies. Therefore, it is applicable to the malaria problem of the country as a whole, and should be emphasized and encouraged by health agencies interested in malaria control.

The Scope of the Problem of Industrial Hygiene.—HAMILTON (*Pub. Health Rep.*, 1922, **37**, 2604) dwells on the extent and complexity of the problem. In discussing dust in relation to mortality and morbidity, it is emphasized that the quality of the dust is largely the determining factor in the hazard. Granite and flint dusts are very dangerous, while marble, sandstone and Portland cement are relatively harmless. Of organic dusts but little is known. Of poisons, benzol causes both acute and chronic poisonings. Specific fields in which our knowledge is very limited are mentioned.

The Responsibility of the Employer for the Health of the Worker.—JACKSON (*Pub. Health Rep.*, 1922, **37**, 2613) considers that the employer should provide: (1) Suitable, safe and healthful working places; (2) well-guarded machinery, tools and processes; (3) suitable foremen and supervisors; (4) suitable placing of each employee to best utilize his or her abilities; (5) protection from communicable diseases; (6) prevention and treatment of injuries; (7) time for rest and recuperation.

The Incubation Period of Typhoid Fever.—MINER (*Jour. Infect. Dis.* **31**, 3, 296) states that the incubation period of typhoid fever is highly variable, ranging in cases studied from three to thirty-eight or forty days. The mean incubation period in different epidemics ranges from 7 plus or minus 0.26 to 19.50 plus or minus 0.31 days, differing significantly from one epidemic to another. The standard deviations range from 1.84 plus or minus 0.18 to 8.85 plus or minus 1.17. The distributions are positively askew. The results obtained are consonant with the belief that the length of the incubation period depends in part on the virulence of the infection. The means of the epidemics due to infected water are 13.81 plus or minus 0.83, 19.38 plus or minus 1.66, and 19.50 plus or minus 0.31, whereas the means for those due to infected food, in which the dose was probably more massive are 7 plus or minus 0.26 and 9.54 plus or minus 0.39.

Detection of Typhoid Carriers.—GEHLEN (*Jour. Am. Med. Assn.*, 1922, **79**, 516) states that the State Board of Health of Minnesota, directly through its own representatives or through the local health officer, gives such instructions to be followed by the carrier and members of his family as are necessary for their protection and that of other associates, and explains the State law, which forbids a carrier to engage in the handling of any part of the public's food supply which may be consumed without being cooked after handling. The local health officer is charged to keep the State Board of Health informed as to any change in the carrier's residence or occupation, and, as long as the carrier obeys directions, all publicity is avoided. In 1 instance only has it been necessary to prosecute a carrier for illegally returning to a forbidden occupation. Three carriers, 1 a dairy woman, another a restaurant keeper, and the third a practical nurse and housekeeper, were forced to abandon their chosen occupations, the nurse-housekeeper having no income aside from her earnings for the support of herself an one dependent. Such restrictions of individual rights and liberty are necessary to protect the public against these innocent distributors of disease and death. Since 1915, the Minnesota State Board of Health has been entrusted by the legislature with the disbursement of a special fund for the support of a typhoid carrier who, after unauthorized newspaper publicity, was unable to obtain work. Should not the State offer compensation to carriers who must give up their chosen occupation in order to protect its citizens?

The Place of Venereal-disease Control in Industry.—The loss of time and efficiency due to venereal diseases is considered by LAWRENCE (*Pub. Health Rep.*, 1922, **37**, 2609), and examples given in which syphilis of employees led to a serious risk to life and property.

Vaccination of Monkeys against Pneumococcus Type I Pneumonia by Means of Intratracheal Injection of Pneumococcus Type I Vaccine.—CECIL and STEFFEN (*Pub. Health Rep.*, 1922, **37**, 2735) show that experimentally in monkeys it is possible to induce immunity against Type I pneumonia by means of intratracheal injections of vaccine. They believe that the immunity is in great part cellular, as the serums of protected animals had almost no demonstrable protective bodies. Spraying with the vaccine was not effective in inducing immunity.

Tuberculosis Among the Ex-service Men.—CUMMING (*Pub. Health Rep.*, 1922, **37**, 2241) discusses the problem of cure for the tuberculous former service men which was presented after the Great War. Approximately the same incidence occurred as was to be expected in the same age group of males of the general population. A surprisingly high incidence of non-pulmonary tuberculosis was noted, chiefly involvement of the bones and joints. The administrative features of the problem are described.

Notice to Contributors.—All communications intended for insertion in the Original Department of this JOURNAL are received only *with the distinct understanding that they are contributed exclusively to this* JOURNAL.

Contributions from abroad written in a foreign language, if on examination they are found desirable for this JOURNAL, will be translated at its expense.

A limited number of reprints in pamphlet form, if desired, will be furnished to authors, *providing the request for them be written on the manuscript.*

All communications should be addressed to—

DR. JOHN H. MUSSER, JR., 262 S. 21st Street, Philadelphia, Pa., U. S. A.

THE

AMERICAN JOURNAL

OF THE MEDICAL SCIENCES

JUNE, 1923

ORIGINAL ARTICLES.

ON SUBCUTANEOUS FIBROID NODULES IN RHEUMATISM.

By E. Bronson, M.D.,

and

E. M. Carr, M.D.,

With a Pathological Report of One Case,

By W. A. Perkins, M.D.,

SAN FRANCISCO, CALIF.

(From the Pediatrics Department of the University of California Hospital and from the Children's Hospital, San Francisco.)

The subcutaneous nodule, as a sign pathognomonic of rheumatic fever, has until recent years scarcely been considered by the American pediatrician. Brennemann,[1] in 1919, published observations on the incidence of these nodules in Chicago. He has given such a clear word picture of them, their size and location, that we need not repeat. He has also summarized their treatment, or rather lack of treatment, by American text-books of pediatrics. The purpose of our paper is to call attention to the fact that fibroid nodules are a frequent accompaniment of severe rheumatic infection in San Francisco, as well as in Chicago and Great Britain, and to emphasize that they are not to be classed as a medical curiosity, but that they are one of our most valuable diagnostic and prognostic signs in rheumatic fever.

Mitchell,[2] in 1888, from Osler's Clinic in Philadelphia, was the

[1] Am. Jour. Dis. Child., 1919, **18**, 179.
[2] Univ. Med. Mag., 1888–9, **1**, 161.

first to report a case in this country. Futcher[3] also, under the inspiration of Osler, quotes the latter as of the opinion that rheumatism occurs much less frequently in Philadelphia and Baltimore than in London, and that the subcutaneous fibroid nodules as a complication of rheumatism are "a great rarity" in the former two cities. It must be recalled, however, that Osler worked chiefly with adults while the British observations were mainly in children and adolescents. In Futcher's paper, Davaine is given as authority for the statement that nodules were known as early as the latter half of the 18th century. Futcher also states that they were associated first with rheumatism in 1843 by Froriep. Hillier,[4] in 1868, appears to have been the first to publish an instance of their occurrence in England. His observations were independent of those previously made on the Continent. In 1871, Jaccoud[5] described fully their character and location. He had seen them in four cases but regarded them as rare.

The paper by Barlow and Warner,[6] at the Seventh Session of the International Medical Congress, 1881, remains to the present the classical exposition of this subject. Their observations over a period of six years were undoubtedly known to their associates before publication. Their paper was followed by Cbeadle's delightful lectures on rheumatism, and thereafter references to rheumatic nodules in British literature became frequent, and the search for nodules, a matter of routine in the examination of the rheumatic child.

Casual references to fibroid nodules are seen occasionally in our journals, sometimes with an unfortunate ambiguity. Riesman,[7] in an otherwise excellent summary of rheumatism, characterizes them in one instance as follows: "Closely aggregated over the buttocks were innumerable reddish papules, pea size and larger, with very little intervening normal tissue. They were movable, not tender and gave the buttock a pebbly feel and appearance. Nodules of smaller size were present on the legs. In addition, there were scars of the same size as the papules scattered over the arms and thighs." This description suggests one of the erythemas not infrequently associated with acute rheumatism, not the fibroid nodule of Barlow and Warner.

On the finding of nodules in several instances, soon after the arrival of one of us* in San Francisco, the suggestion was made that we were dealing with a more severe type of rheumatic infection than was usual in this part of the country. To evaluate this

[3] Bull. Johns Hopkins Hosp., 1895, **6**, 133.
[4] Diseases of Children, Philadelphia, 1868, p. 249.
[5] Traité de Pathologie interne, Paris, 1871, **2**, 546.
[6] Tr. Seventh Internat. Med. Cong., London, 1881, **4**, 116.
[7] Jour. Am. Med. Assn., 1921, **76**, 1377.

* E. B. has to thank Dr. John Thomson of Edinburgh and Dr. G. A. Sutherland of London for calling her attention to this manifestation of rheumatism.

criticism and to estimate how much emphasis is ordinarily put upon this rheumatic sign, we have reviewed the histories of the Pediatric Department of the University of California Hospital from 1914 and of the Children's Hospital from 1917 and analyzed the rheumatic eyele cases. We have separated the cases into those seen before our own observations began and those followed by us. Brief notes on the latter series are tabulated below. We have classified both series, according to our estimation of the severity of the damage following the rheumatic infection, into three groups: Group I, children leaving the hospital with apparently complete recovery or with a slight systolic blow only and no obvious functional disability; Group II, those with a definite carditis but from whom, presupposing no fresh rheumatic infection, one can prognosticate a fairly normal active life; Group III, those with a crippling carditis, such as a progressive mitral stenosis, signs of adherent pericardium, extreme ventricular hypertrophy, as well as those already having the symptoms of chronic cardiac failure.

We realize that in such an arbitrary grouping the personal equation has played an important part. The best of histories does not always give an accurate estimate of the severity of an infection. If we had accepted the diagnosis of mitral stenosis or the mention of a "presystolic murmur and a roughened first sound" as the equivalent of a stenosis, each time so noted, Groups II and III, would have been much greater. We have omitted entirely a considerable number of cases of tonsillitis diagnosed as "mitral disease" on the presence of a slight systolic blow at the apex. In formulating the table we decided that a brief summary of the physical signs would be the simplest and most advantageous method of stating the facts of the history. It will be noticed that cardiac function is relegated to the background and physical signs unduly emphasized. Any other attitude would have been difficult, utilizing routine hospital records. If the history did not mention chorea, we have assumed this to be absent. The omission from our table of a routine reference to tonsillar infections may be criticized. In our experience there has been no correlation between tonsillar involvement and the sign of rheumatic fever which we are discussing. In our "Remarks" column we have endeavored to call attention to instances of infection of a severity which we believe predisposes to the presence of nodules. We have added the group classification, made on as nearly as possible the same basis as we used in the series of cases not seen by us.

These tables are a record of 38 children whom we had the opportunity of observing. We have grouped them as follows:

Group I, 12 cases, or 31.6 per cent, only 1 of whom showed nodules.

Group II, 9 cases, or 23.6 per cent, 3 of whom had nodules.

Group III, 17 cases, or 44.7 per cent, 13 of whom had nodules.

Seven of Group III died and 6 of the 7 showed nodules. Of the total 38 we found nodules on 17, or 44.7 per cent.

Age, sex	Arthritis	Carditis	Chorea	Nodules	Remarks
1[illegible] M	No history.	Systolic murmur which disappeared while under observation	Severe attack tending to become chronic	None	Complete recovery under sedimentive treatment. Group I
13 F.	First attack 1 week before entrance, extensive involvement including small joints	Heart much dilated, loud systolic blow, developed stenosis and pericarditis, general cardiac failure	None	In third week of illness large nodules noted on elbows, patellæ, occiput and spinous processes	A severe infection with recurring arthritis, tonsillitis and crops of nodules, progressive carditis; death in 2 months, no necropsy. Group III
12 F.	First attack 4 years, second attack 1 year before entrance. Entered during third acute attack	Aortic diastolic murmur; mitral systolic blow, cardiac hypertrophy, friction rub of a few days' duration	None	During acute attack small nodules on elbows	In hospital 6 months with slow but steady improvement, has been under constant observation up to present; goes to school and leads fairly normal life; has developed little or no stenosis, shows left ventricular hypertrophy. Group III
1[illegible] M	Definite attacks 8 years and 5 years before entrance, several other mild attacks, none on admission	Heart enlarged, loud systolic murmur	None	None	Present admission for acute nephritis, apparently not related to rheumatic infection. Group I
10 M.	Five previous mild attacks. Entered during sixth	Systolic and presystolic murmurs; no fresh cardiac involvement	None	None	Two previous admissions to University Hospital No. 10679 and No. 11042, second admission 1916 for chorea, at which time nodules stated absent. Little change in cardiac condition since first admission in 1915. Group II
12 M.	Definite attack 2 months before entrance. Convalescing on admission	None	None	None	Made rapid, complete recovery. Group I
10 M.	Entered during acute attack, no previous attack	Systolic murmur, no other abnormal cardiac findings	None.	None	Recovered in 1 month with little if any permanent damage. Group I
11 M.	First attack 5 years before admission. Entered during second with moderate joint involvement.	Heart enlarged, systolic and diastolic murmurs at apex and base; later developed presystolic murmur.	None	None noted on entry; 3 weeks later on head, spinous processes, scapulæ and elbows	Previous entry No. 11006; nodules at that time persisting throughout 2 months' stay in hospital. On present admission an extensive, typical erythema rheumatica circinata. This disappeared and recurred during observation; reëxacerbation of pharyngitis, arthritis and carditis during 3 months' course; discharged little improved. Group III.
5 F.	Mild attack one month before entrance. No involvement on admission	Blowing systolic murmur over precordium.	None.	None.	Severe tonsillar infection with definite arthritis and very little cardiac involvement. Group I

I refers to cases from the Children's Hospital. The cases not thus denoted are from the Pediatrics Department, University Hospital.

L. K. 6087	10 F.	First attack began 3 months before entrance. Entered during exacerbation.	Systolic murmur and enlarged heart on admission; later developed precordial friction and apical diastolic murmur.	None.	Three weeks after entry appeared on occiput, scapulæ, elbows and knuckles. Photograph No. 1.	Temperature 40° C. on admission; several exacerbations of temperature and arthritis during course of 6 weeks in hospital. A steadily progressive carditis; successive crops of nodules; removed against advice and died following month. Group III.
F. R. 7269	9 M.	First attack 2½ years before admission. Entered during second attack.	Blowing systolic murmur. No enlargement.	None.	None.	Recurring joint pains with slight elevations of temperature; discharged after 6 weeks much improved but with persisting systolic blow. Group I.
H. M. 7111	8 M.	Entered during first attack 1 month after onset.	Soft systolic murmur on admission; developed pericardial friction and effusion. Pancarditis.	None.	Developed on head and elbows 5 weeks after onset of arthritis; later on spinous processes and patellæ. Photograph No. 2	Progressive rheumatic infection terminating in death from cardiac failure; no necropsy. Group III.
D. S. 8116	10 F.	Three severe attacks in past 6 years; frequent indefinite joint pains; no acute attack on entrance.	Hypertrophied heart, systolic retraction at apex, presystolic rumble, loud systolic blow.	With first attack of arthritis.	None.	Three previous entries No. 10004, 13215 and 16273. Nodules not mentioned; followed by us since latest admission; marked impairment of cardiac function but no arthritis and no nodules. Group III.
F. B. 06770	11 F	First attack 4 years before admission. Entered during second acute attack.	Heart greatly enlarged; systolic murmur at apex, systolic and diastolic at base; later pericardial and pleural effusions.	With first attack; duration 3 months	On dorsum of feet and elbows.	High septic temperature, progressive carditis, death from cardiac failure after 2 months in hospital; no necropsy. Group III.
L. B. 2327CH	11 M.	First attack very severe, 3 years before entrance and second 1 year before entrance. Entered during third attack.	Heart greatly enlarged, loud systolic blow at apex; later developed typical aortic diastolic at base.	None	None	Cardiac function excellent when seen 5 months after leaving hospital. Group II.
A. A. 2391CH	11 F.	First attack following tonsillectomy 3 years before admission. Entered after second attack.	Soft systolic murmur which disappeared before discharge.	None	None.	A mild rheumatic attack with apparently complete recovery. Group I.
F. W. 2341CH	10 F.	First attack 2 years before entrance; in bed 6 months. Entered during second attack	Heart enlarged; booming first sound and loud systolic blow, later developed apical diastolic.	None.	None.	In hospital 2½ months; since discharge has had several attacks of arthritis and is reported to have mitral stenosis; no nodules at any time when seen by us. Group II.
W. W. 2311CH	11 F.	Entered during first attack, 3 weeks after onset.	Soft systolic apical murmur on admission, later developed into well transmitted murmur of valvulitis	None.	None	Onset with severe tonsillar infection; rapid recovery from arthritis with very little carditis on discharge. Group I.
A. G. 2329CH	13 M	First attack 5 months before entry. Subacute arthritis throughout course in hospital	Systolic and diastolic murmurs on entrance; developed pericardial effusion and extreme cardiac hypertrophy, with definite aortic valvulitis	None.	None	Under observation in hospital for 6 months with signs of cardiac incompetence; died suddenly at home soon after leaving hospital; no necropsy. Group III.
A. N. 2324CH	11 M	None.	Slight transient systolic blow.	Severe attack of 4 months' duration	None	Made complete recovery. Group I.
E. G. 2315	13 F	None	Systolic blow one week after onset of chorea.	Extremely severe attack	Two weeks after onset of chorea nodules developed on spinous processes, scapulæ, elbows, left hamstring tendon	On admission had a typical erythema rheumatica circinata on extensor surfaces of arms. This later appeared on chest and upper abdomen; when seen July, 1921, definite signs of beginning stenosis were present; she reports that she has not been free from nodules since discharge from hospital one year ago, small sago like nodules on elbows and tendons of wrists. Group III

ABLE OF RHEUMATIC CYCLE CASES SEEN BY BRONSON AND CARR BETWEEN SEPTEMBER, 1919, AND SEPTEMBER, 1921.

ise ord, o.	Age, sex.	Arthritis.	Carditis.	Chorea.	Nodules.	Remarks.
L. 90	12 M.	No history.	Systolic murmur which disappeared while under observation.	Severe attack tending to become chronic.	None.	Complete recovery under reëducative treatment. Group I.
P. CH*	12 F.	First attack 1 week before entrance; extensive involvement including small joints.	Heart much dilated, loud systolic blow; developed stenosis and pericarditis, general cardiac failure.	None.	In third week of illness large nodules noted on elbows, patellæ, occiput and spinous processes.	A severe infection with recurring arthritis, tonsillitis and crops of nodules; progressive carditis; death in 2 months; no necropsy. Group III.
L. CH	12 F.	First attack 4 years, second attack 1 year before entrance. Entered during third acute attack.	Aortic diastolic murmur; mitral systolic blow; cardiac hypertrophy; friction rub of a few days' duration.	None.	During acute attack small nodules on elbows.	In hospital 6 months with slow but steady improvement; has been under constant observation up to present; goes to school and leads fairly normal life; has developed little or no stenosis; shows left ventricular hypertrophy. Group III.
J. CH	12 M.	Definite attacks 8 years and 5 years before entrance; several other mild attacks; none on admission.	Heart enlarged; loud systolic murmur.	None.	None.	Present admission for acute nephritis; apparently not related to rheumatic infection Group I.
C. XC	10 M.	Five previous mild attacks. Entered during sixth.	Systolic and presystolic murmurs; no fresh cardiac involvement.	None.	None.	Two previous admissions to University Hospital No. 10679 and No. 11642; second admission 1916 for chorea, at which time nodules stated absent. Little change in cardiac condition since first admission in 1915. Group II.
M. 37	12 M.	Definite attack 2 months before entrance. Convalescing on admission.	None.	None.	None.	Made rapid, complete recovery. Group I.
B. 35	10 M.	Entered during acute attack; no previous attack.	Systolic murmur; no other abnormal cardiac findings.	None.	None.	Recovered in 1 month with little if any permanent damage Group I
F. 73	14 M.	First attack 5 years before admission. Entered during second with moderate joint involvement.	Heart enlarged; systolic and diastolic murmurs at apex and base; later developed presystolic murmur.	None.	None noted on entry; 3 weeks later on head, spinous processes, scapulæ and elbows.	Previous entry No. 11005; nodules at that time persisting throughout 2 months' stay in hospital On present admission an extensive, typical erythema rheumatica circinata This disappeared and recurred during observation; reexacerbation of pharyngitis, arthritis and carditis during 3 months' course; discharged little improved. Group III.
F. 64	5 F.	Mild attack one month before entrance. No involvement on admission.	Blowing systolic murmur over precordium.	None.	None.	Severe tonsillar infection with definite arthritis and very little cardiac involvement. Group I.

* CH refers to cases from the Children's Hospital. The cases not thus denoted are from the Pediatrics Department, University Hospital.

L. K. 6987	10 F.	First attack began 3 months before entrance. Entered during exacerbation.	Systolic murmur and enlarged heart on admission; later developed precordial friction and apical diastolic murmur.	None.	Three weeks after entry appeared on occiput, scapulæ, elbows and knuckles. Photograph No. 1.	Temperature 40° C on admission; several [illegible] of temperature and arthritis during course of 6 weeks in hospital. A steadily progressive carditis; successive crops of [illegible]; removed against advice and died following month. Group III
F. R. 7269	9 M.	First attack 2½ years before admission. Entered during second attack.	Blowing systolic murmur. No enlargement.	None.	None.	Recurring joint pains with slight elevations of temperature, discharged after 6 weeks much improved but with persisting systolic blow. Group I.
H. M. 7441	8 M.	Entered during first attack 1 month after onset.	Soft systolic murmur on admission; developed pericardial friction and effusion. Pancarditis.	None.	Developed on head and elbows 5 weeks after onset of arthritis; later on spinous processes and patellæ. Photograph No. 2	Progressive rheumatic infection terminating in death from cardiac failure; no necropsy. Group III
D. S. 8416	10 F.	Three severe attacks in past 6 years, frequent indefinite joint pains; no acute attack on entrance.	Hypertrophied heart, systolic refraction at apex, presystolic rumble, loud systolic blow.	With first attack of arthritis.	None.	Three previous entries No. 10094, 13215 and 16273. Nodules not mentioned; followed by us since latest admission; marked impairment of cardiac function but no arthritis and no nodules. Group III.
F. B. 9677a	11 F.	First attack 4 years before admission. Entered during second acute attack	Heart greatly enlarged; systolic murmur at apex, systolic and diastolic at base; later pericardial and pleural effusions.	With first attack; duration 3 months.	On dorsum of feet and elbows.	High septic temperature, progressive carditis, death from cardiac failure after 2 months in hospital; no necropsy. Group III.
L. B 2327CH	11 M.	First attack very severe, 3 years before entrance and second 1 year before entrance. Entered during third attack.	Heart greatly enlarged, loud systolic blow at apex; later developed typical aortic diastolic at base.	None.	None.	Cardiac function excellent when seen 5 months after leaving hospital. Group II.
V. A 2304CH	11 F	First attack following tonsillectomy 3 years before admission Entered after second attack.	Soft systolic murmur which disappeared before discharge.	None.	None.	A mild rheumatic attack with apparently complete recovery. Group I.
F. W. 2321CH	10 F	First attack 2 years before entrance; in bed 6 months. Entered during second attack.	Heart enlarged; booming first sound and loud systolic blow; later developed apical diastolic.	None.	None.	In hospital 2½ months; since discharge has had several attacks of arthritis and is reported to have mitral stenosis; no nodules at any time when seen by us Group II.
W. W. 2311CH	11 F.	Entered during first attack, 3 weeks after onset.	Soft systolic apical murmur on admission, later developed into a well-transmitted murmur of valvulitis	None.	None	Onset with severe tonsillar infection; rapid recovery from arthritis with very little carditis on discharge. Group I
A G 2322CH	13 M.	First attack 5 months before entry. Subacute arthritis throughout course in hospital.	Systolic and diastolic murmurs on entrance; developed pericardial effusion and extreme cardiac hypertrophy, with definite aortic valvulitis	None.	None.	Under observation in hospital for 6 months with signs of cardiac incompetence; died suddenly at home soon after leaving hospital; no necropsy Group III.
A. N. 2324CH	11 M.	None.	Slight transient systolic blow	Severe attack of 4 months' duration.	None.	Made complete recovery. Group I.
E. G. 2315	13 F.	None.	Systolic blow one week after onset of chorea	Extremely severe attack.	Two weeks after onset of chorea nodules developed on spinous processes, scapulæ, elbows, left hamstring tendon.	On admission had a typical erythema rheumatica circinata on extensor surfaces of arms. This later appeared on chest and upper abdomen; when seen July, 1921, definite signs of beginning stenosis were present; she reports that she has not been free from nodules since discharge from hospital one year ago; small sago-like nodules on elbows and tendons of wrists. Group III.

F RHEUMATIC CYCLE CASES SEEN BY BRONSON AND CARR BETWEEN SEPTEMBER, 1919, AND SEPTEMBER, 1921.—(*Continued.*)

se ord, o.	Age, sex.	Arthritis.	Carditis.	Chorea.	Nodules.	Remarks
M. CH	13 M.	First attack 3 years, second attack 6 months before admission, none on entrance.	Musical systolic murmur noted after first attack; pericarditis with second; cardiac failure with general anasarca on entrance.	None.	None.	Left [illegible] after 2 months with mitral [illegible]s, adherent pericardium and [illegible] ventricular [illegible]; under observation up to [illegible], no nodules at any [illegible] Group III.
L. CH	10 M.	First attack 4 years before admission. Entered during second attack.	Heart enlarged; blowing systolic murmur.	None.	On admission large nodules on elbows.	Previous admission No 11428; [illegible] not mentioned; 6 [illegible] in hospital on [illegible] entry; no arthritis since discharge; seen J [illegible] 1921, when he had definite presystolic rumble and [illegible] signs of developing stenosis; large [illegible] on right olecranon and small ones on left olecranon. Group II.
I. 68	12 F.	None on first entry; subacute joint pains for past year; acute attack 2 weeks before admission.	Slight systolic blow on first admission; on second pancarditis developing pericardial adhesions and stenosis. Definite signs of aortic insufficiency.	In [illegible] with acute attack one year ago, [illegible] one month, none on present entry.	Present on re-admission; recurring crops on elbows, wrists and spinous processes.	Previous entry No. 6168 for mild chorea; during second stay in hospital, through a period of 7 months, recurring pharyngitis and [illegible] arthritis with [illegible] of temperature; [illegible] crops of nodules with each exacerbation, though improved ultimate prognosis bad Group III.
I 82	14 M.	First attack $1\frac{1}{2}$ years before entry. Entered during second attack.	Apical systolic murmur; diastolic murmur at base; question of adhesive pericarditis.	[illegible]	None.	Left [illegible] after 4 months with definite carditis but with g[illegible]d cardiac fun[illegible]. Group II
L.	12 F.	Entered during first attack.	Dilated heart, loud systolic blow; later developed basal diastolic.	[illegible]	None.	Still u[illegible] observation in hospital; onset of arthritis accompanied by unusually severe tonsillitis. It is impossible at present to say how much cardiac damage will result. Group II
M.	10 F.	Several subacute attacks. Entered during latest.	Soft systolic blow at apex.	None.	Small nodules on elbows, occiput and spinous processes.	After one month's observation with no [illegible] symptoms no [illegible] of temperature over 1° and a [illegible], patient continued to develop nodules Were it not for the presence of [illegible] an excellent prognosis could be giv[illegible] Group I
O'C. CH	7 F.	First attack one year, second 8 months before admission. Entered during third attack.	Loud blowing, systolic murmur and dilated heart on admission; developed presystolic murmur and booming first sound; acute pericarditis second month in hospital.	None.	On both elbows on admission; later developed on spinous processes, tendons of hands and feet and on scapulæ.	Recurring sub[illegible] attacks of [illegible] throughout 3 months' stay in hospital; severe carditis, steadily progressing stenosis and [illegible] pericarditis; crops of large nodules Group III
J. CH	4 F.	Entered during first attack.	Soft systolic blow which progressed into a loud musical murmur, booming first sound, no definite presystolic rumble.	None.	A few small nodules on elbows appeared 2 weeks after onset. These have persisted during past 4 months.	No recurrence of arthritis, yet a gradually i[illegible] ca[illegible] involvement. Group II.

S. S. CH	6 F.	Entered during first attack; very severe.	Very rapid heart; weak first sound; soft systolic blow on admission.	None.	None.	Apparently made a complete recovery within one month from onset Group III
I. D. CH	9 F.	Entered 2 weeks after onset of first attack; joints much swollen, red and fluctuant; very extensive involvement.	While under observation developed systolic blow with slight enlargement and weak first sound.	None.	Three weeks after onset of arthritis nodules appeared on elbows. These increased in size and others appeared on occiput and hands.	A very striking erythema rheumatica circinata and severe tonsillitis a few days after admission After 10 months of observation is still having exacerbations of arthritis and crops of nodules, progressive carditis. Group III
S. M. CH	12 M	Entered during first attack one month after onset.	Systolic murmur which has persisted until present time.	None.	None.	Severe arthritis but with rapid improvement; under constant observation. Group I.
M. P. CH	7 F.	First attack 5 years, second 1 year before admission; both severe; recurring joint pains.	Hypertrophied and dilated heart; signs of mitral stenosis and adherent pericardium	None.	Large nodules on both elbows, spinous processes, scapulæ and wrists.	Symptoms of moderate cardiac failure while in the hospital; a very crippled heart becoming progressively worse Group III
J. B.	12 M	First attack in Italy 6 years ago; in bed 9 months; recurring attacks since, number not known; frequent joint pains.	Extreme cardiac enlargement; presystolic rumble and systolic blow at apex, in aortic area systolic thrill and very rough murmur, diastolic of typical aortic quality.	None.	Large nodules on elbows, forearms, knuckles, spine, knees, and head.	A circinate erythema seen by one of us before admission Patient states he has had nodules for at least 1 year; suffering from chronic cardiac failure Death in hospital, necropsy. Group III.
P. S.	9 M.	Recurrent attacks for 4 years; none on entrance.	History of murmur with first attack of arthritis; heart enlarged, systolic and presystolic mitral murmurs.	Severe attack started 2 months before admission and still present	None.	A moderately severe chorea tending to become chronic, definite carditis. The type of case in which one would expect nodules to develop. Group II.
W. G.	7 M.	Joint pains for 2 months; no severe attack.	Heart enlarged; signs of beginning stenosis but too early in course to predict amount of permanent cardiac damage.	Severe attack started 2 months before entry and still present in hospital.	On occiput one very large nodule with many small ones, large ones on elbows, wrists, scapulæ, tibiæ, patellæ, ankles and spinous processes.	The nodule on the occiput appears to measure 2 cm., but on examination the size is probably due to indurated subcutaneous tissue over a conglomeration of small nodules. The tumor as a whole is soft, the nodules themselves are hard. Group II.
J. P. CH	10 M.	None.	Systolic murmur at apex.	First attack 1 year and second 1 week before admission	None.	Apparently making a complete recovery; still under observation. Group I.
H. M. CH	5 M.	Onset of first attack 8 weeks before admission; none on admission.	Extensive pericardial friction rub; pancarditis; extreme dilation and cardiac failure.	None.	Noted by mother soon after onset; large nodules on occiput, spinous processes, elbows and knuckles.	A very severe acute carditis; died second day in hospital; no necropsy. Group III.

* Death occurred after completion of table, hence this case is not counted in our mortality statistics.
† For pathological report on No. 34, see text:

In the pediatric records of the period before our observations began we have found 45 admissions of rheumatic cycle cases. Four of these were readmissions which we have counted because they were fresh opportunities for the search for nodules. Moreover, in such recurring attacks one is the more likely to encounter nodules. An example is A. L., No. 23 in our table, who has not been without nodules during the nine months we have observed him, yet in whose history for a former admission nodules were not mentioned. D. S., No. 13 in our table, examined at frequent intervals for a year, has had no exacerbation of rheumatic infection and no nodules, though severe cardiac injury. During her preceding hospital admissions she was suffering from some acute phase of rheumatic fever, and at least in a condition to predispose to nodules.

In these 45 histories of rheumatic cycle cases admitted before our series began, nodules were not mentioned in 41, stated absent in 2 and stated present in 2. We have classified the 41 individuals who comprised the 45 admissions as Group I, 23, or 56.1 per cent; Group II, 9, or 21.9 per cent; Group III, 9, or 21.9 per cent. Of the 2 cases in whom nodules were found, 1 was G. F., No. 8 of our own series. Though according to the record of his former admission he is placed in Group II, the present degree of cardiac damage changes him in our series to Group III. Of the other case, T. B., 5122 C. H., the history states, "The mother noticed during the present illness that the child had some small, hard lumps developing upon head and elbows." A careful record was made of these in the hospital. Death occurred two months after these notes were made.

At a glance it would appear that there had been an epidemic of rheumatic fever during the past two years. Of our 38 cases, however, only 14, or 38.8 per cent, were first attacks. Several factors contribute to our comparatively large series. The Pediatric Service of the University Hospital has grown rapidly during recent years. A yearly variation in rheumatic cycle cases is shown, but certain preceding years have a higher ratio to total admissions than has been present during the period we have covered. It should be noted also that the Children's Hospital series begins only in 1917. Another reason for our numbers has been the kind coöperation of our colleagues in affording us an opportunity to examine the largest possible number of cases. We have been invited to see a greater number of severe than mild cases, a factor which has probably swelled the proportion in Group III.

Though our own series shows a greater percentage of severe infection, there are instances in the former histories which parallel certain of ours in the amount of carditis and termination by death. G. A., University of California Hospital, No. 8032, who ran a progressive and finally fatal course in eight months from the onset of the first symptoms, is an example. Fibroid nodules were not mentioned in his history. That nodules are not a necessary accompaniment of fatal cases is shown by the record of A. G., No. 19 of our series, who on no occasion showed them during six months in hospital. He died a month after he was discharged. During the period under observation, however, he was suffering from symptoms of cardiac failure, and at no time had any acute arthritis or fresh cardiac infection. Several of Group III we have followed for nearly two years, at no time finding nodules. They are suffering from inefficient hearts, not from any exacerbation of rheumatism. Such instances illustrate the general fact that the nodules are a sign of some active rheumatic focus, and that they tend to disappear as the infection becomes quiescent. We do not wish to be misinterpreted on this point. Nodules infrequently accompany the high initial fever and stage of swollen joints, circinate erythema, and other signs of acute rheumatism. A reference to our table will show that in our experience they are demonstrable ten days to two weeks from the onset, that is, at the time the more obvious arthritic signs are subsiding, and when a carditis is to be expected. Our observations are in sufficient contrast to the history records of preceding years to justify the statement that in San Francisco the search for nodules has not been a part of the routine in investigating the rheumatic child, or that during the past two years an unusually severe type of rheumatic fever has occurred in this locality.

To reiterate, rheumatic nodules are fibroid tumors varying from the size of a grain of sago to one or more centimeters in diameter. These apparently large nodules are often conglomerations of smaller units. Frequently in a place irritated easily, as the olecranon process or the occiput, the nodules appear much larger than their actual size, due to a chronic thickening of the subcutaneous tissues over and about them. This thickened tissue may be fairly freely movable and should not be confused with the underlying nodules. The nodules themselves are attached to tendon sheaths and aponeuroses. Their movability varies with the tissue to which they are attached. The skin moves freely over them. They are not tender, unless by exigency of size and location, stretching of surrounding tissue occurs. They are not reddened unless by external injury. Their disappearance is macroscopically complete, leaving no discoloration. Early in their development a useful method of detecting them is by moving the skin back and forth over the suspected area. They will appear as little elevations often a bit shiny, not moving with the skin. To verify the presence of a nodule over a bony point, one may compress it between the nails of the forefingers. Even a small nodule gives a feel different from skin and subcutaneous tissue. The growth of individual nodules and the appearance of fresh crops may be rapid, and their disappearance equally so, or they may persist month after month without striking changes.

Histologically, according to Coombs,[8] they are composed of a groundwork of fibrin with multinuclear fusiform cells, together

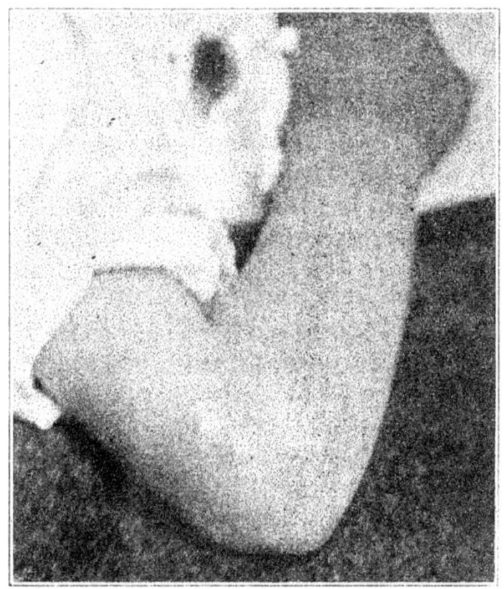

FIG. 1.—L. K., No. 10 of our series.

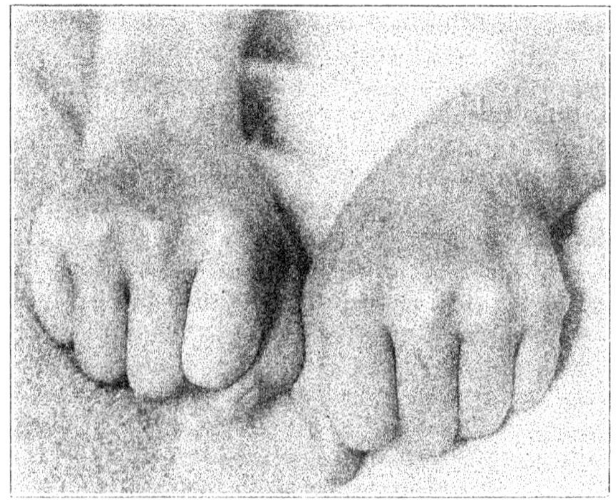

FIG. 2.—H. M., No. 12 of our series.

with leukocytes and plasma cells. Barlow and Warner regarded them as "organizing granulation tissue, homologous with the

[8] Jour. Path. and Bacteriol., 1910, **15**, 489.

inflammatory exudate forming the basis of vegetation on the cardiac valves." According to Coombs and also Jacki,[9] their structure more closely resembles that of the Aschoff bodies in the heart muscle, and, like the latter, they represent a local tissue reaction to the unknown etiological agent of rheumatic fever.

We were able to secure only one necropsy, J. B., No. 34 of our series.

History. An Italian boy, aged eleven years, who came to America one year before his final illness.

Family History. Father and mother and three other children are fairly healthy. No other rheumatic incidence.

Past History. Since he was left in Italy when his people came to this country, the history was obtained chiefly from the boy himself. He stated that his first attack of rheumatism (swollen joints) was seven years ago, when he was kept in bed nine months, and was very ill. He had seven other attacks of arthritis before coming to this country. Once for a few weeks he had, apparently, chorea. He denied ever suffering from sore throat. His relatives stated that the nodules on his elbows had been present on arrival to this country.

Present Illness. He was first seen by one of us (E. B.) July 2, 1921, walking into the office, though looking a very ill boy. He had no fever. He had been in a San Francisco hospital for one month and discharged improved about two weeks previously. The instructions given him had been entirely disregarded, with a rapid return of the signs of cardiac failure. He complained especially of sharp pains occurring almost daily over his left upper chest and inability to sleep.

The signs of venous engorgement in the neck were extreme. His body moved with each cardiac contraction. The carotid and brachial pulsations were visible at a distance, and the blanching and reddening of the lips and nails needed no tests for elicitation. Visible cardiac fluttering impulse and retraction from the third interspace at the right of the sternum to the sixth interspace on the left measured $25\frac{1}{2}$ cm. The ankles pitted on pressure. There was no tenderness. The liver reached nearly to the umbilicus. The pulse counted 148 and was typically aortic. Respirations, 64. Over the aortic area was felt a very striking thrill. None was found over the apex beat. At the apex the first sound was weak rather than exaggerated, and had a gallop rhythm. The second sound was also poorly differentiated. There was a systolic-diastolic blow of no great intensity, and no presystolic rumble. In the aortic area the first sound was accompanied by a rumbling, rough systolic murmur. The second sound was exceedingly sharp and

[9] Frankfürter Ztschr. f. Path., 1919, **22**, 82.

ended in a diastolic blow of typically aortic quality. No extracardial murmur was heard. Though retractions of the interspaces over the precordium accompanied the apex impulse, no retraction of the interspaces over the back could be made out.

Rheumatic nodules of moderate size were present over elbows, knuckles of fingers and spinous processes. There were none over knees and head. He thought they had been bigger than at present.

Progress. Hospital care was refused. He was put to bed and kept quiet with codein. Free catharsis was used. In two days the heart rate dropped to 110 and respirations to 30 to the minute. The venous enlargement in the neck had decreased, and the liver was nearly up to the costal margin. The third day a circinate erythema of rheumatic type appeared, and he complained of pain in knees and ankles, and tenderness to touch. His temperature was around 38° C. No fresh nodules were found.

His family were finally persuaded of the necessity of hospital care, and he was referred to the Children's Hospital, on the service of Dr. Rachel Ash, whom I have to thank for further progress notes:

Blood. Hemoglobin, 60 per cent; red blood cells, 3,296,000; leukocytes, 18,650, of which 75 per cent were polymorphonuclears.

Blood-pressure. Systolic, 105, diastolic: sounds loudly heard to zero.

Urine. Examination negative.

Two days after admission he was put on 20 minims. of tincture of digitalis three times a day. In a week this was increased to four times a day. The pulse record showed no slowing, in fact a slight increase in average rate after digitalis was started. He continued to run a low-grade septic temperature. A troublesome cough and signs of bronchitis developed. The intern's notes stated that the pulse had become irregular, but the type of irregularity was not recorded.

On July 30, about three weeks after admission, the notes say that "Marked dulness was noted over the left posterior chest and also marked impairment of resonance through the right posterior chest." He became very uncomfortable, though he did not complain of pain. The pulse was slow and irregular and became weaker. Friction rubs were heard over the entire chest. Heroin and morphin were given for the restlessness. A thoracentesis was done in the late afternoon and a few centimeters of blood withdrawn. He expectorated blood and died a few minutes afterward.

Clinical Diagnosis. Aortic stenosis and insufficiency, mitral stenosis, adhesive pericarditis.

Pathological Report. Autopsy No. A21, 137, Dr. W. A. Perkins.

The body was that of a very well-developed and nourished boy of eleven years, somewhat above the average in size. The general external examination was negative except for a few small hard nodules about each elbow. Of these one of a symmetrical pair measured about $\frac{3}{4}$ cm. in diameter, and was situated over the posterior border of each ulna about 4 cm. from the tip of the elbow. The others were smaller and were situated over the apex of each internal condyle. All of the nodules were rounded, flattened and firmly fixed to the deeper soft tissues, but not to the bone. An attempt was made to dissect out one of the larger nodules through a small skin incision; as the dissection proceeded the nodule grew less and less distinct until no definite nodule could be made out. A bit of tissue, however, was removed from this region, including the subjacent periosteum and bone, and sections made for microscopic study.

The abdominal cavity was negative. The right pleural cavity contained about 200 cc of dark fluid blood and a small-sized clot, the latter lying between the base of the lung and the diaphragm; there were also several fibrous adhesions at the apex and base. The left pleural cavity was considerably encroached upon by a large heart; there were a few fibrous adhesions at the apex. The pericardial cavity was obliterated by dense fibrous adhesions.

Thymus. Rather large; tissue grossly negative.

Heart. Greatly enlarged, weight with adherent pericardium 1000 grams. The fused parietal and visceral pericardia formed a layer of varying thickness from 3 mm. over the left ventricle to 7 mm. over the right auricle, the two layers being readily distinguished and bound together by a third central thicker layer of translucent, edematous but tough connective tissue. Myocardium hypertrophied throughout and in the following ascending order: Right auricle, right ventricle, left auricle and left ventricle; the right ventricle measured 4.5 mm., the left ventricle 1 cm.; the tissue was rather pale brown, firm, tough and marked with a few small lighter colored depressed fibrous areas. Endocardium showed a slight, irregular, superficial fibrosis just below the aortic valve in the left ventricle. Heart cavities: there was a slight dilatation of the right auricle, a marked dilatation of the left ventricle, the latter encroaching upon the right ventricle. Valves: tricuspid valve-leaflets showed no thickening; the angle between the septal and infundibular cusps was bound down by what appeared to be short anomalous chordæ tendineæ; there was no evidence of any concomitant inflammatory process; the valve measured 10 cm.; Pulmonary valve appeared normal; measured 7.5 cm. Mitral valve showed a marked fairly uniform fibrous thickening of the leaflets, particularly of the anterior leaflet, with a shrinking up and disappearance from the latter of the accessory velum, resulting in the attachment of the chordæ directly on the free border of the cusp; this border appeared finely granular, rounded and somewhat thickened; neither mitral leaflet was much distorted, though there was a relative narrowing of the orifice; this measured 9.5 cm.; the chordæ in several instances, and particularly in the case of those inserted into the anterior leaflet, were moderately thickened. Aortic valve: the cusps were all symmetrically and markedly thickened and retracted with, in addition, fibrous adhesions at the leaflet angles, the whole resulting in a narrowing and an insufficiency of the orifice. Coronary vessels possessed ample lumina no macroscopic sclerosis.

Aorta. The arch appeared moderately dilated, the intima smooth and normal.

Lungs. Right lung: pleural surface smooth except in region of adhesions about apex and base; upper lobe: pink gray in color with the posterior portions somewhat darker; on section the anterior portion of the lobe appeared slightly emphysematous, the posterior portion moderately congested, containing a slight excess of frothy blood-tinged fluid; mid-lobe emphysematous, external and cut surfaces gray, tissue dry, hypercrepitant; lower lobe on the external surface, at about mid-point, just lateral to the posterior border, is a small, roughly, quadrangular dark blue firm area about 1 x 1½ cm., marked by three small puncture wounds; section through this area showed continuation of the dark hemorrhagic discoloration into the lung tissue for a distance of 1½ cm. and ending in the region of a relatively large vein; the lower lobe otherwise resembled the upper but with the appearance of congestion somewhat more marked. Pulmonary vessels: negative; bronchus and branches contained a small amount of blood-tinged mucus; the bronchial branches of the middle lobe contained in addition two or three blood clots. Left lung considerably smaller than the right; pleural surface smooth except for apical adhesions; upper lobe showed a congested anterior portion and a slightly emphysematous posterior border; lower lobe, in addition to congestion, presented a moderate grade of atelectasis owing to compression from the enlarged heart; pulmonary vessels and bronchial branches same as on the right, except that the latter contained no blood clots.

Liver. Enlarged, estimated weight 2000 grams; upper surface roughened by adhesions and marked by a few small scattered seed-like nodules, the latter 1 mm. in diameter, with opaque yellow centers and pale translucent peripheries; cut surface of liver mottled dark red and brown, the lobules large and conspicuous, each with a large reddish center, and a brown periphery; tissue consistency normal.

Gall-bladder. Negative.

Spleen. Enlarged; estimated weight, 200 grams; surface roughened by fibrous adhesions; cut surface a mottled purple and dark red, the pulp soft, increased in amount; considerable scraping away on the knife, the connective-tissue elements conspicuous; the lymphoid elements less prominent; scattered over the cut surface were seen fairly numerous small, hard, calcareous, opaque orange-yellow nodules, similar to those in the liver capsule.

Gastrointestinal Tract. Appeared negative.

Pancreas. Firm; on section there appeared to be a moderate increase in the interlobular connective tissue.

Adrenals. Appeared normal.

Kidneys. About normal size; estimated combined weight 250 grams; right kidney: capsule stripped smoothly leaving a rather dark red lobulated surface; cut surface showed normal markings; cortex, 5 mm. thick; glomeruli present as red points; medulla normal; pelvis negative. Left kidney resembled right.

Bladder. Prostate, testes and epididymes not examined.

Culture from heart's blood was negative.

Thymus. Negative.

Heart. Pericardium: the three layers as described in the gross were readily distinguished, an outer layer of dense hyaline connective tissue, covered superficially with a less dense vascular fatty tissue (the parietal pericardium), an inner layer of areolar connective tissue containing fairly numerous scattered strands of compact hyaline connective tissue and a large number of small injected bloodvessels (the visceral pericardium) and a central layer of edematous granulation tissue containing occasional small, irregular masses of fibrin. All these layers were infiltrated with leukocytes, the inner and central layers particularly. Lymphocytes and plasma cells predominated, though in the central layer polymorphonuclear leukocytes became fairly numerous, while occasionally associated with the fibrin masses were seen large endothelial-like cells with one and sometimes two or three large vesicular nuclei. The cellular exudate extended sparsely into the stroma of the subjacent myocardium. Myocardium: the muscle fibers were generally thickened and hypertrophied and for the most part well preserved; in many places, however, and particularly in the region of the small vessels, fragments only of muscle fibers remained, the rest having been replaced by connective tissue. These replacement scars were comparatively small and irregularly diffuse in their distribution. Furthermore, throughout they showed a moderately extensive infiltration with lymphocytes, plasma cells, eosinophiles, a few polymorphonuclear leukocytes and fairly numerous endothelioid cells. The last named were relatively large, round, oval or more or less elongated cells with abundant cytoplasm and large vesicular nuclei; most of them contained one nucleus; several, however, contained more than one, often appearing as actual giant cells. These endothelioid cells occurred usually in groups and near small bloodvessels, thus forming the so-called Aschoff bodies. (See microphotographs herewith.) The latter are so characteristically present in acute rheumatism involving the heart that the process is called by some rheumatic carditis. The accompanying illustrations show two such bodies, one composed of mononuclear endothelioid cells, the other containing some giant forms as well, and both typically situated in the neighborhood of small bloodvessels. Several of the vessels showed an irregular thickening of the intima, with encroachment on their lumina; there were no thrombi.

Heart Valves. A section through one of the segments of the mitral valve showed this composed of a fairly dense connective tissue in which were seen small bloodvessels that extended well out almost to the free edge of the cusp. There were also present several moderately sized elongated mononuclear cells arranged in a narrow zone near the ventricular surface of the valve while along the auricular surface were seen in one or two places scattered lymphocytes. At the attached border of the cusp there was a fairly abundant infiltration with lymphocytes and larger mononuclear cells and occasional polymorphonuclear leukocytes occurring chiefly as small perivascular foci. A similar cellular infiltration was present in the adjacent myocardium and endocardium. In addition, Aschoff bodies were seen in the myocardium, while a suggestion of such bodies was noted in several places in the endocardium. A second section through another region of the mitral valve showed an inflammatory process similar to the above except that the reaction appeared more acute, as evidenced by the presence of a larger number of polymorphonuclear leukocytes.

The lungs presented the picture of chronic passive congestion with injected tortuous capillaries and alveoli partly filled with serum and moderate numbers of heart failure cells. In addition certain areas showed a slight grade of atelectasis, others a definite emphysema. A section through the lower lobe of the right lung in the region of the puncture wounds mentioned in the gross description showed a marked hemorrhage into all the alveoli, while in the center of this hemorrhagic area several fairly large vessels were noted engorged with blood.

Liver. The central veins and the sinusoids, except those immediately surrounding the portal spaces, were congested, the liver trabeculæ compressed, the portal spaces themselves infiltrated with lymphocytes and a few plasma cells. Section through one of the seed-like nodules in the capsule mentioned in the gross showed concentrically arranged hyaline connective tissue with a softened necrotic center.

Spleen. There was a diffuse increase in connective tissue; the pulp contained an excess of red blood cells, while an occasional nodule similar to that in the liver capsule was found outlined by a band of hyaline connective tissue, but with a relatively large center composed of amorphous material and containing some lime salts. These nodules occurred singly or in groups of two or three. Associated with them was a slight inflammatory reaction consisting of lymphocytes and a rare giant cell, the latter with peripherally arranged nuclei. The process in both liver and spleen probably represents the end result of a previous tuberculous infection.

Pancreas. The vessels were congested, the interstitial connective tissue infiltrated with a moderate amount of hemorrhage, probably artefact.

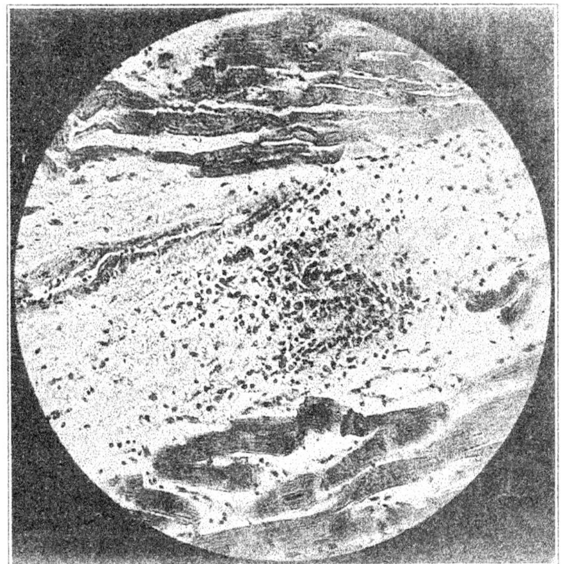

FIG. 3.—Aschoff bodies.

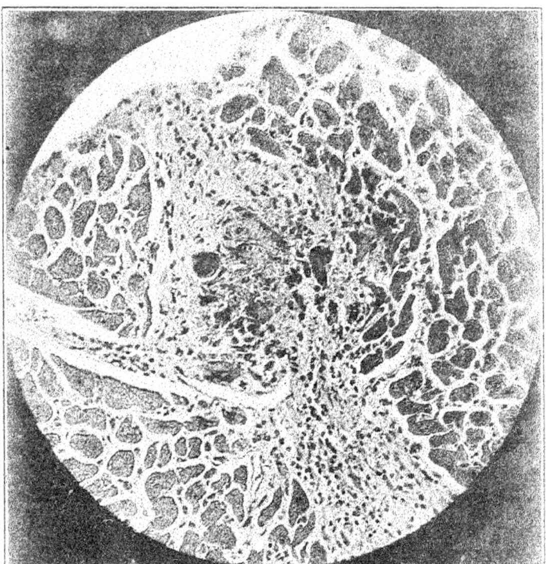

FIG. 4.—Aschoff bodies.

Kidneys. The tubular epithelium showed cloudy swelling; most of the tubules contained a finely granular albuminous material; the vessels were injected; the glomeruli generally were large.

Lymph Node. Congested.

Subcutaneous nodules: sections were negative, showing only normal bone, periosteum and striated muscle. In view of these findings, it is suggested that such nodules be removed "en bloc" without attempted dissection.

PATHOLOGICAL DIAGNOSIS. Subcutaneous rheumatic nodules about elbows; marked subacute and chronic fibrous obliterative pericarditis; diffuse fibrous myocarditis (rheumatic type); chronic mitral and aortic endocarditis, with stenosis and insufficiency; congenital adhesions at the septo-infundibular angle of the tricuspid valve; marked myocardial hypertrophy, especially of the left ventricle; marked dilatation of the left ventricle; general chronic passive congestion; fibrosis of spleen; parenchymatous degeneration of the viscera; multiple miliary calcareous nodules in liver and spleen; bilateral fibrous pleural adhesions; puncture wounds in lower lobe of right lung, with right hemothorax.

Discussion. The presence of a few isolated nodules which disappear with the subsidence of arthritic and cardiac symptoms may or may not be of great significance. Our personal experience is not prolonged sufficiently to pass judgment. We can say, however, that all cases which, while under observation, have had recurring crops of nodules have shown serious and progressive cardiac damage. Fibroid nodules seem to occur frequently in that subacute type of rheumatic infection in which an apparently mild carditis, with little if any rise in temperature, and with no severe joint symptoms, develops into a crippling stenosis, damaged muscle or adherent pericardium. The case with acute onset, high fever, red, swollen joints and rapid heart, with the murmur of regurgitation which responds to treatment and makes a good recovery, remaining without rheumatic symptoms until another similar acute attack occurs, much more rarely shows nodules.

We believe that recurring rheumatic nodules are of more prognostic value than any other one sign in rheumatism. They are our most significant warning that we are dealing with a serious infection which will probably result in great cardiac inefficiency if not in death.*

Summary. In 38 instances of rheumatic cycle cases seen between September, 1919, and September, 1921, fibroid subcutaneous nodules were present in 17, or 44.7 per cent.

Of those patients having nodules, 6, or 35.9 per cent, died during this period. In only one instance did death occur in a patient not having nodules.

* We feel that we owe an apology to such pioneers as Sir Thomas Barlow for attempting to draw conclusions from the study of a rather small selected group of cases observed during the brief period of two years.

Of the 38 cases, 17 were grouped as having serious cardiac damage. Of these 17, 13, or 76.5 per cent, had nodules.

Our series of cases probably includes an abnormally large proportion of a severe type of infection, and should not be judged as entirely representative of the usual incidence of nodules in this part of the world.*

LINITIS PLASTICA—WITH REPORT OF TWO CASES.

By Albert F. R. Andresen, M.D., F.A.C.P.
BROOKLYN, NEW YORK.

(From the Gastro-Enterological Department, Long Island College Hospital.)

The term linitis plastica was first used by Lewis Brinton in 1854 to describe a diffuse or circumscribed increase in the connective tissue of the stomach, involving chiefly the submucosa, and, to a lesser degree, the other layers, with marked thickening of the walls of the stomach, a diminution (rarely an increase) in the size of its lumen, and characterized by an insidious onset, a slowly progressive cachexia, and a fatal termination. Fully twenty-two other terms have been used to describe this condition, the most suggestive of which are: leather bottle stomach, chronic interstitial gastritis, cirrhosis of the stomach, fibroid induration of the stomach and chronic stenosing gastritis.

Although this condition of the stomach had occasionally been described in medical literature before Brinton's time, namely by Lieutaud in 1779, by Andral and Cruveilheir in 1829, and more frequently by other writers after 1829, the credit for recognizing and naming it as a separate disease belongs to Brinton. The most exhaustive study of this disease since Brinton's time was probably that made by H. M. Lyle in 1911, when he described 131 cases gathered from literature, and added 1 case of his own. Since this time not more than a dozen cases have been reported.

Pathology. There has been considerable difference of opinion regarding the classification of cases of linitis plastica. Diffuse carcinoma of the gastric wall produces a condition which is almost identical with the benign type, and some authorities claim that all cases are malignant. Others claim that only the benign cases can rightly be called linitis plastica. Most writers now agree, however, that to both the benign and malignant types the term linitis plastica may properly be applied, Lyle's study, mentioned above, being based on a total of 114 carefully studied cases, of

* We have to thank Dr. William Palmer Lucas, Dr. Florence Holsclaw, Dr. Rachel L. Ash and Dr. Langley Porter for allowing us to study past histories and for inviting us to follow many of the rheumatic cycle cases on their services.

which 62 were benign and 52 malignant. The benign cases of this disease may be of two types, the localized and the generalized. The former type, occurring in the form of small placques, is rare. In the generalized type, except in the rare instances where there is a dilatation as a result of pyloric stenosis, the stomach is found to be hard, rigid and contracted, with thickened and inelastic walls, stomachs as small as 4 inches long, by 2 inches wide, and walls 1 inch thick, with a capacity of not more than 4 ounces, having been reported. The normal stomach is 12 by 5 inches, the wall $\frac{1}{5}$-inch thick, and capacity 40 ounces.

The thickening of the walls usually commences at the pylorus, and spreads toward the cardia. It does not, as a rule, involve the duodenum, but may involve the esophagus. The tissues are grayish in color and there is often an associated adhesive peritonitis. Analogous lesions may be found in the large or small intestines.

Microscopically, the connective tissue of the submucosa is found to be hypertrophied, often causing atrophic, inflammatory or cystic changes in the mucosa. The submucosa shows an interlacing endarteritis, this, with the connective tissue change, producing the weave-like, interlacing effect from the appearance of which the name linitis was coined.

Nests of epithelial cells, possibly portions of gastric glands or mucosa which have become isolated, occur in the submucosa. These closely resemble carcinomatous areas, and may frequently have led to confusion in diagnosis. The connective tissue hypertrophy extends through the muscular coats, causing atrophy of the muscular fibers, and infiltrates the subserosa. The neighboring lymph glands show a fibrosis. In the malignant cases the lesion is an interstitial carcinomatosis, the gross effect being the same as in the benign cases. Gastric syphilis may also occur in the same form.

Etiology. Linitis plastica is a disease occurring in persons of carcinoma age, nearly all cases reported being between the ages of forty and sixty. It affects males twice as frequently as females. Usually there is a history of some previous condition which may have some etiological significance, such as cardiovascular disease, alcoholism, gastric ulcer, syphilis, tuberculosis or occupational trauma.

Symptoms. These are not characteristic, there being a gradually increasing train of dyspeptic symptoms, with anorexia, nausea, upper abdominal discomfort or pain, vomiting attacks, alternate constipation and diarrhea, and a more or less marked secondary anemia—in short, the general symptoms are those of the achylia gastrica which is usually present. Vomiting of blood rarely occurs. A symptom which is very suggestive, being a direct result of the actual diminution in size of the stomach and the inelasticity of its walls, is the feeling of fulness after the ingestion of even very small quantities of food, and the vomiting or regurgitation of any excess above a certain amount; the small quantities may, however, be very frequently repeated without discomfort, due to the rapid emptying of the stomach. Ascites may develop later. The duration of the symptoms before a patient seeks medical advice may vary from a month to a couple of years, during which there has occurred progressive anemia and loss of weight and strength.

Diagnosis. The only symptom which is of aid in the diagnosis is that due to the small capacity of the stomach, mentioned above. In advanced cases a sausage-like tumor may be felt lying transversely in the epigastrium. On inflating the stomach, or injecting water into it through a tube, the air or water may be felt gurgling rapidly through this mass. Even where there is no mass to be felt, the rapid transverse passage of the air or water into the duodenum can often be made out, and is of diagnostic value.

The test-meal examination shows the rapid emptying of the stomach and the absence or reduction of the hydrochloric acid. Lactic acid is present only in the rare cases where dilatation and consequent stasis have occurred. Fluoroscopical examination shows the small size stomach, with marked hypermotility, the barium mixture passing rapidly across the upper abdomen and filling the intestinal coils. Roentgenography will show the small tube-like stomach, its walls rigid, and with no evidence of peristaltic waves.

Although the diagnosis has been rather rarely made before operation or autopsy, the above findings, in a patient of middle age, may justify a presumptive diagnosis of linitis plastica. Whether the condition is benign or malignant can only be determined by microscopical examination, and is of no great importance in the treatment, this being the same in both types.

Linitis plastica must be differentiated from a movable kidney or spleen, pyloric carcinoma or ulcer, pyloric syphilis, malignancy or excessive mobility of the transverse colon, chronic adhesive or tuberculous peritonitis, and portal cirrhosis.

The *prognosis* is not good. The condition is progressive, and even with the removal of the gastric focus there may be progressive changes in the foci in the colon, rectum or small intestine, causing stenosis. The average length of life for the benign cases is four years, for the malignant cases, two years.

The *treatment* is operative. A gastrectomy should be performed, either primarily, or, in advanced cases, after a primary jejunostomy has permitted the patient's nutrition to be improved sufficiently by jejunal feeding, to render him operable.

As a preliminary to operation, where the pylorus is sufficiently patent to permit the passage of a tube, duodenal feeding is indicated. If the tube will not pass, the gastric motor efficiency still remaining should be tested out by injecting into the stomach, through a Rehfuss gastric tube, measured amounts of fluid until the stomach is filled, and then aspirating the fluid remaining after a definite interval, to see the amount the stomach has evacuated during that period of time. The exact amount and frequency of feedings can thus be determined, and concentrated liquid nourishment can thus be given. In the writer's first case, described below, 1½ ounces of a concentrated solution of dextrose, peptones, alcohol and fats was given through the tube or by mouth every fifteen minutes, and easily taken care of by the patient, so that by this method, combined with rectal feeding, 100 to 150 ounces of liquid, containing over 2500 calories was administered every twenty-four hours for several days, until the patient was considered to be in operable condition.

Case I.—A. H., female, aged thirty-eight years, a housewife, married ten years, denied venereal infection, but admitted a few self-induced abortions. She had been in the "show business" for years, and had been more or less addicted to alcohol and late suppers. Except for malarial fever sixteen years before, she had always been healthy, and weighed 180 pounds when, in 1911, at the age of thirty-five, she had an attack of pain, vomiting and jaundice, called gall stones by her physician. After that she had had occasional slight digestive disturbances. She was first seen by me at the Brooklyn Hospital in the early part of 1914, when she was suffering from epigastric pains immediately after eating, going through to the back, vomiting forty minutes after eating, sour regurgitation, constipation, and loss of weight, which symptoms had been persistent for about six months. Examination showed a moderate pyorrhea; head and chest were negative. The abdomen was flabby, distended with gas, and tender in the epigastrium and to the right. No masses were discernible. Pelvic examination was negative. Rectal examination showed an anal fissure and a rectal polyp. The systolic blood-pressure was 105, the diastolic 70. The blood showed a secondary anemia and a negative Wassermann reaction. Repeated test-meals showed a total achylia, with marked hypermotility. The string test was negative. There was no occult blood in the stools. The urine contained an excess of indican. Fluoroscopy showed the stomach small, slightly ptosed, with a very small fundus and a narrow tube-like passage continuous with the duodenum, through which the barium passed with great rapidity, although no peristaltic waves were visible. One hour after the examination the patient took tea and crackers, which were vomited, but no barium was present in the vomitus, showing the rapid emptying of the stomach. The patient at this time was weighing about 100 pounds, being 80 pounds underweight. A provisional diagnosis of hyperperistalsis, due to some reflex irritation, was made, but the possibility of a linitis plastica being present, mentioned. The rectal polyp was removed, to exclude this as a reflex cause, but no relief resulted. On July 1, 1914, Dr. John H. Long performed an exploratory laparotomy. The stomach was found to be somewhat smaller than normal, with greatly hypertrophied walls, thought to be due to hyperperistalsis resulting from the pylorus being bound to the gall-bladder with dense adhesions. The adhesions were freed, but the gall-bladder, being found hard, but patent, was left in. The interior of the stomach was explored through an incision in its anterior wall, but nothing was found. The appendix was removed. The patient improved markedly after this operation, but weighed only 89 pounds on her discharge from the hospital.

In the next six months she gained 25 pounds, and some hydrochloric acid began to appear in the stomach contents. Then she began again to have epigastric pain, vomiting and loss of weight, dropping to 91 pounds in November, 1915. She continued to get worse, and was lost track of until May, 1916, during which time she had been abandoned as an inoperable carcinoma case and reduced to a moribund condition. She was retching and vomiting constantly, urinating a few ounces at a time every twenty-four to forty-eight hours, and having a bowel movement once in ten days, when next seen by me. No mass could be palpated, although emaciation was the most extreme the writer had ever seen. With a duodenal tube in the stomach, it was found that but 1 ounce of fluid could be injected into that organ at one time, any excess being regurgitated through or alongside the tube. This amount of fluid was gone from the stomach, however, in fifteen minutes on repeated tests. The fluid removed from the stomach was anacidic and contained a little occult blood. The tube would not enter the duodenum. Inflation through the tube disclosed the slight distention at the point of the 1 ounce cavity, and then a rapid bubbling of the air across the epigastrium, apparently to another larger cavity, to the right. A diagnosis of linitis plastica, with hour-glass constriction due to scar formation at the point of the gastrotomy, was then made. The patient was too weak for roentgenography. She was fed 1 ounce of a solution of dextrose, peptones and alcohol every fifteen minutes, and as much dextrose solution per rectum as could be retained. She thus received 2500 calories or more per diem for nearly three weeks during which time the capacity of the stomach was increased to 1½ ounces, Dr. Long at this time considering conditions sufficiently improved to warrant the slight amount of shock occasioned by the procedure, did a duodenostomy under local anesthesia, the patient receiving a hypodermocylsis during the operation. He expected to do a gastrectomy later, but the patient died suddenly twenty-four hours after the operation, apparently from uremia.

The principal abnormal findings at autopsy were as follows: The stomach was found buried in adhesions to the liver, gall-bladder, pancreas and abdominal wall. On freeing it, the stomach was found to measure 5 inches in length from cardia to pylorus and $2\frac{1}{2}$ inches in width. The fundus had a capacity of $1\frac{1}{2}$ ounces, and about 2 inches from the cardia the stomach became narrow, with a tough wall $\frac{1}{2}$ inch thick and deep rugæ, this excessively thickened area corresponding to the gastrotomy scar (Fig. 1). The pylorus was fibrous and hard. A finger introduced into the cardia revealed an obstruction at 2 inches, which permitted only a match to pass through it. The microscopical findings were typical of those described for the benign type of linitis plastica. The duodenum was found adherent to the gall-bladder and pancreas, but was otherwise normal. The terminal ileum was reduced to a

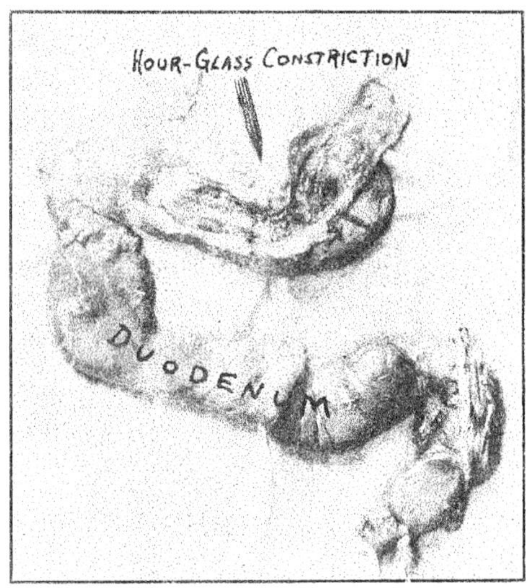

FIG. 1.—Stomach viewed from front. Thickness of wall shown where cut edge is everted. Capacity $1\frac{1}{2}$ oz. Duodenostomy at lower right corner.

fibrous cord, but was patent. The colon was negative. The left ovary was cystic.

This case therefore presented the unusual condition of an hour-glass constriction occurring in the course of linitis plastica.

CASE II.—M. A., female, aged fifty-seven years, Irish, housewife, applied at the Long Island College Hospital for treatment November 20, 1921. She had been married thirty-six years had had seven children and four self-induced miscarriages. Her family history was negative. She had always been healthy except for some minor postpartum infections and an attack of mild arthritis as a young woman. The nervous symptoms of the menopause had been continuous since the cessation of menstruation at age of fifty. She had never eaten much meat, but had indulged moderately in wine and whisky.

In June, 1921, the patient, after a short period of anorexia, had begun to have attacks of diarrhea, with loose watery stools after meals. There was also a pain in the epigastrium, and to the left, increased immediately by taking food or by lying on her back. For two weeks before admission there had been a very marked nausea and the regurgitation of all food taken above a certain moderate amount. There had been a steady loss of weight and strength.

Examination showed an emaciated, weak, pale woman, with all false teeth; infected, cryptic tonsils; normal heart and lungs and no glandular enlargements. Blood-pressure, systolic 122, diastolic 72. Her abdomen was not distended, and there was a sausage-like, hard mass about 1½ by 3 inches, lying transversely across the epigastrium. This mass was movable and not attached to the abdominal wall and was slightly tender on firm pressure. The appendix region was also tender. Pelvic examination showed a lacerated cervic and an old parametritis. There were no other abnormal physical findings.

Laboratory findings were as follows:

Urinalysis and renal function tests negative.

Gastric analysis by fractional method showed a true achylia gastrica with blood present in all specimens removed.

Blood count showed a moderate anemia and the Wassermann reaction was negative. Blood chemistry was normal.

Roentgenological examination showed on fluoroscopy a stomach constricted in its middle portion for about 3 inches, with cardiac and pyloric ends and duodenum somewhat dilated, the barium meal passing rapidly through the constricted area. The roentgenograms showed this deformity with the outline of the constricted area perfectly smooth (Fig. 2). The stomach emptied rapidly and the colon was negative except for some retention of barium in the appendix after forty-eight hours.

Operation, November 16, 1921, by Dr. Emil Goetsch, under local anesthesia, showed at once several large omental glands along greater curvature of stomach, one of which on removal showed carcinomatous changes. The entire stomach, with the exception of slightly dilated portions at the cardia and pylorus, was one large hard mass and there were numerous glands palpable in the omentum, although no liver metastases were found. The abdomen was closed without further procedures.

Following operation, the patient continued to vomit, and a month later began to have gastric hemorrhages every few days. Only small amounts of liquid could be taken at one time and the patient was merely sustained by the use of morphin and alcohol. She died February 16, 1922, three months after operation.

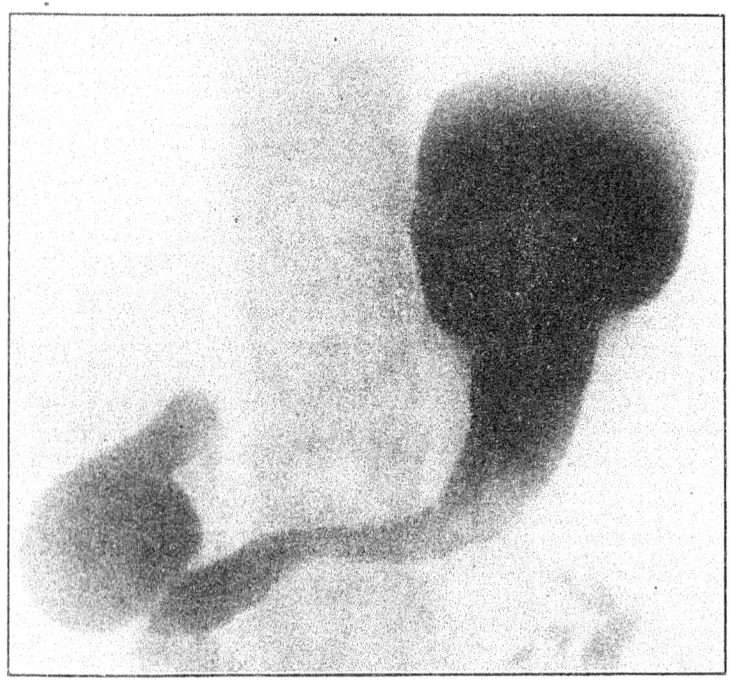

FIG. 2.—Roentgenograph of stomach immediately after barium meal. Pouches of cardia and pyloric antrum, with constricted area.

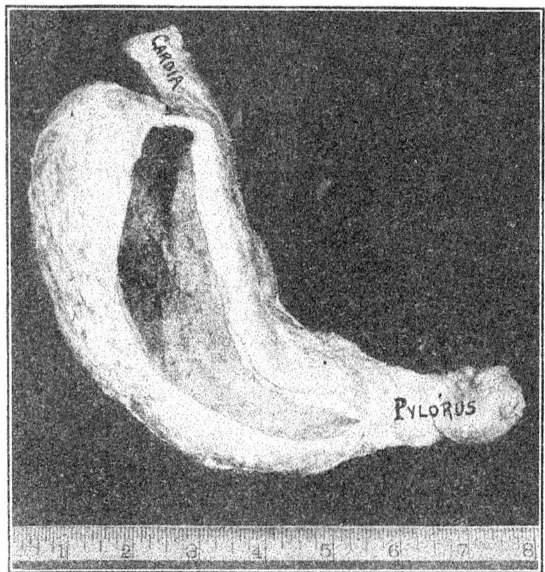

FIG. 3.—Stomach viewed from back. Everted cut edge shows thickness of wall. Dark area in mucosa is vascular, superficial ulcer which caused hemorrhages. Capacity 3 oz.

Autopsy (by Dr. A. Murray): The only abnormal findings besides those in the stomach were a brown atrophy of the heart and a chronic passive congestion of the liver and signs of senile

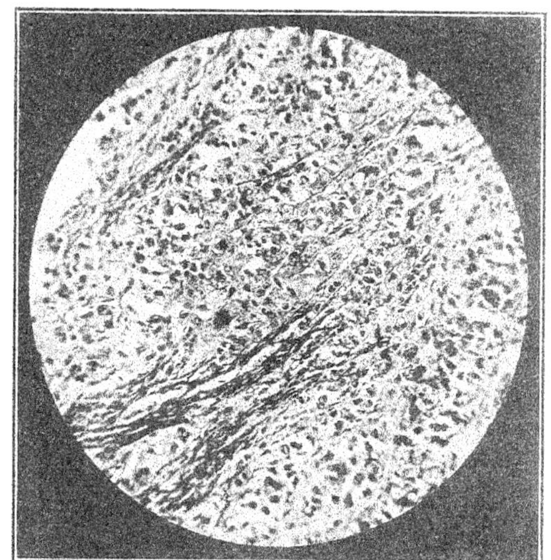

FIG. 4.—Microscopic Section of the Stomach. Low power.

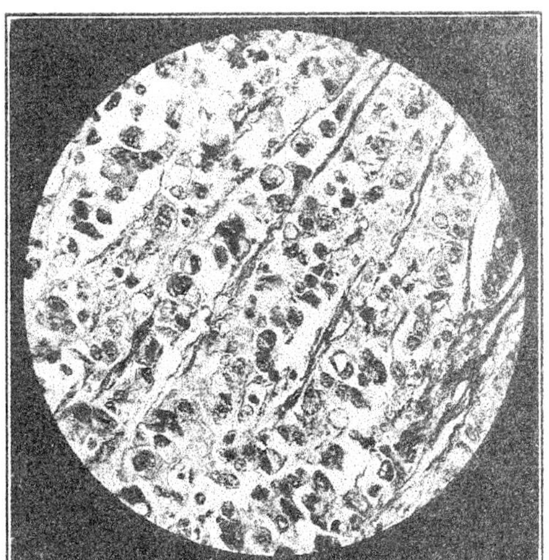

FIG. 5.—Microscopic Section of the Stomach. High power.

atheroma of the aorta. The esophagus was normal. The stomach was 20 cm. long and 8 cm. in diameter and had a normal outline (Fig. 3). Its walls were uniformly infiltrated and made dense by what appeared to be carcinoma. The surface was covered by pearly white nodules loosely adherent to surrounding structures. The mucosa at the cardia was congested and apparently hemorrhagic. A large ill-defined ulcer covered with foul necrotic slough was present on the middle portion of the anterior wall. The distal 3 cm. of the stomach, the duodenum and the rest of the alimentary tract appeared normal. The root of the omentum was densely infiltrated with new growth, as were the retroperitoneal lymph nodes along their entire length. The abdominal aorta was large and replaced by tumor. Microscopical examination of the stomach (Figs. 4 and 5): All layers were uniformly and completely invaded by carcinoma so that only traces of the original structure remained. Nerves, bloodvessels and the islands of the muscularis mucosæ were left intact. The epitheleum was wanting from the mucosa and there were few lymphoid nodules in the submucosa. In the muscular wall, cords of tumor cells had entirely replaced muscle bundles, but had followed their course, so that the tumor cords had the arrangement of the original muscle bundles.

The carcinoma was of the medullary type, with few distinct foci which were composed of columnar epithelial cells.

The heart showed brown atrophy, the liver, passive congestion. and the kidneys were arteriosclerotic.

Diagnosis. Carcinoma of the stomach, linitis plastica.

Summary. Two cases of linitis plastica, confirmed by autopsy, are reported.

BIBLIOGRAPHY.

Moynihan: Abdominal Operations, **1**, 332.
Tilzer, A.: Virchow's Arch., 1893, **122**, 290.
Boas, J.: Arch. f. Verdaungskr., 1898, **4**, 47.
Einhorn, M.: Ibid., 1900, **6**.
Hemmeter and Stokes: Ibid., 1901, **7**, 313.
Jonas, F.: Ibid., 1907, **13**, 591.
Von Sury, K.: Ibid., 1907, **13**, 1.
Lyle, H. M.: Ann. Surg., 1911, **54**, 625.
Johnson, A. B.: Ibid., 1912, **55**, 617.
Krompecher and Makai: Zentralbl. f. Chir., 1912, **2**, 377.
Soper, H. W.: Jour. Am. Med. Assn., 1913, **61**, 2060.
Bland-Sutton, J.: Brit. Med. Jour., 1914, **1**, 229.
Sailer, J.: Tr. Assn. Am. Phys., 1914, **29**, 102.
Northrup, H. L.: Hahnemann Month., 1915, **50**, 432.
Porter, M. F.: Ann. Surg., 1915, **72**, 33.
Sailer, J.: Am. Jour. Med. Sci., 1916, **151**, 321.
McGlannan, A.: Jour. Am. Med. Assn., 1916, **66**, 92.
Barrett, Gilbert M.: Jour. Am. Med. Assn., 1916, **67**, 276.
Handa, E. O.: Northwest Med., 1917, **16**, 197.
LeNoir, Richet and Langle: Abstract, Jour. Am. Med. Assn., 1920, **75**, 1163.
Ousley, J. M.: Jour. Missouri State Med. Assn., 1919, **16**, 53.

ACUTE PERFORATIONS OF STOMACH AND DUODENUM (WITH A REPORT OF SIXTY CASES).*

By Charles L. Gibson, M.D.
SURGEON TO THE NEW YORK HOSPITAL, NEW YORK.

A study of the results of operations for perforations of the stomach and duodenum shows very conclusively the value of prompt recognition and relief of this condition.

The 60 cases reported have been treated on the First Surgical Division of the New York Hospital from February 1, 1913 to April 30, 1922. The operators have been Drs. Gibson, Lee, Hitzrot and Farr. Fourteen of these cases were reported by me[1] in a paper published in 1916, and some of these cases were also reported in a paper by Dr. Farr[2] 1920.

The opinions expressed represent my personal views based on my experience since 1907 when I did my first operation for this condition.

The results obtained in this series confirm my previous belief of the desirability of aiming simply to close the perforation, leaving remote and problematical after results to be taken care of as necessity arises.

The mortality of the whole series, 16.6 per cent (Table I) is not high.

TABLE I.—MORTALITY RATE.

Cases.	Perforations.	Deaths.	Per cent.
43	12 hours	3	6.6 (2.3)
2	18 "		
5	24 "	1	20
10	Over 24 hours	6	60

It is particularly gratifying to note the small per cent, 6.6, in the first eighteen hours, only 3 out of 45 patients succumbing. In fact, the mortality really should be estimated as 2.3 per cent as 2 out of these 3 deaths occurred under conditions which would be thrown out by many writers in reporting their results. The relative benignity when recognized and operated early becomes evident.

Case 210312, male, aged fifty-eight years, gave a gastric history of twenty years duration; perforation of ten hours; showed marked collapse with cyanosis and weak irregular pulse and subnormal temperature on admission; rallied under morphin and operated on under gas-oxygen. The night after operation the patient got out of bed, walked across the ward, drank a glass of cold water and

* Read before the meeting of the American Surgical Association in Washington, May 2, 1922.

[1] Surg., Gynec. and Obst., April, 1916, p. 388.

[2] Ann. Surg., November, 1920.

collapsed. The temperature went to 105° F. and pulmonary edema developed. Death occurred a few hours later (autopsy).

Patient 220548 died forty-five days after operation, twenty-three days after an operation for empyema which could not be demonstrated to follow in any way the results of the first operation.

As will be pointed out later, I have never been in favor of performing a gastroenterostomy as a routine operation, although admitting its occasional necessity, and the low mortality of these early cases strengthens this belief and a study of the late results is also very satisfactory.

The particular points of interest in such a study will be to note: (1) Basis for early diagnosis. (2) Technical procedures, particularly in reference to the performance of gastroenterostomy. (3) After results and particularly bad results requiring further operative measures.

In regard to diagnosis we note in Table II, that the bulk of patients give a previous history of gastric disturbance, most of them of long standing.

TABLE II.—PREVIOUS GASTRIC DISTURBANCE.

	Gastric.	Duodenal.
No previous trouble	9	5
Trouble dating back less than a year	9	3
Trouble of long standing	9	21
Too ill to obtain a history	1	1
One previous attack five years ago, none since	0	1
Time indefinite, slight indigestion at times	0	1
	28	32

We note also that the onset is universally acute and that in all cases pain is given as the chief complaint, usually described as "knife-like." The symptoms in a typical case are unmistakable. Pain "in the pit of the stomach" comes on usually without premonition, is agonizing and often followed by considerable shock. Rather less than half of the patients vomit but vomiting has always been secondary to the pain. The vomitus rarely contains blood.

The patient becomes cold, sweats, and the facial expression reflects the great agony. Soon after these initial symptoms there comes probably quite often a symptom which is seldom described and seldom elicited because of its temporary duration and after it has disappeared the patient forgets about it as his attention is concentrated on the persisting abdominal pain. I refer to severe pain coming on within a few minutes of the perforation and felt in the supraclavicular fossa, usually the left. It lasts only a few minutes, seldom more than fifteen. Given a clear history of this pain with a sudden onset I feel there is no symptom that is more characteristic.

The next most marked feature is a retraction of the abdomen, board like rigidity of the upper half, and great tenderness to pressure. At this stage there are practically no other symptoms worthy of consideration. Much time is wasted by some practitioners at this stage on three perfectly worthless diagnostic features (1) temperature, which may be low, may be normal, or may be slightly increased; (2) changes in the white cell count of the blood, total leukocytosis, percentage of polynuclears and their relation to each other. These changes will not take place until later; (3) obliteration of the liver dulness, a beautiful theoretical symptom which I have never been able to demonstrate in any perforation of the gastro-intestinal tract from any cause and never expect to.

With the progress of the condition we have a sequence of symptoms which are those of a peritonitis. If a patient is seen twenty-four hours after the perforation and a clear history has not been obtained of the previous condition and of the initial symptoms, attention is frequently centered on the possibility of a peritonitis from a perforation of the appendix, and this possibility is emphasized by the mechanical gravitation of the exudate from the upper part of the abdomen down the right gutter, giving tenderness most intense over the right lower quadrant.

The above classical picture is not infrequently modified, symptoms being milder and the onset less clear cut. The alteration of symptoms probably depends a good deal on the physical conditions, being less in a minute perforation with a minimum of extravasation of gastric contents. Moreover, some of these minute perforations become plugged by omentum, greatly modifying the course of the condition.

The conditions which may simulate an acute perforation of the late type are those of an intra-abdominal lesion which would call for interference, particularly appendicitis, acute cholecystitis, acute pancreatitis, and acute bleeding of a gastro-duodenal ulcer. It must also be remembered that occasionally two acute abdominal conditions occur simultaneously. All the conditions just described would justify opening the abdomen even on a mistaken diagnosis as a chance is given to remedy an acute and often dangerous condition.

The most serious mistake and one which I have once personally committed is operating in the face of an impending pneumonia as the signs are often quite identical, the pulmonary physical signs being delayed in their onset and the history misleading. A sign which I have never seen described and have only lately thought of trying is auscultation over the pyloric region with the possibility of recognizing the to and fro passage of air from the stomach into the peritoneal cavity.

Diagnosis of the Condition When the Abdomen is Opened. When operating for a possible perforation or for any acute abdominal lesion that is obscure, I recommend the employment of a procedure which has been of great value to me for many years, namely opening the peritoneum under water. An incision is made down to the peritoneum which is seized between two clamps; the abdominal wound is flooded with water and peritoneum opened. Even the escape of a single bubble of air shows necessarily that there must be a communication with the gastro-intestinal tract.

On the other hand, there may be little or no air in the cavity and the perforation may be temporarily sealed off.

If there is any appreciable amount of fluid in the peritoneal cavity one is usually impressed with the oily or vaseline like character, sour smell, or possibly recognition of food particles, bile or other stomach contents. The administration of a teaspoonful of weak methylene blue solution by mouth just prior to giving the anesthetic is also of value as the stomach contents are easily stained by it.

Anesthesia. Anesthesia is that of the surgeon's choice. Personally I favor open ether, drop method, over all other forms.

Incision. The lesion being in the great majority of cases juxta pyloric, the incision is placed in the upper epigastrium to the right of midline. This should be a large incision, allowing of easy access to the perforation.

Operative Procedure. The perforation having been located usually with the greatest ease, the first thing in order is to close it. This statement may seem unnecessary but I have seen a lot of time wasted in sponging out the abdomen and puttering around while the hole is still discharging gastro-intestinal contents. Some operators report difficulty in closing these perforations; but so far I have been able always to close them securely, usually with mattress sutures or purse-string sutures of catgut. I occasionally feel more secure by fixing the sutured surface with some structure such as omentum or gall-bladder.

While these procedures have been under way, the assistant should have evacuated the abdomen of the extravasated contents. My own feeling is that with rare exceptions, and perhaps only in the later cases, is a drain necessary or even useful.

Cultures. A culture should always be taken and it will be surprising how often an extensive and muddy looking exudate will fail to show a growth.

Dr. E. G. Alexander, of Philadelphia, tells me that he has never obtained a growth within the first eighteen hours.

Closure of Wound. Closure of the wound should be done with much care and accuracy as these wounds do not heal very well and show a tendency to break open.

After-care. I think it extremely important to feed the patient at an early date and push nourishment rather more freely than is the custom.

Gastroenterostomy. In 1916[3] I gave in detail my reasons for not advising the performance of gastroenterostomy as a routine measure. I have had no reason to change my views and the results of the cases here reported, both immediate and remote, justify the belief. Of the 4 gastroenterostomies performed in this series a satisfactory suture was not or could not be made in three of them.

Briefly stated my arguments against routine gastroenterostomy are:

1. It prolongs and complicates what is usually a simple, quick and safe operation.

2. It is only very rarely needed as a technical adjuvant to correct or forestall a stenosis.

3. Few patients have any further trouble with their stomachs after recovery from acute perforation. Moreover, a gastroenterostomy is not a cure all or sure preventative for ulcers, acute or chronic.

4. Gastroenterostomy is an operation which has a certain proportion of recognized drawbacks and dangers.

5. What seems to me the most serious objection is the authority and teaching of particularly successful operators in influencing the unskilled or inexperienced surgeon to do more than he should normally try to accomplish.

End-results. At time of discharge all patients were free of symptoms with the exception of 2 cases that had a little distress after eating; but three months later were entirely well. All patients were reëxamined or reports obtained at variable periods and always three months after operation.* So far the results have been as follows:

Entirely free from symptoms, excellent result	37
Recurrence of symptoms	8
No data	4

Reoperation. We were obliged to reöperate in 16 per cent of our patients. The details are given as they present much of interest.

1. Case 215651. Patient well for eight months. Symptoms then returned. Lost twenty pounds. At operation (two years after first operation), tight constriction of the pylorus found. Moderate amount of thickening on each side but no definite induration or ulcer. Posterior gastroenterostomy. Four months later in excellent health. Gained twenty-three pounds.

[3] Loc. cit.

* Our thanks are due to Dr. Arthur L. Holland, Associate Physician of the New York Hospital for his energy and devotion in investigating the condition of our patients showing poor end-results, particularly by making very accurate fluoroscopic examinations and for his wise counsel in directing the most important after-treatment in all cases.

2. Case 216941. Patient free from symptoms for two years. At operation (two years and one month after first operation) marked duodenal ulcer on superior-posterior surface of duodenum, size of thumb. Pylorus moderately stenosed. Duodenum dilated. Cause adherent gall-bladder. Polya-Mayo resection of pylorus. One year later in excellent health and gained a great deal of weight.

3. Case 202624. Patient perfectly well for five and a half years. Came in for operation three weeks after onset of symptoms. At operation ulcer of duodenum well away from the pylorus, size second phalanx of thumb, very hard and irregular. Wound broke open on second postoperative day. Resutured, but on the twelfth postoperative day again broke open. Did not do well at any time. Vomited and ran constant temperature. Looked the picture of acidosis although urine was negative. Death resulted on twenty-seventh postoperative day.

4. Case 221456. Patient not well since discharge from hospital. Complaints, epigastric pain, loss of appetite, constipation. At operation four months later diffuse adhesions to omentum. Tight stenosis of pylorus due to cicatrization of old ulcer. Posterior no loop gastroenterostomy. Five months later much improved.

5. Case 215114. Return of symptoms one year after operation. Patient came in for operation three months after onset of symptoms. At operation diffuse adhesions, particularly of gall-bladder to duodenum, and of distal section of stomach to abdominal wall. All these were separated. First part of duodenum seat of hard callous ulcer, causing marked stenosis. Posterior no loop gastroenterostomy. Roentgen-ray diagnosis of pulmonary tuberculosis. Never proven from sputum. Died a year after discharge, apparently from pulmonary tuberculosis.

6. Case 229779. Patient readmitted eleven months after first operation. Duodenum is the site of an apparently healed perforation imbedded in solid mass of scar tissue and producing considerable stenosis. On account of technical difficulties thought wisest to do only a gastroenterostomy. Five months after discharge patient in good health and gained weight.

7. Case 232506. Patient readmitted six months after first operation. Numerous adhesions, particularly of gall-bladder to stomach. Stomach is folded over on itself by large adhesion. Ulcer $\frac{3}{4}$ x $\frac{3}{8}$ inch situated on posterior-superior wall. Pylorus turned away from duodenum. In view of mildness of symptoms referable to ulcer decided to do a gastroenterostomy. Five months later condition somewhat improved although still has pain and has been told he has another ulcer. Has been living on a very limited diet. Gained a little weight.

8. Case 207098. Gastric history of long standing. Perforation four and a half years ago—suture. Patient free from symptoms

until six weeks prior to present admission. Then had attack of epigastric pain. Suturing of perforation, two hours old. Perforation occurred in exactly same location as former one, to the duodenal side of the pyloric vein on the anterior aspect. Two years later in excellent health.

Two facts may be noted; that we have a large proportion of saved cases as possible candidates for trouble and if we had performed an "optional' gastroenterostomy on all our patients it is quite probable that 16 per cent or more would have reported more or less serious gastric disturbances.

Two of these cases requiring operation were originally long delayed cases and might have succumbed to a prolonged operation if a gastroenterostomy had been performed.

The conditions found in the 8 reoperated patients were:

5—Stenosis of pylorus.
1—Stenosis of duodenum by cholecystitis.
1—Adhesions.
1—Reperforation.

This gives a 10 per cent sequence of stenosis of pylorus.

Of the cases requiring reoperation the ulcers, with one exception, were situated in the duodenum. Of the results after operation 5 are good, 1 patient is having mild but rather persistent symptoms, 1 patient died and 1 patient died a year later of pulmonary tuberculosis.

The operations performed were gastroenterostomy (5); Polya-Mayo resection (2); suture of acute perforation (1).

We have operated on every patient in whom a possible diagnosis of acute perforation could be entertained. We had 1 case of perforated gastric ulcer revealed at autopsy. The patient was brought in in moribund condition, unconscious, without any history and died one and a half hours after admission.

Additional Data. 1. Location of ulcer.

Gastric, 28; deaths, 6 (1 ten hours; 5 over eighteen hours) 21 per cent.

Duodenal, 32; deaths, 4 (2 ten hours; 2 forty-eight hours) 12 per cent.

2. Sex:

Male, 56.

Female, 4 (3 gastric).

3. Age:

No patient under twenty.

Greatest number between thirty and forty.

4. Operation:

Suture of perforation, 56 cases, 9 deaths.

Suture of perforation and gastroenterostomy, 2 cases, no deaths.

Two gastroenterostomies, 1 without suture, 1 by plugging hole with omentum. Case without suture died.

5. Drainage:
   Cholecystectomy cases, 3.
   Gastroenterostomy, 3.
   Perforation twenty-four hours or over, 6.
   Perforation under twelve hours, 4.

Summary. For the sake of simplicity and because practically all of these ulcers were juxta pyloric, we have considered them as a single entity. A few facts may be emphasized:

1. That the duodenal ulcers, contrary to probability, give severer symptoms and a longer history. Of the patients giving a history of long standing gastric disturbance 30 per cent were gastric, 70 per cent duodenal. Of the patients giving a history of no previous trouble 65 per cent were gastric, 35 per cent duodenal.
2. The mortality from acute gastric perforation is almost double that of duodenal, namely 21 per cent to 12 per cent.
3. Duodenal ulcers give a maximum of conditions requiring further operation, 7 out of the 8 reoperated cases being duodenal. Of the 5 cases of pyloric stenosis found at reoperation, 4 were duodenal.*

TREATMENT OF SPASTIC CONSTIPATION.†

By Charles D. Aaron, Sc.D., M.D.,

PROFESSOR OF GASTRO-ENTEROLOGY AND DIETETICS IN THE DETROIT COLLEGE OF MEDICINE AND SURGERY, DETROIT, MICH.

It was Fleiner who first concentrated professional attention upon the distinction between atonic and spastic constipation. But while many authorities accept this division of chronic constipation into the two groups specified, others strongly dissent from this view on the ground that all the supposedly characteristic signs of spastic constipation are also occasionally observed in the atonic form. It is true that atonic constipation is by far the more common form, and in a considerable number of cases the two forms are associated; nevertheless the existence of a purely spastic type cannot be successfully disputed.

I shall confine this paper to a consideration of cases attributable to functional neurotic causes and the abuse of strong purgatives, disregarding for the present all the other causes of spasms of the colon, such as local inflammatory changes of the intestinal wall, adhesions, and pathological affections of remote organs.

* October 15, 1922; 4 more cases of acute perforations have been successfully operated, 2 duodenal, 2 gastric, all within the twelve-hour period.

† Read before the Annual Meeting of the American Gastro-Enterological Association at Washington, D. C., May 1 and 2, 1922.

In spastic constipation the retardation in the evacuation of the bowel is induced by a spasm (enterospasm) of a few isolated loops of the intestine. This spasm is brought about by an increased irritability of the vegetative nervous system, which may in turn be due to neuropathic conditions associated with diseases of the abdominal viscera or pelvic organs, or to either vagotonia or sympathicotonia from disturbance of the internal secretions.

The normal function of the intestine depends upon the innervation supplied by the two opposing systems of nerves, the vagus acting as the accelerator, while the splanchnics are inhibitory. In a general way we call the two systems, which are so wonderfully well balanced, the vegetative nervous system. Aside from individual variations, which may take place under normal conditions, the several organic functions may undergo far-reaching changes through excess of tonus on the part of one or the other of these sets of nerves. Every increased stimulation of the vagus results in increased activity of the muscles of the intestinal canal. Excessive stimulation, or vagotonia, induces spasm of the circular muscles of the intestine, contraction of the colon, and other phenomena.

Spasms of the colon are observed by means of palpation and roentgenographic examination. They occur most frequently at the transverse colon, hepatic and splenic flexures, sigmoid flexure, rectum, and anus. Spasm of the large intestine is important as the basis of spastic constipation, as distinguished from the atonic form. The characteristic symptoms of spastic constipation are delay in the fecal discharge, and an intestinal colic which usually precedes the defecation. In such cases there are various degrees of abdominal pain, with or without meteorism, which may affect the entire abdomen or only certain portions of the intestine. These pains are often continuous for hours, and finally terminate with the occurrence of defecation, which is often quite voluminous. It is frequently possible to palpate as a thick rope the tender contracting intestinal loops, particularly those of the descending colon and the sigmoid flexure. There is frequent desire for stool, with incomplete evacuation. Spasm may be associated with atony of the distal segments of the colon, and hypermotility or normal tonus of the proximal segments.

Spastic constipation is not to be understood as a mechanical obstruction to the passage of the feces through the intestinal canal; if it were so, hypertrophy and distention of the sections involved would result. High-grade spastic contraction is compatible with the forward movement of the intestinal contents, for it is not a permanent tonic condition. Not infrequently spastic and atonic conditions of the colon alternate or even occur at the same time, as is evidenced by the fact that the retention of feces in the ascending colon is accompanied by excessive tonus of other sections, such as spasms at the beginning of the transverse colon. When functional constipation varies, passing from one form into another, the movements of the colon presenting different conditions at different times, we group these several manifestations together as spastic constipation.

Spastic phenomena of the colon, with or without constipation, occur more frequently in women than in men, probably because of social conditions, the nervous status in the better situated classes, and the causal relation between intestinal function and diseases of the female genital organs. This is the case especially in pronounced neuropathic individuals who are subject to organic disturbances of the gastro-intestinal tract. In the neurasthenic, functional disturbances, among them constipation, usually arise without spastic change of the intestine.

The most varied conditions of the stool coexist with spasms of the colon and of the rectum, as to form, consistency, and frequency. In spasms of the colon with prolonged haustral segmentation, the fecal matter is in the shape of irregular balls, while in proctospasm it is cylindrical or ribbon-like.

By regularly palpating the abdomen and by roentgenologic observation, strongly contracted sections of the colon may be located, especially of the sigmoid flexure and the descending colon. It is easy to distinguish between contracted and filled coils of the intestine by examining the patient repeatedly and at various times of the day. The tonus of the anal sphincter shows the presence of proctospasm, a condition which accompanies spastic contractions of the colon. The characteristic physical sign of this disease is found upon exploration of the rectum, which, instead of being filled with feces, as is common in atonic constipation, fits closely around the examining finger (proctospasm), almost like the finger of a glove. The deciding factor in the diagnosis is the roentgen-ray examination.

In the treatment of spastic constipation, the first care is to provide physical and mental relaxation for these patients, who are usually in an overstrung nervous condition. We recognize that a hypertonic state of the musculature of the stomach and intestine is a constant result in vagotonia. The intestinal canal is unduly constricted. Complete rest in bed or a fresh-air treatment is often sufficient to induce normal defecation. The principal point, however, is the prescription of a suitable diet. I recall the case of a well-known automobile manufacturer who had maltreated his intestine for years with coarse articles of diet and large doses of a variety of purgatives, with the result that he required large doses of cathartics every night. In spite of his objection and to his great astonishment, I immediately stopped all the laxatives, prescribing as a first measure a mild diet, as will be detailed later on. In the morning of the second day there was a spontaneous normal defecation, an event which had not happened in several years.

The diet in the different varieties of constipation is, on general principles, to be formulated in such a manner that a mechanical and chemical stimulation will be produced.

An active diet rich in insoluble residue is particularly indicated in chronic atonic constipation. In such cases there need be no misgivings in advising large quantities of coarse food, so long as the stomach is in normal condition. In spastic constipation the indications point to a chemically acting dietetic regimen exclusively; all kinds of mechanically irritating foods are to be absolutely forbidden. In many cases it may be necessary to occasionally administer vegetables and boiled fruit in purée form, so that our only dependence will be on the mildly laxative chemical effects of appropriate foods.

In chronic atonic constipation a coarse diet, rich in residue, to render the feces more voluminous, is prescribed to incite peristalsis. By this large and bulky diet a mechanical effect is obtained which increases the tonus of the relaxed intestinal musculature. In spastic constipation, however, the treatment is directly opposite. A diet should be selected that will make but slight demands upon the intestine. Soothing, antispasmodic foods should be administered, while the use of water and foods acting mechanically to increase intestinal motility should be excluded. No laxative should be given in the treatment of spastic constipation. Glycerin enemata and glycerin suppositories are to be strictly prohibited.

In spastic constipation raw vegetables and raw fruits containing coarse cellulose, cabbage of all kinds, mushrooms, coarse bread, Graham bread, fruit with small sharp kernels, such as gooseberries, currants and strawberries, should be avoided, as they are unquestionably likely to maintain or even increase the irritable condition of the intestinal mucosa, both mechanically and chemically. Strong spices, strong black coffee, alcohol, or carbonated cold beverages are not allowable. All beverages should be avoided which are known to have a constipating effect, such as strong tea, cocoa, claret, blackberry wine, etc. We must prescribe a soothing diet, endeavoring to render the feces pasty and soft and the intestinal mucous membrane pliant and slippery. Young vegetables, the cellulose of which is comparatively soft and tender, may be allowed, at first in the form of the finest purée and prepared with the yolk of an egg or butter. Fruit should always be stewed. Many dishes are easily made with soluble and easily digestible fats, such as cream, olive oil, almond milk, and butter. Soft fat cheese, cream cheese, and curds mixed with cream are best. Eggs are to be served soft-boiled or raw.

I prescribe a diet as follows:

Breakfast. Orange or grape fruit; porridge boiled in milk and strained, with sugar and plenty of cream and butter; weak or caffein-free coffee, or buttermilk; two ounces of cream; toast, butter, honey, jam, or fruit sauce.

Luncheon. A cup of mucoid soup; sardines in oil; tender vegetables with cream sauce; light egg dishes with vegetable purée and mashed potatoes; jam, stewed fruit (strained), or honey; cream cheese; caffein-free coffee with cream; toast and butter; lemonade sweetened with two tablespoonfuls of levulose.

Dinner. A dish of mucoid soup prepared with butter; three ounces of fowl, veal, pigeon, sweetbread, brain, tongue, tender fillet of pork or tender roast beef, or fish boiled with a free amount of butter sauce; potato purée boiled in milk and mixed with butter; macaroni prepared in butter; plenty of purée of spinach, yellow turnips, young green peas, cauliflower, or artichokes, with butter, cream or the yolk of an egg; purée of stewed fruit, cream candies, or light farinaceous dishes with fruit or cream sauce.

Mucoid soups are made from oatmeal, rice, wheat starch, potato starch, and corn starch. The grains are boiled four to six hours with water, passed through a fine sieve and again brought to the boiling point, butter or cream added, and suitably seasoned ready for use.

An immense variety of fruits must be classed among the laxatives, because of their chemical constitution. These are of particular value in cases of spastic constipation. They stimulate peristalsis partly because of their fruit acids and partly because they contain sugar, which is likely to increase the fermentative processes in the intestine. Oranges, baked apples, grapes and watermelon are valuable. Fruit and its active ingredients may be freely used as jams, jellies, fruit juices, grape juice, cider, etc. Other acids and acid foods are recommended, as citric acid, lactic acid, buttermilk, sour milk, whey, kefir (two days old), sour cream, yoghurt, vinegar, and kraut. The cases of chronic constipation reported cured by the administration of the bulgarian or acidophilus bacillus will on investigation prove to be cases of spastic constipation.

The most useful kinds of the various sugars are the easily broken-up milk-sugar and levulose. Honey induces fermentation and acts well. Easily melted fats, as butter, oil, and cream, not only have a mechanical effect, as has been mentioned, but also act chemically, stimulating peristalsis by means of the great amount of fatty acids they develop. Pure white bread is not irritating and is best. No specific directions, as a rule, need be given concerning the consumption of meat in cases of spastic constipation. Meat may be taken freely, though some authors recommend a restriction or even a prohibition of it on the ground that it induces nervous irritability.

The dietetic therapy may often be advantageously combined with certain medicaments. Large amounts of fat are capable of acting in a beneficial manner, rendering the feces soft and smooth. A. L. Benedict was the first to draw our attention to a similar effect from liquid petrolatum taken internally. These substances may therefore be employed advantageously to increase the effect of the diet. Liquid petrolatum is indicated when we desire to lubricate the entire intestinal tract and facilitate the passage of its contents. The feces are softened and under the microscope are found to contain minute globules of the oil. Too heavy an oil should not be used, for this fails to permeate the fecal material, a desideratum as important as lubrication of the intestinal wall. The oil is not absorbed from the alimentary tract, and even in large doses has no poisonous effect. It is useful not only as a lubricant but also for healing superficial lesions of the intestinal mucous membrane. It may be given in tablespoonful doses three or more times daily.

In spastic constipation atropin or belladonna is our sovereign medicinal remedy. Atropin paralyzes the peripheral ends of the autonomic nerves and relaxes the spastic intestine. The extract of belladonna can be given three times daily in 0.008 gm. ($\frac{1}{8}$ grain) doses. In some cases atropin must be given in full doses. It may also be administered in the form of the less poisonous preparation eumydrin, the methylnitrate of atropin, in 0.001 gm. ($\frac{1}{60}$ grain) doses two or three times daily.

More recently papaverin, which is an opium alkaloid of the isochinolin group, has been recommended. According to Pal's investigations it is said to have an elective paralyzing effect upon the smooth intestinal musculature and therefore has therapeutically valuable antispasmodic properties. This preparation has been superseded by benzyl benzoate. My own experience with benzyl benzoate in doses of 1 to 2 cc (15 to 30 minims) three or more times daily justifies its use.

If the therapeutic treatment, as outlined above, should not have quite the desired effect, recourse may be had to oil enemata, as introduced by Kussmaul and Fleiner. Fleiner's oil enemata are extensively used in the treatment of chronic spastic constipation. Fleiner recommends for this class of cases one injection daily of 250 to 500 cc ($\frac{1}{2}$ to 1 pint) of the purest olive oil. The oil is to be retained in the bowel for a considerable time; it is best to retain it over night if possible. Should discomfort during the night (meteorism, pressure) result, as may occasionally happen, the time of administration should be changed, the enema being given at six or seven o'clock in the morning while the patient is in bed; the oil is then to be retained for three or four hours, thus producing the same laxative effect as if it had been administered at night.

These injections should be continued for several months, at first daily, later every other day, and subsequently twice a week. The results are so good that in many cases of spastic constipation actual recovery is brought about without any other treatment. The oil, by partially breaking up into fatty acids, stimulates peristalsis; and it has a soothing effect on the tense muscular tissue. Besides it lubricates the gut, softens the fecal agglomerations, and forms a protective layer upon any inflamed portion of the mucous membrane.

As a rule no discomfort is caused by the "oil cure," and the patients are at the time hardly aware of the fact that the oil is being introduced. It has not been ascertained definitely whether the oil passes beyond the ileocecal valve in all cases, but some patients experience the taste of oil after receiving a number of enemata. The only inconvenience caused by the oil enemata is the impossibility of avoiding the soiling of the bed and the bedclothes. The patient must remain in bed for at least an hour after the injection, without indulging in much conversation, coughing, or laughter. Should there be no spontaneous action of the bowels in the morning, a small lukewarm sodium-chloride water enema should be given.

Massage is contraindicated in spastic constipation, and all energetic manipulation aggravates the condition. Nor is the use of mechanical vibratory massage of any value in this form of constipation. All abrupt changes of temperature and all forms of mechanical irritation are to be guarded against. Warm applications made to the abdomen frequently overcome the spasms. A Priessnitz abdominal bandage may be applied over night, and a hot water bottle or electric pad placed upon the abdomen several times during the day.

THE DIAGNOSIS AND TREATMENT OF INTESTINAL OBSTRUCTION.[1]

By Alexius McGlannan, M.D.,
BALTIMORE, MD.

Until an antidote is discovered for the toxemia of acute intestinal obstruction, this lesion will remain the most fatal of all acute abdominal crises. The mortality has not been greatly diminished by aseptic surgery and whatever improvement may be noticed in the later statistics can be credited to the performance of an operation in an earlier stage of the condition, rather than to improvement in technical procedure. Recognition of the condition in this earlier stage therefore, becomes the most important factor today in the cure of the patients by prompt operation.

Acute intestinal obstruction is the sudden arrest of the passage of the contents down the intestinal canal. Any one of many causes may be responsible for its development. The position and character of the obstructing force are important factors in determining the severity of the symptoms and the time of the fatal result. It is generally agreed that the higher the obstruction, the more severe the symptoms and the more rapidly fatal the disease. Strangulation, or other interference with the circulation

[1] Read at the meeting of the American Gastro-Enterological Association in Washington, May 2, 1922.

increases the severity of the condition, at the same time adding to the probability of the fatal result. The more serious symptoms appear to be the result of the absorption of toxins from the obstructed bowel. The toxemia and the efforts of the gastro-intestinal organs to overcome the obstruction produce a series of symptoms which are grouped together under the term ileus.

Ileus, therefore, may be the result of many conditions all of which obstruct the flow of the intestinal contents. Reflex and toxic paralyses, spastic contracture, as well as mechanical obstructions, either from within or without the bowel, may be the underlying cause. The mechanical form always requires operation, the paralytic rarely; and the spastic type, while occasionally operated on, probably represents those cases in which spontaneous relief occurs.

The greater intensity of the toxemia in the presence of vascular disturbance is in part due to the resultant change in the intestinal wall. The peculiarities of the mesenteric circulation, especially the results of occlusion or patency of the parallel artery of the small intestine, play a large part in determining the effect of the obstruction.[2]

It is difficult to imagine an obstruction of long duration from any cause in which the intrinsic blood supply has not been affected by the distension and distortion of the bowel wall. Such circulatory change may account for the sudden onset of acute symptoms in cases of long-standing partial obstruction.

Whenever the underlying cause of an obstruction is of such a character that it can be recognized and removed early in the disease, the severity of the toxic symptoms is diminished, or their development is prevented. In strangulated hernia, where a painful external swelling calls direct attention to the obstruction, operation is performed in most cases before toxemia develops. The irreducible external swelling focusses attention on the obstruction and brings the patient to operation without delay. Although certain other conditions may be responsible for the protrusion, these are quickly excluded, or recognized as lesions which require operation for their cure.

Similar reasoning should bring the internal obstructions to early operation. In spite of the fact that there are no signs so distinct as the external hernial swelling, the symptoms of intestinal obstruction are well defined and with proper interpretation it is often possible to make a diagnosis before the onset of grave toxemia.

Symptoms. It is convenient to divide the symptomatology and course of acute intestinal obstruction into three stages:[3]

(1) The stage of onset, when the symptoms are due to the arrest

[2] Murphy, J. B.: Jour. Am. Med. Assn., 1896, **26**, 15.

[3] These stages do not represent any definite period of time. In twenty-four hours a patient may pass through all three and die of toxemia.

of the intestinal current; (2) the stage of compensation, when the gastro-intestinal organs attempt to overcome the obstruction or its results; (3) the stage of sequelæ or complications, when the obstruction has caused secondary destructive changes in the bowel, or in the body as an entirety. The higher and more complete the obstruction the less clearly defined will be the symptoms of the various stages. Vascular injury always intensifies the course of the disease. Gangrene of the bowel may either complicate the compensatory effort, or be present with the toxemia.

The characteristic symptoms of onset are pain, constipation or diarrhea, and vomiting. The pain is paroxysmal, with free intervals, or it may be continuous between the exacerbations. This paroxysmal pain, usually described as cramps, is the most constant initial symptom and becomes increasingly severe during the first hour. The pain of obstruction is not relieved by defecation or by vomiting. Opium brings only temporary ease. Constipation may be absolute, or there may be an initial bowel movement preceding the onset of pain. The constipation resists well given enemas, or an effectual enema does not give relief from the pain. Tenesmus, or diarrhea and pain with blood and mucus in the stools occurs in certain cases of strangulation, with intussusception, and with intestinal tumors.

Vomiting may be the initial symptom, followed by pain and constipation, but the usual sequence is pain, vomiting and constipation. The vomited material may be gastric or duodenal contents. As a rule, however, the material is first gastric, then bilious, and finally intestinal. At the onset it is gastric occurring without regard to the ingestion of food. Lavage does not relieve the symptoms. The initial vomiting is reflex, and may be replaced by hiccough.

The blood-pressure practically always falls as the symptoms develop; occasionally there is a rise in the pressure during this initial stage. A falling pressure indicates the onset of intoxication.

The symptoms of the second stage are local and general. The pain becomes more intense, unless gangrene develops, in which event it may be diminished. The vomitus of the second stage consists of material flowing back into the stomach from the obstructed intestine. The quantity vomited may be extremely large. There is a great increase in the amount of fluid secreted by the obstructed intestine. The fluid is thin, acrid, disagreeable in taste and odor, and is irritating to the mouth, lips and chin. The color seems to darken with the duration of the obstruction, passing from yellow through green to dark brown.

Visible peristalsis or visible and palpable, stiffened intestinal coils are the most characteristic symptoms of the second stage. The stiffened coil is a distended area in which the contractions have reached the tetanic stage, and in which there has occurred an infiltration of the wall with an accumulation of fluid and gases in the interior of the bowel. Visible peristalsis is due to an extraordinary activity of the bowel produced at this time. The movements are vigorous and associated with the presence of the visible stiffened coil. When much small intestine is involved in the process, the spastic distended coils may show as a series of parallel ridges, the ladder pattern. The contractures are accompanied by pain unless the toxemia has become grave.

The early distention is regional and usually asymmetric. Later there will be general distention. Tympanites accompanies distention. The lower the obstruction the greater the distention and tympanites. Local tenderness may indicate the soreness of spastic muscle, or may be from a local peritonitis at the point of obstruction. The blood-pressure falls during the second stage.

In the third stage the symptoms are those of toxemia, gangrene, peritonitis and alteration of the function of the liver and kidneys.

The toxin of intestinal obstruction is a virulent poison, although there appear to be individual variations in resistance to it.

The rate of the pulse and respiration is increased, the blood-pressure falls; there is great prostration and cyanosis with or without clammy skin. The mental condition varies from noisy delirium to unconsciousness. Often there is a subjective sense of well being, contrasting greatly with such objective signs as regurgitation of stercoraceous material, and distended abdomen in which violent peristaltic action is visible.

The development of gangrene is accompanied by collapse, and often sudden and severe increase of pain, although later the pain is diminished. As a result of leakage, peritonitis ensues and with its spread comes movable dulness in the flanks and obliteration of liver dulness.

Peritonitis is the result of invasion by the intestinal bacteria either through gross rupture of gangrenous bowel, or by penetration of the bacteria through an area of intestine whose wall has been altered by distention or constriction. The absorbed toxin probably reaches the circulation through the lymphatics. The liver seems to be involved in the defense of the body, but the changes produced in this way are not yet explained. The kidneys probably make an attempt to excrete the toxin from the blood, and in this way certain changes in their function are brought about. The intestine itself is involved in this process of excretion, which therefore brings about a vicious circle.

Laboratory Studies. Laboratory examinations are not of great value in diagnosis, although the following estimations may prove helpful:

The Blood Count. Usually there is a marked leukocytosis. In a series of 62 cases the average was 16,000; in but 2 was it below

5000, and in 7 others below 10,000. The highest was 46,000 in a case of volvulus of the sigmoid.[4]

The Non-protein Nitrogen in the Blood. In obstruction the quantity of this nitrogen in the blood is increased. Certain variations have been noted by experimenters which indicate that a series of observations made every four or six hours will give better information than a single estimation. If the successive examinations show an increase operation is indicated, while in the presence of a falling or stationary quantity delay seems justifiable.[5]

Unfortunately many of the lesions in which a differentiation from obstruction is difficult give similar changes in the blood nitrogen, or make a diagnosis so urgently necessary that delay for repeated examinations cannot be afforded.[6]

The Urine. Albumin and casts are frequently present from the onset of symptoms and are found in all cases of severe toxemia. The casts disappear from the urine after the obstruction has been relieved.[7] Indol and skatol derivatives are present in the urine in obstruction, but they are also present in so many other conditions that their estimation is of no value in diagnosis.

The foregoing are the general symptoms of intestinal obstruction. No attempt has been made to give signs which will separate the variations in the condition which depend on differences in etiological factors. Such signs exist and usually may be interpreted with ease, but no time should be lost in searching for such differential points. The diagnosis of acute intestinal obstruction as an entity is sufficient indication for operation.

DIFFERENTIAL DIAGNOSIS. The differential diagnosis between intestinal obstruction and other lesions having similar symptoms becomes most important when we are called on to separate the conditions which require operation for their cure from those in which operation is not necessary, or in which it may be even harmful. In the former group of cases it may be impossible to make an accurate diagnosis beyond the recognition of the crisis, which demands immediate intervention. The exact nature of the trouble in such cases must be decided upon after the abdomen is open. Delay for academic accuracy of diagnosis wastes the opportunity for curing the patient before the development of complications which make the use of disagreeable expedients necessary.

Abdominal Symptoms of Thoracic Disease. The onset of pneumonia, of diaphragmatic pleurisy, of pulmonary infarction, of pericarditis, as well as the acute exacerbations of cardiovascular disease may be ushered in by marked abdominal symptoms, which

[4] McGlannan, A.: Jour. Am. Med. Assn., 1913, **60**, 733.

[5] Vaughan, J. W., and Morse, P. F.: Arch. Surg., 1921, **3**, 403. Stone, H. B.: Surg., Gynec. and Obst., 1921, **32**, 415.

[6] Bacon, D. K., Anslow, R. E., and Eppler, H. H.: Arch. Surg., 1921, **3**, 641. Louria, H. W.: Arch. Int. Med., 1921, **27**, 620.

[7] McGlannan, A.: Loc. cit.

may closely simulate those of the first stage of intestinal obstruction, or be accompanied by distention and other signs of the toxic stage.[8] Throat infections in children may simulate abdominal disease.[9]

Rontgen-ray examination of the chest will often show the lung lesion and will aid in recognizing the cardiovascular ones when physical signs are indistinct. Levine[10] notes in the confusing cardiac lesions a small thready pulse with slight increase in rate and a regular rhythm, but quite distant heart sounds. The development of a slow pulse and fainting attacks points directly to a cardiac condition. If the patient is over forty with a history of dyspnea and there are any physical signs of cardiac enlargement, the probability of a thoracic rather than an abdominal cause for the symptoms becomes greater. When the apparatus is available, the electrocardiogram may add to the certainty of the heart lesion.

If the area of pain and tenderness be carefully mapped out, and the patient then be directed to hold his breath, the pain and tenderness will be absent as long as the diaphragm remains quiet.[11] In the absence of other signs of thoracic disease, abdominal pain associated with movements of the alæ nasi during respiration indicates a thoracic and not an abdominal lesion. The anxiety in the case of the thoracic lesion is lethargic and resigned, not terror stricken and active as in the abdominal conditions.[12] If the possibility of thoracic disease as the cause of the symptoms is kept in mind, a mistake in their interpretation is unusual. During an epidemic such mistakes are rare.[13]

The crises of tabes are often associated with distention of the abdomen. The characteristic changes in the pupil and in the other reflexes make the recognition of the tabes definite.

The visceral crises of angioneurotic edema may simulate an acute obstruction. The presence of blood in the stools may lead to the suspicion of intussusception or tumor. The history of previous attacks, or the association with symptoms of hives, of purpura, or other superficial manifestations of the condition will make the diagnosis.[14] Blood in the urine is suggestive of the angioneurotic lesion rather than obstruction. The non-protein nitrogen of the blood is not increased in tabes or in angioneurotic edema.

Acute Dilatation of the Stomach. In this condition the pain is continuous and referred to the chest wall. The distention is epigastric. There is no vomiting, but rather a regurgitation of discolored fluid. Lavage gives immediate relief from the symptoms.

[8] Brooks, Harlow: Med. Record, 1921, **100**, 1103.
[9] Brenneman, J.: Surg., Gynec. and Obst., 1922, **34**, 344.
[10] New York State Jour. Med., 1921, **21**, 382.
[11] Asserson and Rathbun: U. S. N. N. Med. Bull., No. 1, p. 29.
[12] Smith, R. E.: Lancet, 1919, **1**, 421.
[13] McGlannan, A.: Surg., Gynec. and Obst., 1920, **30**, 462.
[14] Dwyer, H. L.: Jour. Am. Med. Assn., 1922, **78**, 1187.

Adrenal Disease. Destruction of the adrenals by disease and experimental removal of these bodies both give rise to certain symptoms resembling those of the toxic stage of obstruction. The action of the toxin of obstruction is almost identical with that of acetylcholin, which substance acts as a physiological antagonist to the suprarenal secretion. The development of analogous toxic symptoms after the destruction of the adrenal bodies points to some antagonism between the substances and indicates the value of epinephrin in the treatment of patients suffering from obstruction with toxemia. The diagnosis between the conditions can only be made by identifying the preëxisting adrenal disease.

Spastic Ileus. Spasmodic contracture of a segment of the bowel occurs in lead poisoning, in certain tabetic crises and as the result of a number of reflex irritations. The obstruction may become so complete as to lead to toxemia and death. As a rule the symptoms are intermittent, but they may be continuous and rapidly progressive. The condition is often observed after operations in or near the peritoneal cavity, for example, after lumbar nephrectomy. Apparently a spastic obstruction may be the beginning of an intussusception, the contracted segment being thrust into the lower loop.[15] The differentiation between spasmodic and mechanical obstruction cannot be made from clinical investigations and therefore in all cases where the symptoms are urgent, operation should be performed and the diagnosis made after the abdomen has been opened. The spasm usually relaxes spontaneously, or as the coils are handled. This fact may account for some of the cases diagnosed as obstruction in which laparotomy has failed to reveal any lesion.

Mesenteric Vascular Occlusion. The occlusion may be arterial or venous, embolic or thrombotic. A combination of injury and infection is the usual cause. The symptoms are very like those of acute obstruction. At the onset the vascular lesion is usually associated with greater shock and there is apt to be a passage of a considerable quantity of blood and fecal material. The distention is general and is seldom as great as in obstruction. Some cases diagnosed mesenteric thrombosis or embolism have recovered without operation, but as a rule it is better to open the abdomen and deal with the condition surgically.

Acute Pancreatitis. The history of long standing gall-bladder disease in an obese individual, who has an acute abdominal crisis, especially if the attack is associated with cyanosis and great collapse, will lead to the suspicion of pancreatitis, but the diagnosis is never certain until the fat necrosis is found after the abdomen has been opened. Therefore no time should be lost in attempting a distinction between this lesion and an acute obstruction. If, as

[15] Freeman, L.: Ann. Surg., 1918, **68**, 196.

Ellis[16] indicates there is a close relation between the toxin of acute obstruction and that of pancreatitis, the differentiation between the lesions approaches the impossible.

Ruptured Abdominal Viscus. After the original collapse, the symptoms of ruptured viscus are those of spreading peritonitis rather than of obstruction. The continuous pain and the board-like rigidity of the abdomen are the best signs for differentiation. Similar symptoms are associated with rupture of an ectopic pregnancy. In this lesion the menstrual history usually helps. The signs are more marked in the lower abdomen, and a pelvic examination may make the diagnosis certain. Bluish discoloration of the umbilicus when present indicates ectopic pregnancy.[17]

Torsion of a pedicled tumor may give symptoms resembling those of obstruction. In the early stage the presence of the tumor will indicate the character of the lesion. In the late stage, a reflex paralytic ileus may complicate the picture. While this condition makes accurate diagnosis doubtful, it gives a clear indication for the necessary treatment, namely operation.

The onset of appendicitis, of cholecystitis and certain types of kidney colic may give symptoms very like those of acute obstruction. With the inflammatory lesions there is usually fever, and there is less shock than in obstruction. The character of the pain is continuous and there is local tenderness and much spasm from the onset of the attack. Appendicitis in older persons is apt to begin with obstructive symptoms.[18]

Kidney colic is associated with blood in the urine, either grossly or microscopically. There are usually other symptoms referred to the urinary tract, as for example, vesical tenesmus.

Peritonitis. The differentiation between peritonitis and intestinal obstruction is usually difficult and often impossible. Laboratory examinations do not help and the clinical signs are likely to be confusing. A local peritonitis by infiltration of the bowel wall can set up an obstruction. The fulminating type of peritonitis causes a paralytic distention of the intestine with stoppage of its contents. A tightly strangulated bowel will allow the passage of infectious material through its damaged wall and thus set up a local peritonitis.

At the onset the continuous pain of peritonitis contrasts with the paroxysms of obstruction. Muscle spasm and rigidity of the abdominal wall are prominent symptoms in peritonitis and are absent in obstruction. Fever is more likely to be present in peritonitis, and peristalsis is lessened. The development of distention in a quiet abdomen indicates peritonitis, and makes a contrast to

[16] Ann. Surg., 1922, **75**, 429.

[17] Cullen, T. S.: Contributions to Medical and Biological Research, dedicated to Sir William Osler, in honor of his seventieth birthday, 1919, **1**, 420.

[18] Bottomley: Ochsner's Surgical Diagnosis and Treatment, 1921, **3**, 55.

the noisy abdomen of obstruction with its visible peristalsis and palpable distended coils. The distinction between peritonitis and obstruction is most important in postoperative cases. Occasionally the nature of the primary operation gives a clue as to the more probable complication. It is possible that a rapidly increasing quantity of non-protein nitrogen in the blood may be characteristic of obstruction rather than of peritonitis.

TREATMENT. With these facts in mind, therefore, how shall we proceed when called on to treat a patient who is suddenly seized with paroxysmal abdominal pain, nausea or vomiting, and disturbance of the bowel movements?

The onset of an acute thoracic lesion, or one of the cardiac upsets should be considered and decided. Unless the lesion above the diaphragm is definitely recognized, the attention should be focussed on the abdomen. Lead colic, angioneurotic edema and tabes are recognized by their extra abdominal symptoms.

The physical examination will determine the presence or absence of masses, tender points, local distention, etc. A ballooned rectum suggests a low obstruction. An empty rectum, or one containing only a little feces, is found with obstruction of the small intestine. The presence of a large quantity of feces, especially if the material be hard, indicates a coprostasis rather than an obstruction. Severe symptoms however are rare in cases of fecal impaction. The obstructed loop may be felt through the rectum.

An enema should be given by a competent person, and the stomach emptied by lavage. If an effectual enema does not bring relief from the pain, the suspicion of a mechanical obstruction becomes very strong. Similiarly gastric lavage which does not bring relief points to an obstruction. If the pain continues, both enema and lavage should be repeated after an hour. If the second enema is retained, or escapes unaltered and with slight force, the presence of an obstruction becomes certain. If the second lavage brings away duodenal contents, the diagnosis is made even more certain. Under such circumstances operation is the proper treatment.

As a rule these tests are sufficient to lead to a diagnosis. In 18 cases of postoperative intestinal obstruction an operation was performed after the diagnosis had been made on these symptoms. In every case a mechanical obstruction was found and relieved and all these patients recovered.

Should the effect of the enema and lavage fail to be convincing, corroborative evidence of obstruction may be furnished by a rise in the quantity of the non-protein nitrogen in the blood. In the doubtful cases repeated blood studies at four-hour intervals are valuable. During this period of doubt the patient should be in the hospital, prepared for operation. The time may be employed in repeating the enema and lavage.

Cathartics are so dangerous that it has become a rule to prohibit their use in the presence of symptoms of obstruction.

Opium is banned, because it may mask symptoms.

In managing the patient in whom an obstruction is suspected, the judicious use of opium or a cathartic may be employed during this period of doubt. After the stomach has been emptied by lavage 2 or 3 ounces of castor oil is poured in through the tube. At the same time $\frac{1}{32}$ of a grain of eserin salicylate, or a dose of pituitrin is given hypodermically. In the presence of mechanical obstruction this treatment intensifies the primary symptoms and hastens the development of the secondary ones to such a degree that the diagnosis becomes certain, and operation imperative. On the other hand, relief of the symptoms ends the uncertainty.

SOME UNAPPRECIATED FINDINGS IN THE LUNGS OF NORMAL CHILDREN.

By Charles R. Austrian, M.D.,

and

Frederick H. Baetjer, M.D.,

Baltimore, Md.

The practical object of diagnosis is to distinguish between healthy and morbid physical conditions. Diagnostic ability depends as much or more upon an accurate recognition of the nonsignificant normal variations in health as upon an appreciation of the manifestations of disease. The latter can evolve only as a corollary of the former.

To Auenbrugger and to Laennec we owe our earliest knowledge of the "physical means of exploration" of the chest. To Wintrich, Skoda, Gerhardt, Flint, Sahli and to a host of others, we are indebted for the elaboration of our understanding of thoracic diagnosis. Yet, even at this late day, all the physiological variations from the normal are not recognized and, as a consequence, an unwarranted diagnosis of disease oftentimes results.

In a clinical and roentgenographic study of normal children, it was found that variations from the usually accepted findings in health were often present, and it is our purpose to emphasize the need of evaluating such findings as physiological and not as evidence of disease.

The clinical data dealt with in this report were obtained by careful examination of more than 200 apparently healthy children between the ages of six and ten years.[1] All children who showed signs of disease were excluded from the series. Individuals from various strata of society were studied: foreign and native born, residents of urban and of rural communities, school children and children residing in institutions, children exposed to tuberculosis and some without a history of such exposure, children with and without a history of previous infectious diseases, all symptom-free, and of an approximately normal height and weight for their ages. A history of each individual was recorded and in making the examination of the chest, care was always observed to have the child relaxed and to see that no cramped or unnatural posture was assumed, for, as is well known, faulty position may lead to findings that cause confusion in interpretation. A roentgen-ray examination of the chest was then made. In addition, a tuberculin test was made on every child. The clinical data were then assembled and after the roentgenologist had interpreted his plate independently, the clinical and roentgenographic findings were correlated.

Our observations disclosed in many the signs generally described as usual in healthy children. In addition, however, we have found on percussion, on auscultation and by examination with the roentgen ray, some changes not generally recognized as within the range of normal before the age of ten years and often incorrectly estimated as indices of pathological change. Only these findings will be considered here.

It is generally stated that the percussion note elicited over the lungs of normal children within the age limits under consideration is fuller, more tympanitic, of higher pitch and more resilient than that noted over those of adults, and that frequently the tympanitic quality is quite outspoken, especially over the lower lobe of the left lung. Although in general our observations confirmed this view, we have been impressed by the fact that in an appreciable number of such children, the note obtained on percussion over the lungs is indistinguishable in quality from that elicited over the lungs of normal adults and that the usual resilience of the note is lacking. These findings in many instances have an analogue in shadows noted in the roentgen-ray films, shadows indicative of increased density along the bronchial tree, similar to those seen in the plates of normal adults. This correlation of the findings on physical examination and on roentgen-ray study is more constantly

[1] The observations reported were made during a period of several years. They have been established in the course of a study undertaken at the suggestion of and under a financial grant from the National Tuberculosis Association. It is part of a report of a Research Committee consisting of Drs. H. R. M. Landis and H. K. Pancoast, of Philadelphia; K. B. Blackfan and K. Dunham, of Cincinnati; and C. R. Austrian and F. H. Baetjer, of Baltimore. The complete report of this committee is to appear in the Transactions of the National Tuberculosis Association for 1922.

possible in studies of the upper half of the chest. When minor changes, similar to those discovered by roentgen-ray examination of the upper lobes, occur in the bases, they usually escape detection by physical examination. In those instances, in which no shadow is found to explain the deviation of the note from the generally accepted one, it is our belief that the lack of resilient quality may be due to a decreased elasticity of the chest wall.

The so-called tympanitic quality of the percussion note over the left base may be increased, decreased or be entirely lacking, depending upon the degree of distention of the stomach or colon, the curvature of the spine, and may likewise vary with the position of the diaphragm or with the posture of the child during the examination. The note over the upper thorax is often the same on the two sides.

A barely detectible diminution of resonance over the spical regions is of no significance unless associated with a modification of the breath sounds in those areas or with other abnormal auscultatory findings.

It is generally accepted that normally in childhood the breath sounds have a harsh, sharp character, with expiration longer and better heard than in the normal adult. This so-called puerile breathing is physiological and though it may seem trite, let it be emphasized that this exaggerated vesiculo-bronchial respiratory murmur, especially well heard in the areas overlying the great bronchi (*i. e.* anteriorly at the level of the first interspace and the second rib just lateral from the sternal margins, and posteriorly, particularly on the right side, at the level of the second to the fourth spine) is often incorrectly interpreted as evidence of pulmonary disease. An auscultatory finding that has not been pointed out, or at least, has not been emphasized, has come forcibly to our attention in carrying out this study. Just as the full, deep note of higher pitch characteristically elicited by percussion of the child's chest is often replaced in health by a note more like that produced when one percusses the normal chest of an adult, so, on auscultation of a child's normal lungs, the exaggerated or puerile breath sounds may be lacking, and instead the so-called vesicular respiratory murmur characteristically present in adult life is heard. This finding, regarded by us as a physiological variation, has been noted as early as the age of four years and may perhaps occur in younger children. It is more readily appreciated and more often found than the variation in the percussion note just described. In more than 50 per cent of the children in which this type of breathing was heard, examination with the roentgen ray gave findings like those obtained by a study of normal adult chests. In fact, the agreement of clinician and roentgenologist was so constant, that on the basis of these variations they are often able to designate the chest of normal children as of "puerile" or of "adult" type. The essential fact to be stressed is that so-called vesicular respiration is heard with great frequency in normal children, and is to be regarded as a variation of normal and not necessarily as an indication of disease.

These variations and those of the percussion note are more generally found in children with a history of infections of the respiratory tract. No satisfactory explanation for this finding is offered. It may be due in part to altered resilience of the chest wall, a suggestion supported by the fact that in some instances in which it was noted, diminished elasticity of the thoracic wall was apparent on percussion. It may depend upon variations of elasticity of the parenchyma of the lung. It may be due to a relative narrowing of the lumen of the bronchial tree. It is hardly to be considered evidence of increased density of respiratory tissue, for, theoretically, at least, that should lead to a modification toward bronchial breathing.

The whispered voice sounds normally are transmitted loudly and often syllabation is heard over the region of the major bronchi. Auscultation of these sounds over the upper thoracic spine of the children has led to the conclusion that d'Espine's sign as indicative of enlarged tracheo-bronchial lymph nodes is, to say the least, of doubtful value. In 23 of the children, this sign was elicited without other signs of a mediastinal mass and without any corroborative evidence on roentgen-ray examination. In 3 children the sign could not be elicited, although from the roentgen-ray plate it might have been inferred that it should be. The presence of this sign, together with a slight diminution of resonance in the interscapular region is all too frequently made the premises for a diagnosis of tuberculosis of the tracheo-bronchial lymph nodes.

Further roentgen-ray examination of normal children within the age limits mentioned has reëmphasized the role that antecedent healed infections may play in the production of areas of increased density within the respiratory tract (bronchial tree, parenchyma of the lungs, etc.). Not only may recognized or remembered infections of the bronchi and lungs be responsible for alteration in these tissues, but other diseases not ordinarily considered of significance in this regard may be the cause of such changes. Our observations indicate that after measles, pertussis or tonsillar infections, areas of increased density radiating from the hilum into the bases especially, often occur. Such lesions generally are not discoverable on physical examination and would be unsuspected but for the use of the roentgen ray. This finding emphasizes the need of a careful history as well as examination in all individuals, before proceeding finally to interpret the findings of the roentgenologist. By way of digression, it may be interesting to point out the fact that though measles and pertussis have been known to produce lesions in the upper air passages, involvement of the lower tract has been considered a complication and was thought to occur only when evidences of bronchitis or of broncho-pneumonia were discovered. Our observations indicate that there may be a mild inflammatory process throughout the respiratory passages in a large percentage of the so-called uncomplicated cases of these diseases. This suggestion warrants further study in relation not only to the infections under consideration but also other infectious diseases. That such shadows, mediastinal and basal, noted in children who give a history of uncomplicated measles and pertussis are evidences of healed processes is evidenced by our experience that similar shadows of like origin have remained unchanged and without the development of clinical symptoms in a series of children observed over a period of from three to five years. Such changes must be properly evaluated as indices, not of present disease, but of lesions past and healed, not as warrants for the diagnosis of present illness and the institution of treatment, but as scars of infections met and overcome.

Conclusions. 1. The data obtained on percussion and auscultation of the lungs of normal children show wide variations from a fixed standard. These variations are usual and are considered to be within normal limits.

2. Failure properly to evaluate these deviations from a fixed standard will often lead to the unwarranted diagnosis of disease and to the institution of even less justifiable treatment.

3. D'Espine's sign as indicative of enlarged tracheo-bronchial lymph nodes is of little value.

4. Inasmuch as shadows noted in roentgenograms of the chest of healthy children are dependent often upon alterations that persist as the residua of past infections of the respiratory tract, it is obvious that a careful anamnesis with special reference to all infections is necessary if diagnostic errors are to be avoided. Even a history carefully taken is often unreliable, as minimal infections are soon forgotten by many and among the unintelligent classes even more significant indispositions are not readily recalled.

5. With a proper appreciation of the widest variations that the normal may present from the ideal, the informed clinician is better able correctly to understand the findings of the roentgenologist, and each, coöperating with the other, is less liable to error.

6. Recognition of and familiarity with the foregoing data is of cardinal and practical importance to every patient, potential and established. Without a proper appreciation of the facts set forth, no intelligent differentiation between a normal and an abnormal respiratory tract can be made.

PLEURO-PULMONARY REFLEX: ITS ETIOLOGY, PREVENTION AND TREATMENT.

By Barnett P. Stivelman, M.D.

MEDICAL SUPERINTENDENT, MONTEFIORE COUNTRY SANATORIUM, BEDFORD HILLS, NEW YORK.

(From the Montefiore Country Sanatorium, Bedford Hills, New York, Dr. M. Fishberg, Chief of Service.)

The general belief that exploratory thoracentesis is a perfectly safe procedure has undoubtedly influenced many of us to resort to this diagnostic measure with a frequency not entirely warranted by the positive results obtained. Indeed, it is a matter of common knowledge that even in the most reputable hospitals a great many exploratory punctures yield negative results and might have been omitted had the clinical data been studied with more care and thoroughness. However, it is not the promiscuous use of this procedure insofar as it betrays wrong diagnoses that prompts this discussion; it is the fact that accidents and even fatal issues may follow ordinary thoracentesis, especially in dry taps, that prompts the serious consideration of this subject.

First and foremost among these distressing occurrences is pleuro-pulmonary reflex, a symptom-complex, characterized by cardio-respiratory failure, tonic and clonic contraction of the body musculature and loss of consciousness which may appear with amazing and dramatic suddenness in the course of pleural puncture and may even cause death.

To Rogers[1] we are indebted for the first description in 1864 of a case of pleural reflex in a girl who, in the course of exploratory pleural puncture was seized with an "eclamptic fit." Raynaud[2] in 1875 recorded 2 similar cases and expressed the belief that such occurrences are more common than the literature on the subject would indicate.

Soon after numerous cases were noted, so that in 1905, Roch[3] was able to collect 39 such cases, and five years later Cordier brought up the total to 84. Dayton,[4] in 1911, in an excellent monograph collected 23 cases in which pleural reflex occurred as a result of ordinary thoracentesis, 15 of which ended fatally. Zesas,[5] in 1914, summarized 54 cases of which 45 exhibited tonic and clonic contractions in addition to cardio-respiratory disturbances. 7 of the 21 fatal issues of this series followed ordinary exploratory puncture.

With the increase in the number of patients treated with artificial pneumothorax there have appeared in recent years numerous reports of the occurrence of this distressing symptom-complex, so that in 1915 Sachs[6] was able to collect 22 such cases among 1122 patients so treated by twenty-four American authors. Forlanini[7] has met with 12 such instances in his 134 cases, and Saugman[8] in seven and a half years encountered 22 such accidents all together; 6 of these were mild and 2 ended fatally. Similar cases were reported by Brauns,[9] Beggs,[10] Lyon,[11] Giese and Conwey,[12] Stivelman,[13] Castle,[14] Unverricht[15] and others.

ETIOLOGY. In estimating the dangers of thoracentesis it is important to take into consideration those instances of severe and fatal accidents which might have occurred without any interference. It has been pointed out by Weill,[16] Brouardel[17] and Lichtenstern[18] that sudden death in pleurisy with effusion is not uncommon. Brouardel records the case of a man who was being prepared for an exploratory thoracentesis, but died as the physician was entering the house. Had he lived a few minutes longer the pleural puncture would have been held accountable for the fatal issue. It must be pointed out, however, that the postmortem examination in such cases reveal pathological processes which are in themselves incompatible with life, namely, extensive thrombosis of the heart or pulmonary arteries, advanced myocardial changes, extreme cardiac displacement and torsion of the larger vessels due to copious effusion and edema of the sound lung.

It is different in the case of pleuro-pulmonary reflex. Here no such pathological lesions are discoverable. Moreover, inasmuch as this reflex most frequently follows thoracentesis yielding negative results, *i. e.*, in the absence of pleural effusion the distressing symptoms attended therewith cannot be explained on the basis of pathological processes due to or resulting from extensive effusions. It is not surprising therefore, that numerous theories have been promulgated in hope of throwing some light on the etiological factors concerned in the production of this distressing symptom complex.

Lemoine[19] is of the opinion that these accidents in the course of pleural puncture are mere coincidences. Brauer[20] still adheres to the idea that gas embolism is the cause of symptoms attributed to pleuro-pulmonary reflex. These views however, seem erroneous, inasmuch as they fail to explain the fact that these symptoms have a tendency to repeat themselves with each succeeding pleural puncture.

Absorption of toxic material has been considered an etiological factor, but as a matter of fact these distressing symptoms frequently occur at the very instant the needle is inserted before absorption of anything is possible.

Status lymphaticus has been suspected as a causative factor,[21] but autopsy findings in children who have died suddenly in the course of thoracentesis fail to lend any support to this view.

Rapid removal of large quantities of pleural exudate may give rise to severe cardio-respiratory embarrassment, but since pleural reflex is particularly liable to follow dry taps, it cannot be explained on the basis of sudden displacement of the mediastinal organs consequent to aspiration.

Those who have encountered the accident in the course of induced pneumothorax have attempted to explain it along different lines. The inflation of the pleural cavity with gas which is below the body temperature has been expressed as a contributory cause,[22] yet this accident occurs most frequently in cases where inflation is not attempted and all methods fail to reveal the presence of air in the pleural cavity. Others maintain that imperfect anesthetization of the needle tract predisposes to pleural reflex. Against this is the fact that this reflex occurs as often after complete anesthetization of the needle tract as when no anesthetic is used at all.

The first intimation of the reflex origin of this symptom-complex was made by Leudet[23] as early as 1876. He recorded the interesting observation that epileptic convulsions, cardiac syncope and coma may follow the introduction of a sound into the pleural cavity of a patient operated upon for the relief of empyema.

von Saar[24] has obtained movements of the upper limb by irritating the parietal pleura, and Davies[25] is of the opinion that syncopal attacks are produced reflexly, as a result of irritation of the pleuro-pulmonary tissue.

Orlowsky and Fofanow[26] express a similar opinion and Langendorf and Zender[27] have succeeded in producing symptoms ordinarily ascribed to pleural reflex by irritating the peripheral ending of the vagus nerve.

Cordier[28] records an interesting experiment. After cutting the right vagus nerve of a rabbit, he injected 4 cc of tincture of iodine into its right pleural cavity. No reaction whatever followed. He then injected 2 cc of tincture of iodine into the left pleural cavity and convulsions occurred almost immediately. Autopsy findings failed to disclose any lesion in the heart, lungs or brain.

Brodie and Russell[29] in extensive experimental investigations have found that the pulmonary nerve fibers at the root of the lung in the bronchial tubes and alveoli would respond to electrical stimulation with a more powerful cardio-inhibitory action than any other of the branches of the vagus. But since they found no effect on the blood-pressure from stimulations of the healthy pleura, they concluded that the irritation of the inflamed pleura will not give rise to reflex phenomena.

In connection with the data just referred to, it occurred to me that the experience gained from pleural punctures in the course of therapeutic pneumothorax might shed some light not only on the symptomatology and frequency but possibly also on the etiology of pleuro-pulmonary reflex. I have therefore analyzed the data accumulated in the last five years during which period there have been performed at our sanatorium 162 thoracentesis for initial pneumothorax and 1824 secondary pleural punctures for gas refills. Careful anesthetization of the needle tract with novocaine-adrenalin preceded all punctures. Primary punctures on the other hand were also supplemented by a subcutaneous injection of morphine, $\frac{1}{8}$ grain, as a sedative and the administration of sp. frumenti as a stimulant. The results of our analysis are shown in the accompanying table (page 840).

Scrutiny of this table discloses the fact that among the 162 primary punctures, pleuro-pulmonary reflex was encountered in 7 patients, in 3 of whom the attacks recurred on subsequent attempts to enter the pleural space. Three of these attacks were mild, 6 were severe, and 1 ended fatally. The most severe and outstanding symptom during the attacks was cardio-respiratory embarrassment. It was present in all. This distressing symptom was of the vago-inhibitory type in 3 and vasomotor in 7, the former being characterized by slowing of respiration and decreased frequency and increased force of the pulse, the latter by rapid, shallow and cessation of respiration, and rapid, feeble and ultimately imperceptible pulse and heart beat.

Unconsciousness was noted in 4, tonic and clonic muscular contractions in 5, and temporary paralysis in 7. Amblyopia was noted in 3 cases and loss of control of sphincters in 1. Precordial pain was severe in 4. *In 7 instances injury to the visceral pleura and underlying lung tissue undoubtedly occurred.* This was evidenced by frank hemopytsis or blood-streaked sputum immediately following the introduction of the needle. In 6 of these cases physical and roentgenological examinations disclosed the existence of extensive pleuro-pulmonary infiltration and fibrosis underlying the point of puncture, and our attempts to induce pneumothorax in these were unavailing.

On the other hand, among the 1824 punctures for refills, *i. e.*, thoracentesis performed in those cases wherein the pleural surfaces were widely separated from each other by pneumothorax so that the needle could not possibly injure the visceral pleura and underlying lung tissue, the accident occurred but twice. In 1 of these cases, on account of the rapid and unexpected reëxpansion of the compressed lung, the needle caused sufficient injury to result in frank hemoptysis, and in the other the cardio-respiratory embarrassment was of the vagotonic or inhibitory type and followed what appeared to be the separation of an adhesion.

Comment. Scrutiny of the clinical data reveals not only suggestive information but point to factors which have a definite etiological relation to pleuro-pulmonary reflex. Dayton,[30] in his excellent monograph on pleural reflex occurring in the course of ordinary exploratory thoracentesis, provides data which are both interesting and instructive. He found that in 17 of his 23 cases there was definite evidence that the visceral pleura had been

TABLE I.—SHOWING SYMPTOMATOLOGY IN GENERAL AND ESPECIALLY BLOOD STREAKED SPUTUM, INDICATING PLEURO-PULMONARY INJURY, IN 13 INSTANCES OF PLEUROPULMONARY REFLEX.

Name.	Side.	Puncture.	Onset of symptoms.	Unconsciousness.	Temporary paralysis.	Muscle contraction.	Cardio-respiratory failure.	Blood in sputum.	Remarks.	Extent of pneumothorax.
H. S. . .	Right	1st	Immediate	No	Right arm; left leg	General severe	Severe vasomotor	Streaked	Precordial pain; amblyopia	None.
H. S. . .	Right	2d	Immediate	Yes	Right arm; left leg	General severe	Severe vasomotor	Streaked	Amblyopia	None.
S. L. . .	Left	1st	Immediate	No	Both legs	Left arm	Vago-inhibitory	Streaked	Amblyopia	None.
M. S. . .	Left	20th	Immediate	Yes	Both legs	None	Vago-inhibitory	Hemoptysis	Disorientation	Fair.
A. K. . .	Left	2d	Immediate	No	None	None	Vago-inhibitory	Streaked	. . . .	Fair.
A. K. . .	Left	3d	Immediate	No	None	None	Vago-inhibitory	Streaked	. . . .	Fair.
I. A. . .	Left	1st	Immediate	Yes	Left leg	None	Vasomotor	Streaked	Precordial pain	None.
I. A. . .	Left	2d	Immediate	No	Left leg	None	Vasomotor	Streaked	Precordial pain	None.
B. D. . .	Left	1st	Immediate	No	None	None	Vasomotor	Streaked	Precordial pain	None.
B. D. . .	Left	5th	Immediate	Yes	None	Left leg	Severe vasomotor	Streaked	Died	None.
A. R. . .	Right	1st	Immediate	No	Right face	None	Vasomotor	None	Cardiac dilatation	None.
E. W. . .	Right	1st	Immediate	No	None	Right arm	Vasomotor	Streaked	Dyspnea	None.
J. B. . .	Right	1st	Immediate	No	None	None	Vasomotor	Streaked	Dyspnea	None.

pierced and the lung underneath injured. In over 75 per cent of these, most of which came to autopsy, the lung underlying the point of puncture was consolidated either on account of uure-solved pneumonia, tuberculosis or compression. He concluded therefore, that pleural reflex is a result of the stimulation of the vagus nerve, probably in the visceral pleura and possibly in the lung and that accidents occur more often in cases with consolidation due to chronic inflammatory changes.

Saugmau[31] has observed that the occurrence of pleural reflex in his wide practice has markedly decreased since he uses all known methods to avoid injury to the lung at the point of puncture.

Our own observations have brought out 4 significant points. (1) That in over 75 per cent of all cases of pleuro-pulmonary reflex there was definite evidence of injury to the visceral pleura and underlying lung tissue. (2) That in these cases the pleuro-pulmonary tissue underlying the point of puncture was the seat of pathological processes of an acute nature. (3) That pleuro-pulmonary reflex practically never followed thoracentesis when the two pleural surfaces were widely separated by induced pneumothorax so that the visceral pleura and lung tissue could not possibly be injured by the needle. (4) That puncture of the parietal pleura when anesthetic is used never causes symptoms ordinarily ascribed to this reflex.

Most of the data derived from experimental investigation are unfortunately vague and even misleading. We will therefore refer briefly only to the excellent investigations of Capps and Lewis which stand out in bold relief against the haze of hypotheses and theories concerning the nature of pleural reflex. These observers differ from Brodie and Russell in that they did obtain pleural reflexes on irritation of both healthy and inflamed pleural surfaces. They maintain that in dogs with induced pleurisy, excitation of the inflamed visceral pleura gives varied results. In some there is no marked change in the blood-pressure, while in others there is a considerable fall in the blood-pressure that may often be fatal. "These reflexes," they say, "conform to two types which, as a rule, occur singly but may be combined. (1) Cardio-inhibitory type, in which the heart is slowed and pulse tracings make violent excursions with great range between systolic and diastolic pressure. Respiration is slowed and inhibited. This type seldom proves fatal. (2) The vasomotor type, in which the pulse tracings show a steady, rapid decline, with no great difference in systolic and diastolic pressure, is frequently fatal. Respiration as a rule is shallow but may be rapid, and in fatal cases the abdominal viscera are much engorged from great vasodilatation. The brain shows no evidence of embolism or hemorrhages. The cardio-inhibitory reflex is central because it is prevented by cutting both vagi. Atropine doses paralyze the cardio-inhibitory fibers and destroy the reflex. The vasomotor reflex may be central or peripheral. If central, they reach the medulla by the way of the thoracic sympathetic nerves and no vago-sympathetics. This is proved by failure of section of the vago-sympathetic cord to alter or abolish the reflex. If peripheral, the reflex goes from the pulmonary fibers to the pulmonary plexus, thence to the thoracic sympathetic nerve, downward to the splanchnic, and celiac plexuses in the abdomen. This reflex is more direct than the central form, but seems inconsistent with views generally accepted as to the cause and direction of impulses in the sympathetic nerve."

It is apparent therefore, that the clinical data above referred to are strongly supported by the results of the experimental investigations of Capps and Lewis, and it seems fair to assume that in many cases it is the injury to and irritation of the inflamed visceral pleura and underlying lung tissue that give rise to the symptom-complex now designated as pleuro-pulmonary reflex.

Methods of Prevention. In the light of our present conception of the etiology of this distressing reflex, it is apparent that definite measures can be taken in its prevention. Indeed, such measures have been taken by most skilled pneumothorax workers, who, like Sangman, have avoided unnecessary injury to the visceral pleura and underlying lung tissue.

It betrays a lack of familiarity with the literature on the subject to argue that cases of pleuro-pulmonary reflex are rare, and those who still maintain this view have either been extremely fortunate or have enjoyed a limited observation. To quote Dayton, "one sudden death is infinitely more convincing than many negative experiences."

A thorough consideration of the clinical history and physical findings will in numerous instances make an exploratory puncture unnecessary and thus prevent accidents, which for obvious reasons are particularly apt to occur in dry taps. The roentgen ray should be used in many doubtful cases in great preference to exploratory puncture. When there is a suspicion of the existence of a small effusion, a delay of a day or two to clear up the diagnosis will do no harm and recent developments in the treatment of empyema point to the fact that even in purulent exudates a little patience on the part of the operator is of unquestionable benefit to the patient.

When there is a definite indication for exploratory puncture, careful anesthetization of the entire needle tract, especially the deeper musculature and parietal pleura, should be carried out to avoid if possible those reflex impulses which may originate in it.

Most observers are in agreement with Sangman that it is only in exceptional cases that a needle longer than 3 cm. is necessary for thoracentesis. We frequently miss the exudate and injure the lung by going in too deep with the larger needles. Furthermore, experience shows that aspiration for diagnostic purposes can be done through the anesthetizing needle in all cases not excluding those in which the exudate is thick and cheesy. Added caution is to be exercised when fluid is not easily obtainable, for it is in dry taps that the chances of injuring the visceral pleura and underlying lung tissue are very great. The mesial portion of the chest should be avoided, even though great care is taken to prevent injury to the larger vessels, the pericardium and its contents, because, as has been shown by Brodie and Russell, injury to the larger nerve trunks at and near the hilus region may result in severe and even fatal accidents. Under no circumstances should the needle be moved laterally after it is inserted into the pleural cavity. Nor should the point of the needle be permitted to inscribe arcs of a circle within the thorax. Such manipulation offers sure means of injuring the lung and pleura. It is far safer, in searching for fluid, to make several punctures at different points in the chest than to move the needle in several directions from one point of puncture. It is important for reasons already recounted, to choose the point of puncture as far away from the inflamed pleuro-pulmonary tissue as possible, and in localized collections of fluid the roentgen ray will indicate the safest point to go into with a certainty far surpassing that of the most skilful diagnostician.

No less caution is to be exercised in the initial inflation in pneumothorax. Indeed, the chances for accident are even greater than in exploratory thoracentesis, because the visceral pleura and lung tissue, not being pushed away by fluid, can very readily be injured by the intruding needle. A point of puncture must be chosen as remote as possible from the main lesion and hilus region. Adhesions must be avoided. And while it is often possible to keep away from the site of the main lesion, no known method can definitely exclude the presence of adhesions at a certain point. Indeed, they are present where we least expect them and the roentgen ray often fails to point to their existence. As a rule, it is safest to go into an area giving a good, resonant note on percussion and fair breath sounds on auscultation; and while it is obvious that a free pleural space may easily be found in an area over which pleural friction sounds are audible, it is certain that punctures at such points are fraught with danger.

A short needle, not longer than 3 cm. and of narrow gauge should be used for anesthetizing purposes and the inflations should be given through the same needle. This can be accomplished in all cases presenting a free pleural space. In the past five years we have not failed to induce all our initial pneumothoraces with the anesthetizing needle. The use of a longer and wider caliber needle is not only unnecessary but distinctly dangerous, and that accidents with these needles are not more common than reported is due either to good fortune, or more probably to the disinclination on the part of their users to divulge.

The old practice of asking the patient to cough while the needle is in the chest cavity so as to augment the manometric oscillations is mentioned here only to be condemned. There is no surer way to injure the pleura and lung tissue.

A needle that is blocked can be made patent by the stilet, or by aspiration with a syringe which should at all times be connected to the pneumothorax needle.

TREATMENT. When symptoms pointing to pleuro-pulmonary reflex make their appearance, the needle should be forthwith withdrawn from the pleural cavity. When the cardiac embarrassment is of the vago-inhibitory type, reassurance of the patient and patience on the part of the operator are all that is necessary. Atropine, to counteract the vagus inhibition, may be administered subcutaneously in fair doses.

On the other hand, should the cardiac embarrassment be of the vasomotor type, adrenalin is urgently indicated and stimulation is at once to be resorted to. Hot coffee, per rectum, and camphor in ether subcutaneously have been strongly recommended. The vast majority of patients recover in from half an hour to one hour, although amblyopia and temporary paralysis may persist for several hours. These however, leave no permanent defects. The patient should remain in bed for a few days or until such time when all symptoms due to the reflex phenomena have disappeared.

It is pertinent to mention that inasmuch as pleuro-pulmonary reflex has a tendency to repeat itself in subsequent pleural punctures for the induction of pneumothorax, most operators are in entire accord with Forlanini who deems it advisable to abandon this form of therapy when the accident occurs with each of the first two attempts to enter the pleural space. Failure to heed this warning may and actually has entailed sad consequences.

Summary. 1. Pleuro-pulmonary shock or reflex may occur with amazing and dramatic suddenness in the course of ordinary exploratory thoracentesis and pleural puncture for the induction of therapeutic pneumothorax.

2. The most constant and distressing feature of this symptom-complex is cardio-respiratory failure. Among other outstanding symptoms are tonic and clonic contraction of the body musculature, amblyopia, temporary paralysis of various parts of the body, and loss of consciousness. Severe cases may end fatally.

3. The cardio-respiratory failure may be of (*a*) the cardio-inhibitory type in which the heart is slowed and the pulse is slow and forceful, with great range between systolic and diastolic pressures, and the respiration greatly inhibited; (*b*) the vasomotor type (the more dangerous) in which the pulse becomes rapid, feeble and imperceptible and respiration is shallow and hurried, and (*c*) a combination of the two types.

4. Clinical and experimental evidence lead us to believe that

injury to the inflamed visceral pleura and lung tissue underlying the point of puncture is a definite factor in the causation of this distressing symptom-complex. It is for this reason that thoracentesis in cases with copious pleural effusion or extensive pneumothorax, that is, punctures in cases where the lung tissue and visceral pleura, on account of their position, cannot be injured by the intruding needle, are rarely if every followed by this accident.

5. Attempts at pleural aspiration in doubtful cases and punctures for initial pneumothorax, because of the fact that the inflamed visceral pleura and lung tissue immediately underlie the point of puncture, should be made with the greatest caution, as it is in such cases that this symptom-complex is most liable to occur.

6. Pleural punctures in such cases should be made as far away as possible from the site of the main lesion. The needle should be of small caliber, held firmly and prevented from moving within the chest cavity. It is safer in order to avoid injury to the visceral pleura to make several punctures at different points on the chest wall than to move the needle in several directions from one point of puncture.

7. In hospital practice it is far safer in cases of doubtful or localized pleural effusions to depend on the roentgenological examinations which will indicate the presence of such effusions with an accuracy far surpassing that of the most skilful diagnostician. This applies to purulent as well as serous effusions.

8. When symptoms pointing to the reflex make their appearance, the needle should be at once withdrawn. If the cardio-respiratory failure is of the cardio-inhibitory type, reassurance of the patient and a little patience on the part of the physician is all that is necessary, although atropine may be given subcutaneously in severe cases, none of which however, have proven fatal. If the cardio-respiratory failure is of the vasomotor type, adrenalin should at once be given subcutaneously and stimulation should be resorted to. Hot coffee, per rectum, caffein and camphor subcutaneously have been found most useful. The temporary paralysis and amblyopia as a rule clear up completely within a few days and require no special treatment.

BIBLIOGRAPHY.

1. Rogers: Bull. Soc. méd. hôp. de Paris, 1864, **6**, 132.
2. Raynaud: Mém. de la Soc. méd. des hôp. de Paris, 1875, **12**, 96.
3. Roch: Rev. de méd., 1905, **25**, 884.
4. Dayton, H.: Surg., Gynec. and Obst., 1911, **13**, 607.
5. Zesas, D. G.: Deutsch. Ztschr. f. Chir., 1912, **119**, 76; Zentralbl. f. Chir., 1914, **12**, 371.
6. Sachs, T.: Jour. Am. Med. Assn., 1915, **65**, 1861.
7. Forlanini, C.: Ergebn. d. inn. Med. u. Kinderh., 1912, **9**, 621.
8. Saugman: Beitr. z. Klin. der Tuberk., 1914, **31**, 571; Trans. 17th Internat'l. Cong. Med., 1913, **6**, 463.
9. Brauns: Ztschr. f. Tuberk., 1912, **18**, 549.
10. Beggs, W. N.: Am. Rev. Tuberc., 1917, **1**, 509.
11. Lyon, J. A.: Boston Med. and Surg. Jour., 1914, **171**, 329.

12. Giese and Conwey: Colorado Med., 1921, **18**, 148.
13. Stivelman, B.: New York Med. Jour., 1919, **109**, 187.
14. Castle, W. F.: Brit. Med. Jour., 1920, **2**, 936.
15. Unverricht: Deutsch. med. Wchnschr., 1921, **47**, 1020.
16. Weill, Ed.: Rev. de méd., 1887, **7**, 33.
17. Brouardel, P.: Death and Sudden Death, 1897 (quoted by Dayton).
18. Lichtenstern, O.: Deutsch. Arch. f. klin. Med., 1880, **25**, 325.
19. Lemoine, G.: Ann. de Policlin. de Paris, 1904, **14**, 243.
20. Brauer, L.: Verhandl. des deutsch. Cong. f. inn. Med., 1913, **30**, 347.
21. Griffiths, J. P.: Am. Med., 1903, **5**, 989.
22. Simon, S.: New York Med. Jour., 1917, **105**, 734.
23. Leudet: Gaz. des hôp., 1876, **106**, 841.
24. Von Saar: Verhandl. deutsch. Gesellsch. f. Chir., 1912, **2**, 361; Arch. f. klin. Chir., 1912, **99**, 243.
25. Davies, H.: Surgery of the Lung and Pleura, P. B. Hoeber, New York, 1920, p. 90.
26. Orlowsky and Fofanow: Tuberkules, Jg. 2 Hg. 386 (quoted by Davies).
27. Langendorf and Zender: Quoted by Davies: Loc. cit.
28. Cordier: Lyon and Paris, 1910. (Des Accidents Nerveux a Cours De La Thoracentese.)
29. Brodie and Russell: Jour. Physiol., 1900, **26**, 92.
30. Loc. cit.
31. Loc. cit.

STUDIES IN RENAL FUNCTION AND METABOLISM IN A CASE OF DIABETES INSIPIDUS.

By David S. Hachen, B.S., M.D.

Assistant in Internal Medicine, University of Cincinnati, College of Medicine; Resident Physician, Cincinnati General Hospital, Cincinnati, Ohio.

(From the Medical Clinic of the Cincinnati General Hospital.)

Diabetes insipidus is a disease concerning the etiology of which we are still largely in the dark. That it bears some relation to disturbed pituitary function seems probable, yet much remains to be done to elucidate the relationship.

During the course of a study of a case of diabetes insipidus admitted to the medical wards of the Cincinnati General Hospital, several unusual findings were made concerning the renal function, blood chemistry and the metabolism of the individual. It was thought wise to report these findings in a further endeavor to aid in determining the principles underlying the cause of the polyuria.

The effect of pituitary extract (posterior lobe) in reducing the urinary output in cases of diabetes insipidus was again demonstrated, as well as its ability to concentrate the urine. A study of the antidiuretic effect of pituitary extract upon other conditions producing polyuria, such as chronic interstitial nephritis and diabetes mellitus, is now in progress.

A review of the subject will be dispensed with because excellent reviews are to be found in the Oxford Medicine,[1] in articles by Barker and Mosenthal,[2] Rabinowitch,[3] and Weir, Larson, and Rowntree.[4]

Case Report.—*Chief Complaint.* A male, white boy, aged twelve years, was admitted December 26, 1921, to the service of Dr. Roger S. Morris, complaining of "water diabetes."

Family History. The family history is essentially negative.

Previous History. Patient had scarlet fever one year ago; the exact time and duration of the disease was not known. Immediately following this, he developed a polyuria.

Present Illness. For the past year the patient had been voiding as frequently as twelve to fifteen times during the day and four to five times during the night. The quantity of urine voided each time was about a pint. There had been no burning upon micturition. He said that frequently there was a feeling of discomfort over the bladder region just before voiding. At times he would become quite thirsty and would void soon after the intake of water. Enuresis was a common occurrence. His appetite was moderate and there had been no loss of weight during the past year.

Physical Examination. Examination made by Dr. Morris revealed a fairly well developed and nourished boy lying quietly in bed. The complexion was fair. Hair was blonde; the texture was fine. No deformities of the head. The skin was soft and clear. There was no abnormal growth of the body hair for a boy of this age. The posterior chain of cervical glands was felt. Epitrochlear glands were palpable. The heart, lungs, and abdomen were normal. The reflexes were equal and active. Blood-pressure: Systolic, 95; diastolic, 55.

Routine Laboratory Record. Blood. Wassermann was negative. Red blood cells, 4,020,000; leukocytes, 11,200; hemoglobin, 80 per cent (Sahli). Differential count: Polymorphonuclear neutrophiles, 61.5 per cent; lymphocytes, 33.5 per cent; eosinophiles, 1 per cent; large mononuclears and transitionals, 3 per cent; unclassified, 1 per cent.

Urine. Clear, pale, acid reaction, no sediment, specific gravity 1.003, microscopical examination negative. Patient voided almost hourly in amounts ranging from 300 to 500 cc. The daily twenty-four hour urinary output ranged between 3 and 9 liters; accurate records could not be kept because patient voided involuntarily during the night. The specific gravity was fixed ranging between 1.001 and 1.003 during the twenty-four hour period. The relationship between the individual voidings and the specific gravity is shown in Fig. 1.

Roentgenogram of Skull. Stereoscopic plates of the skull made with the left side down showed no abnormalities. The sella turcica was slightly shallow.

Treatment. The value of the administration of posterior lobe pituitary extract in cases of diabetes insipidus being known, as demonstrated by R. von den Velden, the patient was started on the dried extract. Increasing doses of the salol coated and non-coated pills up to 3 grains, three times daily failed to produce the desired effect. The intramuscular injection method was then resorted to with immediate and striking results. One cc of obstetrical pituitrin* injected intramuscularly relieved the thirst and decreased the polyuria (Fig. 2). The effects of the extract were noted within ten minutes and lasted over a period of eight to ten hours.. The action of the drug in concentrating the urine, its effect on the phthalein output, blood chemistry and basal metabolism will now be considered in detail.

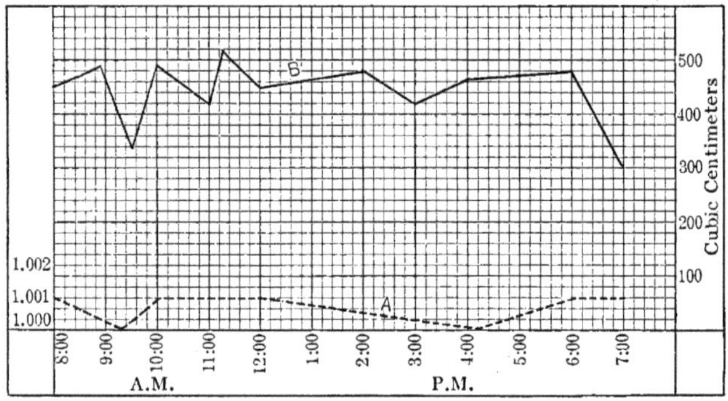

FIG. 1.—A chart showing the specific gravity and individual voidings of a typical twenty-four-hour period before the administration of pituitrin in any form. Note (Curve A) the very low and constant specific gravity.

THE EFFECT OF PITUITRIN ON THE URINARY SECRETION. During his stay in the hospital, the patient was kept on the regular hospital diet. Water was allowed as desired. In Table I is given the volume, specific gravity, chloride and urea nitrogen concentration during a twenty-four hour period.† It will be seen that the patient voided 8,610 cc of urine during twenty-four hours, the quantities voided ranged between 300 and 510 cc. The specific gravity varied between 1.002 and 1.010, the maximum of salt concentration was only 0.165 per cent and that of the urea nitrogen was 0.08 per cent. The total grams of salt secreted was 10 and the total grams of urea nitrogen secreted was 5.88, both of which were normal for the patient under the diet given. Fig. 3 is a graphic representation of the essential features shown in Table I.

In Table II are given the volume, specific gravity, salt, and urea nitrogen concentrations of a twenty-four hour period during which the patient had received 2 cc of obstetrical pituitrin intra-

* An aqueous extract of the posterior lobe of the pituitary prepared by Parke, Davis & Co. for obstetrical use.

† The sodium chloride was determined by the Vollhard principle, and the urea nitrogen by the direct Nesslerization method of Folin. During this period the patient received the dried extract of pituitary gland by mouth.

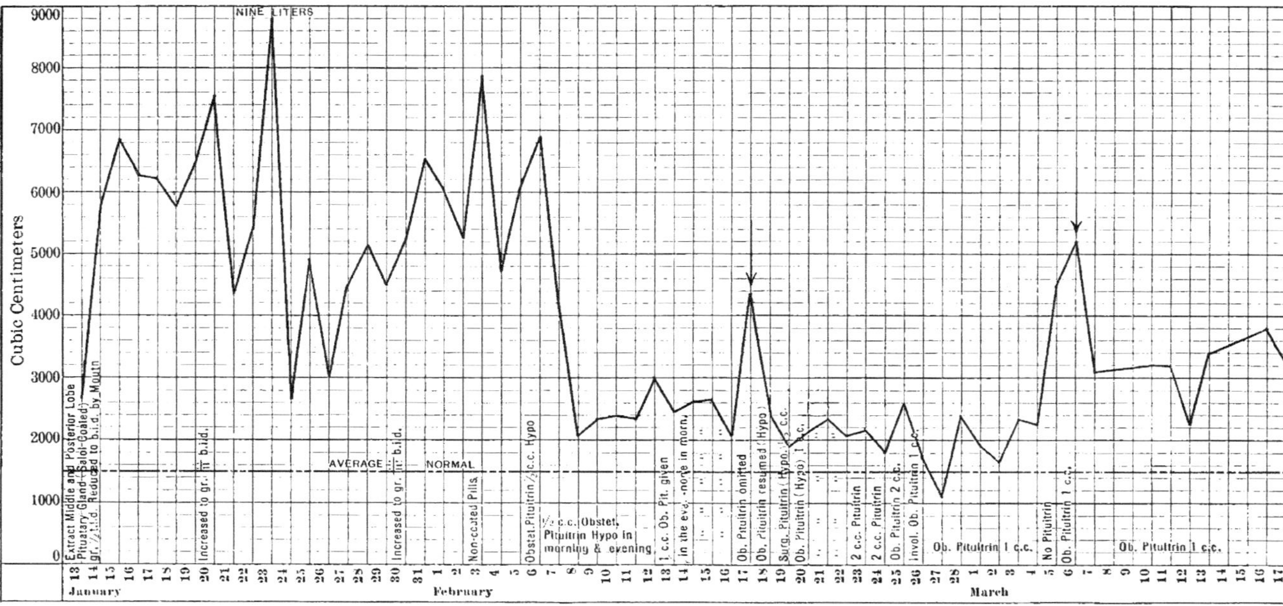

Fig. 2.—A curve showing the daily urinary output over a period of sixty-four days. Note the ineffectiveness of pituitary extract given in various forms by mouth and the marked drop in the urinary output immediately following the hypodermic injections of pituitrin. The arrows point to the increase of the urinary output on two occasions, both of which were due to the temporary omittance of the pituitrin. Note that 1 to 2 cc of the pituitrin had to be given daily to control the polyuria.

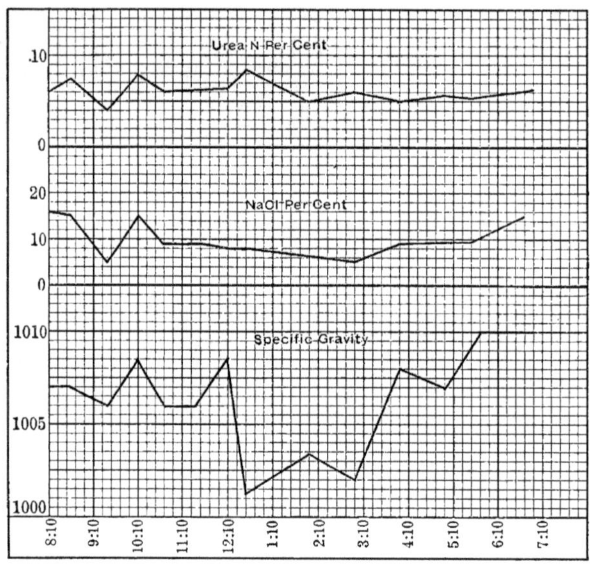

FIG. 3.—Curves showing the urea nitrogen and salt percentage and the specific gravity of individual specimens of urine collected during a twenty-four-hour period before the administration of pituitrin hypodermatically. Note the low specific gravity and the low chloride and urea nitrogen percentages.

TABLE I.—ANALYSES OF URINE DURING ORAL ADMINISTRATION OF PITUITRIN.

No.	Time.	Urine					
		Volume. S.T.	Specific gravity.	NaCl.		Urea nitrogen.	
				Per cent.	Grams.	Per cent.	Grams.
	A.M.						
1	8.10	450	1.007	0.165	0.74	0.060	0.27
2	8.40	480	1.007	0.150	0.72	0.070	0.34
3	9.30	360	1.006	0.045	0.16	0.045	0.16
4	10.10	480	1.008	0.150	0.72	0.080	0.38
5	10.50	420	1.006	0.090	0.38	0.070	0.29
6	11.15	510	1.006	0.090	0.46	0.070	0.36
	P.M.						
7	12.10	450	1.008	0.070	0.31	0.070	0.32
8	1.30	480	1.001	0.070	0.34	0.080	0.38
9	2.00	480	1.003	0.056	0.27	0.050	0.24
10	3.00	420	1.002	0.045	0.18	0.070	0.29
11	4.00	480	1.008	0.090	0.43	0.050	0.24
12	5.00	480	1.006	0.090	0.43	0.060	0.29
13	5.35	480	1.010	0.090	0.43	0.050	0.24
14	7.00	300	1.010	0.150	0.45	0.070	0.21
Total day .	....	6270	....	....	6.02	....	4.01
7 P.M. to 7 A.M.	....	2340	1.007	0.170	3.98	0.080	1.87
Total . .	24 hours	8610	....	....	10.00	....	5.88

TABLE II.—ANALYSES OF URINE FOLLOWING ADMINISTRATION OF 2 CC OBSTETRICAL PITUITRIN HYPO.

No.	Time.	Quanitative urine analysis					
		Volume. Cc.	Specific gravity.	NaCl.		Urea nitrogen.	
				Per cent.	Grams.	Per cent	Grams
	A.M.						
1	7.30	280	1.005	0.165	0.462	0.050	0.140
2	8.50	220	1.004	0.115	0.253	0.054	0.119
3	10.00	200	1.014	0.340	0.680	0.360	0.720
4	11.10	260	1.014	0.650	1.690	0.208	0.541
	P.M.						
5	1.00	300	1.012	0.335	1.005	0.375	1.125
6	2.10	300	1.008	0.160	0.480	0.190	0.570
7	3.00	240	1.007	0.145	0.348	0.125	0.300
8	4.30	200	1.007	0.175	0.350	0.111	0.222
9	6.30	300	1.009	0.155	0.465	0.133	0.399
10	7.10	200	1.006	0.150	0.300	0.077	0.154
Total day .	....	2500	....	....	6.033	....	4.290
7.10 P.M. to 7 A.M.		1000	....	0.200	2.000	0.272	2.720
Total . .	24 hours	3500	....	....	8.033	....	7.010

One cubic centimeter of pituitrin intramuscularly at 8 A.M. and 8 P.M.

muscularly; 1 cc at 8 A.M. and the other cc at 8 P.M. It will be seen that the patient voided 3500 cc during twenty-four hours; the quantities voided ranged between 200 and 300 cc; the specific gravity varied between 1.004 and 1.014, the maximum of salt concentration was 0.650 per cent and that of the urea nitrogen was 0.375 per cent. The total number of grams of salt secreted was 8.033, and that of the urea nitrogen was 7.010. Fig. 4 is a graphic representation of the essential features presented in Table II. Curves are drawn illustrating the variations in the urea nitrogen and salt concentration and the specific gravity from hour to hour. It will be seen that the maximum height of the urea nitrogen, the salt concentration and the specific gravity curve was reached approximately between two and three hours following the intra-muscular injection of 1 cc of pituitrin.

Summary. From these findings it is justifiable to conclude, that in some obscure way pituitrin has the power of concentrating the urine. As shown, both in Table II and in Fig. 4 the maximum of concentration, as indicated by the specific gravity, salt and urea nitrogen percentages, is reached approximately between two and three hours after the intramuscular injection of 1 cc of pituitrin. The specific gravity curve approaches the normal, showing a variation of ten points during the day.

The Effect of Pituitrin upon the Phthalein Output. A further study of renal function was then made by means of the phthalein test of Rowntree and Geraghty. The phthalein test performed a few days after admission showed an excretion of only 26 per cent of the dye in two hours; 18 per cent the first hour; 8

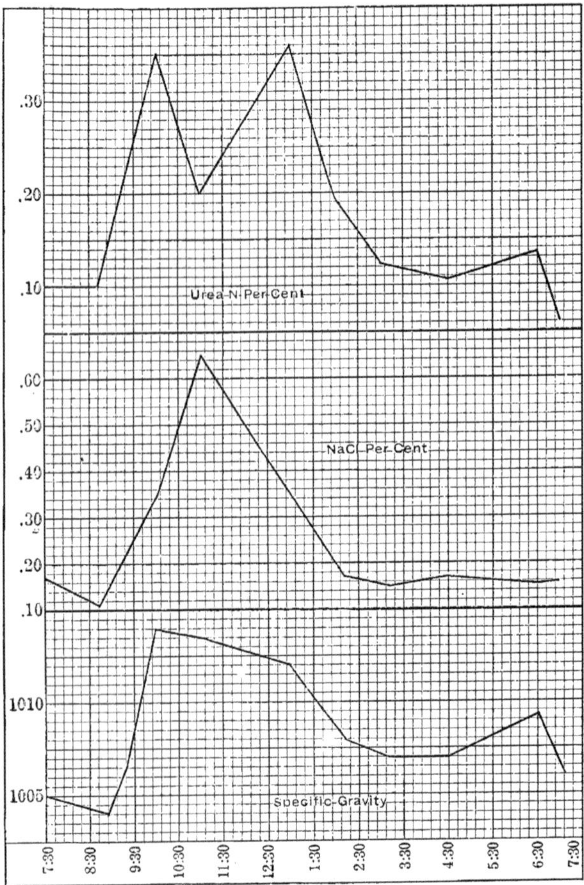

Fig. 4.—Note the rise in the specific gravity and the urea nitrogen and salt percentages. Maximum rise occurred about three hours after 1 cc of pituitrin was given hypodermatically.

per cent the second hour. A few days later, a second phthalein test showed an excretion of 36 per cent of the dye in two hours; 31 per cent the first hour and 5 per cent the second hour.

A similar test was performed during the course of treatment as follows: The patient was given 1 cc of pituitrin intramuscularly at 7.45 A.M. followed by 2 glasses of water. At 8.00 A.M. (fifteen minutes later) 1 cc of phenolsulphonephthalein was administered intramuscularly. The urine passed was collected for the first hour and second hour respectively. Forty-two per cent of the dye was excreted during the first hour and 17 per cent during the second hour or a total of 59 per cent in two hours.

The pituitrin was then discontinued. Thirty-six hours later another phthalein test was performed showing an excretion of 40 per cent of the dye in two hours; 28 per cent the first hour and 12 per cent the second hour. These findings are graphically shown in Fig. 5.

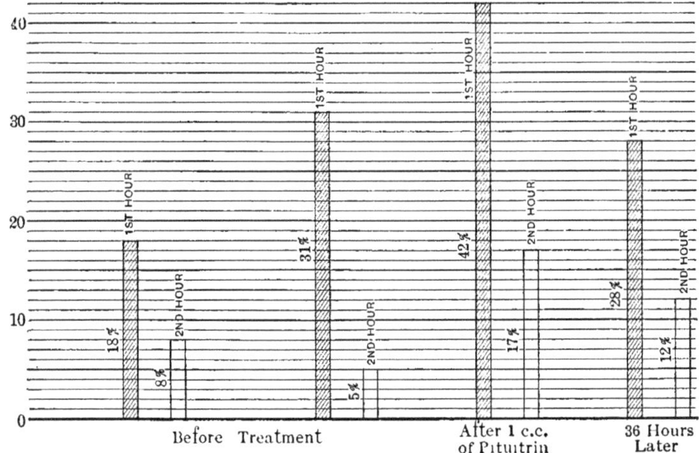

Fig. 5.—Note the increase in the phthalein output immediately following the injection of pituitrin and then the decrease after thirty-six hours of abstinence from the drug.

Summary. From these results one may conclude that pituitrin has not only produced an increase in the salt and urea nitrogen concentration of the urine, but also an increase in the phenolsulphonephthalein output. Thus it is evident that the secretion of the dye and that of the salt and urea are more or less parallel in nature in this case of diabetes insipidus.

Effect of Pituitrin on the Blood Chemistry. Blood analyses* were made before and after the administration of pituitrin intramuscularly. Before treatment the blood analysis was as follows:

	Mg. per 100 cc of blood.
Sugar	87.0
Urea nitrogen	8.3
Uric acid	1.8
Chlorides	515.0

* The blood constituents were determined by the system of Folin and Wu.[7] The blood chlorides were determined by the method of Whitehorn.[8]

A specimen of blood was then taken three hours after the injection of 1 cc of pituitrin intramuscularly. This time was selected because it was shown that urine of maximum concentration (Table II and Fig. 4) was excreted between two and three hours after the intramuscular injection of the pituitrin. The analysis of this blood was as follows:†

	Mg. per 100 cc of blood.
Sugar	111.0
Urea nitrogen	16.0
Uric acid	3.5
Chlorides	370.0

Summary. Thus it will be seen that, although there was some variation in the blood chemical picture before and after the pituitrin treatment, all of the figures were within normal limits. The blood findings were similar in the 15 cases reported by Weir, Larson, and Rowntree.[4] But upon more careful examination it will be seen that there was an increase in the concentration of all the substances with the exception of the chlorides which were markedly decreased.

EFFECT OF PITUITRIN ON THE BASAL METABOLISM. The relation between the basal metabolism and the water excretion of the kidney before and after pituitary administration was studied by Raphael Isaacs. The Sanborn-Benedict apparatus was used. The normal oxygen consumption was taken from Benedict and Talbot's table for normal standards of basal metabolism for boys and girls.[6] Before any treatment was started the basal metabolic rate was—5 per cent. After a month of the administration of pituitary substance in coated and non-coated pills by mouth the rate was —5.68 per cent. After six weeks, during which time the pituitrin was given hypodermatically, the basal metabolic rate was —1.9 per cent twelve hours after the injection of 1 cc of pituitrin. Then 1 cc of pituitrin was given. Forty-five minutes later, the basal metabolic rate was + 1.3 per cent. The calculated urinary output, the vital capacity, and the respiratory and pulse rates were as follows:

TABLE III.

	Before pituitrin.	After pituitrin.
Basal metabolic rate	—1.9 per cent	+1.3 per cent
Urinary output	800 cc per hour	75 cc per hour
Vital capacity	2350 cc	2250 cc
Respiratory rate	14 per minute	16 per minute
Pulse rate	76 per minute	80 per minute

† On this examination, non-protein nitrogen and creatinine determinations were also made with the following results: Non-protein nitrogen, 35.3 mg. per 100 cc of blood; creatinine, 1.5 mg. per 100 cc of blood.

Summary. It will be noted that, although the water output dropped from 800 cc to 75 cc per hour, there was scarcely any perceptible change in the basal metabolic rate. Two interpretations are possible. Either the excretion of water by the kidney does not involve "work" and the consumption of oxygen, or else the decreased oxygen consumption resulting from the lessened urinary output was compensated for by increased oxidations elsewhere.

Conclusions. 1. Two cc of obstetrical pituitrin, administered intramuscularly during a twenty-four hour period decreased the polyuria in a case of diabetes insipidus. The specific gravity was raised and the percentage of salt and urea nitrogen was increased. The maximum concentration was reached within three hours after the injection of the pituitrin. The drug produced its effect immediately (within ten minutes) and was only transient in its action; the effect of 1 cc lasting from eight to twelve hours.

2. Pituitrin injected hypodermatically enabled the kidney to excrete a larger amount of phenolsulphonephthalein.

3. The concentration of the urea nitrogen, uric acid, and sugar in the blood was almost doubled within three hours after the injection of 1 cc of pituitrin. The blood figures before and after injection of the pituitrin remained within normal limits.

4. There was no apparent relation between the basal metabolism and the water excretion of the kidney before and after pituitrin administration.*

* The writer wishes to thank Drs. Cecil Striker, Joseph Ganim, Floyd Hendrickson and Miss Agnes Wolfstein for their help in the completion of this case. He is deeply indebted to Dr. Roger S. Morris for his many suggestions and the privilege of reporting this case.

REFERENCES.

1. Rowntree, L. G.: Oxford Med., London, Oxford Univ. Press, 1921, **4**, 179.
2. Barker, Lewellys F., and Mosenthal, Herman O.: Jour. Urol., 1917, **1**, 449.
3. Rabinowitch, I. M.: Arch. Int. Med., 1921, **28**, 355.
4. Weir, J. F., Larson, E. E., and Rowntree, L. G.: Arch. Int. Med., 1922, **29**, 306.
5. Morris, R. S.: Clinical Laboratory Methods, 1923, p. 113.
6. Benedict and Talbot: Metabolism from Birth to Puberty, Carnegie Institute of Washington, 1921.
7. Folin, Otto, and Wu, Hsien: Jour. Biol. Chem., 1919, **38**, 81.
8. Whitehorn, J. C.: Jour. Biol. Chem., Suppl. II, 1921, **45**, 449.

SPLENIC ANEMIA: A CLINICAL AND PATHOLOGICAL STUDY OF SIXTY-NINE CASES.*

By William C. Chaney, M.D.,
THE MAYO FOUNDATION, ROCHESTER, MINN.

Osler, in his *Principles and Practice of Medicine,* discusses splenic anemia under the heading, "Primary Splenomegaly with Anemia," which he defines as "a primary disease of the spleen of unknown origin, characterized by progressve enlargement, attacks of anemia, a tendency to hemorrhage, and in some cases a secondary cirrhosis of the liver, with jaundice and ascites. That the spleen itself is the seat of the disease is shown by the fact that complete recovery follows its removal." Osler has included the cases of primary splenomegaly which Rolleston prefers to discuss under separate headings, "Chronic Splenic Anemia" and "Banti's Disease."

According to Rolleston, chronic splenic anemia presents the following characteristics: "(1) Chronic splenomegaly which cannot be correlated with any recognized cause; (2) the absence of enlargement of the lymphatic glands; (3) chronic anemia (with low color index); (4) the absence of leukocytosis and usually the presence of leucopenia; (5) liability of copious gastro-intestinal hemorrhages from time to time; and (6) prolonged course without any tendency to spontaneous cure, though splenectomy is usually curative."

Rolleston, in discussing the relation between Banti's disease and splenic anemia, says, "The title, Banti's disease, is now often used as synonymous with splenic anemia even by those who fully recognize that it is a sequel or terminal stage of splenic anemia and does not occur in all cases even when unduly prolonged."

According to Hollins, Banti describes three stages of the disease named for him: (1) the preascitic stage in which splenic enlargement is present with or without anemia; (2) the transitional stage of which the most prominent symptom is diarrhea; anemia and blood changes are found, the liver is somewhat enlarged, and jaundice may be present, and (3) the ascitic stage, or Banti's disease proper.

This report is the result of a study of the pathological findings and clinical records of 69 patients with splenic anemia, on whom splenectomy was performed at the Mayo Clinic from November 14, 1905, to September 1, 1920. Patients who had a distinct hepatic cirrhosis in addition are also considered.

* Abridgment of thesis submitted to the Faculty of the Graduate School of the University of Minnesota in partial fulfillment of the requirements for the degree of Master of Science in Medicine.

The Microscopical Pathology. *Variation in the Normal Spleen.* Before the abnormality of any organ can be correctly investigated, it is essential that the pathologist have a clear conception of the normal. This is especially true in the case of the spleen, for the gross and microscopic picture may vary widely under normal conditions. Such normal changes may be permanent or temporary, as in variations with age or after severe hemorrhage or sepsis. Before the pathological study of splenic anemia was undertaken, therefore, an effort was made to learn of some of the variations that could be ascribed to normal influences.

Terminology. By *sinus endothelium* is meant a specialized form of endothelium and not the lining cells of blood channels as the term is commonly employed. These specialized endothelial cells of the sinuses are probably reticular cells and to be correct should be so designated. The word *pulp* is used to designate the cellular structures lying between the sinuses. *Pulp cords* would probably have been a more suitable term. *Reticulum* refers to all the connective tissue not included in the capsule, trabeculæ, or blood-vessels. Hyaline changes in the capsule and trabeculæ are not included under the term *degeneration* which is reserved for degenerative changes in the reticulum, in the malpighian corpuscles, or within the pulp.

Method of Study. In order to express more accurately the degree of pathological change observed in the study of the spleen, figures instead of descriptive adjectives, have been used. Normal findings were marked zero or simply normal. The degree of increase of the various processes above normal was designated on a scale +1, +2, +3, +4, while the decrease was graded −1, −2, −3, −4; +5 and −5 have been used occasionally in grading very unusual and extreme conditions.

At least three blocks of tissue were taken from each spleen, one containing a portion of the capsule of the diaphragmatic surface, one from near the center of the organ, and one from near the hilus. The last block always included a portion of the wall of one of the large veins.

Microscopical sections were made by the frozen-section method, or by embedding the tissue in paraffin. The routine stain was hematoxylin and eosin, but many of the specimens were also prepared with Dominici's and with methyl-green pyronin stains.

Microscopical Findings. A composite picture of the histo-pathology of splenic anemia is one of generalized fibrosis. There are no very definite and well defined characteristics which will enable the pathologist to say with certainty that the picture is one of splenic anemia (Fig. 1).

The wide variation in the pathological findings in splenic anemia has been one of the arguments used in an attempt to prove that cases so classified belong in closely related clinical groups and do not bear a sufficient clinical and pathological resemblance to justify their being considered as distinct disease entities. From the pathological standpoint, in the case of the spleen, this argument is unfounded, for, while the pathological variations are great, the microscopical and gross studies give results probably as characteristic of splenic anemia as similar studies in the other groups of splenomegaly that present an accepted clinical syndrome, such as pernicious anemia, and hemolytic jaundice.

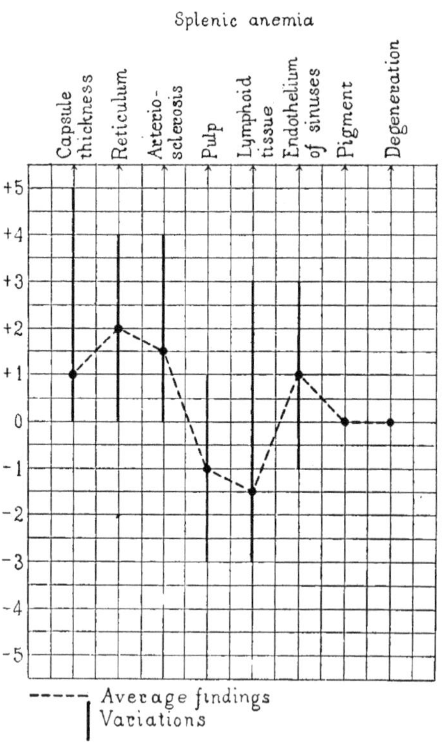

Fig. 1.—Average findings and the variations in the microscopical pathology of splenic anemia.

A great deal of the trouble in distinguishing, microscopically, splenic anemia from the other splenomegalies is owing to the variations encountered in the individual types of splenomegaly. In splenic anemia these variations were found to be quite marked. For example, the thickness of the capsule varied from normal to +5, the reticulum and the arterial walls from normal to +4, the pulp from —3 to +1, the lymphoid tissue from —3 to +3, and the endothelium of the sinuses from —1 to +3. While these variations are great, they are not surprising in view of the factors that may influence the spleen, such as the duration and severity of the disease, the age of the patient, and the changes that may have been caused by previous diseases. These variations, while confusing, nevertheless suggest that the spleen plays an important part in the vital economy of the individual.

The average thickness of the capsule was found to be +1. The variation from +3 to +5 was caused by the extensive hyaline plaques in some of the spleens. For the most part, however, the thickness of the capsule in any given specimen was uniform. As a rule, the more fibrous the capsule the more prominent were the trabeculæ throughout the splenic tissue. Lymphocytic infiltration of the capsule was not seen in any of the sections.

The reticulum may be distinctly prominent either because of marked fibrosis or great cellular activity. The degree of fibrosis of the reticulum seemed to vary in a slight degree with the amount of thickening of the vessel walls, yet many cases were found in which the reticulum was very cellular and the degree of arteriosclerosis marked. The amount of lymphoid tissue present usually varied inversely to the prominence of the reticulum. The average amount of reticulum was found to be +2.

In the study of the degree of arteriosclerosis the artery of the malpighian corpuscle was chosen. It was observed that the more marked the arteriosclerosis, the greater the tortuosity of the vessel, so that it was often found that a malpighian corpuscle might show two to four cross-sections of the same artery. Marked arteriosclerosis was not necessarily associated with extensive fibrosis, and no evidence was found to suggest that fibrosis developed from the vessel wall. Indeed, marked fibrosis was often found in which the fibrous tissue was conspicuously absent in the region of the malpighian corpuscle and the central artery. Arteriosclerosis was, to a slight degree, an exception to the rule that in any given spleen the pathological changes were uniformly distributed. A few spleens showed a variation of from +1 to +3 in the degree of arteriosclerosis in various sections of the organ.

The artery of the malpighian corpuscle was in almost every case eccentrically located, and its position was apparently not disturbed by the thickening process of the vessel wall. There seemed to be at least one factor which helped to determine the size of the malpighian corpuscles, that is, encroaching fibrosis. The fibrosis, in turn, seemed to affect the position of the central artery by reducing, in an irregular fashion, the size of the malpighian corpuscle. It was a fairly constant finding that the greater the fibrosis the more eccentrically located was the artery. The average degree of arteriosclerosis was +1.5.

The degree of thickening of the arterial walls in cases of splenic anemia and in other types of splenomegaly were, syphilis +3, hemolytic jaundice +3, pernicious anemia +2, myelogenous leukemia +2, and splenic anemia +1.5.

No marked abnormality could be detected in the splenic veins, but the veins were usually so closely associated with the trabeculæ that a comparison of their walls was very difficult. In many cases, however, distinct hyaline changes were seen in the walls of the veins, but in no specimen was thrombophlebitis present.

In a spleen in which generalized fibrosis is a prominent feature, it would naturally be supposed that the amount of splenic pulp would be decreased. This was found to be true, and the average was +1. In general, the amount of splenic pulp varied inversely to the degree of fibrosis and the prominence of the sinuses. The proliferative activity of the endothelium of the sinuses, or the true reticular cells, was above normal and was rated +1. In nearly all the microscopical specimens the sinuses were prominent and dilated, but the other types of splenomegaly also showed it. The syphilitic spleens especially resembled those of splenic anemia in this particular. The prominence of the sinuses in splenic anemia averaged approximately +2.

The sinus endothelium or reticulum showed varying degrees of proliferation. In some specimens the cells seemed especially inactive, while in others the cells were very large and, as further evidence of activity, were free within the sinuses.

Downey, in an unpublished article, "The Structure and Origin of Lymph Sinuses of Mammalian Lymph Nodes" makes some very interesting statements: "Both the embryological and anatomical studies have shown, therefore, that the tissue of the splenic sinuses is to be regarded as reticulum rather than endothelium. . . . It is not identical with the endothelium of blood- and lymph vessels." With regard to the relation of the reticular tissue to the sinuses, he says, "The sinuses are closely associated with the reticular tissue of the organs concerned."

The amount of lymphoid tissue was found in many cases to be markedly below normal, but the average was estimated at −1.5. In determining the amount present in any given microscopical specimen, the malpighian corpuscles, perivascular lymphocytic infiltration, and the lymphocytes generally distributed throughout were considered. As a rule, the malpighian corpuscles were fairly well defined and small, but they did not stand out prominently nor were they seen often. Contrary to the findings of certain observers, in this series the so-called germinal centers were very rarely seen and, when found, were small and inconspicious. The intermediate zone of the malpighian corpuscle, "the zone of expansion" which in normal splenic tissue stains deeply and is prominent, was poorly defined and scarcely noticeable.

An attempt was made to study the minute capillaries which are connected with the splenic sinuses (Figs. 2 and 3). In normal splenic tissue these small blood channels consist of but a single layer of endothelial cells, the media and the adventitia disappearing as the vessel approaches the size of a capillary. In splenic anemia and in the other splenomegalies, the spleens showed an increase of fibrous tissue around these vessel walls. Due allowance, however, must be made for the fact that the venules enter

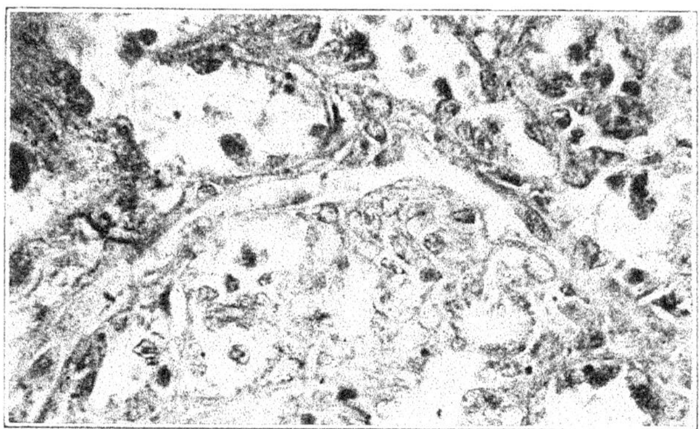

Fig. 2.—Splenic anemia; a capillary is seen.

the trabeculæ soon after their formation. In many instances the walls of these vessels showed a decided hyaline change so that the lumen became quite small and irregular.

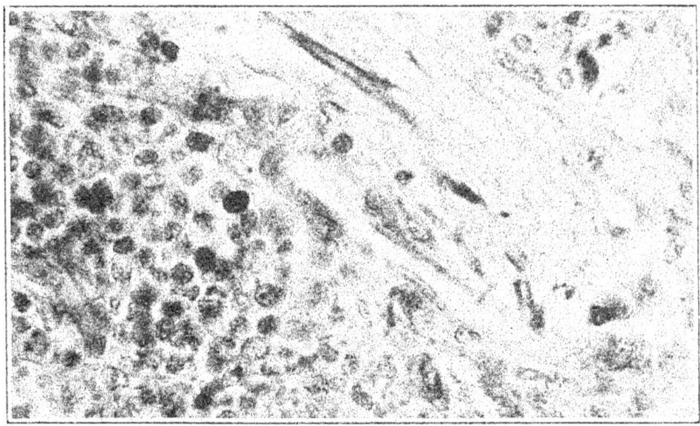

Fig. 3.—Splenic anemia; small capillary near a trabeculum.

In attempting to make a differential diagnosis of the various groups of splenomegaly the greatest difficulty was experienced with syphilitic spleens which resembled those of splenic anemia very closely. The sinuses in the syphilitic spleens were as prominent as those in the spleens of splenic anemia and the fibrosis was as great.

On account of the relative prominence of the malpighian corpuscles and the accuracy with which they can be studied, they were given special consideration, particularly from the standpoint of relative size and number, and general structure. While the malpighian bodies of splenic anemia were fairly prominent in the miscroscopical specimen, and were well circumscribed, they were not so prominent as in the normal, or in cases of pernicious anemia. There were only two or three specimens, however, in which the boundaries of the corpuscles could not be marked out with a fair degree of accuracy.

Contrary to many reports on the subject of splenic anemia, areas of degeneration or fibrous nodules were not found within the malpighian corpuscles. This, however, is entirely in accord with the ideas of Cushing and MacCallum who, in discussing splenic anemia, said, "No progressive sclerotic process, such as Banti described, is seen in these malpighian bodies nor has it been possible to find any fibrous nodules which might have resulted from such a sclerosis."

The larger the malpighian corpuscle, the greater was its tendency to be round or oval in shape and the nearer the center the artery seemed to be. As the generalized fibrosis increased in amount the malpighian corpuscles became smaller and were more irregular in outline.

As the fibrous tissue encroached on the periphery of the malpighian body, it seemed to cut off groups of cells somewhat irregularly. A continuance of this process resulted many times in the malpighian body being composed of a group of cells without a perceptible central artery, the vessel lying entirely outside of the corpuscle.

Before discussing the size of the malpighian body in splenic anemia the size of the normal should be considered. Gray gives the size of the malpighian corpuscles of the spleen as varying from 0.25 to 1 mm. in diameter. Morris gives the average size of the normal as 0.25 to 1.5 mm. Mall says the splenic lobule in a normal spleen is about 1 mm. in diameter and adds, "The malpighian corpuscle usually lies in the proximal end of the lobule, but in case it is very large it may distend the lobule and cause it to bulge."

In order to determine the size of the malpighian corpuscle in splenic anemia a camera lucida was used with the low power of the microscope (Fig. 4). Most of the corpuscles were not exactly round and for this reason the length and breadth were measured and the average was taken. Wheu due allowance had been made for the magnification, it was found that the average size of the malpighian corpuscle was approximately 0.35 mm. in diameter. The variation in size was from 0.2 to 0.6 mm. It is evident, therefore, that the size of the corpuscles in splenic anemia is within the limits of normal, but that the average size is much below the average in the normal.

The next step was the determination of the number of malpighian bodies in a given area of splenic tissue in splenic anemia. The dissecting microscope proved to be very helpful in this work. A square 0.5 by 0.5 cm. was the size of the field chosen and three fields were counted in each spleen in order to get a general average of different portions of the organ. After determining the average for each spleen, the average for 69 spleens was found. The average number of malpighian bodies for each 0.5 cm. squared, or for $\frac{1}{4}$ of 1 sq. cm., was found to be nearly 6. The number of malpighian bodies in a square centimeter was estimated as approximately 23.

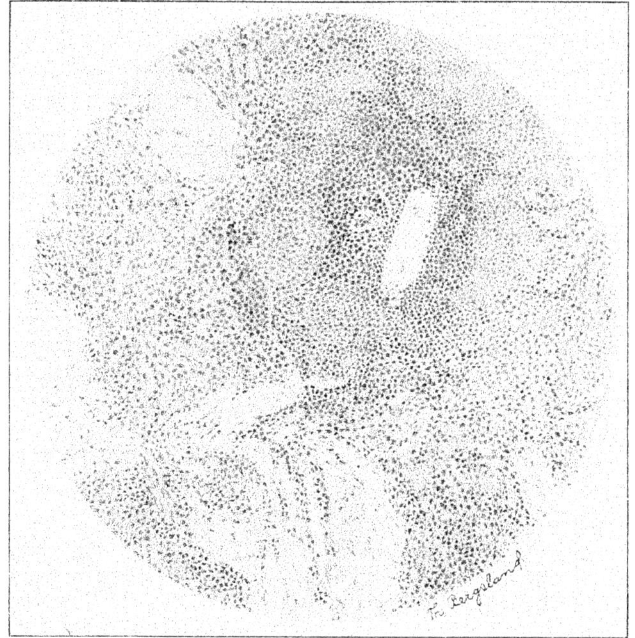

FIG. 4.—A malpighian corpuscle with a great amount of fibrosis around it. The central artery is cut obliquely.

Certainly this number is far less than the number of malpighian corpuscles in the same area in a normal spleen. In a series of about 12 normal spleens (far too few for calculating accurate averages), the number of malpighian bodies for each square centimeter was approximately 40.

The relation of the number of malpighian bodies to the size and weight of the spleens furnishes interesting data. As in all statements concerning the pathology of splenic anemia, however, there are many exceptions. The number of malpighian corpuscles to each square area seemed to decrease as the size and weight of the spleen increased. The size of the malpighian body became smaller as the weight and size of the spleen increased. This was found to be true in 70 per cent of the spleens, and would seem to indicate that the number of malpighian corpuscles in a spleen remains constant until a fibrotic or some other pathological process becomes so marked that many of the corpuscles are completely destroyed or are made so small that they are not recognized.

Gross Pathology. As in the microscopical study, a consideration of the gross pathology consisted in the study of the 69 spleens of splenic anemia and a comparison with 175 specimens from the various other groups of splenomegaly.

The average weight of these spleens was approximately 950 gm., and the variations in weight 120 to 2290 gm. If patients less than ten years of age were excluded, the average weight increased to 1015 gm. Rolleston found the average weight in 21 cases of splenic anemia to be 782.46 gm.

When the average weight of these spleens was compared with that of the other groups of spleens of splenomegaly it was found that those of Gaucher's disease and those in the lymphoma group averaged higher in weight. The spleens arranged according to their number and average weights were: Gaucher's disease, four, 3031 gm.; the lymphoma group, five, 2249 gm.; splenic anemia, sixty-nine, 1015 gm.; pernicious anemia, fifty-three, 940 gm.; myelogenous leukemia, twenty-six, 937 gm.; hemolytic jaundice, thirty-two, 920 gm.; syphilis, six, 778 gm., and tuberculosis, four, 501 gm. It must be borne in mind that all of the spleens here considered were obtained at operation.

An effort was made to ascertain if the weight or size of the spleens varied in any other pathological conditions. Curves were made in order that any slight variation might be detected. When compared with the weight and size, there was no constant change found in the thickness of the capsule in the reticulum, in arteriosclerosis, or in the pulp or endothelium of the sinuses. The heavier spleens showed a slight tendency to have thicker capsules or a greater degree of perisplenitis. The spleen of splenic anemia maintained to a rather remarkable degree the shape of a normal spleen. From the standpoint of perisplenitis, the average was found to be +2. Thirty-eight were +2, eighteen +1, nine +3, and four +4.

Only 5 spleens showed macroscopical infarcts and these were variable in size, the largest being 12 x 8 x 3 cm. and the smallest scarcely perceptible. In these 5 specimens the average arteriosclerosis was +1.2. In 3 cases there was a history of abdominal pain and in 3 of gastric hemorrhage. In 3 cases also, ascites was present. All the changes mentioned, arteriosclerosis, pain, hemorrhage, and ascites were present in 1 case only. There was no constant clinical or pathological finding in the spleen in any of the cases of infarct.

A typical spleen of splenic anemia bears the general shape of a normal spleen, but is about five times as large. When allowed to rest on the table it maintains its shape much better than the normal spleen which flattens out; it is several times as firm as the normal. Its capsule is grayish-white with a slight reddish or a purplish-red tint. Hyaline plaques may or may not be seen on its surface; in the average spleen they would not be present. Perisplenitis is very evident, especially on the diaphragmatic surface.

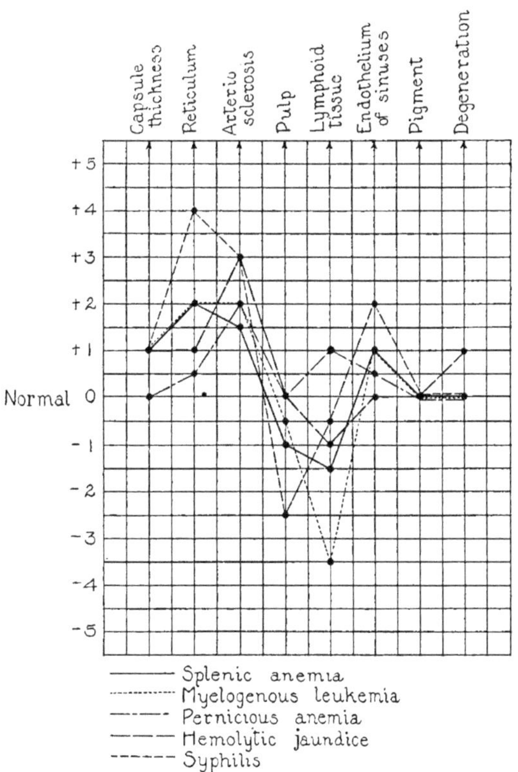

FIG. 5.—Microscopical pathological findings in splenic anemia, myelogenous leukemia, pernicious anemia, hemolytic jaundice and syphilis.

The typical spleen of splenic anemia offers considerable resistance to cutting. The cut surfaces bulge outward and present a red, beefy appearance. Fibrosis is very evident, and the trabeculæ are especially prominent. The malpighian bodies are not seen. The cut surface of a specimen that has been preserved in formalin is quite pink and the trabeculæ, which have become very white, form a prominent network over the surface.

When the results of the pathological study of splenic anemia are summarized and the findings are compared with a similar study of the other groups of splenomegaly, such as pernicious anemia, leukemia, and hemolytic jaundice, the general impression obtained is that there is a very great pathological variation within each group and that while certain conditions seem to be more common in some groups than in others, the findings overlap, to a great extent. The points of similarity in the various groups are rather striking and suggest that the spleen may play a similar part in all of the diseases that produce splenomegaly (Fig. 5).

Clinical Findings. The 69 patients with splenic anemia had been in poor health for an average period of seven years when they came to the Mayo Clinic. Because of the insidious onset of splenic anemia and the unreliability of the patient's memory, the possibility of inaccuracy in this statement is, of course, very great. Moreover, seven years does not indicate the entire duration of the disease, but the period of illness previous to the time of splenectomy.

The average age of the patients was thirty-three years, the youngest being two and one-half and the oldest sixty-nine years. If the average age is thirty-three years and the average duration seven years, the onset must have been about the age of twenty-six. The duration of the illness was in all probability more than seven years, for many of the patients gave a history of "always being delicate." They dated the onset of their illness, however, from the time of some marked disturbance, such as a gastric hemorrhage. The distribution was about equal in the sexes, there being 36 male and 33 female patients.

In no instance was a history of injury obtained as a possible cause, nor did the records show an instance of two or more cases of anemia occurring in the same family. Occupation was apparently not a factor.

Most of the patients complained of more than one abnormal condition which they considered of great importance in their illness. The complaints may be summarized as follows: Enlarged spleen and mass in left abdomen, 29; hemorrhages from the stomach, 20; and weakness, 19. Indigestion, pain in the left side of the abdomen and anemia were each complained of in 6 cases. Diarrhea was mentioned in 3, pallor in 3, pain in epigastrium in 2, shortness of breath in 2, and jaundice in 2; while rheumatism, constipation, palpitation, headaches, bleeding from the bowels, pain and numbness in legs, nervousness, and asthma were each mentioned but once.

The frequency with which hemorrhage occurred was rather surprising. It was not only a very common complaint, but often the severity of it was so alarming that it was a common cause for seeking medical attention. The histories showed that 41 of the

69 patients had hemorrhages. Thirty-eight of these were recognized by the patients as having come from the stomach as they had vomited blood, and 27, besides the vomiting of blood, had recognized blood passed by the bowel. Of the 3 remaining patients 1 noticed blood in the bowel movements only and 2 had quite profuse nasal bleeding. From the standpoint of severity, these hemorrhages may be graded 1, 2, 3, and 4. In 5 patients bleeding was graded 1, in eighteen, 2; in seventeen, 3; and in one, 4. Many of the patients spoke of the alarming nature of the hemorrhages; their prostration was so great that they had to remain in bed from three days to two weeks.

Abdominal pain was rarely mentioned as the chief complaint, probably its relative infrequency caused the patient to consider it of minor importance in his trouble. Nevertheless, on being questioned, 32 patients told of having had one or more attacks of pain, most of which were short, but often rather severe. Four of these patients located the pain definitely over the spleen; 2 had mid-epigastric pain, while 1 located the painful area in the lower right quadrant. There were 25, therefore, who were indefinite with regard to the site of the pain. According to Giffin, "Pain in the region of the spleen in splenic anemia is common and is probably due to perisplenitis which is so often present." Certain patients who complained of pain in the left abdominal area while under observation, presented definite friction rubs over the spleen.

Evidence was found elsewhere than in the spleen that might explain the pain in 15 of the 32 patients who had had pain. Six of those who complained of abdominal pain and one of mid-epigastric pain had gall stones; 4 with abdominal pain had diseased gall-bladders and 4 had chronic appendicitis.

Eight patients gave histories of having had malaria. None of these had had recent attacks nor had the disease lasted long. In all of them a special search had been made in the blood smears for the malarial plasmodia with negative results. Some investigators have taken exception to Banti's cases because they came from malarial districts. Geographical distribution of the patients in this series was: Minnesota 14, Iowa 8, Wisconsin 6, South Dakota 6, Illinois 5, Canada 5, Montana, North Dakota, Nebraska, Michigan, Missouri, and Texas each 2, and 1 each from Oregon, Indiana, Wyoming, New Mexico, New York, Pennsylvania, West Virginia, Kentucky, Tennessee, Mississippi, Alabama, and Arkansas.

Usually the first note made by the clinician in his physical examination was the size of the spleen. There was only 1 patient whose spleen could not be palpated and this might be explained by the presence of ascites; the spleen in this case weighed 390 gm. In 2 patients whose spleens could just be felt below the costal margin, the organs weighed 250 gm. and 425 gm. Another spleen, felt rather indistinctly and described as "a mass in the splenic region," weighed 318 gm. A spleen of 530 gm. was designated as "1 inch below the costal margin." On nearly every history chart a drawing was made by the examiner to show what he considered the relative size of the spleen. The size thus roughly designated varied in a general way with the weight in all except two instances. In these exceptions a spleen of 120 gm. and one of 320 gm. were outlined to suggest a much greater size. Judging from the diagrams on these histories a spleen that extended to the middle line and down to about the level of the umbilicus should weigh approximately 1000 gm. It would seem that the spleen maintained its relative position in the abdomen in spite of the enlarging process.

The adhesions around the spleen were so marked that special mention was made of them in 33 cases. There were, however, few spleens with elongated pedicles. On only one surgical card was reference made to the presence of a twisted pedicle. The spleen in 1 patient who had never had hemorrhages showed one complete turn; the organ weighed 610 gm.

In the physical examination the feel of the spleen was generally described by the clinician as "hard and smooth." A notch was felt in approximately 50 per cent.

Notes in the physical examinations regarding the size of the liver, referred to 24 as enlarged. Some of these organs, however, were apparently just below the costal margin and were marked "questionable enlargement." According to the operative findings, there were 26 patients who had enlarged livers. At operation 30 patients were found to have definite cirrhosis of the liver and in only 13 of these, was the liver larger than normal. The average weight of the spleen in the 24 cases in which the liver was described as enlarged was found to be 1016 gm.

Presumably, the size of the liver in splenic anemia bears no close relationship to the size and weight of the spleen. The findings in this series of cases suggest that there is a steady progressive enlargement of the spleen, but that the liver maintains its normal size until relatively late in the course of the disease. It then enlarges and may remain enlarged, or it may return to its normal size or become even smaller than normal. It cannot be said just how early in the disease cirrhosis of the liver begins. In many respects, therefore, the physical findings in splenic anemia are the reverse of those in portal cirrhosis, for in this latter disease a palpable spleen is usually found relatively late.

Ascites was present in 24 patients, 23 of whom had cirrhosis of the liver. In the other case the liver was enlarged, but apparently not cirrhotic. Allbutt and Rolleston are of the opinion that in splenic anemia ascites may occur in the absence of hepatic cirrhosis.

Only very general statements can be made with regard to weight lost during the progress of the disease. In most cases the disease had lasted so long that the patient was uncertain as to his weight before onset. It would seem, however, that in a series of 22 cases, the average loss of weight was only 5 pounds. The greatest loss was 27 pounds, and 3 patients weighed more than what they considered their normal.

Bronzing of the skin is often mentioned in splenic anemia. In this series 21 patients were described as sallow or pale; 12 showed yellowness of the skin; 7 were described as lemon-yellow, 5 brownish-yellow, 1 tanned skin, 1 cachectic looking, and 1 brownish pigment about the eyes; 27, then, showed some change in the color of the skin; 21 of the remaining 42 patients showed sufficient pallor to attract attention. None of the patients appeared to have definite icterus.

In none of the histories was there a note concerning any enlargement of peripheral veins of the abdomen or chest.

From the standpoint of the laboratory work the blood count was undoubtedly the most valuable, but the reports on the coagulation time, fragility test, Wassermann reaction, and stool tests were not without value. Blood counts were made on all patients with splenic anemia before splenectomy, and on most of them at varying times after the operation.

The Wassermann test was done in 60 instances and was negative in 59. The 1 positive reaction was later discredited as a result of four subsequent negative tests. Four patients gave a history of syphilitic infection, but in none of these could evidence of syphilis be found.

Stool examinations were seldom done. There were apparently two indications; a history of diarrheal attacks, or of residence in the tropics. Thirteen stool examinations were done with the following results: 9 were negative; 2 showed *Amœba histolytica;* 1 *Lamblia intestinalis,* and 1 cercomonads and trichomonas. None of the patients, however, had diarrheal attacks.

The fragility test was done in 29 of the patients. In 15 of these the fragility was normal; only 1 showed a tendency toward an increase in fragility of the corpuscles, while 13 showed an increased resistance.

The coagulation time was determined in only 13 patients. All except 1 were between two and ten minutes. One patient showed a coagulation time of fifteen minutes. In this determination either the Biffi-Brooks coagulometer, the Boggs coagulometer or the Lee and Vincent test-tube method was employed.

A study of the relation between the number of erythrocytes and leukocytes and the hemoglobin before operation revealed a varying degree of anemia. In every case this was of the secondary type, the color index in many cases being relatively low. There was always a relative leucopenia and in some of the counts the number of leukocytes was low in comparison to the number of red corpuscles.

The average erythrocyte count was 3,700,000, the hemoglobin 53 per cent, and the leukocytes 4900. In the 30 patients with definite cirrhosis of the liver, the erythrocytes were about 3,500,000, the hemoglobin 50 per cent and the leukocytes 4600. In the 13 patients with enlargement of the liver but without definite cirrhosis, the erythrocytes were about 4,000,000, the hemoglobin 56 per cent, and the leukocytes 5800. The remaining 26 patients who had approximately normal livers had an average erythrocyte count of 3,750,000, hemoglobin of 55 per cent, and a leukocyte count of 5000.

In many of the patients, changes in the erythrocytes were noted and were usually designated as slight or moderate. These changes were seen in patients with the greatest degree of anemia. Poikilocytosis and anisocystosis were noted in 29 of the 69 patients; anisocytosis, poikilocytosis and normoblasts in 12; and anisocytosis alone in 9. Only occasionally, mention was made of polychromatophilia.

In most of the patients blood counts were made at varying intervals after splenectomy and in every case there was a marked increase in the number of leukocytes. The normal was taken as 8000, and in each case the number of days after operation was considered. A composite chart showed that there was an initial rise in the leukocytes immediately after the operation and that the number gradually increased until about the forty-fifth day. There was then a gradual decrease until the count approached the normal line in seventy-five to one hundred days after splenectomy. An abrupt rise occurred previous to the tenth day after splenectomy. From the tenth to the thirtieth day the increase was more gradual. A very gradual decrease then followed until the normal line was approached.

An attempt was made to determine how long secondary anemia persisted after splenectomy, but the results were rather inconclusive. It is certain, however, that there was an improvement in the hemoglobin and the number of erythrocytes. The degree of improvement varied greatly so that no time relation could be established. In only a very few cases were two or more blood counts made following splenectomy and, while these showed progressive improvement, the number was too small from which to draw conclusions.

A differential cell count was made in 63 of the patients before operation. In the remaining histories the count was noted as normal, and so had to be discarded. If the normal number of polynuclears be considered as varying between 60 and 70 per cent (Piersol), the preoperative counts in these cases were normal in 24 cases, below normal in 10, and there was a relative increase in 29. According to Pappenheim the number of lymphocytes found in a normal differential count is from 20 to 22 per cent. When the lymphocyte counts were compared with these standard figures it was found that 10 were within the limits of normal, 30 above normal, and 25 below normal. A comparison was next made between the preoperative and postoperative differential counts. In 35 patients one of the differential counts had been omitted. Postoperatively 10 patients showed an increase in the polynuclears, and 22 showed an increase in the relative number of lymphocytes. Two patients showed practically no changes in the blood following operation. The length of time that elapsed after splenectomy seemed not to have been an important factor. In patients with an increase in the polynuclear cells, however, the differential count had been made from seven to forty-three days after operation.

Most of the operative findings have already been discussed, but the condition of the gall-bladder as found at operation only has been considered in part. In 11 cases it was described as diseased, markedly distended, or as having a thick wall. In 8 patients the gall-bladder contained stones.

The vermiform appendix was diseased in 7 patients and the extent of disease +2 or +3.

Patients with Cirrhosis of the Liver. There is considerable confusion in the literature with regard to the relation between Banti's disease and splenic anemia. Most American writers choose to consider the two as entirely synonymous, while foreign authors prefer to make a well marked distinction between them.

MacCarty, of the Mayo Clinic, has examined specimens of hepatic tissue obtained at operation is nearly all of the 69 cases of splenic anemia here reported and he is of the opinion that in none of them, no matter how short the duration of the disease, was the liver entirely normal. From the mildest case to the most severe, the liver showed varying degrees of hepatitis. In the more severe types, periportal fibrosis was evident, but there was no sharp line of distinction between those with well defined cirrhosis and those without.

Thirty cases in which there was definite evidence of portal cirrhosis have been grouped together. From the standpoint of morbid anatomy these 30 spleens very closely resembled the remaining 39. Their average weight was a little greater, being 1027 gm. as compared to 1015 gm. of the entire series. There was a slight increase in the amount of fibrosis, but in all other respects no difference could be made out.

This close similarity was found also in the microscopical study. Each pathological finding was graded and averaged as in all the other cases and the results were expressed in a curve. This curve was found to correspond exactly with that for splenic anemia; except that the splenic pulp was −1.4 instead of −1.

The clinical study of this group showed interesting variations from the entire series of cases. The average age was thirty-five;

duration of disease was nine years. As in the other cases, most of the patients dated the origin of the disease, not from the time of the real onset, but probably from the time of some severe manifestation, such as gastric hemorrhage. Nineteen of these patients gave a history of hemorrhage, the severity of which was no greater than that of the remaining 22 patients who also complained of hemorrhages. Eighteen had gastric hemorrhages; 14 had also noticed blood passed by the bowels, and 1 had nasal bleeding; 1 complained of melena only.

In the chief complaints hemorrhages were mentioned 11 times, while enlarged spleen and abdominal mass, if considered together, were complained of 12 times. The less important complaints in order of frequency, were stomach trouble, 5; anemia, 4; abdominal pain, 4; weakness, 4; jaundice, 2; dyspnea, 1; constipation, 1 and pain in the legs, 1.

While most writers consider true Banti's disease to include all patients with definite cirrhosis of the liver, according to Banti there should be ascites besides the cirrhosis. Ascites was rather common in this group, being noted in 24 patients who could, therefore, be classified as cases of true Banti's disease. In 10 of these it was sufficiently marked to be noticed before operation. Thirteen of the 30 patients had enlargement of the liver. An effort was made to find some difference between the 24 cases which showed ascites and the remaining 6 cases of the cirrhosis group. Practically no difference could be made out and for this reason a separate discussion of the group of true Banti's disease would be but a repetition of that given on the group of patients with decided cirrhosis of the liver.

A comparison of the postoperative mortality in patients with cirrhotic livers with that of the remaining patients was interesting. In the 69 patients the highest mortality occurred within forty days of the operation; 12 had died within this period, and 7 of these were patients with marked cirrhosis. If these figures are expressed in terms of percentage, it is seen that 23.3 per cent of the patients in the group with cirrhosis died within forty days of the operation, while only 12.8 per cent of the other patients died within the same length of time.

In splenic anemia the condition seems to be one of under function of the spleen rather than of over function. In the conflict with disease, while all the body tissues suffer, the spleen seems to bear the brunt of the battle. As the normal tissue of the spleen is destroyed it is replaced by fibrous tissues and the organ enlarges in an attempt to keep up its struggle against the disease. Finally, the spleen decompensates and, instead of being a help, it becomes a menace and may be a focus from which the disease is better able to attack the liver and the other organs.

This suggests the question of the most advisable time to perform splenectomy in cases of splenic anemia. From the standpoint of the operative mortality alone the spleen should certainly be removed before definite hepatic cirrhosis has occurred. In the future the development of some test of hepatic function may indirectly be an index to the functional activity of the spleen.

The Mortality and the Postmortem Reports. A general summary of the deaths in this series of patients with splenic anemia has been given by Giffin. There were 9 deaths in hospital and 6 of these patients showed a definite cirrhosis of the liver. It would seem, therefore, that cirrhosis of the liver, especially if associated with ascites, is a very great factor in increasing the operative risk in this disease.

Summary. 1. A composite picture of the pathological findings in the spleen in splenic anemia was found to be one of generalized fibrosis. There were no findings in the splenic tissue that would enable the pathologist to make a positive diagnosis of splenic anemia, yet the abnormality was as characteristic of this disease as in other diseases producing splenomegaly.

2. The degree of fibrosis of the reticulum seemed to vary in a slight degree with the amount of arteriosclerosis. There was no evidence to show, however, that this fibrosis originated in or around the vessel walls.

3. The size of the malpighian corpuscle seemed to be affected by the degree of fibrosis and the greater the fibrosis the more eccentric was the so-called central artery.

4. The splenic veins presented no marked abnormality or evidence of thrombophlebitis.

5. Dilatation of the sinuses was fairly constant and the reticular cells showed a proliferative activity. The syphilitic spleens resembled those of splenic anemia in this respect.

6. The amount of lymphoid tissue present was usually below normal. The malpighian corpuscles were fairly well defined, but the so-called germinal centers were small and seldom seen. Areas of degeneration or fibrous nodules were not found in the malpighian bodies.

7. As a result of an actual measurement it was found that the size of the malpighian corpuscles was within the limits of normal, but that the average size was below the average for the normal. The number of corpuscles for each square centimeter was found to be twenty-three.

8. By actual figures 70 per cent of the spleens showed that the number of malpighian bodies for each square area decreased and the size of the corpuscles became smaller as the size and the weight of the spleen increased.

9. The average weight of the spleens was found to be 1015 gm.

10. The average age of the patients with splenic anemia was

thirty-three years, and the number of males was about equal to the number of females. There was apparently no familial tendency.

11. The most common complaints were mass in the left abdomen, gastric hemorrhage, and weakness.

12. While abdominal pain was rarely given as the chief complaint, the histories brought out the fact that 32 of the patients had attacks at some stage of the disease. In many instances the pain was probably due to perisplenitis.

13. In the physical examination spleens designated as just palpable weighed from 250 to 500 gm., while spleens of approximately 1000 gm. extended to the middle line and almost to the level of the umbilicus.

14. The relation of the size of the spleen, as given by the clinical records, to the actual weight, and the fact that many adhesions were found at operation, suggested that the spleen of splenic anemia maintains its relatively normal position in the abdomen.

15. Physical examination showed 24 enlarged livers, while at the operating table 26 showed a definite cirrhosis, and 13 were larger than normal. The size of the liver seemed to have no relation to the size and weight of the spleen.

16. In the 69 patients the average erythrocyte count was 3,700,000, the hemoglobin 53 per cent, and the leukocyte count, 4990. The coagulation time and the fragility test were normal, and the Wassermann tests and the stool examinations were negative.

17. A composite chart of the blood counts made after the operations showed a gradual increase in the leukocytes up to the forty-fifth day. There was then a gradual decrease until the normal was reached in about seventy-five days. A similar result was obtained in a composite chart in which the number of leukocytes found in the counts made before the operation was taken into consideration.

18. A comparison of the number of lymphocytes in the differential count showed that the average was within the limits of normal. A lymphocytosis did not seem to be a characteristic in this series.

19. In the study of the liver tissue in the cases of splenic anemia, 30 showed a definite cirrhosis, but in none was the liver entirely normal.

20. The chief complaints of the 30 patients that had hepatic cirrhosis were the same as those in the rest of the series; hemorrhage and abdominal mass were the predominating complaints.

21. Twenty-four of the patients with cirrhosis of the liver had ascites.

22. Twenty-three and three-tenths per cent of the patients with cirrhotic livers died within forty days of the operation, while within the same length of time the death rate of the remaining patients was only 12.8 per cent.

BIBLIOGRAPHY.

1. Allbutt and Rolleston: System of Medicine, 1909, **5**, 575.
2. Cushing, H., and MacCallum, W. G.: Two Cases of Splenectomy for Splenic Anemia: A Report on the Pathological Changes in Splenic Anemia, Arch. Surg., 1920, **1**, 1.
3. Downey, H.: The Structure and Origin of Lymph Sinuses of Mammalian Lymph Nodes and Their Relations to the Endothelium and Reticulum (unpublished).
4. Giffin, H. Z.: Present Status of Splenectomy as a Therapeutic Measure, Minnesota Med., 1921, **4**, 132.
5. Giffin, H. Z.: Clinical Observations Concerning Twenty-seven Cases of Splenectomy, AM. JOUR. MED. SCI., 1913, **145**, 781.
6. Gray, H.: Gray's Anatomy, Philadelphia, Lea & Febiger, 1918, 20th ed.
7. Gross, L.: Studies in the Gross and Minute Anatomy of the Spleen in Health and Disease, Jour. Med. Res., 1919, **39**, 311.
8. Hollins, T. J.: Primary Splenomegaly or Splenic Anemia, a Critical Study with Special Reference to the Pathogenesis, Practitioner, London, 1915, **94**, 426.
9. MacCarty, W. C.: Personal communication.
10. Mayo, W. J.: Relation of Chronic Fibrosis and Thrombophlebitis of the Spleen to Conditions of the Blood and of the Liver, Arch. Surg., 1921, **2**, 185.
11. Morris, H.: Human Anatomy, Philadelphia, P. Blakiston's Son Co., 1914, 2d ed.
12. Osler, W.: The Principles and Practice of Medicine, New York, Appleton, 1920, 2d ed.
13. Osler, W.: Splenic Anemia, AM. JOUR. MED. SCI., 1900, **119**, 54.
14. Pappenheim, A.: Clinical Examination of the Blood and Its Technic, Bristol, John Wright & Sons, 1914, **7**, 87.
15. Rolleston, H. D.: Chronic Splenic Anemia and Banti's Disease, Practitioner, London. 1914, **92**, 470.

ELEPHANTIASIS: A CLINICAL REVIEW AND AN ATTEMPT AT EXPERIMENTAL REPRODUCTION.*

BY GEORGE D. MAHON, M.D.

ROCHESTER, MINN.

(From the Divisions of Surgery, and Experimental Surgery and Pathology, The Mayo Foundation, Rochester, Minn.)

VARIOUS definitions of elephantiasis have been given. Practically all refer to the hypertrophy of the skin and subcutaneous connective tissue with vascular disturbances and resulting exudate. The congenital form of elephantiasis usually involves one or more limbs. The pathological picture differs from the true form in that connective tissue hypertrophy and normal cell infiltration are absent.

No one has been able to obtain cultures of bacteria except during the recurring active cutaneous reactions seen in the majority of cases of elephantiasis. It must be remembered, however, that a few cases of elephantiasis occur without local inflammatory manifestations. Sistrunk had several of this type in his series. Bac-

* Abstract of thesis submitted to the Faculty of the Graduate School of the University of Minnesota, in partial fulfillment of the requirements for the degree of Master of Science in Surgery, May, 1921.

teriological studies were made in most of the cases. In one of these in which there had never been local inflammation, Magath was able to grow, in pure culture, a green-producing streptococcus. In another case in which there were local manifestations he was able to isolate practically the same organism from the deep tissues during a period of quiescence.

ETIOLOGICAL FACTORS. Manson has traced the life cycle of the filaria which he considered the etiological factor. Objections have been made because central blockage of the lymphatics cannot produce peripheral edema, and because it has been impossible to find filaria in the blood of patients with well developed elephantiasis, who, at some former time, were known to have been hosts of the filaria. Manson did not attempt to explain the former criticism, but the second issue was well known to him. He believed that the lymph blockage was accomplished by the death of the parent worm, which was caused by the lymphangitis observed in all cases of elephantiasis that he studied. He also believed that trauma to the part harboring the parasite would cause the premature parturition of the ova which, being larger than the embryo filaria and not having power of motion, would cause blockage of the lymphatics.

Blockage of the lymphatics with subsequent edema is not sufficient to explain the connective tissue hypertrophy which is the most characteristic histo-pathological element of the disease. An abundance of experimental proof as well as an enormous amount of clinical material indicate that edema will not excite cell proliferation.

DISTRIBUTION: AGE AND SEX. Elephantiasis has not been recognized as a transmissible disease, although a few reported cases would indicate that it might be. Tuberculosis and syphilis have a questionable relationship to elephantiasis. Operative interference with the inguinal lymphatics has preceded some cases of genital elephantiasis. A preponderance of data favor the idea that the edema and hypertrophy which characterize elephantiasis develop as the result of the action of pathogenic organisms, even though it has not been proved that a specific organism is responsible for the disease. It is the exceptional case that did not begin following lymphangitis, cellulitis, dermatitis, or some manifestation of a local infection. In a few cases onset has been insidious, without symptoms, either local or general, that would lead one to think of an infectious process. This has been observed many times. Webb mentions the same type of case observed by him in India.

Elephantiasis is observed in all parts of the world; but as an epidemic it exists only in certain circumscribed areas in the tropical or subtropical regions. In the United States and Canada, it is uncommon and never epidemic.

In the 33 cases studied in the Mayo Clinic the youngest patient was aged twelve, the oldest fifty-five years. In tropical countries, men are affected more often than women, supposedly on account of injuries and infections to which they are more often subjected. Women and men were affected about equally in the cases reported from the Clinic.

PATHOLOGICAL FINDINGS. Most authors have represented the same pathological findings in elephantiasis. Paget describes elephantiasic tissue as "closely woven and very tough, and on section to exude a whitish fluid." Pusey considers hypertrophy of the subcutaneous tissue the most characteristic feature; he said that the hypertrophy converts the part into a dense fibrous structure in which are usually found dilated lymph spaces. The chorium is greatly thickened, and the matting together of its layers disorganizes its typical arrangement. The epidermis may or may not be thickened. The sebaceous glands, sweat glands, and hair follicles may be unchanged or destroyed. Stelwagon agrees with Pusey that the chief change is hypertrophy of the connective tissue, but he contends that the blood-vessels are also changed, and adds that Mosely and Morrison found an increase in the pigment matter. Hartzell draws attention to a plugging of the veins with a thrombus composed of leukocytes. Elliott believes that there are more changes in the arteries than in the veins. Unna believes that the condition begins quite superficially by a blocking of the veins from the inflammatory process excited by the bacteria. There is a subsequent destruction of some of the vessels, with still more edema, and the ever present bacteria, lying latent in the tissue ready to flare up, produce still more hypertrophy of the tissue, thereby interfering more with the circulation. This chain of events continues until finally there is an enormous tissue hypertrophy, with destruction of many superficial blood-vessels draining the part, and resulting edema.

In the cases of elephantiasis studied, the epidermis was thinned out when the extremity was unusually large. There was always some change in the blood-vessels. Occasionally there was a marked thrombosis and lymphocytic infiltration around the vessel, especially in patients who had had violent cutaneous reactions. The lymphocytic infiltration was always mild in the patient who had not suffered from recurring attacks of erythema; but some of the sections representing the most marked hypertrophy were obtained from patients who had never had erysipelas, cellulitis, or any symptom to indicate inflammation in the part. In such cases there was more evidence of lymphocytic infiltration in the deeper layers, and the aponeurosis was often more thickened; also, there were more changes in the bloodvessels of the deeper tissues than in the chorium. It may be assumed that in many patients who develop elephantiasis, the inflammatory reaction necessary to produce cell proliferation is caused by low-grade organisms confined to the subcutaneous tissue and not of sufficient virulence to produce local or constitutional reactions.

Surgical Treatment. Mann calls attention to the two principles which, at present, are the basis for the surgical treatment of this condition: (1) establishing new lymph paths; and (2) connecting the edematous elephantiasic tissues with the normal musculature below the aponeurosis.

Sistrunk has performed a modified Kondoleon operation on about 40 patients with elephantiasis. He removes, besides the aponeurosis, a wide piece of skin and subcutaneous tissue nearly, though not quite, so wide as the aponeurosis. Recently he has also removed small sections of the aponeurosis in the iliac regions in patients with the disease especially pronounced in the thighs and hips. Sistrunk believes the removal of large pieces of diseased skin and subcutaneous tissue (not capable of functioning because of the destroyed vascular lymph supply) is of great importance.

If these patients are kept in bed for a week or more before operation, the parts will be reduced in size and operation made easier. Morphine given before operation minimizes the shock. In extreme cases, a complete operation cannot be performed at one time, but similar operations on different portions of the extremity may be performed at different times. Operation does not cure elephantiasis, but the condition can be greatly relieved. Better results will be obtained if the patients wear elastic stockings indefinitely, perhaps permanently.

Experiments. Since I believed that the hypertrophy and edema which characterize elephantiasis is caused directly by the action of pathogenic bacteria, I attempted to prove it by experiments on dogs. Bookhardt injected a culture of living organisms (the coccus of Fehleisen) into the tissues of a pedunculated malignant tumor which subsequently took on changes typical of elephantiasis. In a series of experiments on animals, an attempt was made to lower the resistance of the part by interfering with the lymphatics draining the region. Later, the venous return was also partially ligated, further to lower the resistance of the part. The animals were then inoculated with a green-producing streptococcus obtained by Dr. Magath from the subcutaneous tissues of two patients in Dr. Sistrunk's series. Dr. Magath describes the technic used and the type of organism cultured as follows:

"A small piece of tissue taken from the leg (elephantiasis) was introduced directly and immediately into a tube of glucose broth, and incubated for forty-eight hours. At the end of that time a smear made from the broth showed numerous small, short chains of streptococci. Transfers were made by streaking a plate of blood agar; the streptococcus was present in pure culture. The colonies were minute, semi-flattened and circular, growing slowly with the formation of a slight amount of green pigment, less than *Streptococcus viridans* but more than typical pneumococcus. The broth culture was used for the first animal injection, and subcultures taken from this in broth were used for subsequent injections. A similar organism was isolated from a piece of tissue taken from the scrotum of another patient with elephantiasis, and this was used for the last series of animal inoculations."

Twenty animals were used. To favor the development of the organism, the lymphatics of the groin of the leg were dissected out. In others, the femoral vein was also ligated. Controls were used. The injections of the organisms were made intravenously and subcutaneously in different groups of the animals. The intravenous injections were made on the evidence that a blood-borne organism is responsible for the condition. The opposite leg from the one in which the lymphatics or veins, or both, were molested, was used for the injection. We undertook this work with the full understanding that the production of a chronic lesion in an animal offered many difficulties. It is well known that animals may not respond to certain organisms as does man. Moreover, the cultures used must be kept under artificial conditions for a long time and would lose some of their activity.

In some of the experiments neither the operative procedure nor the injected bacteria produced any noticeable effect. In many instances the removal of the lymphatics, and particularly the ligation of the venous return, produced edema of the leg for a variable period. The edema did not persist for any great length of time and a condition resembling elephantiasis never occurred. The effect attributable to the bacteria was obtained. The results of the experiments were negative with regard to the production of elephantiasis.

Conclusions. 1. The characteristic feature of elephantiasis is a hypertrophy of the collagenous connective tissue with some degree of lymph and venous stasis.

2. The hypertrophy of the connective tissue and the corresponding stasis are probably the result of repeated insults from pathogenic bacteria.

3. In one group of cases of elephantiasis, there is an outward manifestation of infection evidenced by erythema and adenitis. This type is more common. There is a second group in which the disease develops insidiously, and without any local manifestation of infection. From the pathological study of these cases, I am convinced that they too have an infection basis, which is confined to the lower layers of the subcutaneous tissue, and of such low grade as not to excite any local symptoms.

4. Anything that causes venous stasis could be considered a predisposing factor in the development of elephantiasis.

5. Central blockage of the lymphatics probably cannot produce permanent peripheral lymph stasis.

6. The parent worm of filaria may excite inflammatory changes, and elephantiasis may be produced in such cases by pathogenic bacteria, the filaria being a predisposing factor.

7. In the Kondoleon operation, we have a means of rendering useful service to patients with elephantiasis, although the operation does not positively cure the disease.

BIBLIOGRAPHY.

1. Bockhart, M.: Zur Actiologie der Elephantiasis Arabum, Monatsh. f. prakt. Dermat, 1883, **2**, 133.
2. Elliott, J. A.: Elephantiasis Nostras; Review of Subject with Report of a Case, Jour. Cutan. Dis., 1917, **25**, 17.
3. Eves, A.: Elephantiasis Successfully Treated by Amputation Above the Knee, Lancet, 1859, **2**, 107.
4. Hartzell, M. B.: Diseases of the Skin, Philadelphia and London, J. B. Lippincott Company, 1917, p. 767.
5. Kondoleon, E.: Die operative Behandlung der elephantiastischen Óedeme, Zentralbl. f. Chir., 1912, **39**, 1022.
6. Magath, T. B.: Personal communication.
7. Mann, F. C.: Personal communication.
8. Manson, P.: Tropical Diseases; A Manual of the Diseases of Warm Climates, London, Cassell & Co., 1898, pp. 623.
9. Mosely and Morrison: Quoted by Stelwagon.
10. Paget, J.:, Lectures on Surgical Pathology Delivered at the Royal College of Surgeons of England, 3d ed., Philadelphia, Lindsay and Blakiston, 1865.
11. Pusey, W. A.: The Principles and Practice of Dermatology, 3d ed., New York and London, D. Appleton & Co., 1917, pp. 1278.
12. Sistrunk, W. E.: The Kondoleon Operation for Elephantiasis; Report of the End-results, Southern Med. Jour., 1921, **14**, 619.
13. Sistrunk: Personal communication.
14. Stelwagon, H. W.: A Treatise on Diseases of the Skin for Advanced Students and Practitioners, 8th ed., Philadelphia and London, Saunders, 1916, pp. 1309.
15. Unna, P. G.: The Histopathology of the Diseases of the Skin, New York, Macmillan & Co., 1896, pp. 1205.
16. Webb: Quoted by Eves.

A STUDY OF URINARY OUTPUT AND BLOOD-PRESSURE CHANGES RESULTING IN EXPERIMENTAL ASCITES.*

BY J. MONROE THORINGTON, M.D.,

AND

CARL F. SCHMIDT, M.D.

PHILADELPHIA, PA.

(From the Presbyterian Hospital, Philadelphia, and the Department of Pharmacology, University of Pennsylvania.)

IN the following paper it is intended to present some simple experimental data dealing with artificially increased intra-abdominal pressure, in the attempt to elucidate the mechanism of some common vascular and renal secretory changes which occur in association with ascites.

* The writers desire to express their thanks to Prof. A. N. Richards for laboratory facilities and valuable suggestions, and to Dr. A. B. Light for technical assistance in connection with these experiments.

The physician who carefully studies patients whose condition is complicated by ascites (the usual case is cardio-renal), will notice that this is accompanied by a diminution of urinary output and that paracentesis abdominalis for removal of a fluid collection is usually accompanied by a slight rise of blood-pressure. The urinary output is in a measure restored to normal by the operation of paracentesis.

These features are not satisfactorily explained, either in text-books on physiology or physical diagnosis. Nowhere does one discover any mention of the influence of ascitic effusions upon either caval circulation or renal output. Krehl[1] makes the following statement, which is quoted as bearing on the problem under consideration: "If the quantity of blood that flows through the kidney be diminished, a small amount of highly concentrated urine is secreted; in other words, the diminution in the total solids is not parallel to that of water. . . , a diminished renal circulation may occur in the absence of any local constriction of the renal vessels, either because the general arterial pressure is reduced or because the pressure in the renal veins is raised. The reduction of the general arterial pressure may result from a wide-spread vasomotor paralysis or from a weakening of the left ventricle. The pressure in the renal veins may be raised by an occlusion of these veins, or of the vena cava inferior; by an increase in the general venous pressure from a weakening of the right ventricle; or by a diminution in the aspirating action of the thorax."

It has been shown by Paneth,[2] and later by de Souza,[3] that every venous obstruction in the kidney lessens the urinary output as soon as it reaches a certain (moderate) degree.

That the presence of fluid in the abdomen causes a diminution of urinary output in cases in which but little renal pathology is demonstrable, is illustrated by the following history.

Case Report. Mary S., aged fifty-three years. Admitted March 27, 1921.

Chief Complaint. Decreasing urinary output. Abdominal swelling.

Present Illness. Patient was well until four weeks ago, when abdominal soreness and swelling began. Urinary output has steadily decreased. No dysuria; never any hematuria. Ankles have not been swollen. No dyspnea nor palpitation. Sleeps poorly. Appetite good. Constipated.

Past Medical History. Always well except for dyspepsia.

Family History. Husband living and well. Seven children living and well.

Social History. Housework. Born in Ireland; in United States thirty years. Drinks tea and coffee, alcohol in moderation.

Physical Examination. Well developed adult white female. The examination of the head, neck, chest and extremities was negative.

Abdomen: Liver and spleen not enlarged. Abdomen much distended and resistance is encountered although no mass is palpable. Dulness in the flanks with coronal tympany. No areas of tenderness.

Gynecological Examination. Bilateral and perineal lacerations. Uterus not enlarged; fixed but not tender.

Diagnosis. Rapidly growing mass; origin undetermined. Advice: Laparotomy.

Clinical Notes. March 28. Has voided only 2 ounces since admission. One ounce of urine obtained on catheterization. Patient feels all right except for abdominal distension.

March 29. Roentgen-ray report: Irregular shadow in lower abdomen, probably due to large mass.

Cystoscopic report: Bladder depressed anteriorly and trigone markedly elevated. Both ureters catheterized for 27 cm. without encountering any resistance. Passage of catheters not followed by any material quantity of urine sufficient to indicate hydroureter or hydronephrosis. Indigo-carmine, right, nine and a half; left, eleven and a half minutes after injection.

Operation. Abdomen opened below umbilicus. Peritoneum thickened and adherent. About 1.5 gallons of straw colored fluid poured out, apparently contained in two or three large cavities formed by intestinal adhesions. Mesentery and omentum were thickened and friable, while a chain of thickened and enlarged glands ran along the mesenteric attachment throughout the length of the small intestine. Diagnosis: Carcinoma; impossible to determine the primary focus. Kidneys on palpation appeared to be normal. Enlarged glands and a piece of thickened omentum were removed for section. Abdomen closed with drainage.

March 31. Patient much more comfortable. Urinary output has greatly increased.

Tissue Diagnosis: Scirrhous carcinoma.

The following are laboratory findings for the first twelve days following the patient's admission to the hospital:

Urine. The specific gravity varied between 1020 and 1030. A very faint trace of albumin was found on the first examination otherwise the results were negative. The volume output in twenty-four hours was between 210 to 270 cc before operation; after operation this was between 500 to 900 cc. The phenolsulphonephthalein was 15 per cent in two hours.

Blood. Wassermann, negative. Urea nitrogen, 19 mg. per 100 cc.

Blood-pressure. March 28, 130 to 65. April 5, 120 to 70.

Abdominal Fluid. Polymorphonuclears 33 per cent, lymphocytes 67 per cent. Negative for tubercle bacilli.

We have here an example of massive ascites, due to rapidly progressing malignancy, in which, with no apparent renal pathology, urine output is greatly cut down; with removal of the ascitic fluid, urinary output immediately returns to a volume approximating the normal.

The intra-abdominal tension required to produce a diminution of urinary output is not great. Two patients whose intra-abdominal tension was measured by means of trocar and attached mercury manometer, registered pressures of 15 to 20 mm. This agrees with the measurements of Quirin,[4] who records 20 mm. as the intra-abdominal pressure in two patients, each with an ascites amounting to about 7000 cc.

Experimental Studies. To obtain further information concerning the conditions which caused such marked changes in urine excretion in this patient, four experiments were performed in which intra-abdominal pressure of dogs was raised by injecting fluid into the peritoneal cavity, urinary output being measured at varying degrees of intra-abdominal pressure.

Procedure. Female dogs, of approximately equal size, were used; to minimize as far as possible suppression of urine due to anesthetic and operation, they were given glucose solution by stomach tube, about twelve hours and again two hours before the experiment began. Anesthesia was induced by intramuscular injection of luminal, as a rule, supplemented by ether inhalation. Carotid blood-pressure was recorded by a mercury manometer. Through a midline abdominal incision, a cannula was inserted into each ureter, and these were connected to a glass tube which passed through the urethra; urine excretion was measured either by volume or in drops. The rectum was divided and a glass tube introduced through the anus; this tube was connected to a pressure bottle containing the fluid to be introduced and to a vertical glass tube which acted as a manometer, the pressure readings being given in millimeters of mercury in the following sections. The abdomen was then closed tightly.

The fluid was kept at 37° to 40° C., and, when it was desired to raise intra-abdominal pressure, was forced into the abdomen by way of the rectum by pumping air into the pressure bottle containing the fluid. In three experiments, 0.9 per cent saline was used; in the fourth, 5 per cent acacia was added, in the hope of diminishing the absorption rate of the fluid. There were no apparent differences in the results obtained with the two solutions.

Results. Urine excretion was always totally suppressed when abdominal pressure was raised to 30 mm. of mercury. Pressures lower than 15 mm. had no constant effect on rate of urine flow, but from 15 to 30 mm. there was always constant diminution. (Figs. 1, 2 and 3).

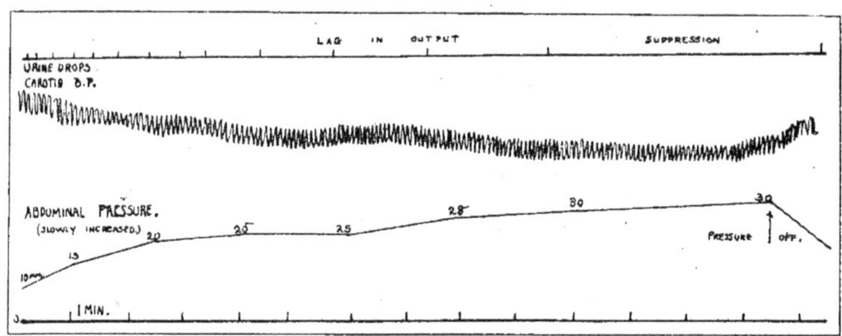

FIG. 1.—Tracing to show decrease in urinary output and suppression of urine which follows a gradually raised intra-abdominal pressure. A slight fall of carotid blood-pressure is also to be noted.

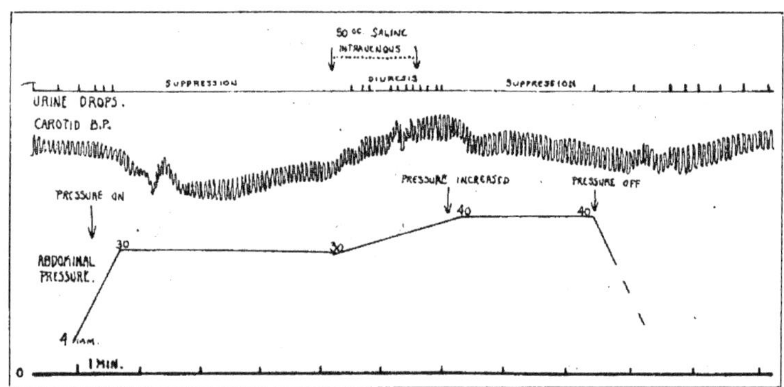

FIG. 2.—Tracing to show urinary suppression following increased intra-abdominal pressure, and the diuresis which may occur, at suppression pressure, when saline is introduced intravenously.

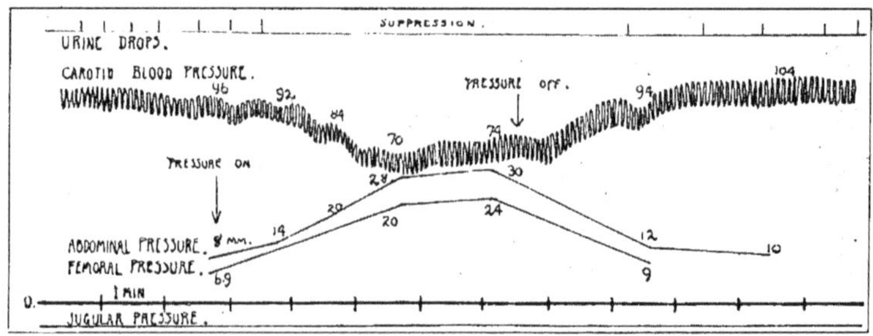

FIG. 3.—Tracing to show the effect of varying intra-abdominal pressure upon urine output, carotid blood-pressure, femoral pressure and jugular pressure.

On releasing abdominal pressure, by allowing fluid to flow back into the bottle, urine usually began to appear promptly; in one experiment there was total suppression at 30 mm. abdominal pressure, while urine reappeared at an intra-abdominal pressure of 28 mm. (Experiment 2), demonstrating the constancy and abruptness of the suppression threshold (Fig. 1 and 2).

Accompanying a rise of intra-abdominal pressure from zero to 30 mm. there was usually a fall of 5 to 10 mm. in carotid blood-pressure (Figs. 1, 2 and 3).

These changes in urine secretion might have been due to pressure on the ureters, to changes in the general circulation, or to pressure on the renal veins.

That the suppression was not due to compression of the ureters, is shown by the results of injecting saline intravenously while urine flow was inhibited by an abdominal pressure of 30 mm. Such an injection was always followed by a profuse flow of urine, which could be readily inhibited by raising intra-abdominal pressure to 35 to 40 mm. (Fig. 2, Experiment 2.)

Changes in the general circulation were not constant, but usually there was a fall of 5 to 10 mm. in blood-pressure when intra-abdominal pressure was raised sufficiently to suppress urine. This fall is scarcely enough to cause total suppression of urine, and urine was often excreted readily at a considerably lower level of blood-pressure, if abdominal pressure was low. Furthermore, blood-pressure might fall less than 5 to 10 mm., and in one instance it rose as abdominal pressure was raised (Experiment 2); often, after a primary fall, blood-pressure rose while intra-abdominal pressure was held at 30 mm. until it was higher than before the fluid was injected into the abdomen, but no urine appeared. In every case, urine was suppressed by an abdominal pressure of 30 mm. regardless of the blood-pressure level.

Of all the structures concerned in the normal renal function, the renal veins are most susceptible to external pressure, since pressure within the inferior cava is normally only a few millimeters of mercury. Consequently, onward flow in this vessel must cease when pressure upon it becomes greater than pressure within it, and could only be maintained by a rise in venous pressure to a point equal to the external pressure.

To determine the presence of a rise in venous pressure, vertical glass tubes, coated with wax, were connected with a femoral and an external jugular vein, while abdominal pressure was raised and lowered. Blood rose in the femoral tube to a height almost exactly equivalent to existing abdominal pressure, and rose or fell proportionately as abdominal pressure was raised or lowered. There was no appearance of blood at any time in the jugular tube, though saline flowed readily and completely from the tube into the vein (Fig. 3, Experiment 2).

The rise in venous pressure must, therefore, have been due to factors operative only below the diaphragm.

In order to determine if this rise in venous pressure was effective at the point of entrance of the renal veins, a small catheter, coated within by means of solid sodium citrate, was connected to a vertical tube and its tip introduced into a femoral vein.

Blood rose in the tube to a height equivalent to the existing abdominal pressure. The catheter was pushed on within the inferior cava, with no change in height of the blood column, until the tip of the catheter reached a point just above the diaphragm, when all the blood flowed rapidly out of the tube (Experiment 3).

The catheter was then introduced into the left external jugular vein and pushed on until its tip was in the inferior cava. There was no rise of blood in the tube as long as the tip of the catheter was above the diaphragm, but as soon as it passed below, blood rose to a height almost equivalent to abdominal pressure.

A rise in intra-abdominal pressure is thus seen to cause a rise in abdominal venous pressure, and this is effective throughout the entire inferior caval system below the diaphragm. Its effect on renal function is directly comparable to the effect of partial occlusion of the renal veins, which uniformly causes partial or complete suppression of urine (Paneth; de Souza).

The first effect of a sudden increase in intra-abdominal pressure is probably a collapse of the inferior cava, for venous pressure is lower here than in its tributaries. Consequently, filling of the heart must be interfered with until venous pressure rises sufficiently to overcome the external pressure, and the fall in blood-pressure which follows a sudden, though comparatively slight increase in intra-abdominal pressure is probably due to this. The ultimate level maintained by blood-pressure when intra-abdominal pressure is held at a high level must depend, to some extent at least, on the proportion of total blood volume required to maintain the higher level of abdominal venous pressure, and which is thereby lost to the effective circulation.

Under such circumstances of increased intra-abdominal pressure, abdominal venous pressure must rise to a point almost, if not exactly, equal to the intra-abdominal pressure, and measurement of the latter is, therefore, an index of the pressure against which the renal circulation is working.

In experiments in which fluid was injected quite rapidly into the abdomen, 750 cc always raised the intra-abdominal pressure to the suppression point of urine (30 mm.) while 1000 cc caused marked respiratory distress.

When fluid was introduced gradually (Experiment 4), so that time was allowed for compensation to occur, 2100 cc was required to raise intra-abdominal pressure to 30 mm., and this relatively enormous volume caused no apparent distress. Beyond this point, however, slight increases in volume of fluid caused marked pressure symptoms, due, apparently, to yielding of the diaphragm, and after 2400 cc had been introduced, blood-pressure fell sharply to zero, the heart giving a few spasmodic beats, but entire recovery occurred promptly when fluid was allowed to escape. It was now possible to reinject rapidly almost 2000 cc of fluid before any symptoms resulted, and at least 300 cc must have remained in the abdominal cavity.

Apparently the abdominal muscles lose their tonicity when gradually distended, and in this way large volumes of fluid can be accommodated in the abdominal cavity without the extreme rise in intra-abdominal pressure seen when much smaller amounts are rapidly injected. The diaphragm seems to retain its tone much longer, but, once it yields, a slight further increase in pressure causes prompt and very marked disturbances of the circulation, these being probably due to an occlusion of the great veins, so that filling of the heart is prevented. Pressure on the ventricles direct would probably not cause so sudden a failure.

Protocols. *Experiment* 1. To determine the effects on urine excretion and blood-pressure of sudden changes in intra-abdominal pressure.

Female fox terrior, 5.8 kilos, was given 400 cc of 5 per cent glucose, by stomach tube, at 9.30 A.M.; luminal, 0.12 gm. per kilo, at 10 A.M. Ether during operation only. Tracheal cannula; left carotid connected to manometer. 0.9 per cent saline was used to raise abdominal pressure. Urine output was measured in cubic centimeters per three minute period.

Time.	Blood-pressure.	Abdominal pressure.	Urine cc per 3 minutes.	Conditions.
4.00–4.12	78	0	0.30	Control.
4.15	72	30	0	750 cc saline injected into abdomen; suppression.
4.18	66	25	0.05	Fluid held in abdomen.
4.30	64	6	0.08	Fluid flowing back into bottle.
4.33	66	4	0.45	Recovery.
4.48	74	4	0.1	Recovery.
4.51	82	30	0	750 cc saline injected into abdomen; blood-pressure rises; suppression.
5.06	82	12	0.1	Fluid flowing back into bottle.
5.12	90	10	0.13	Recovery.
5.18	98	8	0.4	Recovery.

If the injection of fluid be performed more slowly, it causes a progressive lag in urinary output and complete suppression, when the intra-abdominal pressure reaches 30 mm. (Fig. 1).

Experiment 2. A. To determine whether compression of the renal pelvis or ureters by the intra-abdominal pressure is a factor in the suppression; to determine whether, at the intra-abdominal suppression pressure, diuresis may be produced by increasing arterial blood-pressure (Fig. 2).

B. To determine if there is a rise in abdominal venous pressure as intra-abdominal pressure is raised (Fig. 3).

Female fox terrier, 7.5 kilos. 5 per cent glucose, 500 cc at 5.00 P.M., May 23 and at 9.30 A.M., May 24, luminal, 0.12 gm. per kilo, at 10.00 A.M.; ether during operation only. 5 per cent acacia in 0.9 per cent saline used to raise abdominal pressure. Venous pressures recorded later in experiment by cannulas in right femoral and left external jugular.

Time.	Blood-pressure.	Abdominal pressure.	Urine drops per minute.	Conditions.
2.20 / 2.29	72	0	3	Control.
2.30	66	20	1	Acacia injection begun.
2.31	68	30	0	750 cc acacia injected; suppression.
2.35	82	30	0	Fluid held in abdomen.
2.37	90	15	1	Fluid released.
2.40	104	10	4	Recovery.
2.44	100	4	3	Recovery.
2.47	82	30	0	750 cc acacia injected; suppression.
2.52	110	30	8	50 cc saline intravenously (note diuresis).
2.54	102	40	0	More acacia injected into abdomen; suppression.
3.06	104	10	5	Recovery; pressure released.
3.07	96	15	3	Acacia injected slowly.
3.08	90	20	2	Injection continued; lag in output.
3.10	84	25	1	Injection continued.
3.15	84	28	1	Injected continued.
3.20	80	30	0	Injection continued; suppression.
3.28	88	28	1	Pressure released.
3.32	90	20	4	Recovery.
3.36	88	18	4	Recovery.
3.39	80	30	0	Acacia reinjected; suppression.
3.42	80	28	2	Pressure released.
4.20	98	8	3	Control; venous pressure: femoral, 6.9; jugular, 0.
4.25	52	28	0	Acacia into abdomen; venous pressure: femoral, 20; jugular, 0.
4.27	56	30	0	750 cc acacia injected; venous pressure: femoral, 24; jugular, 0.
4.29	74	12	[illegible]	Pressure released; venous pressure: femoral, 9; jugular, 0.

Experiment 3. To determine if pressure is raised in inferior cava at point where renal veins enter, as intra-abdominal pressure is raised.

Female mongrel, 5.2 kilos. Glucose 5 per cent, 500 cc at 5.00 P.M., May 26 and 10.00 A.M., May 27, luminal, 0.012 gm. per kilo. Saline used to raise abdominal pressure. No ether required.

Details of experiment were almost exactly the same as Experiment 2, and results entirely confirmatory.

Catheter used for recording pressure within inferior cava, connected to vertical tube, as manometer.

Abdominal pressure	Catheter inserted (mm)	Venous pressure (mm).	Conditions
4	2	3+	Control; catheter in femoral vein.
19	2	18+	Saline injected into abdomen.
19	10	18+	Saline held in abdomen; catheter pushed on.
19	20	18+	Same.
19	22	0	Blood flowed sharply out of tube.
16	5	0	Catheter in jugular vein; saline held in abdomen.
16	30	0	Catheter pushed on; saline held in abdomen.
16	33	12	Catheter tied in place and animal killed; tip of catheter in inferior cava just below the diaphragm; at 22 cm. from opening in femoral vein, tip of catheter was in inferior cava, just above diaphragm.

Experiment 4. To determine if there is a loss of tonicity of abdominal muscles when intra-abdominal pressure is gradually increased.

Female dog, 8.6 kilos, glucose 5.00 P.M. and 11.00 A.M. as usual. Anesthesia by ether only. Saline injected into abdomen, in 50 cc portions, allowing five minutes between injections. (No urine was excreted at any time during the course of this experiment.)

Total fluid.	Abdominal pressure.	Blood-pressure.	Conditions
0	0.0	120	Control.
100	8.0	112	Sharp fall of blood-pressure followed second 50 cc injection.
500	10.4	116	Blood-pressure did not fall after subsequent injections.
1000	13.8	118	
1500	17.6	118	Abdomen very tense, but no dyspnea.
2000	26.4	120	No apparent change.
2100	30.0	120	Still breathing quietly.
2250	35.0	120	
2300	33.0	116	Fall in abdominal pressure and blood-pressure, with marked dyspnea; lower ribs bulging suddenly.
2350	36.0	114	Very marked respiratory distress.
2400	48.0	?	Blood-pressure fell sharply to zero; then infrequent, spasmodic heart beats and agonal respiration; recovery prompt on releasing pressure.

Conclusions. 1. A rise of intra-abdominal pressure to 30 mm. (mercury) is uniformly followed by complete suppression of urine in dogs; pressures lower than 15 mm. have no constant effect; from 15 to 30 mm., there is progressive diminution in rate of urine excretion. There is usually also a fall of 5 to 10 mm. in arterial pressure.

2. Venous pressure within the inferior caval system below the diaphragm rises with intra-abdominal pressure, and to almost the same extent.

3. Suppression of urine with high intra-abdominal pressure is probably due to the rise in abdominal venous pressure, the effects of which on the renal circulation are comparable to those of partial occlusion of the renal veins.

4. The fall in blood-pressure seems to be due to a temporary collapse of the inferior cava, until the venous pressure has risen to a point equal to intra-abdominal pressure.

5. When fluid is gradually introduced into the abdomen, the abdominal muscles lose their tonus, and much more fluid can be accommodated without pressure symptoms. The diaphragm is the last to yield, and its yielding is following by rapid circulatory failure, while respirations continue.

It is suggested that the loss of tonus in the abdominal musculature occurs as a means of compensating for ascitic collections which would otherwise raise abdominal venous pressure sufficiently to cause urinary suppression.

It is suggested that, since the rise of venous pressure resulting from the presence of an ascitic collection in the abdomen is limited to the venous circulation below the diaphragm, this may be a factor in the comparative limitation of the peripheral edema to the lower extremities in cases of inferior caval obstruction.

Dana and McIntosh[5] report a case of superior caval obstruction. in which edema occurred chiefly in the face, neck and upper extremities; the lower extremities were not involved to any great extent in the edema. This should be contrasted with the inferior caval obstruction type of edema dealt with in the present paper.

REFERENCES.

1. Krehl: The Basis of Symptoms, p. 416.
2. Paneth, J.: Arch. f. d. ges. Physiol., 1886, **39**, 515.
3. de Souza, D. H.: Jour. Physiol., 1900–1901, **26**, 139.
4. Quirin, A.: Deutsch. Arch. f. klin. Med., 1901, **71**, 79.
5. Dana, H. W., and McIntosh, R.: Am. Jour. Med. Sci., 1922, **163**, 411.

SIGNIFICANCE OF THE WILDBOLZ AUTO-URINE REACTION IN TUBERCULOSIS, WITH A REPORT OF 100 CASES.

By Milton Smith Lewis, M.D.,
NEW YORK CITY.

(From the A. Jacobi Division for Children, Service of Dr. A. L. Goodman; from the Medical and Surgical Wards of the Lenox Hill Hospital, New York City.)

The tuberculin test has been regarded by many workers both in surgery and medicine as a certain sign of a tuberculous focus, but its limitations have been found and it is not now regarded as a complete automatic diagnosis but as an indication of the necessity for looking further.

Hence, when Wildbolz and his co-workers published that they believed it was possible to demonstrate the activity of a tuberculous process through the proof of antigens in the urine by means of an allergy reaction of the skin, an added stimulus was given to the efforts to find a positive test which would demonstrate without any doubt the presence of an active tuberculous process.

Wildbolz and his co-workers worked on the theory that when there is an active tuberculous process in the body there must be products of disintegration due to the tubercle bacilli, and that these products of waste or disintegration are antigens or antibodies which are removed by the various secretory organs. The only question was whether the existence of these antigens could be proven.

Wildbolz assumed that if there was an active process in the body then there should be antigens excreted in the urine and that this urine, after certain modifications would, if injected intracutaneously, cause the skin to show infiltration and redness similar to that after the injection of tuberculin. If this reaction was positive then he assumed that as proof that the antigens were in the urine and also that there was an active process in the body producing these. If, however, the reaction was negative then it was assumed that this demonstrated that there were no areas of activity in the body.

Wildbolz stated further that the above reaction would not occur with urines from supposedly healthy individuals or from urines of persons with tuberculous processes that have been healed. Moreover, it never occurs unless the person gives a positive re-spouse to an injection of 1 to 10,000 dilution of tuberculin. Wildbolz first injected tuberculin in a patient to show whether the patient was allergic or not. Then he applied his auto-urine test when, if it did react, he was convinced it was proof of an active process in the person whose urine was used. Hence where there is an anergic person, that is one who would not react to his own urine, the test seemed to be of greater value inasmuch as it could be tried upon some other person who first reacted positively to tuberculin, because a person reacting to tuberculin would react positively to the auto-urine test. The reason for using the tuberculin test first was solely to show whether the person on whom it was performed was hypersensitive, or not.

In demonstrating the superiority of the auto-urine test over the tuberculin, Wildbolz demonstrated that the tuberculin response persisted unmodified for a much longer period than the response of the urine, which fades out completely in seventy-two hours. If the urine reaction persists after the clinical healing of the tuberculin process, then, said Wildbolz, we can be confident that there is some other condition present elsewhere. The specific nature of the urine reaction he demonstrated even more conclusively by the fact that after the subsidence of the urine reaction, if an injection of 1 to 10,000 tuberculin was injected near by, the apparently extinct urine reaction would flare up anew, the infiltration and redness becoming more distinct and more marked again.

The Auto-urine Test. In preparation of the auto-urine test, the first thing to consider is a method by which the antigens can be concentrated from the highly diluted urine in a sufficient quantity for demonstration without destroying the antigens, which are destroyed at a temperature of 60° C. The technic is as follows: 100 cc of morning urine is evaporated to $\frac{1}{10}$ of its volume, or 10 cc, in vacuo, at a temperature not exceeding 50° C. When the urine is concentrated to $\frac{1}{10}$ of its volume, the contents are placed in a sterile test-tube and allowed to stand for twenty-four hours. Then the contents are filtered through sterile filter paper impregnated with 2 per cent phenol. $\frac{1}{10}$ of a cubic centimeter of the filtrated urine is then injected intracutaneously on the anterior surface of the forearm, using exactly the technic of the Schick test. The reaction is manifested by a local infiltration and redness at the point of the injection, which develops within twenty-four to forty-eight hours after the introduction of the urine. The size of the infiltration varies from 5 to 15 mm. In every case a control is injected in the same manner and in the same quanity on the opposite forearm. The control being a 1 to 10,000 solution of tuberculin.

The theory of the auto-urine test sounds very plausible, but is it possible to prove that there is an active tuberculous process in the body by the injection of one's own urine, after certain modifications, and obtaining a response in a local reaction?

We know that the skin of certain individuals is more sensitive than that of others particularly so when these individuals have had previous infections such as tuberculosis, asthma, hay fever, etc. We know that these persons who display an intense reaction to foreign proteins always react to the skin tuberculin test. If this is so, then why should not these persons who react to proteins also react in the same way to the antigens supposedly thrown off in the urine after some infection other than tuberculosis, for if there are antigens given off in the urine from an active tuberculous process somewhere in the body, no matter how remote the focus may be, then there must also be antigens given off in the urine from other infections as well, as in pneumonia, typhoid fever, syphilis, staphylococcemia, and endocarditis? So if the urine from these persons is injected intradermally, why should it not show a similar reaction, and how are we to differentiate these reactions from each other?

In cases of apparently healthy individuals free from any sign or symptom of tuberculosis, I prepared a number of urines and found after injecting these that I obtained reactions similar to those who had tuberculosis. Certainly here there were no specific antigens to cause the reaction. In my series of healthy cases I became doubtful of the specificity of the auto-urine reaction and surmized that the reaction was the result of the traumatic and the chemical qualities of the urine, and that while the urines of tuberculous persons may give a positive reaction, the same reaction may also be obtained from urines of non-tuberculous persons, sometimes on account of the presence of drugs in the urine, but also, in the absence of such a cause, from some unexplainable reason.

The reaction appears to depend not only upon the quality of the urine injected but also on the receptivity of the patient, as the same sample of urine may give a positive, doubtful, or negative reaction in various persons who are in a tuberculous allergic state.

On the whole, therefore, while the presence of antigens in the urine of tuberculous patients is a matter of scientific interest, no diagnosis, and still less an exact appreciation as to the activity of the disease or its clinical prognosis, can be based on this reaction.

According to Petersen, it has been shown that from the time of birth of the individual the organism begins to alter in the reactivity of the skin, which, at first negative to tuberculin, increases progressively with the age of the individual until in adult life a maximum is reached and maintained, but during this period not only does the skin become sensitive to tuberculin, but it becomes increasingly sensitive to a series of other bacterial and plant proteins and extractives as well. We are dealing with a more or less sensitization or allergy of the skin. This allergy may be a more or less specialized property of the skin or may be localized in certain areas of the skin. As a result of it the tissues acquire the ability to react more energetically and more promptly to outside stimuli, whether specific, as with tuberculins, or non-specific as when other proteins are injected in and about an area previously injected. The conclusions, therefore, is that in tuberculous individuals the skin and the body as a whole are hypersensitive not only to tuberculins but to proteins in general. It must always be borne in mind that when the injection is made a certain amount of tissue injury is done and that some of the cells may be injured both by the trauma and the toxic material injected.

From these observations it is apparent that non-specific factors can undoubtedly influence the tuberculin reaction or the other skin reactions, both in the sense of depressing and accelerating the reactivity of the skin.

In performing the auto-urine test in persons with suspected tuberculous processes, how would it be possible to demonstrate the presence of antigens in the urine if there is some renal impairment, for then the antigens would be in such a diluted state that it would hardly be possible to demonstrate their presence by a reaction in the skin? If there is a positive reaction, how can we be sure that the reaction is not due to some chemical substance in the urine that was not altered by the evaporation of the urine?

Reviewing the foreign literature on the subject, I found as follows:

W. Unverricht believed that the sensitiveness of the intracutaneous test is due to the larger area in which the tuberculin and the tissue react, and that the more rapid absorption of the tuberculin is in consequence of the greater pressure with which it is forced into the lymphatics. H. Eliasberg and E. Schiff conclude that the urine reaction may be specific, but it gives no proof as to the activity of the lesion. R. Offenbacher does not believe the test to be reliable, as in a number of instances the tuberculin test was positive and the auto-urine test negative. T. Arlong, Piery, Ledru and Codier consider that the auto-urine test does not differentiate between an active and an inactive lesion. E. Liebhard states that in his series of cases the urine reaction was not intense enough and was too inconsistent to be of great practical significance in its present form. Hanns concludes that an active tuberculous process does not preclude a negative intracutaneous reaction except in fatal rapidly-progressing cases. Parallelism between the intracutaneous tuberculin and the urine reaction was not established. On the contrary, a feeble allergy toward tuberculin was associated with a strong urine reaction and *vice versa.* O. K. Klercher attempted, by means of the intracutaneous test, to differentiate active from inactive tuberculosis, but without success.

G. Farrago and P. Randt conclude that the auto-urine reaction has no value whatsoever in the diagnosis of tuberculosis, as the reaction is due to certain chemical qualities in the urine and the question whether the urine of the tuberculous patient contains specific substances which are valuable in the diagnosis of tuberculosis remains for further investigation.

Reviewing the American Literature on the subject, I found only one article, written by C. B. Gibson and W. E. Carroll. This article working on the same line as Wildbolz worked, gives the data of some 40 cases but does not give conclusions either proving or disproving the efficiency of the auto-urine test.

However, Petersen in his new book on Protein Therapy disproves Wildbolz's statement that many patients with an active tuberculous process do not react to foreign proteins because they have an organic resistance or skin anergy. Petersen states that persons who have tuberculosis, hay fever, or other infections, show a skin allergy or skin hypersensitiveness due to the continual absorption of proteins and that these persons will react to almost every protein injected. This, obviously, is quite contrary to the Wildbolz statement.

Wildbolz also states that the auto-urine test is always negative in non-tuberculous patients, but in my series of cases I cannot agree with this statement as I found a number of healthy persons who gave a positive auto-urine reaction, due, no doubt, either to the hypersensitiveness of the skin, or to some chemical substances in the urine or to traumatism from the injection. The auto-urine reaction was also positive in a number of cases where the tuberculin test was negative and *vice versa*.

Although I considered all these points I was determined to devote enough additional time to try to prove or disprove the efficiency of the auto-urine test for tuberculosis from the standpoint of activity. In my series of anergic cases I injected their urines into persons who were allergic, but found that the result was very inconsistent and unreliable. Neither did those of my injections which were positive flare up again after an injection of tuberculin. In only 5 cases did I get a systemic reaction, whether from the tuberculin or the urine I cannot say. All of the cases complained of a severe burning sensation after the injection of the urine and several had sore arms for a few hours after the injection. No burning sensation or sore arms were noticed following the tuberculin injections.

I was convinced that if this test was reliable, we had at last found something which was a step forward and which would shed some light on the subject of the activity of tuberculosis, all other tests for tuberculosis having been very disappointing and as indicators of activity, valueless.

But I found that the auto-urine test on the whole is one that cannot be performed on every person with the ease with which Mantoux or von Pirquet can be performed. In other words, it is not practical as it requires one who is familiar with the test and who has the time to devote to its preparation, which is considerable, due to the fact that the evaporation of the urines alone require at least one hour. One can readily realize in my series of 100 cases how much time was consumed in the preparation of the urines.

Summary of Results. 1. *Tuberculous Cases.* Result in 48 cases of tuberculosis: In 44 cases of active tuberculosis, 26 resulted in a positive reaction; 18 resulted in a negative reaction; 4 of the 48 cases were classed as inactive or arrested; 3 of these resulted positively and 1 negatively to the auto-urine test.

Cases.	Mantoux.	Auto-urine.
24	Positive	Positive.
8	Negative	Negative.
5	Negative	Positive.
11	Positive	Negative.

2. *Non-tuberculous Pulmonary Conditions.* Result in 24 cases: 14 of these 24 cases gave a positive reaction in the auto-urine reaction; 10 of these gave a negative reaction.

Cases.	Mantoux.	Auto-urine.
9	Positive	Positive.
3	Negative	Negative.
6	Negative	Positive.
6	Positive	Negative.

3. *Apparently Healthy Cases and Various Diseases.* Result in 22 cases: 11 resulted in a positive auto-urine reaction; 11 resulted in a negative auto-urine reaction.

Cases.	Mantoux.	Auto-urine.
13	Positive	Positive.
6	Negative	Negative.
0	Negative	Positive.
3	Positive	Negative.

4. *Allergic Cases with Positive Sputum.* Result in 6 cases: All but 2 patients were negative when their urine was injected into their own skins, but when it was injected into allergic persons, 4 of these gave a positive reaction.

Cases.	Mantoux.	Auto-urine.
0	Positive	Positive.
4	Negative	Negative.
2	Negative	Positive.
0	Positive	Negative.

Summary and Conclusion. 1. Healthy individuals and persons with non-tuberculous diseases may show a positive auto-urine reaction.

2. Persons with healed tuberculous processes may show a positive auto-urine reaction.

3. In allergic persons the auto-urine reaction has no practical value, as proven by inconsistent results obtained from injecting their urines into allergic persons.

4. The auto-urine reaction is not reliable since in a number of cases where the tuberculin test was positive, the auto-urine reaction was neagtive, and *vice versa.*

5. It is not practical for every day use.

6. The reaction appears to be due not only to the quality of the urine injected, but also to the receptivity of the patient, as the same urine may give a positive result in one person and a negative result in another.

7. A positive result is not proof that there are antigens in the urine.

8. In all probability this reaction is due to: The hypersensitiveness of the skin; to chemical properties in the urine; to the traumatism induced by the injection of the urine; to drugs in the urine.

9. From a study of the cases that I have presented I have arrived at the conclusion that the Wildbolz auto-urine test for active tuberculosis has very little, if any significance, in its diagnosis.

I wish to express may appreciation to Drs. A. L. Goodman and Jerome Leopold for their coöperation in making possible my work with the auto-urine test.

BIBLIOGRAPHY.

1. Wildbolz: Corr.-Bl. f. schweiz. Aerzte, 1919, **49**, 793.
2. Unverricht: Berl. klin. Wchnschr., 1920, **57**, 1019.
3. Eliasberg and Schiff: Monatschr. f. Kinderh., 1920, **19**, 5.
4. Offenbacher: Ztschr. f. Tuberk., 1920, **32**, 355.
5. Arlong, Piery, Ledru and Codier: Rev. de Tuberk., 1920, **1**, 183.
6. Liebhard: Ztschr. f. Tuberk., 1921, **34**, 99.
7. Hanns: Ztschr. f. Tuberk., 1921, **33**, 321.
8. Klercher: Zentralbl. f. d. ges. Kinderh., 1920, **19**, 523.
9. Farrago and Randt: Deutsch. med. Wchnschr., 1921, **47**, 219.
10. Gibson and Carroll: Jour. Am. Med. Assn., 1921, **76**, 1381.
11. Petersen and Miller: Protein Therapy and Non-specific Resistance, New York, 1922, p. 130.
12. Nasso: Pediatria, Naples, 1921, **29**, 690.
13. Bosch: Munchen. med. Wchnschr., 1921, **68**, 733.
14. Levi: Med. klin., 1921, **17**, 1926.
15. Fischer: Schweiz. med. Wchnschr., 1921, **51**, 992.
16. Weisz: Med. klin., 1921, **17**, 930.
17. Bezançon and Mathews and Weill: Rev. de Tuberc., Paris, 1921, **12**, 319.

REVIEWS.

CLINICAL DIAGNOSIS AND SYMPTOMS. By ALFRED MARTINET, M.D. Authorized English translation from the third, revised and enlarged edition. By LOUIS T. DEM. SAJOUS, B.S., M.D. Pp. 1388; 895 illustrations. Philadelphia: F. A. Davis Company, 1922.

THIS two-volume work by Martinet, which has been translated by the younger Sajous, offers to the practitioner a fairly thorough discussion of physical diagnosis, laboratory diagnosis and analysis of symptoms. To the reviewer the second volume which contains the analysis of the different symptoms seems to be of greater value than the first volume. The first volume, on the examination of the various organs and portions of the body, seems to be somewhat superficial and to deal with the subject matter non-critically. A certain amount of material in the book is many years old and has not stood the test of time. In the second volume, however, the author has taken up systematically a discussion of symptoms. These are arranged alphabetically and the reader can in a minute, with a minimum amount of difficulty, determine the causes of hematemesis or of hematuria or of jaundice, tremor or any other one of a host of symptoms. The book is profusely illustrated, largely with diagrams, which are well conceived and executed. It can be recommended most highly. M.

DISEASES OF THE EAR, NOSE AND THROAT. By WENDELL C. PHILLIPS. Pp. 881; 572 illustrations. Philadelphia: F. A. Davis Company, 1922.

IN the sixth edition, Dr. Phillips has eliminated much that is obsolete and introduced recent methods in audiometry, bronchoscopy and laboratory diagnosis.

The real test of such a work is its practical adaptability for use by student and practitioner. Its comprehensiveness, especially in minor detail, while somewhat confusing to the former group, will enhance its value to the latter. An increase in the number of basic anatomic illustrations in the nose and throat section would be helpful. The book is more compact in its present form and everything considered is one of our most valuable reference works. B.

PRACTICAL PHYSICS. By J. A. CROWTHER, Sc.D., F. Inst. P., University Lecturer in Physics, as Applied to Medical Radiology, Cambridge University. Pp. 260. London: Henry Frowde, Hodder & Stroughton, 1922.

THIS little book is essentially a laboratory manual for elementary students of physics. It comprises a series of simple experiments, such as are used for teaching in every physics laboratory, so clearly and concisely explained that no student should have difficulty in carrying the work assigned to a successful termination. Its scope is entirely limited to premedical teaching. A.

DIE LUMBALPUNKTION. By DR. MARTIN PAPPENHEIMER, Privatdozent, an der Universität Wien. Pp. 184; 8 illustrations. Wein: Rikola Verlag, 1922.

THE anatomy and physiology of the regions involved, the various methods of examination and their diagnostic, prognostic and therapeutic significance are discussed, in the hope of correcting the serious errors encountered by the author in text-books and in the minds of his acquaintances. W.

A KEY TO THE ELECTROCARDIOGRAM. By LOUIS FAUGERES BISHOP, M.A., M.D., Sc.D., F.A.C.P., Professor of the Heart and Circulatory Diseases, Fordham University, etc. Pp. 94; 43 illustrations. New York: William Wood & Co., 1923.

THE story of electrocardiography has been told simply and in a most interesting manner in this little book, which should be of special value to those who now know nothing of electrocardiography, wish to know something, but are unwilling to devote too much energy to the subject. The author is more optimistic as to the clinical value of electrocardiograms than most workers in this field. Several statements should not be permitted to go unchallenged. The author relates the waves of the electrocardiogram to contraction of the heart and states that the work of the ventricle is recorded by the T-wave. It was demonstrated long ago that the electrical disturbances in the heart precede contraction by measurable intervals and it is now pretty well established that the T-wave records, not work of the ventricle, but subsidence of the excitation wave. Too much dependence is placed upon the electrocardiographic evidence of disproportionate enlargement of one or the other ventricle. The reviewer must dissent from the author's opinion that pulsus alternans is rare, and in view of the statement that he has no example of it in his collection of electrocardiograms, refers him to Fig. 20, page 49. W.

THE MEDICAL CLINICS OF NORTH AMERICA (VOL. VI, No. 4). Pp. 831–1094. Philadelphia and London: W. B. Saunders Company, 1923.

THIS number contains twenty-six clinics from four of Philadelphia's largest hospitals, and numbers among its contributors McCrea, Riesman, Norris, Anders, Musser, Funk, and Pepper. The subjects dealt with vary widely, but there is, on the whole, a preponderance of clinics upon rare conditions, in which diagnostic difficulties afforded the chief interest. Probably to the average reader Pepper's Clinic to the first-year class in medicine, entitled "Diabetes Mellitus with Slight Acidosis: a Discussion of the Buffers of the Blood," and Torrey's discussion of "Aneurysm of the Aorta with Remarks Concerning the Effects of Aneurysm on the Coronary Circulation" will be of the greatest interest. A.

BIOMETRICAL STUDIES IN PATHOLOGY. I. THE QUANTITATIVE RELATIONS OF CERTAIN VISCERA IN TUBERCULOSIS. By RAYMOND PEARL and AGNES LATIMER BACON. Johns Hopkins Hospital Reports, Vol. XXI, Fasc. III. Pp. 72; Figs. II and tables 23. Baltimore: Johns Hopkins Press, 1922.

THIS third emanation from the Statistical Department of the Johns Hopkins Hospital attempts to arouse the medico's interest by considering man in the opening line as one of the higher Metazoa. In spite of the present popularity of biometrics, constitution clinics and such like, however, the pamphlet proved incapable of holding the reviewer's attention. With relief he found a summary of only two and a half pages and there read "the general problem with which this paper, which is the first in a series that as a whole will deal with this problem, is that of the adaptive organic regulation of the normal balance of the parts of the body, operating under pathological conditions." Fatigued by the endless quality of this sentence, he waded irresolutely through the six indices calculated from the data of 5,000 tuberculosis autopsies and the significant and insignificant negative and positive correlations deduced therefrom. When sufficient vigor had returned, he analyzed the analysis and was rewarded in finding that "broadly speaking" no correlation was possible in several of the ratios selected; also that with increasing age the heart tended to be relatively heavier than the other viscera studied and that in active tuberculosis, the heart was relatively to those viscera lighter than in inactive tuberculosis. If the reader's interest is enough greater than the reviewer's, he will turn to the text for the significance of these important facts.

K.

REST AND OTHER THINGS. By ALLEN K. KRAUSE, A.M., M.D., Associate Professor of Medicine, Johns Hopkins University; Director, Dows Tuberculosis Research Fund, Johns Hopkins University; Editor, American Review of Tuberculosis. Pp. 159. Baltimore: Williams & Wilkins Company, 1923.

IN antituberculosis propaganda the author believes that more stress should be laid upon the universal practice of better hygienic habits. Heretofore almost the whole emphasis has been placed upon the well-nigh impossible task of preventing infection with the ubiquitous tubercle bacillus. He makes a plea for the establishment in our medical schools of tuberculosis foundations for purposes of more effectual study and teaching in this field. As in most collections of addresses upon one subject, there is considerable repetition, but the style is forceable, and in the field of tuberculosis the author speaks with undoubted authority. A.

CARRIERS IN INFECTIOUS DISEASES, A MANUAL ON THE IMPORTANCE OF PATHOLOGY, DIAGNOSIS AND TREATMENT OF HUMAN CARRIERS. By HENRY J. NICHOLS, M.D., M.A., Major, Medical Corps, U. S. Army; Instructor in Bacteriology, Parasitology and Preventive Medicine, Army Medical School, Washington, D. C. With a Section on, CARRIERS IN VETERINARY MEDICINE. By R. A. KELSER, D.V.M., M.A., Captain, Veterinary Corps, U. S. Army; in charge, Veterinary Laboratory, Army Medical School, Washington, D. C. Pp. 184; 11 illustrations. Baltimore: Williams & Wilkins Company, 1922.

THIS manual presents a fairly complete consideration of the subject of carriers. Unfortunately, the didactic rather than the monographic style of presentation detracts from the scientific value of the work by permitting the author to introduce personal convictions supported by an incomplete and rather hurried gleaning of the great volume of literature on this important phase of preventive medicine. The section on carriers in veterinary medicine is freer from this than is that on human carriers, and constitutes a very valuable, as well as the first, summarized review of this subject in medical literature. It is to be deplored that the lessons learned from the experiences of the World War in regard to the seriousness of hemolytic streptococcus complications, especially in respiratory diseases, are not emphasized. The introduction of the term phorology may not meet with general acceptance.

S.

Die Pfeilgifte. By L. Lewin. Pp. 517; 75 illustrations Leipzic: J. A. Barth, 1923.

An exhaustive treatise on arrow poisons of all kinds, giving the results of studies and experiments extended over thirty years. The poisoned weapons of the Middle Ages, of India, the Malayan Peninsula, Australasia, Africa and North and South America are all passed in comprehensive review in a manner that makes the book of interest to physicians, naturalists, ethnographers and psychologists alike. If its information is accurate, an estimate beyond the ability of the reviewer, this book should long remain an authoritative one on this subject.

K.

Clinical Laboratory Methods. By R. L. Haden, M.A., M.D., Associate Professor of Medicine, University of Kansas, Kansas City. First edition. Pp. 294; 74 illustrations. St. Louis: C. V. Mosby Company, 1923.

"All discussion of the interpretation of results has been intentionally avoided. The book is in no sense a text-book." On the other hand, it accomplishes well the limited purpose that the author has striven for, namely, to present succinctly a series of "laboratory procedures which have been thoroughly tried out and found to give accurate results." It, therefore, should be of more value as a practical handbook than as a guide to the student of these topics. Going farther afield than clinical pathology in its narrower limits, the author has included chapters on the chemical examination of the blood and other tissues, serology, clinical bacteriology and histological technic that will make the book cover the immediate needs of most clinical laboratories.

Believing the book to be a good one, the reviewer may be permitted to call attention to a few minor desiderata: Goodpasture's oxydase should certainly accompany if not displace the older Schultz method; insufficient emphasis is given to the importance of cyst detection in amebic dysentery; the discription of Wilbur and Addis' quantitative urobilin estimation in stools gives a different calculation from the authors', with resultant figures that are too high (most text-books, however, omit this test entirely!); the method for blood platelets is somewhat antiquated and should at any rate be supplemented by an indirect method; the authors' names on page 113 are incorrect; the inclusion of a thick smear method for malarial organisms would have been desirable. On the other hand, it is up to date in most particulars, has the earmarks of having been written by a capable worker, and the material is offered in very presentable form. The practice of frequently giving the author's reference immediately beneath the title of the test is commendable. Throughout the book are useful tables, presenting valuable information in concrete form, also several laboratory aids of the author's own devising. Altogether it constitutes a welcome addition to the clinical laboratory workshop.

K.

Rules for Recovery from Tuberculosis. By Lawrason Brown, M.D. Fourth edition. Pp. 217. Philadelphia and New York: Lea & Febiger, 1923.

Probably in no disease is a well-considered and well-administered plan of treatment more important than in tuberculosis, and probably nowhere in this country has the system of treating tuberculosis been developed to a higher grade of perfection than at Saranac. From this unique source of experience the author answers the patient's questions in his own language, and tells him not only what he must do to get well, but when and how and why. The book is valuable as a layman's handbook, and may be consulted with profit by the physician as well.

A.

Mind and its Disorders. A Text-book for Students and Practitioners of Medicine. By W. H. B. Stoddart, M.D., F.R.C.P. Fourth edition. Pp. 592; with illustrations. Philadelphia: P. Blakiston's Son Company, 1922.

As is to be inferred from the title, this is primarily a text-book on psychiatry rather than neurology. It is divided into three parts: Part I deals with "Normal Psychology;" Part II, with the "Psychology of the Insane;" and Part III, with "Mental Diseases." The book is refreshing in many respects. It gets away from the straight-laced classifications of many American and German text-books of the period previous to the war. It shows a healthy appreciation of the best things contributed by the psychoanalysts, and of the contributions of such workers as Cannon, Sherrington and others; and, not least of all, it contains some practical though simple hints on usually neglected but necessary topics, such as Case-taking, General Treatment of the Insane and certain Medico-legal Procedures. The last topic, of course, is treated from the British point of view, but this does not discount its value from a general medico-legal point of view. Some of the best chapters under "Normal Psychology," are those dealing with Fatigue, Sleep and Dreams, the Sentiments, Language and the Ego. These are clearly written, brief and to the point. They show a familiarity with the best practical work of recent or current American and English psychologists of accepted standing. Under Part II there is a short chapter on Psychoanalysis. This chapter follows Freud pretty closely, but effectively avoids introducing discussion of material and methods that the best in Freudianism has already discarded. The paragraph on Technic is very explicit and helpful.

In Part III the classification of the Neuroses and Psychoneuroses follows Freud pretty closely. It is pleasing to get a chapter on the Paraphrenias, for which Kraepelin must, of course, be thanked. The chapter on Epilepsy is one of the best written in the book, with possibly the exception of the paragraphs on treatment. It is interesting to note that luminal is not mentioned. The so-called "Organic Insanities" are treated in a rather cursory manner, and evidently with not the same enthusiasm as exhibits itself in the earlier chapters of the book. Their extreme brevity gives one the feeling that perhaps this portion of the book had been better omitted entirely. For a compact, readable, dependable and useful manual of mental disorders, however, the reviewer feels that the beginner, as well as the so-called "busy practitioner," would have to search far to find better. J.

Radio-diagnosis of Pleuro-pulmonary Affections. By F. Barjon. Translated by James Albert Honeij, M.D., Assistant Professor of Medicine in charge of Radiology, Yale School of Medicine. Pp. 183; 27 figures and 50 radiographs. New Haven: Yale University Press, 1922.

This volume is in five parts, taking up: (1) Methods of examination, (2) radiological study of the pleuræ, (3) bronchi, (4) lungs, (5) penetrating wounds of the thorax by war projectiles. The author has attempted one of the most difficult tasks in writing a book on roentgen-ray diagnosis of chest pathology. Part II, dealing with diseases of the pleuræ, is admirably presented. The reviewer, however, feels that the volume is not complete, in that no study of conditions, such as pneumoconiosis and chest signs and pathology, caused by the inhalation of foreign bodies, is included. Then, too, there are quite a few eminent authorities that probably would feel that the chapter on pulmonary tuberculosis is rather weak. The book is well written, and the publishers deserve credit for the printing and the type of paper that is used in the book. The illustrations are fair. The reviewer strongly feels that if the translator were given the privilege of editing the book the weak points would be remedied. P.

Notes on Materia Medica, Pharmacology and Therapeutics for Dental Students and Practitioners. By Frank Coleman, M.C., L.R.C.P., M.R.C.S., L.D.S., Assistant Dental Surgeon St. Bartholomew's Hospital, Dental Surgeon Royal Dental Hospital, etc. Fifth edition. Pp. 308. London: Oxford Medical Publications, 1922.

This little book deals in a concise but reliable manner with the materia medica, pharmacology and uses of the principal drugs employed by the dentist. The names of some of the preparations, being in accordance with the British Pharmacopœia, will be unfamiliar to American students and practitioners. The book contains short chapters on vaccine therapy, organotherapy, electrotherapy and radiotherapy. I.

Exercise in Education and Medicine. By R. Tait McKenzie, M.D., LL.D., Professor of Physical Education and Physical Therapy and Director of Physical Education, University of Pennsylvania. Third edition. Pp. 601; 455 illustrations. Philadelphia: W. B. Saunders Company, 1922.

This book is addressed to students and practitioners, to teachers of youth, medical and physical, hoping to give a comprehensive view of the space exercise should hold in a complete scheme of education and in the treatment of diseased conditions. Exercise has so many points of contact with education, and is so intimately related to mental, moral and social training, that a progressive educator is compelled to study its various phases.

In this, the third edition, the author has inserted the results gained from his experience as, Physical Training Officer in the

British Army at Aldershot, as Medical Officer in Command of Convalescent Camps and as Inspector in such camps in England, Canada and the United States. He shows the part that exercise bears on the treatment of "soldiers" heart; the place Swedish gymnastics has taken in discipling great masses of slow, awkward men in speed, accuracy and alertness. He further shows how the maimed and crippled were and can still be reëducated in their last coördination, their stiffened joints, shattered nerves and atrophied muscles.

Exercise has come to stay. Italy and France have been shown its advantage; England, Germany and Sweden already know it. In the United States already twenty-three states have made physical education part of their school program.

In this work the author shows in most convincing style his thorough knowledge of his subject, and presents it in a most interesting and instructive manner. We all should have the work not only for our patients but for our own use as individuals.

E.

NUTRITION OF MOTHER AND CHILD. By C. ULYSSES MOORE, M.D., M.SC. (PED.), Instructor in Diseases of Children, University of Oregon Medical School; Medical Director of the Coöperative Infant Welfare Society of Oregon. Including menus and recipes by MYRTLE JOSEPHINE FERGUSON, B.S. in H.Ec., Professor of Nutrition, Iowa State College, Ames, Iowa. Pp. 227; 33 illustrations. Philadelphia and London: J. B. Lippincott Company, 1923.

THE reviewer welcomes a book on this most important subject which can be put into the hands of the young mother without feeling that she will be submerged in a maze of, to her, unintelligible scientific phraseology. The same feeling relates to the social worker and the visiting nurse. The author has brought out in a common-sense manner all that vital part of the advances of recent years in nutrition which is necessary for a full understanding of the subject. There is a short discussion of the former and the newer ideas on nutrition. Then a definite statement as to the three known vitamins, their value and their distribution in foodstuffs, and the effects of their omission from the diet. To obstetricians, especially, the chapter of diet during pregnancy and lactation will be of interest. The subject of the diet of the normal baby, of the premature infant, of the older child are gone into in detail. The book makes rather a point of prevention of disease through proper diet than as a book on treatment of disease. The two appendices contain information often sought for in vain in books on nutrition, and add to the usefulness of the book. W.

PROGRESS

OF

MEDICAL SCIENCE

SURGERY

UNDER THE CHARGE OF

T. TURNER THOMAS, M.D.

ASSOCIATE PROFESSOR OF APPLIED ANATOMY IN THE MEDICAL SCHOOL AND ASSOCIATE PROFESSOR OF SURGERY IN THE SCHOOL FOR GRADUATES IN MEDICINE IN THE UNIVERSITY OF PENNSYLVANIA; SURGEON TO THE PHILADELPHIA GENERAL AND NORTHEASTERN HOSPITALS.

Results of the Treatment by Radiation of Primary Inoperable Carcinoma of the Breast.—LEE (*Ann. Surg.*, 1922, **76**, 359) says that primary inoperable carcinoma of the breast has shown good results by radiation. The type of radiation, however, must be properly selected for the individual case, while over-radiation must be avoided. The palliative operation following properly planned radiation is of service in well selected cases. The results to date are very gratifying and encouraging. As the disease itself and the technic of radiation become better understood, it is believed that more satisfactory results will follow.

Diagnosis of Early Breast Tumors: Based on their Clinical Picture or their Gross and Microscopical Picture at the Exploratory Incision.—BLOODGOOD (*Boston Med. and Surg. Jour.*, August 17, 1922, p. 243) says that more attention must be paid to history and to examination by inspection and palpation, first, to exclude the group in which operation is not indicated; second palpation of a definite lump must be developed to a method of greater precision; third, when tumors must be explored, surgeons must learn to recognize the benign type in which excision of the tumor with a zone of breast is sufficient for the protection of the patient. For the present, the mistake that should never be made is an incomplete operation for a malignant lesion. A mistake which is and must be made in a certain group ol benign lesions hard to recognize, is the complete operation. The author feels that trained surgeons can and do recognize cancer of the breast at exploration and also the distinctly encapsulated adenoma and blue-domed cyst.

Autogenous versus Heterogenous Bone Pegs.—TAEMOWSKY (*Surg., Gynec. and Obst.*, 1922, **35**, 342) says that the clinical behavior of a beef bone graft depends entirely on the relative activities of the osteoblasts and osteoclasts. With proliferation of new cells from the living proximal and distal ends of the fractured bone keeping pace with absorption of dead cells from the graft, complete disappearance of the latter coincides with complete union of the fracture or filling-in of defect. With hyperactive new cell formation and sluggish absorption, the graft constitutes a sequestrum which either eburnates and remains in a state of quiescence or acts as an irritant foreign body with sinus formation and periodic extrusion of dead bone spicules. With hyperactive bone absorption and sluggish new bone formation, the graft disappears by combined extrusion and absorption before union or filling-in of defect has taken place. The factors which enable us to attain the ideal, *i. e.*, an even balance of absorption and proliferation are: (1) The thorough trimming off of dead bone proximally and distally with curette and chisel; (2) firm approximation of the bone graft to living bone; (3) absolute asepsis. Finally, it has seemed to the author that the term infection is used too loosely—it is in truth, rapid necrosis of the graft without true infection. In other words, subacute osteomyelitis with no antibody reaction on the part of the individual, should not be classed as an infection, but as an ordinary tissue necrosis.

The Cause of Certain Acute Symptoms Following Gastro-enterostomy.—Haden and Orr (*Johns Hopkins Hosp. Bull.*, 1923, **34**, 26) says that the symptoms and chemical findings (in a short series of patients showing severe reaction after gastro-enterostomy) were characteristic of intestinal obstruction. The authors attribute the symptoms to absorption of poison, probably formed in the duodenum following gastro-enterostomy. These patients showed a high level of non-protein nitrogen of the blood, low blood chlorides and suppression of chloride excretion following gastro-enterostomy. Marked alkalosis was noted in 1 patient; two had a CO_2 combining power at the upper limit of normal when first determined. Very high nitrogen excretion in the urine was also noted. All patients presented clinical symptoms of a severe intoxication, with laboratory findings characteristic of upper intestinal tract obstruction. It is probable that some duodenal obstruction at the site of gastro-enterostomy interferes with drainage of the duodenal loop.

The Lymph Nodes in Carcinoma of Rectum.—McVay (*Ann. Surg.* 1922, **76**, 755) says that rectal carcinomas are the most common form of intestinal neoplasms and make up 4 per cent of all cancers of the body. The majority of patients are in the sixth decade, with males predominating slightly. The location of the growth on the rectal wall varies. About as many occupy the anterior wall as the posterior, with the greatest number of growths from the ampulla to the rectosigmoidal junction. Adenocarcinoma is the commonest type. Metastasis to the glands usually takes place slowly and the liver is the organ most affected, by secondary growths. The size of the growth in the rectum cannot be relied upon as an accurate index of probable lymphatic involvement. Growths without lymphatic involvement, tend to grow into the lumen of the bowel. Growths with slight lymphatic involvement, tend to spread by direct extension and are slow growing. Carcinomas of the rectum with extensive lymph-glandular involvement, tend to metastasize through the lymph stream early. Metastastic lymph-glandular involvement can only be definitely determined by systematic microscopical study of all the regional lymph nodes. The size of the lymph node is not an efficient means of determining whether or not there is metastatic involvement.

Intussusception.—Ellars (*Am. Jour. Surg.*, 1922, **36**, 307) says that intussusception is noted with greatest frequency in children less than one year old, the incidence of the abnormal occurrence gradually decreasing as age advances. It is not a disease *per se*, the intestine ordinarily being normal when invagination begins, later becoming pathological because of strangulation and consequent interference with its blood supply. The actual determining etiological factor of intussusception appears unknown, but there are several anatomical peculiarities incident to infantile life which may be operative as predisposing or contributing causes. All medical and so-called mechanical methods suggested in the treatment of intestinal invagination are unwarranted, for they court disaster. Young children are not invariably unfavorable subjects for operative surgery. The tremendously and unreasonably high mortality of intussusception can be materially reduced by early diagnosis and prompt application of rational surgical principles.

THERAPEUTICS

UNDER THE CHARGE OF

SAMUEL W. LAMBERT, M.D.,

NEW YORK,

AND

CHARLES C. LIEB, M.D.,

ASSISTANT PROFESSOR OF PHARMACOLOGY, COLUMBIA UNIVERSITY.

Voluntal, a New Hypnotic.—Miltner (*Deutsch. med. Wchnschr.*, 1923, **49**, 73) reports that voluntal (tri-chlor-ethyl-alcohol-urethane) has proved, in his hands, an unusually safe and satisfactory hypnotic. It is almost tasteless and is readily administered in water, in which it is freely soluble. It produces a short stage of drowsiness followed by a deep, quiet, dreamless sleep from which the patient awakens fully refreshed. There is apparently a total absence of disagreeable after-effects, such as disturbance of digestion, headache, lassitude, dizziness, etc. No evidence of cumulation was encountered in his rather wide experience of prolonged administration. The hypnotic dose is 0.75 gm., but the factor of safety is apparently large, for no serious or even disagreeable symptoms were noted by the author when he took 2.5 gm. Like most of the other aliphatic hypnotics, voluntal fails to induce sleep in the presence of pain, severe cardiac dyspnea, etc. It is, however, a safe and powerful hypnotic, and in effectiveness stands midway between carbromal (adalin) and barbital (veronal).

The Treatment of Pernicious Anemia.—Though nothing is definitely known of the true cause of pernicious anemia, ROSENOW (*Klin. Wchnschr.*, 1923, **2**, 24) declares that there is little doubt that there is an enormous increase in the destruction of red blood cells and that the regeneration of the erythrocytes by the bone-marrow is quantitatively and qualitatively defective. Therapy may, accordingly, be directed toward decreasing the excessive destruction of the red blood cells or toward stimulating their formation in the bone-marrow. The "hemotoxin" is probably elaborated in the alimentary canal, and many measures have been suggested to limit its production. Rectal and colonic irrigations, as well as those *via* the duodenum, are usually unsuccessful in combatting the formation of the "hemotoxin" or in lessening the severity of any of the symptoms. Certain agents have been recommended as adsorbents of the toxin, but they do more harm than good, since they interfere greatly with the action of the intestinal enzymes. Glycerine and cholesterine have been tried and discarded. Cultures of various bacteria have proved disappointing, despite the abnormal intestinal flora. Such radical operations as the establishment of an artificial anus and subsequent irrigation of the intestinal canal through the artificial opening are of but temporary benefit. One of the most trying features of the treatment of pernicious anemia is the selection of a diet which appeals to the patient and supplies a sufficient number of calories. The anorexia, which is so common, does not yield to bitters, but may disappear after the prolonged use of hydrochloric acid. Large doses of the acid (with or without pepsin) are called for and are most beneficial in the presence of achylia gastrica. A diet rich in protein seems to promote red blood cell destruction, while a diet rich in fats does not. Diseases of the mouth are common and demand careful treatment; glossitis is best treated with tincture of myrrh or some other simple mouth wash; pyorrhea alveolaris and carious teeth are handled along dental lines. Of the drugs that have been tried in pernicious anemia, arsenic is unquestionably the best. It probably does not act directly on the bone-marrow, but acts indirectly by hastening blood destruction and thus inducing an active erythrocyte production. Arsenic may be administered either by mouth or parenterally. For oral use Fowler's solution is the most popular; it is customary to begin with small doses (3 drops three times a day) gradually increasing to full therapeutic amounts (30 drops thrice daily). Arsacetin (0.05 gm. three times a day) has no advantages over Fowler's solution. All arsenic preparations administered by mouth should be given after meals to minimize the local irritation. The arsenic must be continued for months or until saturation is reached; the most common symptom of saturation is paresthesia of the palms and soles. Habituation is readily induced in some patients, so that very large doses are not followed by poisoning. Parenteral administration of arsenic has no advantage over oral. Cacodylate of sodium is less active than Ziemssen's solution (1 per cent sodium arsenite) and is not advised. Atoxyl is altogether too dangerous to warrant its employment. Arsphenamine enjoys no special advantages unless the anemia is associated with lues. Roentgen-rays and radioactive substances are powerful stimulants of the bone-marrow. Thorium-X is more active than radium and is to be preferred. Small "stimulant" doses may be given two or three times a week for a month or two. Iron has always proved quite worthless. Intramuscular or intravenous injections of blood have not proved as helpful as was anticipated when they were first introduced. Extirpation of the spleen is sometimes followed by brilliant results, but the benefit is only temporary. While none of the procedures discussed is curative, some seem to induce remissions and thus prolong life. Among the most valuable measures are arsenic, intramuscular injection of blood and the drinking of thorium-X waters.

The Action of Camphor, Menthol and Thymol on the Circulation.—The reports of the effects of camphor as a circulatory and cardiac stimulant are so contradictory that HEATHCOTE (*Jour. Pharmacol. and Exper. Therap.*, 1923, **21**, 177) deemed it worth while to attempt to clear up the confusion. Thymol is extensively employed in the treatment of ankylostomiasis and is reported to have led to occasional serious circulatory collapse. Menthol is related to camphor chemically and is included in the study for the sake of comparison. It was found that all three drugs (camphor, thymol and menthol) depress the isolated heart of the frog as well as that of the rabbit, and that this effect is due to a direct depression of the cardiac muscle. The strength of the beat is much more affected than the rate of the contraction. None of these drugs acts as an antidote to chloral, and a heart depressed by chloral is further depressed by the perfusion of any one of these drugs. Of the three, camphor is the least toxic and thymol probably the most. The coronary bloodvessels are dilated by all three—least by camphor and most by thymol. In anesthetized animals, camphor in non-convulsive doses does not cause a rise in blood-pressure, whether administered intramuscularly or subcutaneously. In animals deprived of cerebral hemispheres, no rise of blood-pressure is produced by huge doses (1 gm. per kilo). Even such small doses as correspond to those used in clinical medicine, caused a fall in pressure (15 per cent). The lowering of blood-pressure is ascribed chiefly to the depression of the heart muscle, and only to a minor degree to the relaxation of the bloodvessels. There is, therefore, no convincing evidence that camphor possesses any value whatsoever as a cardiac or circulatory stimulant. The unpleasant effects that sometimes follow the administration of thymol are due chiefly to a direct depression of the heart muscle, which is much more marked than with camphor.

On the Sensitivity of Different Nerve Endings to Atropine.—Textbooks on pharmacology frequently state that atropine depresses or paralyzes the nerve endings of the parasympathetic nervous system and the clinician is led to believe that this action is induced by ordinary therapeutic doses. According to HENDERSON (*Jour. Pharmacol. and Exper. Therap.*, 1923, **21**, 99), this is not the case; indeed, the usual therapeutic dose of atropine slows the heart by stimulation of the vagus center and the vagus endings are not paralyzed. He accordingly determined the amounts of atropine necessary to depress the ends of the bulbosacral autonomic outflow and ascertained the amounts necessary to cause so complete a paralysis of the various nerve endings that nerve stimulation with an induced interrupted current became ineffective. The nerve endings are depressed in the following order: Nasal, chorda secretory, cardiac vagus, tonus of pyloric sphincter and small intestine, bladder, oculomotor to the pupil, salivary vasodilator, vagus to intestine for rhythmic and peristaltic movements. The endings are paralyzed in the order: Cardiac vagus, chorda secretory, chorda vasodilator, intestinal vagus. The endings in the bladder cannot be completely paralyzed. In man it was found that 0.2 mgm. caused a decrease in nasal secretion but not marked drying of the mouth, while 0.3 mgm. dried the mouth. This amount relieved griping produced by aloes. Two milligrams are required to increase the heart-rate to 150; this dose caused a submaximal dilatation of the pupil.

The Action of Certain Depressant Drugs on the Sensory Threshold for Faradic Stimulation in Human Subjects and the Effect of Tobacco-smoking on This Action.—Hale and Grabfield (*Jour. Pharmacol. and Exper. Therap.*, 1923, **21**, 77) used the Martin method for determining the effect of the diethylbarbituric acid hypnotics, of antipyrine and of acetphenetidine upon the sensory threshold for faradic stimulation. Parallel observations were made when the subjects were smoking and when they were not. In non-smoking experiments, the barbitals produced a slight transitory decrease in irritability; antipyrine showed its maximum effect at the end of half an hour, when it had decreased irritability by 30 per cent; acetphenetidin was somewhat more depressant, but its greatest effect was not shown till about ninety minutes after its ingestion. In all 3 cases, smoking tended to nullify the effects of these drugs, bringing the threshold observations within normal limits.

PEDIATRICS

UNDER THE CHARGE OF

THOMPSON S. WESTCOTT, M.D., AND ALVIN E. SIEGEL, M. D.,

OF PHILADELPHIA.

Physiology of Exercise in Children.—Seham and Seham (*Am. Jour. Dis. Child.*, 1923, **25**, 1) publish the result of their observations on normal children of school age. They found that the pulse rate in the standing position is invariably higher than in the lying position, the ratio being 1 to 15. The systolic blood-pressure in the lying posture is invariably higher than in the standing posture. The ratio of the blood-pressure in the lying posture to that in the standing equals 1 to 11. The ratio between the systolic blood-pressure in the lying and standing postures is about equal to the ratio between the pulse rate in the standing and the lying postures. All forms of exercise produce an increase in the pulse rate and the blood-pressure, the increase depending mainly upon the type of exercise. Neither the amount of exercise nor the speed determine the time of maximum reading. In the majority of cases the increase of the pulse rate and the blood-pressure as well as the reaction time of the blood-pressure are in direct proportion to the speed and the amount of work performed. Height and weight do not influence the maximum physical output. The maximum physical output is in direct relationship to age, circumference of the chest, circumference of the thigh and the vital capacity. Two formulæ have been computed for calculating the maximum physical output with age as the basis. The first formula, applying to children six to seven years of age, is 1000 (5.45 age minus 25.3). The second formula, applying to children from eleven to fourteen years of age, is 3000 times the age. In exhaustive exercise on the ergometer, the increase of pulse rate varies from 48 to 116 beats irrespective of age. It is not necessarily parallel to the amount of work performed. In exhaustive exercise the rise of blood-pressure is proportional to the increase of work in about 50 per cent of the experiments. The average rise in blood-pressure after exhaustive exercise equals 31 mm. in children aged from six to nine years and 35 to 41.mm. in children who are older. The maximum rise equals 57 mm. and the minimum rise equals 16 mm. In 88 per cent of all the determinations made, the maximum reading of the systolic blood-pressure was seen within thirty seconds, and 12 per cent in from thirty to sixty seconds. In only 2 cases of the entire series was there a true delayed rise. In these experiments delayed rises did not occur after exhaustive exercise nor as the result of "temporary heart insufficiency." The reaction of the pulse is too long to be of any clinical value, as very few pulse rates return to normal within ten minutes. In general the reaction time of the systolic blood-pressure increases with an increase of work. There are exceptions to this.

The Action of Atropine on the Stomach of Infants.—SALOMON (*Monats. f. Kinderh.*, 1922, **24**, 75) found that atropine lowers the tone of the stomach in infants and slows peristalsis. It does not alter the secretion of acid, nor act on the pylorus. The favorable results of large doses of atropine in the treatment of pylorospasm depend on its action on the musculature of the whole stomach. While a normal infant shows a reddening of the scalp after 1 to 2 drops of a 0.1 per cent solution of atropine sulphate when it is indicated, as in vagotonia, the infants may tolerate much greater quantities, and as much as 6 to 8 drops six times a day. Atropine very frequently gives excellent results in the habitual vomiting of infants.

Nutrition and Growth in Children.—EMERSON (*Bost. Med. and Surg. Jour.*, 1923, **188**, 8) says that the forces affecting a child's health, which must be coördinated in order to secure success, are the home, the school and other agencies, medical care, and the child's own interest. The following program is suggested: Weighing and measuring as a means of identification; diagnosis based on complete physical growth, mental and social examinations; removal of physical defects as a prerequisite for successful treatment; measured feeding or a forty-eight hour diet record; mid-morning and mid-afternoon lunches; mid-morning and mid-afternoon rest periods; regulation of physical, mental and social activities; nutrition classes for the treatment of malnutrition; nutrition diagnostic clinics for problem cases; and average weight for height as a minimum standard of nutrition and growth.

Simple, Practical Method for Feeding Infants.—Cowie (*Mich. State Med. Soc. Jour.*, 1923, **22**, 10) states that the normal infant requires 45 calories per pound or 100 calories per kilogram of body weight to maintain its weight. After determining on 1 ounce of sugar as a constant factor, and accepting all sugars as containing 120 calories to the ounce, it becomes a very simple problem to know how much milk was necessary for the balance of the daily food. For example, if an infant weighed 10 pounds, he would require 10 times 45 minus 120, or 330 calories, which must be supplied in the milk. If there are 21 calories in an ounce of milk, 330 divided by 21 equals 15½ ounces as the amount of milk necessary to balance the energy requirements.

The Colloidal-gold Reaction in Acute Poliomyelitis.—Regan Litvak and Regan (*Am. Jour. Dis. Child.*, 1923, **25**, 76) studied 42 cases of acute poliomyelitis, in which a study of the colloidal-gold reaction was carried out on 132 specimens of spinal fluid. There was always a reaction of colloidal-gold solution in the case of every poliomyelitic fluid taken during the acute stage of the disease. This reduction was constantly in the same zone; the zone of low dilutions or the so-called syphilitic zone. In 88 per cent of the spinal fluids examined, the reaction occurred in the first six dilutions between 1 to 10 and 1 to 320. In 14 spinal fluids the reaction extended to the seventh dilution, 1 to 640. These patients more or less characteristically presented marked polyneuritic or meningitic symptoms or else pronounced paralysis. The average curve or reaction showed very similar characteristics in the first and second weeks of the disease. A gradual decline in the curve was then noted. In no instance was a normal reaction encountered before the end of the third week of the illness. In 23 patients the spinal fluid was examined as late as the eighth week, and 15 or 65 per cent had become normal by that time. Cases in which a normal reduction returned early, from the third to the seventh week, were mild types of the disease, while those in which the curve remained elevated beyond the eighth week had usually polyneuritis or extensive and slowly improving paralysis or both. The reaction showed no distinctive points in the fatal cases, and therefore was of no value in prognosis in this regard. The positive reaction bore no constant relation to the presence of globulin in the spinal fluid nor to its disappearance. There was no close ratio between the number of cells per cubic millimeter in the spinal fluid and the test, but as the cell count decreased the colloidal-gold curve subsided, but somewhat more slowly, remaining elevated for several weeks after the cell count was normal. With the subsidence of the colloidal-gold curve there was usually an accompanying improvement in the patient's general condition, the paralysis, the meningitic symptoms, and the polyneuritis. It would seem that the return of a normal reduction of colloidal gold indicates approximately the end of the acute stage of the disease. As this coincides with the improvement noted clinically, this termination of the acute stage can readily be determined by watching the symptoms. In differential diagnosis the colloidal-gold reaction should be utilized in conjunction with history, symptoms and other laboratory data.

Evidence of the Necessity for a Bacteriological Standard for Grade "A" Milk.—Matlick and Williams (*Jour. Hyg.*, 1922, **21**, 33) show the result of two farms producing milk of very different types although both were working under the same system of licensing. In neither case did the results compare with those obtained on a certified milk farm. Similar results were found to occur on certified milk farms when they first undertook production of this type of milk. They are due to the fact that the workers on the farms have to be trained in methods that are necessary for success. The certified farms have in the past been few in number, and have been under the control of those who are very anxious to produce a satisfactory result. These facts coupled with the fact that there is an official bacteriological standard to which the milk must attain, have made it possible to secure efficiency as time went on. There is no official bacteriological standard for Grade "A" milk, so that stimulus to better production is lacking and should be provided. In view of the difficulty, which is sometimes found in bringing the standard of labor on a farm up to the required level, the authors feel that evidence that milk of the required standard of cleanliness is being produced, should be made a condition of licensing. If this is not done, there is a danger that milk not of the required standard of cleanliness may be sold as Grade "A" milk. In that case the consumer may find that the keeping qualities of this milk are no better than those of milk that had previously been purchased. If this is done, grave harm may be done to the milk industry, which is endeavoring to supply the public with milk of uniform quality.

OBSTETRICS

UNDER THE CHARGE OF

EDWARD P. DAVIS, A.M., M.D.,

PROFESSOR OF OBSTETRICS IN THE JEFFERSON MEDICAL COLLEGE, PHILADELPHIA.

Rupture of the Uterine Peritoneum with Premature Separation of the Placenta.—Eufinger (*Monatschr. f. Geburts. u. Gynäk.*, 1922, **59**, 158) describes a case of a multipara who during the first part of labor developed symptoms of separation of the placenta. A physician summoned applied a tampon and brought the patient to the hospital, where she was admitted in a very weak condition. Movements of the child and heart sounds could not be found. Section under local anesthesia was immediately undertaken. On opening the abdomen there was a large quantity of fluid blood. The placenta had almost entirely separated and the patient died shortly after the operation from acute anemia. At the autopsy a longitudinal laceration of the peritoneal coat of the uterus was discovered which penetrated through the upper muscular layer. A considerable part of the bleeding had come from this. On examination it was found that the process known as necrobiosis was present and that blood extravasated when the placenta began to separate had dissected and weakened the muscle fibers. Much of the hemorrhage had come from the rupture of the peritoneum and muscle.

Excretion Through the Mammary Gland.—In the *Journal of the American Medical Association*, February 24, 1923, p. 557, is quoted the result of researches by Taylor concerning the composition of milk. In addition to the group of products manufactured *de novo* in the mammary gland, various substances are present which are also found in the blood and other fluids of the body of the animal. Among these are the so-called non-protein nitrogenous extradines, among which are the amino-acids, urea, creatin, creatinin and uric acid. Very frequently the blood has the same non-protein content as milk. Taylor has presented additional evidence that in the case of a warm-blooded animal during lactation, there is a definite relation between the usual output of nitrogen in the urine and the percentage of non-protein nitrogen in the milk. Both of these apparently depend upon the amount of protein taken in the food. In the blood are found the non-protein nitrogenous catabolites, and their concentration seems to determine the amount excreted in the urine and the percentage present in the milk. There is a distinct function of the mammary gland in this matter and waste non-protein nitrogenous substances evidently pass from the blood to the milk. The degree of concentration in the blood of the end products of protein metabolism determines the percentage in which these substances are found in the milk. When this function of the mammary gland is considered, it may readily be seen that a condition may arise wherein the milk may contain substances which make it unfit for food.

The Treatment of the Pyelitis of Pregnancy.—Rosinski (*Monatschr. f. Geburts. u. Gynäk.*, 1922, **60**, 116) calls attention to the fact that pyelitis complicating gestation may sometimes end fatally. In these cases fever develops soon after labor, which may be rapid and comparatively easy. The fatal issue is often seen about the tenth day after the labor. While it is true that these occurrences are comparatively rare, the author recalls four instances in which the patient became critically ill. The first was a primipara at five months taken suddenly ill with high temperature, two weeks of general medical treatment produced no improvement and the patient's strength failed rapidly. On admission to hospital she was stuporous, complaining of headache. There were symptoms of marked irritation of the peritoneum. The abdomen was distended, the patient vomited frequently and the tongue was dry, there was high fever and rapid pulse. Six days' hospital treatment produced no improvement and therapeutic abortion was practised, followed by recovery. This case occurred twenty-two years ago and the subject of pyelitis was not as commonly understood as at the present time. The second case was that of a young primipara at seven months with high fever, irritafion of the peritoneum, slight jaundice and pain in the right hypochondrium. A diagnosis of gall-stones was made and operation was considered, this was declined although the patient was critically ill. The uterus was emptied and the urine obtained by catheter was loaded with leukocytes. The recovery of the patient followed the termination of pregnancy. His third and fourth cases were similar in severity and recovered after the uterus was emptied. The writer discusses nephrotomy and admits that this deals efficiently in the acute danger, but it leaves the patient with a kidney fistula from which recovery may be long and tedious. Should pregnancy be interrupted after nephrotomy, conditions would not be favorable for healing. In his experience the pyelitis of pregnancy is seldom severe, simple treatment is usually sufficient for these cases, but where the condition becomes threatening the uterus should be emptied. The author describes the case of a young, vigorous woman who during her first pregnancy suffered from pyelitis with high temperature, during the puerperal period the condition of the urine did not greatly improve. The patient suffered little if at all and received no specific treatment for the condition. In the second pregnancy pyelitis recurred more severely and with great pain in the right hypocondrium. When labor came on pain becomes so severe in the region of the right kidney as to require the use of morphine for several days. On the third day of pain three small phosphatic stones were passed. In the third pregnancy the pyelitis became so severe that after a very excessive attack of pain, pregnancy was interrupted at the fourth month.

The Practical Significance of Affections of the Kidneys and Abnormal Conditions of the Urine in Pregnancy.—FINK (*Monatschr. f. Geburts. u. Gynäk.*, 1922, **60**, 229) has studied 215 cases of pregnant women in whom there was some abnormal condition of the kidneys and also an abnormal urine. He believes that the pathology of the kidney in pregnancy divides the condition into three groups: (1) That known as the albuminuria of pregnancy; (2) the nephropathy of pregnancy; (3) the various forms of acute and chronic nephritis complicating pregnancy. The albuminuria of pregnancy is characterized by the presence of serum albumin and hyaline casts of no great number in the urine, and this condition is practically without serious danger to the patient. It is not a disease but the result of the increased susceptibility of the epithelia of the urinary tubules to blood-pressure and altered conditions. This state is to be distinguished from more serious conditions by the absence of edema, increased blood-pressure and other symptoms which are clearly present in more critical states. The so-called pregnancy nephropathy, by some called the kidney of pregnancy, the nephritis of pregnancy and the nephritis of the pregnant, is not a primary kidney affection; it is an edematous state which reflects a similar condition throughout the organism and in common affects the condition of the kidneys. In these cases there is abundant albumen and many casts are in the urine. The principal symptom which distinguishes this from the foregoing, is the presence of edema. This process may go to the point of causing increased blood-pressure and hematuria. From these indications it is natural to treat these patients by limiting carefully the amount of water taken and by giving food which is not rich in water and also in salt. Only those cases which are most acute and accompanied by very high blood-pressure become dangerous, and in these patients eclampsia often develops. Such cases demand hospital treatment. Acute nephritis at any stage of pregnancy is readily distinguished from nephropathy by a careful study of the history. They should be treated during the pregnancy by methods usually employed, with the omission of hot baths. It may be difficult to distinguish them from acute and violent cases of nephropathy but the condition of the blood-pressure should in this particular be of great assistance. Chronic nephritis in pregnancy gives the characteristic history, the long continuance of albuminuria, the presence of many casts and blood in the urine, the presence of fatty casts, of fatty elements in the urinary sediment, chronic headache, increased blood-pressure, a weakened action of the heart, disturbance of vision and cachexia. These cases demand very careful observation and thorough and efficient treatment. Nitrogenous food should be largely withdrawn, blood-pressure and action of the heart should be controlled and the examination of the eye grounds should be utilized as a valuable means of prognosis and the choice of treatment. This condition may clearly indicate the premature interruption of pregnancy.

Roentgen-ray Pictures as a Means of Teaching the Mechanism of Labor.—Warnekros (*Monatschr. f. Geburts. u. Gynäk.*, 1922, **59**, Heft 1–2) contributes a paper drawing attention to the value of this method of illustration in teaching the mechanism of labor. His article is somewhat in reply to a discussion or criticism of Sellheim, who has called attention to the fact that during labor the tissues of the child are subjected to unusual stress and therefore cannot give an accurate picture of conditions present. He illustrates with reproductions of roentgen-ray pictures showing unusual positions of the fetus and drawing attention to the fact that the whole fetal mass is elongated and very much compressed in its progress through the birth canal. The roentgen-ray pictures taken and copied by the author very little resemble those drawn ideally in text-books and are of interest as showing the degree to which the fetus is subjected to pressure during parturition.

An Unusual Complication in Twin Labor, the Entrance of both Heads into the Pelvis.—Described by Mahnert (*Monatschr. f. Geburts. u. Gynäk.*, 1922, **59**, Heft 1–2). The patient in her second labor, aged twenty-nine years, believed herself to be at normal termination of pregnancy. Membranes ruptured without pains which afterward developed and midwife was called. The head of the child was spontaneously born but the remainder of the child, in spite of strong pains and strong contractions of the uterine muscle, was not delivered. Shortly after the birth of the head, the child died. On admission to hospital the mother's temperature was elevated, pulse 120, uterus was in firm contraction, the urinary bladder distended above the symphysis, a contraction ring in the uterus could not be made out. No heart sounds were heard nor could fetal parts be clearly distinguished. The head, already born, lay with the face directed posteriorly. The mucous membranes of the vagina and tissues about the urethra were edematous and suffused with blood. With the catheter 400 cc of cloudy albuminous urine was evacuated. While preparations were made to examine the patient, thoroughly, she had a chill followed by a rise of temperature to 104° F. On examination the membranes of a second fetus containing a little amniotic liquid were detected; the head, with the sagittal suture transverse and occiput behind, was wedged upon the pelvic floor. The chest of the first twin was firmly wedged against the symphysis by the head of the second. Further spontaneous birth was impossible and as both children were dead the remaining membranes were ruptured and the head in the pelvis was perforated, the brain evacuated, and an effort was made through traction upon the head to deliver the second child; this failed and it was necessary to perforate the cranial bones of the second child, and to crush the tissues extensively before its body could be delivered. The perforated head of the second was then extracted by strong forceps. There was profuse postpartum hemorrhage and the placenta was removed manually shortly afterward. On examination of the bodies of the twins, both female in sex, the pressure upon the thorax of one by the head of the other was distinctly evident; at this point the skin was pallid, the neck deeply colored, giving the impression of congenital enlargement of the thymus or thyroid. The first child was 52 cm. in length. The second had also a congenital thyroid enlargement but otherwise well developed, 48.5 cm. long. The placenta was duovular. On measuring the pelvis it was not contracted. The puerperal period was complicated by four severe chills and fever lasting for six weeks with cystitis and pyelitis. On the twelfth day the patient passed urine involuntarily, and a fistula developed between the bladder and the cervix. This was subsequently corrected by operation, and three months after the labor the patient was discharged from the hospital in good condition. The author has collected a number of cases similar to this in the literature, and evidently the importance and severity of the complication will depend considerably upon the size and development of the children. The simultaneous engagement of twins with one child in breech and the other in head presentation is by no means unusual. In 51 such cases of simultaneous engagement, there were 12 where both heads entered the pelvis at practically the same time.

GYNECOLOGY

UNDER THE CHARGE OF

JOHN G. CLARK, M.D.,

PROFESSOR OF GYNECOLOGY IN THE UNIVERSITY OF PENNSYLVANIA, PHILADELPHIA,

AND

FRANK B. BLOCK, M.D.,

INSTRUCTOR IN GYNECOLOGY, MEDICAL SCHOOL, UNIVERSITY OF PENNSYLVANIA, PHILADELPHIA.

Vulvovaginitis.—Vulvovaginitis has been termed a free lance disease by STEIN (*Surg., Gynec. and Obst.*, 1923, **36**, 43), who points out that although the physicians in diverse specialties accept the condition for treatment, there is no uniformity in diagnostic procedure or mode of therapy, nor is there any accepted plan of procedure endorsed by a single. specialty. The treatment of the condition in the hands of various specialists varies from simple hygienic measures to the most painstaking local applications, but is for the most part empirical and frequently irrational. About a year ago, a joint meeting was called of the gynecological and genito-urinary departments of the Michael Reese Hospital Dispensary to discuss the problem of the disposition of the vulvovaginitis patients. No agreement could be reached. One physician claimed that all the cases were gonorrheal, another said that they were never gonorrheal, one held that they always arose from contact, and another believed that filth was the sole cause. With such diversity of beliefs as to etiological factors, naturally no plan of procedure could be outlined, and it was decided to investigate the cause of vulvovaginitis, clinically and bacteriologically. The conclusions which the author has reached as a result of his investigation are that vulvovaginitis is an infection which is frequently gonorrheal in origin, but may even in purulent varieties be non-specific. Filth unquestionably plays a part in predisposing to the infection and may be the chief cause in the milder types. Diagnosis rests upon clinical evidence of the disease and smear examinations made by an expert. Cultures prove positive in about 50 per cent of gonorrheal cases and are therefore not requisite for diagnosis. Purulent vulvovaginitis should be vigorously treated by an approved method and a daily tub bath is an aid to local treatment, and in mild non-gonorrheal cases is all that is required for cure. Determination of cure rests upon the disappearance of clinical evidence of the infection, three negative smears at intervals of one week after suspending treatment and a period of observation equal in time to the duration of the treatment. Summarizing his results of treatment, the author states that gonorrheal vulvovaginitis can be cured by daily injections of 1 per cent mercurochrome ointment into the vagina in an average of 9.7 weeks. Suspicious cases can be cured in 6.5 weeks, and non-gonorrheal cases in 5 weeks. In 2 gonorrheal cases recurrence occurred after contagious disease (chicken pox, measles). In 1 non-gonorrheal case, recurrence occurred from no apparent cause three months after treatment was suspended. It is of interest to note that in six instances sisters were affected at the same time, and in each instance a remarkable similarity in clinical course, bacteriological findings and response to therapy was noted.

Technic of Vaginal Drainage.—In discussing the technic of vaginal drainage of pelvic infections, GIRARD (*California State Jour. Med.*, 1923, **21**, 9) states that in order to make the opening in the posterior fornix a most simple procedure and "fool proof" he has devised a clamp approximately 25 cm. long with a double curve and when closed the end forms an oval ball 3.5 cm. wide and 2.5 cm. high. The anterior surface of the ball is grooved transversely, and this groove the operator feels through the stretched tissues of the posterior fornix, and makes his incision directly down on the ball of the instrument, thus avoiding any possibility of injury to the rectum, which is held posteriorly by the lower half of the ball while the back of the cervix is pushed forward by the upper half. If a large opening is desired, a crucial incision can be made at will, using the ball as a guide. After the incision is made, the clamp is opened by the assistant and the drainage material is placed between the jaws of the guide and withdrawn into the vagina. Gauze drains will cause more outpouring of lymph than rubber tubing or cigarette drains, which is to be desired, but they have the disadvantage of becoming entangled in the tissues when the lymph coagulates and causing injury to the granulations when the guaze is removed. In order to overcome this objectionable feature of gauze, Girard uses paraffine gauze, which can be laid in strips between the plain gauze and the wound or can be used in the form of a casing for a cigarette drain which he has devised, the ends of the paraffine casing being made fan shape so as to cover any large denuded area which cannot be covered by peritoneum and thus protect the denuded area from becoming adherent to omentum, intestines or adjacent organs and which, when removed five or six days later, will not adhere to the protected area which by that time has become well endothelialized.

Cystoscopy in Urinary Tuberculosis.—In commenting upon the value of cystoscopy in the diagnosis of urinary tuberculosis, BALL (*Brit. Jour. Surg.*, 1923, **10**, 326) reminds us that renal tuberculosis is a slowly progressive disease which unfortunately may not give rise to symptoms of a sufficiently definite character to cause the affected person to seek advice until, it may be, considerable destruction of the affected organ has taken place; in fact, the involvement of the bladder, with coincident symptoms, may be the first indication of this serious malady. Symptoms indicating involvement of the kidney are of slow development and may be absent altogether, even when that organ has been completely destroyed, dysuria associated with frequent micturition at night as well as by day being commonly the first evidence of disease. Ability to recognize the appearances seen in the bladder by cystoscopic examination is therefore of great importance in the diagnosis of renal tuberculosis, more especially in demonstrating which kidney is at fault, as in 80 to 90 per cent of cases, so it is stated, one kidney only is affected in the early stages. It is frequently, from the technical point of view, a difficult matter to carry out a satisfactory cystoscopical examination in this condition. Prior to the appearance of tuberculous lesions in the bladder mucosa little difficulty presents itself, but when the latter exist, then, owing either to a spasm in the early stages or to infiltration of the muscle of the bladder wall in the later stages, it is often impossible to make a thorough investigation unless the patient is under a general anesthetic, the distention of the bladder with fluid in sufficient amount causing severe pain. It is the author's practice, whenever a tuberculous infection is suspected, to adopt this procedure; even then, extreme care must be taken to avoid over-distention of the bladder, otherwise hemorrhage may be caused and irreparable damage supervene, such as the lighting up of a latent lesion or the introduction of a secondary infection, results easily induced by even a slight trauma. There is, moreover, a further difficulty in diagnosis from the pathological aspect, namely, that lesions may have assumed such characters, especially in the presence of secondary infection with other bacteria, as to render them indistinguishable from those associated with other forms of cystitis; even in the absence of the latter, the bladder may have become so extensively involved in the tuberculous process as to make it impossible to identify the original site of the bladder lesion, which may be the only clue indicating its possible origin from the kidney. For this reason it is an extremely important matter that an early investigation of the bladder should be carried out in all suspected cases of infection: (1) In order to define the existence of any abnormality in the effluxes from the ureteric orifices or in the bladder mucosa; and (2) to recognize the position of such changes in order to obtain an indication of the site of the primary lesion. The latter point requires emphasizing, for the finding of tubercle bacilli in urine containing blood or pus, with symptoms of cystitis, only indicates the presence of urinary tuberculosis; it offers no suggestion as to the requisite treatment. This the cystoscope alone can give in the absence of localizing symptoms, which may be completely absent, but even if present, confirmation is always necessary. Some authors state that it is unwise to carry out cystoscopical examinations in cases of tuberculous cystitis owing to the liability of causing further damage. It is agreed that it is unwise to employ this method of investigation during the acute symptoms of bladder infection, or more often than is necessary in the chronic stage; but it is obviously important that an exact location of the bladder lesions should be made as soon as possible, in order that the correct treatment may be determined. This information cannot be obtained without a cystoscopical examination, which should therefore be insisted upon. This advice of the author is quoted with the hearty endorsement of the editor in the hope that the forceful dissemination of such knowledge may be the means of saving many lives by bringing to early operation the early cases of renal tuberculosis, which can only be done by the careful investigation of all pyurias and dysurias of more than brief duration.

End-results of Interposition Operation.—Many operations are fascinating to watch or perform, but in the field of gynecology it is doubtful whether any other operation interests the student or the novice more than the interposition operation for prolapse. Whether you would give the credit for the invention of this procedure to Wertheim, Schauta or to our own Watkins (where it properly belongs), the fact remains that it is an ingenious operation *per se*. However, the thinking, conservative surgeon looks at an operation from another angle, namely the end-results. What are the end-results after this operation? Shaw (*Surg., Gynec. and Obst.*, 1922, **34**, 394))has investigated this subject in 118 cases operated upon since 1900 in the gynecological department of the Johns Hopkins Hospital. Of this number he was able to trace 58 patients, 40 of whom were completely relieved of their symptoms, 13 were not improved, 3 had died after leaving the hospital and 2 died in the hospital, 1 from pulmonary embolism on the twelfth day and the other from a hemorrhage of the uterine artery on the tenth day. These results, 13 failures out of 53 cases, the author admits are not brilliant, although he thinks they might be partly due to the fact that most of the patients were of the dispensary type, from whom failures are heard of more readily than successes. With increased experience in selection of cases in which the operation is suitable and with suitable modifications of the technic in the individual case, much better results have been obtained, as there has only been one failure since 1915 in 40 operations, 21 of whom have been followed. The author concludes that the operation is limited to a small group of cases, near or subsequent to the menopause, where an abdominal suspension, combined with a thorough repair of the perineal floor is contraindicated.

PATHOLOGY AND BACTERIOLOGY

UNDER THE CHARGE OF

OSKAR KLOTZ, M.D., C.M.,

DIRECTOR OF THE PATHOLOGICAL LABORATORIES, SAO PAULO, BRAZIL,

AND

DE WAYNE G. RICHEY, B.S., M.D.,

ASSISTANT PROFESSOR OF PATHOLOGY, UNIVERSITY OF PITTSBURGH, PITTSBURGH, PA.

Studies on the Pneumococcus. Acid Death Point of the Pneumococcus.—By seeding 5 cc of an isotonic broth, whose hydrogen-ion concentration ranged in eight steps from pH 4.47 to 7.8, with two drops of a saline suspension of washed living pneumococcus, and by transplanting on blood serum after varying intervals of inoculation, LORD and NYE (*Jour. Exper. Med.*, 1922, **35**, 685) found that at a pH of 4.47 no living bacteria were obtained after an interval of one hour, and at a pH of 5.15 living organisms were obtained after one hour but not after two, while at pH 5.78, they were living after two hours but not after three, whereas at pH 6.33 living pneumococci were encountered after six hours, At a pH of 6.63 to 7.80, the transplants were positive from eight to ten days, indicating that the greater the acidity, the more rapid the death.

In a second communication (*Jour. Exp. Med.*, 1922, **35**, 689) it was learned, from the results of a series of titrations, that suspensions of living pneumococci (Type I, II and III) in approximately isotonic standard solutions and bouillon with pH varying from 4 to 8 after incubation show dissolution of bacteria in those solutions having a pH higher than about 5, the dissolution being most marked at a critical range of about 5 to 7. While some dissolution was encountered toward the more alkaline end, no dissolution occurred at the most acid end of the scale. Although dissolution took place at incubation, room and icebox temperature, it was less marked at the latter. Dissolution also occurred in standard pH solutions with pneumococci allowed to grow and die out in glucose bouillon, but, unlike living organisms, the dissolution was progressive from the acid toward the alkaline end of the scale. Pneumococci killed by heat for one hour underwent less dissolution than living organisms, while those killed by heat at 100° C. for five minutes did not undergo dissolution, and the addition of fresh human serum to the pneumococcal suspensions at varying pH prevented dissolution. Dissolution occurred more rapidly at pH 6.1 in standard solutions in which large numbers of pneumococci had been previously dissolved than in fresh standard solutions at the same pH. The authors believe that this dissolution can be ascribed to an enzyme derived from the bacteria themselves, calling attention to the fact that under similar conditions S. viridans and hemolyticus and S. aureus did not dissolve.

In a third study (*Jour. Exp. Med.*, 1922, **35**, 699) suspensions of Type I, II and III pneumococci were added to the cellular material from a pneumonic lung due to Type I pneumococcus at varying hydrogen-ion concentrations. All types of pneumococci were found to undergo dissolution at a pH of 6.95 and 5.5, but not at a pH of 4.5, whereas S. hemolyticus and viridans do not dissolve. The authors believe that an enzyme derived from the bacteria themselves or from the cellular material may be the cause of the dissolution.

Finally (*Jour. Exp. Med.*, 1922, **35**, 703), the effect of bile at varying hydrogen-ion concentration on the dissolution of Type I, II and III pneumococci was determined by adding pnemococcal suspensions to fresh beef bile. After incubation it was found that the dissolution of the pneumococci occurred most rapidly in the bile at a slight alkaline reaction (pH 6.1). The authors believe "this is probably due to death of the organisms and activation of the endocellular enzymes at the optimum hydrogen-ion concentration."

Melanoblastoma of the Nail-bed (Melanotic Whitlow).—HERTZLER (*Arch. Dermat. and Syph.*, 1922, **6**, 701) reports 2 cases of melanoblastoma of the left thumb nail-beds in women, aged sixty-four and fifty-four years respectively. In 1 case there was a history of slight injury a year and a half previously, while in the other no record of trauma could be elicited, the condition beginning as a black spot under the nail four years previously. In both, too, the nail was absent, having been supplanted by a blue-black ulcerating tumor, which had eventually become painful and sensitive. The border of the tumors was deeply pigmented. No lymphatic involvement was found in either case. Amputation was instituted in each instance, and at the end of two years in the first case and two months in the second, no evidence of recurrence could be demonstrated. The author was able to collect 17 additional similar cases from the literature. He thinks that the term "melanoblastoma of the nail-bed" is more accurate than "melanotic whitlow" and should supplant it.

Experimental Rickets in Rats. IV. The Effect of Varying the Inorganic Constituents of a Rickets-producing Diet.—Having previously shown that rickets could be produced in rats by a diet composed of patent flour, calcium lactate, sodium chloride, and ferric citrate, and that it could be prevented by the substitution of 0.4 per cent basic potassium phosphate for an equal percentage of calcium lactate, PAPPENHEIMER, MCCANN and ZUCKER (*Jour. Exper. Med.*, 1922, **35**, 421) report the above changes which were produced in additional rats by varying the inorganic constituents of the diet. It was found that rachitic bone lesions occurred in rats who had received a diet containing an excess of calcium but deficient in phosphates, while similar lesions followed a diet deficient in calcium but containing an excess of phosphates and that atypical rickets was produced by a diet deficient in both calcium and phosphates, whereas inorganic salts other than calcium or phosphate seemed to be without influence upon the development or prevention of rachitic lesions. The minimal amount of phosphates required for calcification of young growing rats under the conditions of these experiments was about 160 mgm. per 100 gm. of diet. An excess of calcium was not necessary to the production of the rachitic lesions and a reduction of the calcium lactate in a given diet to 0.6 per cent (111 mg. of Ca per 100 gm. of diet) resulted in the development of typical rickets. Adult rats reacted to a deficiency of phosphate in the diet by the production of calcium-free osteoid in abnormal amount about the spongiosa and cortex and there was not produced any alteration of the epiphysial cartilage, as in growing animals.

Experimental Rickets in Rats. V. The Effect of Varying the Organic Constituents of a Rickets-producing Diet.—Under conditions of experimentation similar to those previously employed, PAPPENHEIMER, McCANN and ZUCKER (*Jour. Exper. Med.*, 1922, **35**, 447) continued their investigation of the prevention and production of rachitic bone lesions in rats receiving a diet in which the organic constituents were modified. It was learned that casein phosphorus did not prevent completely the development of rickets when substituted in a given diet in amount equivalent to a protective dose of basic potassium phosphate; that the protection given by lecithin or yeast was proportional to the phosphorus content, and that vitamin A, in the form of butter or butter fat, to the amount of 10 per cent of the diet, neither prevents or cures rickets; that the substitution of 10 per cent of egg albumen in the given diet improved the nutrition but did not prevent rickets, whereas the addition of meat promoted normal growth and bone formation, although a diet of only meat and flour was inadequate for proper growth, leading to bone changes comparable to those observed on a diet low in calcium, but not in phosphorus. The authors state that "a diet has been found which contains the necessary food elements for approximately normal growth and in which the only known deficiency is phosphorus. This leads regularly to the production of rickets."

Do Species Lacking a Gall-bladder Possess its Functional Equivalent?—Some closely related species of animals have a gall-bladder while others do not. It is present in the cow, sheep, goat, hog and wild boar, and absent in the horse, deer and peccary. The hawk and owl possess it, while the dove does not, and among rodents, the mouse is found with the organ, the rat without it. Furthermore, the gall-bladder is not found in the pocket gopher, whereas it occurs in the striped gopher. Again it can be present or wanting in the giraffe. Having previously shown that the gall-bladder concentrates bile greatly and the ducts dilute it slightly, McMASTER (*Jour. Exp. Med.*, 1922, **35**, 127) conducted a series of experiments on rats (animals devoid of gall-bladder) and mice which possess the organ, by determining the amount of pigment normally in the species and after ligating the bile ducts. Both the rat and the mouse were found to secrete larger quantities of bile than the dogs and cats, but less than guinea-pigs and rabbits. Bladder bile of the mouse was found more concentrated than common duct bile and stasis bile showed a great increase in pigment content, whereas in the rat, stasis bile never became more concentrated than normal, indicating that the gall-bladder is absent from the rat not only in form, but in at least one of its important functions, that of a reservoir. On the other hand, although rat bile did not undergo condensation of bulk after leaving the liver, it contained about eight times as much pigment as did liver bile in the mouse, which becomes concentrated in the gall-bladder, so that, in either animal the bile as it reaches the intestine, may not be dissimilar, certainly in pigment, and perhaps in substances useful for digestion, although the author states that little can be said concerning the latter at present.

A Three Months Old Strain of Epithelium.—Although the cultivation of epithelium appeared to be more difficult than that of connective tissue, it seemed probable to FISHER (*Jour. Exper. Med.*, 1922, **35**, 367) that if epithelial tissue could be obtained free from connective tissue cells they could be kept in pure culture indefinitely, Accordingly it has been possible to cultivate, *in vitro*, a strain of pure epithelial cells from that portion of the iris of a chick embryo which adheres to the extirpated lens on the free surface of plasma clot under a film of embryonic tissue juice. The strain is now three months' old and the epithelial cells have not differentiated, growing as a pavement membrane and have retained their epithelial characteristics. The rate of proliferation is increasing, every culture doubling in size after three or four days. Several plates are presented to show numerous mitoses and different stages of amitotic cell division.

Significance of the Hemosiderosis of Pernicious Anemia.—Many believe that pernicious anemia is due to an injurious agent derived from the gastro-intestinal tract, citing the marked siderosis of the liver parenchyma occurring during pernicious anemia as evidence to indicate that pathological blood destruction is localized within the portal tributaries. After experimentation on young rabbits, MCMASTER, ROUS and LARIMORE (*Jour. Exper. Med.*, 1922, **35**, 521) have shown that a similar siderosis can be produced by varying the amount of pigment set free in the general circulation. As a result of these findings, the authors believe that the selective deposition of the hemosiderin in the hepatic parenchyma during pernicious anemia does not constitute evidence that there is a hemolytic cause for the disease located in the portal region. The hemoglobin was prepared from the rabbit corpuscles and was injected six days out of seven in concentrated watery solution, subcutaneously, into the flanks and the abdomen, in doses ranging from $\frac{1}{4}$ to $\frac{1}{150}$ of that normally possessed by the animal over a period from thirteen to one hundred and two days. Blocks from the liver, kidney, spleen and red bone marrow were fixed in alcohol and stained with ammonium sulphide and in duplicate by the combined ammonium sulphide-potassium ferrocyanide method of Nishimura. The criterion employed to gauge the degree of siderosis was the appearance of the tissue under the microscope. When a daily dose less than $\frac{1}{90}$ of the approximate quantity of pigment in circulation was given, even for many weeks, practically no siderosis was found. With slightly larger; long-continued injections, there was a stippling with hemosiderin of the hepatic parenchyma. As in pernicious anemia this stippling was most pronounced near the periphery of the lobule. With still larger inoculations, both the liver and tubular epithelium of the kidneys became equally siderosed, and when the hemoglobin doses were massive the liver was negligibly pigmented in contrast to the heavy deposits in the kidneys, at which times amorphous material giving the iron reaction was seen lying free in the glomerular capsule and in the lumina of the upper tubules. No consequential siderosis was encountered in the spleen or in the bone marrow. Attempts to repeat the work with dogs were not as satisfactory. However, in both dogs and rabbits the renal siderosis affected especially the cells of the proximal convoluted tubules and of the ascending limb of Henle's loop, as seen in pernicious anemia but not in hemochromatosis. The authors point out that many types of blood destruction which are systemic in origin, become portal in completion, a circumstance which may well take place in pernicious anemia, and that no matter how suggestive various factors encountered in this disease may seem, it is "a good policy to box the compass of possibilities in the consideration of so obscure a disease as pernicious anemia, rather than look for enlightenment in a fixed direction."

A Simple Quantitative Precipitation Reaction for Syphilis.—KAHN (*Arch. Dermat. and Syph.*, 1922, **5**, 570) describes a precipitation method based on the employment of syphilitic serum with alcoholic extract antigens of heart muscle. The author has found the test very simple and delicate, having the added attraction that the diluted antigens are quite stable, that the strongly positive serums usually show spontaneous precipitation, the test being complete after three hours in the water-bath and that the end results can be read with relative ease. The antigen consisted of an alcoholic extract of dried pig or beef heart free from ether extractives and cholesterinized by adding 400 mg. of cholesterin to 100 cc of alcoholic antigen. The proper dilution of the antigen was ascertained by adding, rapidly, various amounts of salt solution, that diluted antigen which was milky but opalescent and free from precipitate being the desired one. The serums were inactivated by heating at 56° C. for thirty minutes. To perform the test, 0.3 cc inactivated serum were mixed with 0.1 cc of the diluted antigen in a small tube, gently shaken and incubated at 37.5° C. The results were read after one and three hours incubation, the presence or absence of precipitation determining the positivity or negativity of the reaction. Of 1119 serums examined by the precipitation and Wassermann methods, 213 were positive, 20 were doubtful, and 767 were negative by both methods, giving a total of 1000 specimens or 89.36 per cent showing agreement. 7 positive reactions were doubtful in the precipitation test; 40 doubtful Wassermann reactions were positive; 30 doubtful Wassermanns reactions were negative; 21 negative Wassermann reactions were doubtful; the total 98 specimens (8.75 per cent) showing relative agreement. 14 negative Wassermann reactions gave weakly positive precipitation reactions; 7 weakly positive Wassermann reactions gave negative precipitation reactions, giving a total of 21 (1.87 per cent) specimens which did not check. In not a single instance did a four plus or a three plus Wassermann reaction show a negative precipitation, or a positive precipitation show a negative Wassermann. The author hopes that the simplicity and ease with which the test can be performed will attract others to investigate it in conjunction with clinical studies.

HYGIENE AND PUBLIC HEALTH

UNDER THE CHARGE OF

MILTON J. ROSENAU, M.D.,

PROFESSOR OF PREVENTIVE MEDICINE AND HYGIENE, HARVARD MEDICAL SCHOOL, BOSTON, MASSACHUSETTS.

AND

GEORGE W. McCOY, M.D.,

DIRECTOR OF HYGIENIC LABORATORY, UNITED STATES PUBLIC HEALTH SERVICE, WASHINGTON, D. C.

Pellagra.—Amino-acid Deficiency Probably the Primary Etiological Factor.—GOLDBERGER and TANNER (*United States Public Health Reports*, 1922, **37**, 462) briefly summarize the more important part of the evidence proving diet to be the primary controlling factor in the prevention and causation of pellagra. Cases of pellagra are reported that were observed to occur in individuals who were known to have consumed daily, during a period of not less than two and one-half months immediately before the onset of the distinctive eruption, what is judged to have been a liberal supply of mineral elements and the known vitamines, which would indicate that a deficiency of these dietary factors is not essential in the causation of the disease. These factors having been thus excluded, the dominating role of diet in the prevention and causation of pellagra must be referred primarily to the character of the protein (amino-acid) supply; this being the only other dietary factor at present known to be necessary to physiological well-being. On the assumption that all the dietary factors essential in human nutrition are known, it may be concluded that the essential etiological dietary factor is a specific defect in the amino-acid supply, probably in the nature of a deficiency of some special combination or combinations of amino-acids. There is reason to believe that besides the specific amino-acid defect, pellagra-producing diets may, and probably frequently have other more or less serious faults, including non-specific amino-acid deficiencies, which may operate as accessory etiological factors. In some preliminary therapeutic trials with amino-acids the dermal lesions in each of 2 cases seemed to show a markedly favorable reaction to cystin; and in a third case a steady gain in weight, with some improvement in diarrhea, accompanied the administration of both cystin and tryptophane.

Direct Injection of B. Typhosus into the Gall-bladder.—BECKWITH (*Jour. Infect. Dis.*, 1922, **31**, 458) states that the older idea that presence of B. typhosus within the gall-bladder in a typhoid carrier is due to direct invasion of the bacilli by way of the common and cystic ducts from the duodenum no longer seems tenable. However, there is still strong reason to believe that this may be the path of invasion for Entameba dysenteriæ and for certain parasites. One may conceive that a foreign toxin-producing body within the bile may be able to produce a generalized condition in the body, as the wall of the gall-bladder has been demonstrated to comprise an active permeable and concentrating mechanism. With this possibility in mind it was attempted to learn whether the introduction of B. typhosus within the gall-bladder directly is followed by the appearance of bacilli and of agglutinins in the circulation. The author found that injection of B. typhosus directly into the gall-bladder of the rabbit is followed by prompt appearance of agglutinins within the circulation. This response is stimulated by dead as well as by living organisms. Typhoid bacilli implanted within the gall-bladder pass through the lining epithelium and appear shortly in other organs, such as the spleen, liver, lung and kidney, but they are not isolated from the peripheral circulation. It seems likely that lymph is at least partially responsible for this distribution. Migration of B. typhosus through the epithelium into the tunica is attended after appropriate lapse of time by the formation of lesions which are characteristic of those found in the typhoid carrier.

Experimental Botulism in Dogs.—Graham and Eriksen (*Jour. Infect. Dis.*, 1922, **31**, 402) found that unfiltered type A toxin of Clostridium botulinum proved fatal to dogs in doses of 0.1 cc or more administered subcutaneously. Type A spores, detoxicated by washing and heating, produced no noticeable effects when injected subcutaneously into dogs. Feeding relatively large amounts of unfiltered type A toxin (100 cc) produced illness and death in dogs only when food had been previously withheld for forty-eight hours. The effects of other forms of artificially induced fatigue were not determined. The symptoms of type A intoxication included loss of appetite, muscular weakness, languor, prostration, salivation, congestion of the mucous membranes of the mouth, and respiratory disturbances. Type A antitoxin apparently protected dogs against lethal amounts of toxin. Unfiltered type B toxin of Clostridium botulinum administered intravenously and subcutaneously in liberal amounts failed to induce manifest symptoms. The internal organ and muscle tissues of horses and pigs which had died of type A botulism were consumed by dogs without ill effects. Dogs appear to be satisfactory animals for differentiating A and B toxins of Clostridium botulinum following subcutaneous injection.

Isolation of Anthrax Bacillus from a Shaving Mug.—Vincent (*Jour. Infect. Dis.*, 1922, **31**, 499) reports a case of anthrax of the neck, and concludes from the results of examination of a shaving mug that it is evident that the shaving brush in all probability harbored anthrax bacilli, and that the spores or bacilli adhered to the mug after the removal of the brush, showing again the great resistance of this organism.

Interepidemic Influenza.—Jordan (*Am. Jour. Hygiene*, 1922, **2**, 325) calls attention to the conspicuous place occupied by influenza among the reported causes of death between the epidemics of 1890 and 1918, and brings forward a number of interesting facts. The lack of uniformity in the clinical picture of influenza makes the comparison of the symptoms of epidemic and interepidemic cases of doubtful value.

and the term has undoubtedly been used very loosely. Before 1890 the designation influenza was rare in health reports of American cities, but in that pandemic year it became conspicuous and has remained more or less in evidence since that time. In certain localities there is indicated a tendency to report as influenza deaths that in other localities would be reported as pneumonia or bronchitis. There is no doubt about the comparability of the pandemics of 1890 and 1918. Whether the so-called influenza of interepidemic years is the same disease with these great epidemics is an important question, and until the causal agent or its effects can be recognized a considerable measure of uncertainty will probably continue to exist. But certain kinds of indirect evidence may be interpreted to indicate that the so-called influenza of interepidemic years is at least in part different from the influenza of the great epidemics of 1890 and 1918: (1) In the epidemic of 1918 the greatest mortality was at the ages twenty-five to thirty-five. During the years 1900–1917 less than 10 per cent of the deaths were in this age period, more than 50 per cent being in persons over sixty. (2) In the 1918 epidemic there was a relatively increased mortality in the white race as compared with the negro, in contrast to the higher mortality among negroes in the preëpidemic period. (3) The mortality was higher in white males than in white females, as contrasted with the higher mortality among females in preëpidemic years. (4) There was a relatively increased mortality in colored males during this time as compared with colored females. During 1918 the increase in reported deaths from influenza was accompanied by an increase in deaths from pneumonia, as might be anticipated. In the preëpidemic years (1900–1917) there were notable divergences in the two rates. Too much weight should not be attached to this lack of correspondence between pneumonia and influenza in interepidemic years, since the pneumonia death rate is affected by a number of inconstant factors. The author concludes: Evidently many deaths reported as influenza in interepidemic years are not due to the same microbic causes as those occurring in epidemic years. Is this true of all? May there still be a residuum of cases and deaths from true influenza which keeps a thread of continuity between the great outbreaks? The question probably cannot be answered until the causal agent is identified. Meanwhile local and outbreaks and even individual cases of mild respiratory disease should be given searching study.

INDEX.

Notice to Contributors.—All communications intended for insertion in the Original Department of this JOURNAL are received only *with the distinct understanding that they are contributed exclusively to this* JOURNAL.

Contributions from abroad written in a foreign language, if on examination they are found desirable for this JOURNAL, will be translated at its expense.

A limited number of reprints in pamphlet form, if desired, will be furnished to authors, *providing the request for them be written on the manuscript.*

All communications should be addressed to—

DR. JOHN H. MUSSER, JR., 262 S. 21st Street, Philadelphia, Pa., U. S. A.

INDEX.

A

B

C

S

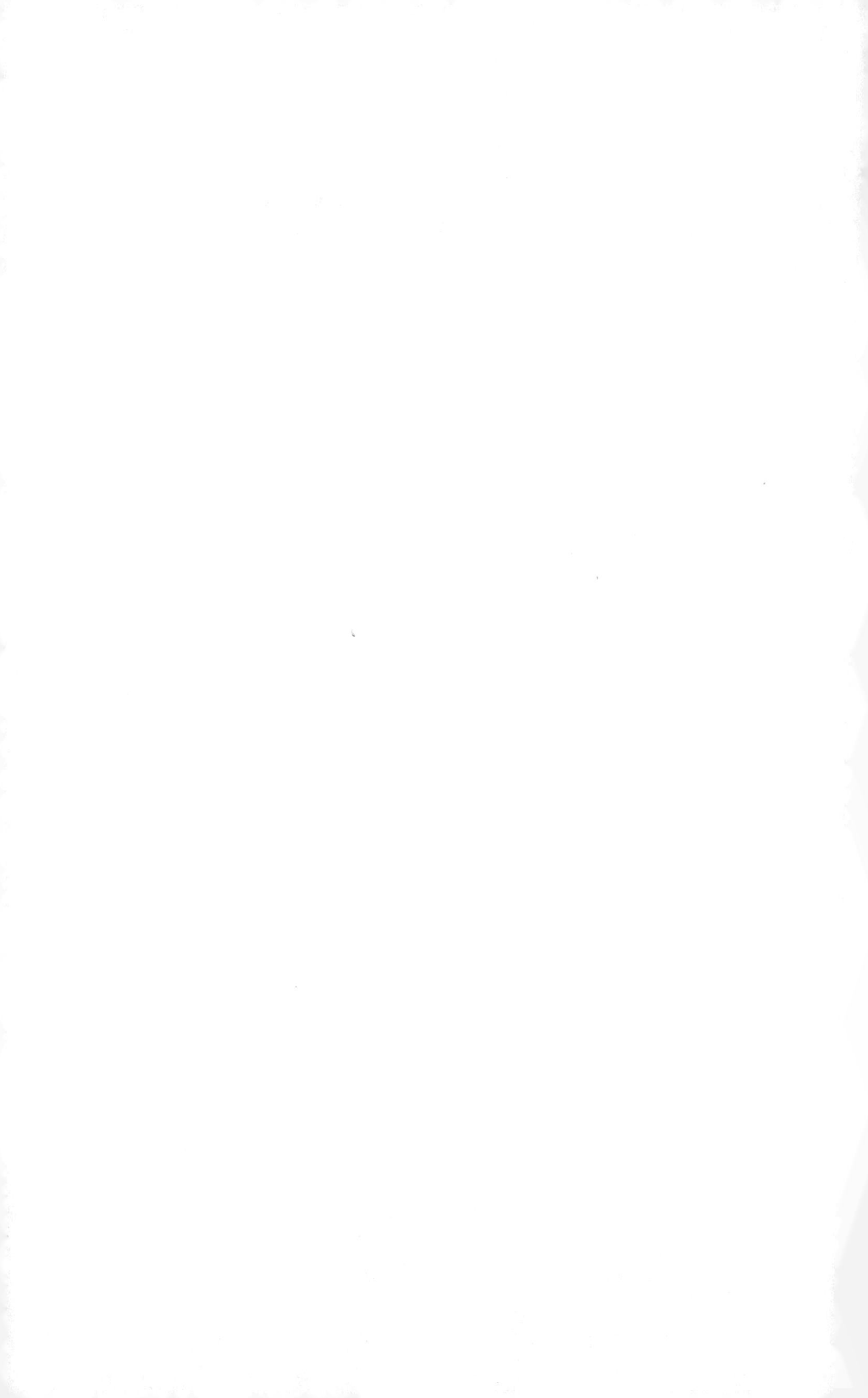

CPSIA information can be obtained
at www.ICGtesting.com
Printed in the USA
BVHW08*1809100918
527043BV00009BA/87/P